Pulmonary Medicine

Pulmonary Medicine

SECOND EDITION

Editor Clarence A. Guenter, *M.D.*
Professor and Head,
Department of Medicine
University of Calgary;
Director, Department of Medicine
Foothills Provincial General Hospital
Calgary, Alberta

Associate Editor Martin H. Welch, *M.D.*
Associate Professor of Medicine
University of Kansas School of Medicine–Wichita
Wichita, Kansas

With Ten Contributors

J. B. LIPPINCOTT COMPANY
Philadelphia London Mexico City New York
St. Louis São Paulo Sydney

The authors and publisher have exerted every effort to ensure that drug selection and dosage set forth in this text are in accord with current recommendations and practice at the time of publication. However, in view of ongoing research, changes in government regulations, and the constant flow of information relating to drug therapy and drug reactions, the reader is urged to check the package insert for each drug for any change in indications and dosage and for added warnings and precautions. This is particularly important when the recommended agent is a new or infrequently employed drug.

Second Edition

For information address J. B. Lippincott Company, East Washington Square, Philadelphia, Pennsylvania 19105.

Library of Congress Cataloging in Publication Data

Main entry under title:

Pulmonary medicine.

Includes bibliographical references and index.
1. Respiratory organs—Diseases. 2. Respiration.
I. Guenter, Clarence A. II. Welch, Martin H.
[DNLM: 1. Respiratory tract diseases. WF 140
P983]
RC731.P84 1982 616.2 81-13728
ISBN 0-397-50444-6 AACR2

3 5 6 4

Printed in the United States of America

Contents

Contributors

ISRAEL BELENKIE, M.D.

Associate Professor of Medicine
University of Calgary
Calgary, Alberta

CLARENCE A. GUENTER, M.D.

Professor and Head,
Department of Medicine
University of Calgary;
Director, Department of Medicine
Foothills Provincial General Hospital
Calgary, Alberta

GARY D. HARRIS, M.D.

Assistant Professor of Medicine
University of Texas Health Science Center at San Antonio
San Antonio, Texas

JAMES C. HOGG, M.D., PH.D.

Professor of Pathology
University of British Columbia;
Director, Pulmonary Research Unit
St. Paul's Hospital
Vancouver, British Columbia

WALDEMAR G. JOHANSON, M.D.

Professor of Medicine
University of Texas Health Science Center at San Antonio;
and Audie L. Murphy Memorial Veterans Hospital
San Antonio, Texas

ALAN K. PIERCE, M.D.

Professor of Medicine and
Chief, Pulmonary Disease Section
University of Texas Southwestern Medical School
Dallas, Texas

JAY J. ROHWEDDER, M.D.
Chief, Pulmonary Disease Section
Veterans Administration Medical Center
Phoenix, Arizona

JOHN G. WEG, M.D.
Professor of Medicine and
Physician-in-Charge, Pulmonary Division
University of Michigan Medical School
Ann Arbor, Michigan

MARTIN H. WELCH, M.D.
Associate Professor of Medicine
University of Kansas School of Medicine–Wichita
Wichita, Kansas

WILLIAM A. WHITELAW, M.D., PH.D.
Associate Professor of Medicine
University of Calgary
Calgary, Alberta

Preface

The abundant advances in pulmonary medicine are well demonstrated by the rapidly proliferating literature in the field. The first edition of *Pulmonary Medicine* was prepared hesitantly, knowing as we did that many exhaustive and highly specialized works were already available. The very warm response from our reviewers and students confirmed the value of an integrated text with a strong clinical emphasis.

Encouraged by our readers, we have thoroughly revised and updated *Pulmonary Medicine* without changing the original format. Contributors have again been selected from a small number of institutions in order to provide a unified approach at a standardized level, with a sharp focus and minimal duplication. Experimental background is explored where it is relevant to the understanding and diagnosis of disease or to management of patients. Themes covered exhaustively elsewhere in the developing literature have been distilled and the selective bibliographies have been updated to assure the reader ready access to the expanded literature on current thinking.

We gratefully acknowledge the support of the staff of the J. B. Lippincott Company, and our indebtedness to our universities and teaching hospitals, which have provided clinical opportunities and the laboratories for our research and contemplation. Finally, we thank our patients and students, who demand that our intellectual exercises maintain clinical relevance.

Clarence A. Guenter, m.d.
Martin H. Welch, m.d.

Preface to the First Edition

This book offers an integrated approach to pulmonary medicine. Consequently, the clinical recognition, evaluation, and management of the diseases of the respiratory system are presented within the framework of lung function, pathophysiology, diagnostic radiology, and microbiology. Within the discussions of clinical recognition, evaluation, and management, the reader will find a strong emphasis upon practical guidelines. Because the spectrum of diseases in patients cared for by the internist and the chest physician today involves new areas of special emphasis, we have included full discussion of environmental factors, pre- and postoperative management, chest trauma, and respiratory failure in all of its aspects.

So that one may approach diagnosis and treatment on the basis of an understanding of functional changes, we begin with an introduction to respirology. In Part I, the respiratory consequences of environmental changes, airways function, ventilatory function, and the respiratory function of the lungs and blood must now more than ever be fully understood prior to the specific management of respiratory illness.

Part II centers upon respiratory disease itself, with the emphasis being placed upon the presenting problem of the patient with respiratory illness. This problem-oriented approach is especially necessary in pulmonary medicine, when the specific etiology is not immediately apparent, and permits reasonable and effective management while the precise cause of the disease is being delineated. Patients with acute respiratory tract infections, chest trauma, or pleural disease commonly present with just those problems.

A number of problems do not fall into a common clinical presentation. These include intrathoracic tumors, chest wall disorders, and pulmonary vascular disease (particularly the ubiquitous process of pulmonary thromboembolism). These are covered in separate sections for ease of comprehension.

In order to provide a sharp focus and unify presentation, the editors restricted contributions to a small number of institutions, availing themselves of the collaboration of authors with recognized eminence in clinical management who could provide standardization and cohesiveness. Each of the contributors also has an ongoing interest in clinical investigation and education in pulmonary medicine.

No attempt has been made in this volume to be exhaustive in areas covered frequently and well in the developing literature. We offer, rather, a distillation of what is known, so that what is presented can be readily understood and effectively applied to patient management.

The bibliographies have been abbreviated and will reveal to the reader an emphasis upon recent articles that offer a further expansion into current thinking and practice. Sufficient documentation of historical work exists to remind us of the heritage upon which our knowledge is based. Consequently, we have not credited individual investigators for many important contributions, even though those contributions are reflected in the information presented herein.

Clinical medicine is an unspecified mixture of scientific fact, judgment, and personal bias. Upon dealing with subjects about which there is recognized controversy, we have made a deliberate effort to point out those aspects which are based on scientific information and those which rely more exclusively upon clinical judgment. It is hoped that the student, recognizing incongruities that are not apparent to us, will himself search for better evidence for clinical approach.

CLARENCE A. GUENTER, M.D.
MARTIN H. WELCH, M.D.

Pulmonary Medicine

Part ONE

Introduction to Respirology

Chapter 1

The Respiratory Environment

CLARENCE A. GUENTER

All living animals are dependent on an environment that permits their energy needs to be supported. Although cellular respiration and energy metabolism have many similarities throughout the animal kingdom, the different mechanisms for extracting oxygen from the environment and eliminating carbon dioxide are intriguing. Through studies of comparative physiology we understand some of the adaptations that permit life to exist in widely disparate environments.[1] The extraordinary diversity of physiological equipment that permits animals to survive, whether as deep-sea cold water fish of the antarctic or vigorously active high flying birds, provides some insight into potential adaptive mechanisms for humans. The human respiratory apparatus is roughly intermediate to the range of equipment in other animals. For example, fluid ventilation through gills is less efficient than air breathing by human lungs, which in turn is less efficient than the countercurrent alveolar ventilation of high-flying birds. Similarly, the high solubility of oxygen in the plasma of cold water fish is a simpler means of oxygen transport than the hemoglobin binding of oxygen in humans or the high oxygen affinity hemoglobin of the llama.

This chapter emphasizes the essential composition of the human respiratory environment, and reviews our understanding of adaptive mechanisms in the human. In addition, it summarizes the rapidly increasing knowledge about our tolerance to changes in the environment.

GASES IN THE RESPIRATORY PATHWAY

Atmospheric Gases

The ubiquitous nature of oxygen, man's most immediately life-sustaining natural resource, may diminish the intrigue of the study of environmental gases. Curiosity is frequently stimulated by the threat of extinction of natural resources, and no satisfactory evidence can be accumulated as to a significant loss of available oxygen in our atmosphere. How the relatively constant concentration of gases (Table 1-1) is maintained in the atmosphere has not been established. Estimates indicate that the proportion of oxygen has been stable for several millennia.[3] The major source of oxygen for environmental replenishment is photosynthesis by plants. The major use of oxygen is by land and marine animals and by the combustion of fossil fuels. The enormous reserves of oxygen in the earth's atmosphere and in the oceans suggest that there will be no global life-limiting oxygen deficiency in the foreseeable future. A recent estimate indicated that if all the fossil fuels were completely burned instantaneously, a decrease of 3% of the earth's global oxygen resources would occur. Variably contested evolutionary hypotheses attempt to explain these atmospheric conditions; however, there are major inadequacies in these hypotheses.

TABLE 1-1. Composition of Atmospheric Gas (Dry, Sea Level)

Gas	mm Hg	% Total
Nitrogen	590	78.09
Oxygen	158	20.95
Carbon dioxide	0.2	0.03
Other inert gases*	7.0	0.93
Water vapor†	—	—
Total	760.2	100.00

* Predominantly argon.

† Water vapor pressure varies greatly with temperature (see Factors Affecting Alveolar Gas Partial Pressures, p 5), but minimally with altitude. Although no figure is included in the preceding table, water vapor is never completely absent from the environment.

(Adapted from Altman PL, Dittmer DS: Biological Handbooks, Respiration and Circulation Federation of the American Society of Experimental Biologists, 1971[2])

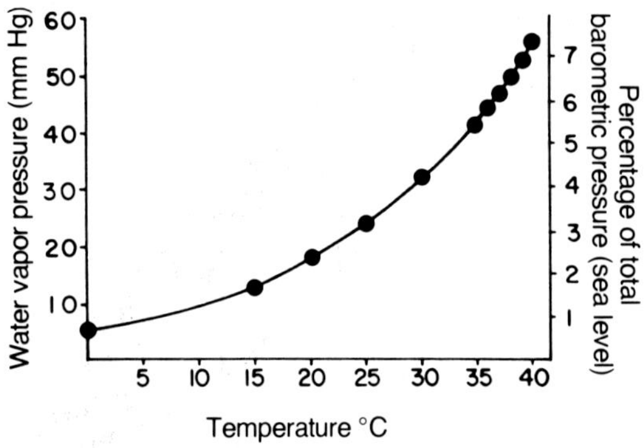

FIG. 1-1. The water vapor pressure, in mm Hg, is plotted on the ordinate on the left, and water vapor pressure as a percentage of total barometric pressure (at sea level) on the ordinate on the right. All values are for fully saturated gas. Note that water vapor pressure in cold environments approaches zero. Sub-zero temperatures frequently encountered in winter in northern climates result in water vapor pressure of less than 5 mm Hg, even when the atmosphere is fully saturated. As a result, warming of such air in heated buildings produces an atmosphere with a relative humidity of approximately 10%. Humidification of air under these circumstances may be a major objective of inside air conditioning. Even when air that is fully saturated with respect to vapor pressure is warmed from room temperature to body temperature (approximately 20° to 37° C), it becomes less than 50% saturated. (Adapted from Altman PL, Dittmer DS: Biological Handbooks. Respiration and Circulation. Federation of the American Society of Experimental Biologists, 1971)

The convenience of unlimited oxygen reserves provides the respirologist with eternal optimism. Fortunately, the other major atmospheric gases are as conveniently arranged. Nitrogen and argon, the chief inert gases, have no known biological effects in concentrations that occur in the atmosphere. Carbon dioxide is suitably present in trace amounts only, permitting the metabolizing body to efficiently discharge its accumulated carbon dioxide into the atmosphere.

Carbon dioxide levels in the environment have increased 15% during this century, largely as a result of combustion of fossil fuels. This may be insignificant to the respiratory apparatus, but may have dramatic effects on climate, with gradual warming of the earth.[4,4a]

At sea level, the barometric pressure is about 760 mm Hg. This pressure is comprised of the pressures of all the gases that are present in the atmosphere, regardless of temperature (see Table 1-1). (Dalton's law of partial pressures states that the partial pressure of each gas in a mixture is independent of the other gases present; therefore, the total pressure equals the sum of the partial pressures of all gases present.)

Whereas man's environment embraces a wide range of atmospheric pressures, functional amounts of the gases are expressed more conveniently as partial pressures than as concentrations. For example, a person traveling from sea level, at a barometric pressure of 760 mm Hg, to

TABLE 1-2. Composition of Respired Gases

	Dry Air		Moist Tracheal Air		Alveolar Air	
Gas	Partial Pressure (mm Hg)	Percent Total	Partial Pressure (mm Hg)	Percent Total	Partial Pressure (mm Hg)	Percent Total
Nitrogen*	600.7	79.02	563.6	74.16	568.0	74.74
Oxygen	159.1	20.95	149.2	19.63	105.0	13.82
Carbon dioxide	0.2	0.03	0.2	0.03	40.0	5.26
Water vapor	0.0	0.00	47.0	6.18	47.0	6.18
Total†	760.0	100	760.0	100	760.0	100

* This value includes other inert gases separately itemized in Table 1-1.

† Values may be calculated for other altitudes by using local barometric pressures (e.g., mean barometric pressure in Denver of 640 mm Hg, or in Calgary, Alberta, 660 mm Hg). For dry gas, the Po_2 at a barometric pressure of 660 mm Hg: 20.95 × 660 = 138 mm Hg. For saturated gas at 37° C: 20.95 × (660 − 47) = 128 mm Hg.

a high altitude, with a barometric pressure of 380 mm Hg, is still breathing 20.95% oxygen; however, the 50% decrease in available oxygen per unit of atmospheric volume is reflected in the partial pressure of oxygen (PO_2), which has decreased from 160 to 80 mm Hg.

Water vapor is a significant variable in atmospheric gas composition. Water vapor pressure (PH_2O) is dependent on available water and H_2O capacity at fixed temperature. Thus, at 0° C air that is fully saturated has a water vapor pressure of 4.6 mm Hg, whereas at body temperature (37° C), the water vapor pressure is 47 mm Hg (Fig. 1-1). In the human body, all gases are saturated with water vapor. When dry air is inhaled, it is warmed and humidified. The increase in temperature in the body increases the capacity of the gases to carry water vapor, while the moist linings of the respiratory airways serve as a source of water, which permits complete saturation of the gases.

Gases in the Body

The interrelationship of atmospheric gases and, in particular, the effect of water vapor pressure on the partial pressures of the gases in the respiratory passages is demonstrated in Table 1-2. Nitrogen and oxygen are the only gases present in noteworthy concentrations in dry air; however, moist, warm tracheal air contains significant amounts of water vapor. Because the total barometric pressure is unchanged in the trachea, water vapor displaces each of the other gases, thereby decreasing their partial pressures. Thus, the partial pressure of oxygen is decreased from 159.1 to 149.2 mm Hg, simply by the warming and humidification of air. As the gas advances to the lower respiratory tract, where gas exchange takes place, there are additional changes in its composition as indicated in the alveolar air column (Table 1-2). These changes in gas composition do not merely reflect physical changes in temperature and water vapor pressure, but result from the actual uptake of oxygen from the alveolar space and the release of carbon dioxide into the alveolar space through the gas-exchanging surfaces of the peripheral lung units (see Chap. 5). Under normal circumstances, oxygen is taken up by the blood in the lungs in proportion to the utilization of oxygen by the tissues; carbon dioxide is released by the blood flowing through the lungs in proportion to the production of carbon dioxide by the tissues.

Figure 1-2 demonstrates the changes in oxygen and carbon dioxide along the entire respiratory pathway under various conditions. Each stage or physiologic compartment is completely dependent on the gas pressures in the stage that precedes it and in the stage that follows it. The gases are predominantly moved by convection from the atmosphere to the alveolar space, and vice versa. Figure 1-2A illustrates the normal progression of oxygen and carbon dioxide partial pressures through the respiratory pathway.

Factors Affecting Alveolar Gas Partial Pressures

1. Inspired PO_2, PCO_2
2. Volume of oxygen uptake and carbon dioxide release in lungs
   a. Oxygen consumption and carbon dioxide production at tissue level (metabolic rate)
   b. Fuel being utilized by tissues and metabolic respiratory quotient
3. Volume of alveolar gas exchange (alveolar ventilation)

The availability of oxygen to the blood is most immediately dependent on oxygen in the alveolar compartment; similarly, the release of carbon dioxide from the blood is most immediately dependent on the level of carbon dioxide in the alveolar compartment. Therefore, an understanding of factors that determine the partial pressures of these gases at the alveolar level is fundamental. Sequentially, the first important factor is the partial pressure of the inhaled gases. It is apparent that if the inhaled PO_2 were decreased, it would necessarily result in a decreased PO_2 of moist tracheal air. This in turn would result in a decrease in alveolar PO_2. High-altitude environments characteristically result in a decreased barometric pressure and a decreased partial pressure of inspired oxygen, compared with sea-level values.

The second important factor determining the

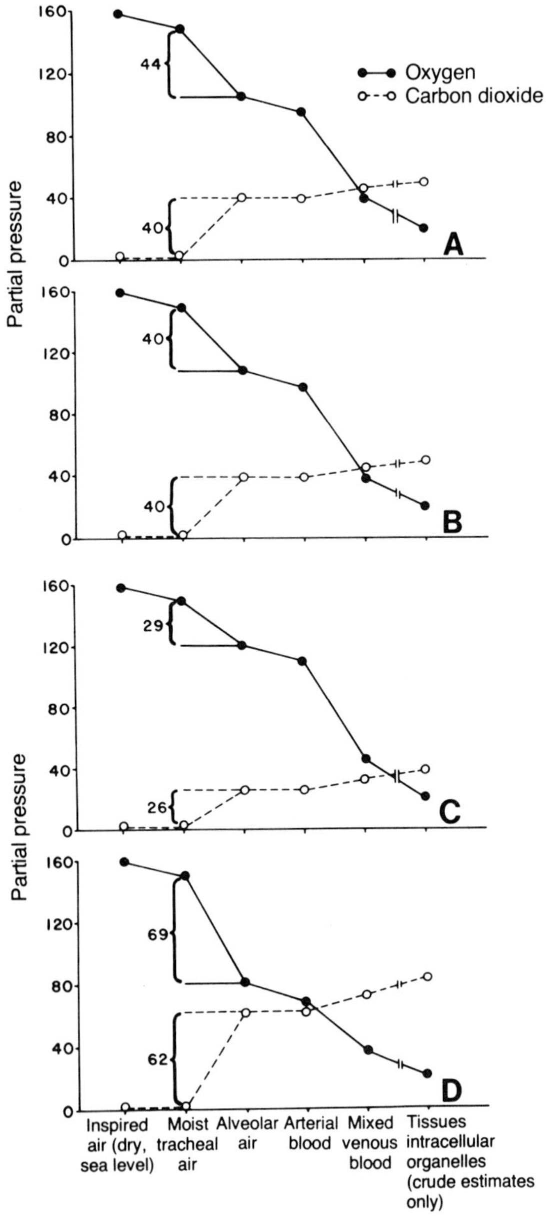

FIG. 1-2. Partial pressures of oxygen and carbon dioxide in the respiratory pathway steady-state conditions. **A.** Normal resting. The solid line indicates the partial pressure of oxygen beginning in the inspired air on the left and progressing to the moist tracheal air, alveolar air, arterial blood, mixed venous blood, and, ultimately, tissues. The values represented indicate the average value in each region of the pathway, but are entirely speculative at the final level of the tissues. Movement of oxygen from the inspired air to the trachea, and from the trachea to the alveolar spaces is almost entirely by convection. Movement of oxygen from the alveolar spaces to the blood is by diffusion. Movement of oxygen within the arterial blood to the systemic capillaries is, again, by convection, as a result of blood flow. Movement of oxygen from the blood to the tissues is by diffusion. The interrupted line demonstrates the partial pressures of carbon dioxide in each region of the respiratory pathway; the same transport processes apply as for oxygen.

B. Normal, resting, metabolic fuel—carbohydrate. The partial pressures for oxygen and carbon dioxide are again illustrated. Note that the alveolar extraction of oxygen and release of carbon dioxide are equal, thus resulting in a respiratory exchange ratio of 1.0. Thus, the alveolar ventilation and the partial pressures of carbon dioxide and oxygen become somewhat dependent on the fuel being metabolized.

C. Effect of increased ventilation without increased metabolic rate. In a hyperventilating individual, the partial pressure of oxygen may be increased throughout the respiratory pathway, and the partial pressure of carbon dioxide decreased. The values illustrated apply only to an individual who has reached a steady state or equilibrium throughout the respiratory pathway.

D. Effect of increased metabolic rate without increased alveolar ventilation. This illustration demonstrates the marked reduction of oxygen and the marked elevation of carbon dioxide throughout the body's respiratory pathways, as a result of the metabolic rate which is in excess of the level of ventilation.

(**B** adapted from Saltzman HA, Salzano JV: Effects of carbohydrate metabolism upon respiratory gas exchange in normal men. J Appl Physiol 30:228, 1971)

alveolar gas partial pressures is the oxygen uptake and carbon dioxide release in the lungs. The metabolic rate of the body is the major factor regulating the volume of oxygen uptake and carbon dioxide release in the lungs. Under most steady-state circumstances, including submaximal exercise, the rate of ventilation is closely matched to the metabolic rate, so that the alveolar gas partial pressures reflect the metabolizing fuel rather than the metabolic rate. It is clear that the decrease in alveolar oxygen would be precisely the same as the increase in carbon dioxide if the oxygen consumption and carbon dioxide production were equal. Most of the time, the alveolar oxygen uptake and carbon dioxide release are not equal. As indicated in Figure 1-2A, the decrease in Po_2 of 44 mm Hg which takes place at the alveolar level is compared with the increase in carbon dioxide of 40 mm Hg. If oxygen uptake and carbon dioxide release were precisely equal, these changes would also be of equal value. This discrepancy between oxygen utilization and carbon dioxide production is a result of the particular fuel being metabolized. The ratio of CO_2 production to oxygen consumption has been termed the *metabolic respiratory quotient*. For example, when pure carbohydrate is metabolized, the oxidation equation may be summarized as follows:

$$C_6H_{12}O_6 + 6O_2 \rightarrow 6CO_2 + 6H_2O \text{ (+ energy).}$$

It is apparent that when glucose is being metabolized, precisely the same amount of carbon dioxide is produced as oxygen utilized. Thus, the metabolic respiratory quotient is 1.0. Similarly, one can calculate the metabolic respiratory quotient for protein (approximately 0.8), fat (approximately 0.7), and ethanol (0.67). The precise fuel being metabolized at any time by the body, or by specific tissues, cannot be ascertained. The oxygen extraction at the alveolar level, and the carbon dioxide washout from the alveoli, however, can be readily assessed. This indirect measurement of the average metabolic respiratory quotient has been termed the *respiratory exchange ratio* (R). It is clear that when the entire respiratory pathway is in equilibrium, this measurement accurately reflects the average of the total body metabolic respiratory quotient. Frequently, however, steady-state conditions do not prevail, and conditions such as transient hypoventilation or hyperventilation alter the respiratory exchange ratio, so that it does not reflect tissue metabolism accurately.

The alveolar gas composition may also be affected by the metabolic fuel through effects on ventilation. When carbohydrate is the major fuel, the carbon dioxide production is higher than with other fuels.[6] This results in a higher alveolar carbon dioxide level, which will result in higher arterial blood carbon dioxide, and stimulate ventilation. Consequently, the alveolar oxygen partial pressure will be increased slightly (Fig. 1-2B).

Several important circumstances that result in altered respiratory exchange ratios should be noted. Completely normal increases in the respiratory exchange ratio are seen at the onset and immediately following cessation of exercise. During these times, alveolar ventilation exceeds tissue metabolic requirements. This does not result in increased oxygen extraction from the alveoli, because oxygen stores cannot be significantly supersaturated. It does, however, result in depletion of carbon dioxide from tissue carbon dioxide stores. Thus, the carbon dioxide washout is greater than the oxygen consumption, and the respiratory exchange ratio may exceed 1.0. Similarly, during transient periods of metabolic acidosis, such as occur with anaerobic metabolism, the oxygen utilization may be relatively fixed, but due to circulating organic acids, body carbon-dioxide stores in the form of bicarbonate and blood carbonic acid are dissociated to H_2O and CO_2, with exhalation of the CO_2. The availability of large body-CO_2 stores thus permits temporary depletion of carbon dioxide, resulting in a respiratory exchange ratio that may exceed 1.0. This abnormal release of CO_2 has been studied as an early indication of tissue hypoxia. The level of exercise (as a determinant of the amount of metabolism) that produces such an increase in the respiratory exchange ratio has been suggested as a sensitive test for metabolic acidosis resulting from limited oxygen delivery (reflecting cardiorespiratory disease).[7] Conversely, circumstances under which ventilation is depressed and the carbon dioxide washout diminished, such as transient alveolar hypoventilation due to breath holding or sudden sedation, result in a respiratory exchange ratio less than that which would be appropriate for the fuel being metabolized at the time, for example, <0.70.

Figure 1-2C illustrates changes in partial pressures of oxygen and carbon dioxide in the respiratory pathway as a result of an increase in ventilation greater than body requirements, under steady-state conditions. Note that under these circumstances, the partial pressures of the inspired gases in moist tracheal air are unchanged. As a result of a marked increase in alveolar ventilation (hyperventilation), an increased amount of oxygen is available at the alveolar level when compared with normal conditions illustrated in Figure 1-2A. Consequently, in this example, the alveolar P_{O_2} is 120 mm Hg. This permits increased oxygen availability for diffusion into the arterial blood and throughout the delivery system, with eventual increased oxygen availability at the tissue level. Carbon dioxide partial pressures are comparably affected. Owing to the increase in alveolar gas exchange, the amount of carbon dioxide remaining in the alveoli is decreased. Thus, the alveolar P_{CO_2} is decreased to 26 mm Hg, the arterial P_{CO_2} is approximately the same, and the tissue CO_2 is washed out to a somewhat lower level than indicated under normal circumstances in Figure 1-2A. Under these steady-state circumstances, the extraction of oxygen from alveolar gas results in a P_{O_2} decrease of 29 mm Hg from inspired air to alveolar gas, and a P_{CO_2} decrease of 26 mm Hg from the alveolar gas to the atmosphere.

The partial pressures depicted in Figure 1-2A represent approximate values seen throughout the respiratory tract, under normal resting steady-state conditions. It is quite clear that if tissue metabolism were suddenly accelerated, as during exercise, oxygen consumption and carbon dioxide production would be increased. Under these circumstances, the body generally responds by delivering more oxygen to the alveoli and removing the carbon dioxide more rapidly by increasing alveolar ventilation. If ventilation were constant, however, the increased extraction of oxygen and production of carbon dioxide would severely alter alveolar gas levels. This situation is illustrated in Figure 1-2D. Now the marked decrease in tissue oxygen tension results in increased extraction of oxygen from the blood at the tissue level, and the mixed venous blood P_{O_2} is diminished. Because alveolar ventilation and, consequently, alveolar oxygen delivery are fixed, there is a decrease in alveolar P_{O_2}. Similarly, the high metabolic rate results in a high tissue P_{CO_2}, increased transport of carbon dioxide from the tissues, and increased mixed venous P_{CO_2}. Because the alveolar ventilation is fixed, removal of carbon dioxide from the alveoli is inadequate, and the alveolar P_{CO_2} is elevated. The P_{CO_2} of blood leaving the alveoli (arterial blood P_{CO_2}) is elevated. This represents an inadequate response to tissue respiratory requirements, and because the response is inadequate primarily with respect to ventilation, it is termed *alveolar hypoventilation*. Note that the alveolar extraction of oxygen results in a drop of P_{O_2} from inspired air to alveolar gas of 69 mm Hg, and the washout of carbon dioxide at the alveolar level results in a decrease in P_{CO_2} from alveolar gas to the atmosphere of 62 mm Hg. This, then, represents a new steady state in which inadequate alveolar ventilation is responsible for marked alterations in alveolar gas partial pressures.

In each of the above circumstances, the person has developed an equilibrium with respect to carbon dioxide and oxygen partial pressures throughout the respiratory pathway. Thus, alveolar gas exchange, blood transport of gases, and tissue metabolism reflect a continuous and stable exchange of oxygen and carbon dioxide. Within wide physiological ranges, once an equilibrium has been established, the actual rate of blood flow (cardiac output) is not a major determinant of the gas levels in the alveoli or respiratory airways.

VARIATIONS IN ATMOSPHERIC CONDITIONS

Decreased Barometric Pressure

Human awareness of adverse effects of the low barometric pressure of high altitudes is recorded in literature regarding the Spanish invasion of the Western Hemisphere. As early as the 1500s, the Spanish complained of the "thinness of the air" in the high mining areas of South America.[8] Their concern about the inability to have offspring suggested that this, too, was a result of environmental hazard. Probably, detailed analysis of folk literature from other high-lying areas in the world would produce additional historical evidence of recognition of these atmospheric problems.[82] Acute mountain sickness, at an elevation of about 3,300 m, was first described in 1671 by the physiologist, Borelli. Subsequently, many additional descriptions of illness were recorded, and we now recognize an entire spectrum, ranging from mild alterations in judgment at relatively low altitudes, to severe acute or chronic altitude disease at higher altitudes. Although persons with previous cardiorespiratory disease may be significantly less well at altitudes as low as 1500 m, more than 3,000,000 persons in South America live above 4000 m, and there are communities in the United States at altitudes above 2300 m. Furthermore, recent wars have been fought between the Indians and the Chinese at altitudes in excess of 4200 m.

The data from the extensive studies of the International Biological Program provide excellent background in this field.[9] Intriguing studies of human adaptation to high altitudes describe life on the Andean Plateau, from Colombia to Chile. This plateau rises above 2400 m and is suitable for human habitation up to the permanent snow line (5300 m). There are more than 10,000,000 persons living in this zone, and historical and archeological records indicate that it has been densely populated for a long time. The Inca Empire had its center in this zone, and it is clear that reproduction by the natives effectively perpetuated the race. Studies of selected communities in this area indicate that although fertility is reasonably maintained (certainly compatible with a population increase), cultural patterns favor reproductive function. The native population has a high birth rate and a high death rate, with peculiarly high prenatal and postnatal death rates for females. This results in a high ratio of males to females in the adult population. Birth weights are low, postnatal growth is quite slow relative to other populations throughout the world, and the adolescent growth spurt is less than that for other groups. A recent assessment of birth weights in Colorado demonstrated normal weights at altitudes of about 3000 m.[9a] Environmental factors appear to be less important than socioeconomic factors in determining the ability of the natives to thrive.

In May 1978 two men first successfully climbed to the summit of Mount Everest (8,848 m, 29,028 ft) without supplemental oxygen. This extreme altitude with a barometric pressure less than 250 mm Hg had been commonly conceded to be beyond human bounds. The feat has since been repeated. No detailed physiological studies have been conducted, but an expedition is now planned for 1981, and will undoubtedly provide many new insights.[10,10a]

Effects of Altitude on Lung Function. In view of the constant concentration of oxygen in air, availability of oxygen to the individual is dependent on barometric pressure. Large changes in barometric pressure are observed with varying altitudes. Figure 1-3 demonstrates the decrease in barometric pressure and the decrease in inhaled P_{O_2} with increasing altitude (an exponential relationship). Thus, the inspired oxygen partial pressure may be predicted on the basis of the change in barometric pressure resulting from the altitude. Figure 1-4 illustrates the approximate values for inspired P_{O_2} at several different altitudes, with approximate changes in P_{O_2} of moist tracheal air, alveolar gas, arterial blood, mixed venous blood, and the directional changes in tissue oxygen partial pressure.

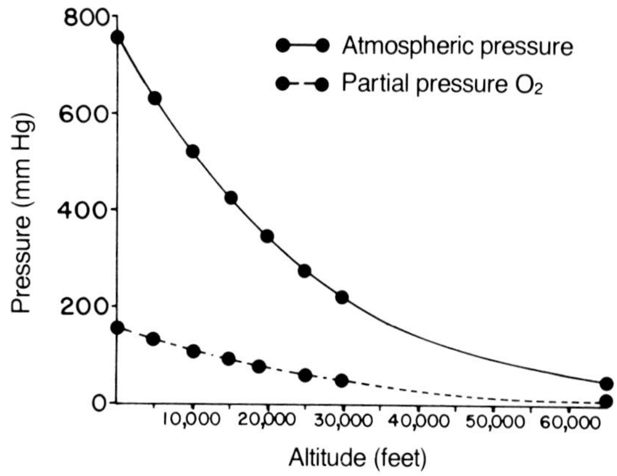

FIG. 1-3. Effect of altitude on barometric pressure and partial pressure of oxygen. The barometric pressure at various geometric elevations is plotted by the solid line. Note the exponential relationship. The partial pressure of oxygen is a fixed proportion (20.95%) of the total barometric pressure and is plotted by the interrupted line. Whereas the atmospheric partial pressure of oxygen at sea level is approximately 160 mm Hg, it is reduced to half that value at 18,000 feet. (Adapted from Altman PL, Dittmer DS: Biological Handbooks. Environmental Biology. Federation of the American Society of Experimental Biologists, 1966)

The immediate effects of a sudden change in barometric pressure have been studied in persons transported to high altitudes and have been simulated in low-pressure chambers. Among the earliest comprehensive studies are those of Hurtado, performed in the Andes. Numerous other important contributions have clarified details of the acute physiological responses to low barometric pressures and have explored adaptive mechanisms that take place early in the sojourner, as well as some of those that appear to take place over generations in inhabitants of high-altitude regions.

Many of the physiological responses of native sea-level inhabitants to sudden exposure to

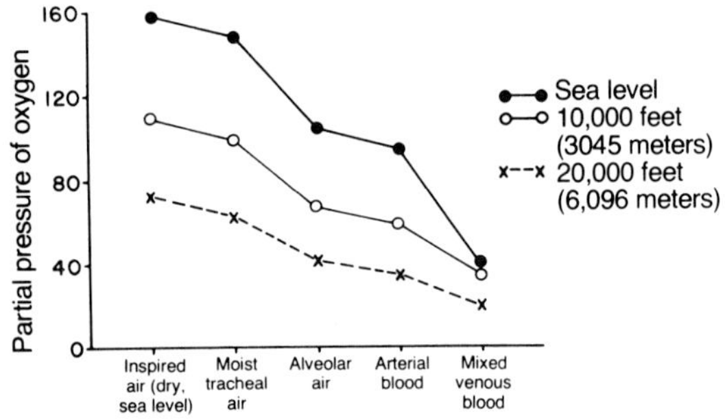

FIG. 1-4. Effect of altitude on partial pressures of oxygen in the respiratory pathway. Average values for partial pressure of oxygen have been plotted at sea level, at a 10,000-foot (3045 m) altitude, and at a 20,000-foot (6096 m) altitude. Considerable individual variation limits the precise application of this data. Note that although the partial pressure of oxygen decreases along the respiratory pathway in approximately the same fashion at higher altitude as at sea level, the adaptive mechanisms are sufficient to minimize the effect on tissue oxygenation. Thus, the mixed venous blood (and the tissues) reflect much smaller changes in partial pressure of oxygen than the arterial blood. (Adapted from Altman PL, Dittmer DS: Biological Handbooks. Environmental Biology. Federation of the American Society of Experimental Biologists, 1966)

higher altitude are illustrated in Table 1-3. A large number of studies with frequently conflicting results are summarized, but it is quite clear that sudden exposure to high altitude, such as occurs with rapid ascent by airplane, results in findings different than the effects of gradual ascent by climbing or slow travel.[12,13] In general, the effects of sudden ascent are quite comparable to exposure to low oxygen partial pressures in gas chambers. The summary data in Table 1-3 refer to responses to sudden ascent to medium altitudes (10,000 to 15,000 ft or 3000 to 4500 m). Although the mechanisms controlling ventilation are complex, it is teleologically noteworthy that the increase in ventilation is proportional to the decrease in the density of the air. Thus, the increase in ventilation is approximately the amount required to produce equivalent delivery of oxygen to the alveolar spaces. This is achieved predominantly through the increase in tidal volume, although in certain instances the respiratory rate may also increase. This elevated minute ventilation is generally sustained throughout the period at higher altitude, although it does not reach its plateau until the second or third day there. As discussed previously and demonstrated in Figure 1-4, the arterial P_{O_2} is decreased as a result of the decrease in alveolar P_{O_2} and inspired P_{O_2}. Although minimal alterations may occur as a result of early adaptive processes, this remains in approximately the same range throughout the time at higher altitude. The arterial hypoxemia results in stimulation of the peripheral chemoreceptors in the aortic and carotid bodies, which are responsible for hypoxic control of respiration. This results in an increase in alveolar ventilation; the carbon dioxide is washed out of the alveolar spaces at a more rapid rate, and the arterial P_{CO_2} is decreased. These circumstances also persist throughout the exposure to higher altitude. This decrease in arterial P_{CO_2} results in a respiratory alkalosis. A major adaptive mechanism, however, comes into play within hours of the arrival at higher altitude, when the decreased arterial P_{CO_2} (and associated increase in arterial *p*H) stimulates the excretion of bicarbonate from the blood by the kidneys. As a consequence, during the ensuing hours to days, the blood bicarbonate is reduced, and a new level appropriate for the degree of hyperventilation is established, with a normal, or nearly normal, arterial *p*H. Thus, the respiratory alkalosis is compensated.

If the person returns from high altitude to sea level within hours of the ascent, ventilation returns to normal. If the individual remains at the higher altitude, ventilation increases for several days. This has been called *ventilatory acclimatization*. Following such ventilatory acclimatization, if the person returns to sea level, mild hyperventilation persists, returning to normal over the next day or so. This ventilatory acclimatization is not purely a result of hypoxemia, and is not satisfactorily explained on the basis of the once-popular theory regarding cerebro-spinal fluid *p*H.[14–16] The ventilatory response to artificially increased CO_2 is higher during the period of ventilatory acclimatization, but the ventilatory response to hypoxia remains unchanged throughout the period at high altitude. At ex-

TABLE 1-3. Physiological Responses to High Altitude Relative to Sea-Level Control Values*

	Immediate	Early Adaptive (72 hr)	Late Adaptive (2 to 6 wk)
Spontaneous ventilation:			
Minute ventilation	↑	↑	↑
Respiratory rate	Variable	Variable	Variable
Tidal volume	↑	↑	↑
Arterial Po_2	↓	↓	↓
Arterial Pco_2	↓	↓	↓
Arterial pH	↑	↑ ↔	↑ ↔
Arterial HCO_3	↔	↓	↓
Evaluation of lung function			
Total lung capacity	↑	↑	↑
Vital capacity	↓	↔	↔
Maximum air flow rates	↑	↑	↑
Functional residual capacity	↔	↔	↔
Diffusing capacity	↑	↑	↑
Ventilatory response to inhaled CO_2	↔	↑	↑
Ventilatory response to hypoxia	↔	↔	↔
Pulmonary vascular resistance	↑	↑	↑
Oxygen transport			
Hemoglobin	↔	↑	↑
Erythropoietin	↑	↔	↔
P_{50}	↓	↑	↑
2,3-DPG	↔	↑	↑
Cardiac output	↑	↔	↔ ↓
Central nervous system			
Headaches, nausea, insomnia	↑	↔	↔
Perception, judgment	↓	↔	↔

* These values apply to native sea-level inhabitants. See text for a discussion of discrepancies with native highlanders.

treme altitude, resulting in arterial Po_2 less than 20 mm Hg, there is profound depression of the central nervous system with suppressed ventilatory drive.

Although these effects on spontaneous ventilation are of considerable interest, additional effects on lung function occur. The vital capacity may be slightly reduced initially, then returns to normal. At high elevations the functional residual volume and total lung capacity are significantly increased, with a shift of the pressure volume curve to the left.[17,19,19a] Maximum air-flow rates (as measured by maximum mid-flow rates, peak-flow rates, and forced expiratory volumes at 1 sec) are increased as a result of decreased density of the gases.[17,19] Numerous complex evaluations of respiratory function have been undertaken; it has been documented clearly that the diffusing capacity for carbon monoxide is increased,[12] and regional distribution of blood flow in the lungs is altered, with an improvement in blood flow to the apical regions.[20,21] Overall matching of ventilation in relation to perfusion, however, does not appear to be improved.[22–24] Pulmonary arterial pressure and pulmonary vascular resistance are increased in proportion to the degree of hypoxia (Table 1-4). As a result, increases in right ventricular pressures over prolonged periods of time produce right ventricular hypertrophy. Predictable elec-

TABLE 1-4. Relationship of Pulmonary Artery Pressure to Altitude*

Location	Altitude (m)	Inspired P_{O_2} (mm Hg)	Mean Pulmonary Artery Pressure (mm Hg)
Boston, MA	2	148	13
Halifax, N. S.	20	148	14
Denver, CO	1,600	121	16
Mexico City	2,400	111	16
La Paz, Bolivia	3,700	92	23
Morococha, Peru	4,600	83	28

* These figures are for natives of these locations.
(Adapted from Cudkowicz L: Mean pulmonary artery pressure and alveolar oxygen tension in man at different altitudes. Respiration 27:417, 1970[25])

trocardiographic changes can be demonstrated, indicating right-axis deviation and right ventricular strain.[26,27]

Effects of Altitude on Oxygen Transport. Teleologically, one might anticipate that all the physiological responses to high altitude would be directed at improved oxygen delivery to the tissues. It is not surprising, then, that most aspects of the oxygen transport system are altered in the direction of improved oxygen delivery. As indicated previously, alveolar ventilation is increased by approximately the amount required to deliver the same molecular amount of oxygen to the alveolar spaces as that which is delivered at sea level.

The oxygen-carrying capacity of the blood is predominantly determined by hemoglobin concentration. When a person travels to a higher altitude, the hemoglobin level initially is unchanged, but within hours it begins to rise. This early rise in hemoglobin is not due to increased red-cell mass, but is a result of hemoconcentration, which is not sustained over prolonged periods at higher altitude.[28,29] The hemoglobin concentration is eventually elevated as a result of increased erythropoiesis and a true increase in red-cell mass. The mean increase in hemoglobin concentration is 1.5 to 2.0 g/100 ml at 3000 m and 3.0 to 4.5 g/100 ml at 4500 m. Erythropoietin levels are elevated within the first hours at high altitude, but the true increase in red-cell mass resulting from increased production takes several weeks.[30] As the red-cell mass and hemoglobin concentration rise, the erythropoietin level decreases. (See also Chap. 5, Polycythemia, a Response to Hypoxia.)

The ability of hemoglobin to transport oxygen is also dependent on hemoglobin affinity for oxygen. (See Chap. 5 for a detailed discussion of oxygen affinity for hemoglobin.) Initially, hemoglobin affinity for oxygen is increased because of the shift of the oxyhemoglobin dissociation curve to the left, which occurs with alkalemia. Since the alkalemia is transient, the curve would be expected to subsequently return to its previous position. Soon after the development of the hypoxic state, there is an increase in production of 2,3-diphosphoglycerate (2,3-DPG), which results in a shift of the oxyhemoglobin dissociation curve to the right. There is conflicting data regarding this shift in oxyhemoglobin affinity as a part of the early acclimatization to altitude. Most studies have demonstrated at least a slight shift in this direction. Recently a group of Sherpas living at 13,000 ft (3,900 m) above sea level were shown to have a 20% increase in 2,3-DPG levels, but overall hemoglobin affinity for oxygen was similar to that of sea level residents.[31] The practical significance of the possible small change in hemoglobin affinity for oxygen has not been established. It might be expected to permit increased unloading of oxygen at the tissue level (at the same tissue P_{O_2}), but, certainly, at very high altitudes it might also interfere with oxygen uptake by the hemoglobin in the lungs.

Cardiac output is characteristically increased initially due to the hypoxic state but has been demonstrated to decrease early in the adaptive phases. Whether this decrease is a result of the increased effectiveness of other components of the oxygen transport system, a mechanism for conserving energy, or a result of myocardial hypoxia, has not been established.[32]

In spite of these adaptive responses to altitude, there is no significant change in resting oxygen consumption, or in the ability to perform vigorous exercise at moderate altitudes. Tolerance of higher work loads is limited by several factors, including tachycardia, hyperventilation, and easy fatigability.[10,33] The capacity to continue vigorous activity is reduced with age as demonstrated by the remarkable sequential studies of D.B. Dill whose most recent data was collected at age 87.[33a]

Effects of Altitude on the Nervous System. At very low levels of altitude, no changes can be demonstrated in central nervous system function. At altitudes varying from 1500 to 2500 m, there may be slight alterations in perception, impairment of judgment, and decreased efficiency of learning.[34] Certainly, these symptoms have been well documented at altitudes over 3300 m. These changes in function were previously ascribed to impaired energy metabolism as a result of tissue hypoxia. Recent studies suggest that mild hypoxia may result in alterations of neurotransmitters in the brain even though oxygen supplies for oxidative phosphorylation remain adequate.[35,36] Headaches, nausea, listlessness, insomnia, and alterations in breathing pattern (Cheyne-Stokes respiration) are all attributed to the effects of altitude. These symptoms have traditionally been ascribed to hypoxia. The symptoms are diminished by gradual ascent, and can be modified or prevented by carbonic anhydrase inhibitors (*e.g.* acetazolamide 250 mg per day for 1 to 3 days prior to ascent). These drugs cause a metabolic acidosis, and prevent the marked respiratory alkalosis, stimulate ventilation, and reduce hypoxemia.[37,38] Fortunately, these symptoms generally improve spontaneously after 48 to 96 hr at higher altitude. Ascending too rapidly to altitudes over 5000 m may be associated with loss of consciousness as a result of the sudden, severe hypoxia.

Studies of climbers on Mt. McKinley in Alaska[39] and Mt. Logan in the Yukon[39a] demonstrated retinal hemorrhages in 36% of climbers above 4200 m and 56% above 5300 m respectively. These hemorrhages were associated with evidence of injury to the microcirculation, but left no residual abnormalities after descent. The severity of retinal hemorrhage was correlated with the severity of headaches. Subjects with a previous history of vascular headache experience a more severe altitude headache, and a more rapid ascent or vigorous exercise predisposed the climbers to more severe hemorrhages and headaches.[39,39a,40]

Miscellaneous Effects of Severe Hypoxia. The acute hypoxia, when severe enough, may be expected to result in interference with function of organ systems in a more profound fashion than indicated above. These manifestations of severe hypoxia are more commonly seen as a result of hypoxia secondary to cardiorespiratory disease. Central nervous system manifestations may present a spectrum of symptoms, including impaired judgment, loss of memory, disorientation, hallucinations, tremor, stupor, coma, and death.[41] The cardiovascular manifestations may include severe hypertension, hypotension, tachycardia, a wide variety of arrhythmias, heart failure (predominantly right ventricular failure due to pulmonary hypertension, but occasionally also left ventricular failure), and alterations in regional blood flow.

Renal manifestations of mild hypoxia are not striking; however, very severe degrees of hypoxia have been associated with a decrease in renal blood flow, with secondary effects including changes in concentrating and excreting capacity, as well as acute renal failure. Severe hypoxia is characteristically associated with development of anaerobic metabolism and metabolic acidosis.[42,42a]

Some studies have dealt with the effects of altitude on a variety of cellular functions and on endocrine function.[37]

Altitude Acclimatization as Seen in the High-Dwelling Native. It is noteworthy that man's capacity to adapt to such austere environments as elevations of 4500 m permits not only productive function, but perpetuation of the race. As indicated previously, the South American Indians' capacity to reproduce is in contrast with the infertility of sea-level dwellers who have moved to those altitudes. In addition, numerous other responses of the body appear to be modified in those who dwell at high altitudes.

Hurtado's studies demonstrated very large lung volumes in natives of the high-altitude plateau in the Andes. The principle of these findings has since been confirmed by animal studies that demonstrated an increase in lung volume and alveolar surface area in experimental animals raised in low-barometric-pressure atmospheres.[43,44] These changes may account for the much higher capacity for diffusing carbon monoxide documented in natives of high altitude when compared with sojourners to these altitudes.[12]

The "highlanders" have a "blunted" respiratory drive in response to hypoxia. As a consequence, they uniformly have a decreased minute ventilation at higher altitude, as compared with sea-level inhabitants ("lowlanders") of the same race, who have temporarily ascended to the same levels.[45] Additional degrees of hypoxia increase the ventilatory drive only minimally in these high-altitude natives. This modified response may be genetic, or it may have developed as a very early response to the environment, since natives of high altitudes sustain the blunted ventilatory response to hypoxia even after prolonged periods at sea level, and sea-level dwellers appear to acquire this response gradually, after prolonged periods at high altitude.[46] This effect may be due to a decrease in sensitivity of the peripheral chemoreceptors to the hypoxic stimulus, or to a decrease in sensitivity of central respiratory control mechanisms to inputs from the peripheral chemoreceptors.[47] The precise advantages of this blunted response to hypoxia are not entirely certain; however, it seems clear that at high levels of exercise, highlanders sustain a low work of breathing because of the lower ventilation.

Tissue adaptation may also take place, and, although convincing evidence in humans is not available, an increase in numbers of systemic capillaries may develop. If appropriate techniques were available, it would not be surprising to find cellular oxygen utilization accomplished more efficiently;[12] however, this remains to be demonstrated in humans.

Chronic Mountain Sickness. Early descriptions of explorations at high altitudes indicated that certain persons develop severe illness not entirely explicable on the basis of predictable responses to altitude.[8,8a,48] These are generally sojourners who demonstrate what appear to be excessive adaptive responses to the altitude. Characteristic findings are plethora, weakness and lethargy, somnolence, and, frequently, evidence of heart failure.[49,50] There is a wide variation in ability to adapt to high altitudes, and some persons, for reasons incompletely explained, may develop much greater increases in pulmonary vascular resistance, modified alveolar gas exchange with more profound hypoxia, and greater elevations in hemoglobin with increased blood viscosity and, ultimately, heart failure (cor pulmonale). A similar syndrome, Brisket disease, has been described in cattle.[51] Until recently this syndrome, known as chronic mountain sickness, was treated effectively only by removal from the high-altitude environment, although long-term therapy with supplemental oxygen may be an alternative. Current studies suggest that at least some patients develop severe sleep hypoxemia, and secondary polycythemia. Treatment with acetazolamide prevents the periodic breathing and excessive sleep hypoxemia,[38] and respiratory stimulants such as medroxyprogesterone acetate improve alveolar ventilation, arterial P_{O_2}, and result in reduced levels of hemoglobin.[52,53] The importance of polycythemia with reduced cerebral perfusion, and adverse effects on blood gas exchange, is under active study.[53a] At least some effects of the polycythemia are maladaptive. (See also Chap. 5 and Chap. 14 for discussion of secondary polycythemia.)

Acute High Altitude Illness. Three clinical presentations of acute high altitude illness can be identified: acute mountain sickness, high altitude pulmonary edema, and high altitude cerebral edema.

The features overlap, often occur together, and probably have similar underlying mecha-

Clinical Characteristics of Acute Altitude Illness

Acute mountain sickness	
Headache	Chest discomfort
Nausea	Peripheral edema
Vertigo	Retinal hemorrhages
Insomnia	Weakness
High altitude pulmonary edema	
Dyspnea	Tachypnea
Cough	Cyanosis
Sputum	Lung crepitations
	Chest roentgenogram infiltrates
High altitude cerebral edema	
Severe headache	Papilledema
Vomiting	Coma
Ataxia	Extensor plantar responses
Abnormal behavior	
Hallucinations	Varied focal neurological deficits

nisms.[54,55] Acute mountain sickness may occur in a benign form (see Effects of Altitude on the Nervous System) but pulmonary edema and cerebral edema have been considered malignant forms, recognizing the life threatening nature of the illness. High altitude pulmonary edema is most frequently seen in dwellers of low lands who ascend to high altitude, but occurs in natives returning to high altitude after several weeks at sea level. It generally occurs within 36 hr of ascending to high altitude. It is frequently referred to by the uninitiated as "nocturnal asthma," or "altitude-induced asthma"; however, the major factor responsible for this condition is an increase of fluid in the lungs, characterized by all the symptomatology, physical signs, and roentgenographic features of acute pulmonary edema. No criteria have been established to predict who will develop high-altitude pulmonary edema. It may occur in persons who have previously been to high altitude without developing it, and it may occur in persons without other manifestations of cardiorespiratory disease, and even in otherwise well-conditioned athletes. The precise altitude at which it will occur is also not certain. It has been suspected at levels as low as 2400 m, but generally does not occur at altitudes under 3000 m. Infection, exertion, age, or sex do not appear to be predisposing factors. In a large military airlift in India, a mean of 5.7 persons out of each 1000 flown to an altitude of 3500 m developed the syndrome.[56] Other studies suggest an incidence of 0.3 to 3.0% in persons going above 3500 m. Manifestations consist of tachypnea, dyspnea, weakness, and nausea, gradually progressing to full-blown pulmonary edema with cough and copious bronchial secretions. The syndrome may progress to death.[57,58]

The mechanisms of production of high-altitude-induced pulmonary edema are not at all clear. It is clear, from the limited number of available hemodynamic studies, that the pulmonary artery pressure is severely elevated, with a normal pulmonary venous pressure. This might be considered evidence against an increase in pulmonary capillary pressure. Pulmonary capillary pressure may, however, be elevated as a result of patchy pulmonary arteriolar constriction, with high capillary pressures in some vessels. On the other hand, there may be increased permeability of lung capillaries, thus producing increased fluid accumulation in the lung. Patients who died with altitude pulmonary edema had limited post mortem examinations by Dr. John Dickinson in Nepal. He noted frequent evidence of lung infection and vascular thrombosis. It is not clear whether these factors contributed to or resulted from the pulmonary edema.

Conventional therapy for pulmonary edema is ineffective, and the only known and absolutely reliable method of control for this condition is administration of oxygen or return to lower altitudes. Acclimatization by spending several days during ascent at 8000 ft (2700 m) appears to reduce the risk of developing pulmonary edema.

High-altitude cerebral edema is the most serious form of acute altitude illness. Progressive headaches, abnormal behavior, focal neurological signs or seizures should all be considered ominous findings requiring immediate descent. Papilledema and retinal hemorrhages are frequently present without these more serious manifestations. Oxygen, diuretics, and corticosteroids have all been recommended, but the mainstay and only proven treatment is return to lower altitude.

Travel at Decreased Barometric Pressures. Early in aviation history, all flights were conducted in nonpressurized planes and, therefore, at decreased barometric pressures. The hazards were proportionate to the altitude, and high-altitude flights required inhalation of supplemental oxygen.[8a] More modern aircraft used for commercial passenger service, flying at high altitudes (30,000 to 40,000 ft), are pressurized to reasonable levels. In general, in-flight cabin pressures are equivalent to 5000 to 8000 ft, though many flights are conducted with cabin pressures near sea-level pressure. Normal persons at rest have no recognizable symptoms at these levels. Not infrequently, however, travelers with cardiorespiratory disease and reduced peripheral oxygen delivery develop symptoms while in flight, including weakness, dizziness, and, occasionally, loss of consciousness.[59] They are generally aided by use of the available oxygen, and such problems may be readily avoided by supplying oxygen to persons at risk. Persons with disease who have severely reduced arterial Po_2 levels should probably be provided with oxygen throughout flight. Aside from hypoxia, patients with pulmonary disease rarely have adverse effects from flying. The presence of a large pneumothorax should be considered a contraindication to flying, because decompression results in expansion of the pneumothorax. Patients with sickle-cell anemia may develop increased sickling and vascular occlusion at high altitudes.

More dramatic problems with atmospheric gases were experienced in the space exploration program. Although fringes of the earth's atmosphere extend 550 to 600 km (approximately 350 miles) above the earth (Table 1-5), the available oxygen diminishes markedly (see Fig. 1-3). Space flights in the outer layers of the atmosphere or interplanetary flights are at barometric pressures that effectively provide no oxygen. After considerable experimentation, most United States manned flights were carried out with cabins pressurized to about one-third atmosphere (barometric pressure 250 mm Hg). Most recent flights have had approximately 67% oxygen (Po_2 150 mm Hg), and the balance of the pressure was made up by nitrogen. Under these conditions, the major additional requirement has been for efficient removal of carbon dioxide. When the cabin pressures are carefully controlled in these ranges, the predominant biological concern relates to problems of weightlessness, nutrition, and isolation. These are under active study.[60–62]

Effects of Latitude on Barometric Pressure. Numerous factors in addition to altitude affect barometric pressures, including atmospheric turbulence, temperature, and latitude. At sea level, barometric pressures have been recorded ranging from 664 to 805 mm Hg, in various latitudes and under widely varying temperature conditions. Although the barometric pressure

TABLE 1-5. Characteristics and Composition of the Atmosphere

Region	Altitude	Temperature
Troposphere	Sea level to 19 km at equator, 9 km at poles (average, 10 km)	Decreases with altitude about 6° C/km rise
Stratosphere	10 to 20 km	Constant at −60°C
Mesosphere	20 to 80 km	Rises to 0° C at 30 to 50 km due to absorption of ultraviolet- and x-radiation
Thermosphere	Greater than 80 km	Rises to 900° C at 200 km
Ionosphere	Greater than 60 km	Constant at 1000° C above 300 km. Temperature rise due to absorption of ultraviolet- and x-radiation, which is strongest at about 150 km
Exosphere	Greater than 550 km	Outer fringe of the atmosphere

(Adapted from Altman PL, Dittmer DS: Biological Handbooks. Environmental Biology. Federation of the American Society of Experimental Biologists, 1966[63])

can be predicted with some confidence from the geometric altitude (as indicated in Fig. 1-3), the actual barometric pressure and thus the available inspired oxygen can be accurately assessed only by measurement of the barometric pressure in that location at a specific time. Thus, it is of interest that studies performed at the geographic South Pole[17] revealed barometric pressures substantially lower than would be anticipated for the geometric altitude of 9280 ft. This decrease in barometric pressure is presumably due to the latitude (90° south) and is equivalent to the geometric altitude of about 11,000 feet in near-equatorial regions.[63]

Increased Barometric Pressure

It is only under water, where the pressure increases approximately 1 atmosphere with each 10 m descent, that man encounters a natural environment in which the pressure is elevated significantly above 760 mm Hg. About three-fourths of the earth's surface is covered by water. The enormous mineral, energy, and potential food resources are now resulting in extensive commercial and recreational underwater exploration.

Effects of Immersion. Simply immersing the human body to the neck results in many important changes in cardiopulmonary function. The total lung capacity, functional residual capacity and residual volume are all decreased. Cardiac output, pulmonary blood flow, and the diffusing capacity are increased and the regional distribution of pulmonary blood flow is reversed. The alveolar–arterial oxygen gradient is generally increased, perhaps related to closing volumes which are higher than the expiratory reserve volume in those persons.[64–66]

Breath-hold Diving. Direct body contact with increased barometric pressure is most commonly encountered during breath-hold diving.[67] Numerous important changes take place in the body during the breath-holding period. Continuous oxygen use by the body results in a progressive pickup of oxygen, eventually reducing available oxygen to critical levels. Similarly, the continuous production of carbon dioxide by the body results in progressively elevated blood and alveolar levels of carbon dioxide.

Under normal circumstances the breath-hold is associated with buildup of carbon dioxide at a rate of 3 to 6 mm Hg per min. This, in conjunction with factors involved in motivation and recently described neuromuscular factors, results in an irresistible drive to breathe. (See Chapter 2). Since hypoxia is a mild stimulus to ventilation, it is a relatively mild stimulus to stop holding the breath. Breath-holding beyond safe intervals is a major hazard in this form of diving, since oxygen is excessively depleted from the alveoli, and serious hypoxia develops. A common and hazardous error is made by swimmers who hyperventilate prior to the dive in order to increase the time of breath holding. This depletes the body carbon-dioxide stores, but the oxygen stores cannot be significantly hypersaturated. Under these circumstances, when a dive is undertaken, the termination of breath holding is considerably delayed. Particularly if exercise is continuing, the available oxygen may be depleted to a dangerously low level before the dive is terminated, and arrhythmias, seizures, or death may occur as a result of hypoxia. This is thought to account for many "swimming pool deaths."

A descent of approximately 10 m (33 ft) in seawater results in an increase of pressure equivalent to 1 atmosphere. Only a few persons can dive while holding their breaths to depths where the pressure exceeds 5 atmospheres; most commonly such diving is confined to pressures of 2 or 3 atmospheres (see Fig. 1-5).

The external pressure exerted on the thorax during a dive results in a marked increase in intrathoracic pressure. This would impair venous return were it not for a concomitant increase in pressure surrounding all other portions of the body, thus compressing blood vessels throughout the body.

Increased intrathoracic pressure results in compression of the air-filled lung. Thus, a lung that was fully inflated as the dive began may be compressed to a very low volume during the dive. For example, if the dive were begun with the lungs inflated to total lung capacity, at a depth of 10 m the volume would be reduced 50%.

It becomes apparent that the person with a large total lung capacity would be capable of dives to greater depths. Several studies suggest that persons particularly suited to diving, such as the diving women of Japan and Korea, have higher-than-normal ratios of total lung capacity to residual volume. Furthermore, divers who begin their dive with low lung volumes may be severely limited when the "lung squeeze" produces volumes near residual volume.

In addition to the net volume changes in the lung during breath-hold diving, the compression of the chest cage results in increased gas pressures in the lung, with resultant increased alveolar P_{O_2} and P_{CO_2}. Increased P_{O_2} merely improves availability of oxygen; however, increased carbon dioxide would be expected to stimulate respiration. The ability to dive in spite of this rise in P_{CO_2} can be cultivated. Submarine escape-training-tank instructors who spent many hours underwater, with prolonged breath holding and frequent periods of increased alveo-

FIG. 1-5. During breath-hold diving the airway is closed, and the compressible intrathoracic volume is subjected to rapidly increasing pressure. Therefore the total lung capacity (and residual volume) decrease severely (*closed circles*). Most such dives are conducted at less than 100 feet (30 m). The same individual using scuba equipment continues to breath, thereby building up the amount of air in his lungs, and maintains his normal lung volume (*open squares*). If the scuba diver fails to breathe during descent he will undergo lung "squeeze" just like the breath-hold diver. If the scuba diver fails to exhale during ascent, the decompression of his thorax will result in rapid expansion of the intrathoracic volume and lung barotrauma (*closed squares*).

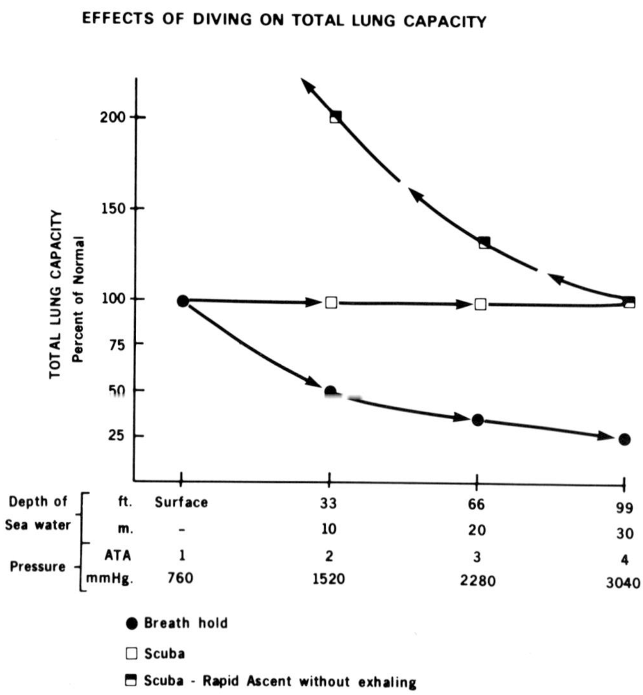

lar (and blood) P_{CO_2}, eventually demonstrated sustained elevations in alveolar P_{CO_2} with appropriate changes in blood electrolytes.[67,68] These chronically elevated CO_2 levels returned to normal during a 3-month layoff period. A significant hazard to the diver develops as a result of the increased P_{O_2} produced by compression, in that the P_{O_2} is relatively high when at depth, but as the diver surfaces and the lung expands, the P_{O_2} decreases. If the lung has been depleted of oxygen by body utilization, the alveolar oxygen may reach critically low levels. The P_{CO_2}, fortunately, decreases as the lung expands when the diver surfaces.

To overcome some of the dangers of breath-hold diving, modern equipment provides for respiration with continuous increased airway pressure, permitting much longer and deeper exposures. Under these circumstances, many of the problems cited below in the discussion of hyperbaric environments become relevant. Hazards of descent, ascent, and barotrauma are much reduced for the breath-hold diver, but the principles are important to consider and are discussed in detail below.

Hyperbaric Diving. Scuba diving is a special case of hyperbaric diving, in which the diver, breathing from a pressurized tank, permits the pressure in his lungs to equilibrate with the pressure of the surrounding water. When the dives are brief, they avoid problems of tissue saturation with inert gases and the potential problems of compression sickness. If the dives take place with slow descent and ascent, problems of barotrauma are few. The commonest cause of serious injury is rapid ascent, with sudden decompression of the thorax and resulting barotrauma.[67]

Preparation of artificial spaces under water frequently requires increased pressure, for example, when compressed air is used to exclude water during construction work in underwater caissons and tunnels. Although submersion in submarines and similar vessels does not normally expose occupants to an elevation of atmospheric pressure, recent use of very deep-sea vessels has required pressurization. Much of our knowledge of the body's responses to high-pressure environments is the result of high-pressure chambers used for experimental simulation of depth.[69] Although depths of 60 atmospheres have been tolerated, there may be severe barriers to diving beyond 60 atmospheres. Studies of sleep, mood, and fatigue suggest that working dives may be limited to about 25 atmospheres.[70]

Early studies of diving under pressurized conditions encountered several important problems: (a) difficulty with adequate extraction of carbon dioxide from the respired gases in a closed environment; (b) high partial pressures of oxygen resulting in oxygen toxicity; (c) inert gas narcosis; and (d) decompression sickness.

Carbon Dioxide Removal. Under normal conditions, adequate alveolar ventilation meets the demands of both carbon dioxide removal and oxygen uptake. The virtual absence of carbon dioxide from the earth's atmosphere conveniently permits alveolar ventilation to be adjusted to the lowest level that will provide optimal oxygenation. Within a closed environment, however, higher levels of oxygen may be present, owing either to compression of atmospheric gases or to supplementation of oxygen, so that the available oxygen is markedly increased. On the other hand, if carbon dioxide removal is not complete, it will gradually accumulate in the environment. Such accumulation of even relatively small amounts of carbon dioxide (*e.g.*, 0.2% at 5 atmospheres of pressure) would result in an increase in inspired P_{CO_2} of 8 mm Hg, with the appropriately increased stimulation to ventilation. The effectiveness of atmospheric carbon dioxide removal systems would, of course, be even more critical at depths of 30 atmospheres or greater. Recent studies suggest that divers have a reduced ventilatory response to CO_2 which may further add to the increased arterial CO_2, but this area requires further clarification.[71,71a]

Oxygen Toxicity. At depths where the pressure is 2 atmospheres, the partial pressure of oxygen rises to 300 mm Hg. This is probably relatively safe even for prolonged periods. At greater depths, however, the partial pressure of oxygen begins to rise excessively. Grand mal epilepsy was first recognized as a central nervous system manifestation of oxygen poisoning in the late nineteenth century. Since that time, it has been well recognized that prolonged exposure to high partial pressures of oxygen, regardless of concentration, may result in numerous other manifestations of oxygen toxicity. It appears likely that partial pressures under 300 mm Hg are not associated with detectable damage, but that increasing levels beyond this will be more likely to cause toxicity. Scuba divers do not suffer from oxygen toxicity, but this may become a major factor in saturation dives.[67] (See Chap. 7 for a discussion of oxygen toxicity.)

Inert Gas Narcosis. The major respired gas, as indicated by volume, is nitrogen. Under normal circumstances, nitrogen does not cause any known chemical reaction in the body and is not produced or used by the body. The high concentration of nitrogen in the atmosphere makes it an important concern in high-pressure environments. Early experiences of divers at depths of from 5 to 10 atmospheres indicated problems arising from the high partial pressures of nitrogen. Its effects on the sensorium and performance are roughly comparable to those of alcohol and are indistinguishable from those of subanesthetic concentrations of nitrous oxide. Although marked individual susceptibility occurs, central nervous system manifestations become apparent at 4 or 5 atmospheres. However, measurable effects on the electroencephalogram and impairment of function may be noted at considerably lower pressures. At pressures in excess of 10 atmospheres, virtually no one can continue to function effectively. Substitution of helium for nitrogen in respired gases avoids the narcotic effects, but at pressures greater than 25 atmospheres, tremors, excitability, and ECG changes develop. This high-pressure neurological syndrome (HPNS) can be modified by rate of pressurization and addition of other inert gases, suggesting it is not a result of a gas narcosis as such.[72]

Decompression Sickness. As a person ascends from a prolonged dive, he may develop illness characterized by itching, bone pain, muscle aches, headache, visual disturbances, and more profound alterations in cerebral function. These clinical features led to the popular use of a descriptive term, "the bends." These manifestations may be a result of the formation of bubbles in blood or tissues previously supersaturated with dissolved gas that was taken up during exposure to the high pressure. The likelihood of these bubbles forming and producing abnormalities of function by interfering with blood flow is dependent on several factors. These include the solubility of the gas, the period of compression, and the rate of decompression. At sea level, approximately 1 liter of nitrogen is dissolved in body fluids; however, at 2 atmospheres of pressure, approximately 2 liters are dissolved, and at 10 atmospheres, approximately 10 liters. The volume of nitrogen released is directly proportional to the partial pressure of the gas at the time of equilibration; this is the hazard of decompression illness. Because the illness associated with decompression was most commonly documented in caisson workers, it was frequently referred to as *caisson workers' disease.* Decompression sickness is a serious and life-threatening problem, best treated by recompression. In addition the use of oxygen and volume expanders has been advocated.[67,73]

In addition to the hazards posed by excessive quantities of gases dissolved at high pressure, the lungs (and other gas-filled organs) are at risk during decompression. So-called barotrauma most commonly results from a large pressure difference across the intrathoracic organs and may result in pneumothorax, pneumomediastinum, mediastinal and interstitial emphysema in the lungs, and occasionally air embolism. Barotrauma in the sinuses (particularly seen in persons with obstructed sinuses during decompression) may result in mucosal damage, with pain and bleeding. The eardrums are occasionally injured by the same mechanism.[67,74]

Effect of Increased Atmospheric Pressure on Lung Function. The resistance to air flow in the bronchial tubes is determined by the caliber of the tubes, turbulence, and viscosity (see Chap. 3 for detailed discussion). Through its effect on turbulence, the density of the gases affects the resistance to air flow, and therefore may modify the maximum flow rate that can be achieved. As illustrated in Figure 1-6, the peak expiratory air flow and the maximum expiratory flow at 50% of vital capacity decrease progressively when the atmospheric pressure is increased from 1 to 7 atmospheres. The greatest change takes place in the range of 1 to 4 atmospheres. These limitations of air flow, when the density of a gas is increased owing to a high barometric pressure, are entirely predictable and also occur with changes in density of gas as a result of a high molecular weight. Similarly, the density may be decreased by substitution of low-molecular-weight gases (for example, helium).[71a,75–78]

Thus, it is perhaps fortuitous that the inert gas helium can be utilized in high-pressure environments, with several distinct advantages: (a) it is less soluble than nitrogen, so that body stores of the gas are diminished, and decompression can take place more rapidly; (b) it has a lower molecular weight, and therefore the rate of diffusion and elimination is increased; and (c) the density is markedly decreased, as compared with nitrogen, thus resulting in improved air flow within the bronchial tubes. Consequently, by substituting helium for nitrogen, ventilatory resistance is minimized, even at very high atmospheric pressures. Studies performed at 33.1 atmospheres of barometric pressure, with gases containing 99.1% helium and 0.9% oxygen, indicate that the density of the respiratory gases is 4.4 times the density of air at 1 atmosphere, and that the impairment of respiratory flow is comparable to that seen at a pressure of 4.4 atmospheres with normal atmospheric gases. Although a slight decrease in respiratory rate and an increase in tidal volume may occur under these circumstances, in order to overcome the increase in resistance to breathing, no clear evidence of significantly increased work of breathing is apparent in resting subjects. It is noteworthy that several subjects have had an increase in arterial carbon dioxide during exercise at these depths, and this may represent an adaptation by the body to the increased work of breathing. Certainly, normal subjects develop diminished ventilatory response to carbon dioxide when the airways' resistance is increased, and patients with sustained elevations of airway resistance

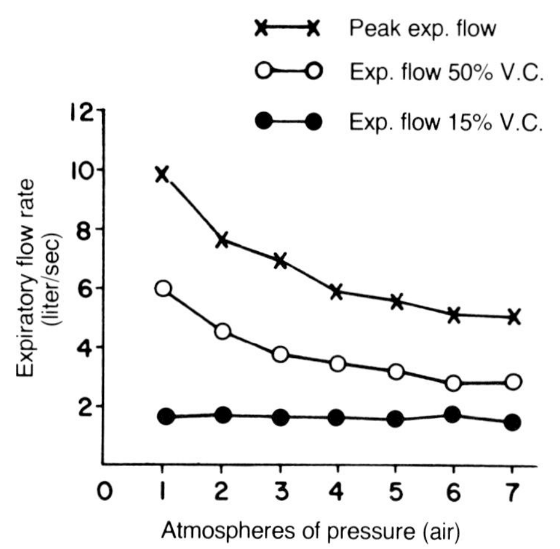

FIG. 1-6. Effect of increased atmospheric pressure on maximum exhaled flow rates. Expiratory flow rates are plotted at ambient pressures of 1 through 7 atmospheres of air. Note that the peak expiratory flow rate of 10 liters/sec at sea level is reduced to approximately 5 liters/sec at 7 atmospheres of pressure. The expiratory flow rates at 50% of the vital capacity are similarly reduced from 6.1 liters/sec to 2.8 liters/sec at 7 atmospheres of pressure. Since the peak flow rate is substantially limited by turbulence, it is not surprising that the increase in density of the gases, as the result of increasing atmospheric pressure, provides increased resistance to flow. Substitution of low-density gas, helium for nitrogen, in respired gases results in flow rates that are maintained at a much higher level at these atmospheric pressures. The observation that the flow rate at 15% vital capacity is relatively unchanged by increasing atmospheric presssures supports the concept that flow is predominantly limited at this lung volume by laminar resistance rather than turbulent resistance. (Adapted from Overfield EM, Saltzman HA, Kylstra JA, Salzano JV: Respiratory gas exchange in normal men breathing 0.9% oxygen in helium at 31.3 atmospheres absolute. J Appl Physiol 27:471, 1969, and Wood LDH, Bryan AC: Effect of increased ambient pressure on flow-volume curve of the lung. J Appl Physiol 27:4, 1969)

frequently develop increased arterial carbon dioxide levels. Normal subjects studied at pressures of 4 atmospheres have been shown to have decreased ventilatory response to carbon dioxide.[71,79]

As a result of these observations, gas combinations are prepared to suit the body's requirements. Generally, the oxygen partial pressure is maintained at approximately 200 mm Hg, carefully avoiding the problems of oxygen toxicity.

Methods of elimination of carbon dioxide are incorporated, with continuous monitoring of the respired atmosphere for traces of the carbon dioxide. The balance of the gas in the atmosphere is made up of helium. Healthy men under these conditions show no important changes in minute ventilation, tidal volume, oxygen consumption, carbon dioxide production, or alveolar gas exchange. They are able to function normally, including performance of mild exercise, for short periods, under these conditions at depths of 450 m below sea level (45 atmospheres).[70]

It is anticipated that the allure of underwater exploration will necessitate the development of increasingly efficient and safe environments for hyperbaric conditions. Many of the preceding generalizations regarding body responses may be modified after experience has been extended beyond the few selected and highly trained experimental subjects that have been studied up to now. A complete understanding of hematological,[80] neurosensory and psychologic,[70,81,82] cardiovascular,[83] and other metabolic factors[84] will be necessary before the ultimate capacity for prolonged high-pressure work has been established. Offshore oil explorations may be expected to stimulate great advances in the technology of underwater hyperbaric physiology. In any event, these exploratory data would support the concept that man is capable of enormous modification of his environment, to provide a unique and life-sustaining microenvironment under high barometric pressures.

Breathing Liquid Atmospheres

Some lines of evidence suggest that all mammalian origins occurred within aqueous environments. Certainly, the variety of animals capable of respiration in fluid environments today is ample evidence that with an appropriate fluid, and adequate exchanging surfaces, fresh- or seawater may serve as a perfectly acceptable source of respiratory gases. In 1962, in a talk entitled "Of Mice as Fish,"[85] Kylstra described the survival of mice in a saline environment specially prepared by oxygenation with hyperbaric oxygen.

The desirability of breathing liquids has several applications to humans. The possibilities of improved versatility during underwater exploration, submarine escape, and improved respiration in diseases where surface tension of the lung lining is severely altered, have encouraged the search for an optimal liquid.[86–89] Obvious problems can be recognized. The viscosity of fluids is greater than that of air; therefore, maximum ventilation rates would be altered. For example, the viscosity of saline solution is approximately 40 times that of air, and therefore a person with a maximum ventilatory rate of 200 liters per minute in air would be expected to have a maximum ventilatory rate of only 5 liters per minute in saline solution. It is not surprising then, that resting animals breathing liquid have very low minute ventilations.[71a,86] Ventilation with air is characterized by gas exchange in which diffusion of gases takes place along pressure gradients, but the gradients are largely maintained by ventilation and perfusion of the lungs. Thus, environmental gas is drawn into the tracheobronchial tree and alveolar spaces by convection where, to a small degree, diffusion within the alveolar space, and, to a much larger degree, diffusion across the alveolar membranes, results in transfer of gas into the blood. Under normal circumstances, the exchange of gas is limited by convective forces. In the liquid environment, on the other hand, particularly with the low alveolar ventilation as a result of increased viscosity, the gas exchange takes place predominantly by diffusion.

The technical complexities of providing ventilation with saline solution that has been hyperbarically oxygenated make this totally impractical. As a result, the search has been undertaken for a more suitable liquid. Such a liquid should have a high solubility for both oxygen and carbon dioxide, but at the same time should permit very rapid diffusion. Since the minute ventilation would be expected to be reduced as a result of the viscosity of the fluid, a very high solubility for oxygen would result in a high oxygen content in the inspired liquid and, consequently, an adequate arterial P_{O_2}. The reduced alveolar ventilation would result in marked accumulation of carbon dioxide. Increases in arterial P_{CO_2}, however, are limited biologically. Therefore, an appropriate combination of high solubility for carbon dioxide and rapid diffusion of carbon dioxide appear necessary for optimal transfer and removal of gases from the lungs.[90]

Particular attention has been focused on fluorocarbon liquids. Several varieties have been developed that appear to be almost biologically inert, are immiscible with aqueous media, have very high solubility for oxygen and carbon dioxide, and permit survival following the period of breathing the liquids. Dogs and rodents have demonstrated that these liquids support life for 1 to 3 hr of breathing the liquid.[86] The solutions are oxygenated by bubbling oxygen through the liquid, and the animal is liquid ventilated by immersion or by a respirator. The solutions contain up to 31 vol % of oxygen at 37° C (more oxygen than is carried by equal volumes of blood), but in general, over a period of time, carbon dioxide accumulates, with marked increases in blood carbon dioxide and respiratory acidosis. These changes are attributable to hypoventilation, but in view of the viscosity of the fluids, it is unlikely that ventilation can be sufficiently increased to overcome these difficulties. It is more likely that increased diffusion rates and altered solubility of carbon dioxide will be necessary as solutions are developed further. These liquids generally have very low surface tension and thus are very effective in wetting all surfaces that they contact. Initially, following a period during which these fluorocarbons were inhaled, the animal tended to have an altered respiratory pattern, and significant arterial hypoxemia. This persisted for days to weeks, but eventually the lungs appeared to be restored to normal. During the early phase after breathing fluorocarbon liquids, there was a considerable increase in numbers of alveolar macrophages and occasional evidence of disruption of alveolar walls, which may have been related to the mechanical trauma of artificial ventilation. The histological abnormalities also improved to normal within 3 wk. In in-vitro and in-vivo experiments, there has been no evidence of alteration of the surface linings of the lungs; in fact, the elastic properties of the lungs and the surface tension characteristics of lung extracts appear to remain normal.[89] The application of breathing liquids to humans has been initiated in the setting of bronchial lavage for alveolar proteinosis.[90]

If a liquid can be developed that is capable of transporting large quantities of respiratory gases, it might also be used as a blood substitute to transport oxygen and carbon dioxide.[87] Fluorocarbon emulsions have been demonstrated to support life by transporting oxygen and carbon dioxide in the circulatory system of animals.

Atmospheric Pollution

In recent years, the presence of significantly increased concentrations of gases or particles in the atmosphere, above generally accepted levels of normal, has come to be known as "air pollution." In present use, this is a sociopolitical term, and not one that can always be associated with scientific evidence of adverse effects.

In general, the gases in the atmosphere are present in predictable concentrations, as illustrated in Table 1-6. The concentration of oxygen appears to be very stable indeed, in spite of the extensive use by combustion of fossil fuels. The concentration of carbon dioxide, on the other hand, has demonstrated measurable changes since the beginning of the nineteenth

TABLE 1-6. Atmospheric Gases

Gas	Concentration
Nitrogen	78.08%
Oxygen	20.95%
Argon	0.93%
Carbon dioxide	0.033%
Neon	18 ppm
Helium	5 ppm
Methane	2.0 ppm
Krypton	1.0 ppm
Hydrogen	0.5 ppm
Nitrous oxide	0.5 ppm
Xenon	0.09 ppm
Sulfur dioxide	0.1 ppm
Nitrogen dioxide	0–0.02 ppm
NH_3	Trace
Ozone	0.07 ppm (winter) 0.02 ppm (summer)

(Adapted from Altman PL, Dittmer DS: Biological Handbooks. Environmental Biology, p 269. Federation of the American Society of Experimental Biologists, 1966[63])

century; it is thought to have increased from 0.029% in 1900 to the present level of 0.033% as a result of fuel combustion.[4] The other gases appear to be present in relatively stable concentrations in the environment in general.

Air pollution may result from increased concentrations of gases, or from airborne particulate matter (aerosols). Many changes in atmospheric composition have no demonstrable adverse effects; furthermore, those adverse effects that are recognized may be related to nonhuman biological changes in plants and vegetables, effects on inanimate objects such as buildings and other structures, or biological effects involving human and animal life. For example, sulfur dioxide at a concentration of 0.5 ppm for 4 hr results in demonstrable injury to numerous vegetables, including alfalfa, lettuce, rhubarb, and spinach. Concentrations in excess of 1.5 ppm produce similar injury in periods of an hour or more. In contrast, citrus fruits are resistant to sulfur dioxide. Many of these biological effects have been reviewed, and new information is acquired rapidly as a result of the renewed societal interest in this area.[91–95]

In addition to direct effects on structure and function of plants and animals and corrosive and destructive processes involving inanimate objects, an indirect, major effect of pollution is change in visibility. This may have important effects on daily sunshine and on aircraft operations, but to many persons, it is more impressive because of its esthetic effects.

TABLE 1-7. Emission of Pollutants from Motor-Vehicle Gasoline Engines*

Carbon monoxide	2,400 lb/1,000 gal
Nitrogen oxide	185 lb/1,000 gal
Hydrocarbons	132 lb/1,000 gal
Particulates	11 lb/1,000 gal
Sulfur dioxide	9 lb/1,000 gal
Organic acids	7 lb/1,000 gal
Aldehydes	4 lb/1,000 gal

* Average emission rates from vehicles, in two large cities, driving at speeds of about 25 miles per hour. (Adapted from Altman PL, Dittmer DS: Biological Handbooks. Environmental Biology. Federation of the American Society of Experimental Biologists, 1966[91])

Gaseous Pollution. *Carbon Monoxide.* This is the most common air pollutant when measured in tonnage and exceeds the amount of all other contaminants added together. Some estimates indicate that the annual world emission is about 250 million tons, and the estimated annual emission of carbon monoxide in the United States is more than 100 million tons. Although the major emission is from the combustion of fuels (in gasoline-powered engines), industrial processes and miscellaneous sources such as forest fires contribute 25 to 30%. Many factors affect the carbon monoxide production of a gasoline engine. The average emission rates listed in Table 1-7 represent random vehicles in city driving, at an average speed of 40 km/hr. Emission rates, however, vary widely with the size of the engine, the speed of operation, the environmental temperature, and, to a certain extent, the fuel. Furthermore, recent advances have permitted the modification of the emission by altering combustion temperature, the air-to-fuel ratio, and other factors. The level of carbon monoxide in the regional environment, thus, is totally dependent on the sources. In a city, high concentrations of carbon monoxide would be anticipated in areas of high traffic density. Atmospheric conditions may influence the rate of dispersion of pollutants.

Carbon monoxide accumulation is a greater problem in areas where wind is minimal, in poorly ventilated buildings, and in heated or enclosed parking lots in northern climates. The odorless and colorless nature of the gas permits it to accumulate undetected.

Fortunately, there has not been a demonstrable accumulation of carbon monoxide in the atmosphere at large. This indicates that the massive quantities of carbon monoxide being dumped into the atmosphere are in some way also being removed. It has not been established by what method carbon monoxide removal occurs but some experiments suggest that soil bacteria are capable of removing carbon monoxide from the air above the soil and thus act as a carbon-monoxide sink. If this mechanism is in effect and is capable of recycling, it is unlikely that carbon monoxide will be a major hazard in terms of general atmospheric pollution.

Urban populations may be exposed to average carbon monoxide levels of 9 to 15 ppm at street level, with peak levels of 30 to 60 ppm.[96] In enclosed parkades, we have observed levels of 50 to 150 ppm commonly, with occasional peak traffic levels as high as 400 ppm. High-rise buildings with no air conditioning demonstrate higher carbon monoxide levels at street level than in upper floors, and buildings with air-conditioning intakes in the upper floors have lower carbon monoxide levels than those with intakes at street level. Buildings heated with oil burners have higher carbon monoxide levels than those with gas or electric heat. A common cause of carbon monoxide poisoning in northern climates is the poorly ventilated tent or camper heated by a low-heat gas or oil heater. The highest occupational levels are seen in fire fighters who may be exposed to over 4000 ppm.[97]

The most predictable and common cause of carbon monoxide inhalation is cigarette smoking. Smoking a single cigarette measurably modifies the level of carbon monoxide in the alveolar gas and in the circulating blood. A person smoking 20 cigarettes per day commonly has 3 to 5% carboxyhemoglobin, and this increases to 10 to 12% for persons smoking 50 to 60 cigarettes per day. Those who inhale deeply have higher levels per cigarette than those who believe they do not inhale.[98] It has been estimated that cigarette smoke contains up to 5% carbon monoxide. A rebreathing technique for analyzing alveolar carbon monoxide levels has been described which permits noninvasive estimation of carboxyhemoglobin levels.[99]

Several studies have emphasized the increased risk of carbon monoxide toxicity in the cigarette smoker who is also exposed to otherwise mild elevations in environmental carbon monoxide levels.[100] When restricted to poorly ventilated areas, even the nonsmoker is at risk from the carbon monoxide generated by the smoker. In one study of subjects in a cigarette-smoke-filled room, carboxyhemoglobin levels of nonsmokers increased from 1.6 to 2.6%, whereas the levels of smokers increased from 5.9 to 9.6%.[101] Air samples from taxicabs with smoking drivers have documented levels as high as 90 ppm. In general, both pipe and cigar smokers have lower levels of inhaled carbon monoxide.

Endogenous sources of carbon monoxide as a by-product of porphyrin metabolism produce negligible levels when compared with exogenous exposures. The average healthy adult produces about 0.4 ml of carbon monoxide per hr, and this value increases in diseases with an increased rate of red-blood-cell breakdown. Normal persons breathing pure air have 0.5 to 0.9% carboxyhemoglobin. Cigarette smokers return to normal levels within 48 hr of cessation of smoking.[102]

The best-understood adverse effect of carbon monoxide is its interference with oxygen transport in the body.[102a] Oxygen binds reversibly with hemoglobin in order to provide adequate transport of oxygen in the blood. Hemoglobin binds reversibly with oxygen and carbon monoxide but has a more than 200 fold greater affinity for carbon monoxide. As a consequence, small amounts of carbon monoxide when in equilibrium with the blood, result in relatively high concentrations of carboxyhemoglobin.

The relationship of inhaled carbon monoxide to carboxyhemoglobin is predictable. It is described over a wide range of inhaled concentrations by the equation

$$\text{Carboxyhemoglobin (\%)} = 0.35 \times \text{carbon monoxide}^{0.8} \text{ (ppm)}.$$

For concentrations of less than 100 ppm, this simpler equation may be used[101]:

$$\text{Carboxyhemoglobin (\%)} = 0.16 \times \text{carbon monoxide (ppm)}.$$

This equation applies only to equilibrium conditions, when the carbon monoxide levels are stable and the gas has been inhaled long enough. At low levels of carbon monoxide and at resting levels of alveolar ventilation, it may require 4 to 8 hr to reach equilibrium. The rate of equilibration is increased when minute ventilation is increased.[104] Table 1-8 compares the levels of carboxyhemoglobin that occur at various levels of inhaled carbon monoxide. Note that the increased ventilation associated with exercise results in higher levels of carboxyhemoglobin after 2 hr, reflecting more complete equilibration of respired gases with the blood. Even this exercise value, however, does not represent complete equilibration. The time necessary for equilibra-

TABLE 1-8. Effects of Exposure to Carbon Monoxide for 2 Hours

CO Concentration Inhaled (ppm)	COHb in Blood of Sedentary Subject %	COHb in Blood with Light Exercise %
20	1.25	2.5
40	2.0	4.0
70	3.8	7.6
100	5.0	10.0
200	10.0	20.0

(Adapted from Bates, DV: A Citizen's Guide to Air Pollution. Montreal, McGill-Queen's University Press, 1972[92])

tion has been worked out for a wide range of inspired carbon monoxide levels.[104,105]

The adverse effects of carbon monoxide on the living organism are summarized below. Impairment of oxygen delivery is of questionable significance in normal persons below levels of 5%. A deficit in "careful-driving" skills has been reported[106] at levels below 5% carboxyhemoglobin. In the range between 5 and 10% carboxyhemoglobin, more definite alterations in perception and mental agility are demonstrable,[107] and in the range of 10 to 20% carboxyhemoglobin, headaches, nausea, and decreased mental acuity occur. As carboxyhemoglobin levels increase beyond 40%, coma develops, and carboxyhemoglobin levels above 50% are commonly associated with permanent cerebral damage or death.

The oxygen transport system is affected in several ways. The binding of carbon monoxide to hemoglobin displaces oxygen, thus leaving less hemoglobin available for oxygen transport. In addition, the remaining hemoglobin is altered so that oxygen is bound with greater affinity, thus decreasing the release of oxygen at tissue levels. The net effect, of course, is to decrease the tissue partial pressure of oxygen in order to facilitate extraction of oxygen from the circulating blood. In chronic carbon monoxide exposure, the hypoxia results in an erythropoietic response, and measurable increases in the red-cell mass.[108,109] Not only does carbon monoxide bind to hemoglobin, but it binds to other porphyrin groups in the body, including myoglobin and the cytochrome oxidase system. These latter groups have a much lower affinity for carbon monoxide than does hemoglobin, and their importance in relation to carbon monoxide toxicity is not clear.

In early studies, it was thought that carbon monoxide exposure resulted in injury to lung tissues. Recently, it has been demonstrated that reduced arterial Po_2 may occur because of modifications in gas exchange in the lungs as a result of the altered oxyhemoglobin dissociation curve.[110] Consequently, patients with ventilation and perfusion imbalance who have arterial hypoxemia develop much more profound hypoxemia when their hemoglobin is partly bound to carbon monoxide. No morphologic change in the alveolar wall is apparent in experimental exposure to carbon monoxide in moderate concentrations.

Adverse Effects of Carbon Monoxide

Normal Persons

1. Decreased oxygen delivery
   a. Less oxygen bound to hemoglobin
   b. Increased affinity of remaining hemoglobin for oxygen with impaired release at the tissue level
   c. Increased red-cell mass
2. Interference with oxygen binding to myoglobin and cytochrome oxidase system
3. Possible increase in atherosclerosis
4. Reduced birth weight and increased neonatal mortality

Persons With Cardiopulmonary Disease

1. Anaerobic myocardial metabolism
2. Increased mortality from myocardial infarction
3. Angina pectoris and intermittent claudication at lower levels of exercise
4. Reduced exercise tolerance in obstructive lung disease

Experimental studies and some evidence in humans have shown an increase in atherosclerotic lesions in the vascular system after exposure to carbon monoxide.[111–113]

The demonstration that the infants of women who smoked during pregnancy had a higher rate of neonatal death and lower birth weights raised the possibility that carbon monoxide was the offending agent. Studies performed on animals with moderate carbon monoxide exposure have demonstrated substantial decreases in birth weight and increases in neonatal mortality. This relationship also requires much further study before it can be established.[114] As might be anticipated, persons with preexisting disease that limits oxygen delivery to specific tissues may demonstrate adverse effects of carbon monoxide at levels lower than those that produce measurable changes in normal subjects. Thus, it was demonstrated that anaerobic myocardial metabolism increased in patients with coronary disease at carboxyhemoglobin concentrations as low as 6%.[115] Exercise tolerance is reduced in patients with obstructive lung disease; angina pectoris and intermittent claudication occur at lower work loads; and the fatality rate due to myocardial infarction may be increased in patients with carboxyhemoglobin levels in the 3 to 6% range.[115–119]

Acute carbon monoxide poisoning may result in demonstrable evidence of tissue hypoxia, ranging from mild alterations in cerebral function to clear-cut evidence of cellular damage in the central nervous system, heart muscle, skeletal muscle, liver, peripheral nerves, and skin. Biochemical evidence of anaerobic metabolism, as reflected by metabolic acidosis and lactic acid accumulation, is present in severe acute toxicity. Liver and muscle enzymes may be severely elevated with myoglobinuria.

The management of acute carbon monoxide poisoning follows entirely from its known effects on oxygen transport. First the subject must be removed from the environment. The urgency of the situation is dictated by the degree of impairment. Mild degrees of intoxication are quickly improved by removal from the environment and the addition of supplemental oxygen. More severe degrees of intoxication require immediate institution of high concentrations of inhaled oxygen. When available in the ambulance or hospital, hyperbaric oxygenation should be immediately instituted. When this is not available, 100% oxygen should be administered.[120] Traditional physiological thinking and early experiments suggested that, since the carbon monoxide was present in small concentrations, it would not affect alveolar or arterial Po_2 and, therefore, would not interfere with the normal respiratory control mechanisms (which act partially through the effect of partial pressure of oxygen on the peripheral chemoreceptors). It is now commonly recognized, however, that sufficient reduction in arterial Po_2 is present to increase the respiratory drive in most patients. This hypoxemia may be the result of central nervous system depression, causing prolonged immobilization with aspiration and infection resulting in ventilation-perfusion imbalance in the lungs. The use of supplemental oxygen raises arterial Po_2, increases dissolved oxygen in the blood, and increases the rate of displacement of carbon monoxide from the hemoglobin.

The washout of carbon monoxide, like the initial accumulation of carbon monoxide in the blood, is dependent on the minute ventilation. Inhalation of carbon dioxide may be utilized to drive ventilation and thus further increase the rate of washout. If adequate ventilation is maintained spontaneously or by an artificial respirator, in the presence of a high arterial Po_2, the carbon monoxide levels of most subjects quickly reduce to a safer range.[120,121] Normal persons breathing ordinary air will have an average half-time of carbon monoxide elimination of about 250 min; if oxygen is substituted, this is reduced to 40 min, and if 5 to 7% carbon dioxide is added, the half-time is further reduced.

Oxides of Sulfur. Sulfur dioxide, which is normally virtually absent from the atmosphere, is a product of burning fuels containing sulfur. The most common source is the burning of coal and oil. Consequently, this, too, is predominantly a problem of urban "progress." Recently processes for eliminating and reclaiming sulfur from fuel oils have been effective in reducing the emission of sulfur dioxide. When combustion of those fuels occurs, sulfur dioxide is oxidized in the air to form sulfur trioxide and sulfates. These form a sulfur oxide-particulate aerosol. Therefore, measurement of sulfur dioxide, sulfates, or particulates may not reflect the effective pollution accurately. Sulfur dioxide is the best studied component of the complex. The oxides of sulfur and of nitrogen, when dissolved in water, form the related acids. When this occurs during natural precipitation, the result is known as "acid rain." Sulfur dioxide therefore has major effects on inanimate substances, such as increased rate of corrosion of metals; substantial deterioration and discoloration of limestone, marble, and slate; and damage to textile fibers, including cotton, rayon, and nylon.

Sulfur dioxide can be detected by most persons by taste, rather than odor, at concentrations in the range of 0.3 to 1.0 ppm. For most persons, the odor threshold appears to be about 0.5 ppm. At levels of 10 to 25 ppm, substantial irritation of mucous membranes is experienced. The high solubility of sulfur dioxide results in almost complete removal from inhaled air, in the upper respiratory passages. The adverse effects of sulfur dioxide on the respiratory tract are potentiated by environmental factors such as humidity, and are additive in the presence of other preexisting diseases.[122,123] Most epidemiological studies that demonstrate increased morbidity and mortality in relation to sulfur oxide pollution indicate that the cigarette smoker is much more susceptible to sulfur dioxide than the nonsmoker. Elderly patients with bronchitis and emphysema are at greatest risk. Asthmatics may have increased bronchospasm, particularly when oxides of sulfur exceed the odor-detection threshold.[124] Excessive acute respiratory disease, including laryngotracheobronchitis, has been reported in children and adults with increased levels of sulfur.[93,125]

The pulmonary effects of sulfur dioxide inhalation have been well defined during acute, high-level exposures.[126,127] Increased airway resistance in the bronchial tubes is reflected in decreased respiratory air-flow rates. The mechanism of the bronchoconstriction has not been established; it is possible that irritation of airway mucous membranes results in reflex increase in bronchial muscle tone. Mucociliary activity is demonstrably impaired by sulfur dioxide, but it should be recalled that this occurs with levels far in excess of those commonly present during peak pollution periods.[123] Acute exposure to extremely high levels results in death with tracheobronchial mucosal necrosis and hemorrhagic alveolar edema.[128]

While there is good epidemiological evidence that periods of high urban pollution due to the sulfur oxide-particulate complex are associated with increased mortality, illness-related absenteeism, and reduced lung function, the dose-effect relationships are poorly defined. Future studies will undoubtedly focus on improved measurement of the components of the oxide-particulate complex.[93–95,129]

Oxides of Nitrogen. Combustion occurring under pressure and with heat is likely to result in the fixation of nitrogen and oxygen, which are normal constituents of air. Initially, most commonly, nitrous oxide is produced, but this quickly becomes oxidized in the atmosphere to become the more irritant nitrogen dioxide. When dissolved, this of course produces the highly corrosive H_2NO_3. The major source of nitrogen dioxide in the environment is fuel combustion, particularly coal and natural gas, and a close runner-up is the production of NO_2 by combustion of gasoline in motor vehicles. In general, the oxides of nitrogen do not achieve high concentrations; the average monthly urban concentrations range from 0.04 to 0.14 ppm, with peak concentrations rarely exceeding 0.5 ppm. Thus, it is uncommon to achieve concentrations that can be demonstrated to cause direct irritation to the tracheobronchial tree.

As with the oxides of sulfur, the health hazards can rarely be attributed to a specific component, and nitrogen dioxide has been best studied. Early evidence of nitrogen dioxide toxicity was provided by silo-filler's disease, which presented as acute bronchitis or pulmonary edema. Current studies suggest reduced lung function, and increased susceptibility to respiratory infections in populations exposed to high ambient levels. Children had reduced vital capacity and expiratory flow rates, while patients with bronchitis and asthma demonstrated increased airway resistance.[92,93,130] The precise level at which nitrogen dioxide becomes a health hazard has yet to be defined.

Hydrocarbons. Twenty-six aromatic hydrocarbons have been identified in the air in several urban areas of the United States. These are produced primarily by automobiles, and the principal compound is methane, which may average 3 parts per million in urban air. Other alkanes and alkenes are produced, and much of the smell of diesel and gasoline exhaust is thought to be the result of the presence of aldehydes. Fortunately, the biological effects of these substances seem to be predominantly related to changes in vegetation, and ethylene appears to have the most direct effect on certain forms of plant life. Small amounts of polycyclic hydrocarbons have been identified, including benzopyrene, which is of particular interest because of its experimentally demonstrated capacity to induce cancer. Concentrations are usually very low, and the measurements are not readily performed.[92] Hydrocarbons are most important as a respiratory hazard because of their contribution to the production of photochemical smog.[93]

Ozone and Photochemical Smog. Ozone is present in the upper atmosphere, where it filters ultraviolet radiation from the sun. There is serious concern that this layer may be depleted by high-flying aircraft exhaust and by excess escape of Freon in propellants and refrigerants. The reduced ozone layer might greatly increase the risk of skin cancer, and could damage plant and animal life.[131]

Ozone is the major oxidant produced during photochemical air pollution. Hydrocarbons and oxides of nitrogen will react in the presence of ultraviolet light to form ozone. This is potentiated in the presence of high humidity and carbon monoxide. Certain cities are uniquely predisposed to this problem as a result of climate. When the chemical reaction produces high concentrations of airborne by-products, it is known as photochemical smog, and contributes to a definite haze.[135]

Ozone produces irritation of the eyes and upper airways. Exercising persons develop evidence of bronchial obstruction acutely[132], but this effect disappears with repeated exposure.[132] Patients with asthma or chronic obstructive lung disease demonstrate deterioration of lung function when exposed to ozone. Animal studies have produced bronchitis, bronchiolitis and emphysema. However, human studies at naturally occurring levels of ozone failed to affect gas exchange in the lungs[134] and have not been established to cause long-term lung injury.[93,95,136]

Particulate Pollution. Soil, dust, and naturally airborne particles will not be considered in this section. Their role as a health hazard is almost totally unexplored. We refer here to solid or liquid matter suspended in air (called *aerosols*).[137] These are comprised of a wide variety of substances with one common feature: a submicron size. Large particulate matter originating as dust from windswept fields tends to be readily deposited owing to its size (in the range of 1 to 10 μ). Smaller particles (less than 1 μ), however, tend to remain suspended for prolonged periods, up to several months under suitable meteorologic conditions. The sources of particulate emission are multiple, but major urban sources include combustion from space heaters, incineration processes (either commercial or domestic), motor-vehicle exhaust, and a variety of sources such as brake linings of vehicles, construction work, road repairs, and so forth. These widely divergent sources of particles contain many common materials, such as carbon and silicon, but also a wide range of metals, such as cadmium, chromium, copper, iron, lead (particularly from leaded gasolines), manganese, nickel, and many others. In addition, asbestos and beryllium play some role. The pulmonary effects of these specific pollutants will be discussed in Chapter 13.

It is of considerable concern that particulate pollution in the urban areas now occurs in the presence of gaseous pollution. Although it has not been clearly established, irritant gases may be adsorbed to particles and deposited in the lungs, with high local concentrations in the lung tissue.

The most important single particulate emitted from the automobile appears to be lead. At present, it has been estimated that approximately 180,000 tons of lead are emitted into the atmosphere in the United States annually as a result of motor-vehicle exhaust. Although little definite evidence of lead toxicity (from this source) has been demonstrated in humans, current studies suggest that the lead has been incorporated into vegetation, which is ultimately consumed by humans, where it may accumulate and the well-recognized deleterious effects of lead become manifest. Current efforts to severely limit the use of leaded gasolines may be early enough to avert some of these consequences.

The adverse effects of particulate pollution may be categorized as follows:[122]

Effects on Health. At the present state of our knowledge, the aerosols are recognized more as potential health hazards than as definite health hazards. The absorption of noxious gases, and the body reactions to deposition of very small particles deep in the tracheobronchial tree all represent areas of concern.

Effects on Visibility. Airborne particles in smog reduce visibility by scattering and absorbing light. Such particulate pollution occasionally requires restriction of aircraft operations. The effects on visibility may be a result of "dust" smog or photochemical smog. These circumstances might be anticipated only in densely populated metropolitan areas; however, the beautiful city of Calgary, Alberta, with a population of half a million persons, located in the foothills of the Canadian Rocky Mountains, has frequent periods of distinct haze, occurring during days in which there is a temperature inversion. Thermal inversions occur in certain geographic areas in relation to wind and surface air mixing. When a warm layer of air overlies a cold layer of surface air, the latter is trapped together with its pollutants, until vertical mixing occurs. When larger cities experience thermal inversions, severe haze and pollution may occur.

Effects on Materials. Substantial evidence has been accumulated showing that the corrosiveness of sulfur dioxide and nitrogen dioxide are increased when absorbed to particulate material.

Undesirable Odor Sources. These refer particularly to motor exhausts, street-paving asphalts, and trash burning.

Effects on Direct Sunlight and Climate. At concentrations ranging from 100 to 150 μg per m^3, where large smoke-turbidity factors persist, particles reduce direct sunlight. The scattering and adsorption of sunlight by airborne particulates reduces the amount of sunlight reaching the ground. Total sunlight is reduced 50% for each doubling of the concentration above 100 μg per m^3, and this reduction is most pronounced for ultraviolet radiation.

Automobile Exhaust. The major emission products of automobile exhaust, as listed in Table 1-7, are carbon monoxide, oxides of nitrogen, hydrocarbons, particulates, sulfur dioxide, organic acid, and aldehydes. The emission rate is dependent on operating temperature of the combustion engine, speed of travel, and, to a certain extent, the type of fuel burned (for example, the emission rate of lead is entirely dependent on the lead content of the gasoline). Furthermore, the precise emission products are modified by pollution-control systems.

The health effects of automobile exhaust are also determined by location. For example, carbon monoxide may accumulate in high concentrations within a motor vehicle that has an unsatisfactory exhaust system. General atmospheric pollution, however, involving carbon monoxide, oxides of nitrogen, hydrocarbons, and the products of photochemical action, predominantly ozone, has adverse effects only when these substances accumulate in sufficiently high concentrations. These factors depend on wind conditions, temperature inversions, and traffic density. The ozone concentration may, of course, increase in the atmosphere considerably later than the peak concentrations of the pollutants, because it is produced by the action of sunlight. Among the most troublesome effects of automobile-exhaust pollution is the emission of lead by combustion of leaded gasolines discussed above under particulate pollution.

Each of the major products of emission and its health hazard have been discussed above. General studies of the overall health effects of motor-vehicle exhaust have failed to demonstrate any additional effects on lung function,[138] or on safety of operation of motor vehicles.[139]

Smoking. "In one year, a typical one-pack-per day smoker takes in 50,000 to 70,000 puffs through the burning column of a unique chemical factory which contains over 2,000 known compounds."[140]

Tobacco is an agricultural crop of the nightshade family, produced in almost all parts of the

TABLE 1-9. Major Toxic Agents in Cigarette Smoke

Gas Phase (90% of total)	Biological Effects	Particulate Phase (less than 10% of total)	Biological Effects
Nitrosamines	C	Nicotine	T
Hydrazine	C	"Tar"	TI
Vinyl chloride	C	Cresols	C
Urethane	TI	Phenol	CoC
Formaldehyde	CT, CoC	DDT*	T, C?
Hydrogen cyanide	CT, T	Hydroquinone	T?
Acrolein	CT	Pyridine	T?
Acetaldehyde	CT	Endrin*	T, C?
Nitrogen oxides	T	Metals	C
Ammonia	T?		
Pyridine	T?		
Carbon monoxide	T		
Acrylonitrile	C		
2-16 tropeopane	C		

* Insecticides used in agriculture.
Key: C—Carcinogen; TI—Tumor Initiator; T—Toxic agent; CoC—Co-Carcinogen; CT—Ciliatoxic.
(Adapted from Smoking and Health: A Report of the Surgeon General. US Dept of HEW, 1979[142])

world and used in almost every country. The contents of tobacco smoke are determined primarily by the physical and chemical properties of the leaf. Various species and strains have been developed to produce wide variations in chemical make-up. This is further influenced by soil, climate, post-harvest handling, and other factors.

The chemical composition of tobacco smoke is conveniently divided into constituents of the gaseous phase and of the particulate phase (Table 1-9). The particulate phase is filterable as particles smaller than 0.1 μ. Mainstream smoke is inhaled by the smoker when he takes a puff. Sidestream smoke drifts from the burning cone into the surrounding air. The involuntary, passive, or non-smoker in the smoker's presence is exposed to sidestream smoke plus the material exhaled by the smoker.

The effects of inhaled tobacco smoke vary tremendously with the nature of the smoking device (cigarette, pipe, or cigar), the presence of a filter, the length of the tube or tobacco through which the smoke is inhaled, and the method of the smoker. Smoke produced by an average cigarette weighs about 500 mg. Five to 10% of this is moist particulate matter; 12 to 15%, carbon dioxide; 3 to 6%, carbon monoxide; and the remainder mainly nitrogen, oxygen, and water. More than 2000 components have been identified in tobacco smoke, predominantly residing in the particulate matter. These include nicotine and the so-called tobacco tar.[141,142]

Cigarette consumption in the western countries has declined about 2% since 1964, when the U.S. Surgeon General's Report first emphasized the health hazards. Many countries and some populations in North America have, however, shown increased use of tobacco.[143] As a result of selective crops, improved curing, reduced use of insecticides and the use of filters, there have been substantial reductions in tar, nicotine and other harmful constituents in recent years.

Effects on the human body are determined by the temperature of the inhaled smoke, the amount of inhalation, the depth of inhalation into the lungs, and the duration of smoking history. As a consequence, cigarette smokers in general have more severe respiratory effects than do smokers of cigars and pipes, and the number of cigarettes smoked relates directly to the health consequences. Table 1-10 indicates approximate carbon monoxide levels for various smoking habits. (see also Carbon Monoxide). So-called tumorigenic agents in tobacco are largely contained in the particulate matter, tar. The well-

TABLE 1-10. Carbon Monoxide Levels in Relation to Smoking*

Category	CO Measured in Expired Air (ppm)	Carboxyhemoglobin (%)
Nonsmoker	3.2	1.2
Smoker		
Pipe and/or cigar only	5.4	1.7
Cigarette:		
Light (less than ½ pack/day)		
Inhaler	17.1	3.8
Noninhaler	19.0	2.3
Moderate (½ to 2 packs/day)		
Inhaler	27.5	5.9
Noninhaler	14.4	3.6
Heavy (more than 2 packs/day)		
Inhaler	32.4	6.8
Noninhaler	25.2	5.6

* The carboxyhemoglobin level tends to remain fairly stable in a habitual smoker. A random blood sample is generally indicative of the approximate level through the day.

(Adapted from Castleden C, Cole P: Variations in carboxyhemoglobin levels in smokers. Br Med J 4:736, 1974[144])

established carcinogenicity of tobacco tar in a variety of animal species makes this a likely offender in the production of lung cancer. Selected carcinogenic polynuclear aromatic hydrocarbons are borne in the particulate component of the smoke. Extensive research is clarifying the role of many of the carcinogens, with clear evidence that some are tumor initiators while others act only as co-carcinogens. Several appear to have organ specific effects such as bladder carcinogens.[142]

The life span of cigarette smokers is reduced in proportion to numbers and duration of cigarette consumption. The mortality ratio for all smokers is about 1.7 when compared to nonsmokers, and 2.0 for two-pack-per-day smokers. A 30-year-old two-pack-per-day-smoker has a life expectancy that is 8.1 years shorter than a non-smoker. Pipe and cigar smokers have much lower death rates than cigarette smokers. Ex-smokers who are well when they quit immediately have a reduced mortality rate, which continues to decline until it reaches the nonsmoker rate 15 years after cessation of smoking. Of course, these overall mortality statistics only hint at the disability and morbidity. The disability varies from minutes, in those who suffer sudden death after acute myocardial infarction, to several years of severe impairment in persons with chronic obstructive pulmonary disease. Specific effects of smoking continue to be elucidated. Epidemiological data provide strong circumstantial evidence for the adverse effects of smoking, but specific mechanisms of tissue injury are not always clear.[145,146]

Involuntary Smoking. The health hazard to the non smoker (involuntary smoking) remains to be completely clarified. Carbon monoxide levels are definitely increased, children of smoking parents have more frequent respiratory infections, and patients with asthma or chronic obstructive lung disease commonly claim respiratory tract irritation.[147,148] There is evidence that airways dysfunction and increased incidence of lung cancer may occur in otherwise normal involuntary smokers.

Smoking and Cardiovascular Diseases. The death rate from coronary heart disease is higher in smokers than in nonsmokers. This higher death rate due to atherosclerotic vascular disease has been confirmed in many studies. Furthermore, there is some evidence that the risk of sudden

Diseases Related to Cigarette Smoking

Cardiovascular Diseases
- Ischemic Heart Disease (Sudden death, acute myocardial infarction, angina pectoris)
- Atherosclerotic peripheral vascular disease
- Atherosclerotic aortic aneurysm
- Thromboangiitis obliterans

Nonneoplastic Bronchopulmonary Diseases
- Abnormal airways function
- Recurrent respiratory infections
- Chronic bronchitis
- Emphysema

Cancer

Lung	Esophagus
Larynx	Urinary bladder and kidney
Oral	Pancreas

Peptic Ulcer Disease

Complications of Pregnancy and Infant Health
- Reduced birth weight
- Increased spontaneous abortion, fetal and neonatal death
- Increased abruptio placentae, bleeding in pregnancy, preterm labor and delivery
- Possible toxic effects of breast milk and atmospheric pollution from smoking mothers upon infant.

(Adapted from Smoking and Health: A report of the Surgeon General, Part I. US Dept of HEW, 1979[149])

death is increased in individuals who are smoking at the time of a myocardial infarction and that this risk is decreased soon after the cessation of smoking cigarettes. Sudden death, acute myocardial infarction, incidence and severity of angina pectoris, atherosclerotic peripheral vascular disease and atherosclerotic aortic aneurysm are all increased in smokers. The literature is divided, but conclusive evidence for increased risk of stroke is not available[149]. The precise mechanism of development of atherosclerosis has not been established. Carbon monoxide has been implicated in experimental development of atherosclerosis, the potential role of nicotine has also been explored, and the effects of smoking on thrombus formation and blood flow have been considered. Aggregation of platelets, increased levels of catecholamine, increased free fatty acids, and mobilization of polymorphonuclear leukocytes have all been demonstrated in various studies of the intravascular circulation.[149,149a]

Smoking and Nonneoplastic Bronchopulmonary Disease. Studies from many countries demonstrate a predictable increase in bronchitis and emphysema related to numbers and duration of cigarettes smoked, and to the reports of degree of inhalation. Recent studies have focused on earlier stages of lung disease and indicate that smokers have measurable abnormalities of lung function, and increased respiratory symptoms at a much younger age than chronic bronchitis and emphysema. Furthermore, children of smoking parents have increased respiratory symptoms when compared to non-smoking parents.[150] It is not yet clear which individuals will develop early abnormalities of lung function, and respiratory symptoms, and whether these always develop chronic obstructive lung disease.[151] A spectrum of abnormalities each with their own natural history, related to individual susceptibility, seems more likely. The precise mechanism whereby cigarette smoke produces lung disease has not been elucidated. Acute inhalation of cigarette smoke produces an increase in central airway resistance and a decrease in lung compliance, but it does not appear to affect the small airways of the lung.[152,153] Cigarette smoke lowers the effectiveness of pulmonary surfactant, thereby increasing the surface-tension properties of the lung lining. It exerts a powerful ciliostatic effect on the bronchial lining under some circumstances, but may actually result in increased mucociliary transport under other circumstances.[154] The metabolism and function of the pulmonary alveolar macrophages and their role in clearing the lungs are impaired by cigarette smoke.[155,156] Each of these factors might play a role in diminishing clearance of noxious agents from the peripheral lung units, thus predisposing to disease. The toxic effects of cigarettes may eventually be separated on the basis of constituents (see preceding chart). Production of phlegm is reduced in those who smoke low-tar cigarettes.[156a] On the other hand, entirely separate lines of evidence indicate that in some persons, other host factors become important. Persons with hereditary alpha$_1$ globulin deficiency (alpha$_1$ antitrypsin deficiency) may lack the inhibitor that prevents proteolytic lung destruction, and they may consequently develop emphysema. This suggests that persons who inhale tobacco smoke may, in some way, increase the concentration of proteolytic enzymes or reduce local inhibitors near critical lung tissues and thereby develop destructive changes in the lungs. Alveolar macrophages, circulating leukocytes, and bronchial leukocytes, as a result of inflammatory reaction, all are potential sources.[150,157,158] It is possible that many persons have a genetic predisposition to lung injury. The pathogenesis of bronchitis and emphysema is discussed in further detail in Chapter 14.

Smoking and Cancer. Lung cancer is the commonest malignant cause of death in North America. The male death rate has increased from 19.9 per 100,000 per yr in 1950 to an estimated 70 per 100,000 per yr in 1980. The rate of increase can be clearly correlated with cigarette consumption, and current rapid increases in female death rates due to lung cancer are probably related to changes in smoking habits. No specific cell type has been consistently linked to the smoking-lung cancer epidemic.[149] Cigarette smoking is considered the major cause of lung cancer in both men and women. Lung cancer is consistently more common in urban than in rural areas, but this can be accounted for by differences in smoking patterns rather than implicating urban air pollution for a significant effect. Ex-smokers' risk of developing lung cancer gradually diminishes, approaching levels of nonsmokers after 15 yr. Perhaps the long-term study of 34,000 British physicians best demonstrates the long-term benefits of smoking cessation.[159]

Current evidence suggests an increased incidence of cancer of the larynx, esophagus, urinary bladder, kidney, pancreas and mouth in smokers. Cancer of the larynx and oral cancer are particularly related to cigar and pipe smoking.[149]

Numerous changes in bronchial epithelium, including hyperplasia, stratification, atypical metaplasia, and carcinoma in situ, are more common in patients who smoke. Direct evidence regarding the specific carcinogenic component and the precise early cytologic change that constitutes neoplasia has not been established. Animal studies have provided ample evidence that certain components of cigarette smoke are potential tumorigenic factors.[149] (See also a detailed discussion of Bronchogenic Carcinoma in Chap. 15).

Smoking and Peptic Ulcer. The prevalence of peptic ulcer is about 1.7 times greater in smokers than in nonsmokers, and the mortality due to peptic ulcer is about twice as high in smokers.[149]

Effects of Smoking on Pregnancy. Although the total health effects of cigarette smoking on pregnancy have not been determined, maternal smoking during pregnancy is associated with decreased infant birth weight and increased incidence of prematurity, spontaneous abortion, stillbirth, and neonatal death. The precise mechanism, again, has not been established; however, carbon monoxide concentrations and nicotine may be important.

Smoking Cessation. Thus, the specific noxious agents in cigarette smoke, their precise site of action, and, in many instances, the actual health hazard and disability have not been established. The enormous impact of this habit on mortality, health-care economy, and human suffering warrants the tremendous research effort currently being exerted. The significant decrease in percentage of smokers and increased numbers of nonsmokers in most age groups may be a response to educational campaigns. The use of filters to substantially reduce tar and nicotine may reduce the health hazards.[160] It is a cause for great disappointment that in the face of such convincing circumstantial evidence, the simplest solution to the cigarette health hazard is proving unsatisfactory to society. Most smokers will not quit! Furthermore, the number of cigarette smokers among teenagers appears to be at least stable or on the increase despite vigorous anti-smoking campaigns.[143] Legislation regarding warning of cigarette health hazards, restriction of cigarette advertising, and enormous tax expenditures in the areas of health-care research have not provided the incentive needed by the masses to deal with this habit. The solution to the smoking problem lies in the understanding of human motivation.[161]

The health benefits of cessation of smoking have been outlined above. Not all studies have demonstrated improvement in obstructive lung disease, and although respiratory symptoms disappear, measurable abnormalities of lung function persist, even in those with small airways disease.[156a,162] The death rate from coronary artery disease is diminished toward normal in exsmokers. This probably does not represent a decrease in atherosclerosis, but other factors responsible for myocardial infarction and sudden death appear to be improved. Cessation of smoking decreases the risk of cancer of the lung several years after the smoker quits.

Cigarette smoking is probably habituating because of the nicotine content. Withdrawal results in hypotension, bradycardia, reduced levels of circulating catecholamines and many other metabolic and physiologic changes. When habitual smokers stop smoking they may experience craving, irritability, restlessness, sleep disturbances, gastrointestinal disturbances, anxiety, and impairment of concentration. Still, it has not been completely accepted as a true addiction.

Many methods for support of the smoker during withdrawal have been used with varying success. None are as effective as initial avoidance. Complete cessation has been more effective than gradual withdrawal.[161]

Problems in Managing Air Pollution. Current epidemiologic approaches have been reasonably criticized because (a) they have frequently depended on analysis of one or two pollutants, when many were present; (b) analytical techniques used limited sampling times; (c) populations at risk were poorly identified; (d) results were interpreted in an advocacy role. Furthermore, studies have attempted to demonstrate either a safe level of pollutants, or a level clearly unsafe, without adequate experimental criteria for either. The scientific community and politicians are required to make decisions that may control pollution at enormous cost, or not control it and permit great health hazards.[163–168]

The retrospective study, the failure to identify multiple variables that may be responsible for effects, genetic population differences, and insensitive techniques for determining early abnormalities all prevent our effective use of large-scale studies to identify health hazards in large populations. Consequently, the purist argues that cigarette tar extracts painted on bald epithelium of rodents may, in spite of their carcinogenic effect, have no bearing on human disease. Similarly, the purist may argue that increased mortality due to myocardial infarction, or chronic obstructive bronchopulmonary disease, relates to other genetic or physiological characteristics of the persons involved rather than the pollutants in cigarette smoke. It is not new to biomedical science that folklore, intuition, and circumstantial evidence provide useful clues regarding health benefits. Biblical prohibition of the eating of pork may well have spared the Israelis from generations of diseased muscles due to trichinosis. While the ultimate in experimental design is being developed and the final mechanisms of histological damage are elucidated, careful avoidance of health hazards, which are identified by strong circumstantial evidence, may prolong active life.[169,170]

REFERENCES

1. WOOD SC, LENFANT C (eds): Evolution of Respiratory Processes, Lung Biology in Health and Disease, Vol 13. New York, Marcel Dekker, 1979
2. ALTMAN PL, DITTMER DS: Biological Handbooks. Respiration and Circulation, p 14. Federation of the American Society of Experimental Biologists, 1971
3. VAN VALEN L: The history and stability of atmospheric oxygen. Science 171:439, 1971
4. EDITORIAL: Costs and benefits of carbon dioxide. Nature 279:1, 1979

4a. MADDEN RA, RAMANATHAN V: Detecting climate change due to increasing carbon dioxide. Science 209:763, 1980

5. ALTMAN PL, DITTMER DS: Biological Handbooks. Respiration and Circulation, p 383. Bethesda, Federation of the American Society of Experimental Biologists, 1971
6. SALTZMAN HA, SALZANO JV: Effects of carbohydrate metabolism upon respiratory gas exchange in normal men. J Appl Physiol 30:228, 1971
7. NAIMARK A, WASSERMAN K, MCILLROY MB: Continuous measurement of ventilatory exchange ratio during exercise. J Appl Physiol 19:644, 1964

8. HOUSTON CS: Lessons to be learned from high altitude. Postgrad Med J 55:447, 1979
8a. HOUSTON CS: Going High: The story of man and altitude; Queen City Printers Inc. Burlington, Vermont, 1980
9. BAKER PT (ed): The Biology of High Altitude Peoples. New York, Cambridge University Press, 1978
9a. COTTON EK et al: Re-evaluation of birth weights at high altitude. Am J Obstet Gynecol 138:220, 1980
10. RENNIE D: High science present and future. N Engl J Med 301:1343, 1979
10a. WEST JB, WAGNER PD: Pulmonary gas exchange at high altitude. Prog Resp Res 16:287, 1981
11. ALTMAN PL, DITTMER DS: Biological Handbooks. Environmental Biology p 350. Federation of the American Society of Experimental Biologists, 1966
12. LENFANT C, SULLIVAN K: Adaptation to high altitude. N Engl J Med 284:1298, 1971
13. DEMPSEY J: Handbook of Physiology. The Respiratory System, Vol 1 (in press)
14. KELLOGG RH: Oxygen and carbon dioxide in the regulation of respiration. Fed Proc 36:1658, 1977
15. CRAWFORD RD, SEVERINGHAUS JW: CSF pH and ventilatory acclimatization to altitude. J Appl Physiol 45:275, 1978
16. DEMPSEY JA et al: Role of cerebrospinal fluid in ventilatory deacclimatization from chronic hypoxia. J Clin Invest 64:199, 1979
17. GUENTER CA et al. Cardiorespiratory and metabolic effects in men on the South Polar Plateau. Arch Intern Med 125:630, 1970
18. CRUZ JC: Mechanics of breathing in high altitude and sea level subjects. Respir Physiol 17:146, 1973
19. KRYGER M et al. Diagnosis of airflow obstruction at high altitude. Am Rev Respir Dis 117:1055, 1978
19a. MANSELL A, POWLES A, SUTTON J: Changes in pulmonary P V characteristics of human subjects at an altitude of 5,366 m. J Appl Physiol 49:79, 1980
20. DAWSON A: Regional pulmonary blood flow in sitting and supine man during and after acute hypoxia. J Clin Invest 48:301, 1969
21. BISGARD G, et al: Distribution of regional lung function during mild exercise in residents of 3100 m. Respir Physiol 22:369 1974
22. HAAB P et al: Ventilation–perfusion relationships during high altitude adaptation. J Appl Physiol 26:77, 1969
23. SPIELVOGEL H et al: Effects of posture on pulmonary diffusing capacity and regional distribution of pulmonary blood flow in normal male and female high altitude dwellers at 3,650 m (12,200 ft). Respiration 35:125, 1978
24. VINCENT J et al: Pulmonary gas exchange, diffusing capacity in natives and newcomers at high altitude. Respir Physiol 34:219, 1978
25. CUDKOWICZ L: Mean pulmonary artery pressure and alveolar oxygen tension in man at different altitudes. Respiration 27:417, 1970
26. BLOUNT SG JR, VOGEL JHK: Altitude and the pulmonary circulation. Adv Intern Med 13:11, 1967
27. VOGEL JHK (ed): Hypoxia, High Altitude and the Heart. Advances in Cardiology, Vol 5. New York, S Karger, AG, 1970
28. KRZYWICKI HJ et al: Water metabolism in humans during acute high altitude exposure (4,300 m). J Appl Physiol 30:806, 1971
29. MYHRE LG et al: Blood volume changes during three-week residence at high altitude. Clin Chem 16:7, 1970
30. WHITCOMB WH et al: Effect of the South Polar Plateau on plasma and urine erythropoietin levels. Arch Intern Med 125:638, 1970. J Appl Physiol 23:531, 1967
31. SAMAJA M, VEICSTEINAS A, CERRETELLI P: Oxygen affinity of blood in altitude Sherpas. J Appl Physiol 47:337, 1979
32. HOON RS, et al: Effect of high-altitude exposure for 10 days on stroke volume and cardiac output. J Appl Physiol 42:722, 1977
33. VOGEL JA, HANSEN JE, HARRIS CW: Cardiovascular responses in man during exhaustive work at sea level and high altitude. J Appl Physiol 23:531, 1967
33a. DILL DB, HILLYARD SD, MILLER J: Vital capacity, exercise performance and blood gases at altitude as related to age. J Appl Physiol 48:6, 1980
34. BLASS JP, GIBSON GE: Consequences of mild, graded hypoxia. Adv Neurol 26:229, 1979
35. SIESJO BK, BERNTMAN L: Cytoplasmic and mitochrondrial redox changes in the brain during hypoxia. Adv Neurol 26:219, 1979
36. DAVIS JN et al: The effect of hypoxia on brain neurotransmitter systems. Adv Neurol 26:219, 1979
37. FRAYSER R et al: Hormonal and electrolyte response to exposure to 17,500 feet. J Appl Physiol 38:636, 1975
38. SUTTON JR et al: Effect of acetazolamide on hypoxemia during sleep at high altitude. N Engl J Med 301:1329, 1979
39. SCHUMACHER G, PETAJAN J: High altitude stress and retinal hemorrhage. Arch Environ Health 30:217, 1975
39a. MCFADDEN DM et al: High-altitude retinopathy. JAMA 245:581, 1981
40. HACKETT PH, RENNIE D: Rales, peripheral edema, retinal hemorrhage, and acute mountain sickness. Am J Med 67:214, 1979
41. CARONNA JJ: Diagnosis, prognosis and treatment of hypoxic coma. Adv Neurol 26:1, 1979
42. KREISBERG RA: Lactate homeostasis and lactic acidosis. Ann Intern Med 92:227, 1980

42a. ROBIN ED: Of men and mitochondria: Coping with hypoxic dysoxia. Am Rev Respir Dis 122: 517, 1980
43. BARTLETT D JR, REMMERS JE: Effects of high altitude exposure on the lungs of young rats. Respir Physiol 13:116, 1971
44. BRODY JS, VACCARO C: Post natal formation of alveoli: Interstitial events and physiologic consequences. Fed Proc 38:215, 1979
45. LAHIRI S et al.: Irreversible blunted respiratory sensitivity to hypoxia in high altitude natives. Respir Physiol 6:360, 1969
46. WEIL J et al: Acquired attenuation of chemoreceptor function in chronically hypoxic man at high altitude. J Clin Invest 50:186, 1971
47. LAHIRI S, EDELMAN NH: Peripheral chemoreflexes in the regulation of breathing of high altitude natives. Respir Physiol 6:375, 1969
48. MOSSO A: Life of Man on the High Alps. London, T Fisher Unwin, 1898
49. MONGE MC: High Altitude disease. Arch Intern Med 59:32, 1937
50. MONGE MC: Life in the Andes and chronic mountain sickness. Science 95:79, 1942
51. HECHT HH et al: Brisket disease. III. Clinical features and hemodynamic observations in high altitude dependent right heart failure of cattle. Am J Med 32:171, 1962
52. KRYGER M et al: Impaired oxygenation during sleep in excessive polycythemia at high altitude: Improvement with respiratory stimulation. Sleep 1:3, 1978
53. KRYGER M et al: Treatment of excessive polycythemia of high altitude with respiratory stimulant drugs. Am Rev Respir Dis 117:455, 1978
53a. CRUZ JC et al: Phlebotomy improves gas exchange in chronic mountain polycythemia. Respiration 38:305, 1979
54. HOUSTON CS: High altitude illness. JAMA 236:2193, 1976
55. DICKINSON JG: Severe acute mountain sickness. Postgrad Med J 55:454, 1979
56. MENON ND: High altitude pulmonary edema. N Engl J Med 273:66, 1965
57. HULTGREN HW, MARTICORENA EA: High altitude pulmonary edema. Chest 74:372, 1978
58. SCOGGIN CH et al: High altitude pulmonary edema in the children and young adults of Leadville, Colorado. N Engl J Med 297:1269, 1977
59. GRAHAM WGB, HOUSTON CS: Short-term adaptation to moderate altitude. JAMA 240:1491, 1978
60. BULLARD RW: Physiological problems of space travel. Annu Rev Physiol 34:205, 1972
61. PACE N: Weightlessness: A matter of gravity. N Engl J Med 297:32, 1977
62. MICHELS DB, FRIEDMAN PJ, WEST JB: Radiographic comparison of human lung shape during normal gravity and weightlessness. J Appl Physiol 47:85, 1979
63. ALTMAN PL, DITTMER DS: Biological Handbooks. Environmental Biology p 269. Bethesda, Federation of the American Society of Experimental Biologists, 1966
64. BEGIN R et al: Effects of water immersion to the neck on pulmonary circulation and tissue volume in man. J Appl Physiol 40:293, 1976
65. PREFAUT CH et al: Influence of immersion to the neck in water on airway closure and distribution of perfusion in man. Respir Physiol 37:313, 1979
66. PREFAUT CH et al: Human gas exchange during water immersion. Respir Physiol 34:307, 1978
67. STRAUSS RH: Diving medicine. Am Rev Respir Dis 119:1001, 1979
68. LANPHIER EH: Man in High Pressure. Handbook of Physiology: Adaptations to the Environment. Bethesda, American Physiological Society, 1964
69. LAMBERTSEN CJ (ed): Underwater Physiology V. Federation of American Society of Experimental Biologists, 1976
70. TOWNSEND RE, HALE DA: Sleep, mood, and fatigue during a 14-day He-O_2 open-sea saturation dive to 850 fsw with excursions to 950 fsw. Undersea Biomed Res 5:109, 1978
71. FLORIA JT, MORRISON JB, BUTT WS: Breathing pattern and ventilatory response to carbon dioxide in divers. J Appl Physiol 46:1076, 1979
71a. GELFAND R, LAMBERTSEN CJ, PETERSON RE: Human respiratory control at high ambient pressures and inspired gas densities. J Appl Physiol 48:528, 1980
72. MILLER KW: The opposing physiological effects of high pressures and inert gases. Fed Proc 36:1663, 1977
73. COCKETT ATK et al: Pathophysiology of bends and decompression sickness: An overview with emphasis on treatment. Arch Surg 114:296, 1979
74. JOHNSON DG, BERGER WD: Injury and disease of scuba and skin divers. Postgrad Med J 49:134, 1971
75. OVERFIELD EM et al: Respiratory gas exchange in normal men breathing 0.9% oxygen in helium at 31.3 atmospheres absolute. J Appl Physiol 27:471, 1969
76. WOOD LDH, BRYAN AC: Effect of increased ambient pressure on flow–volume curve of the lung. J Appl Physiol 27:4, 1969
77. SALZANO J, RAUSCH DC, SALTZMAN HA: Cardiorespiratory responses to exercise at a simulated seawater depth of 1,000 feet. J Appl Physiol 28:34, 1970
78. LORD GP, BOND GF, SCHAEFER KE: Breathing under high ambient pressure. J Appl Physiol, 21:1833, 1966
79. DOELL D, ZUTTER M, ANTHONISEN NR: Ventilatory responses to hypercapnia and hypoxia at 1 and 4 ATA. Respir Physiol 18:338, 1973
80. JACEY MJ, GONZALES A, TAPPAN DV: Hematologic changes after 2 exposures to 6.7 ATA air at 3 day intervals. J Appl Physiol 42:838, 1977
81. WILSON JM et al: Human EEG changes during

prolonged hyperbaric exposures breathing N_2-O_2 mixtures. J Appl Physiol 42:614, 1977

82. SPENCER J et al: Tremor and somatosensory studies during chamber He-O_2 compressions to 13.1, 25.2, 37.3, and 49.4 ATA. J Appl Physiol 47:804, 1979
83. SMITH RV et al: Hana Kai II: A 17-day saturation dive at 18.6 ATA. Undersea Biomed Res 4:267, 1977
84. NEUMAN TS, et al: Urinary excretion of water and electrolytes during open-sea saturation diving to 850 fsw. Undersea Biomed Res 6:291, 1979
85. KYLSTRA JA, TISSING MO, VAN DER MOEN A: Of mice as fish. Trans Am Soc Artif Intern Organs 8:378, 1962
86. Symposium on inert organic liquids for biological oxygen transport. Fed Proc 29:1696, 1970
87. Symposium on artificial blood. Fed Proc 34:1428, 1975
88. MODELL JH et al: Oxygenation by ventilation with fluorocarbon liquid (FX-80). Anesthesiology 34:312, 1971
89. MODELL JH et al: Effect of fluorocarbon liquid on surface tension properties of pulmonary surfactant. Chest 57:263, 1970
90. SCHOENFISCH WH et al: Liquid breathing: expiratory flow and CO_2 elimination using fluorocarbon and aqueous solutions. In Lambertsen CJ (ed): Underwater Physiol V, p 91. FASEB, 1976
91. ALTMAN PL, DITTMER DS: Biological Handbooks. Environmental Biology, pp 270–315. Bethesda, Federation of the American Society of Experimental Biologists, 1966
92. BATES DV: A Citizen's Guide to Air Pollution. Montreal, McGill-Queen's University Press, 1972
93. FERRIS BG: Health effects of exposure to low levels of regulated air pollutants. J Air Pollut Control Assoc 28:482, 1978
94. MITCHELL RS et al: Health effects of urban air pollution. JAMA 242:1163, 1979
95. Health effects of air pollution. Statement by ATS Scientific Assembly on Occupational and Environmental Health, ATS News, 1978
96. GODIN G, WRIGHT G, SHEPHARD RJ: Urban exposure to carbon monoxide. Arch Environ Health 25:305, 1972
97. BARNARD RJ: Carbon monoxide: A hazard to firefighters. Arch Environ Health 38:255, 1979
98. WALD N, IDLE M, BAILEY A: Carboxyhemoglobin levels and inhaling habits in cigarette smokers. Thorax 33:201, 1978
99. SMITH NJ: End-expired air technique for determining occupational carbon monoxide exposure. J Occup Med 19:766, 1977
100. GOLDSMITH JR: Contribution of motor vehicle exhaust, industry, and cigarette smoking to community carbon monoxide exposures. Ann NY Acad Sci 174:122, 1970
101. RUSSELL MAH, COLE PV, BROWN E: Absorption by non-smokers of carbon monoxide from room air polluted by tobacco smoke. Lancet 1:576, 1973
102. DAVIES JM et al: Effects of stopping smoking for 48 hours on oxygen availability from the blood. Br Med J 2:355, 1979

102a. TURINO GM: Effect of carbon monoxide on the cardiorespiratory system. Circulation 63:255A, 1981

103. GOLDSMITH JR, LANDAW SA: Carbon monoxide and human health. Science 162:1352, 1968
104. ROUGHTON FJW, ROOT WS: The fate of carbon monoxide in the body during recovery from mild carbon monoxide poisoning in man. Am J Physiol 145:239, 1945
105. ROUGHTON FJW: Kinetics of gas transport in the blood. Br Med Bull 19:80, 1963
106. LATIES VG, MERIGAN WH: Behavioral effects of carbon monoxide on animals and man. Annu Rev Pharmacol Toxicol 19:357, 1979
107. MCFARLAND RA: Low level exposure to carbon monoxide and driving performance. Arch Environ Health 27:355, 1973
108. SAGONE AL JR, LAWRENCE T, BALCERZAK SP: Effect of smoking on tissue oxygen supply. Blood 41:845, 1973
109. SMITH JR, LANDAU SA: Smokers polycythemia. N Engl J Med 298:6, 1978
110. BRODY JS, COBURN RF: Effects of elevated carboxyhemoglobin on gas exchange in the lung. Ann NY Acad Sci 174:255, 1970
111. ASTRUP P: Some physiological and pathological effects of moderate carbon monoxide exposure. Br Med J 4:447, 1972
112. WALD N et al: Association between atherosclerotic diseases and carboxyhemoglobin levels in tobacco smokers. Br Med J 1:761, 1973
113. TOPPING DL: Metabolic effects of carbon monoxide in relation to atherogenesis. Atherosclerosis 26:129, 1977
114. ASTRUP P et al: Effect of moderate carbon monoxide exposure on fetal development. Lancet 2:1220, 1972
115. AYRES SM, GIANNELLI S JR, MEULLER H: Myocardial and systemic responses to carboxygemoglobin. Ann NY Acad Sci 174:268, 1970
116. ARONOW WS, ISBELL MW: Carbon monoxide effect on exercise-induced angia pectoris. Ann Intern Med 79:392, 1973
117. ARONOW WS, FERLINA J, GLAUSER F: Effect of carbon monoxide on exercise performance in chronic obstructive pulmonary disease. Am J Med 63:904, 1977
118. COHEN SI, DEANE M, GOLDSMITH JR: Carbon monoxide and survival from myocardial infarction. Arch Environ Health 19:510, 1969
119. KULLER LH et al: Carbon monoxide and heart attacks. Arch Environ Health 30:477, 1975
120. LARKIN JM, BRAHOS GJ, MOYLAN JA: Treatment of

carbon monoxide poisoning: Prognostic factors. J Trauma 16:111, 1976
121. NORMAN JW, LEDINGHAM IMA: Carbon monoxide poisoning: investigation and treatment. Prog Brain Res 24:101, 1967
122. STOKINGER HE: Toxicity of airborne chemicals: Air quality standards—a national and international view. Annu Rev Pharmacol 12:407, 1972
123. ANDERSEN I et al: Human response to controlled levels of sulfur dioxide. Arch Environ Health 28:31, 1974
124. JAEGER MJ: Effect of 0.5 ppm sulfur dioxide on the respiratory function of normal and asthmatic subjects. Lung 156:119, 1979
125. FRENCH JG et al: The effect of sulfur dioxide and suspended sulfates on acute respiratory disease. Arch Environ Health 27:129, 1973
126. FRANK NR, SPEICER FE: Effects of acute controlled exposure to sulfur dioxide on respiratory mechanisms in healthy male adults. J Appl Physiol 17:252, 1962
127. NADEL JA, SALEM H: Mechanisms of broncho-constriction during inhalation of sulfur dioxide and cigarette smoke. Arch Environ Health 16:651, 1968
128. CHARAN NB et al: Pulmonary injuries associated with acute sulfur dioxide inhalation. Am Rev Respir Dis 119:555, 1979
129. AUBRY F, GIBBS GW, BECKLAKE MR: Air pollution and health in three urban communities. Arch Environ Health 37:360, 1979
130. DAWSON SV, SCHENKER MB: Health effects of inhalation of ambient concentrations of nitrogen dioxide. Am Rev Respir Dis 120:281, 1979
131. Editorial: Ozone in smog. Lancet 2:1077, 1975
132. HAZUCHA M et al: Pulmonary function in man after short term exposure to ozone. Arch Environ Health 27:183, 1973
133. FARREL BP et al: Adaptation in human subjects to the effects of inhaled ozone after repeated exposure. Am Rev Respir Dis 119.725, 1979
134. LINN WS et al: Effect of low-level exposure to ozone on arterial oxygenation in humans. Am Rev Respir Dis 119:731, 1979
135. Photochemical Air Pollution: Formation Transport and Effects. National Research Council, No NRCC 14096 Canada, 1975
136. MELLICK PW et al: Short term morphologic effects of high ambient levels of ozone on lungs of rhesus monkeys. Lab Invest 36:82, 1977
137. BRAIN JD, VALBERG PH: Deposition of aerosol in the respiratory tract. Am Rev Respir Dis 120:1325, 1979
138. SPEIZER FE, FERRIS BG: Exposure to automobile exhaust. Arch Environ Health 26:319, 1973
139. URY HK, PERKINS NM, GOLDSMITH JR: Motor vehicle accidents and vehicular pollution. Arch Environ Health 25:314, 1972
140. Smoking and Health: A report of the Surgeon General. Preface, No 79-50066 p xii, US Dept HEW, 1979
141. WYNDER EL, HOFFMAN D: Tobacco and Health. N Engl J Med 300:894, 1979
142. Smoking and Health: A report of the Surgeon General. Chapter 14: Constituents of Tobacco Smoke, No 79–50066 US Dept of HEW, 1979
143. HANLEY JA, ROBINSON JC: Cigarette smoking and the young: A national survey. Can Med Assoc J 114:511, 1976
144. CASTLEDEN C, COLE P: Variations in carboxyhemoglobin levels in smokers. Br Med J 4:736, 1974
145. Smoking and Health: A report of the Surgeon General. Chapter 2: Mortality, No 79–50066 US Dept of HEW, 1979
146. Smoking and Health: A report of the Surgeon General. Chapter 3: Morbidity, No 79–50066 US Dept of HEW, 1979
147. WHITE JR, FROEB HF: Small airways dysfunction in nonsmokers chronically exposed to tobacco smoke. N Engl J Med 302:720, 1980
148. Smoking and Health: A report of the Surgeon General. Chapter 11: Involuntary smoking, No 79–50066 US Dept of HEW, 1979
149. Smoking and Health: A report of the Surgeon General, Part I: The health consequences of smoking, No 79–50066 US Dept of HEW, 1979
149a. ZALOKOV JB, RICHARD JL, CLAUDE JR: Leucocyte count, smoking and myocardial infarction. N Eng J Med 304:465, 1981
150. Smoking and Health: A report of the Surgeon General. Chapter 6: Non-neoplastic bronchopulmonary diseases, No 50066 US Dept of HEW, 1979
151. DOSMAN J et al: The relationship between symptoms and functional abnormalities in clinically healthy cigarette smokers. Am Rev Respir Dis 114:297, 1976
152. NADEL JA, COMROE JH JR: Acute effects of inhalation of cigarette smoke on airway conductance. J Appl Physiol 16:713, 1961
153. DASILVA AMT, HAMOSH P: Effect of smoking a single cigarette on the "small airways." J Appl Physiol 34:361, 1973
154. WANNER A: State of the Art. Clinical aspects of mucociliary transport. Am Rev Respir Dis 116:73, 1977
155. GREEN GM, CAROLIN D: The depressant effect of cigarette smoke on the in vitro antibacterial activity of alveolar macrophages. N Engl J Med 276:421, 1967
156. WARR GA, MARTIN RR: In vitro migration of human alveolar macrophages: Effects of cigarette smoking. Infect Immun 8:222, 1973
156a. HIGGENBOTTOM T et al: Lung Function and symptoms of cigarette smokers related to tar yield and number of cigarettes. Lancet 1:409, 1980

157. MITTMAN C et al: Smoking and chronic obstructive lung disease in $alpha_1$ antitrypsin deficiency. Chest 60:214, 1971
158. GUENTER CA, WELCH MH, HAMMARSTEN JF: $Alpha_1$ antitrypsin deficiency and pulmonary emphysema. Annu Rev Med 22:283, 1971
159. DOLL R, PETO R: Mortality in relation to smoking: 20 years' observations in male British doctors. Br Med J 2:1526, 1976
160. Smoking and health: A report of the Surgeon General. Appendix: Cigarette smoking in the United States 1950–1978, No 79–50066 US Dept of HEW, 1979
161. Smoking and Health: A report of the Surgeon General, Part II: The behavioral aspects of smoking, No 79–50066 US Dept of HEW, 1979
162. BUIST AS, NAGY JM, SEXTON GS: The effect of smoking cessation on pulmonary function: A 30 month follow-up of two smoking cessation clinics. Am Rev Respir Dis 120:953, 1979
163. GOLDSMITH JR: Air pollution epidemiology: A wicked problem, an informational maze, and a professional responsibility. Arch Environ Health 18:516, 1969
164. BRAUN DC, JURGIEL JA, GROSS P: Establishing environmental criteria: Medical perspectives. Arch Environ Health 27:121, 1973
165. BATES DV: Air pollution: Political initiative, scientific reality, and the process of decision-making. Lung 156:87, 1979
166. DE NEVERS N: Human health effects and air pollution control philosophies. Lung 156:95, 1979
167. TAYLOR JK: The status of chemical analysis in environmental research and control. Lung 156:109, 1979
168. BOUHUYS A, BECK GJ, SCHOENBERG JB: Priorities in prevention of chronic lung diseases. Lung 156:129, 1979
169. WILSON R: Risks caused by low levels of air pollution. Yale J Biol Med 51:37, 1978
170. KNELSON JH: Evidence for the influence of sulfur oxides and particulates on morbidity. Bull NY Acad Med 54:1137, 1978

Chapter 2

The Respiratory Pump

WILLIAM A. WHITELAW

Most of this book is concerned with the lungs themselves, their normal function, and the diseases that affect them, but the passive lungs cannot work without the neuromuscular pump that expands and contracts them. The physician dealing with respiratory problems must have an understanding of how this pump functions and how it can be altered in disease, either as an adaptive response or because of disease of the pump itself. Research in control of breathing during the past two decades has improved our understanding of the pump and brought forward many ideas with which a physician should be acquainted in order to recognize and analyze these problems.

Unlike the heart, which beats rhythmically by itself, the lungs are expanded by the action of ordinary skeletal muscle contracting upon impulses from motoneurons from the spinal cord. Knowledge of this system falls into the provinces of neurophysiology, neurology, and kinesiology.

NORMAL FUNCTION

Studies of control of breathing, combined with rapidly expanding knowledge of neurophysiology in recent years, have shown that the traditional textbook description of respiratory control is in fact a simplification that only partly explains the majority of clinical observations. Although the new approaches have not yet solved all the problems or led to a full understanding, they have made the major step of forcing us to accept that the respiratory control system has many complexities, and that parts of it that were previously regarded as unimportant may sometimes be of overriding importance. Many features of this system and its disorders are open to new interpretation and new observation.

The traditional physiology of respiratory control concentrates narrowly on the principle of homeostasis of P_{CO_2} and P_{O_2} by means of "negative feedback loops." Arterial blood is sampled by chemoreceptors which in turn stimulate the respiratory center to increase or decrease alveolar ventilation, restoring P_{CO_2} or P_{O_2} to a predetermined level.[1,2] It is convenient to begin by explaining how such a simple system operates. Breathing is in fact regulated much better than would be predicted by this theory, and the following sections show how the chemical control theory may be made more sophisticated, and how accessory, nonchemical control loops further help to stabilize ventilation. Finally, the elements of the pump—the respiratory centers, the muscles, and the chest wall—are described in more detail.

The Chemical Control System

The purpose of the respiratory control system is to maintain body acid–base balance and oxygen supply.[3] It is not surprising, therefore, that a major element of the system is a set of receptors that measure levels of P_{O_2}, P_{CO_2}, and hydrogen ions and stimulate the respiratory centers in a way that tends to restore these values to normal if they are altered by an extraneous process. Of these, the P_{CO_2} receptors have the most potent effect on breathing. A brief description of how a "negative feedback system" works to stabilize CO_2 illustrates some important principles.

Simple Feedback Control. Figure 2-1 is an engineer's schematic diagram of the respiratory "chemostat," so called because its principle of operation is analogous to that of a simple household thermostat.

The lungs must remove carbon dioxide from the blood stream at the same rate as this gas is produced by metabolism. If carbon dioxide is made faster than it is removed, alveolar P_{CO_2} will rise and acidosis will ensue; the reverse process will lead to alkalosis. The amount of CO_2 exhaled per minute is given by the concentration of CO_2 in alveoli multiplied by the volume of alveolar air exhaled per minute.

$$\dot{V}_{CO_2} = \dot{V}_A \times F_{ACO_2} = \dot{V}_A \times \frac{P_{ACO_2}}{P_B - 47} \quad \text{(Equation 1)}$$

where $\dot{V}_A$ = Alveolar ventilation per minute
F_{ACO_2} = Fraction of alveolar CO_2
P_{ACO_2} = Alveolar P_{CO_2}
$P_B - 47$ = Barometric pressure minus water vapor pressure
$\dot{V}_{CO_2}$ = Carbon dioxide production per minute

As long as metabolic rate is constant, alveolar ventilation and P_{ACO_2} are reciprocally related by the equation

$$P_{ACO_2} = \frac{(P_B - 47)\dot{V}_{CO_2}}{\dot{V}_A} \quad \text{(Equation 2)}$$

To maintain P_{CO_2} constant when CO_2 production increases, the controlling system must somehow recognize a change in $\dot{V}_{CO_2}$ and adjust $\dot{V}_A$ to match it, keeping the value of the fraction $\frac{\dot{V}_{CO_2}}{\dot{V}_A}$ always the same. Since arterial blood is equilibrated with alveolar gas, arterial P_{CO_2} is approximately equal to alveolar P_{CO_2}. If the rate of CO_2 production increases (as in exercise, for example) but alveolar ventilation remains the same, venous blood will deliver carbon dioxide into alveoli faster than it is being removed, and P_{ACO_2} will rise. If an arterial P_{CO_2} detector is arranged so that when P_{CO_2} rises it will stimulate the respiratory centers to increase $\dot{V}_A$, then $\dot{V}_A$ will go up and P_{ACO_2} will drop back towards normal. The effectiveness of this kind of controller depends on how big a change in $\dot{V}_A$ follows a given change in P_{ACO_2}. This can be seen quantitatively in the graph of Figure 2-2. Figure 2a shows the graphic form of equation 2 for two different values of $\dot{V}_{CO_2}$. At rest, P_{ACO_2} is related to $\dot{V}_A$ by a hyperbola. In exercise, $\dot{V}_{CO_2}$ is higher and there is a new hyperbola where, to maintain the same P_{CO_2} as at rest, $\dot{V}_A$ must be much higher. Figure 2b shows how the controller reacts to an increase in P_{CO_2}. This sort of graph is obtained in human subjects by having them breathe gas mixtures that include carbon dioxide in various concentrations, and plotting ventilation against alveolar P_{CO_2}. As the carbon dioxide level is artificially raised, respiratory centers are stimulated and $\dot{V}_A$ goes up. The slope of the line is said to describe the sensitivity of the respiratory system to CO_2. Figure 2c shows how such a system reacts when $\dot{V}_{CO_2}$ rises. A resting subject starts at point A with normal $\dot{V}_A$ and P_{ACO_2}. When exercise begins he must move to some point on the exercise curve. If ventilation did not increase at all he

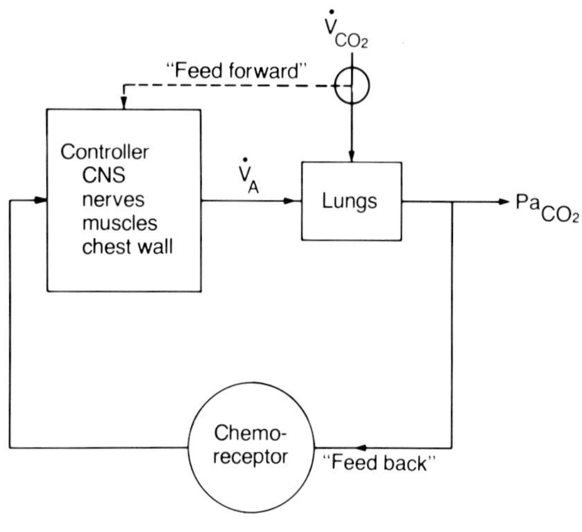

FIG. 2-1. Conceptual model of a body "chemostat," or automatic control system, to stabilize arterial P_{CO_2}. In a "feedback" system the controller sets the level of alveolar ventilation ($\dot{V}_A$) according to information it receives from the chemoreceptor sampling arterial blood. If metabolic rate ($\dot{V}_{CO_2}$) increases, P_{CO_2} rises, and chemoreceptors tell the controller to increase $\dot{V}_A$. In a "feed forward" system the controller is informed directly about changes in $\dot{V}_{CO_2}$ and increases $\dot{V}_A$ accordingly, so there is no need for P_{CO_2} to rise.

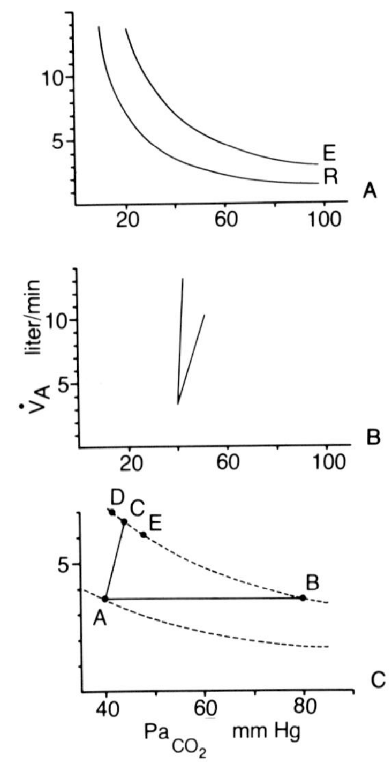

FIG. 2-2. Quantitative aspects of feedback control. See text for a full explanation. **A.** Relation between alveolar ventilation and P_{CO_2} at rest ($\dot{V}_{CO_2}$ = 200 ml/min) and light exercise ($\dot{V}_{CO_2}$ = 400 ml/min). **B.** Two carbon dioxide response curves. In each case a subject began at resting P_{CO_2} of 40 mm Hg, and normal resting ventilation. When CO_2 is artificially raised, ventilation may increase rapidly in a sensitive subject (*steeper line*) or slowly in an insensitive one (*less steep line*). **C.** Magnified graph of relations between ventilation and P_{CO_2} (see text).

would go to point B, with a P_{CO_2} of 78. Because the CO_2 receptor stimulates breathing exactly as described in Figure 2b, however, he moves up the CO_2 response line to point C. $\dot{V}_A$ is increased and the new value of P_ACO_2 is higher than normal, but not a great deal so. How much the P_{CO_2} rises depends on the sensitivity of the respiratory system to P_{CO_2}. If the response is very steep the subject will move up to point D with even higher ventilation and P_{CO_2} more nearly normal. On the other hand, a patient who is relatively insensitive to P_{CO_2} will move up to point E, allowing P_{CO_2} to rise rather than increase ventilation. The sensitivity of this respiratory controller has been assessed in many normal subjects and patients. There is a wide range in normal, roughly between the extremes shown in the examples of Figure 2-2. The sensitivity increases when hypoxemia or metabolic acidosis is present but decreases in sleep, in anesthesia, and when sedative or narcotic drugs are given.

Principles that apply to this kind of negative feedback controller are (a) by its nature it can defend the respiratory system only against stresses that actually change P_{CO_2}; (b) it does not regulate P_{CO_2} perfectly (the only stimulus to increase $\dot{V}_A$ is the abnormal CO_2, so that ventilation does not increase unless P_{CO_2} is at least a little bit elevated); (c) for the same reasons it never over-corrects P_{CO_2}; (d) it can be assessed by measuring the ventilatory response to CO_2. Another important point is (e) that the removal of carbon dioxide depends on *alveolar* ventilation, *not* minute or total ventilation. As the respiratory center increases its output and steps up the pumping action of the lung, the total flow of air is important but so also is the pattern of breathing because of the effect of dead space. Alveolar ventilation equals minute ventilation minus dead space ventilation, as defined in the following equation.

$$V_A = (V_T - V_D) \times f$$
$$= V_E - (V_D \times f) = V_E (1 - V_D/V_T)$$
(Equation 3)

where V_A = Alveolar ventilation per min
V_T = Tidal volume
V_D = Dead space per breath
f = Respiratory rate (frequency)
$\dot{V}_E$ = Total ventilation per min (minute ventilation)

Thus, an important aspect of pump activity is the ratio of dead space to tidal volume. When the chemoreceptor works correctly and the respiratory center "throttle" is turned on appropriately, giving the correct minute ventilation, the removal of carbon dioxide from blood can still be impaired if (1) dead space is abnormally high, or (2) the pattern of breathing is changed to one of rapid small breaths.

There are additional chemical feedback mechanisms, one that increases ventilation in response to hypoxemia, another responding to changes in *p*H. The way in which they work is very similar to the CO_2 mechanism. Because *p*H and Po_2 can vary independently of Pco_2, it is useful for each to be able independently to stimulate alveolar ventilation to protect the organism from hypoxemia and to stabilize *p*H in the case of metabolic acidosis. The response of normal subjects to hypoxemia is shown in Figure 2-3. As Po_2 drops, ventilation rises but the change is small before Po_2 reaches about 50 mm Hg. Sensitivity to Po_2 depends on Pco_2. When Pco_2 is high, a much smaller drop in Po_2 will stimulate $\dot{V}_A$. On the other hand, when Pco_2 is below normal there is almost no response, even to severe hypoxemia.

In some clinical situations the three chemical feedback mechanisms act in the same direction. For example in asphyxia the drop in *p*H, the rise in Pco_2, and the drop in Po_2 all work together synergistically to stimulate respiration, the low Po_2 increasing sensitivity to Pco_2 and vice versa. In other situations, the different mechanisms may antagonize each other, for example in pneumonia, where hypoxemia stimulates breathing but the increased ventilation lowers Pco_2, raises *p*H, and reduces sensitivity to a low Po_2, thus vitiating the original effect of hypoxemia.

Chemoreceptors. Two sets of receptors are recognized. The peripheral receptors in major arteries include the carotid and aortic bodies and measure Po_2, Pco_2, and *p*H in arterial blood. The central receptors are in the cranium and behave as if they were mainly sensitive to *p*H of the cerebrospinal fluid (CSF). Carbon dioxide equilibrates rapidly between blood and CSF, changing *p*H and stimulating both carotid bodies and central receptors, but the central effect is the more important. Hypoxemia acts almost entirely through the carotid bodies. For *p*H the situation is more complex because the arterial and the central chemoreceptors are more or less equally sensitive to it. Hydrogen ions do not easily cross the blood-CSF barrier, and it may happen that the *p*H sampled by central receptors is radically different from the arterial *p*H sampled by the carotid bodies. These two *p*H receptors may then act in opposite directions, creating a confusing clinical picture. Examples of this are discussed below (see Metabolic Acidosis).

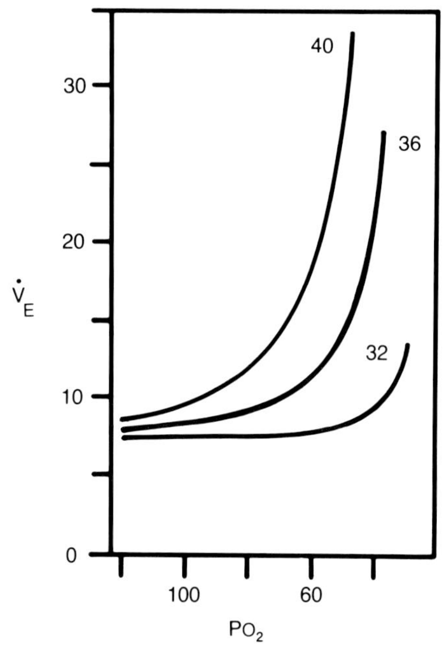

FIG. 2-3. Ventilatory response to hypoxia of a normal subject. This graph describes what happens to total ventilation ($\dot{V}_E$) when a subject is made hypoxic by breathing a gas mixture low in oxygen. Carbon dioxide is added to the inspired gas to keep arterial Pco_2 at some fixed level. The three curves are done at different Pco_2 levels, as indicated in milimeters of mercury.

The carotid bodies, the principal oxygen sensors, are found very close to the carotid sinus at the bifurcation of the common carotid artery. They are small, highly vascular structures which have been isolated in animal experiments and thoroughly studied. They receive arterial blood from the carotid artery and send afferent neural information to the respiratory centers through the glossopharyngeal nerve. The ratio of blood flow to oxygen uptake in the carotid body is very high, so that the venous blood draining from them has a Po_2 nearly the same as that of arterial blood. The receptors are clearly sensitive to Po_2, not to oxygen concentration or saturation. Being quite insensitive to loss of oxygen-carrying capacity, they fail to stimulate breathing in anemia or carbon monoxide poisoning except when these are very severe. When carbon dioxide tension is high the carotid body sensitivity to oxygen is enhanced, and vice versa.[3a]

Experiments in which carotid bodies are perfused with blood at different oxygen tensions while recordings are made from afferent nerve fibres show that these tiny organs have a steady low-level discharge when Po_2 is in the normal range, and increase their firing rate progressively as Po_2 falls. A graph of carotid body discharge against Po_2 very closely resembles the graph of ventilation against Po_2 found in normal people (see Fig. 3). In such preparations discharge from the carotid body can be altered by stimulating its sympathetic nerve supply or by applying autonomic drugs like atropine and phenoxybenzamine, but such manipulations are not known to have any clinical significance. Under the microscope the carotid body is seen to consist of nests of cells that contain neurosecretory granules and are connected to each other by synaptic junctions. Although it is small, self contained, and simple in structure, it has not so far yielded up the secret of how it operates.

The carotid body increases its discharge when arterial pressure falls, which accounts for part of the hyperpnea of shock. It is stimulated by cyanide, giving rise to marked hypernea in cases of poisoning. It is also stimulated by nicotine and mediates some of the effects (tachycardia, vasoconstriction) of this drug. Increased temperature causes an increase in carotid body discharge, but the hyperpnea of fever is likely mediated by central as well as peripheral mechanisms.

Aortic bodies,[3,3a] similar to carotid bodies in structure, are scattered over the surface of the aorta but are not known to be of importance in humans.

Central Chemoreceptors. Most of the response to change in Pco_2 is mediated by receptors within the cranium.[4] Ventilation does not seem to correspond directly to the level of carbon dioxide or hydrogen ion in intracranial arteries, but when cerebrospinal fluid is examined, minute ventilation is found to correlate very well with CSF *p*H, no matter whether this *p*H is altered through changes in Pco_2 of arterial blood or changes in bicarbonate concentration of CSF. From these observations it is concluded that central chemoreceptors are exposed to brain interstitial fluid or CSF, and are exquisitely sensitive to *p*H.[5] Hyperventilation can be produced by perfusing the ventricles with acid solutions or by diseases which make CSF acid. Since hydrogen ion concentration seems to be the immediate stimulus, changes in Pco_2 affect ventilation by shifting hydrogen ion–bicarbonate equilibrium, governed by the Henderson-Hasselbalch equation.

$$pH = pKa + \log \frac{(HCO_3^-)}{\alpha \, Pco_2} \quad \text{(Equation 4)}$$

If CSF bicarbonate is large, as in chronic respiratory acidosis or metabolic alkalosis, a given change in Pco_2 will produce a smaller-than-normal change in CSF *p*H. The central receptors will therefore receive a smaller-than-normal stimulus and the ventilatory response of arterial Pco_2 will be attenuated. This mechanism accounts for part of the loss in CO_2 sensitivity found in chronic CO_2 retention.[6] The receptors appear to be close to the surface of the medulla oblongata on its ventrolateral aspect.[7] Some observations indicate that these, or possibly a separate set of intracranial receptors are also responsive to arterial *p*H or Pco_2. Thus, ventilation can be affected to some degree by arterial gases, even when CSF values are held constant. Much remains to be learned about the location, mechanism of action and physiological role of the central receptors. In some circumstances, (at altitude, for example) ventilation goes in a direction opposite to that predicted by measuring CSF *p*H.[8] This implies that the powerful central chemoreceptor drive to breathe can be overridden by some other control system, and cautions a wary approach to any analysis of ventilatory response to chemical stimuli. However, some otherwise perplexing clinical situations can be understood by considering changes in CSF.

Although the chemical control system has been very thoroughly studied for several decades, using very sophisticated techniques, much remains to be learned about it. As described here, chemical feedback does not satisfactorily explain the fact that P_{CO_2} remains completely within normal limits in the face of the huge changes in metabolic rate that occur in exercise. (Reference to Figure 2c shows that to treble or quadruple ventilation by negative feedback requires that P_{CO_2} rise above normal even in subjects with the steepest response lines.) Nor does it explain how patients with extreme muscle weakness or severe airways obstruction contrive to keep their CO_2 normal, making near-maximal respiratory efforts without any more than normal chemical stimulus. There are many refinements of the chemical feedback theory that attempt to explain the increased ventilation of exercise:

1. The carotid bodies are sensitive to the changes in P_aCO_2 and P_aO_2 that occur with each breath, as well as to the mean value. The amplitude of these fluctuations increases in exercise and could constitute an added stimulus.[9]

2. The sensitivity of the controller to CO_2 seems to be temporarily enhanced in exercise, the ventilatory response curve of Figure 2 becoming more vertical.

3. A "feed-forward" system has been postulated in which the body measures $\dot{V}_{CO_2}$ directly, and adjusts ventilation to suit, without waiting for P_aCO_2 to change. (One way the body could do this would be to measure mixed venous P_{CO_2} and multiply this by cardiac output, but no evidence can be found for the existence of CO_2 receptors in the venous circulation.) A feed-forward system would very nicely explain the wide variety of circumstances (exercise, hyperthyroidism, muscle weakness) in which $\dot{V}_{CO_2}$ and $\dot{V}_A$ are closely coupled.

None of these factors has yet been shown to explain convincingly the hyperpnea of exercise, but the remarkable fact that P_{CO_2} does stay within a very narrow range in almost all circumstances argues forcibly that a chemical regulatory system must be involved, at least as a final reference.

Nonchemical Stimuli

It would not be reasonable to confine the regulation of such a crucial life support system as breathing to a single mechanism consisting of a few chemosensitive cells in the medulla and the tiny carotid bodies. In fact, the respiratory system is provided with an interlocking set of accessory control devices designed to stabilize or adjust ventilation in the face of many kinds of interference that can be anticipated in the course of everyday life or common illness. Some of these mechanisms are probably unknown and others poorly understood, but they are effective enough to maintain stable ventilation for minutes, hours, or days while ignoring signals from chemoreceptors. Additionally, they can anticipate and prevent changes in ventilation due to changes in mechanical load on the respiratory system, and increase ventilation before planned exercise begins. Examples of the influence of nonchemical control systems are: (a) conscious subjects continue to breathe normally for a long time when the most potent chemical stimulus, P_{CO_2} is removed by hyperventilation[10]; (b) while talking, normal people maintain nearly constant normal ventilation in spite of a substantial increase in P_{CO_2} induced experimentally by raising P_{CO_2} of inspired gas[11]; (c) in REM sleep, ventilation remains close to normal although ventilatory response to P_{CO_2} is severely attenuated[12]; and (d) treated patients with such diseases as pneumonia and pulmonary edema hyperventilate in spite of normal oxygen, low P_{CO_2}, and high *p*H.

Numerous reflex mechanisms have been identified in animals and probably have counterparts in humans. They come from various receptors and seem well designed to stabilize ventilation in various conditions. In the lung are three kinds of receptors with axons in the vagus nerve:[13]

Stretch receptors located in the smooth muscle of trachea and mainstem bronchi fire when the lungs expand, sending a signal that is closely related to lung volume. In animals, stretch receptors are responsible for the Hering–Breuer reflex; their role in normal breathing is to switch off inspiration at a certain level, causing expiration to begin, and thus accelerating respiratory rate.[14] Steady inflation of the lungs, as in positive end-expiratory pressure, elicits reflex tonic activity of expiratory muscles through this mechanism. It has been hard to demonstrate that these receptors influence breathing in humans, although recordings from vagus nerves exposed at operation show that they are active. Conceivably, they may be important in patients on mechanical ventilators, who often synchronize their own breathing efforts with the breathing cycle of the machine. This could come about through stretch-receptor activity in the following way. As the lungs are passively inflated, the receptors send an inhibitory discharge to the inspiratory neurons. The inhibition is maximal at end-inspiration and switches off the patient's own inspiratory effort just as the respirator enters its expiratory phase. As the lungs deflate, inhibition is removed, and the patient begins to inspire again at about the same time as the machine delivers its next impulse of positive pressure.

Irritant and cough receptors are unmyelinated fibers located just beneath the epithelium of larynx, trachea, and bronchi. Upper and lower airway receptors are morphologically identical but have different effects. Stimulation of tracheal and laryngeal "cough receptors" by dust or toxic chemicals leads to cough and bronchoconstriction. The same stimuli applied to "irritant" receptors within the lung lead to tachypnea and increased ventilation. In experimental animals, irritant receptors have been shown to fire in response to atelectasis, bronchoconstriction, pneumothorax, and microembolism. Clearly, they may be invoked to explain hyperventilation in many clinical situations.

"J" receptors found in the periphery of the lung are stimulated by accumulation of fluid in the interstitial space and cause rapid shallow breathing. They may be involved in the increased ventilation of pulmonary edema.

Receptors in the muscles and joints are well disposed to idenufy movements and stresses in the respiratory system and help make adjustments to unexpected loads on muscles. Thus, spindles and tendon organs in intercostal muscles and the diaphragm probably regulate length and tension in these muscles, making sure that appropriate breathing efforts are made even when extra mechanical loads, changes in postural stress, or unexpected chest deformations occur. Joint receptors of the rib cage may inform the respiratory centers about changes in lung volume. In exercise, joint and muscle receptors in the limbs may transmit information about the amount of work being done, allowing the respiratory system to anticipate needs for ventilation.

The effect of nonchemical mechanisms can be seen in the "loading response." If a normal subject or patient is obliged to breathe through a small tube with high resistance, simulating added airways obstruction, he immediately increases his inspiratory efforts, managing to maintain nearly normal tidal volume and ventilation even if resistance is raised to two or three times normal. While some of this response could be attributed to chemoreceptors (the load leads to reduction in ventilation, which in turn leads to increased carbon dioxide and increased chemically stimulated effort to breathe), most of it occurs even when changes in blood gases are prevented by manipulating inspired gas tensions.[15] The loading response varies in importance from one subject to the next and is abolished by sleep or anesthesia. The receptors mediate it are unknown, but probably lie in the chest wall.

Another observation of interest is that ventilation tends to remain constant independent of P_{CO_2}, as if subjects become accustomed to a certain way of breathing and tend to perpetuate it out of habit, at least over a short term of minutes to hours. Thus, most subjects at the end of a period of the voluntary over-ventilation tend to keep on over-ventilating, only very gradually allowing their ventilation to drop to normal even though P_{CO_2} is well below normal, so that they have a greatly reduced chemical stimulus to breathe.[10] Similarly, partially paralyzed patients who have been artificially over-ventilated for a few hours struggle to maintain ventilation above normal when left to themselves and complain of dyspnea when P_{CO_2} starts to rise towards normal.[16]

The Respiratory Centers

It is not at all certain that respiratory activity is confined to very small discrete areas of the brain. By respiratory centers we mean all the parts of the central nervous system that mediate between stimuli and respiratory responses. Many parts of the brain including the cortex, hypothalamus, pons, medulla, and cerebellum are able to influence breathing, but the way in which the various parts cooperate to generate normal breathing patterns is poorly understood. It is everyday experience that breathing occurs automatically in waking and sleep, that all the breathing muscles can be voluntarily activated or put at rest, that emotions affect the amount and pattern of breathing, and that the regular to-and-fro of quiet breathing is frequently interrupted as the respiratory muscles are diverted to the performance of specialized acts including speech, singing, swallowing, sighing, coughing, hiccuping, and defecation. As well, some respiratory muscles have a postural function. Each of these functions is probably served by a different neural circuit in the brain. Each uses slightly different combinations of respiratory muscles (for example, speech and singing are controlled largely with intercostals) and each of the circuits may be differently affected by sleep or drugs. The respiratory centers that have drawn the attention of most researchers are the circuits that are most active during general anesthesia or after decerebration of experimental animals. These circuits generate a steady rhythmic breathing pattern, respond to changes in blood P_{CO_2} and P_{O_2}, and are quite likely the ones that govern breathing during sleep and quiet breathing in wakefulness.

Even in the anesthetized experimental animal (usually a cat) from which most of our information is drawn, there seems to be a hierarchy of respiratory rhythm generators, just as there is a hierarchy of rhythm generators in the heart (the ventricles, AV node, and SA node). A primitive rhythm generator in the spinal cord may be capable of carrying on if all higher centers fail. The medulla can generate a rather irregular rhythm by itself if all higher areas are destroyed. When the pons (which includes the pneumotaxic center) is intact, rhythm is faster and more finely controlled. In awake animals, cortical centers become important and may either influence lower centers or bypass them to control respiratory muscles directly. Most clinical observations can be explained satisfactorily by a simple scheme in which there are two major control circuits.[17,18] One, called the metabolic system, is located in the pons and medulla. It seems to control breathing in sleep and anesthesia and to be mainly responsive to changes in gas tensions of blood or CSF. It has a descending pathway that lies in the anterolateral cord close to the reticulospinal tract. The other, called the behavioral system, includes circuits in the cerebral cortex, governs complex integrative breathing acts such as speech, may control breathing during much of the day, can supersede the metabolic system in many circumstances, and has its own separate descending pathway close to the corticospinal tract. Damage to either of these systems can occur in isolation (Fig. 2-4B).

The medullary and pontine centers have been extensively studied in animals and several recent reviews provide good summaries of the physiological data.[19–21] Because little of this information has direct clinical relevance, only a few salient features will be described here. Although most of this information is derived from studies of cats, there is no reason to doubt that analogous circuits exist in humans.

By successively cutting off pieces of the central nervous system until breathing is finally stopped, older experiments located the irreducible minimum of brain required for breathing in the medulla. Extensive exploration of this region with modern electrophysiological techniques has shown two major pockets of neurons that fire in synchrony with breathing (Fig. 2-4A). One of these lies in or alongside the nucleus of the solitary tract, beneath the floor of the fourth ventricle. This nucleus is the receiving station for visceral sensory information including taste, touch, and other stimuli from the tongue, pharynx, larynx, and lungs. The other lies near the

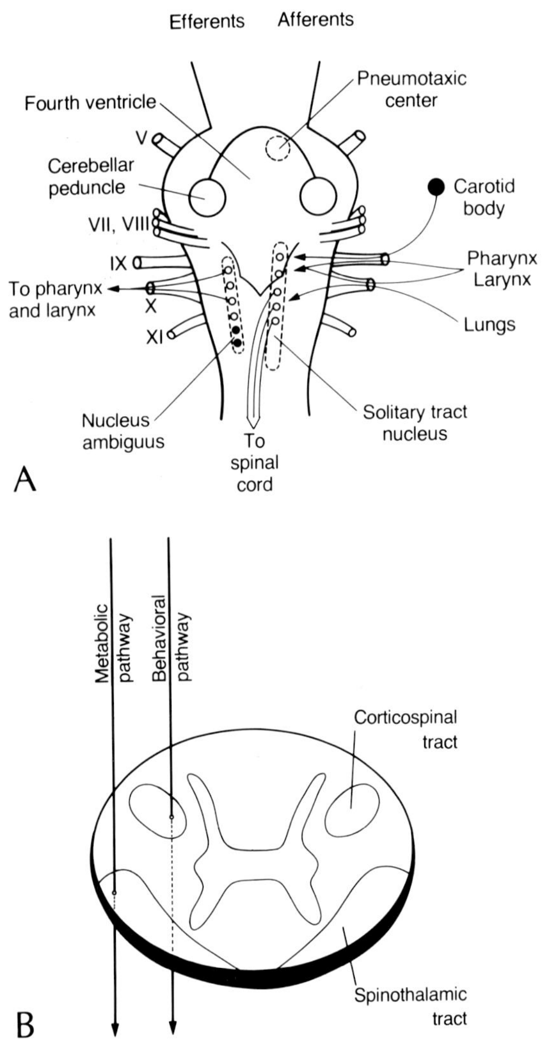

FIG. 2-4. A. Scheme of the anatomy of the brainstem respiratory centers. Open circles in the solitary tract nucleus and nucleus ambiguus represent inspiratory neurons; solid circles are expiratory neurons. Connections between neurons are not shown, but some are described briefly in the text. **B.** Scheme of the separate descending pathways for metabolic and behavioral systems.

nucleus ambiguus, which is the visceral motor nucleus of the tenth cranial nerve. The neurons beside the nucleus of the solitary tract are called the dorsal respiratory group (DRG), fire in inspiration, and send axons directly to alpha motoneurons of the phrenic nerve. Some of them also receive afferent information from vagal pulmonary stretch receptors. When lungs expand, these receptors fire and the discharge, feeding directly to DRG cells, inhibits them. This simple circuit provides the neural mechanism for the Hering-Breuer reflex found in animals, where inflation of the lungs can interrupt inspiration.[22] Although this reflex controls respiratory rate and tidal volume in some mammals, it has not been shown to be very important in normal humans. Inspiratory neurons in the DRG also receive inhibitory impulses from receptors in the upper airways. The physiological role of these is not clear but they may be responsible for the diving reflex, swallowing reflexes, or the exaggerated tendency of newborn infants to slow their breathing when stimulated in the nose or face. In each of these cases, upper airway stimulation leads to apnea. The respiratory neurons of the nucleus ambiguus (called the ventral respiratory group or VRG) include some motoneurons that supply pharyngeal and laryngeal muscles, which contract on inspiration, as well as others whose connections are not known. Some of the neurons in this area fire on expiration.

The "pneumotaxic center" has been localized to the nucleus parabrachialis medialis in the upper pons. Its connections are not clear but stimulation of the area can shut off inspiration and start expiration, just as can stimulation of vagal stretch receptors or upper airway receptors.

In the lower pons are neurons that exert a steady tonic discharge, generally inspiratory. They may play a role by setting the end-expiratory level. That is, if there is a constant inspiratory tone, inspiratory muscles will still be active when all the phasic variation is gone at end-expiration and functional residual capacity (FRC) will be above the resting level.[23] When higher centers are destroyed, the balance of tonic activity may be altered and an overriding tonic inspiratory activity arising from this area may cause the form of breathing called apneusis. However, the idea that cells of this "apneustic center" play an important part in generating basic respiratory rhythm has been abandoned for the present.

The generation of breathing rhythm is now thought of in terms of two interacting processes.

One is a growing and spreading of excitation in a pool of inspiratory neurons, building up from zero in a ramp, recruiting more and more neurons and motor units, and thus steadily increasing the force of contraction of inspiratory muscles and progressively expanding the lungs. The other is a switching circuit that interrupts inspiration at some point, letting the inspiratory muscles relax. The whole cycle then recurs. Neither the site or mechanism for generating the rising ramp of excitation are known but they probably lie somewhere within the medulla, close to or within the DRG or VRG. The pneumotaxic center, the vagal, and other inhibitory afferents that work through the switching circuit have little effect on minute ventilation, but change tidal volume and frequency. Hypercapnia and hypoxia accelerate the rise in inspiratory excitation and increase minute ventilation no matter what happens to tidal volume and frequency.[22]

The Respiratory Muscles

Action of the Muscles. The diaphragm is the principal muscle of respiration.[24–26] It is attached by its edges to the lower borders of the rib cage and arches up under the lungs as shown in Figure 2-5. When its fibers contract, they generate tension in the whole curved sheet of muscle plus the central tendon. This tension results in a pressure gradient across the diaphragm according to LaPlace's Law:

$$(P_{abd} - P_{pl}) = \frac{2T}{R} \qquad \text{(Equation 4)}$$

where T = tension
R = radius of curvature

Contraction thus generates negative pressure in the pleural space and causes the lungs to expand. The tension is also applied to the attachments of the diaphragm. The result of the tension depends on which part is fixed and which is movable. If the rib cage were solidly fixed in one position, contraction would draw down the dome of the diaphragm. On the other hand, if the diaphragm dome were fixed in position, tension would pull up the rib cage. Whether the diaphragm dome is fixed or can move depends on

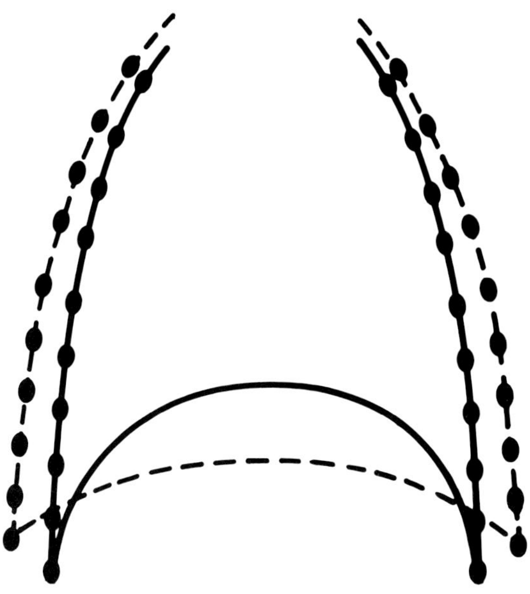

FIG. 2-5. Action of the diaphragm. The diaphragm is shown as a curved line across the bottom of the rib cage. At end-expiration, indicated by solid lines, rib cage diameter is small and the dome of the diaphragm is sharply curved. As the diaphragm contracts, the dome descends and becomes flatter, while the lower border of the rib cage is simultaneously pushed upward and outward.

pressure in the abdomen, which in turn depends on the activity of abdominal muscles. In descending, the diaphragm must displace the contents of the abdomen; this displacement can only be outward, by distention of the anterior abdominal wall. If tense abdominal muscles prevent such motion, diaphragm contraction must raise the rib cage.

It is clear that the muscles of the abdominal wall can act as synergists of the diaphragm. They remain relaxed in quiet breathing, but there is enough positive pressure in the relaxed abdomen to cause the rib cage to be lifted up to some degree while the dome of the diaphragm descends.

The line of pull of diaphragm fibers is upward and inward, but the rib cage usually moves up and outward when pulled by diaphragm contraction. This is because the rib cage is quite rigid, although hinged at its spinal attachments. Like a door, it seems to swing in the same direction whether it is pushed straight on or tangentially. The complex interaction between diaphragm, abdominal muscles, and rib cage is discussed in a recent symposium.[26]

Part of the rigidity of the rib cage seems to depend on active contraction of intercostal muscles. When these are not functioning, the rib cage is more deformable, and the pull of the diaphragm does draw the lower ribs slightly inward. It must also be remembered that the negative pressure generated in the pleural space by diaphragm descent and rib cage expansion tends, in itself, to collapse the rib cage. When this negative pressure is very high, as when the lungs are very stiff or obstructed, it may become the major factor determining motion of the chest wall.

The exact way in which intercostal muscle contraction manages to expand the rib cage is not known, but electromyography shows that the muscles close to the sternum in the upper intercostal spaces are usually activated on inspiration during quiet breathing. Inspiratory activity spreads downward mainly in external intercostal muscles as ventilation increases. Internal intercostals in the posterior and lateral parts of the chest are more commonly involved with postural activity and expiration.

General Principles of Respiratory Muscle Function. The respiratory muscles are similar in their behavior to other skeletal muscles. The distance a respiratory muscle moves or the volume it displaces when it contracts depends not only on the neural stimulus applied to it but also on many other factors. These include the mechanical load against which it is working (in the case of the respiratory muscles the resistance and compliance of the lungs and chest wall), the resting length of the muscle (through the force–length relationship, similar to the "preload" in cardiac mechanics), the speed of contraction (through the force–velocity relationship), the mechanical advantage of the muscle attachments on the chest wall, the co-operation of other muscles, and muscle fatigue and training.

Both force–length and changes in mechanical advantage make inspiratory muscles less effective at high lung volume than at FRC. This is easiest to visualize in the case of the diaphragm which becomes very short as it descends but also changes shape from that of a dome towards that of a flat membrane stretched across the bottom of the rib cage. In the latter position its contraction will tend to draw the ribs inward, reducing lung volume rather than expanding it. Similarly, the expiratory muscles are most effective at high lung volume.

The importance of muscle synergy is shown by patients with quadriplegia due to high spinal cord lesions.[27,28] Without contraction of the intercostal muscles during inspiration the rib cage loses its rigidity, so that contraction of the diaphragm, instead of lifting the rib cage as one unit and expanding it, tends to draw in the lower part of the rib cage and decrease thoracic volume. Breathing is thus bound to be less efficient.

The amount of useful work performed by the whole set of respiratory muscles acting together can be estimated from measurements of pressure and volume through the respiratory cycle (pressure × volume, like force × distance, has the dimensions of work or energy).[25] The work done in moving the lungs and in moving the chest wall can be calculated separately. "Work of breathing" has been used to estimate the overall activity of the respiratory centers and respiratory muscles, and one way of looking at the respiratory control system is to suppose that it tries to optimize its own performance (in the engineering sense) by achieving required ventilation with the minimum possible work. This attractive hypothesis is difficult to study in practice because "work of breathing" as usually calculated does not include all the work done by respiratory muscles. The hypothesis predicts that patients with pulmonary fibrosis would breathe quickly and shallowly (which they do), whereas patients with airways obstruction would breathe slowly and deeply (which they seldom do).

The efficiency of the respiratory muscles is defined as the amount of "work of breathing" divided by the oxygen consumption of the respiratory muscles. If the muscles contract vigorously and consume oxygen but fail to generate pressure because they waste effort distorting the chest, or cannot generate volume because of obstruction or restriction of the respiratory system, they are inefficient. The oxygen consumption of the respiratory muscles is difficult to measure accurately, but a good estimate can be made by measuring the total oxygen consumption of a subject at rest, then getting him to increase the effort of his breathing muscles alone (by voluntary overventilation or breathing through a resistor). The increase in total oxygen consumption can then be attributed entirely to the respiratory muscles, and the calculated increase in work of breathing, divided by the increase in oxygen consumption, gives efficiency of the same muscles. When the respiratory muscles are very inefficient and when excessive work is required to achieve normal ventilation, a considerable proportion of total body oxygen uptake may be consumed by the respiratory muscles. This may be one of the factors limiting exercise in patients with chronic airways obstruction, who have inefficient respiratory muscles, increased work of breathing, and in addition, have higher than normal ventilation for any given level of exercise.[29]

Muscle Fatigue. The idea that muscles can become fatigued is a familiar one from everyday experience. Clinicians have often wondered whether patients who appear exhausted in the final stages of respiratory failure due to emphysema or fibrosis may actually have fatigue of respiratory muscles. It has been difficult to define, detect, or measure fatigue in any satisfactory way, but recent interest in this subject promises to bring a better understanding. In general, fatigue may be said to be present when, after repeated hard contractions, a muscle gets into a state where it can no longer generate a certain force. When this happens the failure might be in the metabolic machinery of muscle contraction, in excitation contraction coupling, at the neuromuscular junction, in the spinal cord, in the motor cortex, or elsewhere in the central nervous system.[30] It has been shown that it is possible to fatigue the inspiratory muscles of normal subjects by having them breathe repeatedly through a very high resistance until they are no longer able to generate a prescribed inspiratory pressure.[31] Fatigue appears sooner if the effort is greater or if hypoxemia is present. Eventual fatigue, manifested as failure to maintain the required pressure, is preceded by changes in the electromyogram of the diaphragm.[32] The meaning of these EMG changes is still obscure but they seem to be associated with fatigue in various muscles and may eventually allow respiratory muscle fatigue to be detected in patients. The neural or metabolic processes that underly fatigue are not yet known.

Just as they can be fatigued, respiratory muscles can be trained. Specific exercises such as breathing against an inspiratory resistor lead to improved strength and endurance of inspiratory muscles.[33] Exercises can be directed specifically at strength or endurance. It might be hoped that specific training would prepare patients with serious lung disease to cope better with episodes of acute respiratory embarrassment, and this principle is being applied to patients with quadriplegia and children with cystic fibrosis.[34,35] General exercise incidentally trains respiratory muscles and this may be an unsuspected but important benefit of exercise programs. It has been proposed that fatigue of respiratory muscles may give rise to dyspnea. If this is true, it may help to explain how physical conditioning can improve exercise tolerance in patients with lung disease when there is no detectable change in lung function.[36,37]

The Pattern of Normal Breathing

Breathing is a complex coordinated act involving simultaneous and sequential activation of many muscles. It is orchestrated by a central pattern generator in the central nervous system and can be adapted to suit many circumstances. Polygraphic tracings of two typical respiratory cycles of a normal seated subject are shown in Figure 2-6, one at rest and one at moderate exercise. At the top, a volume tracing shows inspiration and expiration. In quiet breathing the cycle begins at the end of a relaxed expiratory plateau with all muscles inactive. The diaphragm begins to be stimulated and its activity rises in a more or less straight ramp to the end of inspiration. Intercostal muscles turn on at about the same time to stabilize the rib cage against diaphragm tension and to expand the ribs outward, while the posterior

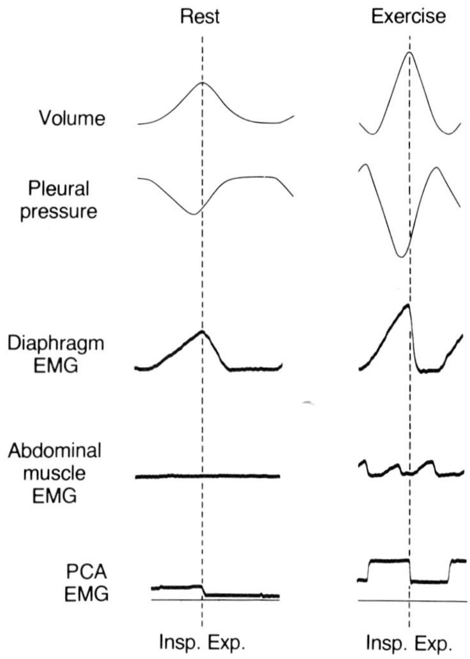

FIG. 2-6. Normal breathing. Volume is shown with inspiration up, pleural pressure with positive up. Pleural pressure and volume are slightly out of phase because of the flow resistance of the respiratory system. Instantaneous electrical activity of the diaphragm, external oblique muscle of the abdomen, and posterior circoarytenoid muscle (PCA) of the larynx are shown.

cricoarytenoid muscle contracts to open the glottis. (Recordings of many other upper airway muscles would show similar activity as they contract to stiffen the walls of the oropharynx and keep it patent. Even the alae nasae have phasic activity in quiet breathing.) During the inspiratory phase the diaphragm descends and the belly expands, but the rib cage also expands. At the end of inspiration diaphragm activity does not stop abruptly but declines gradually, so that the diaphragm lets volume out slowly. Activity in posterior cricoarytenoids decreases, allowing the larynx to close partially and slowing expiration by increasing the resistance to flow. Exhalation is thus not passive but is actively braked.[38] The volume is monitored by stretch receptors and joint receptors, while tension and length of respiratory muscles are measured continuously by tendon organs and muscle spindles and the information sent back to the central nervous system. Additional phasic motor output is sent to numerous muscles of the trunk to make minor postural adjustments as the mass of abdominal contents moves downward and upward.

This pattern can be modified in many situations. The whole pattern may be preempted by a cough, a sigh, or speech. If the subject lies down, subtle adjustments of individual muscle tone will compensate for the new geometry, and upper airway muscles will become more active to counteract the increased tendency of the tongue to fall back in the throat and the pharynx to collapse. The second polygraphic tracing (Fig. 2-6) shows what happens when ventilation is increased by the stimulus of exercise or increased carbon dioxide. Tidal volume is increased, as is respiratory frequency, shown by a decrease in the duration of the single breath. Diaphragm activity rises more steeply and reaches a higher peak. It then falls much more sharply at the beginning of expiration, while the laryngeal adductors remain more active, keeping the larynx wide open and allowing faster expiratory flow. Abdominal muscles that were silent during quiet breathing are now active in expiration. They may accelerate expiratory flow, but the more important effect of their activity at the end of expiration is to force the thorax below resting FRC and thus to increase tidal volume. Abdominal muscle activity is also seen in inspiration, when abdominal muscle contraction assists inspiration by increasing abdominal pressure, thus supporting the diaphragm and allowing it to lift up the rib cage.

Attention has recently turned to studying some simple details of the pattern of normal breathing in the hope that this may give clues to the stimuli that are driving respiration or to the state of the respiratory centers.[39,40] These details are the ratio of duration of inspiration (TI) to duration of expiration (TE), respiratory frequency, tidal volume, and the relative contribution to tidal volume of rib cage expansion and descent of the diaphragm (assessed by abdominal expansion). The pattern of resting breathing is easily disturbed. If the patient knows he is being observed, for example, he tends to breathe more slowly with larger tidal volumes, and subjects breathing through a mouth piece are known to have artificially low respiratory rates. With this proviso, data collected from a large number of subjects show that normal resting respiratory rate falls as children grow, reaching a minimum of 12 at age 25. Through adult life, it rises slowly again to 20 at age 80. Ventilation remains constant as a result of reciprocal changes in tidal volume.[41] The normal ratio of inspiratory time: total breath duration is about 0.4 and falls with exercise. Normal subjects expand their rib cage and abdomen more or less equally in inspiration. There is no truth to the legend that women breathe preferentially with their rib cages as compared to men.

Specialized Acts Involving the Respiratory Pump

Coughing is a complex act that can be initiated voluntarily but is usually set off by stimulation of cough receptors within the larynx and trachea.[42,43] Neural integration of the reflex probably occurs in the pons and medulla. A deep inspiration is followed by brief closure of the glottis while expiratory muscles compress thoracic gas up to two or three hundred centimeters of water. The glottis then opens and the gas is expelled. Dynamic compression of the large airways occurs, their cross-sectional area becomes very small, and the speed of gas expelled is very high, near the speed of sound. Cough remains reasonably effective when the larynx is bypassed by laryngectomy or endotracheal tube. A cough is followed by a period of reflex bronchoconstriction lasting about one minute.

In defecation, following a deep inspiration, both diaphragm and abdominal wall muscles contract simultaneously to generate large positive intraabdominal pressure.

Singing, and playing wind instruments require very precise control of intrathoracic pressure. This seems to be achieved mainly with intercostal muscles, since most of the inspired air is taken in by expanding the ribcage, rather than the abdomen.[44] The glottis is then nearly closed, and constant subglottal pressure is maintained by gradually relaxing the intercostal muscles.

"Output" of the Respiratory Centers

When considering patients who appear to have some disorder of the ventilatory pump, it is convenient to keep in mind a simple scheme of the processes that take part in transforming the rhythmic discharge of respiratory neurons into movement of air (Fig. 2-7).[44] Neural discharge is transmitted down the spinal cord, integrated at the anterior horn cell, and leaves the spinal cord and brainstem in numerous peripheral nerves. These can be grouped into the nerves to laryngeal and pharyngeal muscles, phrenic nerves, and segmental nerves to intercostal and abdominal muscles. The impulses then cross neuromuscular junctions, depolarize muscle cells, and set off muscle contraction. Tension generated by muscle metabolic machinery depends on fiber length and velocity. It pulls on muscle attachments, generating an amount of pressure that depends on the geometry of the thorax. The pressure in turn causes expansion of the respiratory system, but the speed and extent of the volume change depends on the resistance and compliance of both lungs and chest wall. Resistance of the upper airway can be changed by the muscles located there. At various stages, neural feedback loops can modify the output so that net output depends on peripheral sensory activity as well as respiratory center activity.

Disease can interfere with this process at any stage along the way, but careful dissection of the various elements can usually pinpoint the problem. The output takes several forms as it moves from brain to lungs. It can be measured as electrical activity in muscles, as pressure, and as minute volume. The distribution of output among various respiratory muscles can be assessed by measuring separately the volume expansion of rib cage and abdomen. The temporal pattern of inspiratory and expiratory times, tidal volume, respiratory frequency, and the "shape" of the inspiratory effort (whether the subject breathes in sharply at first and slows down toward the end of inspiration, or tends to breathe with a steady flow rate throughout) may all give useful information.

Assessment of the Respiratory Pump

Resting arterial P_{CO_2} indicates whether there is correct matching of alveolar ventilation and carbon dioxide production and demonstrates a significant derangement if it is abnormal. Substantial respiratory pump problems may be present

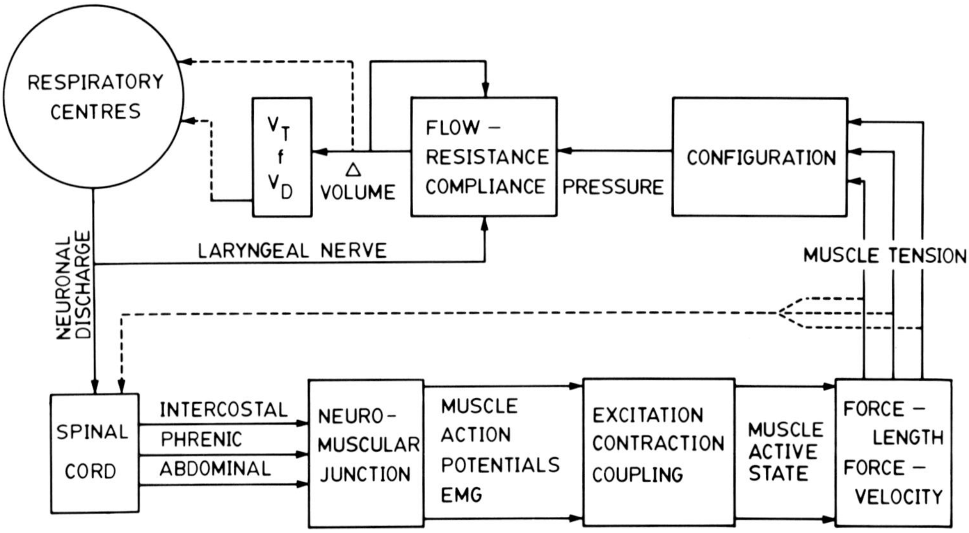

FIG. 2-7. A scheme of the "output" of the respiratory centers. Neural discharge from the medullary or higher centers is integrated in the spinal cord and sent out along peripheral nerves, then goes through a series of transformations (indicated by boxes) before emerging as flow or volume. Along the way, output can be measured as electromyogram voltage, as intrathoracic pressure, or as flow or volume. At several points the output modifies itself through reflex feedback loops (indicated by dashed lines). Muscle spindles and tendon organs are stimulated by muscle length and tension, and modify activity at both the spinal and central levels. Lung volume directly affects lung airway resistance, and can affect neural output through stretch receptors. Ventilation changes blood gas levels and feeds back through the chemoreceptor reflexes.

in spite of a normal carbon dioxide level, however. They may be brought out by imposing stress on the system, or by assessing the function of separate components.

Commonly used stresses are high carbon dioxide, low oxygen, and exercise. Each of these stimuli should increase ventilation in a predictable way. Failure to change overall ventilation may be due in each case to failure of appropriate receptors to recognize the stimulus, to unresponsiveness of the central rhythm generator, or to a defect somewhere along the output chain. Methods and normal values for stimulation with carbon dioxide,[45–47] oxygen,[48,49] and exercise are available,[50,51] and the tests are relatively simple to perform.

If it is certain that no pulmonary or chest wall disease is present, measurement of lung volumes and flow rates offers information about strength of respiratory muscles. Total lung capacity is reduced if inspiratory muscles are too weak to expand the lungs completely, and residual volume is increased if expiratory muscles are weak. This is an insensitive test because considerable loss of strength must occur before volumes are affected; this is because the pressure-volume curve of the respiratory system is nearly flat at the extremes of volumes (Fig. 2-8).

To test inspiratory muscle force more directly, maximum inspiratory pressures can be measured. The patient makes a maximal inspiratory effort against a closed valve and pressure is recorded. Since inspiratory muscles are more effective at low lung volumes and less so near TLC, the absolute lung volume at which pressure is measured must be noted. Normal values for this test are available.[52,53] At residual volume, normal men can generate about 120 cm H_2O negative pressure, and women about 90 cm H_2O. The test is clearly effort-dependent and requires good cooperation from the patient. Care must be taken to make sure the negative pressure is not being generated by the cheeks, which can make very high negative pressure in the mouth by sucking. Similarly, expiratory muscle strength can be assessed from maximal positive pressures. Since maximal pressures are generated by all the inspiratory muscles in concert, a reduction does not help to pinpoint individual muscle failure. Interpretation is further complicated by the synergy of respiratory muscles. Failure of one muscle, as well as removing that muscle's direct contraction, renders the other muscles less effective. The diaphragm can be tested separately by measuring transdiaphragmatic pressure. If pressure is recorded simultaneously in esophagus and stomach during breathing or voluntary inspiratory effort, transdiaphragmatic pressure will change if the diaphragm contracts and generates tension. This gives semiquantitative information about diaphragm strength. For a given level of stimulation, pressure will vary with diaphragm length and shape. The result must therefore be interpreted in the light of information about absolute lung volume, configuration of the chest wall at the time the test is performed, and changes in configuration that occur as a result of intercostal muscle activity. Starting from the relaxed position at functional residual capacity, normal men can generate more than 50 cm H_2O of transdiaphragmatic pressure, but a wide variation in normal can be expected.

The contribution of rib cage expansion and diaphragm descent to tidal volume can be measured separately with magnetometers[54,55] or other devices that quantitate body surface movements.

Electromyographic activity of the diaphragm can be analyzed quantitatively using recordings from an electrode swallowed into the stomach and pulled back up and secured by a balloon in the cardia, at the diaphragmatic hiatus.[56,57] Abdominal and intercostal recordings are made with appropriate surface or needle electrodes. "Occlusion pressure" quantitates the effect of inspiratory muscle contraction, more or less independently of lung mechanics, and can be used to assess output in patients whose minute ventilation is impaired by airways obstruction or reduced compliance of lung or chest wall. The patient's airway is blocked briefly just as inspiration is beginning, and the pressure generated by inspiratory effort against the block is measured.[58]

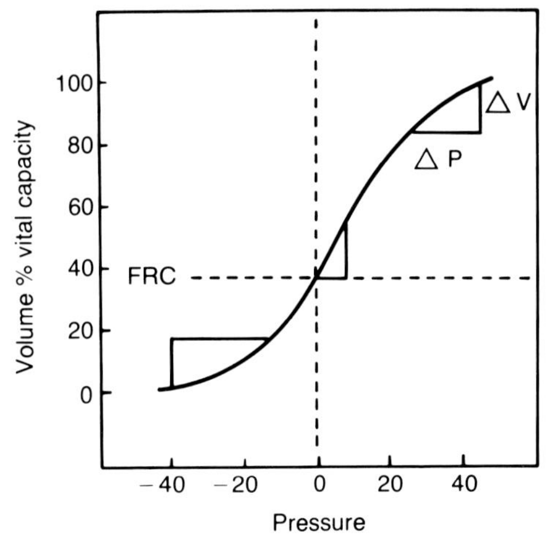

FIG. 2-8. The normal pressure-volume curve of lungs plus chest wall. The pressure (in cm H_2O) required to produce a given change in volume is much higher near residual volume or total lung capacity than it is in the tidal volume range.

Few pulmonary function laboratories are equipped to test the components of the respiratory pump in detail, and a sensible interpretation of the results requires very thoughtful appraisal of the clinical data as well as a detailed understanding of respiratory muscle function. Nevertheless, the tests are technically not very difficult, and can be done with ordinary instruments for recording pressures, volumes, and electromyograms. Maximum inspiratory pressures can be measured with a mercury or aneroid manometer and are extremely helpful in separating muscle weakness from restrictive lung disease. The application of special tests is discussed in Chapter 6.

DYSPNEA

Dyspnea or "shortness of breath" is a common complaint, useful in directing the attention of the physician to disease of the respiratory or cardiovascular system. A careful history of dyspnea can be invaluable in pinpointing the diagnosis and in assessing the duration and severity of the disease. In general, dyspnea can be defined as a distressing sensation associated with breathing, but it means different things to different patients and to different clinicians. Shortness of breath and labored breathing often seem necessary for homeostasis, but there are many patients in whom the symptom causes much distress without any apparent benefit. Useful information about the sources and character of dyspnea comes from conversation with patients, from examination of patients with clear-cut neurologic lesions and dyspnea, and from reports of physiologists who have experienced dyspnea, usually during breath-holding or experiments where mechanical loads have been added to the respiratory system. Dyspnea is not often discussed at length in textbooks but occupies an important part of everyday activities of chest physicians. Many ideas and information about shortness of breath are to be found in two symposia on the subject which gathered together respiratory and neurophysiologists and psychologists.[59,60]

It is customary to separate dyspnea from other readily defined feelings of discomfort in the chest. These include angina pectoris (which may in practice be difficult to separate from dyspnea on exertion), pleural or chest-wall diseases that cause pain on inspiration, awareness of normal breathing or of normally increased ventilation as in exercise, and neurotic over-concern with patterns of breathing. Clinicians and physiologists who have experienced dyspnea have tried to classify the distressing sensations associated with breathing. Although there is no general agreement it seems likely that dyspnea may include several quite different sensations: (1) a vague feeling of tightness in the chest associated with irritation of airways; (2) a discomfort felt in the rib cage during breath-holding experiments and breathing against heavy mechanical loads; (3) anxiety provoked by hypoxemia; (4) dizziness and headaches due to high P_{CO_2}; (5) a conscious fear of not breathing enough—found, for example, in chronic respirator patients when the respirator is turned off while they are awake. Physiologists have directed most of their attention to the first two of these.

Although the neurophysiology of dyspnea is not agreed upon, it is clear that it is not analogous to pain in that there are not specific dyspnea receptors projecting to the central nervous system. Stimuli arising from many different sources appear to give rise to similar sensations. In what part of the central nervous system these are collected and how they reach the conscious level are not known. A list of the possible sources of stimuli giving rise to dyspnea is provided below.

Possible Mechanisms for Dyspnea

Increase in normal breathing movements
Abnormal blood chemistry
Decrease in breathing movements
Stimuli arising in lung receptors
Stimuli arising from the chest wall
Added mechanical loads

When patients are experiencing dyspnea, they might report one of the following:

1. Awareness of increase in normal breathing movements. When exposed to increased inspired carbon dioxide levels, subjects are unable to detect the increased excursion of their respiratory muscles until minute ventilation is twice its resting value.[59] Subjects rebreathing CO_2 do not find breathing uncomfortable until they reach about 50 liters per min. During exercise normal subjects reach very high ventilation before becoming aware of their breathing. Patients with Cheyne-Stokes breathing are often not aware of their unusual breathing pattern. The ability to detect increased breathing movements thus seems to be limited and awareness of them is not at all distressing until very large volumes are reached.

2. Awareness of abnormal blood chemistry. Most people imagine that hypoxemia and hypercapnia are sensed directly as unpleasant stimuli and interpreted as shortness of breath. This does not seem to be true. Inadequate oxygenation of the brain first causes loss of judgement and sometimes euphoria. Lower oxygen levels often cause serious confusion without drawing the victim's attention to the respiratory system as the source of the trouble. Similarly, hypercapnia causes sweating, faintness, and stupor without focussing attention on breathing. Unconsciousness and death from inadequate oxygenation can therefore occur without warning. The poor correlation between abnormal blood gases and dyspnea can result in death in aviators, underwater swimmers and divers. Ignorance of this principle on the part of physicians and nurses can lead to death in patients with hypoxemia if lack of dyspnea is interpreted as proof of adequate oxygenation. Hypoxemia and hypercapnia are more likely to cause dyspnea indirectly by causing an increase in breathing effort and thus stimulating receptors that measure effort. This kind of indirect mechanism may explain why exertional dyspnea occurs at lower work loads in the presence of hypoxemia than when oxygen levels are normal.

3. *Awareness of decrease in breathing movements.* The ability of normal subjects to notice when their ventilation is reduced has not been measured. Most patients who underventilate without having obstructive or restrictive lung disease appear to be relatively free of distress. When a normal subject was paralyzed with curare, he was not made uncomfortable by the lack of breathing movements.[61] Paralyzed patients seem to suffer little dyspnea while underventilating, although they are subject to unpleasant sensations due to hypoxia and hypercapnia. After a period of overventilation on a respirator such patients may become distressed when they are removed from the respirator and minute volume is lowered and P_{CO_2} raised to normal. Such patients often cannot tolerate normal levels of CO_2 after becoming accustomed to too-low levels; the sensation in these cases seems to arise from the chemical stimulus.[62]

4. *Awareness of stimuli arising in lung receptors.* Hyperpnea and dyspnea are often seen in patients whose airways or lung parenchyma is diseased and whose vagal receptors, particularly irritant or "J" receptors, could be assumed to be overactive. Howell[59] has argued on clinical grounds that the special complaint of tightness in the chest may be specifically caused by lung receptors. Vagal blockade has abolished this symptom in acute asthma and has reduced dyspnea in patients with restrictive lung disease, pulmonary artery obstruction, and pulmonary lymphatic carcinomatosis.[63] Vagal blockade also lengthens the time that normal subjects are able to hold their breath.[64] In this situation, however, the blockade results in a decrease in the involuntary muscle contractions that occur during breath-holding, and it may be that the sensation of dyspnea comes from these movements of the chest wall rather than directly through the vagus.[65]

5. *Awareness of stimuli arising from the chest wall.* Muscle spindle receptors which seem ideally placed to transmit information about movement, position, and tension in muscles are apparently not responsible for providing any conscious sensation. Joint receptors, on the other hand, probably inform the conscious subject about the movement and position of his respiratory muscles.[66] Patients with high spinal cord sections are often unaware of their breathing movements even though the vagus nerve remains intact. The role of tendon organs in conscious sensation is not known. A case has been described in which severe dyspnea was relieved by local anesthesia of segmental nerves supplying an area of the lower rib cage previously affected by disease.[59]

6. *Awareness of added mechanical loads.* A number of experiments, begun by Campbell,[66] showed that normal subjects are capable of detecting very small changes in respiratory system impedance when these are produced by adding external mechanical loads to stimulate increased airways resistance or decreased compliance. Receptors for this are probably located in the chest wall, although pharyngeal pressure sensations may contribute.[67] Such experiments prove that information about mechanical loads can reach the conscious level and make it reasonable to assume that mechanical changes could produce dyspnea.

Many examples of dyspnea can be brought together by postulating that the distress comes from awareness of unexpected or undue strain upon the respiratory muscles or the chest wall. As the muscles contract against an unusually high load (or against a thorax in an unusual shape) they generate high tensions within themselves, as well as pulling on the ribs and altering their shape. These strains might be detected by tendon organs or joint receptors. Stimuli such as high P_{CO_2}, low P_{O_2}, and drive from pulmonary receptors, can act through this mechanism. Instead of directly stimulating the sensory cortex they may act by stimulating respiratory centers, causing stronger contraction of respiratory muscles and large strains in the chest wall which secondarily give rise to dyspnea.[68] Such a theory can explain why patients with damaged respiratory centers or weak muscles usually do not complain very much of dyspnea. Similarly it would predict that subjects who try harder to breathe against obstruction would have more dyspnea, the dyspnea being secondary to effort rather than the other way around.

Voluntary breath holding is a convenient way to produce dyspnea in normal subjects and illustrates some of the principles above. In breath holding, or apnea of any cause, alveolar and arterial gas tensions change in a predictable way, but not as quickly as most people imagine.[69] The rates of change of oxygen and carbon dioxide depend on the rates of production of carbon dioxide and consumption of oxygen, on the starting volume of gas available as stores, and on the interaction of Po_2 and Pco_2 through the Haldane and Bohr effects. As it turns out, the storage space for carbon dioxide is large, and Pco_2 rises only about 5 mm Hg per min during breath holding after oxygen breathing, and about 15 mm Hg per min after air breathing. The body's oxygen stores are smaller, being confined to the oxygen in alveolar gas and hemoglobin, so that oxygen falls at a rate of about 1 mm Hg per sec in a breath-hold following air breathing.

Breath holding becomes uncomfortable long before gas tensions reach a level that causes distress; the discomfort seems to be related to involuntary contractions of the respiratory muscles. Soon after the beginning of a breath-hold the diaphragm begins to make contractions, after which breathing is prevented only by closing off the upper airway. The contractions become stronger and stronger, generate large negative pressures in the thorax, and distort the chest wall, probably causing dyspnea by stimulating chest-wall receptors. If the contractions are prevented by administering curare, apnea can go on for several minutes without significant discomfort. In breath holding, the abnormal blood-gas tensions thus seem to cause dyspnea indirectly, by causing respiratory muscle contractions which in turn act on some sensory mechanism in the chest wall.[65]

The physiology of breath-hold diving[69] is more complex because of the change in ambient pressure with depth, and because oxygen consumption increases with exercise. At 10 meters beneath the surface, thoracic gas is pressurized to nearly two atmospheres, and the partial pressure of all the gases is also doubled. If a swimmer stays down until his alveolar Po_2 drops far enough to cause dyspnea (*e.g.*, 40 mm Hg) he may black out as he returns to the surface, and his Po_2 falls to half of that value (*e.g.*, 20 mm Hg). The risk of this accident may be increased if the diver hyperventilates before going down, because by doing so he removes the carbon dioxide stimulus that should warn him that it is time to resurface before the oxygen tension is too low (see Chap. 1).

Patients who complain of dyspnea may require laboratory evaluation in attempts to demonstrate objectively whether they have abnormal lung function, and quantify the severity of abnormalities. The laboratory approach to the evaluation of dyspnea is presented in Chapter 4.

REFERENCES

1. RAHN H: Gas transport from the external environment to the cell. In de Rueck AVS, Porter R (eds): Development of the Lung. Boston, Little, Brown & Co., 1967
2. PURVES MJ (ed): The Peripheral Arterial Chemoreceptors: Proceedings of an International Workshop. London, Cambridge University Press, 1975
3. COMROE JH: Physiology of Respiration. Chicago, Year Book Medical Publishers, 1974

3a. WHIPP BJ, WASSERMAN K: Carotid bodies and ventilatory control dynamics in man. Fed Proc 39:2668, 1980

4. BERGER AJ, MITCHELL RA, SEVERINGHAUS JW: Regulation of respiration (3). N Engl J Med 297:194, 1977
5. PAPPENHEIMER JR: The ionic composition of cerebral extra-cellular fluid and its relation to control of breathing. In The Harvey Lectures, Series 61, p 71. New York, Academic Press, 1967
6. FLENLEY DC, MILLAR JS: Ventilatory response to oxygen and carbon dioxide in chronic respiratory failure. Clin Sci 33:319, 1967
7. BERGER AJ, MITCHELL RA, SEVERINGHAUS JW: Regulation of respiration (1). N Engl J Med 297:92, 1977

8. FORSTER HV, DEMPSEY JA, CHOSY LW: Incomplete compensation of CSF [H+] in man during acclimatization to high altitude. J Appl Physiol 38:1067, 1975
9. BLACK AMS, MCCLOSKEY DI, TORRANCE RW: The responses of carotid body chemoreceptors in the cat to sudden changes of hypercapnic and hypoxic stimuli. Respir Physiol 13:36, 1971
10. FINK BR: Influence of cerebral activity in wakefulness on regulation of breathing. J Appl Physiol 16:15, 1961
11. PHILLIPSON EA et al: Interaction of metabolic and behavioral respiratory control during hypercapnia and speech. Am Rev Respir Dis 117:903, 1978
12. BULOW K: Respiration and wakefulness in man. Acta Physiol Scand (Supp) 209:1, 1963
13. FILLENZ M, WIDDICOMBE JG: Receptors of the lungs and airways. In Neil E (ed): Handbook of Sensory Physiology, Vol III. Springer-Verlag, Berlin 1972
14. CLARKE FJ, VON EULER C: On the regulation of depth and rate of breathing. J Physiol 222:267, 1972
15. ALTOSE MD et al: Effects of hypercapnia and inspiratory flow-resistive loading on respiratory activity in chronic airways obstruction. J Clin Invest 59:500, 1977
16. SMITH AC, SPALDING JMK, WATSON WE: Ventilation volume as a stimulus to spontaneous ventilation after prolonged artificial hyperventilation. J Physiol 160:22, 1962
17. BERGER AJ, MITCHELL RA, SEVERINGHAUS JW: Regulation of respiration (2). N Engl J Med 297:138, 1977
18. PLUM F: Neurological integration of behavioral and metabolic control of breathing. In Porter R (ed): Breathing. London, J & A Churchill, 1970
19. COHEN MI: Neurogenesis of respiratory rhythm in the mammal. Physiol Rev 59:1105, 1979
20. MITCHELL RA: Neural regulation of respiration. In Williams MH (ed): Disturbance of respiratory control, Vol I, No. 1, of Clinics in Chest Medicine. Philadelphia, WB Saunders, 1980
21. NEWSOM DAVIS J: Control of the muscles of breathing. In Widdicombe JG (ed): Respiratory Physiology. London, Butterworth & Co, 1974
22. WYMAN RJ: Neural regulation of the breathing rhythm. In Knobil E (ed): Annual Review of Physiology p 417. Palo Alto, Annual Reviews Inc, 1977
23. SEARS TA: The respiratory motoneuron and apneusis. Fed Proc 36:2412, 1977
24. DERENNE J-PH, MACKLEM PT, ROUSSOS CH: The respiratory muscles: Mechanics, control and pathophysiology. Parts I, II and III. Am Rev Respir Dis 118:119, 373, 581, 1978
25. CAMPBELL EJM, AGOSTONI E, NEWSOM DAVIS J: The respiratory muscles. London, Lloyd-Luke, 1970
26. International symposium on the diaphragm. Am Rev Respir Dis (Suppl), 119, 1979
27. MORTOLA JP, SANT'AMBROGIO G: Motion of the rib cage and abdomen in tetraplegic patients. Clin Sci Mol Med 54:25, 1978
28. DANON J et al: Function of the isolated paced diaphragm and the cervical accessory muscles in C-1 paraplegics. Am Rev Respir Dis 119:909, 1979
29. LEVISON H, CHERNIACK RM: Ventilatory cost of exercise in chronic obstructive pulmonary disease. J Appl Physiol 25:21, 1968
30. EDWARDS RHT: Physiological analysis of skeletal muscle weakness and fatigue. Clin Sci Mol Med 54:463, 1978
31. ROUSSOS CS, MACKLEM PT: Diaphragmatic fatigue in man. J Appl Physiol 43:189, 1977
32. GROSS D et al: Electromyogram pattern of diaphragmatic fatigue. J Appl Physiol 46:1, 1979
33. LEITH D, BRADLEY M: Ventilatory muscle strength and endurance training. J Appl Physiol 41:508, 1976
34. KEENS TG: Ventilatory muscle endurance training in normal subjects and patients with cystic fibrosis. Am Rev Respir Dis 116:853, 1977
35. GROSS D et al: The effect of training on strength and endurance of the diaphragm in quadriplegia. Am J Med 68:27, 1980
36. GRASSINO A et al: Inspiratory muscle fatigue as a factor limiting exercise. Bull Eur Physiopathol Respir 15:105, 1979
37. PERESS L: Ventilatory muscle training in obstructive lung disease. Bull Eur Physiopathol Respir 15:91, 1979
38. BARTLETT D, REMMERS JE, GAUTIER H: Laryngeal regulation of respiratory airflow. Respir Physiol 18:194, 1973
39. MILIC-EMILI J: Drive and timing components of ventilation. Chest [Suppl] 70:131, 1976
40. REMMERS JE: Analysis of ventilatory response. Chest [Suppl] 70:134, 1976
41. JAMMES Y et al: The ventilatory pattern of conscious man according to age and morphology. Bull Eur Physiopathol Respir 15:527, 1979
42. WIDDICOMBE JG: Respiratory reflexes. In Fenn WO, Rahn H (eds): Handbook of Physiology, sect 3: Respiration, Vol I, p 585. Washington, D.C. American Physiological Society, 1964
43. MACKLEM PT: Physiology of cough. Ann Otol 83:761, 1974
44. MILIC-EMILI J, WHITELAW WA, GRASSINO AE: Measurement and testing of respiratory drive. In Hornbein T (ed): Regulation of Breathing New York, Marcel Dekker, 1981
45. READ DJC: A clinical method for assessing the ventilatory response to carbon dioxide. Australasian. Ann Med 16:20, 1967
46. HIRSHMAN CA et al: Normal values for hypoxic and hypercapnic ventilatory drives in man. J Appl Physiol 38:1095, 1975
47. CHERNIACK NS et al: Workshop on assessment of respiratory control in humans. I. Methods of measurement of ventilatory responses to hypoxia

and hypercapnia. Am Rev Respir Dis 115:177, 1977

48. WEIL JV et al: Hypoxic ventilatory drive in normal man. J Clin Invest 49:1061, 1970
49. KRONENBERG RS et al: Comparison of three methods for quantitating respiratory response to hypoxia in man. Respir Physiol 16:109, 1970
50. JONES NL et al: Clinical Exercise Testing. Philadelphia, WB Saunders, 1975
51. WASSERMAN K, WHIPP BJ: Exercise physiology in health and disease. Am Rev Respir Dis 112:219, 1975
52. BLACK LF, HYATT RE: Maximal respiratory pressures: normal values and relationship to age and sex. Am Rev Respir Dis 99:696, 1969
53. RINQUIST T: The ventilatory capacity in healthy subjects. An analysis of causal factors with special reference to respiratory forces. Scand J Clin Lab Invest 88(Suppl) 18:5, 1966
54. KONNO K, MEAD J: Measurement of the separate volume changes of rib-cage and abdomen during breathing. J Appl Physiol 22:407, 1967
55. SHARP JT et al: Use of the respiratory magnetometer in diagnosis and classification of sleep apnea. Chest 77:350, 1980
56. GRASSINO A, WHITELAW WA, MILIC-EMILI J: Influence of lung volume and electrode position on the electromyography of the diaphragm. J Appl Physiol 40:971, 1976
57. LOPATA M, EVANICH MJ, LOURENCO RV: Quantification of diaphragmatic EMG response to CO_2 rebreathing in humans. J Appl Physiol 43:262, 1977
58. WHITELAW WA, DERENNE JP, MILIC-EMILI J: Occlusion pressure as a measure of respiratory centre output in conscious man Respir Physiol 23:181, 1975
59. HOWELL JBL, CAMPBELL EJM (eds): Breathlessness. Oxford, Blackwell Scientific Publications, 1966
60. PORTER R: Breathing. Ciba Foundation Symposium. London, J & A Churchill, 1970
61. CAMPBELL EJM et al: The effect of muscular paralysis induced by tubocurarine on the duration and sensation of breath holding. Clin Sci 32:425, 1967
62. SMITH AC, SPALDING JHK, WATSON WE: CO_2 as a stimulus to spontaneous ventilation after prolonged artificial ventilation. J Physiol 160:32, 1962
63. GUZ A et al: Experimental results of vagal block in cardiopulmonary disease. In Porter R (ed): Breathing. London, J & A Churchill, 1970
64. GODFREY S, CAMPBELL EJM: The role of afferent influences from the lung and chest wall in respiratory control and sensation. In: Porter R (ed): Breathing. London, J & A Churchill, 1970
65. NOBLE MIM, EISELE JH, TRENCHARD D et al: Effect of selective peripheral nerve blocks on respiratory sensations. In Porter R (ed): "Breathing". London, J & A Churchill, 1970
66. CAMPBELL EJM, NEWSOM DAVIS JN: Respiratory Sensation. In Campbell EJM, Agostoni E, Newsome Davis J (eds): "The Respiratory Muscles". London, Lloyd Luke, 1970
67. NEWSOM DAVIS J: The effect of upper spinal cord lesions on the detection of increased airway resistance in man. J Physiol 179:25, 1965
68. GODFREY S, CAMPBELL EJM: Mechanical and chemical control of breath holding. Q J Exp Physiol 54:117, 1969
69. MITHOEFFER JC: Breath-holding. In "Handbook of Physiology", Sect 3: Respiration, Vol II. ed. W.O. Fenn and H. Rahn American Physiological Society, Washington, DC, 1965

Chapter 3

The Respiratory Airways

JAMES C. HOGG

In this chapter, two basic approaches will be taken in an attempt to present the normal structure and function of the airways and to discuss the changes that occur in them with disease. The first approach will be to present theoretical concepts concerning aerodynamics and mechanics that are useful to the understanding of airways function. These basic principles are fundamental to the analysis of many physiological measurements and commonly used clinical techniques. The second section will deal with airway anatomy, the morphological changes that occur with disease, and the relationship of disordered morphology to function.

THEORETICAL ASPECTS OF AIRWAYS FUNCTION

Ideally, to understand airflow in the lung, one should be able to describe the characteristics of flow through an irregularly branched system of distensible tubes, where the geometry of the system changes considerably during inflation and deflation of the lung. Unfortunately, the mathematical approach to such a system is poorly developed, and an adequate description of the recent attempts at such an analysis is beyond the scope of this presentation. A more simplified approach to fluid mechanics, however, can still provide us with information necessary for a minimum understanding of airflow in the lung. The basic concepts describing the relationships of flow to pressure, resistance, and dimensions of the conduit are presented.

POISEUILLE'S LAW

An empirical law governing the flow of a viscous liquid through a fine tube was reported by Poiseuille in 1842. He found that the volume of liquid passing through a tube per unit of time was proportional (a) to the difference in pressure at the two ends of the tube, (b) to the fourth power of the radius of the tube, and (c) to the reciprocal of the length. Hagenbach later defined the coefficient of viscosity (μ) and worked out the formula now referred to as Hagen-Poiseuille's law:

$$\dot{V} = \Delta P \frac{\pi}{8} \times \frac{r^4}{l} \times \frac{1}{\mu} \quad \text{(Equation 1)}$$

($\dot{V}$ = flow, r = radius, l = length of tube, μ is the viscosity of the liquid, and ΔP is the difference in pressure at the inlet and outlet of the tube).

Although this relationship is often applied to flow through the airways, it has definite limitations because it is valid only for laminar flow. Furthermore, the geometric factor r^4/l does not take branch points and bends into account, or allow for the fact that changes in driving pressure (ΔP) also change the transmural pressure of the airways, thereby changing their diameter and altering the geometric relationship.

One important factor in considering the flow through a parent tube and its two daughter branches is that the pressure drop along the two daughters will be greater than that along the parent until the cross-sectional area of daughters exceeds that of the parent by a factor of $1/\sqrt{2}$.

CONTINUITY EQUATION

Under conditions of steady flow through a tube of changing dimension (Fig. 3-1), the law of conservation of matter is expressed by the equation

$$A_1V_1W_1 = A_2V_2W_2 \quad \text{(Equation 2)}$$

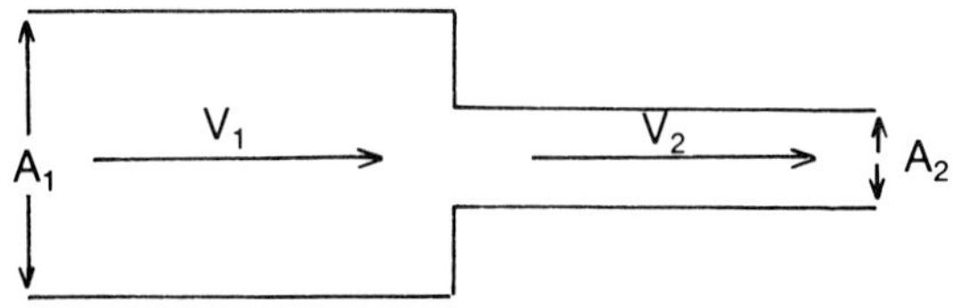

FIG. 3-1. When flow is constant and incompressible, the rate of flow through the tube of large diameter is exactly equal to the rate of flow through the tube of small diameter. (See text, Equation 2.)

(A is the area in cm^2, V is the velocity in cm/sec, and W is the specific weight of the substance in grams/cm^3).

Since the units are in grams/sec, the equation states that the weight rate of flow is the same in both diameter tubes. When the flowing gas is not compressed, the W term is dropped, and the volume rate of flow is constant.

MOMENTUM EQUATION

Newton's first law states that the momentum of a body is constant unless it is acted on by an external force, and his second law states that the external force acting on a body is equal to the time rate of change of its momentum. Therefore, it follows that if a liquid loses velocity as it flows through a tube, there will be a loss of momentum. The force (F) acting on the liquid to change its momentum will be

$$F = m\frac{V_1 - V_2}{t} \text{ or } F = m\frac{dv}{dt} \quad \text{(Equation 3)}$$

(where m is the mass of the liquid, V_2 and V_1 are the initial and final velocities, and t is the time during which the velocity changed.)

The work done to accomplish this change in momentum will be the force (F) times the distance through which it acts.

ENERGY EQUATION

The energy of a body is defined as the capacity for doing work, where work is the product of force and displacement. The total force resulting from the movement of the liquid that is available to do work can be found by integrating the momentum equation and is equal to $^1/_2\, mv^2$. A liquid also has potential energy in proportion to its height above some arbitrary datum and has hydrostatic energy in proportion to its depth below the same point. By the law of conservation of energy, as a liquid flows through the tube the loss in energy will equal the work done on the liquid plus the heat produced, when the heat equivalent of work has a definite value (1 BTU = 778 ft lbs). Under conditions of constant temperature there is no heat lost by the fluid, so that the loss in energy is equal to the work done. If flow occurs through a pipe of varying diameter, it is obvious that as the velocity of the fluid increases, there will be a rise in kinetic energy and a fall in hydrostatic energy, because the total energy is constant. The fall in hydrostatic pressure that accompanies an increase in kinetic energy when a continuous flow passes through a narrowing in a tube is referred to as the *Bernoulli effect*.

INTERNAL FRICTION

When liquid or air flows through a pipe, the thin layer of liquid that adheres to the pipe wall has zero velocity. The velocity of concentric rings of fluid toward the center of the pipe gradually increases. The distance between the ring with zero velocity and that with the greatest velocity is referred to as the *boundary layer*, and it is in this boundary layer that all the viscous forces are concentrated. Figure 3-2 shows that if a column of fluid enters a pipe with uniform velocity, the effect of friction is initially limited to the layer of liquid closest to the pipe wall. As a parabolic or laminar flow profile is established, the boundary layer can be seen to grow, so that the frictional forces become distributed throughout the liquid.

A force is required to overcome the internal friction of viscosity between layers. The dynamic viscosity between the layers of the fluid may be assessed as follows:

$$\text{dynamic viscosity} = \frac{\text{shear stress}}{\text{rate of shear stress}} \quad \text{(Equation 4)}$$

(Shear stress equals the force divided by the area

of contact between the layers; the rate of shear strain is the velocity of the layer divided by its thickness.)

The unit of dynamic viscosity is the poise, and its symbol is μ. Therefore,

$$\mu = \frac{\frac{\text{dynes}}{\text{cm}^2}}{\frac{\text{cm/sec}}{\text{cm}}} = \frac{\text{dynes/sec}}{\text{cm}^2} \quad \text{(Equation 5)}$$

$$\text{and since a dyne} = \frac{1 \text{ gram/cm}}{\text{sec}^2},$$

$$1 \text{ poise} = \frac{\text{gram}}{\text{cm/sec}}$$

Kinematic viscosity is the ratio of dynamic viscosity to density, and its unit is the stoke.

$$\text{Kinematic viscosity} = \frac{\frac{\text{gram}}{\text{cm/sec}}}{\frac{\text{grams}}{\text{cm}^3}} = \frac{\text{cm}^2}{\text{sec}} \text{ or } \textit{stoke}$$

(Equation 6)

The viscosity of viscous fluids such as glycerine is about 15 poise, whereas that of water is about 0.01 poise, and air, 0.0001 poise. Once motion of a liquid begins, the forces acting to slow it down are frictional, and one might think that those which were the most viscous would slow at the fastest rate. This is not so in practice, as one can demonstrate by the fact that stirred air slows much faster than stirred water, after the stirring force is removed. Dividing the viscosity by the density takes into account the momentum of the stirred air, and we find that the kinematic viscosity of air is 0.162 stoke, whereas that of water is 0.01 stoke.

REYNOLD'S NUMBER

When the flow through a tube is laminar, the interaction between concentric layers of fluid is dependent on friction alone, so that only viscous forces are exerted between layers. When flow becomes turbulent, however, there is an actual transfer of fluid mass between concentric layers, so that inertial forces interact between layers. The exact nature of turbulent flow has not been completely determined, but flow can be described in terms of the ratio between inertial and viscous forces in the liquid. This ratio is known as the Reynold's number.

The Reynold's number for flow in a tube

$$= \frac{\text{inertial forces}}{\text{viscous forces}} = \frac{2\rho v}{\pi r \mu} \quad \text{(Equation 7)}$$

where ρ = the density of the fluid in $\frac{\text{grams}}{\text{cm}^3}$

v = the velocity of the fluid $\frac{\text{cm}^3}{\text{sec}}$

r = the radius of the tube (cm)

μ = the viscosity of the fluid in poises or $\frac{\text{gram}}{\text{cm/sec}}$

If all units are inserted into the equation as indicated below, all the units cancel, and the Reynold's number is dimensionless:

$$\frac{\frac{\text{gram}}{\text{cm}^3}\ \frac{\text{cm}^3}{\text{sec}}}{\text{cm}\ \frac{\text{gram}}{\text{cm/sec}}}$$

Flow is found to be laminar when the Reynold's number is less than 2000, transitional between 2000 and 3000, and turbulent when the Reynold's number is above 3000.

ENTRANCE LENGTH PHENOMENA

If the velocity of a fluid entering a tube is uniform (see Fig. 3-2), a boundary layer is set up in the tube. The concentric laminae near the tube wall decelerate, and the concentric laminae at the center of the tube accelerate to satisfy the conservation of momentum. The boundary layer grows during the period, so that viscous forces become more widely dispersed. During the development of a laminar profile, liquid mass exchanges between laminae, so that energy is required to overcome both inertial force and viscous forces. The length of the tube required for a laminar profile of flow to develop is called the *entrance length*. It follows that the pressure

FIG. 3-2. During the development of laminar flow, the inertial forces developed by fluid exchange between layers fall to a minimum, and the boundary layer, where viscous forces are concentrated, expands throughout the liquid.

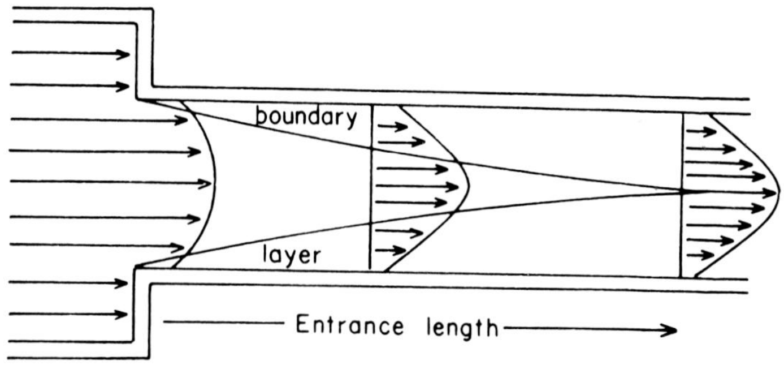

drop along the entrance length is greater than the pressure drop along an equal length of tube when laminar flow is fully established, because in the former, energy is required to overcome both inertial and viscous forces, whereas in the latter, only viscous forces must be overcome. In the normal human lung, entrance length phenomena are observed primarily in the central airways, whereas in the peripheral airways, fully developed laminar flow prevails. This fact has been used to determine sites of airways resistance. In the normal subject, the cross-sectional area of the central airways is small in relation to that of the peripheral airways (see Fig. 3-8D), so that the velocity is greater in the central airways than in the periphery. Under these circumstances, one would expect the flow profiles to be turbulent in large airways and laminar in the small airways.

Reviewing Equation 7, it is clear that decreasing gas density or increasing viscosity results in a decrease in the Reynold's number.

Breathing a helium-oxygen mixture, which is much less dense and only slightly more viscous than air decreases the resistance by this mechanism (primarily in the central airways), so that normal persons achieve increased flow rates under these circumstances. If the major site of resistance is in the peripheral airways, where flow is laminar, however, breathing a helium–oxygen mixture does not have this effect.

Several authors[1,2] have recently taken advantage of this property of helium to localize the site of airways obstruction. For example, asthmatics who have primary disease in the central airways increase their maximum flow rates with helium–oxygen mixtures; whereas chronic bronchitics who have primarily peripheral airways obstruction do not.

THE APPLICATION OF THEORY TO THE LUNG

GENERAL PRINCIPLES

The Swiss physiologist, Rohrer, was the first to apply Newtonian mechanics to the lung. By making two assumptions, he wrote an equation of motion for the lung that related its elastic, viscous, and inertial properties to the applied force. Although his analysis was not appreciated during his lifetime, it was so thorough that in a modern review of lung mechanics, Mead[3] stated that a bibliography combining Rohrer's name with those of his pupil Neergaard and a few contemporaries would encompass most of the ideas and techniques in this field. Therefore, prior to reviewing the measurements of mechanical properties of lungs, this analysis and its underlying assumptions will be discussed.

The assumptions that have to be made in order to write an equation of motion for the respiratory system are that the system behaves as a rectilinear system of one degree of freedom, in which the elements are nonlinear. This means that when a force is applied, the lung should move in only one dimension. To make this clear, let us consider a point in three-dimensional space. Such a point has three degrees of freedom, because it is free to move in any of three dimensions. If the point were a block of wood fastened to a stick held in the hand, the block would be free to move in three dimensions and therefore would have three degrees of freedom. If the block is placed in a groove on a flat surface, however, any force applied by the hand can only move the block up and down the groove, so that it moves in a single dimension and therefore has only one degree of freedom. It follows that in one-dimensional systems, the single degree of movement can be characterized by a linear change; in two-dimensional systems, by an area change; and in three-dimensional systems, by a volume change. Lung motion can be described by volume change, and the lung can be considered to be a system with one degree of freedom if the motion at each position in the lung bears a fixed relationship to the total motion of the lung. The evidence that suggests that this is so in the lung relates to the fact that the distribution of air along the various pathways within the lung is normally independent of breathing frequency, and this fact suggests that the motion of each unit always has a fixed relationship to the motion of the whole lung.[4] Because the lung behaves as a system of one degree of freedom, it follows that its motion can be described by a single variable, lung volume. When a force is applied to the lung, it must overcome elastic, viscous, and inertial forces that are developed by the lung. It can be shown that the elastic forces are proportional to the volume change, the viscous forces to the rate of volume change ($\dot{V}$) or flow, and the inertial forces to the rate of change in flow ($\ddot{V}$), which is the acceleration.[5] The equation of motion can then be written

$$F\ (\text{applied}) = K1V + K2\dot{V} + K3\ddot{V} \quad \text{(Equation 8)}$$

(K1, K2, and K3 are constants; the applied force (F) is the transpulmonary pressure; and V, $\dot{V}$, and $\ddot{V}$ are volume, flow, and volume acceleration, respectively.) This equation can be written more simply:

$$P_L = P_{CL} + P_{RL} + P_{IL} \quad \text{(Equation 9)}$$

(P_L is the instantaneous value for the pressure drop from the airway opening to the outer pleural surface; P_{CL} is the component of P_L required to overcome elastic forces; P_{RL} is the component of P_L required to overcome flow-resistive forces; and P_{IL} is the component of P_L required to overcome inertial forces.)

This simply states that the sum of elastic, flow-resistive, and inertial forces equals the total force developed by the lung to oppose the force applied to it and that these forces are proportional to the volume, flow, and volume acceleration that occur when the force is applied.

The phase relationship of these forces can be examined by determining these parameters during breathing. These relationships are shown in Figure 3-3. A full inspiration from RV (residual volume) to TLC (total lung capacity) and back to FRC (functional residual capacity) is shown in the volume tracing for orientation. By comparing the tracings during a sinusoidal pattern of respiration that approximates tidal breathing, it can be seen that the flow tracing is 90°out of phase with volume and that volume acceleration lags behind flow by another 90°, so that it is 180° out of phase with volume. When the frequency of breathing is increased at a constant tidal volume, both flow and volume acceleration increase.

Figure 3-3B shows the relationship between P_{CL} and P_{IL} as breathing frequency is increased. It is clear from Figure 3-3A that the pressures required to overcome elasticity remain the same at a higher frequency because tidal volume is constant. The pressures required to overcome inertia, however, increase with increased breathing frequency, because volume acceleration increases. This means that at some frequency, inertial and elastic forces will be equal, and because they are 180°out of phase, they cancel. This is known as the resonant frequency of the lung, and at this frequency the applied force has to overcome only the resistive properties of the lung. This relationship can therefore be used to measure airways resistance of normal lungs, and equipment has been devised to take advantage of it.

This resonant frequency method is useful in assessing lung mechanics, because the lung has a

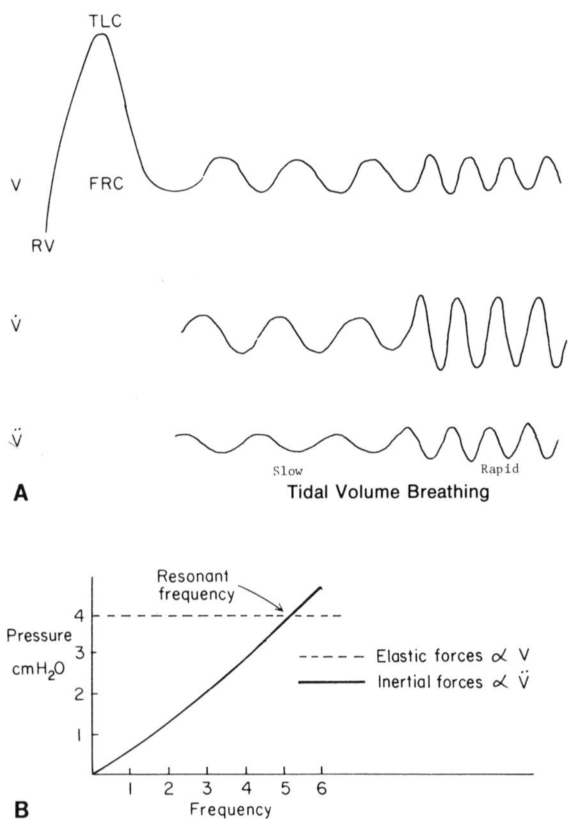

FIG. 3-3. A. These graphs show that volume (V) is 90° out of phase with the flow (V) and 180° out of phase with volume acceleration (V), when the breathing pattern is a sine wave. When frequency is increased at a constant tidal volume, the inertial forces increase. When the inertial forces equal the elastic forces, they cancel, because they are 180° out of phase. **B.** The elastic forces remain constant in spite of an increased rate of breathing; they are proportional to lung volume. The inertial forces are proportional to the rate of acceleration; therefore, they are increased at rapid breathing frequencies. Since these forces are 180° out of phase, they cancel, when equal.

high degree of viscous damping, and therefore it approaches the resonant frequency in a stable fashion. The stability of a mechanical system as it approaches resonance is a function of damping. Figure 3-4 shows the magnitude of the response to a particular applied force as the frequency with which the force is applied is increased. With an underdamped system the magnitude of the response increases dramatically near the resonant frequency, because as the elastic and inertial forces cancel, the applied force has only the resistive forces to overcome. Thus, a singer's note can shatter a wineglass under appropriate conditions. Damping decreases the amplitude of this response in the manner indicated, and with an overdamped system, the amplitude of the response decreases as soon as the frequency is increased. In a critically damped system, the amplitude of the response to an applied force remains constant as the resonant frequency is approached. This fact is often alluded to by manufacturers of measuring instruments such as pressure transducers, who describe the frequency response of their instruments as being flat to so many cycles/second. It follows that in order to measure the flow and volume changes that occur in the lung, the frequency response of the measuring devices must be such that they remain flat well beyond the cycling frequencies at which the measurements are made.

MEASUREMENT OF TOTAL PULMONARY RESISTANCE

Pulmonary resistance measurements, then, require an analysis of the flow-resistive forces reflected in the pressure gradient from the alveolus to the mouth, and an analysis of elastic and inertial forces reflected in total transpulmonary pressure (mouth pressure minus pleural pressure). At zero flow, the flow-resistive and inertial forces are zero, and the only force is elastic, which is easily measured (Equation 9).

Total lung resistance can be assessed during flow by construction of a pressure volume diagram during respiration,[3] and with minor changes in technique and instrumentation this can be readily applied clinically[5,6] to differentiate elastic from flow-resistive components. These techniques are discussed in relation to clinical applications in Chapter 4.

The study by Dubois and associates[7] of the oscillatory mechanics of the lungs and chest wall led to the ingenious method of measuring the resistance of the respiratory system by using an oscillating system. They found that the lung and chest wall constituted a highly damped system, with a resonant frequency of from 4 to 6 cycles per sec. As we have seen, inertial and elastic forces cancel at the resonant frequency, so that the pressure required to drive the lung at this frequency has to overcome only the flow-resistive components (see Fig. 3-3). In the initial studies with this method, a pump was used to drive flow in a sine-wave frequency. Mead and his associates modified the technique by using a loudspeaker in an enclosed box to produce the oscillations, and this method is now in common use in many laboratories to measure airways resistance.

The introduction of a satisfactory body plethysmograph[8,9] allowed alveolar pressure to be estimated for the first time. This permitted a direct analysis of flow resistance, because the mouth-to-alveolus pressure gradient could be assessed. The clinical applications of this method are discussed in Chapter 4

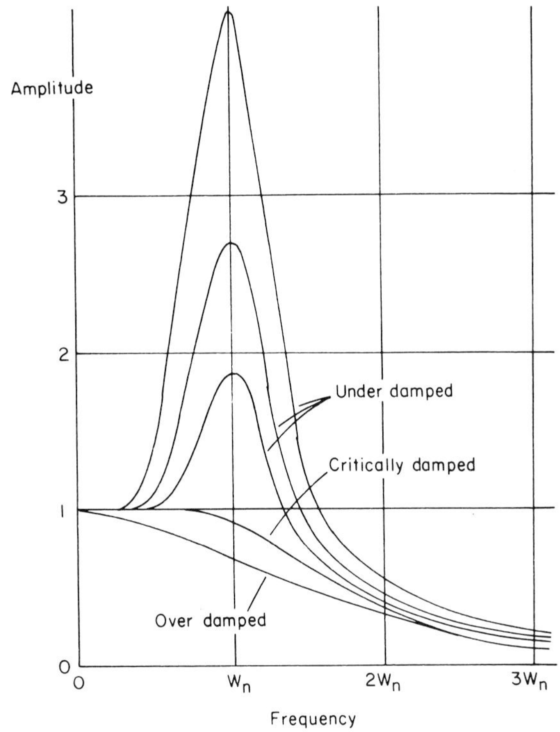

FIG. 3-4. The amplitude of a response to a constant input in relation to frequency and damping. The maximum response occurs at the resonant frequency (W_n), but increasing the damping decreases this response. If the system is over-damped, the response decreases as soon as the frequency is increased, but when critical damping is achieved, the response is the same at all frequencies up to the resonant frequency.

THE EFFECT OF LUNG INFLATION AND LUNG SIZE ON PULMONARY RESISTANCE

As we have seen, resistance refers to the relationship between the pressure drop from the alveoli to the atmosphere divided by the instantaneous airflow. With increasing rates of airflow, the relationship between pressure and flow becomes curvilinear. Fry and his associates[10,11] have shown that there is a specific pressure flow curve for each lung volume and introduced the term *isovolume pressure flow curve* to describe them. At high lung volumes, much higher expiratory flow rates can be achieved than at low lung volumes, because the airways are larger. The relationship between resistance and lung volume has been thought to be hyperbolic,[12] so that the smallest values for resistance occurred at the highest lung volumes. Macklem and Mead[13] have shown that the minimal value for resistance actually occurred at about 70% VC (vital capacity). These authors found it difficult to ascribe the increase in the resistance that occurred in both central and peripheral airways at higher lung volumes to change in airway length. They suggested that the pressure-to-area relationship of the airways might change as the airways lengthened, so that the airways might narrow somewhat at high lung volumes.

Briscoe and Dubois[14] have studied the effect of lung size on airway conductance and have shown that there is a linear relationship. Although their number of cases studied is small, their results indicate that for adults of similar age but different size, the linear dimensions of the lungs and airways change nearly equally.

THE EFFECT OF LUNG GROWTH ON PULMONARY RESISTANCE

In comparing lungs of persons of different ages, it is helpful to use the inverse of resistance (*i.e.*,

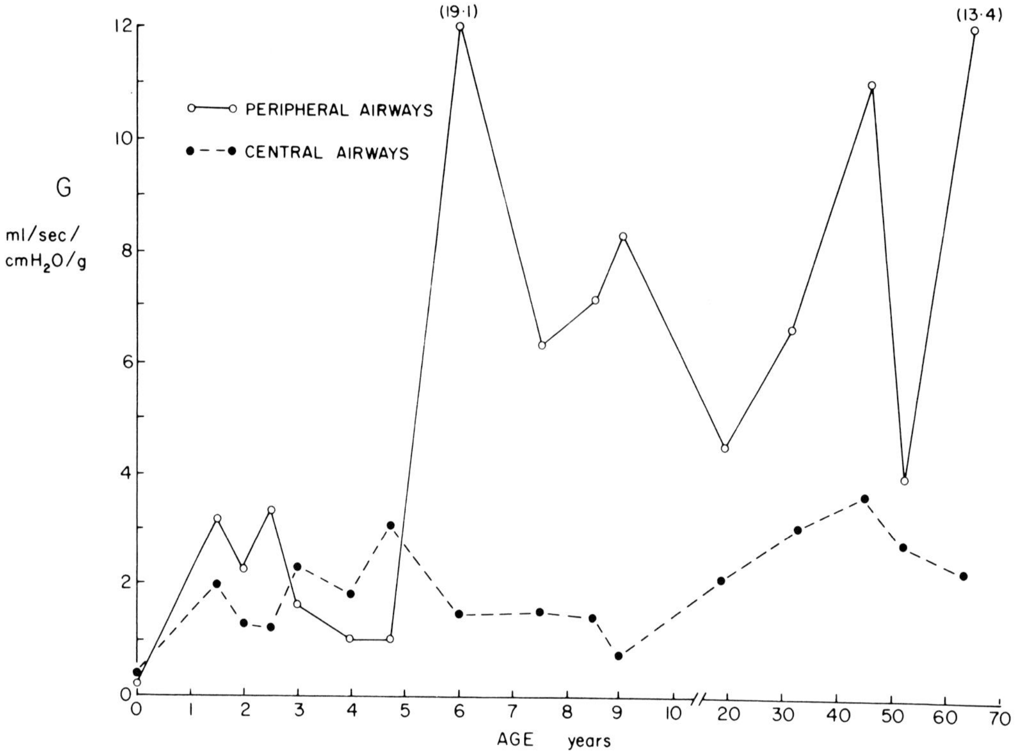

FIG. 3-5. Airways conductance of lungs from subjects of varying ages. The central and peripheral airways are plotted separately. Although the central airways conductance remains uniform at all ages, the peripheral airways conductance increases markedly at about age 5. This is thought to be due to the fact that the peripheral airways increase their radii relatively slowly during the first few years of life, but later, these increase very strikingly.

pulmonary conductance), because conductance is positively correlated with increases in volume. In examining the relationship between airways conductance and lung volume in the data of Briscoe and Dubois,[14] and Cook and associates,[15] Mead[3] drew attention to the fact that between the ages of 9 and 15, lung volume increases at a greater rate than conductance, whereas between 15 years and adulthood, conductance increases at a much faster rate than does volume. Mead suggested that this might mean that initially the size and number of alveoli increase out of proportion to the size of the airways, whereas later on in life, the airways more than catch up. It has been shown that the number of conducting airways is complete at birth,[16] whereas the number of alveoli increase rapidly after birth and approach the adult number at between 5 and 8 years of age.

In the normal adult lung, the bulk of the resistance is in the central airways, and the resistance beyond the twelfth generation of airways is very small. (See the section on lung anatomy for a further description, and see Fig. 3-9.) This relative distribution of airways resistance is different in early life, because the growth of the conducting airways lags behind during the period of rapid alveolar multiplication, from birth to age 5. Indeed, a series of experiments in our laboratory indicated that significant changes in airway resistance occur at the lung periphery about the same time that the number of alveoli reach the adult value.[17,18] Figure 3-5 shows the data from these experiments. A catheter was carefully placed in the same position in the airways of lungs of persons of various ages so that airways conductance could be measured. In the adult lung the conductance of the peripheral airways was much greater than that of central airways, and this relationship held true down to about 6 or 7 years of age. In the younger children, however, the peripheral airways conductance fell off markedly.

This observed increase in peripheral airways conductance after about age 5 could be explained if the total number of conducting airways in the periphery of the lung increased, or if their size increased at a more rapid rate than the central airways. We know that the number of conducting airways is fixed by the third month of intrauterine life[16]; therefore, it is likely that the peripheral airways increase in size at a more rapid rate than the central airways, beginning at about age 5. When the number of alveoli is nearly complete at age 5, further lung growth, due to an increase in alveolar dimensions, is probably associated with an increase in small airways diameter.

To understand why a tiny change in airways caliber causes such an increase in conductance requires a return to our previous consideration of flow through tubes. If a single tube branches and if the total cross-sectional area of the two daughter branches is exactly equal to that of the parent, the pressure drop along the daughters is greater than the pressure drop along the parent. However, when the ratio of cross-sectional area of parent to daughters becomes greater than $1/\sqrt{2}$, the pressure drop along the daughters is less than that along the parent. Weibel[19] has shown that in adult lungs, the total cross-sectional area increases with each generation at a rate that is much greater than $1/\sqrt{2}$ (see Fig. 3-8D). Our data suggest, however, that the same may not be true in children under 5 years of age. Indeed, Charles Bryan and his colleagues* have shown that the ratio is less than $1/\sqrt{2}$ in this age group. This disproportionately high peripheral airways resistance in children is an important concept because it relates to their lung pathology, a point to which we will return later.

CHANGES IN AIRWAY RESISTANCE WITH THE RESPIRATORY CYCLE

In 1892, Einthoven[20] predicted that airway resistance would change during breathing because of dynamic widening of the airways during inspiration and narrowing during expiration. He reasoned that if the pressure outside the airways is equal to the pleural pressure, then when no air flow occurs, the pressure across the wall of the airways is equal to the difference between atmospheric pressure and pleural pressure.

During the respiratory cycle there is a gradient of pressure across the airway wall, as well as a gradient from trachea to alveoli, to produce air flow. During inspiration the pressure at the outer wall becomes more negative, and a gradient in pressure is introduced at the inner wall, varying from atmospheric pressure near the airway opening to a value less than atmospheric pressure in the alveoli. The distending pressure difference across the airway wall is, therefore, greater in the large airways than in the small airways. During expiration the pressure at the outer wall of the airway increases toward atmospheric and the gradient of pressure on the inner wall of the airways is reversed, with pressure falling from greater than atmospheric near the alveoli to atmospheric pressure at the airway

FIG. 3-6. Inspiratory and expiratory flow volume curves. The solid line represents a maximal effort, from TLC to RV. The dotted line represents a submaximal effort.

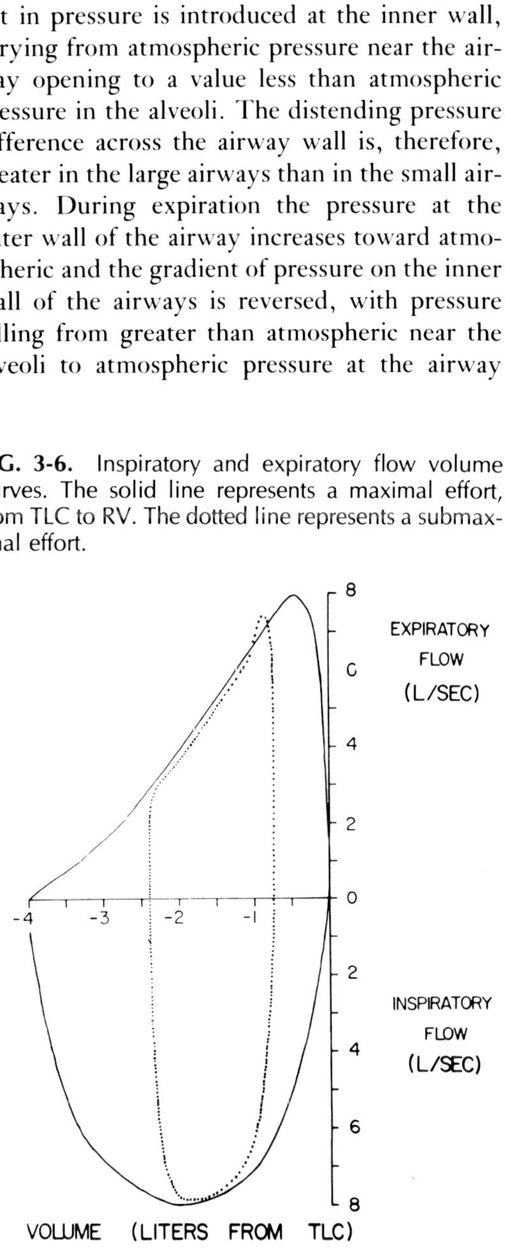

* Personal communication.

opening. Therefore, when the airways near the airway opening are compared with those near the alveoli, the large airways have a greater distending force exerted on them during inspiration and a lesser distending force exerted on them during expiration than do the small airways. Much later, Dayman[21] measured a variation in airway resistance during the breathing cycle in normal subjects and independently proposed the same mechanism that Einthoven did. Dekker and associates[22] measured intrabronchial pressure directly during voluntary wheezing in normal subjects and showed that the major obstruction during expiration was in the large bronchi. Fry and Hyatt[11] have shown that when flow is plotted against volume during inspiration, flow increases with each increase in effort throughout the inspiration (Fig. 3-6). During forced expiration, however, the maximum flows over the lower two-thirds of the vital capacity are extremely reproducible, uninfluenced by external resistances and independent of effort once maximum flows are reached. To further clarify this, they showed that when transpulmonary pressure is plotted against different flow rates at a particular lung volume in the range of the vital capacity, expiratory flow could not be increased beyond a certain maximum value by increasing driving pressure. This suggested that flow was being limited during expiration by dynamic compression of the intrathoracic airways, and led Fry[10] to develop the concept of flow-limiting segments of the airways. The analysis of these segments has proved extremely complex because of the difficulty in characterizing events in the compressed airways.

Mead and associates[23] avoided the compressed segment entirely when they introduced the "equal pressure point" theory in their analysis of expiratory flow. During forced expiration, alveolar pressure drives flow. Because alveolar pressure is made up of the static recoil pressure of the lung and the pleural pressure, it follows that as the pressure drops from the alveolus to the atmosphere, there are points along the airway where the pressure outside the airway (pleural pressure) and the pressure inside the airway are equal. The driving pressure for the segment from the alveolus to the equal pressure points is, therefore, the static recoil pressure of the lung. The equal pressure point (EPP) divides the airways into an upstream segment (alveolus to EPP), where the transmural pressure is positive, and a downstream segment (EPP to mouth), where the transmural pressure is negative. Flow through the upstream segment can be characterized by the resistance of the small airways and the elastic recoil pressure, both of which can be measured. Because the upstream and downstream segments act as resistances in series, characterizing flow through one of them characterizes the flow through the entire system. Using this approach, Mead and co-workers theorized that the equal pressure point is at the airway opening when pleural pressure is atmospheric. As the pleural pressure becomes more positive than atmospheric pressure, the equal pressure point moves upstream (toward the alveoli) and shortens the upstream segment, decreasing its resistance, so that flow increases. When the equal pressure point becomes fixed, the resistance of the upstream segment is fixed. This coincides with the observation that further increase in pressure results in little increase in flow (the flat part of the isovolume pressure flow curve). The disadvantage of the theory is that it ignores the compressed downstream segment and therefore cannot be used to attempt to explain the mechanisms that actually limit flow.

A third attempt to explain flow limitation on forced expiration, based on the model of a starling resistor, has been put forward by Pride and associates.[24] A starling resistor is a collapsible tube whose resistance depends on the relationship between inlet pressure and surrounding pressure, as long as surrounding pressure is greater than the outlet pressure. Pride and coworkers have applied this to the lungs, where pleural pressure is the surrounding pressure, alveolar pressure is the driving pressure, and outlet pressure is atmospheric pressure. By their analysis, flow continues to increase at a particular volume until the transmural pressure at some point in the airways causes the airway to narrow. They refer to this pressure, which is just sufficient to limit flow, as PTm' and suggest that it is the same as the transmural pressure required to close the airway under static conditions.

It is important to note that the compression of

intrathoracic airways, which limits flow, presents a problem for each of these three theories and that they are not mutually exclusive, but rather focus on one or another part of a complex mechanism. It is of interest that the airway narrowing produced during forced expiration is of greater significance than flow limitation; airway narrowing markedly increases the velocity of the air flow, which is an important feature of the clearance of the airways by the cough mechanism.

SINGLE-BREATH ANALYSIS OF DISTRIBUTION OF VENTILATION

Considerable information can be obtained about the distribution of gases in the ventilated lung regions by analyzing a single respiratory cycle. If nitrogen is measured in the expirate after a single inspiration of pure oxygen, a rapid increase in the amount of nitrogen is observed as the dead space is washed out, followed by a gradually increasing alveolar plateau (Fig. 3-7B). Krogh and Lindhard[25] thought that this plateau was due to the fact that gas mixing was slow enough to leave a gradient in nitrogen within the lungs. Rauwerda,[26] however, calculated that diffusion in the lungs is rapid enough to make this gradient unlikely and concluded that Krogh and Lindhard's explanation of the alveolar plateau was incorrect. This led to the consideration that the plateau could be explained by regional inhomogeneity in the distribution of the inspired air.

The relative importance of compliance over resistance in the distribution of ventilation was first suggested by Fowler.[27] He estimated that the time constant (*i.e.*, the product of resistance and compliance) of the lower airways and lung was about 0.15 sec. He concluded, from theoretical considerations, that the threefold changes in the time constant produced by changes in resistance would have little effect on ventilation distribution. He therefore analyzed single expired breaths obtained after the introduction of argon and calculated the effective compliance of the well-ventilated and poorly ventilated spaces. When the expired air is analyzed for argon after a single inspiration of the argon mixture, a downward-sloping plateau is observed. This indicates that the flow from the space receiving the least amount of argon is greatest at low lung volumes. By introducing boluses of argon at RV, FRC, and near TLC in separate tests (see Fig. 3-7A), he observed that the argon concentration in the expired breath was upward sloping, flat, and downward sloping, respectively. He concluded that the poorly ventilated space received the highest flow near RV, whereas the well-ventilated space received the highest flow between FRC and TLC. Because of the location of the cardiac oscillations during these expired breaths, he speculated that the well-ventilated space was in the lower lung and the poorly ventilated space in the upper lung.

The introduction of radioactive gas methods made it possible to demonstrate the topographical difference in the distribution of ventilation between lung regions. Milic-Emili and associates[28] showed that at RV the upper lung regions expand to about 35% of their total capacity, whereas the lower lung regions expand to only about 10%. During the initial expansion of the lung above RV, the upper regions expand rapidly, with very little expansion in the lower zones. At lung volumes above 40% of TLC, however, the expansion is greatest in the lower regions, and this relative distribution of regional expansion remains the same up to TLC. They assumed that there was no difference in the pressure–volume characteristics of lung regions and attributed the differences in expansion that they observed to the pleural pressure gradient. It followed that because the pleural pressure is more negative at the lung top, the upper lung regions would expand more at RV, and because they were on the steep portion of the pressure–volume curve, they would expand most rapidly close to RV. The lower regions would be much less expanded, so that closure of the lower airways would explain the fact that these regions expand little during the initial phase of respiration. Above FRC, the upper lung regions approach the flatter, less compliant portion of the lung pressure–volume curve and expand slowly, whereas the lower lung regions remain on the steep, more compliant portion of the curve and expand rapidly. Dolfuss and associates[29] used the bolus technique with radioactive xenon as the test gas. This allowed the distribution of gases in the inspired breath to be studied

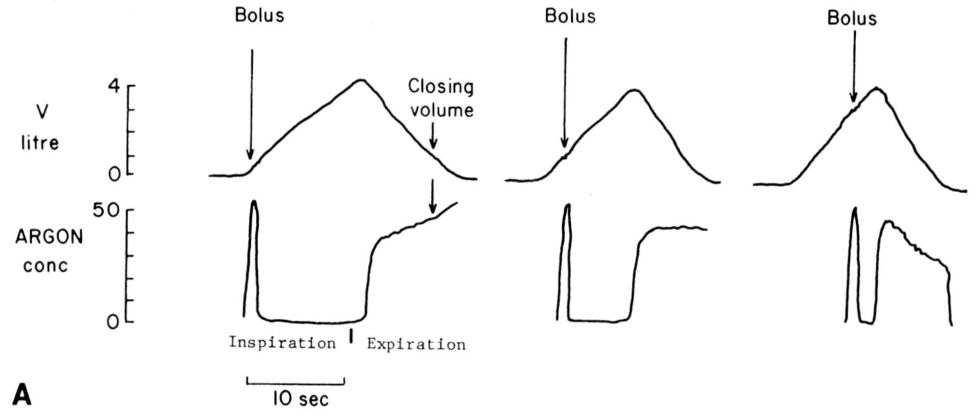

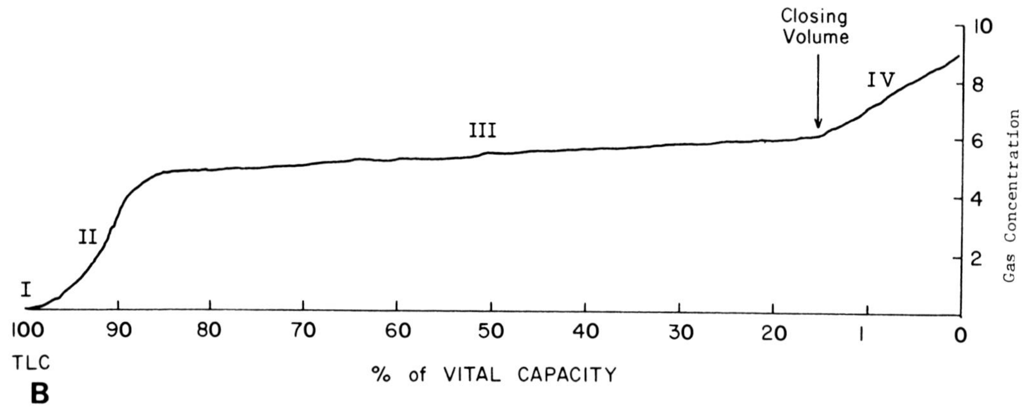

FIG. 3-7. A. The continuous analysis of expired breaths following an inhalation of bolus of argon. When the bolus is inhaled near residual volume, the argon trace slopes upward throughout expiration, with an inflection and a steeper upward slope as residual volume is approached. When the bolus is inhaled higher in inspiration, the argon trace is flat throughout expiration, and when it is inhaled near TLC, it slopes downward. (Data modified from Fowler K: Relative compliances of the well and poorly ventilated spaces in the normal human lung. J Appl Physiol 19:937, 1964) **B.** This shows the tracer gas plotted against the vital capacity. The bolus is introduced at RV; the subject inhales to TLC; and the expired breath is analyzed at the mouth. Phase II represents the washout of mixed alveolar and dead-space gas. Phase III represents alveolar gas, which is upward-sloping because of the continuous addition of gas from poorly ventilated spaces. Phase IV represents the contribution from the poorly ventilated space following closure of the airways. The point of inflection of this trace is labeled *closing volume* and can also be seen on the argon trace of the RV bolus in Fowler's data **(A)**. A similar curve is obtained for nitrogen, when a single breath of oxygen is inhaled from RV to TLC. (Adapted from Dolfuss R, Milic-Emili J, Bates D: Regional ventilation of the lung studied with boluses of xenon. Respir Physiol 22:760, 1967)

both by examination of the expired breath and by external counting of the xenon over the chest. They tied together the observations of Fowler and of Milic-Emili and associates by demonstrating a gradual progression from the poorly ventilated upper lung regions to the well-ventilated lower lung regions. The slope of the alveolar plateau (Phase III, Fig. 3-7B) was found to be consistent with small progressive increases in the contribution of alveolar gas from the upper lung regions, and the steep rise in the slope of Phase IV (Fig. 3-7B) was found to be consistent with lower airway closure, so that all of the remaining expired breath came from the upper regions.

Analysis of single-breath expirates has been popular in recent years in the diagnosis of lung disorders. By displaying volume on one axis and gas concentration on the other axis of an X-Y recorder. (Fig. 3-7B), a tracing of the washout curve can be easily obtained. The measurement of both the closing volume and the slope of Phase III are popular tests for minimal airways obstruction, and this is discussed further in relation to the early detection of disease on page 182.

THE ANATOMY OF THE AIRWAYS AND THEIR RESPONSE TO INJURY

In this presentation, we will not provide a description of the segmental anatomy of the airways, because this has been adequately covered in numerous other texts. This omission will allow us to concentrate on the quantitative anatomy of the airways and the alterations that occur in the lung in response to injury.

ANATOMY OF THE CONDUCTING AIRWAYS

A great deal of pertinent information concerning the nature and branching of the airways can be gained by looking at a normal bronchogram. Careful examination of the tracheobronchial tree (Fig. 3-8A) shows that it is slightly asymmetrical, because the branches are not always equal in size. It also shows that it is possible to reach the alveolated structures from the trachea by traversing a different number of branch points, depending on the pathway followed. The exact number of branch points or generations traversed as different pathways are followed has been computed by Horsfield and Cumming,[30] who showed that the path from the trachea to the alveolated structures may traverse as few as eight or as many as twenty-four branch points (Fig. 3-8B). This means that airways of a particular size are found at a variety of positions along the length of the airway, because they narrow at different rates. For example, Weibel[19] (Fig. 3-8C) has shown that 2-mm airways may be found anywhere from the fourth to the fourteenth bronchial divisions. The size of the total cross section of airways of different generations is also of interest, because this information is crucial in understanding the distribution of airways resistance. For many years it was thought that the peripheral airways (*i.e.*, 2 mm and smaller) constituted the narrowest point in the tracheobronchial tree. This information was based on the work of Rohrer, who measured with calibrated bougies the diameter of airways in excised uninflated lungs. Much more recently, Weibel[19] measured the diameter of these airways from casts of human lungs and found that Rohrer had grossly underestimated both the number and the total cross-sectional area of these small airways Weibel showed that as one progressed towards the peripheral generations of airways, the total cross-sectional area increased markedly (Fig. 3-8D). This information has important physiological implications, because it means that the peripheral airways should account for a very small proportion of the total airways resistance. This was shown to be the case by Macklem and Mead,[13] who introduced an ingenious method for measuring pressure in the small airways, so that peripheral airways resistance could be measured. Similar data[17] have also been obtained using this technique in human lungs (Fig. 3-9). An important corollary of this is that disease must be very severe in these airways before it can be detected by measuring total airways resistance.

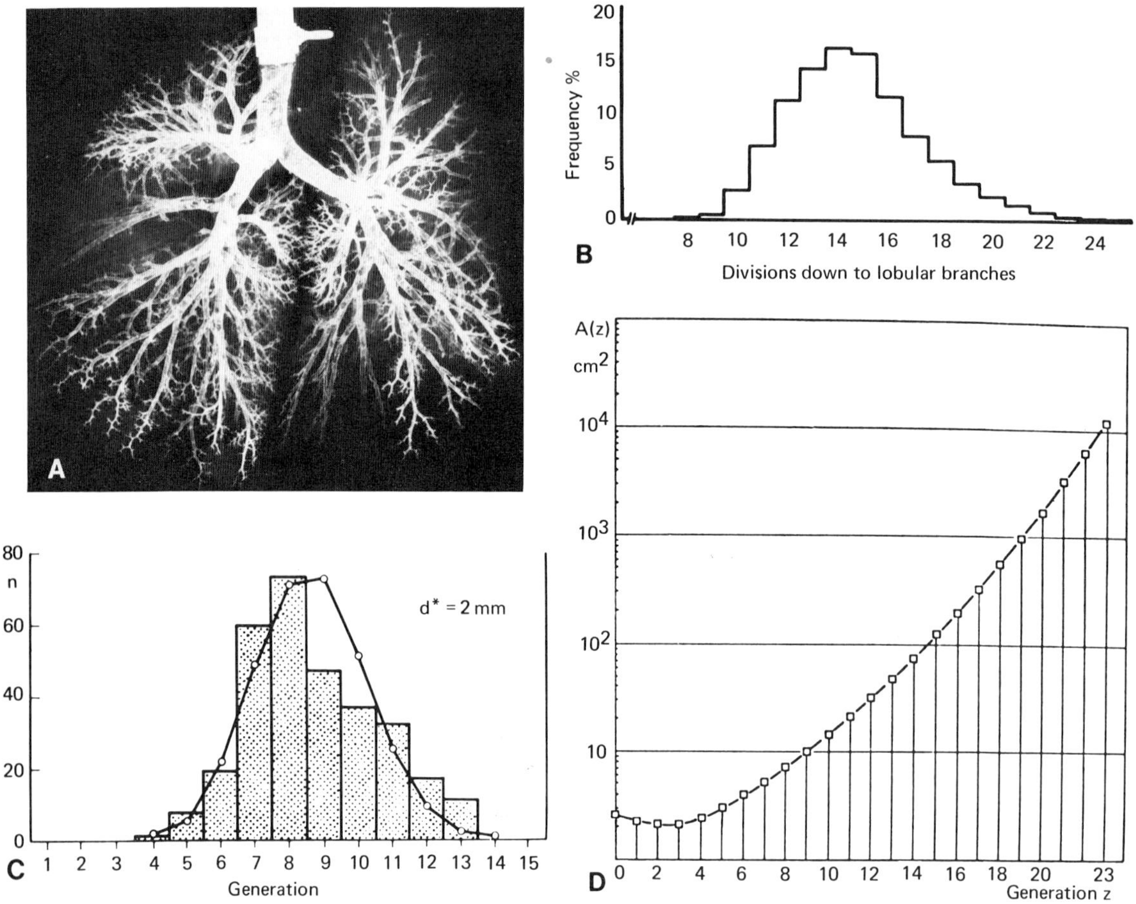

FIG. 3-8. A. A normal human bronchogram. Note the differing size of bronchi and the varying number of branches. **B.** The number of branches along the bronchial tree. Eight to twenty-four branches may occur, depending on the lung region. The most frequent number is fourteen. **C.** The distribution of small airways may occur after a highly variable degree of bronchial branching. This graph demonstrates the number of divisions of bronchi that result in 2-mm diameter airways. Although they are found after four to fourteen divisions, they most commonly occur after eight. **D.** The cross-sectional area of the airways may decrease slightly at the time of the first or second division. Thereafter, it progressively increases to the most distal degeneration of bronchi. (*B* adapted from Horsfield K, Cumming G: The morphology of the bronchial tree in man. J Appl Physiol 24:373, 1968. *C* and *D* reproduced with permission from Weibel E: Morphometry of the Human Lung. New York, Academic Press, 1963)

Returning to our discussion of lung growth, it is possible that the airways cross-sectional area of children's lungs, from trachea to alveoli, increases at a slower rate than the rate Weibel has shown for adult lungs. If this is so, it would explain why the peripheral airways resistance in children's lungs is disproportionately high and perhaps why airways disease can be so devastating in the younger child.

MICROSCOPIC ANATOMY OF THE AIRWAYS

The airways are made up of cartilage, smooth muscle, mucus-producing glands, connective tissue, and epithelium. The relative amounts of cartilage, smooth muscle, and mucous gland that make up the walls of the airways are shown in Figure 3-10. Cartilage makes up about 30% of

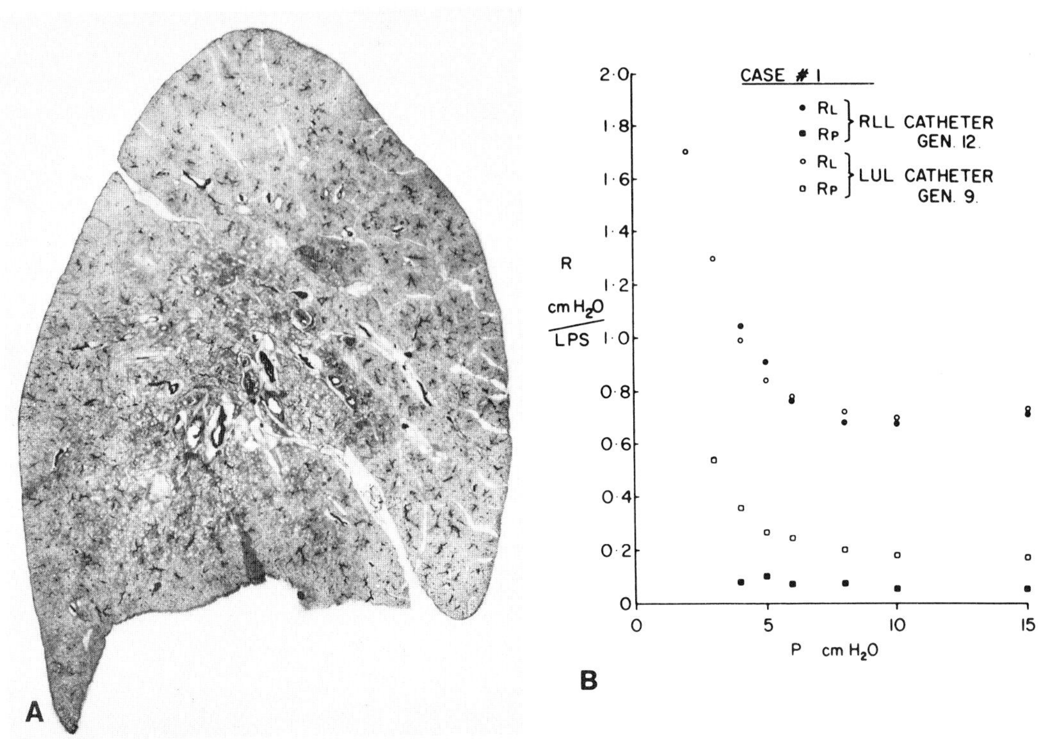

FIG. 3-9. A. A normal, paper-mounted, whole lung section. **B.** The distribution of airways resistance in an excised normal human lung. R_L is total airway resistance, and R_P is the resistance of the peripheral airways. Total resistance at a transpulmonary pressure of 4 mm Hg is about 1 cm of water per liter per second; about 10% of this is located in airways distal to generation twelve. This compares favorably with values in life, which are about 2 cm of water per liter per second, with the remainder being accounted for by the larynx, which was not present in these experiments. (*B* adapated from Hogg J, Macklem P, Thurlbeck W: Site and nature of airways obstruction in chronic obstructive lung disease. N Engl J. Med 278:1355, 1968)

the wall thickness in the mainstem and lobar bronchi and gradually decreases. By definition, the bronchioles are airways that do not contain cartilage in their walls. The bronchial mucous glands make up about 12% of the wall thickness in the mainstem bronchi, and then these, too, gradually diminish as the more peripheral airways are reached. The bronchioles contain no mucous glands in their walls. Smooth muscle, on the other hand, represents only about 5% of the airway thickness in the mainstem airway, but this increases along the airways. The wall thickness of the bronchioles, which are the most muscular airways, is composed of about 20% muscle.

The Bronchial Epithelium

The epithelium in the airways is a pseudostratified columnar type. The cells of which it is primarily comprised are the goblet cell and the ciliated cell. Other cells such as the nonciliated bronchial epithelial cell (Clara cell) and the representatives of the APUD system have also been described, but their function is less certain.[31] The major functions of the epithelium are to protect the lung from injurious agents and to trap and clear particulate matter from the airways. The two major cell types responsible for these functions are the ciliated epithelial cell and the goblet cell. These cells are responsible for

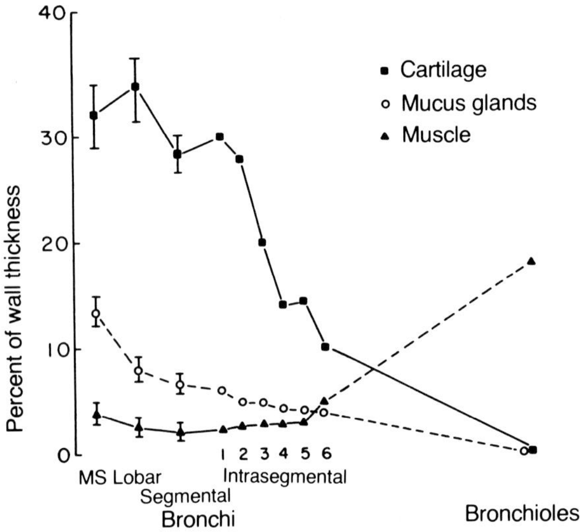

FIG. 3-10. The distribution of cartilage, mucus glands, and muscle, from main-stem bronchi to bronchioles, in the tracheobronchial tree. Note that bronchioles have no cartilage but are muscular.

maintaining the mucociliary blanket that serves to protect the tracheobronchial tree by trapping and removing foreign material. The mucous layer is produced by both the goblet cells and the bronchial mucous glands. Reid has shown that the number of cells producing mucus in the glands is greater than the number of goblet cells, and it has been assumed that the glands are more important as a source of mucus than are the goblet cells. Study of the physical characteristics of the mucous layer shows that the superficial layer is more viscous than the deep layer. This is important with respect to the ciliary function, because the cilia are allowed to recover rapidly in the less viscous lower layer, whereas they attach to the highly viscous superficial layer during their power stroke to propel this layer toward the mouth. The cilia beat in unison to provide an effective escalator type of mechanism to clear the airway. The structure of cilia is similar in all biological species, in that they all have a characteristic 9 + 2 structure. This means that there are nine pairs of microtubular structures arranged in doublets around the periphery of each cilia, with one central pair of microtubules that are separated from each other (see also Chap. 8). The structure and function of the microtubules in many cell types are presently under active investigation, but their specific function in the ciliated epithelial cell of the tracheobronchial tree is only beginning to be studied. The fact that the cilia maintain a constant length in both the power and recovery strokes, however, suggests that the microtubules move as a system of sliding filaments, with a powerful winding of the filaments during the slow power stroke, followed by a quick release and rapid unwinding during the higher-velocity recovery stroke.[32,33]

The recognition that cilia have abnormal structure and function in several different airways disease states is a recent development.[34] Further elucidation of their role in obstructive lung diseases, particularly those associated with bronchiectasis, is likely to shed new light on our understanding of these diseases in the years ahead, as discussed in Chapter 14.

In addition to the mucous layer, the epithelium provides a further protective mechanism by the arrangements of the cell junctions. The junctional complexes of most epithelial cells have three components that succeed one another, proceeding from the luminal surface to the base of the cell. The zonula occludens provides membrane-to-membrane contact around the periphery of the cells at the luminal surface. This function represents a fusion of the outer leaflet of the membranes of adjacent cells. This fusion is not continuous but represents a series of fusions arranged in parallel. The number and extent of these fusions appear to determine the permeability of the junctional complexes and vary with epithelia in different organs. The second component of the junctional complex is the zonula adherens, where the membranes of the adjacent cells are separated by a space of about 200Å, which is filled by protein filaments. The third component of the functional complex is the desmosome or macula adherens, where the adjacent cell membranes are separated but are joined by an intermediate line that may represent condensation of the material of the cell coat.

In addition to the junctional complex, the epithelial cells are joined at various other sites by the nexus or gap junction. This junction provides direct communication between cells without communication with the intercellular space, but its function is unknown. Whether or not these communications are important in controlling the unformity of the ciliary beat remains to be investigated, but it is worth noting that these junctions are thought to be important in the electrical coupling of cells and in the passage of small molecules between cells. Of great interest is the fact that these junctions have been shown to decrease in number during the development of squamous-cell carcinoma of the cervix and to be related to the phenomenon of contact inhibition of cells growing in tissue culture. The investigation of the precise structural and functional relationships will provide intriguing questions for the investigator interested in the biology and pathology of the airway epithelium.

The Bronchial Glands

The secretory portions of the mucous glands are embedded in the submucosa. The ducts from these glands extend to the luminal surface of the airway, where they empty their contents onto the mucociliary blanket. Their secretion can be influenced by the autonomic nervous system, in that stimulation of the vagus or injection of acetylcholine can cause beads of secretion to appear where the duct opens onto the epithelial surface. Just what part the autonomic nervous system plays in the normal function of the glands is more difficult to determine.

Airway Cartilage

The trachea and the extrapulmonary bronchi consist of a framework of incomplete rings of hyaline cartilage united by fibrous tissues and nonstriated muscle. The trachea has from sixteen to twenty horseshoe-shaped cartilages that open posteriorly. Two or more of these cartilage plates often unite either partially or completely; they may calcify and sometimes contain bone in advanced age. The cartilages are enclosed by an elastic fibrous membrane, with a dense layer passing over the outer surface of the rings and a less dense layer over the inner surface. These layers fuse to form a tough membrane both between the rings and in the posterior part of the trachea and mainstem bronchi, where the rings are deficient.

The horseshoe-shaped rings of cartilage in the trachea and extrapulmonary bronchi are replaced by irregularly-shaped cartilage plates in the intrapulmonary bronchi. Although their irregularity in shape suggests that they might not encircle the bronchus, Miller showed, by reconstruction, that these cartilage plates are positioned to encircle the lumen of the airway completely in many instances. The cartilage, like the mucous glands, decreases in amount with successive generations of airway, until it disappears completely in the bronchioles.

Smooth Muscle

Muscle is present only in the posterior part of the trachea and extrapulmonary bronchi, where it is located within the fibrous membrane. The longitudinal fibers are external and consist of a few scattered bundles, whereas the transverse fibers form the tracheal muscle, which extends between the ends of the cartilage and passes across in the intervals between them.

In the intrapulmonary airways, the muscle lies between the epithelium and cartilage in a layer that encircles the lumen. It is formed by two sets of fibers, one rotating around the airway in a counterclockwise fashion. The function of this muscle is not at all clear, but it is influenced by the autonomic nervous system. Stimulation of the parasympathetic nervous system causes contraction, and stimulation of the β-adrenergic system causes dilation. The contribution of the α-adrenergic system to bronchoconstriction is controversial.

Bronchial Circulation

The various elements of the airways that have been described all receive their blood supply from the systemic circulation. The tracheal blood supply is variable but usually arises from the inferior thyroid vessels and drains into the inferior thyroid venous plexus. The bronchial arteries supply the extrathoracic airways, and these usually arise from the descending thoracic aorta and form the upper posterior intercostal arteries. In the bronchi they form a capillary plexus that supplies the muscle and submucosa of the airways. This plexus communicates with branches of the pulmonary artery and empties into the pulmonary veins. Other branches supply the interlobular tissue and the pleura, and these drain into the bronchial veins, which empty into the azygos vein on the right side and into the superior intercostal or superior hemiazygos vein on the left side.

THE PATHOLOGY OF TRACHEOBRONCHIAL INJURY

ACUTE TRACHEOBRONCHIAL INJURY

Tracheitis and Bronchitis

Acute tracheitis and bronchitis are very common afflictions. Indeed, most persons suffer these illnesses many times during their life. A wide variety of agents can produce laryngotracheobronchitis; these include noxious gases, particulate irritants, and a variety of living organisms. The conducting airways have a limited way in which to respond, in that the common denominator of all of the agents is that they induce an inflammatory response. This response follows a typical usual sequence: initial vasoconstriction, followed by vasodilation, and transudation of fluid from capillaries into the interstitial space and on to the luminal surface of the airways. Because most irritants also increase mucus production, the fluid has a characteristically sticky white appearance until the polymorphonuclear cells migrate from the capillaries into the mucous exudate and change it to the characteristically yellow-green sputum of purulent tracheobronchitis. The exfoliation of superficial bronchial epithelial cells is increased by this process and if the injury is severe, ulceration of the mucosa may develop and bleeding may occur, so that the sputum becomes blood-tinged.

The extent and degree of the injury depend on the distribution of the agent and its concentration at various levels of the tracheobronchial tree. The factors determining this are very complex. For example, nitrogen dioxide gas is extremely soluble in water and is therefore absorbed rapidly in the airways, so that it damages primarily the upper airways, trachea, and main bronchi. The bacteria and viruses that infect the tracheobronchial tree are carried in water droplets. The deposition of these aerosol droplets depends on the droplets' weight, size, velocity, and settling time. Large droplets tend to impact by inertial forces, so that they leave the flowing stream of air at bends and branch points in the nose and larynx. Smaller particles remain in the stream and penetrate deeper into the lung. Differences between the agents producing disease in the airways and those producing disease in the alveoli may relate to the physical characteristics of the agents, which determine how they are delivered to the lungs. The responses of the airways and parenchyma could differ, because the conducting airways are supplied by the bronchial circulation, where a higher capillary pressure might result in exudates that are sticky and remain localized, as in the so-called bronchopneumonic processes; whereas the lung parenchyma is supplied by the pulmonary circulation, where capillary injury might produce a transudate that would spread quickly through the alveolar spaces, as in the early stages of pneumococcal pneumonia. Direct evidence in support of these hypotheses, however, is difficult to come by.

Bronchiolitis

There probably is involvement of the bronchioles in most cases of airway injury. In adults, however, this has relatively little effect on airways resistance, and since it is usually not life-threatening, we seldom have the opportunity to observe the pathology of this condition. Quite the reverse is true in children, where the peripheral airways make up a significant proportion of total resistance, and disease in the bronchioles can be serious. Bronchiolitis has been defined as an acute illness, mainly affecting infants, in which the principal lesion is an inflammatory obstruction of the small airways.[35,36] It is usually preceded by several days of mild upper respiratory infection, followed by an acute onset of respiratory distress when the lower respiratory tract becomes involved. Physical examination at this time reveals a rapid respiratory rate; a hyperinflated chest, with marked activity of the accessory muscles of respiration; a dry, unproductive cough; and a low-grade fever.

In a study of forty-one cases, High[36] found that twenty-one cases occurred in children less than 6 mo of age, ten cases in children between 6 mo and a year, and eight of the remaining ten cases in children in the second year of life. Only two of the forty-one cases were in older children, and the oldest was 4 years of age.

Laboratory investigation reveals signs of overinflation on the chest reontgenogram, with little or no parenchymal change. Bacterial pathogens are often isolated from the throat and sputum of these patients and are thought to represent secondary invastion rather than a primary cause. The etiological agent in the disease is generally thought to be of viral origin.[37] Further information on this topic is included in the section on viral infections, Chapter 8.

The most consistent disorder of anatomy in bronchiolitis is a lymphocytic infiltration of the bronchiolar wall, with a proliferation of the basal cells and extrusion of the columnar cells toward the center of the lumen. This produces a marked thickening of the bronchiolar wall and a narrowing of the lumen, but actual plugging of the lumen with inflammatory mucus is a less obvious feature of the disease.[35,36] It is of interest that even though upper respiratory infections with later involvement of the lower respiratory tract are common in adults as well as in children, this sequence of events rarely has a serious effect on older children and adults. Studies done on human lungs obtained at autopsy have shown that bronchiolitis does occur in adults, but that it probably goes unrecognized, because it produces little effect on total airway resistance. Results from two postmortem studies shown in Figure 3-11A and B illustrate this point. Both cases had morphological evidence of bronchiolitis (Fig. 3-11C, D), and both had physiological evidence of increased central and peripheral airways resistance. The 6-month-old child, however, died from the disease, whereas the 63-year-old patient had only minor respiratory symptoms at the time of sudden death from a cerebrovascular accident. One possible reason for this could be the anatomy of the airways. In the child, the peripheral airways are disproportionately narrow, and collateral ventilation is poorly developed, so that airway closure with overinflation might easily occur. This could result in defective gas exchange and a life-threatening situation. On the other hand, in the adult, the peripheral airways total cross-sectional area is large, and collateral ventilation is well developed, so that the interference with gas exchange may be minimal.

CHRONIC BRONCHIAL INJURY

When the tracheobronchial tree is subjected to injurious agents over long periods of time, fundamental changes occur in the airways. The ciliated cells of the epithelium are replaced by either goblet cells or squamous cells, as a result of a metaplastic process. This change, which must be an attempt at protection, leads to difficulty by both increasing the production of and decreasing the clearance of the mucus. In the later stages of chronic bronchitis, the inflammatory process becomes less impressive, with the striking pathological features being enlargement of the bronchial mucous glands and some increase in the number of goblet cells. Study of postmortem lungs has shown that the greatest degree of obstruction with chronic disease occurs in the peripheral airways, and this seems to be due to mucus plugging the lumen of these small airways, chronic inflammation of their walls with fibrosis, and even obliteration of the small airways in some cases.

Chronic Bronchitis

This condition has been defined as persistent excess mucus in the tracheobronchial tree that is not caused by other specific conditions such as bronchiectasis.[38] It is recognized clinically by excessive sputum production, which is usually associated with cough. (For a complete clinical definition, see Chap. 14.) The morphological criteria for diagnosis involve a description of the mucous glands and the mucosal goblet cells. Because the mucous glands have been estimated to have 100 times the volume of the goblet cells, their size has been taken as a morphological criterion for the diagnosis of chronic bronchitis. Although the Reid index, or ratio of gland thickness to wall thickness, offered some promise in separating patients with bronchitis from those without bronchitis, it is now apparent that there is a considerable overlap in the values obtained for this ratio between these two groups. Thurl-

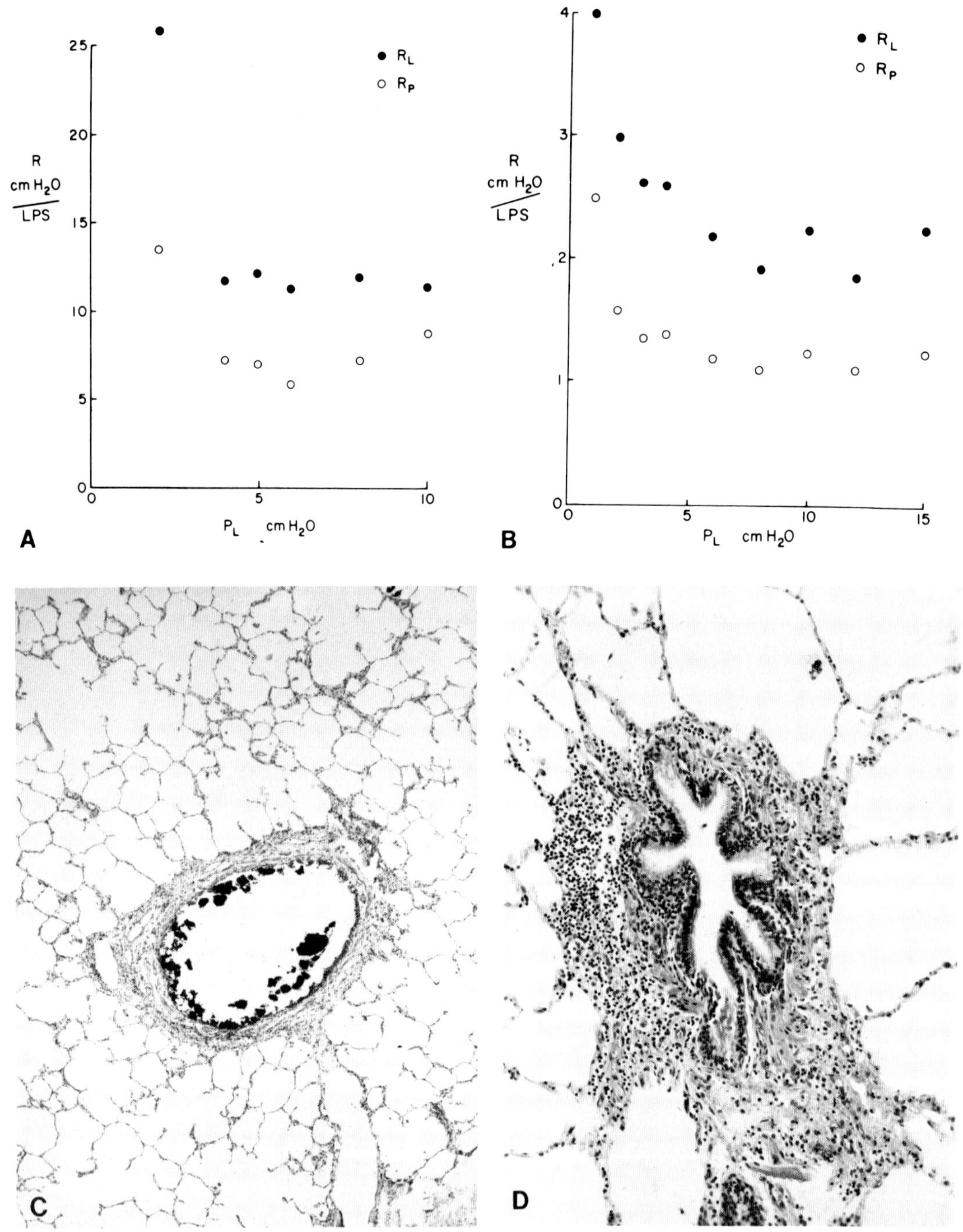

FIG. 3-11. The distribution of airways resistance in a 6-month-old child **(A)** and in a 63-year-old adult **(B)**, both of whom have bronchiolitis. In both cases, the total airways resistance (R_L) is high, with a large portion of the resistance being accounted for by a increase in peripheral airways resistance (R_P). Compare this with the normal lung in Figure 3-9B. The morphological features of the child **(C)** and the adult **(D)**. In both cases, note the thickening of the airway wall due to the inflammation of the wall. The surrounding parenchyma is normal in both cases.

beck and Angus[39] have shown that the distribution curve of the Reid index in the general autopsy population is bell-shaped, where those subjects with values less than 0.35 usually did not have symptoms of bronchitis during life, and those with values greater than 0.55 usually had clinical evidence of bronchitis. The bulk of the values for the patients in their study fell in the intermediate range, however, where there was a varying incidence of bronchitis. They suggested that because the clinical criterion of sputum production is open to considerable error, it may be more realistic to consider a continuum from normal to bronchitis, without an arbitrary separation of the two distinct groups (bronchitics and nonbronchitics), based on rigid morphological criteria.

The possibility that decreased bronchial clearance might result in excessive tracheobronchial mucus has not been adequately investigated. Although the use of radiopaque and radioactive materials shows promise for the study of clearance mechanisms in the lung, these mechanisms have not been satisfactorily characterized. The morphology of the bronchial cilia and the excessive mucus found in the airways at autopsy, however, suggest that abnormal clearance may be of great importance in this disease.[40] The physical properties of mucus in health and disease are of equal importance; even though descriptions of "viscid, sticky, highly viscous and thick" mucus abound in the literature, the study of the exact visco-elastic nature of the material has proved to be difficult.

Pulmonary Emphysema

Emphysema has been defined as an increase, beyond normal size, of the air spaces that are distal to the terminal bronchioles, accompanied by destructive change.[38] The relative importance of overinflation and actual destruction of lung tissue in emphysema has been controversial. The published works supporting each side of the controversy are very extensive, and a discussion of them is not relevant here. Laennee[41] provided the first lucid amount of the condition in 1819 and gave excellent gross descriptions of air-dried specimens of lungs from patients who had died of the disease. In his review of the morbid anatomy of emphysema, Strawbridge stated, "Since the original microscopic description of chronic emphysema by Rainey in 1848 there has been virtually complete agreement that the basic lesion is destruction of the alveolar walls by the process of fenestration."[42]

Etiology. The present working hypothesis for the mechanism of alveolar wall distruction is based on the possibility of an imbalance between the proteolytic and antiproteolytic forces acting on the lung parenchyma. The fact that both proteolytic and antiproteolytic forces come into play during an inflammatory reaction has been known since the classic study of Opie[43] just after the turn of the century. The relevance of this to the pathogenesis of emphysema became apparent in the 1960s when Laurell and Eriksson[44,45] found that some patients with emphysema had markedly depressed levels of the antiprotease α_1 antitrypsin, and Gross[46] showed that the proteolytic enzyme papain produced emphysema in animals. These studies have been rapidly extended and it is now established that experimental emphysema is produced by enzymes that attack elastin, that α_1 antitrypsin has anti-elastase capability, and that human leukocytes are the major source of elastase.[47]The role of cigarette smoke in disturbing the elastase–antielastase balance may be substantial because cigarette smoke may both increase the available elastase by recruiting[48] and activating blood neutrophils and decrease the anti-elastase activity on the lung surface by depressing the activity of the α_1 antitrypsin.[49,50] These factors and the relationship to hereditary α_1 antitrypsin deficiency are discussed in detail in Chapter 14.

Morphological Types of Emphysema. *Centrilobular Emphysema.* A renewal of interest in the morphology of emphysema was brought about by the description of centrilobular emphysema by Gough.[51] He and Leopold[52] showed that centrilobular emphysematous spaces are respiratory bronchioles, arising from more than one of the terminal bronchioles within a lobule, that have enlarged and become confluent. In the classic case, the alveolar ducts and sacs at the rim of the lobule are preserved, so that the cut surface of

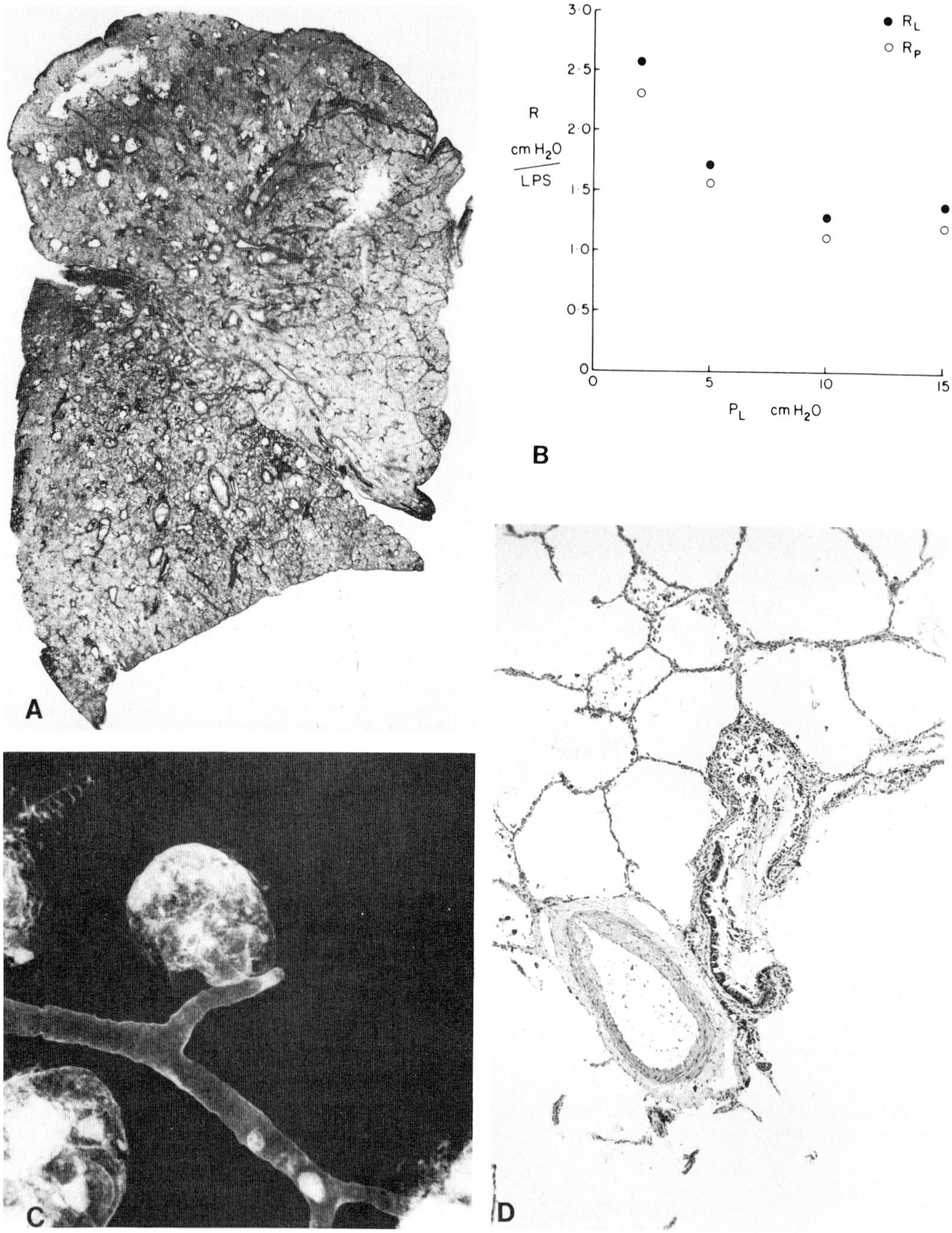

FIG. 3-12. **A.** A paper-mounted, whole lung section with centrilobular emphysema. **B.** The distribution of airways resistance in a case of centrilobular emphysema. In this case, the total airways resistance is increased (R_L), primarily because of the increase in peripheral airways resistance (R_P). **C.** A bronchogram of the centrilobular emphysematous space. **D.** Histological section of the airways near a centrilobular emphysematous space, showing narrowing and mucus plugging.

the lung appears to have punched-out holes that are separated by relatively normal-appearing alveolated structures. In many instances, however, the parenchyma at the rim of the lobule is not normal, and arbitrary decisions have to be made concerning the type of emphysema that is present. In general, the disease is more severe in the upper zones of the lung (Fig. 3-12).

Panlobular Emphysema. In this form, the entire acinus is involved. In the early stages, effacement of the alveoli produces a loss of the sharp distinction between alveoli and ducts, so that some scientists have referred to this as *alveolar duct emphysema.* As the disease progresses, however, there is a gradual destruction of the entire acinus. Panlobular emphysema is more or less random in its distribution within the lung, but there is a tendency for more frequent occurrence in the anterior basal segment and the tip of the lingula (Fig. 3-13).

Other Types of Emphysema. Heard and Izukawa[53] have described a form of emphysema that selectively involves the periphery of the lobule, and because of its relationship to the lobular septae, it was referred to as *paraseptal emphysema.* Since the lobular septae are often incomplete, some prefer to call this *periacinar*, *linear*, or *superficial* emphysema.

Emphysema that shows no particular localization within the acinus is termed *irregular emphysema*, and as this is often seen in relation to scars, it is also referred to as *scar emphysema.*

Incidence of Emphysema. If examples of scar emphysema are included, emphysema can be demonstrated in 80 to 90% of random adult necropsies.[54] Only about 50%, however, show well-defined panlobular or centrilobular forms. The disease occurs from the third to the ninth decade, with the majority of cases occurring in the sixth, seventh, and eighth decades, and although all forms of emphysema are more common in men than women, panlobular emphysema is more common than centrilobular emphysema in women.

Measurement of Emphysema. There have been many attempts to quantitate the extent and severity of emphysema in lungs obtained at autopsy. Thurlbeck[55] has recently reviewed the methods that have been used and pointed out that because most of them are subjective, it is difficult to compare observations obtained by one method to those obtained by another. The type of measurement selected depends on the exact correlation between structure and function that is being attempted.

The extent of emphysema is usually assessed on the cut surface of a whole lung fixed in inflation. Heard and Izukawa[53] divided the surface of the lung into six zones and assessed the extent separately in each zone. Sweet and colleagues[56] covered the lung with a grid 1 cm square and assessed the amount of emphysema in each square. Dunnill[57] used a grid with holes in it and assessed the lung he could see through the holes, using the Delesse principle to quantitate the amount of emphysema in the lung. Pratt and coworkers,[58] on the other hand, planimetered the area of the lung and the area of the surface that was involved with emphysema. Thurlbeck[55] assessed the amount of emphysema in each of ten zones in the lung and graded the emphysema in each zone on a 0-to-3 scale, depending on its severity. This gave a possible score ranging from 0 emphysema to 30 units of emphysema in extremely severe cases. His attempt to grade both extent and severity of the disease has an advantage over the methods that only measure the extent of the condition. For practical purposes the severity and extent of emphysema can now be established by comparing the lung to a standard set of photographs.[59]

Peripheral Airways Disease in Emphysema. Recent quantitative assessments of disease in the peripheral airways are of interest with respect to the relationship of airways disease to emphysema. Cosio and associates[60] developed an index of pathological change in the airways that was based on all of the known pathological lesions. Their study showed that deterioration in small-airways function correlated best with inflamatory lesions of the peripheral airways; Petty and co-workers[61] have recently confirmed this observation. Cosio and associates also showed that while emphysema increased with increasing air-

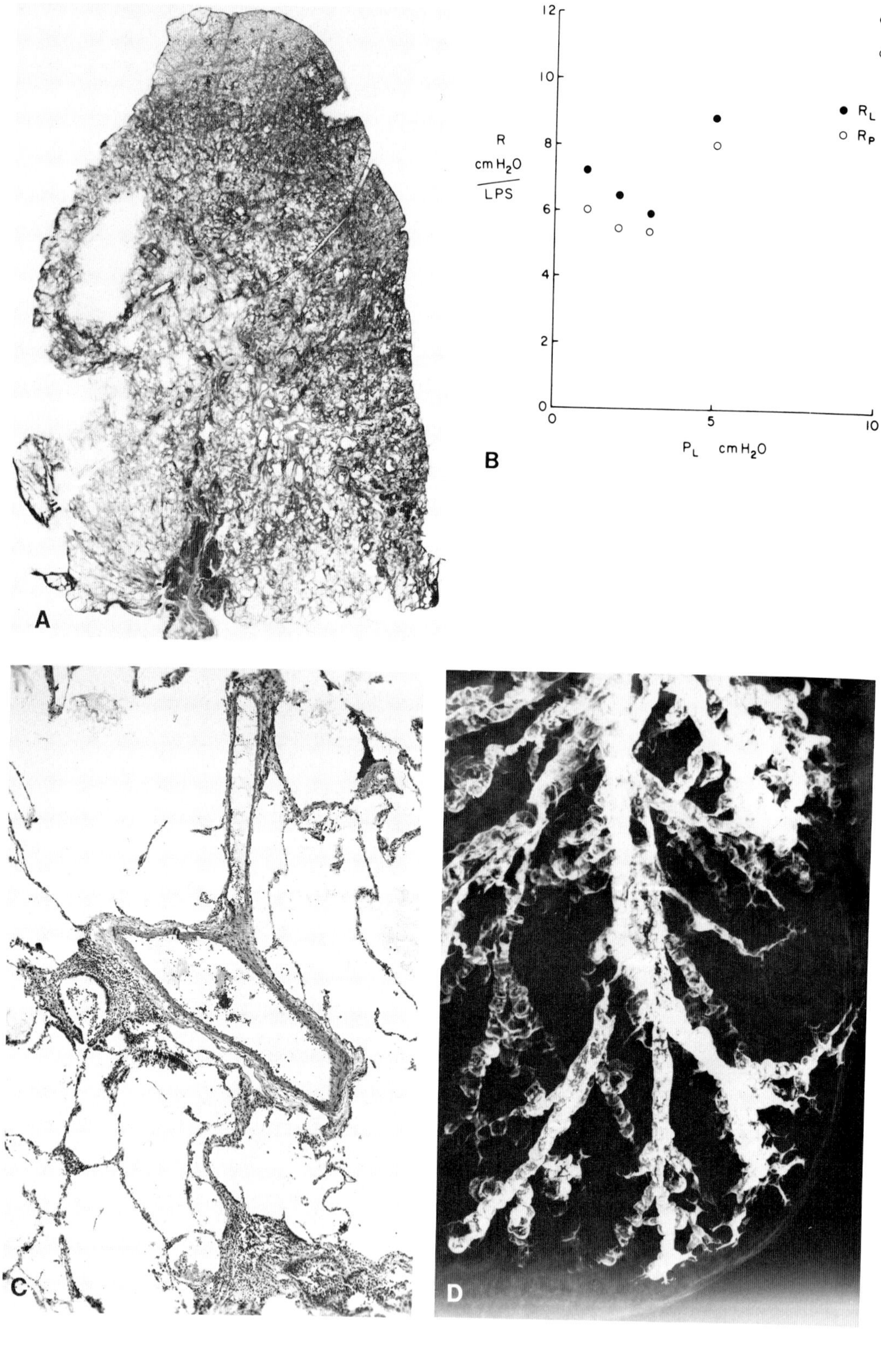
A
B
R
cm H_2O
LPS
R_L
R_P
P_L cm H_2O
0
2
4
6
8
10
12
5
10
C
D

ways disease, it did not occur in all cases that had severe small-airways pathology and disordered function. It is of interest to consider this fact in relation to the hypothesis that emphysema results from an imbalance between proteolytic and antiproteolytic processes in the inflammatory reaction in the distal airways. It seems possible that there could be extensive inflammation of the small airways and no emphysema as long as the antiproteolytic mechanisms prevail, and that emphysema would result from the balance shifted in favor of proteolysis.

Another interesting feature of the relationship of emphysema to chronic bronchitis can be found in Cosio and associates' study. Although excess mucus production is the hallmark of chronic bronchitis and the Reid Index of bronchial mucus gland size[62] has been thought to be a yardstick for bronchitis, Cosio and associates found that mucous plugging of the airways correlated poorly with decreasing airways function. This suggests that although mucus hypersecretion may be a symptom of the inflamation of the airway mucosa, it may not be an important cause of airways dysfunction.

Mechanical Properties of the Lung in Emphysema. *Lung Compliance.* In 1934, Christie[63] observed that patients with emphysema had a much smaller elastic recoil pressure at a given lung volume than did normal persons. Since that time, it has been well documented that these patients have an increased static compliance and that this falls rapidly with breathing frequency.[64] The work of Otis and associates[4] has shown that the fall in compliance with increased breathing frequency is due to an inequality of the time constants of the various parallel pathways.

The fact that static lung compliance is increased means that in advanced cases it is impossible to determine whether inequality in time constants is due to changes in the resistance of the airways or changes in the elastic property of the parenchyma. In early disease, when the lung's elastic properties are normal and airways resistance is not increased, the frequency dependence of compliance has been taken as evidence of disease in the peripheral airways.

Pulmonary Resistance in Emphysema. An increase in total pulmonary resistance is a characteristic finding in patients with clinical emphysema, but the site and nature of this increase have been centers of controversy. Laennec[39] attributed the airway obstruction to mucous plugging of the small bronchi and bronchioles and felt that the inspiratory muscles could overcome this obstruction but the expiratory muscles could not. Dayman[21] showed that the tendency for the pulmonary resistance to rise during expiration was increased in emphysema, and he attributed this to the fact that emphysema destroyed the peribronchiolar supporting structures, causing the bronchioles to act as a check valve. Butler and associates[66] proposed a third mechanism, stating that the decrease in elasticity, which is characteristic of emphysema, causes the small airways to be narrower at the particular lung volume than they normally would be.

The introduction of bronchial pressure measurements by Koblet and Wyss[67] enabled the lower airway resistance to be partitioned. Using such a technique, Macklem and co-workers[68] found that there were two sites of obstruction in patients with emphysema. The airways central to the segmental branches accounted for the increased resistance during forced expiration, and the airways beyond this point accounted for a fixed proportion of the resistance that was the same in both inspiration and expiration.

The contribution of large and small airways has also been studied in excised lungs; this study showed that the major site of obstruction was the peripheral airways (Figs. 3-12, 3-13) and that the resistance of these airways was the same on

FIG. 3-13. A. Paper-mounted, whole lung section with panlobular emphysema. **B.** A case of panlobular emphysema, with a marked increase in total airways resistance (R_L) caused by the disease in the peripheral airways (R_P). **C.** Panlobular emphysema, with marked narrowing of the airways, seen in a histological specimen. **D.** Panlobular emphysema, with narrowing of the small airways, seen in a bronchogram.

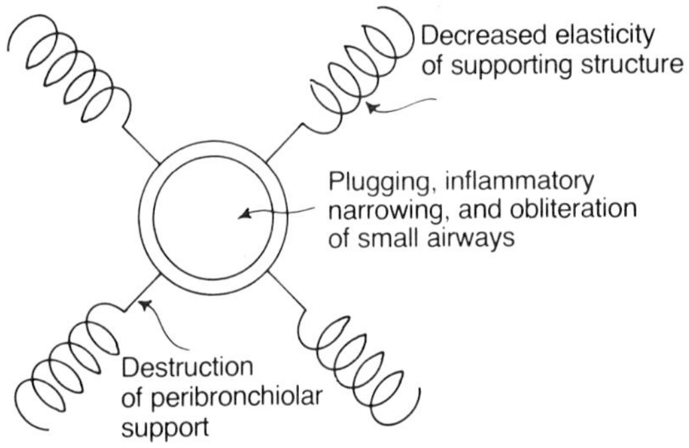

FIG. 3-14. The mechanisms that have been suggested for peripheral airways obstruction.

both inflation and deflation. It follows from the foregoing discussion of normal airways that the introduction of a fixed resistor in the small airways would require a markedly increased alveolar pressure to produce flow. This would be transmitted to the bronchial wall, causing dynamic compression of the large airways in forced expiration, which would severely limit maximum flow.

The nature of the peripheral airways disease that is responsible for the fixed resistance in the small airways has been a subject of debate, and the various sites and mechanisms of obstruction that have been proposed are summarized in Figure 3-14. Leopold and Gough[52] were unable to demonstrate significant obstruction of airways leading to the centrilobular spaces. McLean[69] and Anderson and Foraker[70] found evidence to support Laennec's original notion that organic obstruction of the small airways by mucous plugging and inflammatory narrowing and obliteration was important. Liebow[71] has been attracted by Dayman's hypothesis[21] that emphysema destroys peribronchial support, leading to a check-valve obstruction in the small airways. Butler and colleagues[66] postulated that diminished elastic recoil caused the peripheral airways to be narrower at a given lung volume than they would be in a normal lung at the same volume.

In our studies of postmortem lungs, the peripheral airways constituted the major site of airways resistance in both centrilobular and panacinar emphysema (Fig. 3-12, 3-13). These studies also showed that there was significant organic disease in the small airways and this has been borne out in our more recent studies of surgical specimens[60] where inflammation of the small airways correlated best with deteriorating airways function. The measurements of the peripheral airways obstruction in COPD also showed that the increased peripheral resistance was the same on both inspiration and expiration,[17] suggesting that the marked increase in airways resistance seen on forced expiration during life is due to dynamic compression of the large airways rather than a check-valve mechanism in the small airways.

Cystic Fibrosis

Cystic fibrosis is a disease of infancy and childhood, originally described by Andersen[72] in 1938 as being a rare, uniformly fatal, pancreatic disorder. The generalized nature of the disease was pointed out by Farber[73] in 1944, and he suggested the name *mucoviscidosis* because there seemed to be widespread involvement of the mucus-secreting glands. A recent review[74] of the advances in the understanding of the condition has shown that it is not rare; that survival into adulthood can be achieved; that it is transmitted as a Mendelian recessive; that it affects the respiratory system in all cases; and that the cause of death is most often related to pulmonary involvement. The term *mucoviscidosis* has now lost favor because abnormalities of the sweat glands have been demonstrated.

Pathological Anatomy of the Lung in Cystic Fibrosis. At autopsy the trachea and bronchi are generally filled with muco-purulent material. The lungs are large and do not completely deflate, and bullae are sometimes seen on the lung surface. The cut surface of the lung shows widespread plugging of large and small airways with purulent mucus.[75] In a study of eighty-four autopsies on infants and children with fibrocystic disease, Esterly and Oppenheimer[76] reported that bronchiectasis was present in fifty-three cases and that hypertrophy and hyperplasia of the bronchial mucous gland layer, with evidence of chronic inflammation of bronchial walls with follicle formation, were common features in nearly all cases. They also found evidence of chronic inflammation of the bronchioles, which was severe and often obliterative in character. Evidence of emphysema in the children that Esterly and Oppenheimer studied, however, was sparse, and diffuse interstitial fibrosis was not an important feature.

The primary features of the pathology of the lung in fibrocystic disease of the pancreas are, therefore, bronchitis, obliterative bronchiolitis, and bronchiectasis, which is chronic and progressive in nature (Fig. 3-14). Atelectasis, pneumonia, and abscess formation, when present, are probably secondary to airway obstruction; whereas emphysema and diffuse pulmonary interstitial disease do not appear to be important features of the disease.

Mechanical Properties of the Lung in Cystic Fibrosis. The abnormalities in lung mechanics in fibrocystic disease have been studied by Mellins and co-workers.[77,78] Routine pulmonary function tests on patients with cystic fibrosis showed a reduction in vital capacity; a less reduced peak flow rate; increased air flow resistance, on both inspiration and expiration, which is reflected in a reduced maximum breathing capacity; and a reduced dynamic compliance. They also presented cineradiographic evidence of dynamic collapse of the proximal portion of bronchiectatic airways and single-breath nitrogen washout curves, which would fit well with collapse of lower lobe airways because they have a markedly increased Phase IV. This is, however, not clearly interpretable in view of other evidence of airway disease.

Mellins and associates stressed the fact that patients with the abnormalities they have demonstrated have an ineffective cough, because the large airways collapse during cough, so that bronchial secretions are retained. They then interpreted their data to mean that cystic fibrosis is a patchy disease of large airways, but in a later study[78] they suggested that the small airways were probably the major site of obstruction. This is much more consistent with the pathological evidence,[75,76] which shows that the most severe disease is in the small airways. Indeed, studies of the distribution of airways resistance carried out in our laboratories[18] on postmortem in lungs from patients dying with cystic fibrosis (Fig. 3-15) showed that the major site of airway obstruction in these lungs was in the small airways. It therefore seems likely that the airway obstruction is primarily due to fixed organic disease in peripheral airways and that the increased resistance seen on forced expiration is due to dynamic compression of the central airways.

Bronchiectasis

Anatomical Types of Bronchiectasis. As the name implies, bronchiectasis occurs when there is a permanent dilation of one or more bronchi. The word *permanent* is important, because it excludes the acute reversible dilation of bronchi that often accompanies pneumonia.[79] Because an increase in the diameter of a bronchus can result from a variety of conditions, the term describes a disorder of anatomy rather than a single disease.

There have been many attempts to classify this condition, but none of these has been completely satisfactory. Lynne Reid[80] attempted to classify bronchiectasis on the basis of the appearance of the bronchi and on the number of branches of airways in the lung segment containing the bronchiectatic lesions. In the *cylindrical* form she found that the number of branches identified in the specimen by dissection was within normal limits, although plugging of the airways by secretions often prevented the filling of the small airways on the bronchogram. In the *varicose* type of bronchiectasis she found that the number of bronchi in the segment was reduced, both on the bronchogram and when the lung was dissected and the bronchi counted. She also found that discrete cords could be seen beyond the point at which the bronchial lumen was obliterated by fibrous tissue. In the *saccular* type she found the least number of bronchial branches, with only a few generations of airway being demonstrable by careful dissection of the specimen.

Whitewell[81] classified bronchiectasis into follicular, saccular, and atelectatic forms on the basis of the pathology and clinical features of 200 surgically resected specimens. In follicular bronchiectasis (14% of his cases), the main lesion occurred in the smaller bronchi and bronchioles

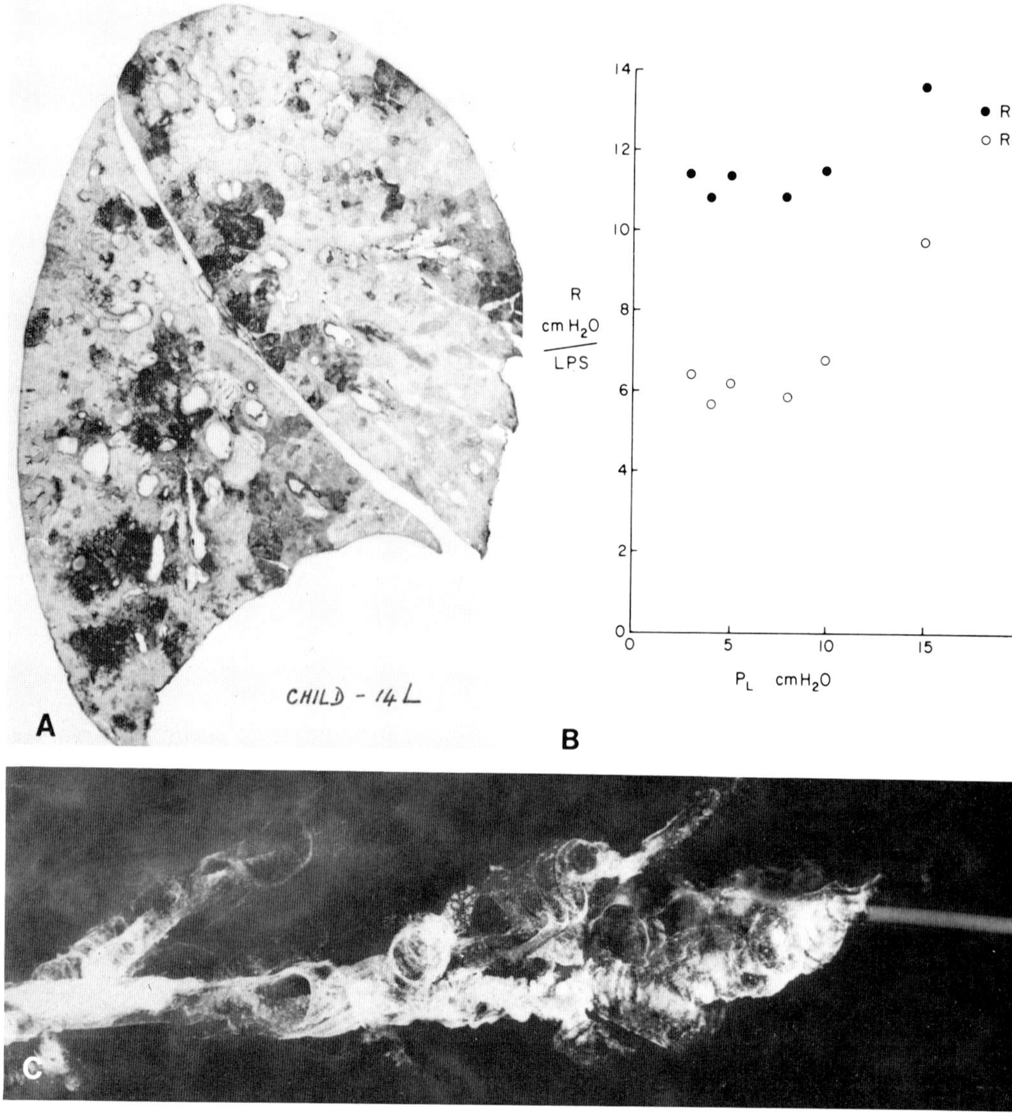

FIG. 3-15. From a case of fibrocystic disease of the pancreas. **A.** Paper-mounted, whole lung section with marked bronchiectasis. **B.** The marked increase in total airways resistance (R_L) is due to disease in the peripheral airways (R_P). **C.** Bronchogram demonstrating marked bronchiectasis. (*B* modified from Hogg J et al: Age as a factor in the distribution of lower airways conductance and in the pathologic anatomy of obstructive lung disease. N Engl J Med 282:1283, 1970)

in the early stages, but as the condition became more severe it extended towards the trachea, with gradual obliteration of the distal bronchial tree. The lesion initially consisted of thickening of the bronchiolar walls due to edema and lymph-follicle formation, with destruction of the elastic tissue near the follicles. More advanced lesions showed a diffuse mural bronchiolitis, with destruction of the elastic tissue. The clinical fact that this form of bronchiectasis usually begins in early childhood and either starts insidiously or follows illnesses thought to

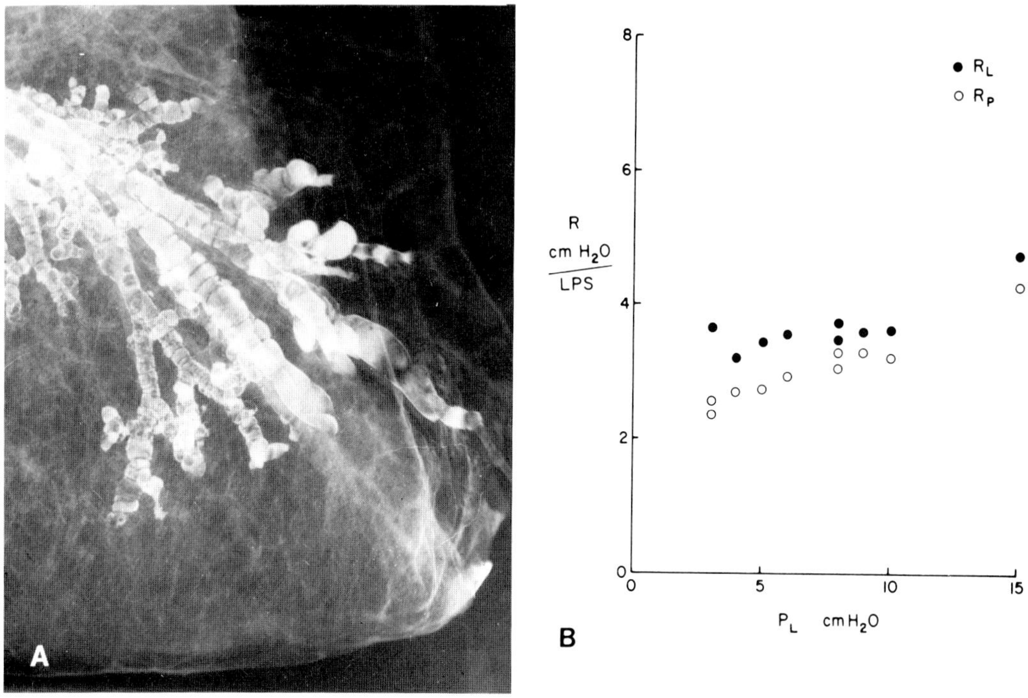

FIG. 3-16. **A.** Bronchogram demonstrating severe varicose bronchiectasis. **B.** The physiological data demonstrate a marked increase in peripheral airways resistance (R_P), causing a high total airway resistance (R_L).

be associated with viral disease led Whitewell to speculate that this form of bronchiectasis was a sequel to acute viral infections.

Seventeen percent of his 200 cases were classified as saccular bronchiectasis, and he showed that the bronchial sacs were fibrous structures lined by cuboidal epithelium, without elastic tissue muscle or cartilage in their walls. No dilation occurred in the presaccular bronchi, but there was an inflammatory reaction in their walls, with polyposis of the bronchiolar epithelium. Although the dilations often ended blindly, atelectasis was not a feature of either follicular or saccular bronchiectasis; collateral ventilation apparently kept the parenchyma inflated. Ten percent of Whitewell's cases were classified as atelectatic bronchiectasis, because the lung around the bronchiectatic sac was not well aerated. In these cases, there was a generalized distribution of collapse and bronchiectasis in the lobes, and no obstruction in the airways, but enlarged hilar nodes were always found around the lobar bronchus. Whitewell suggested that this condition was due to obstruction of the lobar bronchus, caused by external compression by the surrounding lymph glands, and that atelectasis occurred because collateral ventilation could not take place between lobes.

It is important to note that the majority of the cases that Whitewell described could not be classified under the headings that he chose. In fact, it seems that the capability to defy a particular classification is one of the most common features of any study of bronchiectasis. The disorder, however, seems to have many features that are common in a majority of individual cases. These include evidence of onset in early childhood, previous lower respiratory tract infections that are often recurrent, chronic productive cough, and poor general health that extends over many years. The bronchial dilatations tend to involve the lung segmentally, with the segments of the

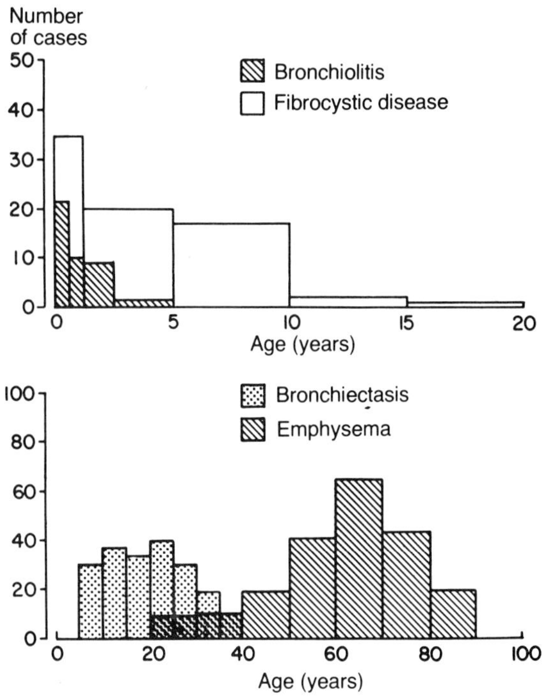

FIG. 3-17. Age distribution of obstructive lung diseases. Note that bronchiectasis (*bottom*) occurs primarily in the younger age period, whereas bronchitis and emphysema (*bottom*) occur primarily during the last third of life. Bronchiolitis (*top*) occurs primarily in the first few years of life, and fibrocystic disease (*top*) has a high mortality in the first 20 years.

left lower lobe being the most commonly affected. The lingula of the left upper lobe is involved more often than the right middle lobe. The reason for the tendency for involvement of the left side is presumably less adequate drainage, caused by the angle at which the left main bronchus branches off the trachea, but this has not been proven.

Mechanical Properties of the Lung in Bronchiectasis. In 1971, Bates and Christie[82] reviewed the available information on pulmonary function in bronchiectasis. They found that the total lung capacity was close to the predicted value, but that there was a marked reduction in vital capacity, with increases in the residual volume and the functional residual capacity. Maximum expiratory flow rates were markedly reduced, and there was evidence of hypoxia, and a reduced diffusing capacity in most cases. Cherniack and Carton[83] demonstrated a reduced vital capacity, increased residual volume, and evidence of airway obstruction in more than half of their cases. This was directly proportional to the number of lobes involved.

Fraser and associates[84] studied twenty cases of bronchiectasis by combining bronchial pressure measurements with cinebrochography. They clearly demonstrated that the marked reduction of flow seen on forced expiration in the varicose and cystic forms of the disease was associated with dynamic collapse of segmental airways. They also showed that the bronchial dilatations change little in size during forced expiration and cough, and they pointed out the deficiency in bronchial clearance that results because the dilated airways fail to narrow during cough. Figure 3-16 shows postmortem data from a case of varicose bronchiectasis seen in a 39-year-old female. The bronchogram demonstrates the severity of the bronchiectasis, whereas the physiological data show that the severity of the peripheral airways disease resulted in a marked increase in peripheral resistance. These data also showed that the obstruction in the peripheral airways was unchanged on inspiration and expiration, which again suggests that the marked increase in resistance seen in living persons during forced expiration is due to dynamic collapse of the central airways.

AN INTEGRATED VIEW OF AIRWAYS DISEASE

Among the variety of obstructive lung diseases, there are many common features. For example, bronchiolitis in children and acute bronchitis in adults are quite similar morphologically, although their outcomes may be very different. The fact that acute airways disease causes a life-threatening illness in the young child is probably related to the child's peripheral airways being more vulnerable during the development of the conducting airways, which lags behind the development of the gas-exchanging portion of the lung in the first few years of life. It also seems clear that the major site of airways obstruction is in the small airways in cystic fibrosis, bronchiectasis, bronchitis, and emphysema, and that the peripheral airways obstruction is the same on both inspiration and expiration in these conditions. This means that the markedly increased resistance seen on forced expiration is best attributed to dynamic compression of the central airways. This abnormal compression of the central airways can also interfere with the cough mechanism because segments of the airways will collapse.

The separation of bronchiectasis, bronchitis, and emphysema by age (Fig. 3-17) is of interest because it suggests that the age of the patient may have something to do with the anatomical disorder. For example, when chronic airways disease begins early, as with fibrocystic disease and bronchiectasis, the mature lung growth may explain why the anatomic disorders are similar. The disproportion between conducting airways and parenchyma and the decreased collateral ventilation in children's lungs would cause disease in small airways to lead to alveolar collapse and infection, so that the central airways dilate and fill with secretions to produce the anatomic disorder we call bronchiectasis. Similarly, if the chronic peripheral airways inflammatory disease begins because of excessive smoking after the lung is fully developed, collateral ventilation of the obstructed units may play a role in the fenestration of the pores of Kohn, so that emphysema develops. If this were so, one could think of the insult of airways inflammatory disease in the same way that the orthopedic surgeon thinks of the result of a fall on an outstretched hand, wherein the site of the lesion is determined largely by the age of the patient. Recent epidemiological evidence suggests that children with recurrent bronchiolitis may be predisposed to chronic bronchitis and emphysema as adults. This may be interpreted as bronchiolitis having an etiologic role, or the childhood and adult conditions demonstrating continuing susceptibility to disease in that patient.

REFERENCES

1. DESPAS PJM, LEROUS M, MACKLEM PT: Site of airway obstruction in asthma as determined by the maximal expiratory flow breathing air and a helium–oxygen mixture. J Clin Invest 51:3235, 1972
2. DOSMAN J et al: The use of a helium–oxygen mixture during maximum expiratory flow to demonstrate obstruction in small airways of smokers. J Clin Invest 55:1090, 1975
3. MEAD J: Lung—mechanical properties of the lungs. Physiol Rev 41:281, 1961
4. OTIS AB et al: Mechanical factors in distribution of pulmonary ventilation. J Appl Physiol 8:427, 1956
5. CLEMENTS J et al: Estimation of pulmonary resistance by repetitive interruption of outflow. J Clin Invest 38:1262, 1959
6. MEAD J, WHITTENBERGER J: Physical properties of human lungs measured during spontaneous respiration. J Appl Physiol 5:779, 1953
7. DUBOIS A et al: Oscillation mechanics of the lungs and chest in man. J Appl Physiol 8:587, 1956
8. DUBOIS A, BOTELHO S, COMROE J JR: A new method of measuring airway resistance in man using a body plethysmograph. J Clin Invest 35:327, 1956
9. DUBOIS A et al: A rapid plethysmographic method for measuring thoracic gas volume. J Clin Invest 35:322, 1956
10. FRY D: Theoretical considerations of the bronchial pressure-flow-volume relationship with particular reference to the maximum expiratory flow volume curves. Phys Med Biol 3:174, 1958
11. FRY D, HYATT R: Mechanics—a unified analysis of the relationship between pressure–volume and gas flow in the lungs of normal and diseased human subjects. Am J Med 29:672, 1960
12. DUBOIS A: The resistance of breathing. In Fenn WO, Rahn H (eds): American Physiological Society. Handbook of Physiology. section 3, Vol 1, Baltimore, Williams & Wilkins, 1964–1965
13. MACKLEM P, MEAD J: The resistance of central and peripheral airways measured by a retrograde catheter. J Appl Physiol 22:395, 1967
14. BRISCOE W, DUBOIS A: Relationship between airways resistance, airway conductance and lung volume in subjects of different age and body size. J Clin Invest 37:1279, 1958
15. COOK C, HELLIESEN P, AGATHEN S: Relation between mechanics of respiration, lung size and body size from birth to young adulthood. J Appl Physiol 13:349, 1958
16. REID L: The embryology of the lung. In A CIBA Foundation Symposium: Development of the Lung. London, J & A Churchill, 1967
17. HOGG J, MACKLEM P, THURLBECK W: Site and nature

of airways obstruction in chronic obstructive lung disease. N Engl J Med 278:1355, 1968

18. HOGG J et al: Age as a factor in the distribution of lower airways conductance and in the pathologic anatomy of obstructive lung disease. N Engl J Med 282:1283, 1970
19. WEIBEL E: Morphometry of the Human Lung. New York, Academic Press, 1963
20. EINTHOVEN U: Ueber die Wirkung der Bronchialmuskeln nach einer neuen Methode untersucht und uber Asthma Nervosu. Arch Ges Physiol 5:367, 1892
21. DAYMAN H: Mechanics of airflow in health and in emphysema. J Clin Invest 30:1175, 1951
22. DEKKER E. DEFARES J, HIEMSTRA H: Direct measurements of intrabronchial pressure. Its application to the localization of the check valve mechanism. J Appl Physiol 13:35, 1958
23. MEAD J et al: The significance of the relationship between lung recoil and maximum expiratory flow. J Appl Physiol 22:95, 1967
24. PRIDE W et al: Determinants of maximal expiratory flow from the lungs. J Appl Physiol 23:646, 1967
25. KROGH A, LINDHARD J: The volume of the dead space in breathing and the mixing of gases in the lungs of man. J Physiol 51:59, 1917
26. RAUWERDA P: Unequal Ventilation of Different Parts of the Lung and the Determination of Cardiac Output. The Netherlands, University of Groningen, 1946
27. FOWLER K: Relative compliances of the well and poorly ventilated spaces in the normal human lung. J Appl Physiol 19:937, 1964
28. MILIC-EMILI J et al: Regional distribution of inspired gas in the lung. J Appl Physiol 21:749, 1966
29. DOLFUSS R, MILIC-EMILI J, BATES D: Regional ventilation of the lung studied with boluses of xenon. Respir Physiol 22:760, 1967
30. HORSFIELD K, CUMMING G: The morphology of the bronchial tree in man. J Appl Physiol 24:373, 1968
31. SAID S: Metabolic events in the lung. In Frohlich ED (ed): Pathophysiology: Altered Regulatory Mechanisms in Disease, 2nd ed Philadelphia, JB Lippincott, 1976
32. COHEN A, GOLD W: Defense mechanisms of the lungs. Annu Rev Physiol 37:325, 1975
33. SATIR P: How cilia move. Sci Am 231:44, 1974
34. STURGESS JM et al: Cilia with defective radial spokes. N Engl J Med 300:53, 1979
35. WOHL MEB, CHERNICK V: Bronchiolitis: State of the art. Am Rev Respir Dis 118:759, 1978
36. HIGH R: Bronchiolitis. Pediatr Clin North Am 4:183, 1957
37. COATES H, CHANOCK R: The clinical significance of respiratory syncytial virus. Postgrad Med 35:460, 1964
38. CIBA Guest Symposium. Thorax 14:286, 1959
39. THURLBECK W, ANGUS G: A distribution curve for chronic bronchitis. Thorax 19:436, 1964
40. SIMONSSON B, TELA E: Experimental studies on bronchial secretions [Int Symposium]. Scand J Respir Dis [Suppl] 90, 1974
41. LAENNEC R: A Treatise on the Diseases of the Chest and on Mediate Auscultation, 3rd ed, pp 167–168. New York, SS & W Wood, 1838
42. STRAWBRIDGE H: Chronic pulmonary emphysema (an experimental study). I. Historical review. Am J Pathol 37:161, 1960
43. OPIE EL: Enzymes and anti-enzymes of inflammatory exudates. J Exp Med 7:316, 1905
44. LAURELL CB, ERIKSSON S: The electrophoretic $alpha_1$ globulin pattern of serum in $alpha_1$ antitrypsin deficiency. Scand J Clin Lab Invest 15:132, 1963
45. ERIKSSON S: Pulmonary emphysema and $alpha_1$ antitrypsin deficiency. Acta Med Scand 175:197, 1964
46. GROSS P¿ et al: Enzymatically produced pulmonary emphysema: A Preliminary Report. J Occup Med 6:481, 1964
47. KARLINSKY JB, SNIDER GL: Animal models of emphysema: State of the art. Am Rev Respir Dis 117:1109, 1978
48. KAZMIEROUSKI JA, GALLIN JI, REYNOLDS HY: Demonstration and partial characterization of alveolar macrophage chemotactic factor with preferential activity for polymorphonuclear leukocytes. J Clin Invest 59:273, 1977
49. JANOFF A, et al: Cigarette smoking decreases $alpha_1$ antitrypsin activity in rat lung. Science 206:1313, 1979
50. GODEK JE, FELLS GA, CRYSTALL RG: Cigarette smoke induces functional antiprotease deficiency in the lower respiratory tract. Science 206:1315, 1979
51. GOUGH J: Discussion in the diagnosis of pulmonary emphysema. Proc R Soc Med 45:576, 1952
52. LEOPOLD J, GOUGH J: The centrilobular form of hypertrophic emphysema and its relation to chronic bronchitis. Thorax 12:219, 1957
53. HEARD B, IZUKAWA T: Pulmonary emphysema in fifty consecutive male necropsies in London. J Pathol Bacteriol 88:423, 1964
54. THURLBECK W: Chronic Obstructive Lung Disease. Pathology Annual, pp 367–368. New York, Appleton-Century-Crofts, 1968
55. THURLBECK W: Measurement of pulmonary emphysema. Am Rev Respir Dis 95:752, 1967
56. SWEET J, WYATT J, KINSELLA P: Correlation of lung macrosections with pulmonary function in emphysema. Am J Med 29:277, 1960
57. DUNNILL M: Quantitative methods in the study of pulmonary pathology. Thorax 17:320, 1962
58. PRATT P, JTABHA O, KLUGH G: Quantitative relationship between structural extent of centrilobular emphysema and post mortem volume and flow

characteristics of lungs. Med Thorac 22:197, 1965

59. THURLBECK W et al: A comparison of three methods of measuring emphysema. Hum Pathol 1:215, 1970
60. COSIO M et al: The relationship between structural changes in small airways and pulmonary function tests. N Engl J Med 298:1277, 1978
61. PETTY TL et al: Small airways pathology is related to increased closing capacity and abnormal slope of Phase III in excised human lungs. Am Rev Respir Dis 121:449, 1980
62. RESTRIPO G, HEARD B: The size of the bronchial glands in chronic bronchitis. J Pathol Bacteriol 85:305, 1963
63. CHRISTIE R: The elastic properties of the emphysematous lung and their clinical significance. J Clin Invest 13:295, 1934
64. MEAD J, LINDGREN I, GAENSLER E: The mechanical properties of the lungs in emphysema. J Clin Invest 34:1005, 1955
65. WOOLCOCK A, VINCENT N, MACKLEM P: Frequency dependence of compliance as a test for obstruction in small airways. J Clin Invest 48:1097, 1969
66. BUTLER J et al: Physiological factors affecting airway resistance in normal subjects and in patients with obstructive airway disease. J Clin Invest 39:584, 1960
67. KOBLET H, WYSS F: Das klinische und functionelle Bild des genuinem bronchial Kollapses mid lung Emphysem. Helv Med Acta 23:553, 1956
68. MACKLEM P, FRASER R, BROWN W: Bronchial pressure measurements in emphysema and bronchitis. J Clin Invest 44:897, 1965
69. MCLEAN K: The pathogenesis of pulmonary emphysema. Am J Med 25:62, 1958
70. ANDERSON A, FORAKER A: Population of non-respiratory bronchioles in pulmonary emphysema. Arch Pathol 83:286, 1967
71. LIEBOW A. Pulmonary emphysema with special reference to vascular changes. Am Rev Respir Dis 80:67, 1959
72. ANDERSEN D: Cystic Fibrosis of the pancreas and its relation to celiac disease. Am J Dis Child 56:344, 1938
73. FARBER S: Pancreatic function and disease in early life, pancreatic changes associated with pancreatic insufficiency in early life. Arch Pathol 37:238, 1944
74. SHWACHMAN H: Cystic fibrosis. In Kendig EL Jr (ed): Disorders of the Respiratory Tract in Children. Philadelphia, WB Saunders, 1967
75. ESTERLY J, OPPENHEIMER E: Cystic fibrosis of the pancreas: Structural changes in peripheral airways. Thorax 23:670, 1968
76. ESTERLY J: Observations in cystic fibrosis of the pancreas. III. Pulmonary lesions. Johns Hopkins Med J 122:94, 1968
77. MELLINS R et al: Obstructive disease of the airways in cystic fibrosis. Pediatrics, 41:560, 1968
78. MELLINS R: The site of airways obstruction in cystic fibrosis. Pediatrics 44:315, 1969
79. BACHMAN A, HEWITT W, BEEKLEY H: Bronchiectasis, a bronchographic study of sixty cases of pneumonia. Arch Intern Med 91:78, 1953
80. REID L: Reduction in the bronchial subdivisions in bronchiectasis. Thorax 5:233, 1950
81. WHITEWELL F: A study of the pathology and pathogenesis of bronchiectasis. Thorax 7:213, 1952
82. BATES D, CHRISTIE R: Respiratory Function in Disease. Philadelphia, WB Saunders, 1971
83. CHERNIACK N, CARTON R: Factors associated with respiratory insufficiency in bronchiectasis. Am J Med 41:562, 1966
84. FRASER R, MACKLEM P, BROWN W: Airway dynamics in bronchiectasis, a combined cinefluorographic–manometric study. Am J Roentgenol Radium Ther Nucl Med 93:821, 1965

Chapter 4

Ventilatory Function of the Lungs

MARTIN H. WELCH

EVALUATION OF THE PATIENT WITH VENTILATORY DYSFUNCTION

The clinical pulmonary-function laboratory offers help to the physician with patients in five basic categories (see list below). Tests of both ventilation and respiratory gas exchange are of importance in each of these circumstances. This section deals with the role of ventilatory tests in the evaluation of respiratory function.

Uses of the Clinical Pulmonary-Function Laboratory

- Initial evaluation of the patient presenting with the complaint of breathlessness
- Initial evaluation of the patient with known respiratory disease
- Following the course of disease in a patient with an established diagnosis of respiratory disease
- Preoperative evaluation of the patient with a high risk of respiratory complications
- Screening for subclinical disease

Evaluation of Breathlessness. Ventilatory tests play an especially important role in the evaluation of the patient undergoing investigation of the complaint of shortness of breath, or dyspnea. This common symptom occurs in association with a wide range of conditions and defies a unifying concept of its pathogenesis.[1–5] It is a reasonable generalization to state that dyspnea, when it occurs as a manifestation of organic disease, correlates better with abnormal results of tests of ventilatory function than with respiratory gas exchange.

Factors Affecting Dyspnea. Dyspnea is a subjective sensation, by definition, and cannot be equated with any objective sign. It may be absent in the face of apparently labored, abnormally rapid, or deep breathing; and it may be present in a subject who appears normal. Breathlessness occurs as a normal phenomenon in exercise; and it is a common, benign manifestation of anxiety and excitement. To be considered a symptom worthy of investigation, it must occur with less exertion than is normally required to produce it. Some investigators require that a sensation of breathlessness be experienced as unpleasant to warrant application of the term *dyspnea*.

Dyspnea is best understood in terms of the relationship between the factors that stimulate tidal breathing and the resistances that must be overcome in the act of breathing. Some knowledge of the control of ventilation is therefore essential to a discussion of dyspnea. The reader is referred to Chapter 2 for details of neural and chemical control of ventilation.

Conditions that produce breathlessness as a symptom include those resulting primarily in an abnormally increased stimulus to breathe; a greater-than-normal effort required to breathe; and most mysteriously, an inability to respond to a ventilatory stimulus because of respiratory muscle weakness (see list below). Conditions in which dyspnea is primarily related to an increased effort required for ventilation are clinically the most frequent. These include a wide range of pulmonary diseases in which ventilatory abnormalities can be readily characterized by the pulmonary laboratory. The correlation between dyspnea and abnormal results of tests of ventilation is generally good in this category. Complex and poorly understood combinations of these three categories are probably common in clinical practice; but a simplified consideration of relatively pure examples is informative.

Factors Associated With Dyspnea

Increased stimulus to breathe
- Exercise
- Anxiety
- Excitement
- Hypoxemia
- Acidosis
- CNS disease

Increased effort required to breathe
- Obstruction to air flow
- Decreased lung or chest-wall compliance

Decreased ability to exert effort required to breathe
- Disease of neural supply to muscles of respiration
- Primary muscle disease
- Asynchronous breathing

Increased Ventilatory Stimulus. Increase respiratory drive in the presence of normal lungs and chest wall results in increased respiratory rate and depth; with a widely variable threshold, individual persons may become aware of this change in ventilatory pattern and interpret this awareness as shortness of breath. Most surprising, perhaps, is the relative mildness of dyspnea of this sort in most circumstances. Indeed, some investigators would not apply the term *dyspnea* to this sensation, but would refer to it only as breathlessness, because it generally is not experienced as unpleasant. The hypoxemia incurred at high altitudes causes an increased drive to ventilation through stimulation of carotid and perhaps aortic body chemoreceptors; but if increased ventilation proceeds without mechanical hindrance, the subject breathes more rapidly and deeply with little awareness that he is doing so. Inadequate oxygenation of the brain causes confusion and euphoria, often before the drive to ventilate becomes intense enough to cause disproportion between sensed ventilatory need and ventilatory ability. Unconsciousness and death may therefore occur without apparent warning. This poor correlation between hypoxemia and dyspnea can result in death in aviators, underwater swimmers, and divers. Similarly, ignorance on the part of physicians and nurses can lead to the death of patients with hypoxemia, if lack of dyspnea is interpreted as proof of adequate oxygenation.

The hyperpnea of metabolic acidosis is another commonly encountered circumstance in which an increased ventilatory stimulus may occur in a subject with normal ventilatory reserve. In such a patient, increased hydrogen ion concentration produces increased ventilation. Objectively dramatic hyperpnea in a patient with metabolic acidosis often occurs with minimal or no awareness on the patient's part. When metabolic acidosis supervenes in a patient with impaired ventilatory reserve, it appears more likely to produced the subjective complaint of dyspnea.

One of the most fascinating of respiratory aberrations associated with dyspnea is the "hyperventilation syndrome." This functional disturbance seems to be an exaggeration of the normal ventilatory response to anxiety and occurs acutely and sometimes chronically in susceptible subjects. The alkalosis of hyperventilation, which occurs so commonly in acute anxiety, may be accompanied by marked dyspnea and may produce dizziness, perioral and peripheral paresthesias, and sometimes bronchospasm and spasms of voluntary muscles, as discussed in Chapter 6.

Increased Effort Required to Breathe. The dyspnea of most patients with organic respiratory disease has a mixed pathogenesis but is probably chiefly related to this mechanism. The effort required to breathe is known to be increased in these patients because of mechanical abnormalities of the lungs and chest wall. In diseases associated with obstruction to air flow through central or peripheral airways, the resistive work required to breathe is increased. In a wide range of disorders of the lung interstitium, pleura, and chest wall, stiffness (decreased compliance) of the diseased structures causes an increase in elastic resistance during breathing and, therefore, an increase in elastic work.

Dyspnea may not correlate so perfectly with the volume of air moved by the chest bellows or even with effort exerted in an attempt to accomplish ventilation, but it may correlate better with the relationship between the volume of air moved and effort exerted. This relationship could well be expressed in terms of volume and pressure changes measured during ventilation. Because the relationship might most logically be expected to be sensed by intercostal muscle spindles, Campbell expressed it in terms of length and tension.[1,2] Because his experiments demonstrated a remarkable ability of normal persons to detect changes from normal in the effort required to move a given volume of air, he formulated the theory that dyspnea is most closely related to changes from normal (inappropriateness) in the ratio of length to tension. His concept of length-to-tension inappropriateness has become the theory under consideration by many investigators at present.[4]

The clinical pulmonary laboratory offers no direct measurement of length-to-tension inappropriateness, and work of breathing is difficult to measure. The importance of this discussion to the clinician is to emphasize the relative importance of measurement of mechanical abnormalities, as opposed to arterial blood gases, in the assessment of patients with dyspnea. As a final example emphasizing this point, the patient with severe dyspnea due to respiratory insufficieny should be considered. In many such cases, arterial P_{CO_2} is normal or even decreased, and hypoxemia is easily corrected or overcorrected by oxygen administration alone. In such cases, persistence of dyspnea is common and certainly is best explained in terms of mechanical abnormalities.

What measurements of abnormal ventilatory mechanics are readily available, and how well do they correlate with dyspnea?

Measurements of total or effective ventilation actually achieved during rest or exercise are rather easily accomplished but are of limited application. Normal values vary considerably, obscuring the slight changes that may occur because of inefficient ventilation in early lung disease. A significant, measurable decrease in total ventilation occurs chiefly in advanced disease, and serial measurements may be helpful in assessing the patient with severe respiratory failure, prior to the institution or discontinuance of mechanical ventilation.

A widely available, simple measure of ventilatory reserve, known as *maximum voluntary ventilation*, has broad application in the assessment of exertional dyspnea. This "sprint test" quantitates the amount of air that can be moved by the chest bellows during a brief (12 to 15 sec) maximum effort. It normally exceeds the ventilation required under resting conditions by a factor of about twenty—a functional reserve so great that ventilation itself is not normally a limiting factor in exercise. Breathlessness is generally experienced by normal and abnormal subjects during exercise that requires a minute ventilation in excess of 50% of the subject's maximum voluntary ventilation. This rule of thumb is useful in estimating the limitation of exercise tolerance due to decreased ventilatory reserve, if allowances are made for considerable normal variation and for the increased ventilation required in disease because of decreased efficiency of ventilation. Twenty to 30 liters of ventilation are generally needed each minute in normal subjects to provide 1 liter of oxygen for metabolic needs; the ratio may be as high as 40:1 in diseased subjects.[87]

Vital capacity is a limited measurement of ventilatory reserve that has a somewhat narrower application, because it correlates quite differently with maximum voluntary ventilation in restrictive, as opposed to obstructive, diseases. It is a simple measurement to perform and is of great value in following individual patients on successsive occasions. In patients with neuromuscular disease, as well as other restrictive diseases of the lung and chest wall, it often correlates very well with dyspnea, and marked decreases may occur before blood gas abnormalities become evident.

The mechancial abnormalities that presumably are most directly responsible for dyspnea are increased airways resistance and decreased lung and chest-wall compliance. As pointed out in subsequent pages, these measurements can be carried out, but with some technical difficulty. Normal values for various populations are not well established. Consequently, measurements of airways resistance and compliance are not readily available or useful to clinicians in most communities.

Abnormalities in more readily available tests of lung mechanics generally accompany changes in airways resistance and compliance. Flow-rate measurements during the maximum-effort expiratory maneuver have a close enough relation to airways resistance to be of great use. Most commonly available measurements of flow rates include the forced expiratory volumes, at 0.5 and 1.0 sec, and the forced expiratory flow rate, from 25 to 75% of the forced vital capacity. As described in more detail elsewhere, these measurements are theoretically imperfect reflectors of airways resistance, because the pressure differential generated to produce flow is not taken into account but is simply defined as *maximum* during the maximum-effort expiratory maneuver. This does not detract substantially from their practical usefulness.

Compliance changes in disease are rather well reflected by changes in the various compartments of lung volume. Reduction in vital capacity, particularly, is an easily measured change that usually accompanies reduced compliance. The lung diseases characterized by stiffness (decreased compliance) of lung parenchyma are characterized by a rather symmetrical decrease in lung volumes (restriction), except for residual volume and functional residual capacity, which may be normal or even increased. Likewise, the restrictive chest-wall diseases cause decreased lung volumes, except perhaps for residual volume and functional residual capacity. The obstructive diseases also show decreased vital capacity and increased RV and FRC but show normal total lung capacity, except for emphysema, in which TLC is increased, presumably owing to increased lung compliance.

It should be apparent, then, that measurement of lung volumes may serve as a helpful reflector of changes in lung or chest-wall compliance, but that interpretation must be made cautiously and with knowledge of the patient's clinical, radiological, and physiological profile. There can be no simple, quantitative relationship expressed between dyspnea and lung volumes, except perhaps for vital capacity in carefully defined circumstances.

Decreased Ability to Exert Effort to Breathe. Shortness of breath due to neuromuscular disease is intriguing in that it represents a third category of dyspnea that is not readily explained by an abnormal stimulus to breathe or by an increase in effort required to breathe. Campbell has questioned whether the type or degree of distress in this setting is the same as that experienced by patients with mechanical hindrance to ventilation.[1,2] He has carried his curiosity to the point of inducing the two forms of distress in himself by curarization and by mechanical loading and found the former less unpleasant.

The problem of dyscoordination of respiratory muscle function has recently attracted increasing interest for its apparent contribution to ventilatory insufficiency in various settings. A case has been reported in which asynchronous breathing was the only mechanical disturbance observed in a patient with dyspnea.[5]

Whatever may be the nature or degree of distress in neuromuscular respiratory paralysis, it is clear that in patients with progressive disease such as Guillain-Barré syndrome, measurement of vital capacity is an excellent way to document deterioration or improvement. This measurement often correlates well with the patient's subjective complaints. Dyspnea and a decrease in vital capacity ordinarily occur before blood gas deterioration. (See Chap. 6).

Evaluation of Patients With Respiratory Disease. A second important role of the pulmonary-function laboratory is the initial evaluation of patients with respiratory disease, regardless of the presence or absence of dyspnea. In such patients quantitation of simple parameters of lung function is a desirable routine. Such an evaluation may be of some help in diagnosis, because most diseases produce characteristic, though not specific, physiological profiles of abnormalities. In addition, quantitation of the amount of dysfunction produced by a disease is often helpful in planning therapy, especially in providing a baseline for following the results of therapy.

Following the Course of Disease. Serial testing to follow progression of disease or results of therapy is a third valuable function of the pulmonary laboratory. Demonstration of stability or progression of physiological abnormality may be essential in such decisions as whether or not to treat pulmonary sarcoidosis with corticosteroids. Improvement in function may provide support for a decision to continue or discontinue such therapy. Similarly, the degree of success achieved with bronchodilators and other forms of therapy can be assessed with some objectivity by pulmonary-function testing. A change of 20% from baseline spirometric values is often suggested as a minimum acute change in response to bronchodilator administration to be considered significant; but in an excellent laboratory, testing a cooperative and well-informed patient, reproducibility may be possible within 5% for simple spirometric tests. Therefore, measurement of vital capacity and expiratory flow rates alone may be adequately discriminating to follow the course of diseases that affect them and the response to therapy in such diseases.

Preoperative Evaluation. Preoperative testing of patients at high risk of respiratory complications in association with the operative procedure is a fourth role of the pulmonary-function laboratory.[6–10] Ventilatory failure may occur in patients with decreased ventilatory reserve following preoperative sedation or during recovery from anesthesia. Increased risk of this complication can be predicted by simple spirometry. Of course, patients with chronic carbon dioxide retention are at great risk of acute decompensation in this setting, so arterial blood gases should be measured in patients with decreased ventilatory reserve. Postoperative atelectasis with infection occurs with increased frequency in patients with obstructive lung disease, and its identification can enable the physician to provide appropriate measures to prevent it. Hypoxemia when identified preoperatively, is in itself easily dealt with by oxygen administration. A history and physical examination, spirometry, and measurement of arterial blood gases, then, provide an adequate assessment for preoperative respiratory evaluation of most patients prior to surgery of virtually any kind, except thoracic and cardiovascular procedures. In fact, pulmonary resection is the only major procedure that commonly requires a more extensive workup, which may include evaluation of distribution of ventilation and blood flow, with reference to the portion of the lung to be resected. Preoperative pulmonary evaluation is discussed further in Chapter 11.

Screening of Patients for Subclinical Disease is a fifth role of the pulmonaryfunction lab and may require more discriminating tests than simple ventilatory measurements. Populations at risk from special environmental hazards, such as miners, foundry workers, and others exposed to industrial hazards, may require periodic testing of a sort designed specifically to detect early effects of the injurious agent involved. Screening programs to detect early obstructive airways disease in the population at large have not as yet been proven useful. This subject is considered in greater detail later in this chapter.

FORCE AND RESISTANCE IN SPONTANEOUS VENTILATION

The mechanical factors governing the flow of air into and out of the lungs during various spontaneous ventilatory maneuvers must be understood prior to undertaking a discussion of abnormalities of ventilation. Especially important is the recognition that factors that produce and limit air flow differ during resting tidal breathing, exercise, and maximum-effort ventilatory maneuvers that are widely used in pulmonary-function laboratories to assess ventilatory reserve (Table 4-1).

The Resting Expiratory State. The mechanics of the thorax and lungs during the resting expiratory state (Table 4-1A) are of basic interest. At this level of inflation, referred to as *functional residual capacity*, a balance exists between two opposing forces: the tendency of the lungs to further collapse and the tendency of the chest cage to further expand. These forces are independent of effort on the part of the subject; they result from the elastic properties of the lungs and chest cage. This resting expiratory level of inflation will be assumed, then, at the bottom of a normal resting tidal breath. At this level, the respiratory muscles are least active, and elastic forces determine the level of lung inflation. The magnitude of the opposing elastic forces of the lungs and chest wall can be measured as intrapleural pressure, which is negative at functional residual capacity (FRC). The unopposed effect of these elastic forces is observed at surgery or autopsy,

TABLE 4-1. Mechanical Characteristics of Spontaneous Ventilatory Maneuvers (Normal Subjects)*

	Volume per Breath	Respiratory Rate	Minute Ventilation	Mechanical Forces at Work	Forces To Be Overcome†	Alveolar Pressure‡	Elastic Recoil Pressure	Pleural Pressure	
A. Resting expiratory state	N/A	N/A	N/A	Elastic forces of chest tending to expand Elastic forces of lungs tending to collapse		0	+	−	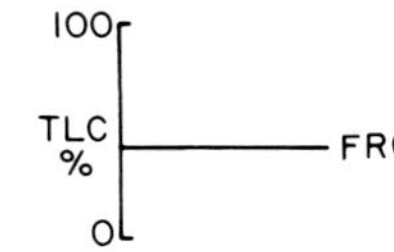
B. Tidal breathing at rest	500 ml	16/min	8 l/min	*Inspiration:* active, contraction of inspiratory muscles	Air flow resistance Elastic recoil	−	+	−	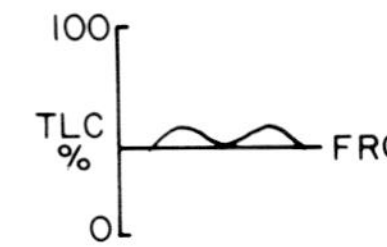
				Expiration: passive, elastic recoil of lungs and chest wall	Air flow resistance	+	+	−	
C. Tidal breathing during heavy exercise	2000 ml	50/min	100 l/min	*Inspiration:* active, contraction of inspiratory muscles	Air flow resistance Elastic recoil	−	+	−	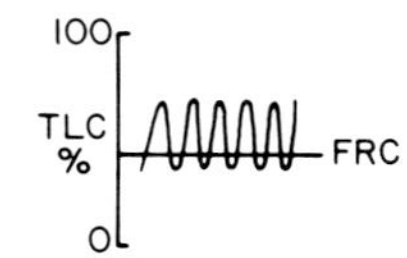
				Expiration: may be passive or active. Elastic recoil of lungs and chest wall, and contraction of expiratory muscles	Air flow resistance	+	+	+ or −	
D. Maximal voluntary ventilation	2000 ml	80/min	160 l/min	*Inspiration:* active, contraction of inspiratory muscles	Air flow resistance Elastic recoil	−	+	−	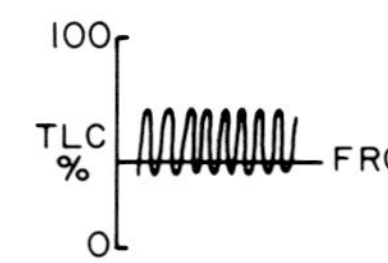
				Expiration: active, elastic recoil of lungs and chest wall, and contraction of expiratory muscles	Air flow resistance	+	+	+	
E. Maximal-effort expiratory maneuver	5000 ml		N/A	Active contraction of expiratory muscle	Air flow resistance	+	+	+	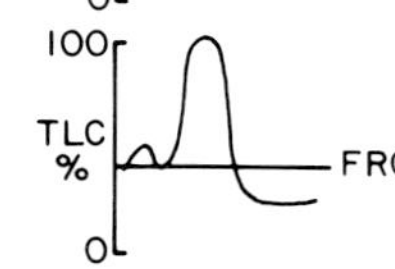

* N/A = not applicable.
† Tissue viscous resistance and inertia must be overcome during any active ventilatory maneuver, but are negligible.
‡ Pressures: 0 (atmospheric); − (negative); + (positive).

when the chest is opened: the lungs collapse further, and the chest inflates slightly, but perceptibly (see Chap. 2 and 6 for further details).

The volume of air in the chest at FRC, then, is determined by the elastic properties of the lungs and chest (which may be altered in disease) but is independent of the subject's effort. Inflation or deflation above or below FRC requires contraction of the muscles of respiration and results in alterations in intrapleural and alveolar pressures, as discussed in the following paragraphs.

Tidal Breathing at Rest. Normal resting tidal breathing (Table 4-1B) consists of repetitive inflation to a level about 500 ml above FRC (in the normal adult male), followed by deflation to FRC. Inflation is a result of active contraction of inspiratory muscles; deflation occurs passively, owing to elastic forces returning the chest to the resting level of inflation. During inflation, expansion of the chest cage produces increasingly more negative intrapleural pressure, which overcomes the elastic recoil pressure of the lung, and causes it to expand. During passive expiration, the lungs recoil, drawing the chest cage to FRC. During all phases of resting tidal breathing, intrapleural pressure remains negative (less than atmospheric), keeping the visceral and parietal pleura in intimate apposition.

Alveolar pressure, on the other hand, is less than atmospheric during inspiration, resulting in air flow into the lungs, and is greater than atmospheric during expiration, resulting in flow out of the lungs. Alveolar pressure during any phase of respiration is the algebraic sum of elastic recoil pressure of the lung and pleural pressure. Pleural pressure, in turn, is due to a combination of elastic forces and positive or negative forces created by contraction of the muscles of respiration.

These relationships are complicated by the fact that frictional as well as elastic forces must be overcome to produce lung inflation, and by the fact that frictional resistance must be overcome while elastic forces contribute to deflation. The frictional resistances to be overcome include viscous resistance of the tissues and flow resistance of the airways. Tissue viscous resistance and inertia are negligible in health and disease, whereas airways resistance is of major importance in normal and abnormal physiology. The latter topic has been extensively reviewed by Macklem.[11]

The chest bellows are capable of moving considerably larger volumes of air at much higher flow rates than those that occur during resting tidal breathing. In other words, the normal "ventilatory reserve" is great, and ventilation can increase to support a metabolic rate as much as twenty times the resting level.

Voluntary inflation of the lungs to levels above those reached during resting respiration can be readily attained by contraction of inspiratory muscles, achieving more negative pleural pressures. The maximum attainable level of inflation is referred to as *total lung capacity*. Deflation to FRC occurs passively, owing to elastic forces, when inspiratory muscles are relaxed. During such a passive expiration, pleural pressure remains negative. Expiration can be speeded up by voluntary contraction of expiratory muscles, in which case positive pleural pressures may be attained. Expiration below FRC requires contraction of expiratory muscles and results in positive pleural pressure, beginning at a level slightly below FRC. The minimum level of inflation that can be achieved by contraction of expiratory muscles is called *residual volume*.

Tidal Breathing During Exercise. During exercise, greatly increased flow rates, tidal volumes, and respiratory rates can be achieved (Table 4-1C). The mechanics of ventilation, as described previously, remain operative, with certain exceptions. Inspiration results in inflation greater than at rest, and expiration may result in deflation below FRC. Expiration may become active, rather than passive, with contraction of expiratory muscles increasing air flow. Normally, sustained exercise does not tax the ventilatory apparatus quite to its maximum, so that flow rates during inspiration and expiration remain below those that are the greatest achievable during a brief maximum voluntary effort.

Breathing During Maximal Voluntary Ventilation. Measurement of minute ventilation during a brief maximum effort is a useful test of ventilatory reserve (Table 4-1D). The mechanics of breathing in this "sprint" test are similar to those operative during exercise. The MVV is customarily carried out for only 12 to 15 sec, however, so that higher values are obtained for minute ventilation than those that can be sustained for long periods or during maximal exercise.

Ventilatory Mechanics During the Maximal-Effort Expiratory Maneuver. Pulmonary-function testing that measures tidal ventilation at rest and during exercise may be diagnostically useful, because ventilation may become inefficient due to disease and because tidal ventilation required for a given level of exercise may increase. Ventilatory tests have been designed, however, that are more sensitive and discriminating. Measurements of certain ventilatory parameters during a single maximum expiratory effort can be used to tax the ventilatory apparatus to its mechanical maximum, thus contributing information about ventilation in health and disease that can be approached in no other way.

Analysis of the maximal-effort expiratory maneuver (Table 4-1E) has contributed to the basic understanding of normal and abnormal ventilatory function.[12,13] The maneuver consists of a full expiration from full inspiration, performed as rapidly and completely as possible. It has been recognized since the early use of clinical spirometry that this maneuver is quite reliable and reproducible and can be used to detect and quantitate obstructive lung disease. This knowledge has been refined, and special characteristics of the maneuver have been clarified in recent years.[14,15]

The most conventional analysis of the maximal-effort expiratory maneuver is carried out from a volume–time curve, as described in this book's section on clinical spirometry. More sophisticated equipment is needed for an analysis of flow–volume curves. Considerable experience with these techniques has shown that the midportion of a maximal-effort expiratory volume–time or flow–volume curve in any individual subject is remarkably reproducible and is sensitive to mild obstructive lung disease. The initial and terminal portions are poorly reproducible, and less discriminating.

The relative effort-independence of flow during the latter portion of a maximum-effort expiration can be demonstrated and quantitated by measuring both flow and effort during such a maneuver. Flow can be measured easily by use of a simple watersealed spirometer. Effort can also be measured, indirectly, as esophageal pressure. The contraction of expiratory muscles during forced expiration contributes to air flow by producing a positive pleural pressure, which is transmitted to the alveolus, resulting in flow from the alveolus to the mouth. Pleural pressure cannot be measured without invasive techniques, but intra-esophageal pressure approximates pleural pressure. It can be measured by passing a small rubber balloon, connected by polyethylene tubing to a manometer, into the esophagus.

By this technique, it can be shown that increasing effort produces increasing expiratory flow up to only about one-fourth of maximum effort. Greater effort does not produce greater flow.[12,13] Maximum expiratory flow declines during the course of expiration; for a given lung volume, a maximum flow can be defined. Therefore, for any cooperative normal or abnormal person, the latter portion of a volume–time or flow–volume curve performed with greater than one-fourth maximal effort is precisely reproducible. Current theory attempting to explain this phenomenon is summarized on page 115.

Such a relationship between effort and flow does not exist during forced inspiration. Increasing effort, up to maximal for an individual person, produces increasing inspiratory flow.

Physical Findings in Ventilatory Dysfunction
Shape of the thorax
Character of movement of the thorax
Movement of the diaphragm
Percussion note
Auscultatory findings
Measurement of respiratory rate
Estimation of tidal volume
Estimation of expiratory flow rates

BEDSIDE EVALUATION OF VENTILATORY FUNCTION

Obstructive lung disease is often easily diagnosed at the bedside in the patient who is so severely afflicted that he is dyspneic at rest. Such a patient may assume a characteristic posture, usually the sitting position, bending slightly forward and bracing his hands or elbows against a table or upon his knees. His breathing may be obviously labored, with his chest moving poorly in spite of use of accessory muscles of respiration. A barrel-shaped chest, with intercostal and supraclavicular retraction on inspiration, is common. Expiration may be obviously prolonged, accompanied by wheezing, and carried out against pursed lips. The disordered ventilatory function in such a patient is easily appreciated.

Less severely diseased persons or those with a less classic clinical presentation may be difficult to assess. Early emphysema may produce dyspnea only on exertion, and cursory examination at rest may reveal no abnormalities. Dyspnea due to left ventricular decompensation may be accompanied by wheezing and may resemble obstructive or restrictive lung disease in clinical presentation. Mixed pulmonary and cardiac disease may be especially difficult to assess. The following paragraphs provide some suggestions to assist in the detection and identification of ventilatory dysfunction, especially that due to obstructive lung disease.

Observation of respiratory rate and depth are basic to physical diagnosis, but they are often misused and misinterpreted. Rapid rate and increased tidal volume in the hyperventilation syndrome or in severe metabolic acidosis are easily recognized, but are often interpreted as respiratory distress due to heart or lung disease. Rapid rate and diminished tidal volume in lung disease with decreased alveolar ventilation can easily be mistaken for overbreathing, because the adventitious sounds in such a case may create the illusion that normal or increased volume is being exchanged with each breath. Often such a patient is described as "hyperventilating," when, in fact, his alveolar ventilation is diminished, or at least inadequate for his metabolic rate, as reflected by an elevated arterial carbon dioxide tension. Observation of breathing rate and depth should always be carried out, but with the knowledge that tidal volume is difficult to quantitate in this fashion.

The shape of the chest and the extent and character of its movement during respiration is another basic but sometimes deceptive part of the clinical examination. There is general agreement that the "barrel chest" configuration of the thorax, with increased anteroposterior diameter of the chest, is a classic finding in advanced chronic obstructive lung disease, but that this finding is not a sensitive indicator of mild disease and may be seen in persons without obstructive disease, especially elderly persons.

Related findings referable to the thorax have been examined in a study to detect correlation with presence and severity of airway obstruction.[16,17] One study was carried out on a group of patients with "stable" obstructive disease. Airway obstruction was quantitated as "specific conductance," a measurement that is the reciprocal of airway resistance, corrected for lung volume. Rhonchi and rales at the bases, and diminished breath sounds, although frequently present, were not correlated significantly with specific conductance. Other signs that did not correlate were paradoxical inward movement of the costal margin with inspiration; loss of lateral and upward bucket-handle movement of the upper ribs, with exaggeration of forward and upward (pump handle) movement; and shortening of the length of the trachea, from cricoid cartilage to sternal notch. These findings do occur in obstructive lung disease but are not sensitive indicators or reliable indicators of severity of disease.

In the same study, correlation was found between specific conductance and the time required to perform a complete forced expiration from maximum inspiration. This finding was not unexpected, because velocity of air flow is inversely proportional to airways resistance. Correlation of specific conductance was also found with a group of signs related only indirectly to resistance of airways *per se.* Increased resonance to percussion showed significant correlation, though it is due to the secondary effect of increased lung volume. Another secondary effect, disordered muscle activity, produces tracheal descent (due to downward pull of the depressed diaphragm) and contraction of the scalene and sternocleidomastoid muscles during inspiration. These findings correlated with specific conductance, as did excavation of the supraclavicular fossae on inspiration, a result of wide intrathoracic pressure swings required to produce air flow through a highly resistant system of airways.

A more recent study examined the reliability of subjective complaints and physical findings in assessing the severity of acute attacks of bronchial asthma.[18] The investigators studied subjective dyspnea and wheezing at rest, retraction of the sternocleidomastoid muscles, and wheezing audible through the stethoscope during tidal breathing. These complaints and findings were correlated with plethysmographic measurements of airways resistance and lung volumes and with spirometric measurements of forced expiratory flow rates. The results are interesting and useful.

Only retraction of the sternocleidomastoids correlated closely with severity of functional derangement. When this sign was present, specific conductance, maximum mid-expiratory flow rate, and forced expiratory volume at 1 sec were always severely reduced, the latter usually to less than 1 liter. Subjective wheezing and dyspnea, and wheezing audible through the stethoscope on tidal breathing were always present with functional derangement, but did not correlate well with its severity.

During improvement a definite order of disappearance of signs and symptoms was the rule. Retractions disappeared first, then symptoms, then wheezing on stethoscopic examination. At the time of disappearance of signs and symptoms, lung function remained abnormal, with most parameters only 60 to 70% of normal.

The findings of these two studies serve well to remind us that the classic symptoms and physical findings of obstructive lung disease, although useful, are not perfectly discriminating. A more sensitive technique is often needed for detection of mild obstructive disease. Even in moderate disease, more quantitative techniques may be needed to distinguish obstructive disease from other causes of dyspnea, such as cardiac decompensation.

One popular bedside test that roughly quantitates the severity of obstructive airways disease is the match test. Several variations of this test of ability to extinguish a match with a forced expiration have been described.[19–21] Snider and colleagues described a technique in which the subject was directed to blow out a match held 15 cm from his open mouth.[19] Ability to perform this test correlated well with a maximum voluntary ventilation of 60 liters per min and a forced expiratory volume at 1 sec of 1.6 liters.

Of the 52 subjects who could not blow out the match, 80% had a maximum voluntary ventilation below 60 liters per min, and 85% had a forced expiratory volume at 1 sec below 1.60 liters. Of the 74 who could extinguish the match, 80% had a maximum voluntary ventilation above 60 liters per min, and 85% had a forced expiratory volume at 1 sec above 1.60 liters.

In a similar study, Olsen found that 94.8% of 327 subjects who could blow out a match 8 cm from the open mouth had MVV values of 40 liters per min or greater.[20] Eighty-nine % of the 26 subjects who could not extinguish the match had MVV values below 40 liters per min.

Approaching the match test somewhat differently, Carilli and Henderson studied 146 subjects, including normal persons and those with assorted forms of ventilatory defect.[21] They determined the maximum distance at which a match could be extinquished with a forced expiration through a standard mouthpiece and 8 cm of Collins spirometer tubing. They found that the predicted MVV in percentage was approximately equal to the match distance in centimeters.

Another useful bedside technique for clinical estimation of severity of airway obstruction is the measurement of forced expiratory time.[22,23] To perform this test, the subject is instructed to inspire maximally, then exhale as rapidly, forcefully, and completely as possible to residual volume, as when performing a forced vital-capacity maneuver. The cessation of expiratory flow can best be detected with a stethoscope placed at the lung base or over the trachea; and the duration of time required for the maneuver can be measured with a second hand of a conventional watch, or more precisely with a stopwatch. Rosenblatt and Stein[22] and Lal and associates[23] have correlated the forced expiratory time with clinical spirometric indices in two separate studies. It appears that virtually all normal subjects can complete the forced expiratory maneuver in less than 4 sec, whereas most subjects with moderate to severe obstructive disease require more than 6 sec. More precise quantitation of airway obstruction appears impractical by this technique, and it should be emphasized that the subject must be vigorously coached in order to perform the test well.

Regional alterations of ventilation may also be recognized clinically.[24] The findings are summarized in Chapter 5.

CLINICAL SPIROMETRY

Volume–Time Analysis of Air Flow

In the preceding section we considered parameters of chest-wall and lung mechanics according to a classification designed to help the reader better understand ventilatory function. Not all of the parameters considered are equally susceptible to measurement in the usual clinical pulmonary-function laboratory. Subsequent discussion will consider measurements of ventilatory function in a more practical way, with reference to their availability to the clinician.

A group of measurements of ventilatory function that are easily performed with inexpensive equipment will be discussed first. This group of measurements, performed and displayed in a stereotyped fashion, is highly recommended as a basic ventilatory profile with which the clinician should become thoroughly familiar, and which should be obtained on all patients entering the laboratory. This battery of tests can be performed with a simple recording spirometer that is inexpensive enough to be standard equipment in the diagnostic laboratory of even the smallest hospital caring for patients with respiratory disease. Recommended criteria for a satisfactory spirometer have recently been published by the American College of Chest Physicians[25–27] and the American Thoracic Society, along with recommended techniques for performance. Normal values have been established for these parameters in a spectrum of subjects of both sexes, varying ages, and varying sizes.[28–39] Patterns of abnormality in a wide range of diseases have been characterized during the past 20 years.

The tests are heavily dependent on patient understanding and cooperation and must be carried out by an informed technician who is able to communicate instructions well. Extensive training however, is not required. Properly performed and interpreted, the ventilatory profile thus obtained provides a large return in information essential for diagnosis and patient care, with a very small investment.

Clinical spirometry for volume–time curve analysis consists of the recording of volume change plotted against time during a series of ventilatory maneuvers by the patient. This permits the determination that the patient has either normal ventilatory reserve or an abnormal pattern characteristic of obstructive, restrictive, or mixed ventilatory abnormalities. Although most diseases are rather predictable in the type of ventilatory defect that they produce, it should be emphasized that such patterns are nonspecific. Spirometry alone is never sufficient to enable a physician to make a diagnosis of a specific disease; however, the volume–time curve is sufficiently reproducible to be useful in following the course of many disease processes. An estimation of the degree of exercise limitation due to a ventilatory defect is possible from volume–time studies; and the patient who is likely to incur ventilatory failure owing to lung or chest wall disease can be identified.

As with any clinical measurement, sensible interpretation of ventilatory testing requires a clear understanding of its limitations. Spirometry does not provide a measurement of the amount of air contained in the chest at the completion of a full expiration (residual volume) and therefore does not permit calculation of the other lung compartments containing residual volume (functional residual capacity, total lung capacity). Likewise, it does not provide direct assessment of the resistance to breathing (lung and chest-wall elastance and airways resistance). It provides no information about control of ventilation, distribution of ventilation, or respiratory gas exchange. Because it is effort-dependent, it cannot be performed usefully on patients who are unable or unwilling to cooperate. Furthermore, the range of normal values for volume–time indices is high. Nevertheless, in combination with measurement of arterial blood gases, spirometry provides sufficient information for intelligent care of patients with respiratory disease in almost every case. More sophisticated tests, requiring far more complicated instrumentation, often provide a fuller understanding of pathophysiology.

To provide volume–time curves, the patient breathes in and out through a mouthpiece, with a nose clip in place, displacing the air within a reservoir of some sort. The excursions of the reservoir are recorded as volume change (on a vertical axis) against time (on a horizontal axis). Many satisfactory devices are commercially available for carrying out simple spirometry. Water-sealed spirometers are inexpensive and reliable. Air is displaced from a container suspended in a water seal, and an attached pen inscribes vertical movement on a drum that revolves at a predetermined speed. The patient is instructed to perform three breathing maneuvers: (a) the vital capacity maneuver, (b) the forced expiratory maneuver and (c) maximum voluntary ventilation. It has been recommended that the forced expiratory maneuver be repeated three times, and the best curve chosen on the basis of the FVC and $FEV_{1.0}$.[26,27,40]

Vital Capacity and Other Static Lung Volumes. Early in the development of clinical spirometry, only static lung volumes were measured. The usefulness of dynamic ventilatory measurements in obstructive disease was recognized later. Of the static lung volumes defined by the Pappenheimer Committee in 1950,[41] vital capacity was most routinely measured as a clinical reflection of ventilatory reserve.

In the vital capacity maneuver, the patient is instructed to inhale as deeply as possible and then exhale fully, taking as much time as he requires. The measurement sought from this maneuver is a single volume measurement. An alternative way of arriving at this measurement is to add two of its components. The patient first exhales maximally from resting expiration, to record expiratory reserve volume. After a few breaths, he then inspires fully from resting expiration, to record inspiratory capacity. These two measurements are added, giving a "combined vital capacity." Normally, and in most patients, the vital capacity and the combined vital capacity are equal. Occasionally, a severely obstructed patient is unable to complete a conventional vital capacity maneuver without interrupting it because of air hunger or fatigue. In this case, the combined vital capacity appears larger than the vital capacity.

The pathophysiological significance of the vital capacity can best be appreciated by referring to the diagram of the subdivisions of lung volume defined by the Pappenheimer report (Fig. 4-1). This 1950 report summarized the terminology agreed upon by the country's leading respiratory physiologists.

Consideration of this diagram readily reveals that each of the volumes here defined can be recorded and measured by a simple spirometer as described earlier, except those containing residual volume. This volume, remaining in the thorax at the end of a maximum expiration, can be measured only by indirect means (*e.g.*, helium dilution, nitrogen washout, or body plethysmography). Also readily apparent is the fact that vital capacity can be reduced in two different ways: reduction of total lung capacity and increase in residual volume. These two mechanisms can be differentiated clearly only by measurement of residual volume and calculation of total lung capacity. Subsequent experience has shown that significant elevation of residual volume is the mechanism by which vital capacity is limited in the "obstructive diseases": asthma, chronic bronchitis, and emphysema. Diseases that cause infiltration or edema of the interstitium, or volume displacement of lung tissue, cause a decrease in vital capacity chiefly by a decrease in total lung capacity. The demonstration of marked reduction in expiratory flow rates may support a clinical diagnosis of one of the obstructive diseases and may permit the clinical in-

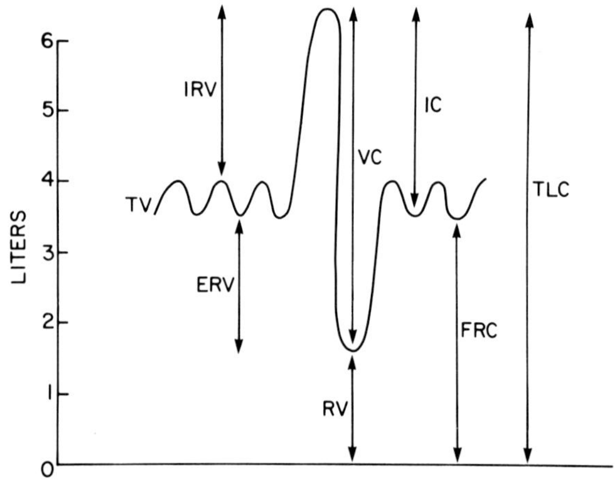

FIG. 4-1. Subdivisions of lung volume. Key: TV-tidal volume, IRV-inspiratory reserve volume, ERV-expiratory reserve volume, RV-residual volume, VC-vital capacity, IC-inspiratory capacity, FRC-functional residual capacity, TLC-total lung capacity.

terpretation that vital capacity is limited by high residual volume. Conversely, relatively normal flow rates may rule out obstructive disease and may permit a presumption that a severe decrease in vital capacity is due to decreased total lung capacity.

The measurement of reduced vital capacity alone, then, provides a very inadequate, nonspecific assessment of decreased ventilatory reserve. The performance of complete clinical spirometry provides additional clarification of the mechanism and severity of a ventilatory defect with satisfactory clinical accuracy. The additional measurement of residual volume, at greater inconvenience and expense, provides convincing proof of the presence or absence of lung overinflation or underinflation.

The Maximal-Effort Expiratory Maneuver. During the years following 1950, interest in physiology began to move toward clinical application. It soon became apparent that measurement of vital capacity had severe limitations in the assessment of ventilatory abnormalities. In particular, patients with significant disability from obstructive lung disease were often noted to have a relatively normal vital capacity. Demonstration of decreased flow rates during breathing, especially during forced expiration, correlated well with clinical disability, however. The maximal-effort expiratory maneuver was therefore developed. Extensive literature soon appeared that centered on the analysis of measurements obtained during performance of this maneuver by normal subjects and by patients with various respiratory diseases. Efforts to extract information from this simple maneuver by a host of different analytical approaches continue to the present.

In performing the maximal-effort expiratory maneuver, the subject is instructed to exhale as rapidly and forcefully as possible, from a full inspiration. When this maneuver is performed as a part of conventional clinical spirometry, volume is recorded on the vertical axis of recording paper, and time is recorded on the horizontal axis; the curve so obtained is referred to as a *forced vital capacity curve.*

In analyzing the volume–time curve obtained during a maximal-effort expiratory maneuver, three types of measurements can be readily performed. The volume exhaled during a defined time interval (forced expiratory volume, timed) following initiation of the maneuver can be measured; the ratio of such a volume to the total forced vital capacity can be computed; and average flow rates during defined portions of the curve can be obtained. During the early years of clinical spirometry, many variations of these three types of measurements were performed and their relative merits touted. Terminology was confusing and poorly standardized.

In 1963, the Section on Pulmonary Function Testing, Committee on Pulmonary Physiology, American College of Chest Physicians, outlined a format for clinical spirometry that incorporated an analysis of the maximal-effort expiratory volume–time curve and maximal voluntary ventilation, in addition to vital capacity.[42] Table 4-2 summarizes the committee report concerning definitions and terminology, which has since been reviewed and confirmed.[43]

"To warrant diagnostic acceptance, the expiratory spirogram should exhibit a reproducible configuration which reflects the underlying physical state of the respiratory tract."[44] Various

TABLE 4-2. Terms Used for Spirometric Measurements

Description	Term Used	Symbol	Other Previously Used Terms
The largest volume measured on complete expiration after full inspiration	Vital capacity	VC	
The vital capacity performed with expiration being as forceful as possible (*i.e.*, forced)	Forced vital capacity	FVC	Timed vital capacity Fast vital capacity
The volume of gas exhaled over a given time interval during the performance of a forced vital capacity	Forced expiratory volume (qualified by subscript indicating the time interval in seconds)	FEV_t (e.g., $FEV_{1.0}$)	Timed vital capacity
FEV_t expressed as percentage of the forced vital capacity (*i.e.*, $\frac{FEV_t}{FVC} \times 100$)	Percentage expired (in t sec) (e.g., $FEV_{1.0}$)	$FEV_t\%$	Timed vital capacity
The average rate of flow for a specified volume segment of the forced expiratory spirogram. (Most commonly used segment in adults is between 200 and 1200 ml)	Forced expiratory flow qualified by subscript indicating volume segment	FEF_{V1-V2} (e.g., $FEF_{200-1200}$)	Maximal expiratory flow rate
The average rate of flow during the middle two quarters of the volume segment of the forced expiratory spirogram (*i.e.*, from 25–75% of the volume)	Forced mid-expiratory flow	$FEF_{25-75\%}$	Maximal mid-expiratory flow
The volume of air that a subject can breathe with voluntary maximal ventilatory effort for a given time	Maximal voluntary ventilation	MVV	Maximum breathing capacity

(Adapted from Kory RC: Clinical spirometry: recommendations of the Section on Pulmonary Function Testing, Committee on Pulmonary Physiology, American College of Chest Physicians. Dis Chest 43:214, 1963)

portions of the curve have differing diagnostic characteristics. The mid-portion of the maximal-effort expiratory curve is the most effort-independent portion, and it may be most sensitive to early disease of peripheral airways. The early portion of the curve is more effort-dependent; and is perhaps more sensitive to obstruction in large central airways, as due to tumor in the trachea or tracheomalacia. The terminal portion is sometimes poorly recorded when a dyspneic patient terminates the maneuver prematurely because of air hunger.

More recently, analysis of flow–volume curves has been popularized as a method of studying the maximal-effort expiratory maneuver and is discussed in more detail below. This method requires somewhat more complex instrumentation but is thought by some investigators to contribute superior diagnostic information in certain cases.[39]

Forced Expiratory Volume, Timed. The forced expiratory volume at 1 sec ($FEV_{1.0}$ sec) is the dynamic volume (or flow) measurement that has been most often used, along with the vital capacity, in an abbreviated form of spirometry. It incorporates the early, effort-dependent portion of the curve but also enough of the mid-portion to make it reproducible, and sensitive enough to be clinically useful. It has an advantage of simplicity, because it can be easily read from a permanently recorded spirogram, or it can be read automatically by a variety of inexpensive spirometers with timing devices. The literature indicates a large experience with this measurement. Normal values for a variety of populations are available, as well as correlation with the degree of clinical disability and long- and short-term prognoses for impairment due to a variety of clinical value. Forced expiratory-volume measurements at 0.5 sec and 0.75 sec incorporate more of the effort-dependent portion of the curve and that portion which has been alleged to better reflect large central-airway obstruction. The latter property is not reliable enough to be of clinical value. Therefore, the $FEV_{1.0}$ sec is more useful than the $FEV_{0.5}$ sec or $FEV_{0.75}$ sec, and the addition of one of the latter measurements serves chiefly as a validity check to the complete spirogram. The $FEV_{2.0}$ sec and $FEV_{3.0}$ sec add very little additional information.[27]

Forced Expiratory Volume, Timed, as a Percentage of Forced Vital Capacity. The forced expiratory volumes expressed as a percentage of the total forced vital capacity have a limited value.[45] Prior to the availability of satisfactory prediction tables for the volumes themselves, these ratios were useful as crude indicators of airways obstruction. Normally, the $FEV_{0.5}$/FVC should exceed 50%, and the $FEV_{1.0}$/FVC should exceed 75%. (A recent study by Morris and associates[38] defined the latter ratio more precisely in normal subjects and indicated decline with age.) Lower values reliably indicate airways obstruction. Normal or greater ratios, however, do not reliably exclude airways obstruction, especially when the FVC is reduced. When reduction of the FVC is due to interstitial disease or chest-wall restriction, with the airways being normal, FEV/FVC ratios are increased. Failure of the ratio to increase in this clinical setting may actually result from concomitant airways disease. Interpretation of the spirogram in mixed disease may then be facilitated by looking at the forced expiratory volumes in absolute terms as a percentage of FVC. Flow rates are volume-dependent and do decrease in restrictive disease without airways obstruction, but precise quantitation of this phenomenon in various pure restrictive diseases is not available. Measurement of airways resistance may be helpful in sorting out this kind of problem.

In summary, then, a decreased FEV/FVC ratio reliably indicates airway obstruction; a normal ratio does not reliably exclude it if the FVC is reduced.

Average Forced Expiratory Flow Rates. Two measurements of average flow rate over portions of the expiratory curve have been widely used. The forced expiratory flow between the first 200 and 1200 ml of the forced vital capacity ($FEF_{200-1200}$) was originally called the *maximal expiratory flow rate* (MEFR) and was introduced to evaluate that portion of the curve that is most affected by obstruction of the larger airways and that is most responsive to bronchodilation. These properties have not stood the test of time well, and the test is declining in popularity. The forced expiratory flow between 25 and 75% of the forced vital capacity was introduced by Leuallen and Fowler[29] as the maximal mid-expiratory flow rate (MMF). It was intended to select the most effort-independent portion of the curve and that portion most sensitive to obstructive disease of the smaller airways. These properties have gained support from both clinical experience and recent theory, and the $FEF_{25-75\%}$ is currently widely used, especially as an indicator of early disease of peripheral airways in asymptomatic subjects with otherwise normal spirometry. It should be noted that both the $FEF_{200-1200}$ and $FEF_{25-75\%}$ demonstrate wide variation in normal populations studied. Therefore, 95% confidence limits for normal values are wide.

The availability of computers has resulted in many programs which measure various other and poorly standardized portions of the expiratory flow curve. None of these has been shown superior to the $FEF_{25-75\%}$.

Peak Expiratory Flow Rate and Other Instantaneous Flow Measurements. Instantaneous flow-rate measurements cannot be read from a conventional volume–time spirometric tracing. The moment of most rapid expiratory flow occurs early in the maximum-effort expiration and is brief. Peak flow as an isolated measurement is easily assessed with a Wright peak flow meter.[46]

Because the peak flow occurs during an effort-dependent portion of the expiratory maneuver, it has been criticized as potentially unreliable. Great effort by a patient with obstructive disease can produce a relatively normal peak flow by expulsion of air from compressable airways, creating an impression of better ventilatory ability than is actually the case. It has been pointed out, however,[47] that in practice, peak flow can be reproducible even though effort-dependent, and the convenience of the Wright peak flow meter makes it useful for following results of therapy in some settings.

The peak flow rate and the flow rates when 25, 50, or 75% of forced vital capacity have been exhaled can be easily read from a flow–volume curve, and will be discussed in more detail later in this chapter.

Relative Effort-Independence of the Maximal-Effort Expiratory Maneuver. It has been mentioned that certain portions of the FVC curve are remarkably effort-independent and therefore reproducible in the same person. This is a rather surprising observation and deserves further comment. Experimental data support the observation, and theoretical considerations provide an intriguing explanation.[12–15]

Expiratory flow rate from the lungs during a FVC maneuver can be viewed as resulting from driving force created by lung elastic recoil and intrapleural pressure. That is, air is expressed from the lungs by the tendency of the lungs to collapse, owing to their elastic properties, and by pressure exerted on them by the thoracic cage (during active expiration)—measured as intrapleural pressure. These forces are opposed by the resistance of the airways and, of less importance, the resistance and inertia of lung tissue, opposing deformation. The degree of patient effort in a FVC maneuver is reflected by pleural pressure, and close approximation of pleural pressure can be obtained by measurement of intra-esophageal pressure. This can be done by having the patient swallow a tiny balloon, connected by polyethylene tubing to a manometer. It can be shown that increasing effort creates increasing expiratory flow rates only up to about one-fourth the effort that can be exerted by a normal person. This is true over the lower two-thirds of vital capacity. Maximum flow for a given lung volume may be reached by effort resulting in as little as 10 or 20 cm of water pleural pressure. Increases in pressure to as high as 60 or 80 cm of water do not result in further increases in flow rate.[14,15] Thus, the clinical observation of relative effort-independence of a portion of the FVC curve is firmly supported and quantitated.

It has been suggested that critical narrowing or collapse of airways occurs at the flow maxima.[14,15] Intrapleural pressure created during active expiration not only creates flow by elevating alveolar pressure, but also is transmitted to the walls of intrathoracic airways, tending to collapse them. Collapse is prevented by airway pressure, which gradually drops from alveolus to mouth, as well as by stiffness of airway walls themselves. At some point along the airways the pressure inside is equal to the pressure outside, and narrowing or collapse may occur. The location of these equal pressure points[14] is a function of the mechanical properties of the subject's lungs: elastic recoil, as well as airways resistance. The location of the equal pressure points changes during the course of expiration; but so long as they occur within the thorax, flow maxima may occur. Increasing intrapleural pressure results in increased driving force to create flow, but also in equal force to narrow airways and oppose flow.

It can be readily imagined that disease might alter any of the determinants of expiratory flow rate, as hypothesized by this model, and therefore might alter the maximum flow achievable at any lung volume. Bronchospasm, edema, and obstructing secretions might increase the magnitude and alter the location of resistance limiting to air flow. Emphysema might contribute to the collapsibility of airways by the loss of supportive alveolar walls. Infiltrative interstitial diseases might increase recoil pressure and decrease airway collapsibility, with a resultant increase in maximum flow rates. For a detailed theoretical discussion, see Chapter 3.

Maximal Voluntary Ventilation (MVV). This test was introduced in 1933 by Hermannsen[48] and was known for many years as the *maximal breathing capacity*. It is defined as the maximal volume of air in liters that can be moved by voluntary effort during 1 min. Patients are instructed to breathe as rapidly and deeply as possible for 12 to 30 sec; the ventilatory volumes are recorded; and the result is expressed in liters per min. When the longer periods of time are used, fatigue may result in diminution in ventilation toward the end of the test in patients with cardiopulmonary or other disease. If the test is carried out for longer periods, even normal persons are unable to maintain the initial levels of ventilation, because of fatigue. Diagnostic usefulness of the test may be increased by analyzing the breathing frequency chosen by the patient.

The MVV is a performance test that is heavily dependent on patient cooperation and effort. It is sensitive to loss of muscular coordination, musculoskeletal disease of the chest wall, neurologic disease, and deconditioning from any chronic illness. Values are reduced in patients with airways obstructive disease, but less so with mild or moderate restrictive disease, because a rapid, shallow breathing pattern can be chosen that compensates effectively for the mechanical defect.

In spite of these serious drawbacks, the MVV can be useful in special circumstances. It correlates well with subjective dyspnea; it is useful in evaluating exercise tolerance; and it has prognostic value in the preoperative workup, because the extrapulmonary factors to which it is sensitive are important in the patient's recovery from a surgical procedure.

Interpretation of Volume–Time Studies

The range of normal values for spirometric indices is rather wide, (Table 4-3). For static lung volumes and forced expiratory volumes (timed), there are good correlations with sex, age, and height. Larger values are normally seen in males and in taller subjects, and values normally decline with age after adulthood. When these variables are taken into account, a mean value for a normal population can be found that has 95% confidence limits (approximately two standard deviations), extending 20 to 30% above and below the mean. That is, for a group of normal persons of a stated sex, age, and height, 95% have lung volumes and expiratory flow rates that are within a range of, for example, 20% above and below the mean value for that measurement.

The range of normal for certain of the midflow measurements has been even more difficult to define. Correlations with sex, age, and height are poor, and even a recent study that was confined to healthy nonsmoking adults demonstrated wide variation in normal subjects.[36]

This wide range of normal values places certain limitations on spirometric interpretation.[50,51] If the spirometric values of a person studied at a given point in time are in the very low normal range, they may represent normality for that subject, or they may represent significant functional derangement in a person whose vital capacity or flow rates were higher than average prior to the onset of disease. A discrepancy between static and dynamic volume measurements, expressed as a percentage of that predicted, can be a clue to this sort of circumstance. For instance, a normal person seldom would have a vital capacity of 115% of predicted and a forced expiratory volume of 85% of predicted. A person with such values probably has obstructive airways disease. Statistical data to support such an interpretation are not available, however, and in general it is wise to avoid overinterpretation of spirometric measurements. As with all laboratory tests, sensible clinical correlation is essential if spirometry is to be helpful rather than misleading.[50,51] Imperfect agreement among interpreters of spirometry has been shown to emphasize this point.[45,52]

Although the range of normal values is wide, reproducibility of spirometric measurements in the same subject is possible within very close limits. Beyond the point of a modest learning effect, spirometry in a cooperative subject should be reproducible to within at least 5 to 10% of the initial values obtained. Gaensler[50] has indicated

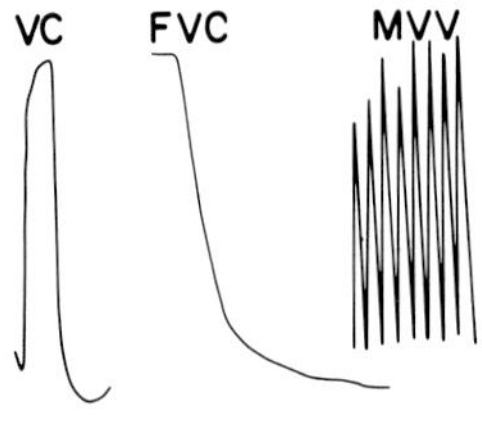

Interpretation: Mild Restrictive Ventilatory Defect

	Predicted Normal	Performed	Percent of Predicted
VC	3.72 L	2.84	76
FVC	3.72 L	2.84	76
$FEV_{0.5}$	2.21 L	2.28	103
$FEV_{0.5 (\%FVC)}$	50%	80%	
$FEV_{1.0}$	2.92 L	2.50	86
$FEV_{1.0 (\%FVC)}$	75%	88%	
$FEF_{25-75\%}$	3.6 L/sec	4.33	
MVV	129 L/min		

FIG. 4-2 Restrictive ventilatory pattern. Age, 51; sex, M; height, 159 cm.

that with optimal cooperation, variation as small as 2 to 3% can be achieved. If a subject is unable or unwilling to cooperate fully, a valid spirogram cannot be obtained. Certain patterns of abnormality are characteristic of poor effort, and malingering or inability to cooperate can be suspected from such patterns, as will be described later.

There are two basic patterns of spirometric abnormality in disease: restrictive and obstructive. Typical examples of these two patterns are easily recognized and interpreted. From a classic spirogram demonstrating predominant obstruction or restriction, it may be possible to infer validity and adequate patient cooperation, and even to predict exercise tolerance and likelihood of supervening ventilatory failure with some degree of confidence. Mixed patterns are common and may be difficult to interpret, because a combination of slow flow rates and reduced vital capacity may occur in many clinical settings. Muscular weakness and suboptimal patient effort and cooperation may contribute to such a mixed pattern and may be difficult to recognize.

Restrictive Ventilatory Defect. "Restriction" to ventilation, as defined spirometrically, is simply reduction in vital capacity; that is, limitation of the extent of excursion of the chest bellows. A classic "restrictive pattern" on spirometry consists of reduced vital capacity (to less than 80% of the predicted values); little or no reduction in expiratory flow rates; and relative preservation of the maximum voluntary ventilation (see list below and Fig. 4-2). A patient whose spirogram shows a restrictive pattern can be considered to be suffering from one of the *restrictive diseases*—conventionally referring to a group of disorders in which the vital capacity is reduced, primarily due to reduction in total lung capacity rather than to increase in residual volume.

The Restrictive Pattern

Characteristics of restrictive ventilatory defect
- Decreased vital capacity
- Relatively normal expiratory flow rates
- Relatively normal maximal voluntary ventilation

Supplementary data confirming restriction
- Decreased total lung capacity

The "restrictive diseases," which result in a typical restrictive spirometric pattern and reduction in vital capacity due to low total lung capacity, are quite variable in etiology and pathology (see list below). They include a variety of interstitial lung diseases: the diffuse interstitial pneumonias, pulmonary edema, interstitial granulomas, and fibrosis, which can result from any of the foregoing. Any localized parenchymal disorders that occupy volume and displace lung tissue, such as tumors, may be included. Pleural diseases (including effusion, pneumothorax, and fibrosis) limit chest bellows expansion and are included in the group of restrictive disorders. Numerous diseases of the central and peripheral nervous system, muscle, joints, and bone interfere with movement of the chest wall and diaphragm and are classified as restrictive disorders. Although the ventilatory defect as demonstrated by spirometry may be identical in these diseases, the effects on blood-gas exchange may be quite variable.

Common Causes of Restrictive Ventilatory Defect

- Interstitial lung diseases
  - Interstitial pneumonitis
  - Fibrosis
  - Pneumoconiosis
  - Granulomatosis
  - Edema
- Space-occupying lesions
  - Tumors
  - Cysts
- Pleural diseases
  - Pneumothorax
  - Hemothorax
  - Pleural effusion, empyema
  - Fibrothorax
- Chest-wall diseases
  - Injury
  - Kyphoscoliosis
  - Spondylitis
  - Neuromuscular disease
- Extrathoracic conditions
  - Obesity
  - Peritonitis
  - Ascites
  - Pregnancy
- Upper abdominal surgery

In patients with restriction due to parenchymal lung disease, the forced expiratory volume, timed, as a percentage of the forced vital capacity (*e.g.*, $FEV_{1.0}/FVC$) is characteristically increased. This may result from relative dilatation of the airways owing to traction by the stiff lungs. In other restrictive disorders, there is some degree of slowing of expiratory flow rates. This decrease in flow rates is minimal and is easily recognized as being secondary to low lung volumes, unless the restrictive disorder is extremely severe or airway obstruction coexists. Several causes for the slowing of expiratory flow, other than obstructive airways disease, may be operative in the restrictive diseases. Altered action of respiratory muscles and smaller diameter of airways at low lung volumes; altered tissue viscous resistance and elastance; and decreased fitness of respiratory muscles may all play a part.

The relative preservation of the maximal voluntary ventilation in restrictive disease may be diagnostically helpful. Reduction of vital capacity can be moderately severe before it impinges upon the volume of the tidal breath that the patient usually adopts when instructed to breathe as rapidly and deeply as possible. In addition, a subject with decreased vital capacity has the option of selecting a very rapid and shallow breathing pattern in order to perform a MVV maneuver, if his maximum flow rates are not reduced. The MVV helps to distinguish most patients with true restriction from subjects who have muscular weakness or who are not cooperating fully, because the latter usually have reduced vital capacity and MVV, with relatively normal flow rates.

A subject with restrictive disease, then, characteristically has a reduced vital capacity but relatively normal expiratory flow rates and MVV.

Obstructive Ventilatory Defect. Although the diagnosis and quantitation of airway obstruction is one of the most important uses of clinical spirometry, it is important to realize that airway resistance cannot be directly measured by spirometry. The spirometric parameters used to infer elevated airway resistance are simply expiratory flow rates that are achieved with an effort that is presumed to be the patient's maximum. Because the "maximum" effort is not quantitated, the observer can only presume, without solid evidence, that a decrease in flow is due to increased resistance to flow rather than to a decrease in the driving force that creates flow.

Nevertheless, reproducible patterns of spirometric values in normal subjects (Fig. 4-3) and in diseased persons are sufficiently characteristic that a valid maximum effort can usually be assumed. The diagnosis of increased airway resistance can be made with reasonable assurance, and correlation is reasonably good with body plethysmographic measurement of airways re-

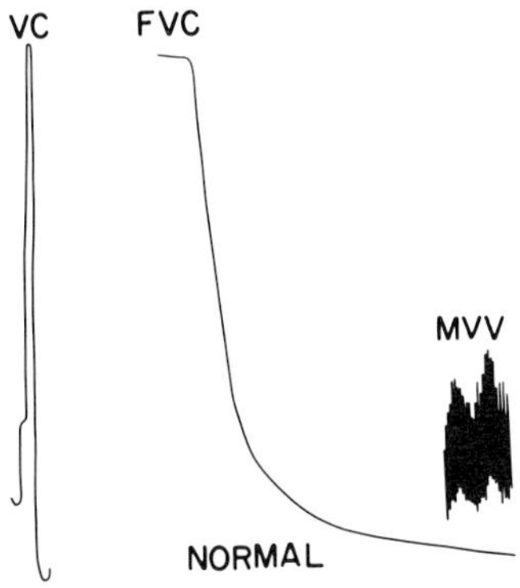

Interpretation: Normal Ventilatory Study

	Predicted Normal	Performed	Percent of Predicted
VC	4.52 L	4.89	108
FVC	4.52 L	4.89	108
$FEV_{0.5}$	2.60 L	2.67	103
$FEV_{0.5\,(\%FVC)}$	50%	55%	
$FEV_{1.0}$	3.55 L	3.82	108
$FEV_{1.0\,(\%FVC)}$	75%	78%	
$FEV_{25-75\%}$	4.3 L/sec	4.11	
MVV	152 L/min		

FIG. 4-3. Normal spirogram. Age, 47; sex, M; height, 173 cm.

sistance in bronchitis and asthma, as well as in obstruction of the trachea or upper airways due to tumor, stenosis, collapse, or foreign body.

In subjects with emphysema a decrease in maximum expiratory flow rates is thought to be chiefly due to decreased elastic recoil of the lungs and, therefore, to decreased driving force rather than increased resistance to flow. Nevertheless, it is customary to speak of emphysema (along with bronchitis, bronchiectasis, asthma, and bronchiolitis) as one of the *obstructive* lung diseases. According to one school of thought, there is a collapse of the airways in emphysema owing to loss of elastic recoil of the alveolar tissue that normally supports the walls of the airways by radial traction. To the extent that this actually occurs, emphysema may truly be an obstructive disease in the more usual sense.

In emphysema and in other diffuse "obstructive" diseases, it is common for a decrease in expiratory flow rates to be accompanied by a decrease in vital capacity. This decrease is a result of increased residual volume, that is, an inability to empty the lungs normally. Measurement of residual volume is necessary to unequivocally document that this "air trapping" phenomenon is the mechanism of decreased vital capacity, rather than a decrease in total lung capacity, which occurs in the "restrictive" diseases. Typically, however, the decrease in vital capacity in obstructive diseases is relatively less severe than the decrease in flow rates. This relation can be readily observed by comparing the values recorded in the column labeled *percent predicted* on the display form recommended. The observation of this "obstructive pattern" of ventilatory defect permits the inference that the relatively mild decrease in vital capacity is due to increased residual volume (see list below and Fig. 4-4). This inference is usually correct.

The Obstructive Pattern

- Characteristics of obstructive ventilatory defect
  - Normal or decreased vital capacity
  - Decreased maximum expiratory flow rates
  - Decreased MVV
- Supplementary data confirming obstruction
  - Increased residual volume
  - Increased airway resistance

The obstructive pattern is relatively nonspecific, however, and usually permits no inference to be made as to the disease process producing it (see list below). A relatively greater decrease in flow rates over the early portion of the curve may suggest major airway obstruction, whereas diffuse peripheral obstruction may be reflected by a more severe decrease in mid-flow rates. These findings are not entirely clinically reliable, however. When central airway obstruction is suspected, repeated studies may establish reproducibility, suggesting adequate patient cooperation. Because central airway obstruction is manifested by a considerable decrease in inspiratory as well as expiratory flow rates, performance of a forced inspiratory ma-

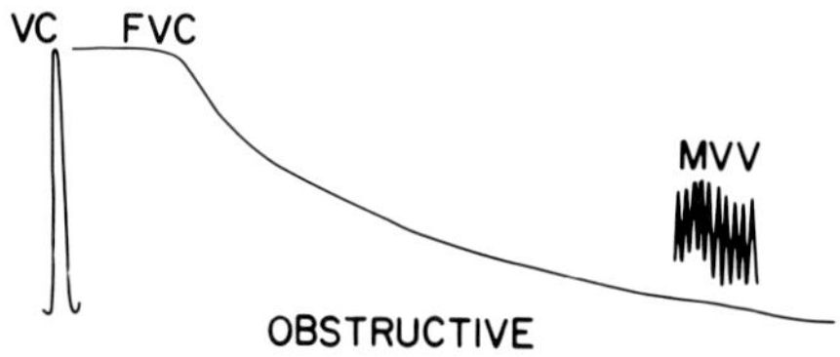

Interpretation: Very Severe Obstructive Ventilatory Defect

	Predicted Normal	Performed	Percent of Predicted
VC	4.60 L	2.33	51
FVC	4.60 L	2.33	51
$FEV_{0.5}$	2.70 L	0.54	20
$FEV_{0.5\,(\%FVC)}$	50%	23	
$FEV_{1.0}$	3.68 L	0.85	23
$FEV_{1.0\,(\%FVC)}$	75%	36	
$FEF_{25-75\%}$	4.3 L/sec	0.39	
MVV	158 L/min		

FIG. 4-4. Obstructive ventilatory pattern. Age, 41; sex, M; height, 171 cm.

neuver may be of help in distinguishing central from peripheral airway obstruction. The ratio of the forced expiratory volume at 1 sec to the forced inspiratory volume at 1 sec is approximately 0.85 in normal subjects. The ratio is decreased in peripheral airways obstruction and is increased in central obstruction. A ratio greater than 1 in a subject with a decreased $FEV_{1.0}$ suggests that the obstruction may be central.[53] This topic is discussed below, along with other aspects of flow–volume relationships.

Common Causes of Obstructive Ventilatory Defect
Upper airway disease
Pharyngeal and laryngeal tumors, edema, infections
Foreign bodies
Tumors, collapse, and stenosis of trachea
Peripheral airway disease
Bronchitis
Bronchiectasis
Bronchiolitis
Bronchial asthma
Pulmonary parenchymal disease (loss of airway support and of elastic recoil)
Emphysema

Another convenient index of central airway obstruction can be obtained by measurement of the peak expiratory flow rate (PEFR) with a Wright peak flow meter and comparison with the forced expiratory volume at 1 sec. The ratio of the FEV_1 (in milliliters) to PEFR (in liters per min) usually exceeds 10 in upper airway obstruction and is less than 10 in normal subjects or those with diffuse peripheral obstruction.[54]

Assessment of reversibility of impaired expiratory flow rates may be useful. Diagnostically, reversibility implies exclusion of emphysema, at least as a cause of the reversible component of the impairment. Reversibility may occur acutely in response to bronchodilator administration; chronically in response to an assortment of treatment modalities; or spontaneously during remissions of bronchial asthma. Reversibility implies a better prognosis than fixed impairment of expiratory flow and may have considerable significance in planning a therapeutic program.

Laboratory techniques for assessment of acute reversibility of airways obstruction in response to bronchodilator administration must vary according to the needs of the individual patient and laboratory logistics. Ideally, chronic bronchodilator administration should, of course, be discontinued several hours before testing; but this may not be feasible in some patients. An aerosol bronchodilator should be administered in the appropriate dose, which varies from one patient to another, and testing should be carried out after an interval appropriate to the time of onset and duration of action of the drug selected. No amount of care in standardizing dose and route of administration can really ensure that each patient will receive a maximally effective nontoxic dose, or a comparably effective dose, so individualization is necessary. Interpretation of test results should be made rather cautiously, appropriate to the difficulties inherent in standardizing such a test.

The Committee on Emphysema of the American College of Chest Physicians has suggested that the forced vital capacity, the forced expiratory volume at 1 sec, and the maximal mid-expiratory flow rates are the simplest and most available tests reflecting severity of airways obstruction.[55] The committee members have recommended that a significant change in two of these three tests be required as evidence of improvement. A 15 to 25% change is considered slight reversibility; 25 to 50% improvement is moderate reversibility; and a greater than 50% change reflects marked reversibility (see list below).

Criteria for Reversibility of Airways Obstruction

- Significant improvement in two of these three parameters indicates reversibility
  - Forced vital capacity
  - Forced expiratory volume at 1 sec
  - Forced expiratory flow rate from 25–75% of forced vital capacity
- Degree of reversibility
  - Slight: 15–25% change
  - Moderate: 25–50% change
  - Marked: greater than 50% change

These rather rigorous criteria are useful as guidelines for interpretation and are certainly appropriate for comparison of populations for investigative purposes. For clinical purposes in individual patients, bronchodilator therapy should not be withheld simply on the basis of failure of one spirometric test to meet arbitrary criteria. Bronchodilator therapy is commonly useful in patients with less demonstrable acute response than these criteria demand. The forced vital capacity is sometimes the only spirometric parameter that shows improvement (reflecting a decrease in residual volume) in patients who have subjective and arterial blood-gas improvement from a bronchodilator. In some patients, improvement is demonstrable after weeks of drug therapy, when initial tests administered before and after bronchodilator showed no significant change.

The "Poor-Effort" Pattern of Spirometric Abnormality. As stated previously, spirometry is heavily dependent on the cooperation of the subject being tested. For this reason, excellent laboratories have traditionally demanded that the physician who is responsible for interpretation of the test results observe the patients as they perform effort-dependent tests. In addition, some such laboratories have considered that interpretation of pulmonary-function tests should be carried out by specialists in pulmonary disease only as a part of a complete clinical evaluation, including history and physical examination.

Such requirements place undesirable restrictions on the use of the pulmonary-function laboratory, and the benefits of wider application of simple ventilatory tests outweigh the disadvantages of less careful quality control. When a competent and conscientous technician carries out the test procedures and when a recording of the tracings obtained accompanies the battery of measurements recommended, interpretation of the data may render a satisfactory judgment of validity in most cases. The "poor-effort" spirogram can usually be identified (see list below).

"Poor-Effort" Pattern

- Characteristics of "poor-effort" ventilatory defect
  - Decreased vital capacity
  - Relatively normal expiratory flow rates
  - Decreased maximum voluntary ventilation
- Supplementary data confirming invalid test results
  - Uneven, slurred, or notched curve on direct examination
  - Poor reproducibility on repeated testing

Interpretation should be carried out with some caution, avoiding terms that imply that a morphological or etiological diagnosis can be made from these test results alone. A specific diagnosis must be made in the final analysis by the physician caring for the patient, using all the available knowledge at his disposal, interpreting test results in the light of other clinical findings.

Certain portions of the data collected during performance of spirometry are more likely to be abnormal with poor effort than others. The vital capacity and maximal voluntary ventilation are rather heavily effort-dependent. Early portions of the forced vital capacity curve are somewhat less effort-dependent, and the mid-portion of the forced vital capacity curve is much less effort-dependent and highly reproducible. As would be expected from this, a poor effort in a normal subject commonly results in a reduced vital capacity; a somewhat reduced forced expiratory volume at 0.5 sec; and a less reduced volume at 1.0 sec, since the latter measurement incorporates relatively more of the effort-independent portion of the curve. A poor-effort spirogram almost invariably shows a reduced maximal voluntary ventilation.

A submaximal effort is poorly reproducible and is characterized by an uneven, slurred forced expiratory curve, which may be terminated before reaching a plateau. Whether the poor effort is due to inadequate understanding, muscular weakness, neurasthenia, or malingering often cannot be determined readily by examination of test data.

A valid restrictive spirogram generally differs from the "poor-effort" test in being reproducible; showing relatively normal forced expiratory volumes at both 0.5 and 1.0 sec, with expiratory curves appearing smooth on direct examination; and demonstrating a normal or nearly normal maximum voluntary ventilation.

The validity of any normal spirogram can be inferred from close reproducibility on repeated performance and from the appearance of smooth expiratory curves, without continued notching or slurring, until a plateau is achieved. Comparable decrease in forced expiratory volumes at 0.5 and 1.0 sec usually accompanies the appearance of a smooth curve when obstruction is present, except that central airway obstruction or central airway collapse may produce a greater decrease in the volume at 0.5 sec than at 1.0 sec. In a normal or abnormal subject, a maximum effort produces a value for maximal voluntary ventilation that is about 40 times the forced expiratory volume at 1.0 sec. Achievement of this value for the MVV is excellent evidence of validity of the spirogram in terms of patient cooperation.

The Mixed Pattern of Ventilatory Impairment. In most cases of ventilatory impairment, a decrease in vital capacity and a decrease in expiratory flow rates coexist, but one or the other often clearly predominates. If decreased vital capacity predominates, restriction is inferred, and obstruction need not be considered in order to explain a milder decrease in flow rates. A predominant decrease in expiratory flow rates suggests obstruction, with an accompanying decrease in vital capacity due to increased residual volume. Restriction need not be considered in order to explain the decreased vital capacity in such a case.

Clear guidelines are not available to suggest what degree of predominance must be present in order to infer pure obstruction or restriction and exclude a mixed pattern of impairment. For purposes of uniformity and simplicity, it is suggested that the forced expiratory volumes at 1.0 sec, expressed as a percentage of predicted values, be used as an index of obstruction, and that vital capacity be used as an index of restriction. When the percentage of predicted values differs by more than 15%, the more severely abnormal one indicates predominance of obstruction or restriction. A smaller difference often indicates a mixed ventilatory defect (see list below). The observation of a mixed or indeterminate defect is an indication for further pulmonary-function testing if the defect is to be more precisely defined.

Mixed or Indeterminate Pattern

Characteristics of Mixed Ventilatory Defect
- Decreased vital capacity
- Decreased expiratory flow rates
- Decreased maximal voluntary ventilation
- Lack of predominance of obstruction or restriction

Supplementary tests
- Lung volume determination
- Repeat tests after bronchodilator administration
- Diffusing capacity
- Compliance
- Airways resistance

An impression of the overall severity of the defect in terms of its impairment of the patient's ventilatory function can be gained from the forced expiratory volumes, whether or not the character of the defect is clearly defined. The forced expiratory volumes at 0.5 sec and at 1.0 sec, expressed as a percentage of predicted normal values, may be used to categorize the severity of a ventilatory defect.[56] Arbitrarily, values from 65 to 79% of predicted reflect a mild defect; 50 to 64% characterize a moderate abnormality; and 35 to 49% reflect severe impairment. Other sets of criteria preferred by some interpreters are likewise arbitrary.[57–59] Values below 35% are categorized as very severe ventilatory impairment (see list below).

Criteria for Severity of Ventilatory Defect

Tests utilized to reflect overall severity of ventilatory defect
- Forced expiratory volume at 0.5 sec
- Forced expiratory volume at 1.0 sec

Degree of severity
- Mild: 65–79% of predicted value
- Moderate: 50–64% of predicted value
- Severe: 35–49% of predicted value
- Very severe: below 35% of predicted value

(Adapted from data in Snider GL, Kory RC, Lyons HA: Grading of pulmonary function impairment by means of pulmonary function tests. Recommendations of the Committee on Pulmonary Physiology, American College of Chest Physicians. Dis Chest 52:270, 1967)

If better characterization of a mixed defect than can be obtained from spirometry is desired, measurement of lung volumes, airways resistance, and compliance may be indicated (see The Restrictive Pattern, and The Obstructive Pattern).

TESTS OF LUNG MECHANICS THAT SUPPLEMENT VOLUME–TIME ANALYSIS

As described previously, volume–time curve analysis provides an inexpensive, simple approach to pulmonary-function testing that can be provided by small hospital laboratories or even in the physician's office. Along with arterial blood-gas and *p*H measurements, volume–time curves provide sufficient physiological information for sensible care of patients with clinically significant respiratory disease in virtually every instance. Normal values for measurements obtained from volume–time curves are available, obtained from relatively large populations of varying ages and both sexes.

Additional measurements of lung mechanics require substantially more expensive and complex instrumentation. The information obtained often provides additional insight into the pathophysiology of disease in the patient tested and occasionally may result in significant alterations in therapy. Normal values for many of these measurements are inadequately established, however, and in some cases, the techniques are sufficiently cumbersome to cast doubt on the accuracy of results obtained in laboratories that perform the tests infrequently.

Table 4-3 summarizes references containing normal values for both volume-time parameters of ventilatory function and the more complex measurements of lung mechanics.

Flow–Volume Relationships

Flow–Volume Curves and Loops in Normal Subjects. Conventional spirometric analysis has been developed around the plot of volume against time, because this sort of spirogram can be obtained with simple, inexpensive equipment. The development of sophisticated electronic gadgetry has led to an interest in analysis of various other parameters, plotted in numerous ways. One of the most popular has been the flow–volume curve,[60–65] which is obtained by having the subject inspire and expire fully, with maximum effort, into an instrument that measures flow and volume change simultaneously. These parameters are plotted on the two axes of an X-Y recorder or oscilloscope. Such a curve actually presents no information not contained in a conventional display of volume plotted against time, because flow, after all, is simply a function of these two parameters. Consideration of similar data displayed in a different fashion, however, often leads to advances in understanding. Accordingly, flow–volume curve analysis has contributed to our basic understanding of

(*Text continues on P. 126*)

TABLE 4-3. Commonly Used References for Predicted Normal Values for Ventilatory Tests

Year of Publication	Ref. No.	Authors	TLC	FRC	RV	VC	FEV 1.0	FEF 25–75	MVV	Age* (years)	Sex	Smokers Specifically Excluded	Method for RV and FRC	omments	Number of Subjects
1948	28	Baldwin, et al	✓	✓	✓	✓			✓	16–69	Both	No	Nitrogen washout	Regression equations incorporating height and age for VC and MVV	92
1955	29	Leuallen and Fowler						✓		Men 20–79 Women 17–62	Both	No		Normal values for men and women grouped according to age by decade	140
1959	30	Goldman and Becklake	✓	✓	✓	✓			✓	Men—mean, 44.3 (SD, 16.6) Women—mean, 38.5 (SD, 16.3)		No	Helium dilution	Regression equations incorporating height and age	94
1961	31	Kory, et al				✓	✓	✓	✓	18–66	Males	No		Regression equations incorporating height and age, except for $FEF_{25-75\%}$	468
1962	32	Bates, et al	✓	✓	✓	✓		✓						Regression equations incorporating height and age	
1965	33	Ferris, et al				✓	✓			25–74	Both	Smokers and nonsmokers tested and compared		Regression equations incorporating height and age	1,167

1966	34	Cotes, et al				✓	✓			20–64	Males	No		Regression lines incorporating height and age	275
1969	35	Weng and Levison	✓	✓	✓	✓	✓	✓	✓	4–18	Both	No	Helium dilution	Regressions are for height, with boys and girls combined	139
1971	36	Morris, et al				✓	✓	✓		20–80	Both	Yes		Regression equations incorporating height and age	988
1972	37	Cherniack and Raber				✓	✓	✓	✓	15–79	Both	Yes		Regression equations incorporating height and age	1,331
1966	49	Boren, et al	✓	✓	✓	✓	✓		✓	20–66	Males	Partially excludes smokers	Nitrogen washout and helium dilution	Regression equations incorporating height and age	422
1976	39	Knudson, et al				✓	✓	✓		8–90	Both	Yes	NA	Regression equations incorporating height and age	746

* SD = standard deviation.

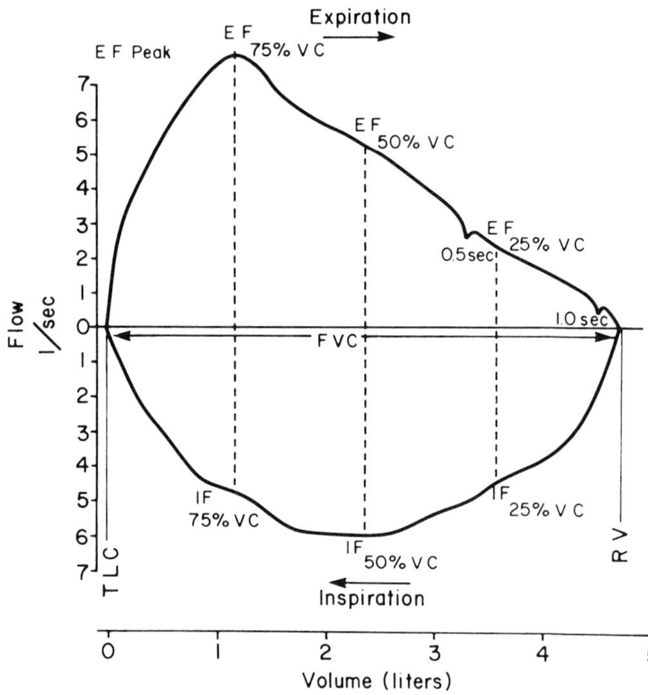

FIG. 4-5. Normal maximal-effort flow-volume loop. Note that the recorded maneuver begins after a maximal inhalation. The subject is asked to exhale as rapidly and forcefully as possible, and the expiratory curve is inscribed by the recording pen. Expiratory flow (EF) can be measured at its peak, or at various volumes of expired air (e.g., 75%, 50%, 25% of the vital capacity). Furthermore, the volume exhaled in 0.5 sec or 1.0 sec can be plotted as indicated by the time markers on the expiration curve. The total air exhaled is, of course, the vital capacity (VC). Immediately following the maximal expiration, the subject is asked to inhale as quickly and deeply as possible, and then inspiratory flow (IF) is measured.

the mechanical events that occur during ventilatory efforts. In particular it has emphasized the dependence of maximum achieveable flow on lung volume. For every point on the lower two-thirds of the volume axis of an expiratory curve, a maximum flow exists that cannot be exceeded, regardless of the effort exerted (see also Chap. 3). It logically follows from this observation that maximum flow must be dependent on mechanical characteristics of the lungs. Elucidation of some of these mechanical characteristics has resulted from flow–volume curve analysis. In addition, flow–volume curves constitute an informative way of displaying ventilatory data for clinical diagnostic purposes,[66] and some investigators predict that this type of analysis of the maximal-effort expiratory maneuver will prove to be more useful than conventional spirometry as more experience with it is accumulated.

The initial portion of a flow–volume curve during a forced expiratory maneuver describes flow during exhalation of approximately the first one-third of the vital capacity (Fig. 4-5). The curve shows a rapid ascent to "peak flow" and then begins a slow descent. This initial portion of the curve is effort-dependent; that is, increasing transpulmonary pressure results in increasing flow. It can be readily demonstrated that as a subject exerts increasing effort during exhalation, this is reflected by increasing intrathoracic pressure, and therefore increasing flow is generated, as displayed on the initial phase of the flow–volume curve. This portion of the curve is of limited diagnostic use, then. Its appearance depends chiefly on the subject's muscular effort rather than on the mechanical characteristics of the lung as altered by disease.

Shortly after the development of peak flow, a remarkably reproducible portion of the flow–volume curve can be identified as a slow descent continues to residual volume. As discussed in the section on volume–time analysis, this portion of the curve has been shown to be relatively effort-independent. For each point on the volume axis, a maximum flow exists, which cannot be exceeded, regardless of the pressure generated. Maximum flow is reached at about one-quarter of the maximum muscular effort that can be generated. In fact, flow at a given volume may decrease as pressure increases above the optimum value.

The effort-independent portion of the expiratory curve is very reproducible in a given subject from time to time but is altered in a characteristic way as disease changes the mechanical properties of the lung.

The recording of flow plotted against volume during forced inspiration as well as expiration is referred to as a *maximal-effort flow–volume loop* (Fig. 4-5). The inspiratory limb of this loop is entirely effort-dependent; that is, no maximum flow has been defined for any portion of it. The shape of the inspiratory limb is rather symmetrical, with flow increasing to a peak about midway through inspiration, then decreasing as inspiration proceeds to total lung capacity.

The inspiratory limb of the maximal-effort flow–volume loop is more sensitive to major central airway obstruction than is the expiratory limb. The inspiratory limb is relatively little influenced by diffuse peripheral airway or parenchymal disease. Flow–volume loops including the inspiratory limb therefore have major practical usefulness when central airway obstruction is suspected, and ordinary spirometry demonstrates a nonspecific obstructive pattern.

Flow–Volume Analysis in Screening for Asymptomatic Obstructive Disease. Abnormalities of flow–volume loops in clinically manifested disease have been well defined, and this type of analysis is comparably useful to conventional spirometry in the usual types of obstructive and restrictive pulmonary disease. It has been hoped that special advantages might become apparent with further experience, especially in the area of screening for early asymptomatic obstructive disease, because maximum expiratory flow rates at low lung volumes are thought to be sensitive to resistance in small peripheral airways. In order for subtle abnormalities to be identifiable in flow–volume loops, normal values for these parameters must be established, with rather narrow confidence limits. A few studies are available providing normal values and assessment of various sorts of analyses of the flow–volume curve for screening purposes.[65,67,68–71]

The Flow–Volume Loop in Airways Obstruction. Normally the descending limb of the curve is relatively linear, with only a slight upward concavity. In patients with obstructive lung disease[61,62,64,72–74] and indeed in some normal persons, especially when initiating the forced expiration from a low lung volume, this linearity is disrupted by an initial sharp, downward deflection of the curve. This deflection corresponds to a "tracheobronchial collapse" pattern sometimes seen on a conventional spirogram. More consistently, obstructive disease produces simply an exaggerated upward concavity of the descending limb of the curve (Fig. 4-6). The descending limb usually follows a diminished peak flow in subjects with obstructive disease. Peak flow is often less impaired than flows at lower lung volumes, because peak flow appears to occur before the flow-limiting mechanism becomes operative. In addition, it is probable that abrupt emptying of the airways, during a vigorous expiratory maneuver that causes them to collapse, can result in a very brief period of high flow.

Emphysema seems to have the greatest tendency to produce early downward bowing of the descending limb of the curve. This tendency is not entirely consistent, however, and downward bowing relates to severity of obstruction as well as type of disease.

Shortening of the volume axis of the curve in both obstructive and restrictive disease indicates decreased vital capacity. This shortening is relatively less in obstructive than restrictive diseases, so that the characteristic obstructive flow–volume loop appears oriented along the horizontal axis.

Flow–Volume Loops in Central Airways Obstruction. Flow–volume loops may be especially helpful in identifying tracheal or upper-airway disease as a cause of obstruction. Central airway obstruction tends to produce a blunted, upwardly bowed appearance of the descending limb of the maximum-effort expiratory flow–volume curve. This appearance of a high flow "plateau" takes the place of the usual rapid rise to and descent from peak flow.[75–77] When a characteristic expiratory curve or clinical information such as an audible inspiratory stridor suggests central airway obstruction, particular attention should be given to the inspiratory limb of a flow-volume loop.

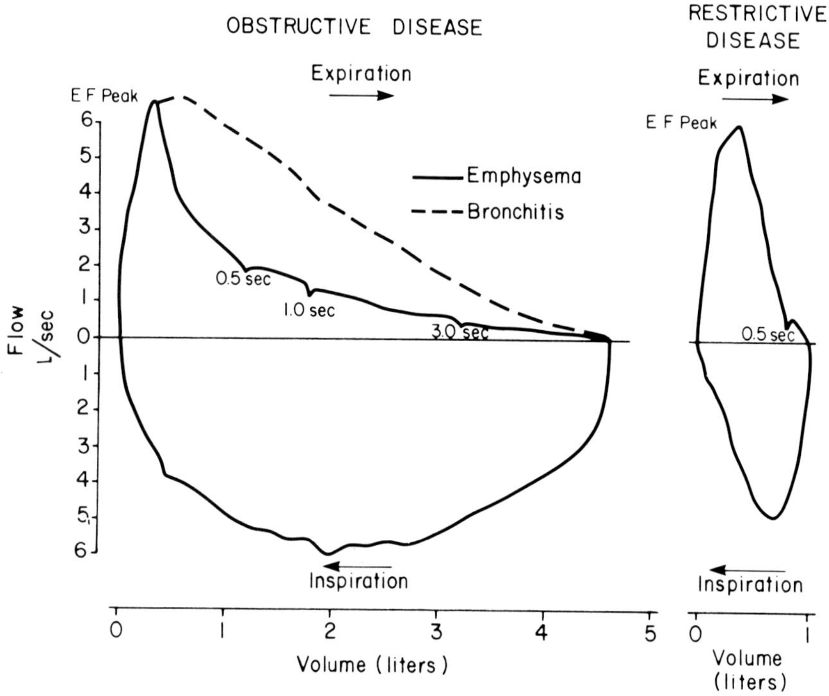

FIG. 4-6. Maximum-effort flow-volume curves in obstructive and restrictive disease. Typical flow-volume loops for a patient with obstructive disease (*left*) and a patient with restrictive disease (*right*). Note that patients with obstructive disease have reduced expiratory flow rates, particularly at low lung volumes. In emphysema, with obstruction primarily due to loss of elastic recoil, there is an early peak flow as the airways collapse, followed by severely reduced flow rates during sustained expiratory effort. This "collapsing" expiratory flow curve is typical of advanced emphysema.

Miller and Hyatt[76,77] described characteristic flow–volume loop abnormalities occurring in central airway obstructions of three types: fixed obstruction, variable extrathoracic obstruction, and variable intrathoracic obstruction. The type of pattern produced depends on the location and character of the lesion, as well as the rigidity of the adjacent tracheal wall.

In fixed obstruction the diameter of neither the obstructed lumen nor the proximal or distal trachea is altered by changes in transmural pressure. Such an obstruction, whether intrathoracic or extrathoracic, produces a similar decrease in inspiratory and expiratory flow rates. This proportionate obstruction to both phases of respiration is in contrast to the predominant expiratory slowing seen with diffuse peripheral airways obstruction. The ratio of mid-vital capacity flow rate during expiration to that during inspiration permits quantification of this phenomenon.

When central airway obstruction is variable, the flow–volume loop produced depends on location of the lesion. The extrathoracic trachea has a negative intraluminal pressure (relative to atmospheric) during inspiration and a positive pressure during expiration. This may result in a tendency to collapse during inspiration and to dilate on expiration. Extrathoracic obstruction is therefore commonly worse during inspiration than expiration. The intrathoracic trachea, however, is subjected to the intrathoracic pressure swings. These tend to dilate the trachea during inspiration and to collapse it during expiration. Obstructing lesions of the intrathoracic trachea, therefore, impair inspiration to a lesser degree than expiration.

The pattern of variable extrathoracic obstruction, then, consists of a predominant decrease in inspiratory flow rates. Variable intrathoracic obstruction predominantly affects expiratory flow, in a pattern similar to that of diffuse peripheral obstruction, but often characterized by a plateau following a peak flow, rather than by downward bowing of the expiratory limb.

Flow–Volume Loops in Restrictive Ventilatory Disorders. Because restrictive disorders are characterized by a predominant decrease in vital capacity and less impaired flow rates, the typical flow–volume curve in restriction is tall and narrow.[73,74] (Fig. 4-6). Peak expiratory flow is relatively preserved, and the descending portion of the expiratory limb is straightened, falling sharply downward from peak flow to residual volume. The loop often maintains a nearly normal shape, appearing miniaturized in all dimensions.

Measurement of Lung Volumes

Conventional terminology for the subdivisions of lung volume has been discussed elsewhere (Fig. 4-1).[43] All of these subdivisions can be measured directly with simple spirometry, except those containing residual volume. Residual volume is the quantity of air contained in the lungs at the end of a full expiration and can be measured only by special techniques. These generally utilize the body plethysmograph or inert gas dilution or washout,[78–81] or planimetric measurement of chest roentgenograms[82–86] (see list below). Functional residual capacity and total lung capacity both contain residual volume and therefore cannot be measured without these techniques.

Methods for Measurement of Subdivisions of Lung Volume

- Methods that underestimate lung volume in obstructive disease and bullous disease
  - Nitrogen washout[78]
  - Helium dilution[80]
- Methods that accurately measure lung volume in obstructive disease and bullous disease
  - Plethysmography[79]
  - Planimetry of chest roentgenograms[82–86]

These techniques can be adapted to measure any quantity of gas contained in the lungs at the time the test is initiated. That is, one could measure RV by initiating the test at maximum expiration; FRC by initiating the test at resting expiration; or TLC by initiating the test at full inspiration. One such measurement would be sufficient, because vital capacity, inspiratory capacity, and expiratory reserve volume, measurable from simple spirometry, can be added or subtracted to compute the remaining volumes.

By convention, FRC is selected for measurement by inert gas or body box; RV is calculated by subtracting ERV; and TLC is calculated by adding IC. The reason for this selection is simple: FRC is the most effort-independent and reproducible of the volumes. To achieve RV by exhaling fully requires effort, understanding, and cooperation. To achieve TLC by inhaling fully also requires effort, understanding, and cooperation. FRC is attained normally at the end of each tidal breath and requires no patient cooperation. An alert technician can initiate the test at the end of a normal breath simply by observing the patient.

Inert gas techniques usually used to measure FRC are nitrogen washout[78] (Fig. 4-7) and helium dilution[80] (Fig. 4-8). These two gases are harmless and are neither produced nor used by the body. Their concentrations can be measured simply and rapidly by equipment that is commercially available at moderate cost.

Nitrogen normally represents 79% of the total gaseous atmospheric constituents. It exists within the lungs at approximately the same level (approximate because oxygen utilization and carbon dioxide production slightly alter the concentration, but not the amount, of nitrogen). To measure FRC by nitrogen washout, pure oxygen is inhaled in order to wash the nitrogen from the lungs. The exhaled gas is collected and its volume measured, and the nitrogen concentration is analyzed. Knowing the amount of nitrogen that was washed out and the concentration in which it was present in the lungs, one can calculate the lung volume in which it was contained. To determine FRC accurately by this technique, the washout process must be initiated properly at resting expiration by a quick

$$V_1C_1 = V_2\,C_2$$
$$V_1 = \frac{V_2\,C_2}{C_1}$$

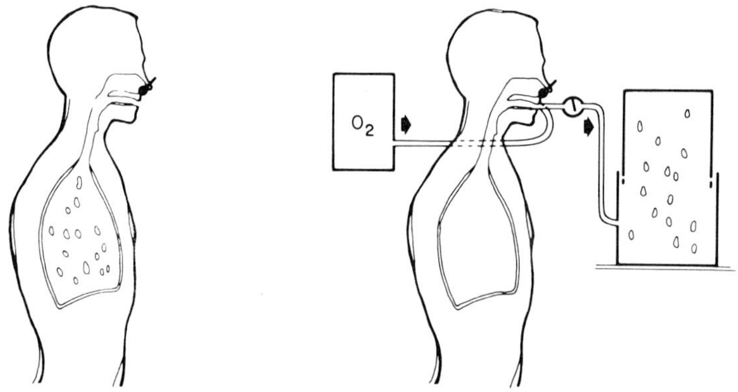

A B

FIG. 4-7. Lung volume determination by nitrogen washout. **A.** Resting expiration prior to test. **B.** Resting expiration at end of test. V_1 = volume of lungs (to be determined); C_1 = concentration of nitrogen in lungs at beginning of test (assumed to be 79%, as in room air); V_2 = volume of gas in spirometer at end of test (measured); C_2 = concentration of nitrogen in spirometer at end of test (measured).

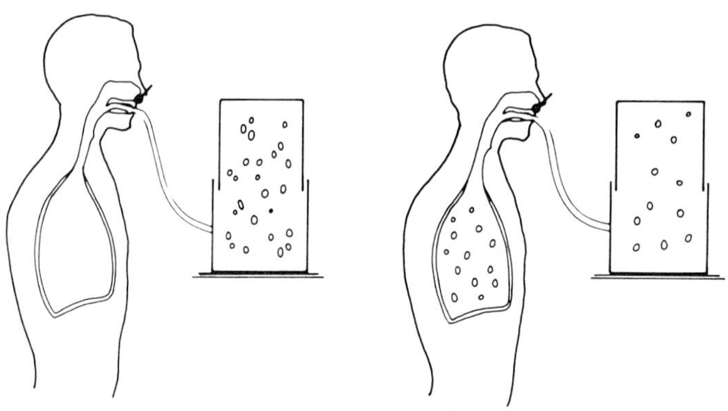

$$C_1\,V_1 = C_2\,V_2$$
$$V_2 = C_1\,V_1\,\frac{C_1\,V_1}{C_2}$$
$$FRC = V_2 - V_1$$

A B

FIG. 4-8. Lung volume measurement by helium dilution. **A.** Resting expiration at beginning of test. **B.** Resting expiration at end of test. Helium is now evenly distributed throughout lungs and spirometer. C_1 = concentration of helium in spirometer at beginning of test (measured); V_1 = volume of gas in spirometer (measured); C_2 = concentration of helium in spirometer and in patient's lungs at end of test (measured); V_2 = volume of gas in spirometer and in patient's lungs combined (to be calculated).

turn of a valve in the circuit. The washout must be continued until nitrogen is emptied from all parts of the lung. This process is normally completed in less than 7 min but may require 20 or 30 min in patients with obstructive disease who have abnormal distribution of ventilation. The washout must take place within a completely closed system, with a well-fitting mouthpiece and a nose clip in place; and it must be uninterrupted, because the addition of nitrogen to the system from room air invalidates the calculation.

Helium dilution is performed by introducing the patient into a circuit containing a known volume and concentration of helium. Carbon diox-

$$
\begin{aligned}
P_1 V_1 &= P_2 V_2 \\
P_1 V_1 &= P_2 (V_1 + \Delta V) \\
P_1 V_1 &= P_2 V_1 + P_2 \Delta V \\
P_1 V_1 - P_2 V_1 &= P_2 \Delta V \\
V_1 (P_1 - P_2) &= P_2 \Delta V \\
V_1 &= \frac{P_2 \Delta V}{P_1 - P_2}
\end{aligned}
$$

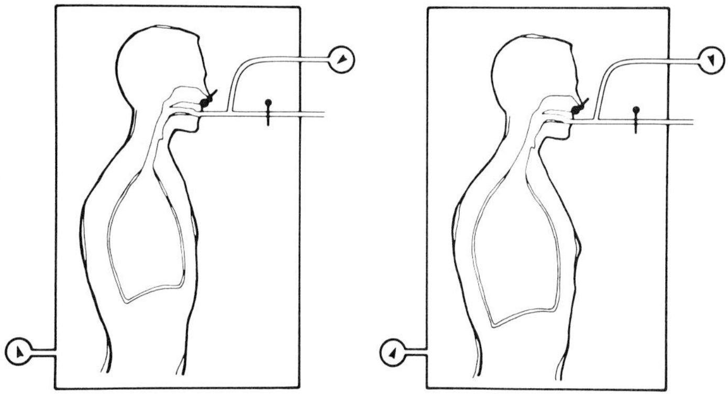

A B

FIG. 4-9. Measurement of lung volume by plethysmograph. **A.** Resting expiration. **B.** Inspiratory effort. P_1 = alveolar pressure during resting expiration (measured at the mouth); V_1 = volume of lungs during resting expiration (to be determined); P_2 = alveolar pressure during inspiratory effort (measured at the mouth); V_2 = volume of lungs during inspiratory effort (unknown); $\Delta V = V_1 - V_2$ (measured as box pressure change).

ide is removed from the system by an adsorbent, and oxygen is added at the rate at which it is consumed. After an appropriate time for equilibration of helium throughout the system (7 to 30 min), the study is terminated. Equilibration is assumed to have occurred when the helium concentration within the circuit, which is continually monitored, stabilizes. The helium concentration at the end of the test is lower than the initial concentration, in proportion to the volume of the FRC by which it has been diluted.

These two techniques, nitrogen washout and helium dilution, have similar limitations. Patients with blebs or bullae that are very poorly ventilated may not have equilibration of these areas of the lung with the helium or nitrogen circuit during the time the test is carried out, and therefore falsely low values for FRC may be obtained.

Plethysmography. The body plethysmograph overcomes this handicap by utilizing Boyle's law, and measurements of pressure and volume change during ventilatory efforts against a closed shutter to measure FRC[79] (Fig. 4-9). This technique employs more expensive instrumentation than the inert gas techniques. Total gas volume within the chest at the initiation of the test sequence is measured, however, and air spaces in poor communication with airways are included. Prior to surgery to remove bullae, FRC determined by inert gas techniques can be subtracted from FRC determined by plethysmography, in order to provide an estimate of the volume occupied by bullae that are functionally not in communication with the airways. A discrepancy between values obtained by the two techniques does not prove the presence of discrete bullae, however, because diffuse emphysema or small-airways disease may produce such a discrepancy.

For determination of FRC by plethysmography, the subject is placed in a large, sealed chamber, with a mouthpiece in place that can be occluded by a remotely operated shutter. A sensitive pressure transducer measures pressure at the mouth, proximal to the shutter. This pressure, under conditions of no air flow, is assumed to reflect pressure within the thorax. Another pressure transducer measures pressure in the chamber, outside the subject's thorax. As inspiratory and expiratory efforts are made by the subject against the closed shutter, volume changes within the thorax cause volume changes in the chamber and are reflected by pressure changes in the chamber. Pressure change in "the box" is thus employed to measure volume change within the thorax. We thus have a system in which a subject can attempt to breathe against a closed shutter, expanding and contracting the air within his chest. Two parameters can be measured during this maneuver: pressure in the chest and volume change within the chest. Note that chest pressure can be measured against atmospheric pressure during both attempted inspiration and attempted expiration. Volume in the chest cannot be measured, but volume change from inspiratory to expiratory effort can be measured. These data are sufficient to calculate lung volume at the initiation of the test according to Boyle's formula, relating pressure change to volume change. This system, a constant-volume, variable-pressure plethysmograph, is replaced by a constant-pressure, variable-volume unit in some laboratories.[13]

Roentgenography. Planimetric measurement of total lung capacity, using posteroanterior and lateral chest roentgenograms, has been demonstrated to be an acceptable substitute for inert gas and plethysmographic methods.[82–86] Logistical considerations may favor the selection of a roentgenographic method in some hospitals (Fig. 4-10).

Measurement of the subdivisions of lung volume is of greatest interest when a ventilatory defect is mixed or indeterminate, as demonstrated by simple volume–time spirometry. Extreme elevations of residual volume and an increase in total lung capacity strongly support a diagnosis of an obstructive disorder, especially emphysema. A decrease in residual volume and total lung capacity defines a restrictive defect and may force strong consideration of a group of disease processes of entirely different etiology. The additional information gained from measurement of compliance and airways resistance may complete the physiological profile in a subject with mixed disease, clarifying the relative contributions of each disorder to the ventilatory dysfunction.

Satisfactory estimation of predicted values for normal populations has been carried out in order to facilitate the interpretation of measurements performed in individual patients.[30,35,49]

Abnormalities of Ventilation at Rest and During Exercise

Tidal breathing at rest requires far less than a normal person's maximum ability to ventilate. Therefore, ventilatory impairment due to disease must be extremely severe before it significantly reduces minute ventilation at rest. Disease can alter mechanics sufficiently, however, to change the pattern of tidal breathing, as discussed in Chapter 2. Obesity tends to produce a reduced tidal volume and increased rate, as do interstitial edema, fibrosis, and other parenchymal and chest disorders that decrease compliance of the lungs or thorax. Disorders that increase airways resistance often produce a relatively slow, deep breathing pattern, though not consistently. Disorders of regulation of respiration produce characteristic patterns of breathing which may be diagnostic; these are discussed in detail in Chapter 6.

Ventilatory efficiency also can be altered by disease, so that increased minute ventilation at rest is required for normal gas exchange (Table 4-4). Normal variation in ventilatory patterns and efficiency is so great, however, that the diagnostic usefulness of such alterations is limited. Measurement of alterations in ventilation during exercise may be somewhat more informative.[51,87]

An average-sized normal adult male at rest breathes about 16 to 18 times each minute, exchanging about 500 ml of air during each breath. Of each breath, about 150 ml is "wasted," ventilating only airways (anatomical dead space) and poorly perfused areas of lung (alveolar dead space). The total of this wasted ventilation is referred to as *physiological dead space* ventilation. The remainder of each breath takes part in gas exchange by coming into intimate contact with pulmonary capillaries, contributing oxygen to and removing carbon dioxide from the blood. This portion is referred to as *alveolar ventilation*.

Because there is considerable normal variation in blood flow and ventilation distribution, the amount of physiological dead space varies from person to person, and the amount of each breath that contributes to gas exchange (alveolar ventilation) varies. Variation in depth of respiration also varies normally from person to person. For purposes of gas exchange, slow ventilation is more efficient than rapid, shallow ventilation, because a greater portion of each breath contributes to alveolar ventilation (Table 4-5).

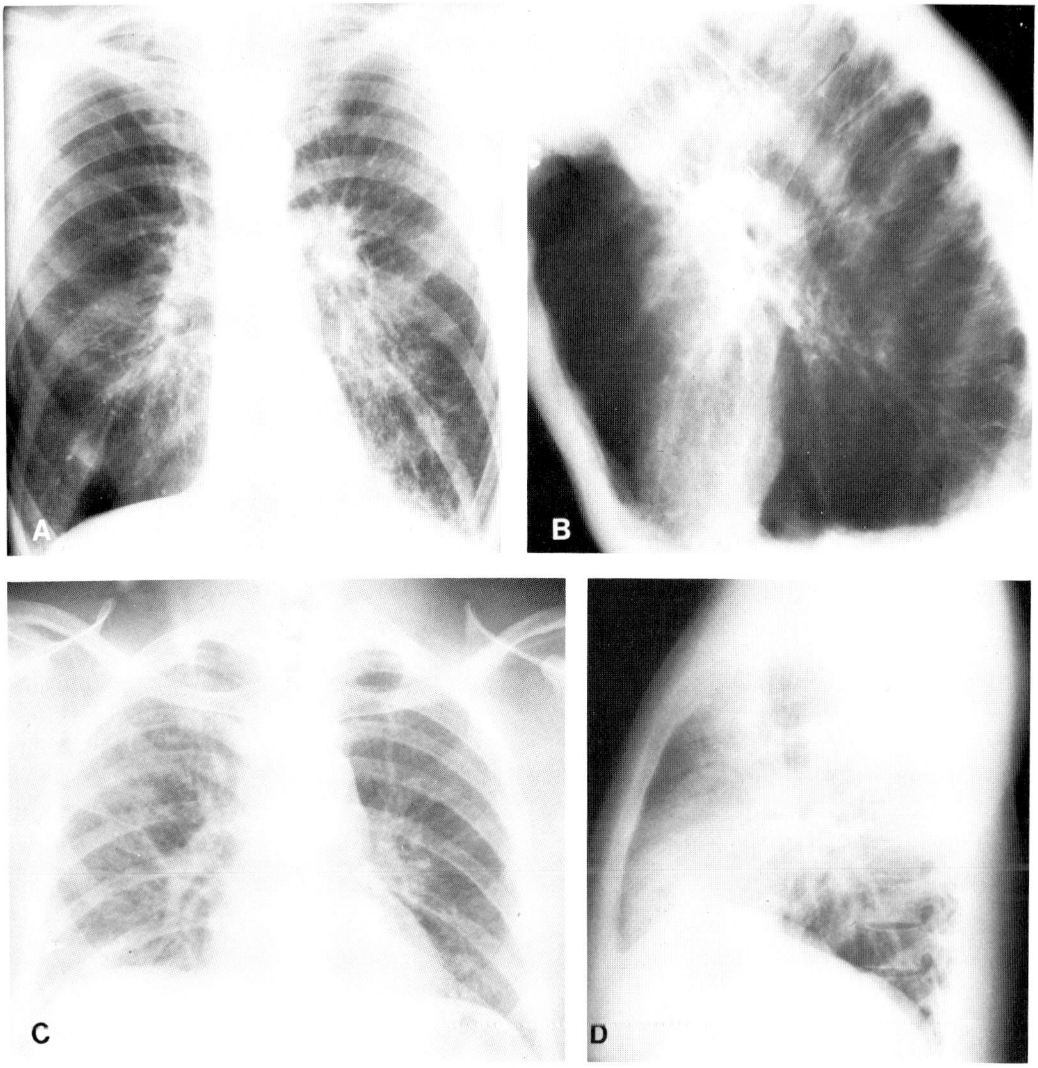

FIG. 4-10. Chest radiographs of patients with abnormally large and small lung volumes. **A, B.** Patient with emphysema. Total lung capacity = 14.6 liters (194% predicted). **C, D.** Patient with sarcoidosis. Total lung capacity = 4.5 liters (71% predicted).

Because of these factors (variation in physiological dead space and variation in ventilatory pattern), efficiency of ventilation varies from one normal person to another. Minute ventilation required to provide adequate gas exchange for a given metabolic demand is therefore inconstant.

Efficiency of ventilation can be expressed conveniently in terms of minute ventilation required per liter of oxygen consumed (ventilatory equivalent of oxygen consumption). The normal ventilatory equivalent ranges from 20 to 30 liters of ventilation for each liter of oxygen consumed.[87] A reciprocal of this measurement, percentage of oxygen extraction, is an equally convenient expression of ventilatory efficiency. Ventilatory equivalent of oxygen extraction can be assessed simply by measuring minute ventilation and oxygen consumption; or the latter can be estimated rather closely, knowing body size and level of activity and referring to tables readily available.[88] As mentioned previously, however, the wide range of normal values limits the

TABLE 4-4. Methods of Assessing Ventilatory Impairment as a Factor Limiting Exercise Tolerance

Method	Requires Measurement of
1. Efficiency of ventilation	
Ventilatory equivalent of oxygen consumption	Minute ventilation and oxygen consumption
Ventilation required for exercise	Minute ventilation and exercise load (treadmill, bicycle ergometer)
Oxygen extraction	Oxygen concentration of inspired and expired air
2. Maximum exercise load clinically tolerated	Exercise load, observation of clinical distress, pulse, blood pressure. If available, electrocardiogram, arterial blood gases, and oxygen consumption may be useful
3. Maximum voluntary ventilation	Minute ventilation during brief stint of maximum effort
4. Maximum oxygen consumption	Oxygen consumption at increasing exercise loads until plateau is reached
5. Predicted maximum oxygen consumption	Ventilatory equivalent of oxygen consumption at submaximal exercise and maximum voluntary ventilation

TABLE 4-5. Relationship of Dead Space to Alveolar Ventilation*

Total Minute Ventilation	Respiratory Rate	Tidal Volume	Physiological Dead Space	Alveolar Ventilation
(A) 8 l/min	16	500 ml	150 ml	5.6 l/min
(B) 8 l/min	8	1,000 ml	250 ml	6.0 l/min
(C) 8 l/min	16	500 ml	250 ml	4.0 l/min

* Note that the same minute ventilation may result in widely varying alveolar ventilation. A normal relationship of about one-third dead space ventilation is illustrated in A. This is contrasted with a larger tidal volume in B. Dead space increases normally with increased tidal volume, but not directly proportionately. In C, an abnormally high dead space results in reduced alveolar ventilation.

diagnostic usefulness of such information. Change in ventilatory efficiency, especially during exercise, can be demonstrated in an individual person over a period of time, however. Improvement due to breathing retraining and physical conditioning can be demonstrated and quantitated in this way.[89]

The most predictable change in ventilatory efficiency occurs at altitude. Ventilation is increased approximately proportional to the reduction in molecular oxygen available per unit volume. Therefore, when the atmospheric pressure is reduced to half normal, the ventilation at rest would be approximately double for the same level of oxygen consumption (see Chap. 1).

The deterioration in ventilatory efficiency that occurs in disease is chiefly due to the mechanism of ventilation–perfusion imbalance. Increased physiological dead space occurs whenever redistribution of ventilation and perfusion results in decreased blood flow to well-ventilated areas or in increased ventilation to poorly perfused areas. Ventilation in excess of perfusion is wasted ventilation, because it does not result in increased gas exchange. Therefore, total minute ventilation for a given metabolic demand is increased, to provide adequate alveolar ventilation in the face of increased wasted ventilation. When altered mechanical characteristics of the lung and chest wall result in a rapid, shallow breathing pattern, efficiency of ventilation is further reduced, owing to the increased proportion of dead space per breath. Ventilation–perfusion imbalance results to some extent from most disorders that alter the mechanical properties of the lungs: airways disease, interstitial disease of various sorts, pneumonia, and neoplasms. Chest-wall diseases may alter ventilatory patterns to such an extent that ventilation–perfusion imbalance occurs. Chronic obstructive lung disease is one of the most common and most important of the diseases that cause increased physiological dead space. Improvement in this physiological dysfunction occurs whenever the basic disease process is reversed; but even in the face of irreversible disease, some physiological improvement may occur. Breathing training, with development of a slow, deep ventilatory pattern, may be especially useful.

Ventilatory efficiency is, in fact, the major ventilatory parameter that can consistently be demonstrated to improve over time through rehabilitation programs that incorporate breathing retraining and physical conditioning.[89] For simplicity of measurement in such a program, minute ventilation is usually measured during a given level of exercise without measurement of oxygen consumption. Standardized exercise on a treadmill or bicycle ergometer is carried out on successive occasions. Minute ventilation is measured: a decrease in the ventilation required for a specified work load reflects improved efficiency.

The exercise test is a very complex tool for evaluating physical performance.[88,90–98] The interpretation of the results must include consideration of cardiovascular status because claudication, fixed low cardiac output, arrhythmias, or angina may be limiting factors. Altitude, anemia, or carboxyhemoglobin may limit exercise by reducing oxygen availability. A clear understanding of the role and physiology of physical training or conditioning is essential; reduced maximum tolerated work, inordinate fatigue, or tachycardia may not represent disease, but merely a low level of fitness.[95–97] In asthmatics, exercise may be used as a diagnostic provocative test.[98]

Exercise testing may play a future role in assessing other organ systems. Altered levels of endorphins, profound effects on the hypothalamic–pituitary axis, changes in levels of clotting factors, and immune mechanisms are all under study. In some diseases of muscle metabolism, such as phosphorylase deficiency, exercise may be diagnostic in eliciting metabolic defects.

Clinical Applications of Exercise Testing

- Assessment of respiratory dysfunction
  - Evaluation of dyspnea
  - Quantitation of disability
  - Provocative test for bronchospasm
- Assessment of cardiovascular disease
  - Evaluation of dyspnea
  - Assessment of arrhythmias
  - Assessment of peripheral vascular disease
  - Assessment of ischemic heart disease
  - Hemodynamic evaluation
- Assessment of fitness (conditioning)
  - Specific muscle groups
  - Total performance
- Evaluation of other organ systems' response to exercise (immune, endocrine, central nervous system, hematopoietic, musculoskeletal)

Exercise evaluation in the laboratory must be tailored to provide the clinical and physiological data required for each patient. This may range from simple observation of the patient, with measured pulse and ventilatory rate at known exercise loads, through various levels of sophistication, to include measurements of blood gases, alveolar–arterial oxygen gradients, diffusing capacity, cardiac output, mixed venous blood gases, estimates of oxygen debt, anaerobic metabolism, use of blood nutrients and assays of metabolites, and multiple-lead electrocardiograms. Various stages of exercise evaluation have been established in some laboratories.[94]

The pulmonary laboratory is often called upon to quantitate exercise capacity in a patient with respiratory dysfunction. Direct and indirect means are available to carry out this request. A simple, direct approach consists of observing the subject perform standardized exercise on a treadmill or bicycle ergometer. Pulse rate, respiratory rate, and the patient's appearance and subjective complaints of distress usually provide a reasonable guide to the maximum amount of exercise he is able to perform and sustain. It has been suggested[88] that exercise testing not be pressed to levels of intensity that result in heart rates above 170 per min for subjects aged 20 to 29 yr, decreasing to 130 per min for subjects age 60 to 69. Signs or symptoms of circulatory insufficiency, including inappropriate bradycardia for a given level of exercise, should signal cessation of the test. The level of exercise achieved can be related to various activities of daily living by reference to published tables.[90] The specific physiological function that limits exercise in a given patient may not be readily apparent. Malingering is usually easy to recognize, though it may be difficult to prove.

A simple, indirect approach to assessing ventilatory impairment during exercise is the measurement of maximal voluntary ventilation.[51] This reflects a subject's ability to perform a brief stint, not a sustained level of ventilation. It is a reasonable rule of thumb that most persons can sustain a level of exercise requiring a minute ventilation of 35 to 50% of their MVV. Considering that 30 liters of ventilation is the upper limit of normal required to sustain a liter of oxygen consumption and that diseased persons may have somewhat less efficient ventilation, it is possible to roughly estimate the degree of exercise limitation, in terms of oxygen consumption. The oxygen requirements for common activities of daily living can then be obtained from tables such as those available through the American Heart Association.[90] In this way, exercise limitation can be translated into readily understandable terms. It is evident that a person with a normal MVV may have severe exercise impairment due to other causes (see list below).

Some Factors That May Limit Exercise Tolerance in Disease

- Decreased ventilatory reserve
- Hypoxemia, anemia, carboxyhemoglobin
- Cardiovascular disease: angina, limited cardiac output, arrhythmias, peripheral vascular disease
- Musculoskeletal disorders
- Dyspnea in absence of objective ventilatory impairment
- Malingering

Measurement of maximum oxygen consumption in the sense intended by physiologists implies repeated measurement of oxygen consumption at successively increasing exercise loads until a plateau is reached, above which increased exercise no longer results in increased oxygen consumption. This sort of measurement is neither safe nor practical for clinical purposes in patients with cardiorespiratory disease. Measurement of oxygen consumption at a maximum exercise load that is clinically well tolerated, however, is a practical and useful measurement.

Armstrong and colleagues,[93] using data compiled by Wright, suggested an approach to quantitating exercise impairment due to ventilatory limitation. Their technique consists of the measurement of the ventilatory equivalent of oxygen consumption at a submaximal exercise level, and the measurement of maximum voluntary ventilation. A predicted maximum oxygen consumption is then calculated from the following formula:

$$\dot{V}O_2 \text{ max} = 0.018 \text{ MVV (L/min)} - 0.044\ O_{2\ \dot{V}E} + 2.14$$

Assessment of gas exchange in the lungs and the effects of lung disease on arterial blood gases during exercise are discussed in Chapter 5.

Airways Resistance

Air flow into and out of the airways of the lungs, like flow of fluid through any system of tubes, is dependent on driving pressure across the system and on the resistance of the system. In the case of the respiratory tract, driving pressure is the difference between pressure in the alveoli and the atmospheric pressure at the mouth; and resistance of the system of tubes is airways resistance as defined by the formula

$$\text{airway resistance (cm } H_2O\text{/L/sec)} = \frac{\text{alveolar pressure (cm } H_2O) - \text{mouth pressure (cm } H_2O)}{\text{flow (L/sec)}}$$

Tissue viscous resistance is quantitatively small but contributes to the total frictional resistance of the lungs. Resistance of such a system in turn depends on length and cross-sectional area, as well as on flow characteristics of the fluid.[13,99]

Theoretical concepts that have application to air flow in the pulmonary airways are considered in depth in Chapter 3.

The usual clinical approach to diagnosis and quantitation of obstructive disease of the airways is the measurement of expiratory flow during maximum effort. It is tacitly assumed that effort, hence the alveolus-to-mouth pressure gradient, is constant and that decreased flow is evidence of increased resistance of airways. With some qualifications, this simplified approach can be clinically useful, but of course it is not physiologically correct. Determination of actual airways resistance is more informative but requires measurement of alveolar pressure, and this measurement presents technical problems.

Methods of Measuring Air-Flow Resistance

Techniques used to measure total pulmonary resistance
- Transpulmonary pressure (esophageal balloon)[100]
- Forced oscillations[101]

Techniques used to measure only airways resistance
- Estimation of alveolar pressure by momentary flow interruption[102]
- Panting technique with plethysmography and sustained shutter closure[103]

In fact, analysis of pressure–flow characteristics of breathing presents complications beyond the technical problem of measuring alveolar pressure.[99] The diameter and length of the airways are not constant; they are continually changing during respiration. In addition, the intricate branching of the system of airways results in a changing combination of laminar and turbulent flow, which influences pressure–flow relationships. In spite of these problems, the measurement of airways resistance has been tackled with some degree of success by techniques briefly described below. In each case, the description concentrates on the problem of measurement of alveolar pressure, because flow can be easily obtained by flow meters or as volume change per unit of time, measured with a conventional spirometer.

Techniques of Assessing Airways Resistance. Alveolar pressure in any phase of respiration is the algebraic sum of pleural (esophageal) pressure and lung elastic recoil pressure. This relationship is true throughout the respiratory cycle but is most easily understood by considering active expiration. During a forced expiration, the positive alveolar pressure that drives air from alveolus to mouth is the sum of elastic recoil pressure (tending to deflate the lungs) and positive pleural pressure (compressing the lungs). Elastic recoil pressure can be measured as the reciprocal of negative pleural (esophageal) pressure when there is no air flow. During active expiration, positive pleural pressure is created by respiratory muscle contraction and is measured as positive esophageal pressure. Therefore, alveolar pressure at any level of lung volume during a forced expiratory maneuver is the sum of two different pressures: elastic recoil pressure (measured under static conditions at that lung volume) and pressure created by active muscle contraction under dynamic conditions. To arrive at alveolar pressure, then, two separate measurements must be carried out. A static pressure–volume curve must be constructed from numerous measurements of esophageal pressure at different levels of inflation. A dynamic pressure–volume curve must be traced during forced expiration. The alveolar pressure at any level of inflation can be obtained by adding the two pressure measurements taken at that level during the two maneuvers. Alveolar pressure during tidal breathing can be calculated by measuring compliance as "dynamic" compliance, taking esophageal pressure measurements at points of no flow, at end inspiration and expiration.[100] This technique actually measures total flow resistance, including tissue viscous as well as airways resistance. A newer method of measuring flow-resistive forces, utilizing forced oscillations generated from a loudspeaker,[101] is described in Chapter 3.

Another technique (simpler, but perhaps not entirely valid) is the flow-interruption technique, in which a forced expiration is carried out through a mouthpiece, and momentary shutter closure interrupts flow.[102] Pressure at the mouth is measured during flow interruption and is assumed to equal alveolar pressure. In patients with airways obstruction, it is believed that equilibrium of pressure from alveolus to mouth may be sufficiently delayed to invalidate this technique. This technique measures only the resistance of the airways.

A fourth technique, using the body plethysmograph, is currently popular, and commercially available automated instrumentation has been designed around it.[103] It consists of a two-part test, carried out during a rapid, shallow, panting maneuver in order to minimize phase lag and the changes in airways resistance that occur with change in the level of inflation. Panting is carried out with similar effort with an open shutter, and then against a closed shutter. The entire test is carried out within a sealed cabinet. Pressure change within the chamber is monitored during the maneuver, as chest expansion and contraction displace volume and alter chamber pressure. With the shutter open, flow is plotted against chamber pressure on an X-Y recorder or oscilloscope. With the shutter closed, mouth pressure is plotted against chamber pressure. Under conditions of no flow, imposed by the shutter, mouth pressure is assumed to be equal to alveolar pressure. In this way, two relationships are measured: flow to chamber pressure, and alveolar pressure to chamber pressure. From these two relationships, a third relationship can be calculated: flow to alveolar pressure. This third relationship is, in fact, airways resistance. This method of measuring airways resistance appears to be theoretically valid; is reproducible; and changes predictably with diseases and drugs that would be expected to alter airways resistance. It provides a single estimate, at only one lung volume, of airways resistance during the artificial circumstance of the panting maneuver.

It has been demonstrated that in the normal lung, most of the resistance to flow is in airways central to those that are 2 mm in diameter and less.[104] So little resistance occurs in the smaller peripheral airways that considerable narrowing due to disease must occur before total airways resistance is significantly altered. Because these airways appear to be the site of most of the pathological changes in chronic obstructive lung disease, airways resistance is an insensitive test for identifying early disease of this sort (see Chap 3). Severe asthma and bronchitis, however, are associated with elevation of airways resistance, which improves with bronchodilator drugs. It appears that emphysema without bronchospasm or bronchitis can cause significant slowing of maximum expiratory flow rates without causing elevation of airways resistance. Two factors may explain this phenomenon. The major cause of slowed flow in this situation may be the loss of the contribution of elastic recoil to lung deflation, and the airways may be unaffected. On the other hand, loss of elastic support may permit the airways to collapse, and pressures in the alveoli distal to the collapsed segments may not be transmitted to the mouth, thereby invalidating the alveolar pressure measurement.

Compliance

Compliance of the lungs and chest wall is, for most clinicians, a rather nebulous physiological concept, with little application to practice. In fact, compliance is a rather simple mechanical property that undergoes major alterations in disease and can be easily measured.[13,99,105–109]

Compliance is simply distensibility. Physiologically, it is defined as volume change (in milliliters) produced by pressure change (in centimeters of water). By definition, compliance is a static quality or measurement and is not influenced by frictional forces or inertia. Compliance of the lungs, or lungs and thorax, might be defined as the pressure required to maintain a given level of inflation. Elastance, or elastic recoil, is the reciprocal of compliance and is the tendency of the lungs, or lungs and thorax, to return to a given level of inflation.

Because elastic forces are stored, an inflated chest contains energy to return it to FRC; hence, active work is not usually required for tidal exhalation. Exhalation is ordinarily passive, requiring little or no contraction of muscles of respiration, except to overcome resistive forces, which are normally small during tidal breathing.

Compliance of the lungs can be measured clinically with the use of an esophageal balloon (Fig. 4-11); compliance of the lungs and chest

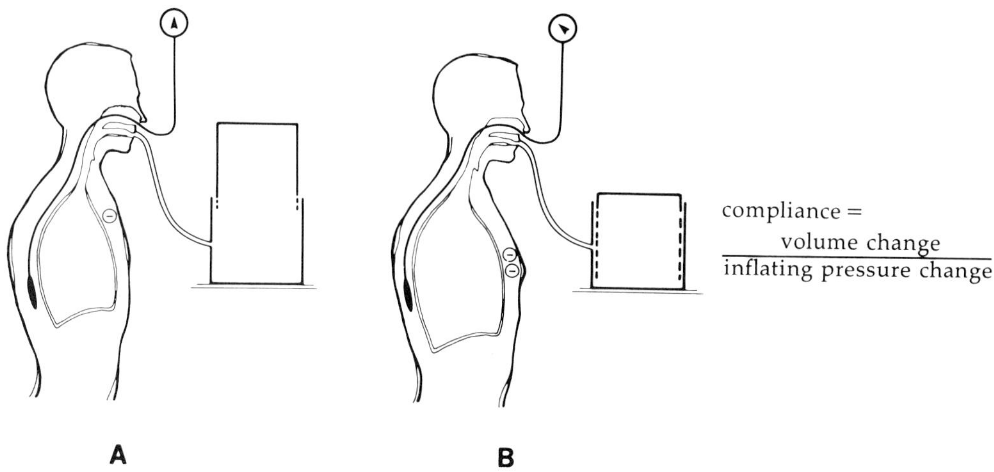

FIG. 4-11. Lung compliance. **A.** Resting expiration. **B.** Breath-holding during inspiration, with glottis open. Change in lung volume is measured with a conventional spirometer. Change in inflating pressure (intrapleural pressure) is measured with an intraesophageal balloon.

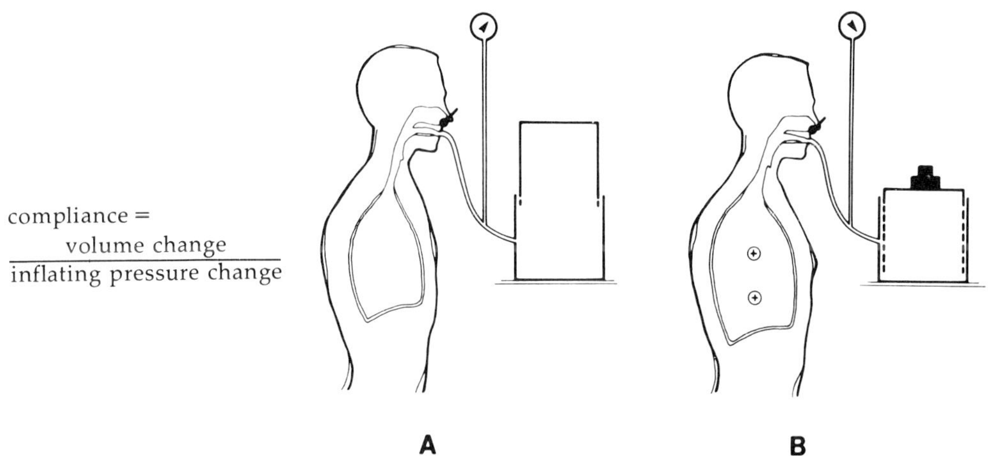

FIG. 4-12. Total respiratory compliance. **A.** Resting expiration, with weightless spirometer. **B.** Resting expiration with weighted spirometer. Change in lung volume is measured with a conventional spirometer as change in the level of FRC. Change in inflating pressure is measured as positive alveolar (mouth) pressure created by weights on the spirometer bell.

wall in concert can be measured by assessing the difference between alveolar pressure and atmospheric pressure required to maintain a known level of inflation (Fig. 4-12). These techniques will be described subsequently. Chest compliance cannot be measured directly but can be calculated from the difference between reciprocals of lung and total thoracic compliance, according to the formula

$$\frac{1}{\text{total compliance}} = \frac{1}{\text{lung compliance}} + \frac{1}{\text{chest-wall compliance}}$$

Measurement of Static Compliance of the Lung. As the lungs are suspended within the chest at any given level of inflation, it is the difference between alveolar pressure and pleural pressure that maintains that level of inflation. Whether the negative pleural pressure or the relatively positive atmospheric pressure in the alveoli is viewed as being responsible is immaterial; the difference between them is the same. Intrathoracic pressure is measured by an intraesophageal balloon, which reflects intrapleural pressure with reasonable accuracy.[105,106]; this measurement is plotted against chest volume. The volume change created by a given change in negative intrathoracic pressure, measured under conditions of no flow, is compliance. Although data for the prediction of normal values for lung elasticity are somewhat limited, normal lung compliance over the tidal volume range is about 200 ml per centimeter of water.[108] At higher levels of inflation, near the elastic limits of the lungs, compliance is reduced. Interpretation of a compliance measurement therefore requires knowledge of the level of inflation at which it is taken. An abnormally high value results when emphysema destroys alveolar walls; compliance characteristically increases with age. An abnormally low value reflects "stiffness" of the lung, caused by infiltrative diseases of the lung parenchyma, such as interstitial fibrosis.

Elastance has similar significance; specific compliance and specific elastance are those measurements corrected for the level of inflation at which they are obtained. A compliance curve can be constructed over the vital capacity range to provide a complete representation of elastic properties of the lung, or a single simplified but less informative measurement called *elastic recoil* can be obtained. Recent analysis of pressure –volume curves indicates that a slope can be established which permits more discriminating analysis than single points.[110] Elastic recoil is a term commonly applied to the maximum negative esophageal pressure that can be generated at the end of a full inspiration.

Measurement of total respiratory compliance requires knowledge of the difference between alveolar pressure and atmospheric pressure at various levels of inflation. This can be estimated in a trained subject by maintaining inflation at various levels of a passive deflation against a closed shutter or by maintaining inflation with negative pressure outside the chest, as with a Drinker respirator. These techniques require a trained and relaxed (or anesthetized) subject, to avoid interference with the test by respiratory-muscle activity. An alternative technique involves the use of a water-sealed spirometer with a weighted bell.[107] The subject is directed to breathe normally, and changes in FRC are noted to occur as the weights on the bell are changed. Because FRC occurs at a moment of chest-muscle relaxation and no flow, pressure at the mouth at FRC is equal to alveolar pressure. The change in FRC in response to changes in alveolar pressure induced by the weighted bell is in effect a measure of total thoracic compliance. Normal total compliance over the tidal volume range is about 100 ml per centimeter of water pressure.

Abnormalities of Compliance. Clinically significant abnormalities of compliance are common in disease of the lungs and chest wall.[13,109] Pulmonary emphysema is the major recognized cause of abnormally increased lung compliance. At first glance, increased compliance would not appear to be a physiological disadvantage, because it implies less effort required to inflate the lungs; however, increased compliance involves loss of the ability to store elastic energy, thus impairing the ability of the lung to recoil passively to FRC. In addition the loss of elastic support of the airways permits them to collapse during expiration, which further interferes with lung emptying.

Interstitial diseases (whether resulting from edema, inflammatory infiltrate, granulomas, or fibrosis) cause a decrease in lung compliance. In these disorders, increased effort is required to inflate the lungs, but emptying occurs readily. A shallow rapid, ventilatory pattern results, and severe exertional dyspnea may be a concomitant of decreased compliance, as chest-wall stretch receptors recognize the increased tension required for ventilation.

Unfortunately, these approaches to the assessment of compliance involve an averaging effect. Almost certainly, variations in compliance of some lung units take place in disease, long before the average changes, thereby limiting the diagnostic usefulness. Similarly, when certain lung units are damaged (*e.g.*, large emphysematous bullae), they may reduce the average lung compliance even though many lung units are normal. Assessment of regional lung compliance is not yet possible.

A measurement known as *dynamic compliance* can be made during tidal breathing. This measurement and its significance are discussed further under the heading, Laboratory Screening for Subclinical Respiratory Disease.

Distribution of Ventilation

Even in the normal young adult, ventilation is not entirely equal throughout all areas of the lungs.[111] In the upright posture, the lower, dependent lung zones are best ventilated during tidal breathing at rest. The reason for this is that the lung parenchyma in the upper zones supports the weight of the lung beneath it, producing a more negative pleural pressure in the upper thorax and stretching the lung nearer to its elastic limit. A given change in intrapleural pressure during respiration therefore produces little change in the volume of the already distended upper lung zones but produces greater change in the volume of the lower zones. Interesting phenomena occur with deeper breathing above and below the tidal volume range, however.

During an inspiration to TLC, ventilation is distributed preferentially to upper zones, beginning at some point above tidal volume after the lower zones have been filled. During exhalation below FRC, ventilation to and from dependent lower zones ceases, owing to functional, if not anatomical, closure of the airways. The volume at which this occurs is referred to as *closing volume*. The principles underlying this measurement are discussed in detail in Chapter 3.

In the recumbent posture, airway closure occurs chiefly in the posterior lung zones, which are now dependent.[112] Closing volume increases with age[113,114] after maturity, and with the onset of chronic obstructive lung disease. The increase is more functionally significant in the recumbent posture than in the upright posture, because FRC is less in the supine position than in the sitting position. When airway closure occurs above FRC (that is, within the tidal-volume range), dependent lung zones cease to be ventilated but continue to be perfused, and ventilation-perfusion imbalance ensues, with physiological shunting and arterial hypoxemia. Closing volume above FRC occurs with normal aging, first in the recumbent and later in the upright posture, accounting for at least part of the drop in arterial oxygen tension that occurs with age. Obstructive lung disease accelerates these changes with age, which presumably are related to loss of elastic recoil, at least in part.

In addition to these changes in regional distribution of ventilation, patchy unevenness of ventilation occurs in emphysema, bronchitis, and asthma, owing to uneven changes in compliance and airways resistance. These changes have long been recognized and studied by single-breath[115,116] and multiple-breath nitrogen washout techniques.[117] Single-breath nitrogen washout is carried out by continuous measurement of nitrogen concentration at the mouth during a full exhalation from total lung capacity, following a single inhalation of pure oxygen. Normal distribution of ventilation results in an "alveolar plateau" of uniform nitrogen concentration in the gas leaving all portions of the lung parenchyma. Uneven distribution disrupts the alveolar plateau. The closing volume measured by the nitrogen washout technique is a refinement of the traditional single-breath technique and appears to be sensitive to early, asymptomatic obstructive disease (see Fig. 3-7B). During multiple-breath nitrogen washout, the nitrogen concentration is monitored at the mouth during tidal breathing of pure oxygen, which slowly replaces nitrogen. Normal distribution of ventilation is indicated by a smooth, rapid (exponential) decrease in expired nitrogen concentration; uneven ventilation is indicated by a delayed and irregular decrease. The decrease in nitrogen concentration with each succeeding breath proceeds slowly and unevenly in obstructive disease, contrasted with the smooth, rapid washout in a normal person. Multiple-breath washout is rather insensitive to mild disease.

Radioactive-isotope ventilation studies provide an especially graphic way of evaluating regional ventilation.[118,119] Radioactive xenon may be inhaled and its distribution mapped out by quantitating radioactive counts over the surface of the thorax. Numerical counting or scintiphotography may be used. Patchy distribution of ventilation occurs in most forms of obstructive lung disease, and a defect in ventilation predominantly affecting the lower zones is characteristic of panacinar emphysema.[120] As carried out in most clinical isotope laboratories, these techniques provide reliable topographical mapping of distribution of ventilation, but quantitation in absolute terms of ventilation to each zone may be performed for investigative purposes. Regional distribution of ventilation, especially with reference to matching of ventilation and perfusion, is discussed in Chapter 5.

LABORATORY SCREENING FOR SUBCLINICAL RESPIRATORY DISEASE

Laboratory detection of early, subclinical pulmonary dysfunction is of great interest for persons at risk in various occupations, cigarette smokers and those exposed to their smoke, and people living in areas of air pollution. Methodology for screening individuals and groups continues to be refined.

Aberrations in lung function can be detected in smokers who do not have disabling pulmonary disease, at a stage when normal values are obtained in conventional tests of ventilation, such as vital capacity and forced expiratory volumes.[121] Furthermore these subtle abnormalities can be reversed by treatment.[121,122]

This knowledge is exciting to the physician interested in preventive medicine. It raises the possibility of detecting obstructive lung disease early in susceptible persons, and of planning and instituting preventive measures. Such an approach implies, however, a link, as yet unproven, between these subtle laboratory findings and disabling obstructive lung disease. Are the asymptomatic patients who have laboratory evidence of airways obstruction those who will develop severe chronic bronchitis and emphysema? If so, can the course of the disease be altered if detected early? Only carefully designed, prospective, longitudinal studies can answer these questions; and such studies are urgently needed.[123,124]

The place that screening tests for airways obstruction may ultimately find in clinical practice, then, remains unclear. A description of currently available techniques is warranted, however, because the need for widespread clinical evaluation of their usefulness is clear. It is notable that the discussions below deal with sensitivity and avoid the question of specificity, because this problem has not yet been solved conclusively. Pathological correlations are not available for the physiological abnormalities in very early peripheral-airways obstruction, and long-term follow-up is not available, of course. Correlation among decreased maximum mid-expiratory flow rate (MMF), abnormal closing volumes, and frequency dependence of compliance has been demonstrated, however[121,123]; and these parameters have been shown to coexist in many cases with elevated residual volume,[122,123] physiological dead space-to-tidal-volume ratio, and alveolar–arterial oxygen-tension difference.[122] When frequency dependence of compliance is due to changes in the elastic properties of the lung, altered static compliance might be expected. Therefore, normal static compliance in a subject with frequency dependence of dynamic compliance is generally interpreted as evidence of obstructive disease of small peripheral airways. A morphological study of the lungs of young (average age, 25 yr) smokers and nonsmokers who died from traumatic causes provides support for this interpretation.[125] The smokers had a characteristic finding: respiratory bronchiolitis associated with clusters of pigmented alveolar macrophages. The investigators suggested that this lesion may be a precursor of centriacinar emphysema and may cause the changes in dynamic compliance and closing volume that have been found in some young smokers.

The evidence is attractive, then, though not conclusive, that physiological tests may be capable of detecting airways disease very early in its course. The prognostic implications for the patient with such physiological abnormalities are uncertain. Evidence has recently been cited to show that if the forced expiratory volume at 1 sec is normal in a 40-year-old patient, he will never be seriously disabled by chronic obstructive lung disease, so slow is the progression of this disorder.[124] A similar analysis[126] has suggested that the FEF_{25-75} will probably be abnormal by age 30 in a subject who will be severely disabled at age 50. If this is true, then more sensitive screening tests would need to be performed in subjects under the age of 30 in order to justify their use.

Although debate continues,[127–130] the future role of screening and the techniques that will be employed will probably be determined by reports such as the eight-year study of the British Medical Research Council, recently reported by Fletcher and associates.[131,132] This study suggests that the smoker at risk of early mortality from chronic airflow obstruction can usually be detected within early middle age simply by an abnormal forced expiratory volume at one sec. The specificity of one such simple determination could be improved upon by more discriminating tests of function, or by repeated tests to evaluate rate of decline. Smoking cessation would prevent premature disability and death, according to Fletcher's analysis.

Frequency Dependence of Dynamic Compliance

The cumbersome technique of measuring frequency dependence of dynamic compliance has gained acceptance as being the most sensitive physiological indicator of obstructive disease involving airways smaller than 2 mm in diameter.[121,133,134] Because the measurement is difficult to carry out, it is impractical for widespread use. It is, however, regarded as the standard to which simpler techniques for detection of early obstructive disease are compared. The concept of dynamic compliance requires some explanation, because compliance is ordinarily defined as a static measurement, taken under conditions of absence of flow rather than during tidal breathing.

When esophageal pressure and lung volume are plotted against each other during normal respiration, with no attempt to interrupt flow, the relation becomes nonlinear, and a pressure–volume (P-V) loop is traced. Because flow stops momentarily at the end of inspiration and at the end of expiration, the line drawn through these points normally has a slope identical to a compliance slope that is constructed from a series of no-flow points. This slope remains identical over a wide range of breathing frequencies in normal lungs of a normal person. Therefore, the measurement expressed as *compliance* is identical whether it is obtained from a series of points taken during breath holding (static compliance) at several levels of inflation or whether taken from the tangent drawn through a P-V loop inscribed during breathing (dynamic compliance) over a wide range of frequencies.

This tendency of dynamic compliance to be independent of breathing frequency is due to uniformity of the mechanical properties of the normal lung and, hence, synchronism of all portions of the lung on inflation and deflation. When disease alters the lung nonuniformly, rapid breathing rates may result in failure of some portions to fill and empty. Dynamic compliance is then measurably reduced, progressively so with each increase in respiratory rate. This may occur when disease alters the elastic or resistive properties nonuniformly. Dynamic compliance is then "frequency-dependent."

It seems likely that when nonuniform changes in elastic properties of the lung become severe enough to result in frequency dependence of dynamic compliance, static compliance will also be altered. On the other hand, there is evidence to show that it is possible for nonuniform alterations of small-airways resistance to occur and to result in frequency dependence of dynamic compliance, without causing any measurable changes in other physiological parameters. Small airways normally contribute so little to total airways resistance that such early changes might be expected not to affect measurements of total airways resistance or maximum expiratory flow rates.[11]

On the basis of these considerations, persons with normal static pressure–volume curves, airways resistance, and conventional spirometry, who exhibit frequency dependence of dynamic compliance, are thought to have early obstructive disease of small peripheral airways.

Mid-Expiratory Flow Rate

It has been recognized since early in the development of the technique of simple spirometry that the midportion of the forced expiratory volume–time curve has the special characteristic of relative independence of patient effort, as compared with the initial portion of the curve. More recently, another special characteristic of the midportion of the curve has appeared: it is relatively sensitive to alteration caused by obstructive disease in small peripheral airways.[122]

The maximum mid-expiratory flow rate (MMF) or "forced expiratory flow rate from 25 to 75% of forced vital capacity" has been most extensively studied.[29,36] (See the section on volume-time curve analysis, p. 116.) This measurement is simple to carry out, with inexpensive equipment and minimal patient discomfort. The patient is instructed to perform a forced expiratory maneuver into a spirometer (*i.e.*, he exhales completely from full inspiration, as rapidly as possible). Volume is usually plotted on the vertical axis and time on the horizontal axis of the recording device. The portion of the curve from 25 to 75% of the volume expired (forced vital capacity) is chosen for analysis. The average rate of flow over this portion of the curve is calculated by drawing a straight line between the two points, defining its extent and determining its slope.

A recent study has focused on a group of smokers with normal spirometry, except for a reduction in MMF, and with normal airways resistance and static compliance. These persons had frequency dependence of dynamic compliance, supporting the interpretation that they did have obstructive disease of small peripheral airways. Bronchodilator therapy and cessation of smoking resulted in improvement of these functional abnormalities in many, and return to normal in some of these subjects.

It seems clear from these investigations and others that this simple test can detect peripheral airways disease earlier than most other spirometric indices, sometimes at a stage of complete reversibility. Other evidence suggests, however, that this test detects only half of the subjects identified as abnormal by demonstration of frequency dependence of compliance.[121] The wide range of values for this determination in normal subjects may account for this relative insensitivity.[36] If Bates' analysis of the time course of the disease[126] is correct, however, insensitivity may not be a serious handicap to the use of the MMF for practical clinical screening. Perhaps the abnormalities detected only by more sensitive tests are of no importance as a cause of disabling disease, at least if they do not occur until after the age of 30 or 40.

Flow–Volume Curves

When expiratory flow is plotted against volume (Fig. 4-5) during a maximum-effort expiratory maneuver, the flow rate rapidly reaches its peak, dependent to a large extent on effort; then as lung volume decreases, the flow rate approaches zero at RV.

Expiratory flow rates late in the maneuver, at low lung volumes, have characteristics that would suggest that their measurement would provide a useful means of identifying mild peripheral small-airways obstruction.[67] Flow rates during the later portion are relatively effort-independent and are more sensitive to narrowing in small airways, where the changes of chronic obstructive pulmonary disease are most marked.

Either flow–volume or volume–time curves can be used to evaluate abnormalities of this sort. Flow–volume curves, however, logically provide a more convenient and potentially more precise method, because a reproducible maximum flow rate can be defined for each point on the volume axis of such a curve for a given person. This maximum flow rate is dependent on elastic and resistive properties of the lung at each lung volume.

The full potential usefulness of flow–volume curves in the quantitation of peripheral airways obstruction cannot be realized until normal values are well established. Further studies of flow–volume curve parameters in larger normal populations are needed.[65,68–71] As such data become available, it should be expected that flow-volume curve analysis will be more widely used.

Closing Volume

Promising techniques for identifying early obstructive airways disease, which combine simplicity and sensitivity, are those that determine closing volume.[135–140] This determination has been defined as "the lung volume at which the dependent lung zones cease to ventilate, presumably as a result of airway closure." Alterations in closing volume occur with obstructive disease of small airways and can be detected with a sensitivity approaching that of frequency dependence of dynamic compliance. The mechanisms that cause alterations in closing volume are a matter of some debate as is the significance of such alterations.[136] Recent studies would suggest that airway closure does occur,[141] but not precisely at "closing volume" as it is ordinarily determined.[142]

Techniques for determining closing volume employ any of a group of inert gases that can be inspired without harm and whose concentration can be easily measured. Changes in the expired concentration of any of these gases can be plotted during a vital capacity maneuver and can be interpreted in light of regional differences in ventilation summarized below.

Ventilation to or from dependent lung zones is greater during normal tidal breathing than that of upper zones. A given change in intrapleural pressure during breathing therefore produces little change in the volume of the already distended upper lung zones, but a greater volume change in the lower zones.[111]

At low lung volumes, however, functional closure of small airways in dependent lung zones occurs, and ventilation of these zones ceases. The level at which this closure occurs is called *closing volume* and is detected as the lung volume at which an abrupt shift in ventilation from dependent to upper lung zones occurs.

Closing volume can be detected by any of several variations of this technique: a patient is connected by means of a mouthpiece to a spirometer, and a detector sensitive to argon concentration is placed at the mouthpiece. The patient is instructed to exhale maximally and then slowly inhale maximally.

As inhalation begins, a bolus of argon is introduced into the mouthpiece. Because the dependent airways are closed at the beginning of the inspiration, the argon is distributed mostly to the upper zones. As the dependent airways open, the subsequently inspired room air enters the dependent lung zones. As full inspiration is reached, the recording of volume and argon concentration on two axes of an X-Y recorder is begun, and the patient is instructed to begin a slow, full expiration. Argon concentration at the mouthpiece rises in four stages during expiration (see Fig. 3-7).

1. Dead space gas contains little argon.
2. Mixed dead space and alveolar gas contains a higher concentration.
3. Alveolar gas from lower lung zones contains a slightly higher concentration, which gradually increases (slope of Phase III).
4. Near the end of expiration, airway closure occurs in the dependent lung zones, and the final portion of the breath contains a high concentration of argon from the upper lung zones.

This final sharp rise in argon concentration is interpreted as coinciding with dependent airway closure, and the volume at which it occurs is recorded as closing volume.

Variations in the closing volume technique utilize argon detected by a mass spectrometer; xenon (^{133}Xe) detected by its radioactivity; helium detected by conventional rapid analyzers available in most pulmonary laboratories; and nitrogen concentration as altered by breathing pure oxygen and detected with a conventional rapid nitrogen analyzer.

Closing volume increases with advancing age and increases in obstructive diseases of small peripheral airways. As normal values for closing volume in different age groups continue to be developed, and as further data are collected about alterations in disease, this measurement may find usefulness as a screening technique for early obstructive lung disease.[136–140]

A further variant, analysis of the slope of the "alveolar plateau" or Phase III of the single-breath test, may also be used to study airways function. Abnormal results of this analysis are believed to be an early manifestation of airways disease, and may be equally or more sensitive.

Helium–Oxygen Breathing

The resistance of the pulmonary airways to flow is influenced by the physical properties of the gas which passes through them, as well as by the mechanical properties of the lungs themselves. Therefore, observations of the changes in results of ventilatory tests produced by substituting various gas mixtures for the air which is breathed can provide certain inferential information about the mechanical properties of the airways. A mixture of 20% oxygen in helium has been most often used for this purpose. This mixture differs from air chiefly in being only 36% as dense. It is also slightly (12%) more viscous than air.[143]

A gas of low density flows more readily under turbulent conditions than does a denser gas. Laminar flow is not influenced by density, however. Within the respiratory airways, turbulent flow is characteristic of larger, and laminar flow of smaller airways. Therefore, expiratory flow at the mouth is density-dependent when the resistance of the large central airways is flow-limiting. When expiratory flow is limited by small peripheral airways in which laminar flow predominates, it is not density-dependent.

In normal humans, air flow at the mouth during a forced vital capacity maneuver is limited by the large airways at high lung volumes (see Chapter 3). Toward the end of expiration the flow-limiting segment of the airways moves upstream to the small peripheral airways. Therefore, flow is density dependent at high, but not at low lung volumes. The volume at which density dependence is lost can readily be shown by superimposing forced expiratory flow–volume curves done in a subject first breathing air, and then breathing a helium–oxygen mixture. The volume at which the curves become superimposed is referred to as the volume of isoflow (Viso$\dot{V}$).

From our understanding of factors controlling the location of the flow-limiting segment (Chapter 3), it would follow logically that an increase in upstream resistance or a decrease in elastic recoil would cause the flow-limiting segment to move upstream and the volume of isoflow to increase. It has been shown that smokers, who presumably have emphysema or small airway obstruction, do have a relative increase in the volume of isoflow.[144,145,146] The test appears, in fact, to be very sensitive in its ability to separate smokers from nonsmokers. Another measurement taken from superimposed flow–volume curves breathing air and breathing a helium–oxygen mixture is the difference in maximum flow at 50% vital capacity ($\Delta \dot{V}_{max\text{-}50}$). This parameter is said to be relatively specific for detection of change in location of the flow-limiting segment due to small airways obstruction rather than elastic recoil.[146]

Maximal expiratory flow studies breathing helium–oxygen mixture have also been used to identify the location of airway obstruction in asthmatics, and showed it to be variable, involving both large and small airways.[143] A diagnostic use of such studies has recently been demonstrated in identifying severe upper-airway obstruction when it is clinically difficult to separate from ordinary chronic obstructive pulmonary disease.[147]

REFERENCES

1. HOWELL JBL, CAMPBELL EJM (eds): Breathlessness: Proceedings of an International Symposium. Oxford, Blackwell Scientific Publications, 1966
2. HOWELL JBL, CAMPBELL EJM: Breathlessness in pulmonary disease. Scand J Respir Dis 48:321, 1967
3. LUKAS DS: Dyspnea. In MacBryde CM, Blacklow RS (eds): Signs and Symptoms: Applied Pathologic Physiology and Clinical Interpretation, 5th, ed, pp 341–357. Philadelphia, JB Lippincott, 1970
4. BURKI NK: Breathlessness and mouth occlusion pressure in patients with chronic obstruction of the airways. Chest 76:527, 1979
5. MOISAN TC, CHANDRASEKHAR AJ, SHARP JT: Asynchronous breathing: A possible etiology for dyspnea in a patient with normal lungs. Chest 75:624, 1979
6. TISI GM: Preoperative evaluation of pulmonary function. Validity, indications and benefits. Am Rev Respir Dis 119:293, 1979
7. CAIN HD, STEVENS PM, ADANIYA R: Preoperative pulmonary function and complications after cardiovascular surgery. Chest 76:130, 1979
8. GRACEY DR, DIVERTIE MB, DIDIER EP: Preoperative pulmonary preparation of patients with chronic obstructive pulmonary disease: A prospective study. Chest 76:123, 1979
9. LEFRAK SS: Preoperative evaluation for pulmonary resection. Chest 72:419, 1077
10. BOYSEN PG et al: Prospective evaluation for pneumonectomy; using the 99m technetium quantitative perfusion lung scan. Chest 72:422, 1977
11. MACKLEM PT: Airway obstruction and collateral ventilation. Physiol Rev 51:368, 1971
12. HYATT RE: Dynamic lung volumes. In Fenn WO, Rahn H (eds): Handbook of Physiology, Section

3: Respiration. Baltimore, Williams & Wilkins, 1964, 1965
13. BATES DV, MACKLEM PT, CHRISTIE RV: Respiratory Function in Disease. Philadelphia, WB Saunders, 1971
14. MEAD J et al: Significance of the relationship between lung recoil and maximum expiratory flow. J Appl Physiol 22:95, 1967
15. PRIDE NB et al: Determinants of maximal expiratory flow from the lungs. J Appl Physiol 23:646, 1967
16. CAMPBELL EJM: Physical signs of diffuse airways obstruction and lung distention. Thorax 24:1, 1969
17. GODFEY S et al: Clinical and physiological associations of some physical signs observed in patients with chronic airways obstruction. Thorax 25:285, 1970
18. MCFADDEN ER, KISER R, DEGROOT WJ: Acute bronchial asthma: Clinical and physiologic relations. N Engl J Med 288:221, 1973
19. SNIDER TH et al: Simple bedside test of respiratory function. JAMA 170:1631, 1959
20. OLSEN CR: The match test: A measure of ventilatory function. Am Rev Respir Dis 86:37, 1962
21. CARILLI AD, HENDERSON JR: Estimation of ventilatory function by blowing out a match. Am Rev Respir Dis 89:680, 1964
22. ROSENBLATT G, STEIN M: Clinical value of the forced expiratory time measured during auscultation. N Engl J Med 267:432, 1962
23. LAL S, FERGUSON AD, CAMPBELL EJM: Forced expiratory time: A simple test for airways obstruction. Br Med J 1:814, 1964
24. PARDEE NE, MARTIN CJ, MORGAN EH: A test of the practical value of estimating breath sound intensity; breath sounds related to measured ventilatory function. Chest 70:341, 1976
25. MORGAN WKC, BRANSCOMB BV: The assessment of ventilatory capacity. Statement of the Committees on Environmental Health and Respiratory Physiology, American College of Chest Physicians. Chest 67:95, 1975
26. PERMUTT S, CHESTER EH (Co-Chairmen): Office spirometry in clinical practice: Statement of the American College of Chest Physicians committee on clinic and office pulmonary function testing. Chest 74:298, 1978
27. American Thoracic Society statement: Snowbird workship on standardization of spirometry. Am Rev Respir Dis 119:831, 1979
28. BALDWIN E DEF, COURNAND A, RICHARDS DW JR: Pulmonary insufficiency. I. Physiological classification, clinical methods of analysis, standard values in normal subjects. Medicine 27:243, 1948
29. LEUALLEN EC, FOWLER WS: Maximal midexpiratory flow. Am Rev Tubercul 72:783, 1955
30. GOLDMAN HI, BECKLAKE MR: Respiratory function tests: normal values at median altitudes and the prediction of normal results. Am Rev Tubercul 79:457, 1959
31. KORY RC et al: The Veterans Administration Army cooperation study of pulmonary function. I. Clinical spirometry in normal men. Am J Med 30:243, 1961
32. BATES DV, WOOLF CR, PAUL GI: Chronic bronchitis. A report on the first two stages of the coordinated study of chronic bronchitis in the Department of Veterans Affairs, Canada. Med Serv J Can 18:211, 1962
33. FERRIS BG JR, ANDERSON DO, ZICKMANTEL R: Prediction values for screening test of pulmonary function. Am Rev Respir Dis 91:252, 1965
34. COTES JE, et al: Average normal values for the forced expiratory volume in white caucasian males. Br Med J 1:1016, 1966
35. WENG TR, LEVISON H: Standards of pulmonary function in children. Am Rev Respir Dis 99:879, 1969
36. MORRIS JF, KOSKI A, JOHNSON LC: Spirometric standards for healthy nonsmoking adults. Am Rev Respir Dis 103:57, 1971
37. CHERNIACK RM, RABER MB: Normal standards for ventilatory function using an automated wedge spirometer. Am Rev Respir Dis 106:38, 1972
38. MORRIS JF, TEMPLE WP, KOSKI A: Normal values for the ratio of one-second forced expiratory volume to forced vital capacity. Am Rev Respir Dis 108:1000, 1973
39. KNUDSON RL et al: The maximal expiratory flow-volume curve: Normal standards, variability and effects of age. Am Rev Respir Dis 113:587, 1976
40. NATHAN SP, LEBOWITZ MD, KNUDSON RJ: Spirometric testing: Number of tests required and selection of data. Chest 76:384, 1979
41. PAPPENHEIMER JR (committee chairman): Standardization of definitions and symbols in respiratory physiology. Fed Proc 9:602, 1950
42. KORY RC (committee chairman): Clinical spirometry: Recommendations of the Section on Pulmonary Function Testing, Committee on Pulmonary Physiology, American College of Chest Physicians. Dis Chest 43:214, 1963
43. BURROWS B (committee chairman): Pulmonary terms and symbols. Chest 67:583, 1975
44. DAYMAN H: The expiratory spirogram. Am Rev Respir Dis 83:842, 1961
45. CARY J et al: Variability in interpretation of pulmonary function tests. Chest 76:389, 1979
46. WRIGHT BM, MCKERROW CB: Maximum forced expiratory flow rate as a measure of ventilatory capacity. Br Med J 2:1041, 1959
47. SOBOL BJ: Effort independence and forced expiratory flow; end of an era? Chest 73:566, 1978
48. HERMANNSEN J: Untersuchungen über die maximale Ventilationsgrosse (Atemgrenzwert). Z Gesamte Exp Med 90:130, 1933
49. BOREN HG, KORY RC, SNYER JC: The Veterans Administration—Army cooperative study of pul-

monary function. II. The lung volume and its subdivisions in normal men. Am J Med 41:96, 1966
50. GAENSLER EA: Clinical pulmonary physiology. N Engl J Med 252:177–184, 221–228, 264–271, 1955
51. GAENSLER EA, WRIGHT GW: Evaluation of respiratory impairment. Arch Environ Health 12:146, 1966
52. COLP R: Interpretation of pulmonary function tests. Chest 76:377, 1979
53. CLARK TJH: Inspiratory obstruction. Br Med J 3:682, 1970
54. EMPEY DW: Assessment of upper airways obstruction. Br Med J 3:503, 1972
55. SNIDER GL, et al: Criteria for the assessment of reversibility in airways obstruction. Report of the Committee on Emphysema, American College of Chest Physicians. Chest 65:552, 1974
56. SNIDER GL, KORY RC, LYONS HA: Grading of pulmonary function impairment by means of pulmonary function tests. Recommendations of the Committee on Pulmonary Physiology, American College of Chest Physicians. Dis Chest 52:270, 1967
57. GAENSLER EA, WRIGHT GW: Evaluation of respiratory impairment. Arch Environ Health 12:146, 1966
58. ELLIS JH JR, PERERA SP, LEVIN DC: A computer program for calculation and interpretation of pulmonary function studies. Chest 68:209, 1975
59. KANNER RE, MORRIS AH (eds): Clinical Pulmonary Function Testing—A Manual of Uniform Laboratory Procedures for the Intermountain Area. Salt Lake City, Intermountain Thoracic Society, 1975
60. HYATT RE, SCHILDER DP, FRY DL: Relationship between maximum expiratory flow and degree of lung inflation. J Appl Physiol 13:331, 1958
61. FRY DL, HYATT RE: Pulmonary mechanics: A unified analysis of the relationship between pressure, volume and gasflow in the lungs of normal and diseased human subjects. Am J Med 29:672, 1960
62. HYATT RE: The interrelationships of pressure, flow, and volume during various respiratory maneuvers in normal and emphysematous subjects. Am Rev Respir Dis 83:676, 1961
63. JORDANOGLOU J, PRIDE NB: Factors determining maximum inspiratory flow and maximum expiratory flow of the lung. Thorax 23:33, 1968
64. JORDANOGLOU J, PRIDE NB: A comparison of maximum inspiratory and expiratory flow in health and in lung disease. Thorax 23:38, 1968
65. HYATT RE, BLACK LF: The flow-volume curve: A current perspective. Am Rev Respir Dis 107:191, 1973
66. MACKLEM PT: Current concepts: Tests of lung mechanics. N Engl J Med 243:339, 1975
67. GELB AF, MACANALLY BJ: Early detection of obstructive lung disease by analysis of maximal expiratory flow-volume curves. Chest 64:749, 1973
68. BLACK LF, OFFORD K, HYATT RE: Variability in the maximal expiratory flow volume curve in asymptomatic smokers and in nonsmokers. Am Rev Respir Dis 110:282, 1974
69. WEBSTER PM, ZAMEL N, BRYAN AC, KRUGER K: Volume dependence of instantaneous time constants derived from the maximal expiratory flow-volume curve: A new approach to the analysis of forced expiration. Am Rev Respir Dis 115:805, 1977
70. KNUDSON RJ, BURROWS B, LEBOWITZ MD: The maximal expiratory flow-volume curve: Its use in the detection of ventilatory abnormalites in a population study. Am Rev Respir Dis 114:871, 1976
71. KNUDSON RJ, LEBOWITZ MD: Comparison of flow-volume and closing volume variables in a random population. Am Rev Respir Dis 116:1039, 1977
72. GAZIOGLU K et al: Study of forced vital capacity and maximal expiratory flow-volume curves in obstructive lung disease. Am Rev Respir Dis 98:857, 1968
73. LORD GP, GAZIOGLU K, KALTREIDER N: The maximum expiratory flow-volume in the evaluation of patients with lung disease. Am J Med 46:72, 1969
74. CARILLI AD et al: The flow-volume loop in normal subjects and in diffuse lung disease. Chest 66:472, 1974
75. SHIM C et al: Pulmonary function studies in patients with upper airway obstruction. Am Rev Respir Dis 106:233, 1972
76. MILLER RD, HYATT RE: Obstructing lesions of the larynx and trachea: Clinical and physiological characteristics. Mayo Clin Proc 44:145, 1969
77. MILLER RD, HYATT RE: Evaluation of obstructing lesions of the trachea and larynx by flow-volume loops. Am Rev Respir Dis 108:475, 1973
78. DARLING RC, COURNAND A, RICHARDS DW JR: Studies on the intrapulmonary mixture of gases. III. An open circuit method for measuring residual air. J Clin Invest 19:609, 1940
79. DUBOIS AB et al: A rapid plethysmographic method for measuring thoracic gas volume: A comparison with a nitrogen washout method for measuring functional residual capacity in human subjects. J Clin Invest 35:322, 1956
80. MENEELY GR et al: A simplified closed circuit helium dilution method for the determination of the residual volume of the lungs. Am J Med 28:824, 1960
81. SCHAANING CG, GULSVIK A: Accuracy and pre-

cision of helium dilution technique and body plethysmography in measuring lung volumes. Scand J Clin Lab Invest 32:271, 1973

82. O'SHEA J et al: Determination of lung volumes from chest films. Thorax 25:544, 1970
83. GREENE R: Radiographic measurement of thoracic gas volume. Radiol Clin North Am 9:63, 1971
84. HARRIS TR, PRATT PC, KILBURN KH: Total lung capacity measured by roentgenograms. Am J Med 50:756, 1971
85. MARMORSTEIN BL, CIANCIULLI FD: Planimetric measurement of total lung capacity in asthma. Chest 66:378, 1974
85a. PIERCE RJ et al: Estimation of lung volumes from chest radiographs using shape information. Thorax 34:726, 1979
86. BARRETT WA et al: Computerized roentgenographic determination of total lung capacity. Am Rev Respir Dis 113:239, 1976
87. DEJOURS P: Control of respiration in muscular exercise. In Fenn WO, Rahn H (eds): Handbook of Physiology, Section 3: Respiration. Baltimore, Williams & Wilkins, 1964
88. FOX SM III, NAUGHTON JP, GORMAN PA: Physical activity and cardiovascular health. Part II. The exercise prescription: intensity and duration. Mod Concepts Cardiovasc Dis 41:21, 1972
89. PIERCE AK et al: Responses to exercise training in patients with emphysema. Arch Intern Med 113:28, 1964
90. FOX SM, III, NAUGHTON JP, GORMAN PA: Physical activity and cardiovascular health. Part III. The exercise prescription: frequency and type of activity. Mod Concepts Cardiovasc Dis 41:25, 1972
91. JONES NL: Exercise testing in pulmonary evaluation. N Engl J Med 293:541, 647, 1975
92. WASSERMAN K, WHIPP BJ: Exercise physiology in health and disease. Am Rev Respir Dis 112:219, 1975
93. ARMSTRONG BW et al. Clinicophysiologic evaluation of physical working capacity in persons with pulmonary disease. Am Rev Respir Dis 93:90 (Part I); 223(Part II): 1966
94. JONES NL et al: Clinical Exercise Testing. Philadelphia, WB Saunders, 1975
95. DAVIS JA et al: Anaerobic threshold alterations caused by endurance training in middle aged men. J Appl Physiol 46:1036, 1979
96. MACDOUGAL JD et al: Biochemical adaptation of human skeletal muscle to heavy resistance training and immobilization. J Appl Physiol 43:700, 1977
97. CLAUSEN JP: Effect of physical training on cardiovascular adjustments to exercise in man. Physiol Rev 57:779, 1977
98. MCFADDEN ER JR, INGRAM RH JR: Exercise induced asthma. Observations on the initiating stimulus. N Engl J Med 301:763, 1979
99. MEAD J: Mechanical properties of lungs. Physiol Rev 41:281, 1961
100. MEAD J, WHITTENBERGER JL: Physical properties of human lungs measured during spontaneous respiration. J Appl Physiol 5:779, 1953
101. FISHER AB, DUBOIS AB, HYDE RW: Evaluation of the forced oscillation technique for the determination of resistance to breathing. J Clin Invest 47:2045, 1968
102. OTIS AB, PROCTOR DF: Measurement of alveolar pressure in human subjects. Am J Physiol 152:106, 1948
103. DUBOIS AB, BOTELHO SY, COMROE JH: A new method for measuring airway resistance in man using a body plethysmograph: values in normal subjects and in patients with respiratory disease. J Clin Invest 35:327, 1956
104. HOGG JC, MACKLEM PT, THURLBECK WM: Site and nature of airway obstruction in chronic obstructive lung disease. N Engl J Med 278:1355, 1968
105. MEAD et al: Measurement of intraesophageal pressure. J Appl Physiol 7:491, 1955
106. MILIC-EMILI J et al: Improved technique for estimating pleural pressure from esophageal balloons. J Appl Physiol 19:207, 1964
107. CHERNIACK RM, BROWN E: A simple method for measuring total respiratory compliance: Normal values for males. J Appl Physiol 20:87, 1965
108. TURNER JM, MEAD J, WHOL ME: Elasticity of human lungs in relation to age. J Appl Physiol 25:664, 1968
109. SCHLUETER DP, IMMEKUS J, STEAD WW: Relationship between maximal inspiratory pressure and total lung capacity (coefficient of retraction) in normal subjects and in patients with emphysema, asthma, and diffuse pulmonary infiltration. Am Rev Respir Dis 96:656, 1967
110. GREAVES IA, COLEBATCH HJN: Elastic behavior and structure of normal and emphysematous lungs post mortem. Am Rev Respir Dis 121:127, 1980
111. MILIC-EMILI J, HENDERSON JAM, KANEKO K: Regional distribution of pulmonary ventilation. In Cumming G, Hunt LB (eds): Form and Function in the Human Lung. Edinburgh, E & S Livingstone, 1968
112. CRAIG DB et al: "Closing volume" and its relationship to gas exchange in seated and supine positions. J Appl Physiol 31:717, 1971
113. LEBLANC P, RUFF F, MILIC-EMILI J: Effects of age and body position on "airway closure" in man. J Appl Physiol 28:448, 1970
114. ANTHONISEN NR et al: Airway closure as a function of age. Respir Physiol 8:58, 1969
115. FOWLER WS: Lung function studies. III. Uneven pulmonary ventilation in normal subjects and in

patients with pulmonary disease. J Appl Physiol 2:283, 1949
116. BRODY AW et al: Standards and significance for three tests of the distribution of ventilation. The time to equilibration, the forced equilibrating expiration, and the Fowler Single Breath Test. Am J Med 48:424, 1970
117. COURNAND A et al: Studies on the intrapulmonary mixture of gases. IV. The significance of the pulmonary emptying rate and simplified open circuit measurement of residual air. J Clin Invest 20:681, 1941
118. WEST JB: Ventilation–perfusion relationships. Am Rev Respir Dis 116:919, 1977
119. WAGNER HN JR: The use of radioisotope techniques for the evaluation of patients with pulmonary disease. Am Rev Respir Dis 113:203, 1976
120. MEDINA JR et al: Use of the scintillation Anger camera and xenon Xe^{133} in the study of chronic obstructive lung disease. JAMA 208:985, 1969
121. MACKLEM PT: Obstruction in small airways—a challenge to medicine. Am J Med 52:721, 1972
122. MCFADDEN ER JR, LINDEN DA: A reduction in maximum mid-expiratory flow rate: A spirographic manifestation of small airway disease. Am J Med 52:725, 1972
123. MACKLEM PT: Workshop on screening programs for early diagnosis of airway obstruction. Am Rev Respir Dis 109:567, 1974
124. BURROWS B: Early detection of airways obstruction. Chest 65:239, 1974
125. NIEWOEHNER DE, KLEINERMAN J, RICE DB: Pathologic changes in the peripheral airways of young cigarette smokers. N Engl J Med 291:755, 1974
126. BATES DV: The prevention of emphysema. Chest 65:437, 1974
127. SOLOMON DA: Are small airways tests helpful in the detection of early airflow obstruction? Chest 74:567, 1978
128. MACKLEM PT, BECKLAKE MR: Is screening for chronic limitation of airflow desirable? Chest 74:608, 1978
129. PERMUTT S: Pulmonary function testing and the prevention of pulmonary disease. Chest 74:608, 1978
130. KRONENBERG RS, NIEWOEHNER DE: Screening for early obstruction of the airways; a 1978 reappraisal. Chest 74:610, 1978
131. FLETCHER C et al: The Natural History of Chronic Bronchitis and Emphysema. Oxford, Oxford University Press, 1976
132. FLETCHER C, PETO R: The natural history of chronic airflow obstruction. Br Med J 1:1645, 1977
133. MCFADDEN ER et al: Small airway disease: an assessment of the tests of peripheral airway function. Am J Med 57:171, 1974
134. WOOLCOCK AJ, VINCENT NJ, MACKLEM PT: Frequency dependence of compliance as a test for obstruction in the small airways. J Clin Invest 48:1097, 1968
135. MANSELL A, BRYAN C, LEVISON H: Airway closure in children. J Appl Physiol 33:711, 1972
136. HYATT RE, RODARTE JR: "Closing volume," one man's noise—other mens' experiment. Mayo Clin Proc 50:17, 1975
137. MCCARTHY DS et al: Measurement of "closing volume" as a simple and sensitive test for early detection of small airway disease. Am J Med 52:747, 1972
138. BUIST AS, VANFLEET DL, ROSS BB: A comparison of conventional spirometric tests and the test of closing volume in an emphysema screening center. Am Rev Respir Dis 107:735, 1973
139. BUIST AS, ROSS BB: Predicted values for closing volumes using a modified single breath mitrogen test. Am Rev Respir Dis 107:744, 1973
140. BUIST AS: Early detection of airways obstruction by the closing volume technique. Chest 64:495, 1973
141. ENGEL LA, GRASSINO AE, ANTHONISEN NR: Demonstration of airway closure in man. J Appl Physiol 38:1117, 1975
142. FORKERT L, DHINGRA S, ANTHONISEN NR: Airway closure and closing volume. J Appl Physiol 46:24, 1979
143. DESPAS PJ, LEROUX M, MACKLEM PT: Site of airway obstruction in asthma as determined by measuring maximal expiratory flow breathing air and helium–oxygen mixture. J Clin Invest 51:3235, 1972
144. HUTCHEON M et al: Volume of isoflow; a new test in detection of mild abnormalities of lung mechanics. Am Rev Respir Dis 110:458, 1974
145. DOSMAN J et al: The use of helium–oxygen mixture during expiratory flow to demonstrate obstruction in small airways in smokers. J Clin Invest 55:1090, 1975
146. GELB AF, KLEIN E: The volume of isoflow and increase in maximal flow at 50 percent of forced vital capacity during helium–oxygen breathing as tests of small airway dysfunction. Chest 71:396, 1977
147. LAVELLE TF JR, ROTMAN HH, WEG JG: Isoflow volume curves in the diagnosis of upper airway obstruction. Am Rev Respir Dis 117:845, 1978

Chapter 5

Respiratory Function of the Lungs and Blood

CLARENCE A. GUENTER

ARTERIAL BLOOD GAS ANALYSIS

The major function of the lungs is the exchange of oxygen and carbon dioxide. It is convenient that this function can be assessed by measurement of oxygen and carbon dioxide in systemic arterial blood. Techniques for rapid and simple analysis of gases in the blood have become widely available since the early 1960s and have had enormous impact on the diagnosis and treatment of respiratory insufficiency. Arterial blood gas analysis is the final yardstick of overall adequacy of lung function.

OBTAINING ARTERIAL BLOOD

Selection of an Artery. Arterial puncture for sampling of blood has been established as a relatively safe and simple procedure (see list below). Although any artery in the body could conceivably be used, the radial, brachial, and femoral arteries are most accessible to percutaneous cannulation.[1,2] Generally, the complications of puncture of the radial artery are less severe than those of the brachial or femoral artery.

Most major complications of arterial puncture have occurred when the femoral artery has been utilized. In that artery, (a) atherosclerotic plaques may be dislodged, resulting in distal occlusion of the artery; (b) hemorrhage may occur, occasionally dissecting upward retroperitoneally, with major blood loss occurring before it is apparent; and (c) thrombosis at the site of the puncture may result in distal ischemia. These problems are more likely to arise in patients with clinical evidence of atherosclerosis (such as tortuous vessels, aneurysms, or bruits) or in patients with clotting abnormalities. All of these complications are relatively rare when a small needle is used for a single arterial puncture, placed well below the inguinal ligament in the femoral region. In view of the potential for complications, however, the femoral artery should be used only as a last resort.

Requirements for Safe Arterial Blood Sampling

Sterile needle, heparinized syringe
Aseptic technique
Palpable artery
Understanding of the anatomy of the region
Identification of the risk factors
- Hypertension
- Local disease (atherosclerosis, aneurysm)
- Anticoagulants or bleeding diathesis

Compression of artery after puncture

Venous blood is not an acceptable substitute for arterial blood when respiratory function is being assessed. The blood draining the tissues reflects the metabolism of the particular tissue that the vein drains. Mixed venous blood provides useful information regarding net oxygen availability to the body and acid–base balance. "Arterialized" capillary blood can be obtained after warming a capillary bed for approximately 10 min; the vasodilation results in an increased rate of blood flow, minimizing the effects of local tissue metabolism. The preferred puncture sites include the heel pad, earlobe, and finger tip. Although arterialized capillary blood values only approximate arterial blood values, they may be sufficiently accurate for major therapeutic considerations, particularly in infants with inaccessible arteries.[3]

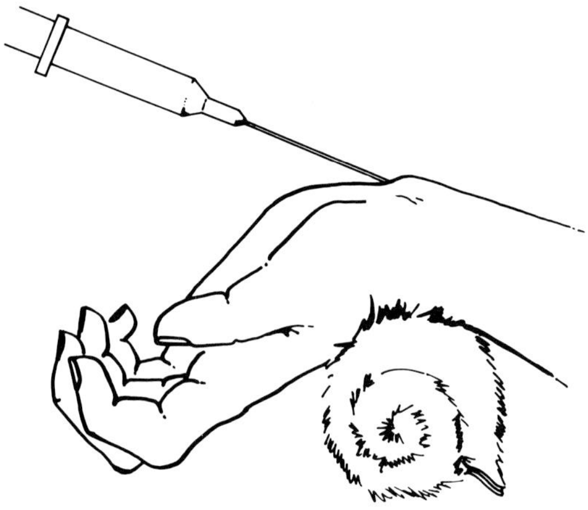

FIG. 5-1. Optimal position for radial artery puncture. Note the extension of the wrist and the angle of entry of the needle.

Single puncture of the radial artery is performed readily as follows. The patient is comfortably seated or preferably allowed to lie down (to minimize the likelihood of a vasovagal faint). The forearm is extended, and the wrist is dorsiflexed about 30 degrees. The radial artery should then be carefully palpated proximally from the wrist crease as the artery passes medial to the styloid process of the radius, and for about 5 cm (2 in) up the forearm. After the course of the artery has been well defined, a needle (21 or 22 gauge) is inserted through the skin approximately 2.5 cm proximal to the wrist crease (and immediately over the pulsating vessel). The needle is then advanced at an angle almost parallel to the artery, but to a sufficient depth to actually enter the artery (Fig. 5-1). This oblique angle provides a longer vessel pathway for the needle to traverse. When the needle enters the artery, a slow but pulsatile flow of blood occurs. Occasionally, the artery is completely traversed, and the needle passes through the opposite wall. When this occurs, if the needle is withdrawn gradually, the tip will again enter the lumen, and blood can be obtained. When a free flow of definite arterial blood is apparent through the hub of the needle, a 5-ml heparinized syringe is attached, and blood is withdrawn. When a glass syringe with a well-lubricated barrel is used, the pressure of the blood generally causes the syringe to fill. When plastic syringes are used, withdraw gently on the plunger. Introducing the needle without the syringe attached permits definite identification of arterial flow. This may not be important in well-oxygenated patients, whose arterial blood is bright red; however, it is particularly important in patients with hypoxemia, whose blue arterial blood may be indistinguishable from the dark color of venous blood.

Many physicians prefer to inject a small amount of topical anesthetic in the skin and infiltrate locally along each side of the arterial wall prior to arterial puncture. This may decrease the pain if multiple punctures are necessary before the artery is entered, but it is just as painful as a single direct arterial puncture performed by a skilled technologist, and does not significantly improve the reflection of a steady state.[3a]

The cleaning of the skin need not be elaborate; swabbing with an alcohol sponge generally is as effective for this procedure as for a venipuncture.[4] After withdrawal of the required volume of blood (generally 3 to 5 ml), any air bubbles should be expressed, the syringe capped, and the sample placed on ice until analysis is carried out. Direct pressure should be applied to the puncture site for at least 3 to 5 min, or longer if the patient is anticoagulated or has other bleeding diatheses. The puncture site should be rechecked within 5 min after releasing pressure, to be sure that a hematoma is not gradually forming. The swelling of a hematoma is easily apparent at the site of a radial artery puncture. Although hematomas at the site of radial artery puncture rarely cause major complications, they result in pain and discomfort. A hematoma in the fascial plane of the wrist rarely may cause median nerve compression. Multiple punctures of an artery can be safely carried out in the course of a day if skill and care are exerted.

Insertion of an indwelling arterial cannula into the radial artery may be desirable to provide multiple sequential sampling. This technique is also desirable when acute effects of breath holding or hyperventilation in response to the procedure need to be avoided. The artery is identified and its course determined in the same manner as for a single arterial puncture. The overlying skin is swabbed with alcohol, and an indwelling arterial cannula (of which many commercial varieties are now available) is inserted into the artery. The polyethylene or Teflon sheath is advanced proximally to a secure position well within the lumen of the artery. The cannula may then be attached to a stopcock and may be kept open by flushing intermittently with heparinized saline. Alternatively, a pressure-sensitive valve may be introduced, preventing any flow except during the time of sampling, with intermittent injection of heparin to prevent thrombosis. The cannula may be safely left in position for 24 to 48 hr. The incidence of infection and thrombosis tends to increase with prolonged cannulation.

Complications of single arterial needle punctures are infrequent. In our experience, with more than 10,000 radial arterial punctures performed predominantly by ancillary medical personnel (respiratory technologists and nurses), only two major complications occurred. Both of these consisted of extensive bleeding into the fascial planes of the wrist, with median nerve compression. Paresthesias were transient, relieved after 5 to 7 days. One of these patients had been on anticoagulants.

Several anticoagulated patients have developed compression neuropathy following brachial artery puncture. Surgical decompression and drainage may be necessary.[5]

On the other hand, cannulation of the radial artery frequently results in obstruction to blood flow[6]; 35 to 40% of patients who had radial artery cannulation developed evidence of thrombosis as assessed by ultrasonic measurements of flow, and this was markedly reduced when smaller (20 gauge) cannulae were used instead of 18 gauge.[7] Gangrene of the hand requiring amputation followed cannulation with 18 gauge catheters in 2 patients.[8] In view of this rate of vascular occlusion, it is recommended that prior to the insertion of a cannula into the radial artery, flow through the ulnar artery be demonstrated by means of the Allen's test. This test is performed by having the patient make a fist, to drain the palmar vascular bed of blood, then occluding the radial and ulnar arteries by local pressure. The hand is then opened, while the radial and ulnar arteries are occluded. Pressure is first released from the ulnar artery, permitting flow to the hand. The blanched palmar vascular beds should give place to erythema if the ulnar artery is patent. Although it is not certain that cannulation of the radial artery in the face of an occluded ulnar artery causes complications, the risk is probably increased.[9] Embolization from an indwelling arterial cannula to the pulp spaces of the fingers occurs commonly, but this is generally of minor significance if care is taken to maintain a clot-free arterial cannula.[3,10–12]

The widespread use of arterial catheters for hemodynamic monitoring has resulted in serious infections arising at the site of insertion. In one series, 18% had evidence of local infection and 5% developed septicemia. The most severe infections occurred when catheters were left in place for more than 4 days.

It is generally considered reasonable to train respiratory technologists, intensive-care-unit nurses, and pulmonary laboratory technologists to obtain samples of arterial blood, although the medicolegal implications have not been uniformly established.[14,15] A system of training, supervision, and certification of competence must be established in each institution, as for other procedures, to protect the patient.

Processing the Blood. Because arterial blood is deliberately sampled to assess the effects of equilibration of alveolar gas with the blood passing through the lungs, it is of utmost importance that no other gas be permitted contact with the blood. Every effort must be made to prevent air from entering the syringe. A discrete bubble may be expelled immediately, but multiple small bubbles generally cause a modification of blood gases. When air contaminates the sample, the oxygen and carbon dioxide of the blood are altered in the direction of the partial pressures of those gases in air; therefore, the blood P_{CO_2} decreases, and, in a sample from a normal or hypoxic person, the P_{O_2} increases.

The sample should be cooled as rapidly as possible in order to lower the metabolic rate of the erythrocytes and leukocytes, which utilize oxygen and produce carbon dioxide and metabolic acids at sufficiently rapid rates to alter the gas partial pressures and pH. An iced sample, tightly sealed, may be analyzed in 30 to 45 min with barely measurable changes, and for as long as 2 hr after sampling with only minor degrees of alteration in the gases.

Diffusion of carbon dioxide and oxygen is sufficiently slow through plastic so that disposable syringes may be used if prompt analysis is available. An exception should be made when collecting blood with high oxygen tension (greater than 300 mm Hg), because the high pressure gradient between blood and room air increases the rate of diffusion; under this circumstance, glass syringes are preferable.

When the patient is febrile or hypothermic, errors in gas values may be introduced by analyzing the blood at the usual instrument temperature of 37° C. Blood from a hypothermic patient analyzed routinely at 37° C results in falsely high Po_2 and Pco_2 values and a low pH. Conversely, blood from a hyperthermic patient has low Po_2 and Pco_2 values and a high pH, compared with the true values *in vivo*. Nomograms have been developed that permit corrections back to the values at the patient's temperature, particularly the pH and the Po_2 values. Such corrections take into account the difference in hydrogen ion concentration with varying temperature, and shifts in the oxyhemoglobin dissociation curve.[16,17] For example, blood analyzed with a normal pH and Pco_2, with a Po_2 of 50 mm Hg, may reflect a patient Po_2 of 40 mm Hg if the body temperature is 34° C, or a Po_2 of 62 mm Hg if the body temperature is 40° C. These changes are even more significant at lower levels of oxyhemoglobin saturation, or when hemoglobin is completely saturated.

Severely elevated blood leukocyte counts (greater than 50,000 per cm^3) may result in rapid oxygen consumption in the blood sample with a spuriously low blood Po_2. This most commonly occurs in patients with leukemia and has been called "leukocyte larceny."[18]

Instruments for measuring arterial blood pH, Po_2 and Pco_2 are relatively inexpensive and readily available. These instruments should be available in any institution that accepts the responsibility for oxygen therapy, general anesthetics, care of comatose patients, or respiratory care. The mere presence of a technician willing to perform arterial blood gas analysis on an available instrument does not assure a high standard of quality in the analytic technique. Reliable systems of quality control must be established, yet they are frequently lacking in apparently smoothly functioning laboratories.

Pitfalls in Interpretation of Blood Gas Values

- Blood from vein or hematoma rather than artery
- Patient status not noted (e.g., breathing oxygen, on respirator)
- Blood contaminated by air (bubbles or unsealed syringe)
- Patient temperature significantly different from 37° C.
- Blood stored too long prior to analysis
- Severely elevated blood leukocyte count
- Analytic error (faulty calibration or faulty handling of specimen or instrument)

FACTORS AFFECTING ARTERIAL BLOOD Po_2 AND Pco_2

The sum of the pressures of each of the gases in the atmosphere equals the total atmospheric pressure. As discussed in Chapter 1, the fraction of the total that each gas represents may be expressed as its *partial pressure*. For example, at sea level, the average barometric pressure is 760 mm Hg (sometimes expressed as *tension* or *Torr*, according to the Torricelli scale[19]); the amount of oxygen is 20.95%, and the partial pressure of oxygen (Po_2) is 159 mm Hg. When the air equilibrates with a liquid such as blood, the gas partial pressure in the blood is the same as in the air.

The volume of gas that may be present in a liquid varies with each gas and the specific liquid. The volume of gas in a liquid is determined by (a) the solubility of the gas in the liquid, (b) the partial pressure of the gas, and (c) the presence of additional binding mechanisms in the liquid (*e.g.*, hemoglobin in blood). It is of utmost importance to bear in mind that analysis of blood Po_2 and Pco_2 reflects only the partial pressure of the gases and not the volume. If the solu-

TABLE 5-1. Mechanisms of Reduced Arterial Po_2

	Arterial Gas Tensions		Alveolar–Arterial Oxygen Gradient	
	Pao_2	$Paco_2$	Room Air	100% Oxygen
Reduced atmospheric oxygen (high altitude)	↓	↓	N	N
Alveolar hypoventilation	↓	↑	N	N
Altered intrapulmonary gas exchange				
Regionally decreased ventilation compared with perfusion	↓	↓ N or ↑	↑	N or ↑
Intrapulmonary right-to-left shunt	↓	N or ↓	↑	↑
"Diffusion block"	↓	N or ↓	↑	N
Anatomical right-to-left shunt (intrapulmonary or intracardiac)	↓	N or ↓	↑	↑

bility and other binding mechanisms are known, relationships between partial pressures and volumes of the gases may be predicted. This extrapolation is frequently useful in medical practice, as long as its limitations are kept in mind.

Arterial blood analysis for Po_2 and Pco_2 primarily reflects the effect of blood coming into contact with gases in the lungs. This analysis of gas exchange in the lungs reflects oxygen delivery to the tissues only if other aspects of the transport system are normal. Abnormalities in oxygen transport are discussed below. The factors that result in arterial hypoxemia are listed in Table 5-1.

Atmospheric Oxygen. When a normal person is transported from sea level to an altitude of 1000 m, his environment changes from a barometric pressure of approximately 760 to approximately 660 mm Hg. The Po_2 in the inspired air (P_IO_2) decreases from about 159 to 138 mm Hg. Therefore, air breathed into the terminal air units produces a lower level of alveolar oxygen. Blood perfusing the lungs with this reduced level of oxygen necessarily equilibrates at the lower level, and there is a reduced Po_2 in the arterial blood (see Chap. 1). This mechanism produces predictable decreases in arterial Po_2 whenever environmental Po_2 is reduced. Conversely, when the environmental oxygen is increased (either as a result of oxygen supplements or hyperbaric environments), the alveolar Po_2 normally increases in a predictable fashion. Because the equilibration of blood with alveolar gas is not perfect, alveolar ventilation is variable, and the transport of oxygen in the blood is complex (the relationship of environmental oxygen to arterial blood oxygen content is not simple, direct, or linear). The normal arterial Po_2 at sea level (P_IO_2 = 159 mm Hg) is about 90 mm Hg. At Calgary, Alberta, altitude 1000 m (P_IO_2 = 138), arterial Po_2 is about 79 mm Hg.[20] At sea level, breathing pure oxygen (P_IO_2 = 760), the arterial Po_2 is about 600 mm Hg.

Changes in inspired oxygen do not affect arterial Pco_2 directly, but may result in altered levels as a result of secondary effects on alveolar ventilation. Generally, hypoxemia stimulates respiration.

Alveolar Ventilation. The next phase of the respiratory pathway that may result in reduced blood oxygen levels is the bellows function of the lung. If ventilation of the alveolar spaces is reduced, the amount of oxygen available to the pulmonary blood is reduced. Consequently, a greater proportion of alveolar oxygen is removed, resulting in a decreased alveolar oxygen partial pressure.

The effects of alveolar hypoventilation are illustrated in Table 5-2. In Subject A, with normal ventilation, the alveolar ventilation is approximately 5 L per min. At rest, the oxygen consumption is 250 ml per min. Knowing these factors, it is possible to calculate the rate of extraction of oxygen from the air as breathing goes

TABLE 5-2. Mechanism of Arterial Hypoxemia in Alveolar Hypoventilation

	Subject A Normal Ventilation	Subject B Severe Hypoventilation
Alveolar ventilation	5 L/min	2.5 L/min
Oxygen consumption	250 ml/min	250 ml/min
Oxygen content		
Inspired air	210 ml/L (21% of atmospheric gas)	210 ml/L (21%)
Alveolar air	160 ml/l (16% alveolar gas)	110 ml/L (11%)
Po_2 Alveolar gas	114 mm Hg (0.16 × 713)*	78 mm Hg (0.11 × 713)*
Po_2 Arterial blood	95 mm Hg (approx.)	65 mm Hg (approx.)

* Corrected for water vapor pressure (47 mm Hg at 37° C).

on. The oxygen content (21% of the air) will be 210 ml per liter of air. Because the subject has 5 L per min of alveolar ventilation, he will have to extract 250 ml per min from the 5 L of air, thus extracting 50 ml per liter. Subtracting 50 ml from the 210 ml that are present in air leaves 160 ml per liter in the alveolar gas (16% of the alveolar gas). Compare this with Subject B, who has severe hypoventilation, with 2.5 L per minute of alveolar ventilation; it is clear that the same amount of oxygen will have to be extracted from a much smaller amount of air. By the same calculations, one can demonstrate that the oxygen left in the alveolar gas will be 110 ml per liter, or only 11%. It follows, then, that with less oxygen in the alveolar gas, there will be less oxygen available to the arterial blood, and arterial hypoxemia will result. These figures may now be readily corrected to partial pressures. If the total barometric pressure is 760 mm Hg, a fixed proportion of this will be composed of water vapor when inside the body at the alveolar level. At body temperature (37° C), this is 47 mm Hg. For Subject A, the fraction of oxygen (0.16) times the corrected barometric pressure (713 mm Hg) will be the Po_2 of the oxygen in the alveoli. The calculated decrease in alveolar Po_2 from 114 to 98 mm Hg is thus accounted for purely on the basis of alveolar hypoventilation.

Conversely, a hyperventilating subject has an increased alveolar oxygen content and alveolar Po_2, with a resultant rise in arterial Po_2 (see list below). In fact, this is the only mechanism whereby an individual can have an elevated arterial Po_2 without an increased inspired Po_2.

Mechanisms of Increased Arterial Po_2

- Hyperventilation (always associated with reduced Pco_2; Po_2 generally at least 20 mm Hg below inspired Po_2)
- Increased environmental oxygen (Po_2 increased in proportion to P_IO_2)
- Contamination of blood by air (Po_2 never higher than environmental Po_2)

Changes in alveolar ventilation directly influence the level of carbon dioxide as well. This relationship has been defined as follows:

$$PaCO_2 \cong \frac{0.863\ (CO_2\ \text{production})}{\text{alveolar ventilation}}$$

A decrease in alveolar ventilation, therefore, results in elevated $PaCO_2$, and, conversely, hyperventilation results in reduced arterial Pco_2.

Altered Intrapulmonary Gas Exchange. The most common cause of arterial hypoxemia in patients with pulmonary disease is altered intrapulmonary gas exchange. The elegant mechanism whereby air is distributed throughout the tracheobronchial tree to terminal lung units is discussed below (see Effects of Abnormalities of

Regional Ventilation or Perfusion on Gas Exchange). Ideally, every terminal lung unit that receives air also is serviced by an appropriate allotment of venous blood. In the average alveolus, the ratio of the flow of air to that of blood at rest is approximately 0.8. Total alveolar ventilation is approximately 4 L per min, and the total pulmonary perfusion is approximately 5 L per min.

In the ideal alveolus, with appropriate matching of ventilation and perfusion, the blood is fully arterialized, and the Po_2 of the blood leaving the alveolus is virtually the same as the Po_2 of alveolar air. The very thin alveolocapillary wall normally presents no significant barrier to diffusion. Not all alveoli, however, function in this ideal fashion; in fact, the mixed arterial blood has a Po_2 approximately 10 mm Hg lower than the alveolar Po_2,[21–25] known as the *alveolar-arterial (A-a) gradient*. This is a result of three contributing factors: (a) venous blood that enters pulmonary veins and the left heart (*i.e.*, thebesian veins and bronchial blood flow); (b) anatomical arteriovenous communication in the lungs (these factors normally account for a 2 to 5% shunt, or approximately 50% of the A-a oxygen gradient)[21,22,24]; and (c) mismatching of ventilation in relation to perfusion. The latter mechanism has been estimated to contribute about half of the A-a gradient in normal persons, and the contribution of any of these may be increased in disease.

Even in normal persons, there are marked regional disparities in the distribution of air and blood. For example, in the upright position, while breathing spontaneously at a normal resting volume (functional residual capacity), more air is distributed to the alveoli in the lower lung zones than the upper lung zones.[26] There is also significantly more blood distributed to the lower zones than the upper zones, however, so that the proportion of air to blood is greater than 1.0 in the upper zones and less than 0.8 in the lower zones. This general mismatching of air in relation to blood flow results in some alveoli receiving excessive amounts of blood in the lower lung zones, resulting in inadequate gas to fully arterialize the blood; whereas in the upper zones, with an excessive amount of air, the blood is more

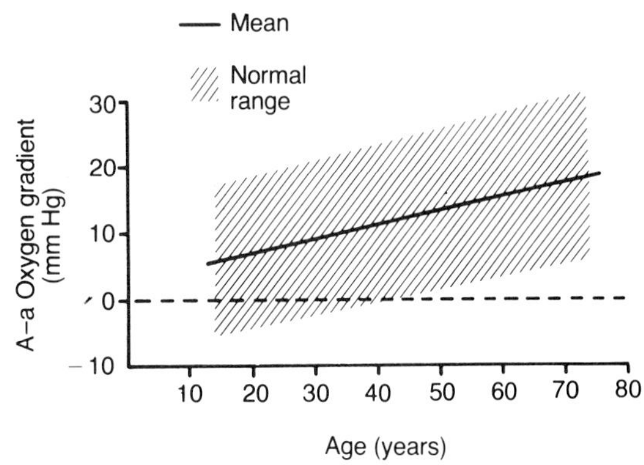

FIG. 5-2. Alveolar-arterial (A-a) oxygen gradient in normal subjects at various ages. Mean value for $P_{(A-a)}O_2$ = 2.5 + 0.21 (age) in mm Hg. Shaded areas indicate 2 standard deviations. (Compiled from data in Mellemgaard K: The alveolar-arterial oxygen difference: its size and components in normal man. Acta Physiol Scand 67:10, 1966)

than fully arterialized, and there is wasted ventilation.

Normal persons probably have increased A-a oxygen gradients with prolonged recumbency.[27] In one study, healthy young men had an increase from 9 mm Hg to 19 mm Hg after 10 days of imposed recumbency. This elevated gradient resulted in a decreased arterial Po_2, because the alveolar Po_2 remained normal. The mechanism was not established but probably relates to mismatched ventilation in relation to perfusion. This was not observed in a shorter study of 24 to 48 hr of recumbency.[28] Furthermore, the A-a gradient is increased with age, as illustrated in Figure 5-2. This, too, is probably due to uneven matching of ventilation and perfusion,[29] and results in a reduced arterial Po_2.

The alveoloarterial oxygen gradient is characteristically increased in diseases involving lung parenchyma, pulmonary airways, the pleural space, and the chest wall. As indicated in Table 5-1, when gas exchange is altered, with decreased ventilation compared with perfusion, the arterial Po_2 is reduced, and the alveolar-arterial oxygen gradient is increased while room air is breathed. In patients with regions of lung that are inadequately but partially ventilated, administration of high levels of inspired oxygen may provide sufficient alveolar oxygen to completely arterialize the perfusing blood. Therefore patients with low (but not zero) ventilation–perfusion ratios characteristically achieve a normal or near normal A-a gradient when breathing pure oxygen.[30] This is in contrast to conditions in which there is complete absence of ventilation, resulting in an intrapulmonary right-to-left shunt. Under these circumstances, the administration of 100% oxygen has no effect on the abnormal regions, and a high A-a gradient will be observed.

A diffusion block is characterized by a decrease in the arterial P_{O_2}, with an increased A-a oxygen gradient while room air is breathed. When high oxygen concentrations are administered, the diffusion gradient is unchanged, the A-a gradient generally falls within the normal range, and high levels of arterial P_{O_2} are observed.

An anatomical right-to-left shunt, such as a pulmonary arterial-venous fistula, or an atrial septal defect with reversed shunt has the same gas-exchange characteristics as an intrapulmonary right-to-left shunt that results from a complete lack of ventilation of some lung regions.

In general, the mechanism of the hypoxemia can be defined on the basis of the alveoloarterial oxygen gradient and the response of that gradient to inhalation of 100% oxygen. The arterial P_{CO_2} is elevated only in alveolar hyperventilation or in severe disturbances of ventilation–perfusion relationships, where some regions of the lung are critically underventilated. All other causes of hypoxemia tend to stimulate ventilation, which results in normal or reduced arterial P_{CO_2} levels.

Exercise at modest levels is associated with mild hyperventilation and no significant change in the alveolar-arterial oxygen gradient in normal persons. In patients with alveolar hypoventilation due to primary pulmonary disease, the arterial gas abnormalities are generally aggravated. When abnormal intrapulmonary gas exchange is present, exercise produces widely varying effects on arterial blood gases. Patients with regionally decreased ventilation, compared with perfusion, may have arterial P_{O_2} further reduced, unchanged, or actually improved, depending on the regional effects on ventilation and perfusion during exercise. Patients with "diffusion block" characteristically have further reduced arterial P_{O_2} as the rate of pulmonary blood flow is increased and the time available for diffusion in the pulmonary capillaries is reduced. Patients with intrapulmonary right-to-left shunts may have variable changes in blood gases during exercise; those with anatomical right-to-left shunts vary with the site and nature of the shunt. Patients with pulmonary arteriovenous fistulas have been reported to have increased, decreased, or unchanged arterial P_{O_2} with exercise; this is presumably dependent on the balance between flow through the defect and other regions of the lungs. Patients with intracardiac right-to-left shunts generally aggravate their shunt because during exercise pulmonary artery pressure is increased in the rigid pulmonary vascular bed and systemic vascular resistance is reduced. Therefore, their arterial hypoxemia is generally more severe during exercise.

ASSESSMENT OF INDIVIDUAL COMPONENTS OF THE RESPIRATORY GAS EXCHANGE SYSTEM

The optimal test of respiratory gas exchange would be an analysis of arterial blood gases through the entire spectrum of a person's bodily requirements. If arterial gases were normal, not only in the laboratory while at rest, but also during a full range of physical activity, during sleep, in various body positions, and when exposed to whatever environments the person might find himself in, pulmonary gas exchange would be adequate for clinical purposes. Screening tests of pulmonary function should include the assessment of arterial blood gases at rest and during laboratory-induced exertion. In selected instances, the response to inhaled irritants, to change in posture, or to sleep may be evaluated. If no abnormalities are identified in the gas analysis, further studies are not necessary. On the other hand, if abnormalities are identified, additional studies may be warranted in order to elucidate the underlying mechanism.

ALTERED ENVIRONMENTAL GASES

The effects of altered environmental gases (*e.g.*, at high altitude) have been dealt with in detail in Chapter 1.

ASSESSMENT OF ADEQUACY OF VENTILATION

The arterial Pco_2 is the best criterion for evaluating overall alveolar ventilation. Normally, at sea level, the arterial Pco_2 is maintained in a narrow range, from approximately 38 to 42 mm Hg. Anxiety with transient hyperventilation, transient breath holding, and other factors that modify the rate of ventilation also modify the gases in the arterial blood. Therefore, measurements should be sought with the person in a "steady state." An increase in arterial Pco_2 above this range (*e.g.*, greater than 45 mm Hg) indicates alveolar hypoventilation. Conversely, a decrease below 35 mm Hg indicates alveolar hyperventilation.

Assessment of the mechanisms which regulate breathing is dealt with in detail in Chapter 2, and the mechanisms of hyperventilation and hypoventilation in Chapter 6 (Table 6-1, 6-2).

ASSESSMENT OF INTRAPULMONARY GAS EXCHANGE

The factors affecting the ventilatory function of the lungs were reviewed in detail in Chapter 4. The effectiveness of the lung as a gas exchange unit requires more than overall ventilation in appropriate quantities. Regional distribution of that air through each of the peripheral lung units must be exquisitely balanced with the blood flow. Too much air will be wasted by ventilating units in excess of blood flow. On the other hand, too little air fails to arterialize the blood perfusing those units.

DISTRIBUTION OF VENTILATION

Regional differences in pleural pressures, along with gravity acting on the lung, result in dependent (lower) lung regions being less expanded than the upper regions of the lung. While breathing at normal resting levels (FRC), there is greater respiratory movement in the dependent regions. In the upright position, then, the lower regions of the lung receive more air per breath than the upper regions of the lung (Fig. 5-3). Patients with respiratory disease may have dramatically impaired regional distribution of ventilation to any size of lung unit. For example, a large pneumothorax, pleural effusion, or total atelectasis of the lung may completely prevent ventilation of a hemithorax. Similarly, conditions affecting smaller portions of the airways, such as obstruction due to secretions or bronchospasm in bronchial asthma, a foreign body, aspiration of foreign material, or pulmonary edema affecting bronchial walls, may all decrease the size of the airway to a given region of the lung and thereby diminish the ventilation to that region. In addition, a partially destroyed lung unit may be hyperinflated, as occurs in emphysema, but may not be ventilated with each breath and therefore may receive inadequate ventilation. In each of these circumstances, ventilation may be reduced, as compared with the pulmonary blood flow, and there will be insufficient ventilation to permit arterialization of the blood flowing through the lung units.[26,30]

Conversely, persons with thromboembolic disease resulting in pulmonary vascular occlusion, or regional spasm of the pulmonary arteries due to hypoxia, or acidosis may have some areas of the lung receiving poor blood supply, compared with the level of ventilation. Such regions of the lung may be relatively overventilated and contribute to wasted ventilation.

The list on p. 162 shows the methods that may be used to identify abnormalities of regional ventilation. When patients have gross abnormalities, bedside examination may reveal marked changes. With the patient positioned comfortably and symmetrically, unilateral lag of chest wall movement may be the most striking clinical manifestation of obstruction of a bronchus, atelectasis, pneumothorax, pleural disease, pneumonia, kyphoscoliosis, or localized chest wall disease. Similarly, reduced diaphragmatic motion with respiration may indicate phrenic paralysis or the characteristic decrease in diaphragmatic motion after abdominal sur-

Methods of Assessing Regional Ventilation

- Abnormal movement of the chest wall
  - Reduced diaphragmatic motion
    - Phrenic paralysis
    - Postoperatively
    - Upper abdominal disease
  - Asymmetrical movement of the chest wall
    - Atelectasis
    - Pneumothorax
    - Pleural disease
    - Pneumonia
    - Kyphoscoliosis
    - Chest wall pain
- Auscultation
  - Regional abnormalities of breath sounds
  - Rhonchi (inspiratory or expiratory)
- Chest film
  - Regional hyperlucency
  - Parenchymal disease
  - Abnormal bronchial walls
- Tests of distribution of inhaled inert gases
  - Single-breath nitrogen washout
  - Multiple-breath nitrogen washout
  - Mixing efficiency (helium)
  - Closing volume
- Assessment of physiological dead space or alveolar-arterial oxygen gradient
  - Exercise
- Lateral position test
- Radioisotope inhalation with lung scanning
- Bronchospirometry

gery. The latter results in reduced ventilation, particularly in the lower lung zones. When motion of the thoracic cage in all its diameters appears to be approximately normal, abnormalities of regional ventilation may still be identified by physical examination. Auscultation frequently demonstrates evidence of underlying airways disease. The dramatically reduced breath sounds in the periphery of the lung in patients with emphysema, the presence of widespread inspiratory and expiratory rhonchi in the asthmatic, terminal expiratory rhonchi in the patient with bronchitis, and the respiratory rales commonly heard in pulmonary edema all provide sound clinical suspicion of abnormalities of regional distribution of air.

The plain chest film is commonly helpful in identifying abnormalities associated with alterations in regional ventilation. Hyperlucency may indicate the parenchymal destruction of emphysema. Densities indicating parenchymal disease may suggest areas of decreased compliance that will be poorly ventilated. Thickened bronchial walls may indicate airway abnormalities, as in bronchitis or bronchial asthma. Each of these should alert the physician to the possibility of abnormal gas exchange. Some centers take inspiratory and expiratory films, with sequential films during a forced expiratory maneuver. The changes in lung volume measured in specific lobes and in the entire lung fields, particularly in relation to expiratory time, can provide substantial evidence regarding the regional distribution of gases.

Numerous tests have been designed to assess the evenness of distribution of air in the lungs. These have been discussed in detail in Chapter 4. In symptomatic patients, they are required only to confirm or quantitate clinical impressions. In mild or early disease, these tests may provide the only objective evidence for abnormal function. It is of utmost importance to recognize that all of these tests only indicate abnormalities in ventilation. No assessment of perfusion in relation to the regions of altered ventilation can be obtained by these methods.

Bronchospirometry, a technique that measures the ventilation of each lung by direct cannulation of the bronchi with a tracheal tube, has been less popular since the introduction of indirect and less traumatic tests of distribution of ventilation.[31]

A pragmatic approach to evaluation of regional lung function before surgical resection is presented in Chapter 11.

DISTRIBUTION OF PERFUSION

It is now well established that the patterns of blood flow in the lung can be generally divided into four zones.[31–34] This distribution of blood flow through the lungs is normally predominantly determined by simple pressure relationships as follows.

Zone 1, which is in the apical regions of the lung in the upright position, is too high for the hydrostatic pressure in the pulmonary artery to perfuse. At this level, the pressure in the alveolus (atmospheric) is greater than the pressure in the artery, and consequently the capillaries remain collapsed. This arbitrary zone is, of course, obliterated when the person lies down, or during exercise, when pulmonary artery pressure rises. Furthermore, there is no sharp division between Zone 1 and the next lower zone, because slightly lower regions of the lung have portions of the cardiac cycle during which pulmonary artery pressure is greater than atmospheric, therefore distending the capillaries at least during systole, resulting in small amounts of pulsatile flow.

In the next lower zone, Zone 2, pulmonary artery pressure is greater than atmospheric and therefore greater than the alveolar pressure, and there is a driving pressure for forward flow through the pulmonary capillaries. Progressing to lower regions of the lung, the pulmonary artery pressure increases linearly with the distance, but the alveolar pressure is still atmospheric. Therefore, the hydrostatic driving pressure increases linearly, and blood flow increases proportionately with distance down the lung. This second zone is roughly in the upper portion of the midlung field and again is not sharply demarcated from the next lower zone.

The third zone, representing the lower lung regions, is also characterized by linear increases in blood flow proportionate to the distance down the lung. At this level in the lung, the pulmonary venous pressure and the pulmonary arterial pressure are both greater than atmospheric. Therefore, the driving pressure is determined by pulmonary arterial pressure minus pulmonary venous pressure. Because both pressures increase linearly with descent down the lung, intravascular hydrostatic driving pressure does not explain the progressive increase in blood flow. A more likely explanation is the increase in both arterial and venous pressure, resulting in high intracapillary hydrostatic pressures that produce distention of pulmonary capillaries in this lower zone. In fact, studies of capillary volume have indicated that the capillaries in the apices of the lung are collapsed throughout the cardiac cycle, whereas capillaries in the base of the lung are widely distended. The progressive increments in blood flow in Zones 2 and 3 are illustrated in the upper, middle, and lower thirds of the lung (see Fig. 5-3).

A fourth zone is of little clinical significance at the present time in normal persons. In this small region at the inferior aspect of the lung, flow is limited by interstitial pressure, owing to the effects of gravity on the parenchyma of the lung and pleural pressures, and in this region blood flow is again reduced.

It is clear from this physiological zoning in the lung that changes in alveolar pressure, pulmonary arterial pressure, or pulmonary venous pressure all affect the hydrostatic pressures in the pulmonary vasculature and modify the distribution of blood flow. Similarly, changes in the person's position modify the dependent region (Zone 3) and the upper region (Zone 1). The zones can be entirely reversed in the normal subject who stands on his head.

Symmetrical changes in the distribution of perfusion are seen in both lungs in patients with elevated venous pressure. For example, patients with mitral stenosis shift the region of maximum blood flow in their lungs from the bottom upward and may do so approximately proportionally to the increase in venous pressure.[35,36] Patients with elevated pulmonary artery pressures also have symmetrically altered perfusion, predominantly characterized by increased perfusion of the apical lung regions and somewhat decreased perfusion in the lower lung regions.[37]

Regional changes in perfusion occur in a number of disease states. Pulmonary embolism results in obstruction of vessels of varying sizes and in various locations, with decreased blood flow beyond the region of the obstruction. Severe defects of perfusion are seen in congenital absence or hypoplasia of the pulmonary artery, the uncommon syndrome of the unilateral hyperlucent lung,[38,39] and patients with central lung tumors. Transient modifications in pulmonary vascular tone, due to hypoxia, acidosis, or perhaps inflammation, may result in regional deficits of perfusion, and patients with destructive changes of emphysema characteristically lose blood supply to areas of the lung.[40] Ventilation is less evenly distributed in the older age groups.[41] Whenever these lung regions continue to be ventilated out of proportion to the lung blood flow, the ventilation is wasted.

The list below summarizes the methods of evaluating regional distribution of perfusion. Here the physical examination is not nearly as

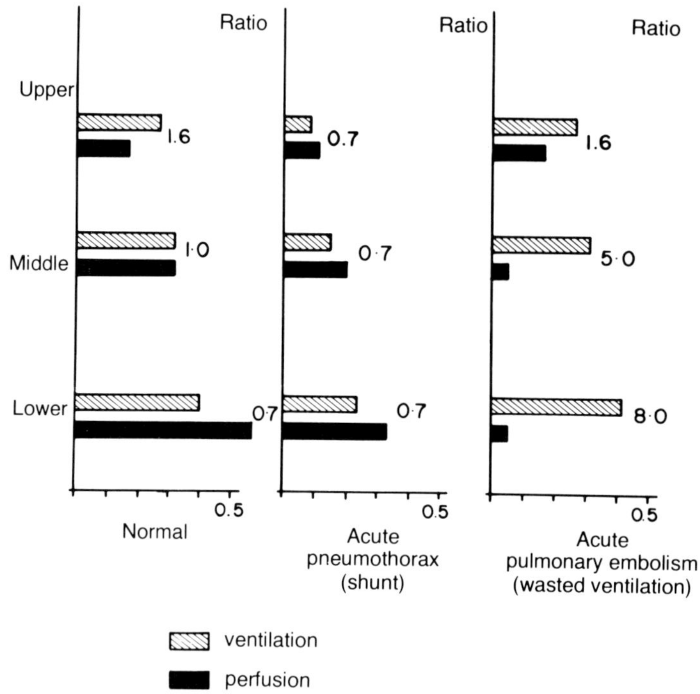

FIG. 5-3. Ventilation-perfusion relationship in the lung. (*Left*) Bar graphs indicate the proportion of normal total ventilation and perfusion for the upper, middle, and lower thirds of the lung. These arbitrary divisions are not precisely quantitative and do not coincide with the physiologically sound division into Zone 1, Zone 2, and Zone 3. As indicated in the text, Zone 1 has no perfusion and would therefore be even higher than the upper zone indicated in this graph. (*Center*) Bar graphs demonstrate the effect of a pneumothorax on ventilation and perfusion in the affected lung. During the acute phase ventilation would be strikingly reduced. As a compensatory mechanism, the perfusion is eventually also shunted to the opposite lung (which is being ventilated). This takes minutes to hours, however, to become established. As is apparent, perfusion in excess of ventilation in this lung will result in physiological shunt. (*Right*) The third set of graphs demonstrates the effect of a massive pulmonary embolism involving vessels to the middle and lower zones of the lung. Note that the perfusion is strikingly reduced, but ventilation is initially near normal. This, then, will result in wasted ventilation or physiological dead space. Later in the course, the distribution of ventilation and perfusion is affected by more complex factors.

rewarding as when evaluating ventilation. The physical examination is helpful only in those circumstances where modified flow results in turbulence with the production of murmurs. Consequently, the continuous murmur heard in the region of a pulmonary arteriovenous fistula or the systolic murmurs heard peripherally in the lung with peripheral pulmonary artery stenosis may draw attention to these uncommon abnormalities of regional distribution of perfusion. The chest film may be somewhat more helpful, because striking decreases in vascularity are seen with pulmonary embolism, and increased vascularity is seen with acute elevations in pulmonary venous pressure or in high pulmonary blood flow, as noted in congenital left-to-right shunts. The nodular densities seen in pulmonary arteriovenous fistulas generally require additional evidence, such as angiography, to confirm the nature of the lesion.

Methods of Assessing Regional Perfusion

- Auscultation
  - Continuous murmur with pulmonary A-V fistula
  - Systolic murmurs with pulmonary artery stenosis
- Chest film
  - Decreased vascularity (pulmonary embolism)
  - Increased vascularity (congenital left-to-right shunt)
  - Nodular densities (pulmonary A-V fistulas)
- Assessment of physiological dead space or alveolar-arterial oxygen gradients
- Tests of distribution of blood flow
  - Intravenous, inert, insoluble isotopic gases with lung scanning
  - Intravenous isotope-labeled macroaggregates with lung scanning
  - Pulmonary angiography
- Bronchospirometry

In general, definitive demonstration of abnormal regional distribution of blood in the lungs is dependent on more sophisticated techniques. Lung scanning by use of radioisotopes may be performed following injection of gaseous isotopes that are insoluble and that cross the alveolar membrane into alveolar tissues in the lungs. Appropriately timed counting of radioactivity over the lungs permits imaging.[42] Clinically, more commonly macroaggregated proteins are labeled with isotopes and injected intravenously. They are distributed wherever blood flow goes in the lung, trapped in pulmonary capillaries, and emit their radioactivity. Lung tissues may then be mapped according to the amount of radioactivity in the capillaries. Regions with decreased radioactivity indicate decreased blood flow. This technique is particularly applicable to the study of the microcirculation of the lung, but as might be expected, only fairly large lung units can be analyzed; terminal lung units cannot be identified individually by this technique. Pulmonary angiography is useful when identifying the structure of the large vessels and, if sequentially performed, can demonstrate approximately where blood flow is distributed. Large abnormalities in the amount of blood flow can be established from the density of the radiopaque dye.

Bronchospirometry permits estimation of blood flow by analyzing the oxygen uptake and carbon dioxide release of a lung that is ventilated.

Determinants of Pulmonary Artery Pressure (Pulmonary Hypertension)

The factors that result in elevated pulmonary artery pressure are indicated in the list below.[43–49]

Factors Affecting Pulmonary Artery Pressure

- Increased pulmonary blood flow
  - Exercise
  - Fever
  - Congenital heart disease with left-to-right shunts
- Increased pulmonary venous pressure
  - Left ventricular failure
  - Mitral valve disease
  - Pulmonary vein thrombosis
- Increased pulmonary vascular resistance
  - Vasospasm
    - Hypoxia
    - Hypercapnia
    - Acidosis
    - Histamine
    - Angiotensin
    - Serotonin
    - Vasoactive peptides (S.R.S.A.)
    - Prostaglandins ($F_{2\alpha}$)
  - Vascular wall hypertrophy
    - Long-standing hypoxia
    - Long-standing increase in PA pressure
  - Perivascular edema
  - Vascular thromboemboli
  - Destruction of vascular bed
    - Emphysema
    - Fibrosis
    - Surgical resection

In general, these can be classified according to the well-known formula that describes the inter-

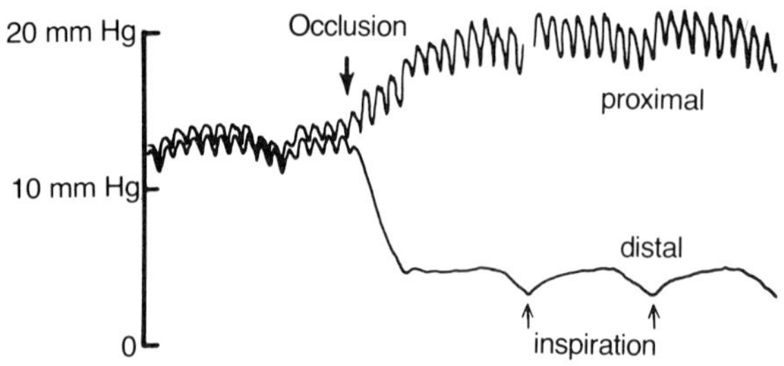

FIG. 5-4. Effect of occlusion of one pulmonary artery on pulmonary artery pressure. The graph demonstrates the pressure in the pulmonary artery proximal and distal to an inflatable balloon. At the time of occlusion, the pressure distal to the balloon drops to the pressure in the pulmonary veins and left atrium. The pressure proximal to the balloon rises because of the reduced total vascular bed. The mean increase in pressure demonstrated here, from 12 to 18 mm Hg, is a normal pulmonary artery pressure response to doubling the blood flow to the lung. Because the pulmonary artery pressure did not double, the pulmonary vascular resistance in the perfused lung has decreased to accept the additional blood flow.

relationships of flow, driving pressures, and resistance:

$$\text{resistance} = \frac{\text{driving pressure}}{\text{flow}}$$

For the majority of blood flow, in the pulmonary vascular bed, the driving pressure equals the pulmonary artery pressure minus the pulmonary venous pressure. Therefore, the formula can be rearranged as follows:

$$\text{resistance} = \frac{\text{pulmonary artery pressure} - \text{pulmonary venous pressure}}{\text{flow}}$$

or:

$$\text{pulmonary artery pressure} = [\text{resistance} \times \text{flow}] + \text{pulmonary venous pressure}$$

It is apparent that any factors that increase pulmonary blood flow, pulmonary vascular resistance, or pulmonary venous pressure will produce elevated pulmonary artery pressures. The pulmonary vascular bed is very distensible, and consequently increased pulmonary blood flow accounts for only small changes in pulmonary artery pressure. Exercise that results in a two- to threefold increase in pulmonary blood flow increases the pulmonary artery pressure only to a small degree. Further increases in the rate of flow, however, result in a striking increase in pulmonary artery pressure.

Blood flow through a given lung can also be increased by occlusion of the artery to the opposite lung. When this is done by inflation of a balloon catheter positioned in one of the pulmonary arteries, the pressure in the artery perfusing the opposite lung rises slightly (Fig. 5-4). As is apparent, this small rise in pressure that occurs with the relatively large rise in blood flow must be associated with an actual drop in pulmonary vascular resistance. This is generally attributed to recruitment of additional vessels that may not have been perfused, or to distention of vessels in this relatively compliant vascular system. Such compliance is lacking, however, in patients whose vascular beds have become rigid owing to disease (as occurs with sustained pulmonary hypertension, chronic obstructive lung disease, and diffuse pulmonary parenchymal disease), and their pulmonary artery pressure rises much more quickly during exercise or times of increased cardiac output. The increase in pulmonary artery pressure that results from increased pulmonary venous pressure is seen characteristically in patients with left ventricular failure or mitral valve disease. During the early phase, the rise of pulmonary artery pressure is approximately proportionate to the rise in pulmonary venous pressure.

The above mechanisms of increasing pulmonary pressure are readily evaluated. A more comprehensive understanding of pulmonary vascular physiology is required to elucidate the mechanisms of increased vascular resistance. In general, this may be caused by vasospasm, vascular wall hypertrophy as a result of long-standing vasospasm, perivascular edema, vascular thrombi or emboli, or destruction of the vascular bed by parenchymal disease. Of this group of causes, those which are physiologically reversible bear additional consideration. Alveolar hy-

TABLE 5-3. Comparison of Responses of Systemic and Pulmonary Vascular Beds

Vasoactive Factor	Systemic	Pulmonary
Hypoxia	Dilates	Constricts
Acidosis	Dilates	Constricts
Hypercapnia	Dilates	Dilates
Isoproterenol	Dilates (β adrenergic)	Dilates
Angiotensin	Constricts	Constricts
Histamine	Dilates	Constricts

poxia,[43,48–50] hypercapnia, and acidosis[51,52] are common causes of pulmonary hypertension during episodes of acute respiratory failure. Many times, however, the above mechanisms are not so clearly active,[53] and numerous other factors affecting pulmonary vasomotor tone have been well documented. Histamine, serotonin, and various prostaglandins have all been incriminated at one time or another, but none of these has been clearly demonstrated to be the specific mechanism of pulmonary vasomotor changes in a given disease. It is to be hoped that active investigation in this area will clarify additional factors that are clinically important.[43,54–56] Finally, increased blood viscosity (particularly at hematocritis above 55 and under conditions of high pulmonary blood flow) may raise the resistance to perfusion.[57,58]

It is noteworthy that several factors affecting the pulmonary circulation have quite different effects on the systemic circulation, as itemized in Table 5-3.

The administration of oxygen, theophylline, isoproterenol, or acetylcholine may result in reduced pulmonary vascular resistance in persons in whom it was elevated. This evidence of reversibility may be particularly important when planning therapy. Prolonged administration of oxygen may further reduce pulmonary vascular resistance in those whose primary problem is related to hypoxia. These factors are discussed in detail in Chapter 14.

The vasospasm that takes place in pulmonary vessels during hypoxia seems teleologically appropriate in the fetus, where blood should be shunted to the systemic circulation. Furthermore, if the ductus arteriosus remains patent, increased pulmonary vascular resistance in the neonate may modify the degree of shunting of systemic blood through the pulmonary circulation. In the adult, the advantages of diminished blood flow through lung regions that are not ventilated (and have a low Po_2) are also apparent. This diminishes the amount of wasted perfusion or shunt-like effect in the lung and thereby permits diseased regions of the lung to autoregulate the impact on oxygen exchange in the lungs. The generalized vasoconstriction that occurs in persons with respiratory failure or at high altitude, however, cannot be rationalized to the same degree.

EFFECTS OF ABNORMALITIES OF REGIONAL VENTILATION OR PERFUSION ON GAS EXCHANGE

DECREASED VENTILATION IN RELATION TO PERFUSION

When ventilation is reduced in relation to perfusion, blood flowing through these areas of the lungs will leave without adequate exposure to respiratory gases and will be partially venous. This has the same effect as an anatomical shunt. Most diseases that affect the airways do not affect the vasculature of the lungs in precisely the same location or to the same degree; therefore, a wide variety of airway diseases result in some regions with ventilation decreased in relation to perfusion. Such persons generally have arterial hypoxemia (see above, Factors Affecting Arterial Po_2 and Pco_2).

The presence of arterial hypoxemia raises concern regarding regional hypoventilation (Fig. 5-5). This can be further defined by calculation of the alveoloarterial gradient. The average alveolar Po_2 can be calculated by using the alveolar gas equation as follows.[59]

$$P_AO_2 = P_IO_2 - P_ACO_2\left[F_IO_2 + \frac{1 - F_IO_2}{R}\right]$$

$$\underset{\text{unknown}}{\downarrow} \quad \underset{\text{known}}{\downarrow} \quad \underset{\text{measured}}{\downarrow} \quad \underset{\text{correcting factor}}{\downarrow}$$

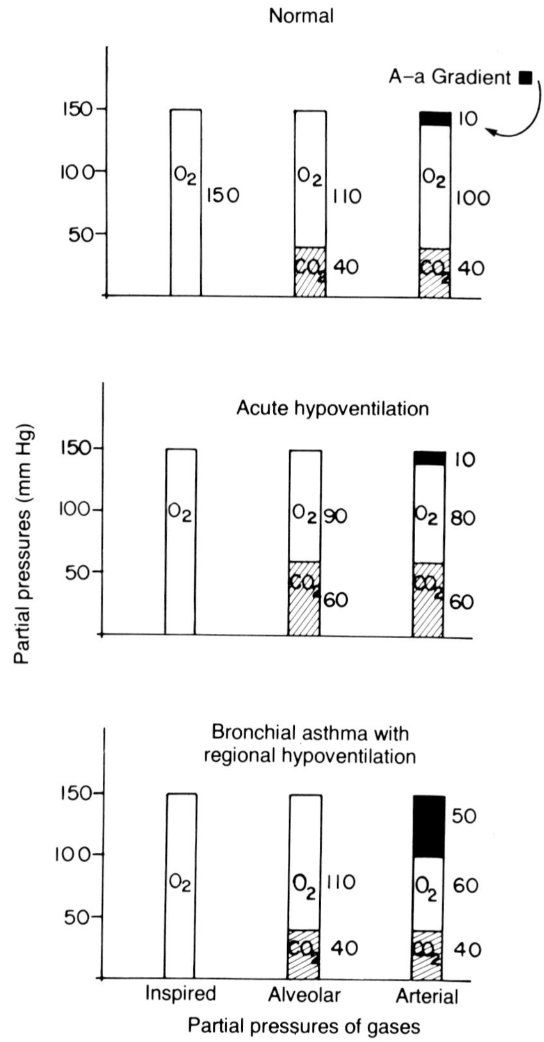

FIG. 5-5. Alveolar–arterial oxygen gradient. (*Top*) Bar graph demonstrates the normal gas partial-pressure relationships in inspired, alveolar, and arterial compartments, respectively. At sea level, the inspired oxygen (corrected for water vapor pressure) is 150 mm Hg. As the air is inhaled, the gas partial pressures in the alveolus must add up to barometric pressure. Because nitrogen is neither utilized nor produced by the body, the partial pressure of nitrogen is approximately the same in the alveolus as in the inspired air. When the respiratory quotient is 1, the oxygen removed from the alveolus equals the carbon dioxide delivered to the alveolus (*i.e.*, if 40 mm Hg of oxygen are removed, 40 mm Hg of carbon dioxide will be added). Because alveolar carbon dioxide is approximately equal to the arterial carbon dioxide, the inspired Po_2 minus the arterial Pco_2 equals the alveolar Po_2, and the alveolar Po_2 minus the arterial Po_2 equals the alveoloarterial gradient. Although under highly controlled conditions this gradient is less than 10 in most normal subjects, when these crude calculations are used, a range of up to 20 should probably be accepted as normal. (*Center*) Graph demonstrates the effect of a high arterial (and alveolar) Pco_2 on alveolar Po_2. This patient with acute hypoventilation cannot possibly have an arterial Po_2 greater than 90; with a gradient of 10, his arterial Po_2 is 80. This, then, is a normal gradient in spite of a reduced arterial Po_2. (*Bottom*) Graph demonstrates a patient with a normal arterial (and alveolar) Pco_2, a normal alveolar Po_2, but an unusually low arterial Po_2. The alveolar Po_2 (110) is 50 mm higher than the arterial Po_2, indicating a very high alveoloarterial gradient. Simple construction of these plots for hypoxic patients permits reasonably accurate delineation of the mechanism of reduced arterial Po_2. When the arterial Po_2 is reduced as a result of high altitude, the inspired Po_2 would be less than 150 mm Hg, and each subsequent compartment would reflect this reduced inspired oxygen.

The partial pressure of inspired oxygen (P_IO_2) can be calculated as outlined in Chapter 1. The partial pressure of alveolar CO_2 is almost identical to arterial Pco_2, and thus they can be used interchangeably. The correcting factor is introduced because of the variation in tension of alveolar gases under conditions with different respiratory quotients. The effect of the respiratory quotient on alveolar gases was discussed in Chapter 1. This can be determined simply by measuring oxygen consumption and carbon dioxide production. The average respiratory quotient is 0.8. For clinical purposes, this equation can be simplified to

$$P_AO_2 = P_IO_2 - \frac{PaCO_2}{0.8}$$

Furthermore,

$$\text{A-a gradient} = P_AO_2 - P_aO_2$$

Then one can calculate the alveoloarterial oxygen gradient by subtracting this alveolar gas Po_2 from the measured arterial Po_2. For practical clinical purposes, gradients greater than 20 mm Hg are abnormal. In the older age groups, perhaps 25 mm Hg should be considered abnormal (see Fig. 5-2).

Additional tests to elucidate the mechanism of an increased alveolar-arterial gradient may be directed at understanding whether the region is underventilated (but still ventilated) or has the effect of an absolute shunt (perfused areas of lung that are totally without ventilation).[30] If there is some (although inadequate) ventilation, the administration of oxygen to the inhaled air may dramatically improve the oxygen available to the pulmonary capillary blood flow, and the arterial Po_2 will approach normal values. When there is a complete absence of ventilation, as may occur with atelectasis, administration of increased inhaled oxygen will not improve the arterialization of blood in that region of the lung, and the arterial blood Po_2 value will remain much lower than that predicted for the inspired oxygen. The list below shows factors that affect the A-a gradient.[30,60]

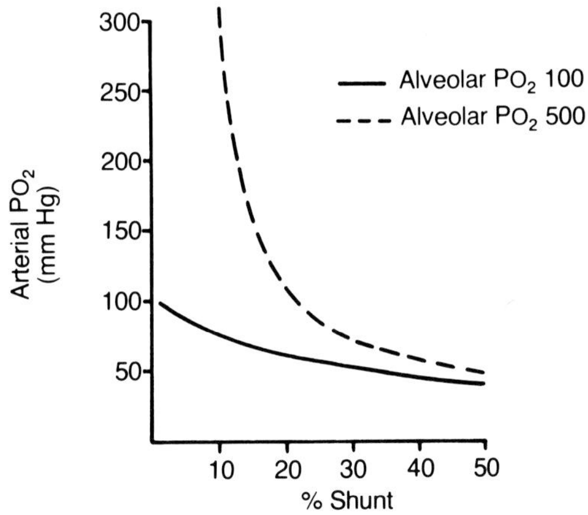

FIG. 5-6. Effect of true physiological shunt on arterial Po_2. This figure demonstrates the magnitude of shunt required to produce various levels of arterial Po_2, breathing room air (alveolar Po_2 100) or breathing 75% oxygen (alveolar Po_2 500). Note that an arterial Po_2 less than 50 mm Hg, with a normal alveolar Po_2, indicates approximately 30% physiological shunt. When breathing high concentrations of inspired oxygen, the Po_2 is regularly greater than 100, except where the shunt is quite large (greater than 20%). (Adapted from Pontoppidan H, Geffin B, Lowenstein E: Acute respiratory failure in the adult. N Engl J Med 287:743, 1972)

Factors That Influence the Alveolar-Arterial Oxygen Gradient

- Right-to-left shunt
- Inspired oxygen levels (ventilation-perfusion inequalities have a greater role at lower inspired Po_2)
- Mixed venous oxygen content
- Oxygen consumption (through its effect on mixed venous oxygen content)
- Cardiac output (through its effect on mixed venous oxygen content)
- Oxyhemoglobin affinity

It is impossible to tell from this data whether a high A-a gradient on 100% oxygen is due to an anatomical intracardiac or intrapulmonary shunt or merely to blood flowing through regions of the lung that are totally without ventilation.

The amount of blood flowing through shunt pathways may be determined by having the patient inhale 100% oxygen until all the nitrogen is washed out of the lungs. At this point, the alveolar Po_2 equals barometric pressure minus arterial Pco_2 minus water vapor pressure. At sea level, this would be 760−40−47, or 673, mm Hg.[60]

The deficiency of oxygen exchange can be estimated from this alveoloarterial gradient and expressed as a quantitative shunt. In a normal person at rest, the portion of blood "shunted" ranges from 2 to 5% of the cardiac output. A 50% shunt is compatible with life only if the person is breathing nearly 100% oxygen. Figure 5-6 illustrates the effect of increasing inspired oxygen tensions on the A-a gradient with different degrees of shunt. The following parameters permit quantitation of the shunt.[30,60]

$$\frac{\text{shunt blood flow}}{\text{cardiac output}} = \frac{\text{arterial oxygen content} - \text{pulmonary venous oxygen content}}{\text{systemic venous oxygen content} - \text{pulmonary venous oxygen content}}$$

Application of this shunt calculation in detail requires measurement of cardiac output, mixed venous oxygen content, arterial oxygen content, and the assumption that pulmonary venous blood is ideally oxygenated. If inhalation of 100% oxygen does not raise the arterial P_{O_2} above 100 mm Hg, the shunt is greater than 20%.

Precise localization of the area of shunt (*e.g.*, anatomical vascular or pulmonary parenchymal) may require cardiac catheterization or angiography.

INCREASED VENTILATION IN RELATION TO PERFUSION

Under normal circumstances, ventilation of the nasal passages, oropharynx, trachea, and bronchi, down to the gas-exchanging units, has been termed the *anatomical dead space*. This dead space ventilation is "wasted." When peripheral lung units contribute to wasted ventilation, this is in excess of the anatomical dead space, and the entire functional dead space has been termed the *physiological dead space*.

The physiological dead space can be readily measured during normal breathing. The following equation indicates the components that must be known:

$$\text{dead space ventilation} = \frac{(\text{arterial } P_{CO_2} - \text{expired } P_{CO_2}) \times \text{minute ventilation}}{\text{arterial } P_{CO_2}}$$

This simply requires measurement of arterial P_{CO_2}, collection of timed samples of expired air, calculation of minute ventilation, and analysis of the expired gas for carbon dioxide. When the rate of respiration is known, this may be converted to dead space per breath.[59] (Dividing minute ventilation by the respiratory rate yields tidal volume; dividing dead space ventilation by the tidal rate yields dead space per breath.) Dead space is normally increased approximately proportionally to body size and tidal volume. The ratio of physiological dead space (per breath) to tidal volume permits an estimate of the wasted ventilation. In general, this ratio should not exceed 0.3 in normal persons.

The techniques of assessing the alveoloarterial oxygen gradient and the physiological dead space are useful in demonstrating functionally significant ventilation–perfusion inequalities. (See also Chap. 7.)

Diffusion Across the Alveolocapillary Membranes

Normally, blood perfusing the pulmonary capillaries is in contact with aerated alveoli long enough to permit almost complete equilibration of gases. In fact, carbon dioxide diffuses readily, so that the major portion of diffusion is completed within the first 20% of the transit time through the pulmonary capillary. Oxygen, on the other hand, is only 95% equilibrated within the first 30% of the time the blood is in the capillary. The rate of diffusion of oxygen may decrease when the alveolocapillary membrane is thickened, thus increasing the length of the diffusion path. When the time required for equilibration exceeds the time available in the capillary, the blood leaving the capillary is incompletely arterialized. Conditions in which there is a reduced pulmonary capillary transit time include lung disease with reduced capillary bed and maximum exercise.[20,61] At extreme altitudes, diffusion may become a critical factor, owing to the short pulmonary capillary transit time and the narrow arteriovenous oxygen difference.[61a] In view of the very rapid diffusion of carbon dioxide, this does not influence arterial P_{CO_2} significantly. It is apparent, then, that in a patient with an increased barrier to diffusion, anything that speeds up the rate of blood flow through the pulmonary capillary consequently shortens the time for equilibration and amplifies the degree of hypoxia. Consequently, hypoxia that results from a diffusion block is always worse during exercise, fever, and other circumstances with an increased rate of pulmonary blood flow. At present, there is no widely accepted technique for assessing the rate of diffusion as such. Although the rate of diffusion might be easily calculated if the lung were composed of a single alveolus, analysis of gas exchange throughout millions of terminal lung units becomes much more complex. Methods have been established for calculating the diffusing capacity of oxygen, but these are not readily applicable clinically.

The most popular methods use the rate of transfer of carbon monoxide. Carbon monoxide is readily measurable; its diffusion characteristics are approximately comparable to those of oxygen; and it is bound by hemoglobin, as is oxygen. Therefore, many of the factors involved in oxygen transfer are comparable to those of carbon monoxide. Two general methods have been developed for the assessment of carbon monoxide "diffusion capacity."[61] Steady-state techniques assess the average rate of transfer of tracer amounts of carbon monoxide from inhaled air to the blood, over a period of several minutes. The amount of carbon monoxide inhaled minus the amount exhaled indicates the amount that has been transferred. Estimates of the alveolar carbon monoxide partial pressure then permit calculations of the amount of carbon monoxide transferred per mm Hg partial pressure of carbon monoxide, per minute. Single-breath techniques require an inhalation of tracer amounts of carbon monoxide with a timed period of breath holding, during which carbon monoxide is transferred to pulmonary capillary blood. Although the principles are similar, these single-breath techniques generally estimate higher levels of carbon monoxide diffusing capacity than do steady-state techniques. In fact, neither of these methods measures the diffusion characteristics of the alveolocapillary membrane as such. Both methods are affected by regional distribution of ventilation, alveolocapillary surface area, pulmonary vascular back pressure of carbon monoxide (which may be present as a result of environmental pollution or smoking), pulmonary capillary blood flow, alveolar oxygen partial pressures, hemoglobin of the perfusing blood, and other factors. Thus, although the diffusing capacity is characteristically reduced in patients with diffuse interstitial disease from any cause, it is also reduced in patients with pneumonectomy, pulmonary emphysema with parenchymal destruction, pulmonary embolic disease with widespread vascular occlusion, pulmonary vascular disease associated with connective-tissue disorders, and conditions that severely alter ventilation–perfusion relationships.

There is no pure test for diffusion, and it has not yet been established that a clinical situation exists in which a barrier to diffusion alone is responsible for abnormalities of gas exchange.[62] Diseases in which the diffusing capacity is most consistently abnormal are listed below. Tests of diffusing capacity may have their greatest value in following the course of certain diseases sequentially.

Conditions Commonly Associated with Reduced Diffusion Capacity*

- Diffuse interstitial disease
  - Pulmonary edema
  - Interstitial pneumonia
  - Lung fibrosis
- Reduced lung volume
- Parenchymal destruction (emphysema)
- Reduced pulmonary vascular bed (thromboembolism)
- Pulmonary resection

* Anemia and carboxyhemoglobin may result in low values not related to the lung.

TRANSPORT OF OXYGEN AND CARBON DIOXIDE

Oxygen Transport

Arterial Oxygen Content

The cardiac output of an average person at rest is about 5 L per min. The body oxygen consumption is approximately 250 ml per min. Therefore, the requirement of oxygen by the tissues is approximately 5 ml per 100 ml of blood flow per min. During strenuous exertion, the cardiac output may rise to 20 L per min and the oxygen consumption to 2500 ml per minute. At this level the requirement of oxygen by the tissues is approximately 12.5 ml per 100 ml of blood flow. To provide the requirements during exercise, the arterial blood must contain at least 12.5 ml of oxygen. Because the body is unable to function at very low levels of blood oxygen, additional reserve oxygen is carried. In fact, the arterial blood contains approximately 20 ml of oxygen per 100 ml of blood.

The solubility of oxygen in plasma at body temperature is low (0.3 ml dissolved in 100 ml per 100 mm Hg partial pressure of oxygen). Therefore, only about 0.3 ml of oxygen is carried in the dissolved state. The remainder of the oxygen is carried in combination with hemoglobin. Normal hemoglobin, when fully saturated, binds with 1.39 ml of oxygen per gram. A person with a normal hemoglobin value of 14 to 15 g per 100 ml of blood has a potential binding capacity of approximately 20 ml.

The list below summarizes the factors that determine the transport of oxygen to the tissues. The oxygen content of the arterial blood is not the only important factor.

The Oxygen Transport System

- Oxygen content of arterial blood, determined by:
  - Po_2 (dependent on pulmonary gas exchange)
  - Hemoglobin content
  - Hemoglobin affinity for oxygen
    - Physiological variables
    - Abnormal hemoglobin
- Blood flow to tissues
  - Cardiac output
  - Regional distribution
- Tissue factors
  - Vascularity
  - Diffusion characteristics
  - Intracellular mechanisms

Total blood flow to the tissues, regional distribution of blood flow in the tissues, and numerous poorly defined tissue factors are also important.

Hemoglobin is bound to oxygen in a relationship that is peculiarly suited to the body's wide range of physiological requirements. The relationship of dissolved plasma oxygen (Po_2) to the hemoglobin-bound oxygen is curvilinear (Fig. 5-7). The affinity of hemoglobin for oxygen permits almost complete saturation at the level of the pulmonary capillary ($Po_2 \cong 100$), with the release of about 30% of this oxygen in the tissues, as reflected in mixed venous blood (Po_2 approximately 40). The structure of the hemoglobin molecule, changes in configuration related to its state of oxygenation, and the intricate effects of hydrogen ions, CO_2, and other constituents of the red cells are now well understood.[63,64] Under normal circumstances the relationship of hemoglobin affinity for oxygen to the partial pressure of oxygen in the plasma is highly predictable. The affinity of hemoglobin for oxygen is popularly defined by the Po_2 required to produce 50% saturation. This so-called P_{50} is readily measured by modern technology.[65–69] At sea level, in normal persons, it is approximately 26 mm Hg, with more than 95% of the population having values between 24 and 28 mm Hg. Increased affinity for oxygen results in a shift of the curve to the left and a decrease in the P_{50}. Decreased affinity for oxygen results in a shift of the curve to the right or an increase in the P_{50} (Figs. 5-7, 5-8). Table 5-4 lists the factors that influence the affinity of hemoglobin for oxygen.

Cyclic circulation from the tissues to the lungs is associated with blood changes that affect oxygen's affinity for hemoglobin, improving both the unloading of oxygen in the tissues and the loading of oxygen at the pulmonary capillary level. As the blood flows through the tissues, several factors contribute to a reduced hemoglobin affinity for oxygen and improved oxygen release to the tissues. Carbon dioxide is released from the tissues, and combines with hemoglobin to produce carbamino groups. Some CO_2 is dissolved, and dissociates to form increased hydrogen ions. Metabolic acids released at the tissue level further reduce the *p*H, and contribute to reduced hemoglobin affinity for oxygen. Highly metabolically active tissues may have a higher temperature, which also results in decreased affinity of hemoglobin for oxygen and improved release of oxygen. This release of oxygen at the tissue level (or extraction by the tissues) determines the arteriovenous oxygen difference. Although the factors listed above have clear effects on oxygen availability to the tissues, few studies have systematically explored the factors that may facilitate oxygen extraction from blood at the tissue levels. When the blood returns to the pulmonary capillary, carbon dioxide is diffused

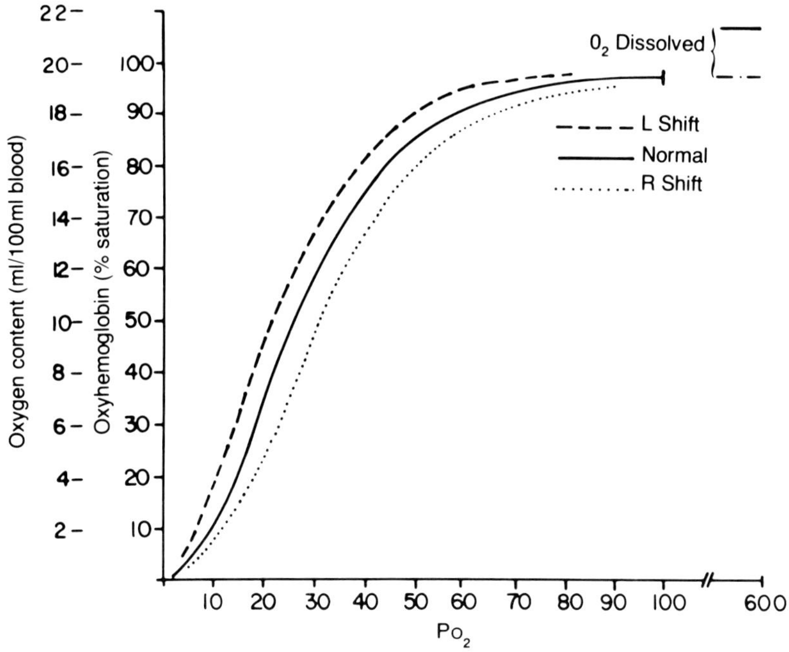

FIG. 5-7. Oxyhemoglobin dissociation curve. The oxygen content increases in proportion to the oxyhemoglobin saturation. When the hemoglobin is 95% saturated ($Po_2 > 80$), further increases in Po_2 produce small increases in oxygen content. Increasing the Po_2 from 100 to 600 results in a small additional increase in oxygen content (about 1.8 ml/100 ml, almost all in dissolved form). As the Po_2 is reduced from arterial blood values (80 to 100) to mixed venous values (about 40), the saturation is reduced from 97% to 70%. This permits a high oxygen content in the venous blood in spite of a relatively low extracting partial pressure at the tissue level. As discussed in the text, factors that shift the curve to the right facilitate the unloading of oxygen, and factors that shift the curve to the left facilitate the loading of oxygen. For example, normal blood provides an oxygen content of 15 ml per 100 ml of blood with a Po_2 of 40; the curve shifted 5 mm to the right provides 15 ml of oxygen at a Po_2 of 46; the curve shifted 5 mm to the left provides 15 ml of oxygen at a Po_2 of 36. Factors that determine the position of the curve are listed in Table 5.4.

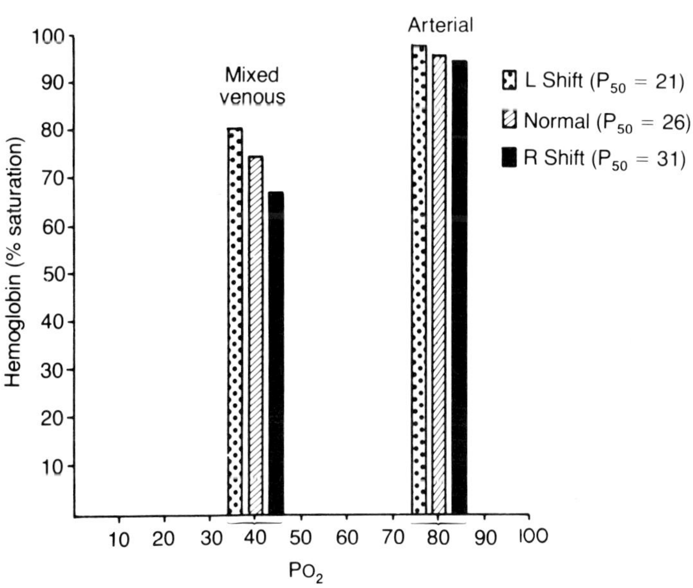

FIG. 5-8. Bar graph demonstrates oxygen content at the mixed venous level and at the arterial level for a normal curve (P_{50} equals 26 mm Hg), for a right-shifted curve (P_{50} equals 31 mm Hg), and for a left-shifted curve (P_{50} equals 21 mm Hg). Note that when the arterial Po_2 is normal, the major effect is on the unloading of oxygen. If the arterial Po_2 is less than 60 mm Hg, these changes in hemoglobin affinity for oxygen affect the uptake of oxygen in the lungs almost as much as the unloading in the tissues (see Fig. 5-7).

TABLE 5-4. Factors Affecting Hemoglobin Affinity for Oxygen[58,70–74]

Physiological Factors Affecting Persons With Normal Erythrocytes		
	Increased Affinity (↓ P_{50}) *(Shift of the curve to left)*	*Decreased Affinity* (↑ P_{50}) *(Shift of the curve to right)*
*p*H	Increased	Decreased
Pco_2	Decreased	Increased
Temperature	Decreased	Increased
2,3-DPG	Decreased	Increased
	Stored blood	Alkalosis
	Acidosis	Hypoxemia
	Hypophosphatemia	Hyperphosphatemia
Other Factors		
	Increased Affinity (↓ P_{50})	*Decreased Affinity* (↑ P_{50})
	Fetal hemoglobin	
	Acquired abnormalities of hemoglobin	
	Carboxyhemoglobin	
	Methemoglobin	
	Increased hemoglobin A_{1c}	
	Enzyme abnormalities	Enzyme abnormalities
	Pyruvate kinase excess	Pyruvate kinase deficiency
	Hexokinase deficiency	
	Diphosphoglycerate mutase deficiency	
	Abnormal hemoglobins	Abnormal hemoglobins
	Chesapeake, Little Rock, Creteil, McKeese-Rock, others	Kansas, Seattle, S, others

to the alveolus and exhaled. This results in a rise in *p*H, with a resultant increase in affinity for oxygen and improved uptake at the pulmonary capillary level. For each of these circumstances, it can be readily understood how the changes in hemoglobin affinity for oxygen are advantageous for tissue oxygenation.

Other factors that result in modified hemoglobin affinity for oxygen are not so obviously beneficial. For example, chronic hypoxemia (as a result of pulmonary disease, high altitude, or congestive heart failure) may be associated with reduced affinity of hemoglobin for oxygen. This seems reasonable as an adaptive mechanism to improve oxygen unloading; however, most of these states are also associated with reduced arterial blood Po_2, and reduced pulmonary capillary oxygen loading may cancel out any benefits of improved unloading of oxygen at the tissue level.[75–77]

Human studies suggest that in conditions of reduced available inhaled oxygen (altitude), a left-shifted oxyhemoglobin dissociation curve may be advantageous even though most people develop a shift to the right.[78] A shift to the left would be expected to impair oxygen unloading at sea level, but small shifts are tolerated without adverse effects.[79] Animals have been shown to tolerate hemorrhagic shock less well with a left-shifted curve,[80] but unstressed animals maintained normal oxygen consumption without evidence of anaerobic metabolism.[81] A right-shifted curve resulted in improved tissue extraction of oxygen.[81a]

In recent years, a great deal of interest has focused on the intracellular organic phosphate, 2,3-diphosphoglycerate (2,3-DPG), which apparently enters the hemoglobin molecule, modifying its affinity for oxygen.[82,83] Increased levels of 2,3-DPG are associated with reduced affinity for oxygen, and decreased levels of intraerythrocytic 2,3-DPG are associated with increased af-

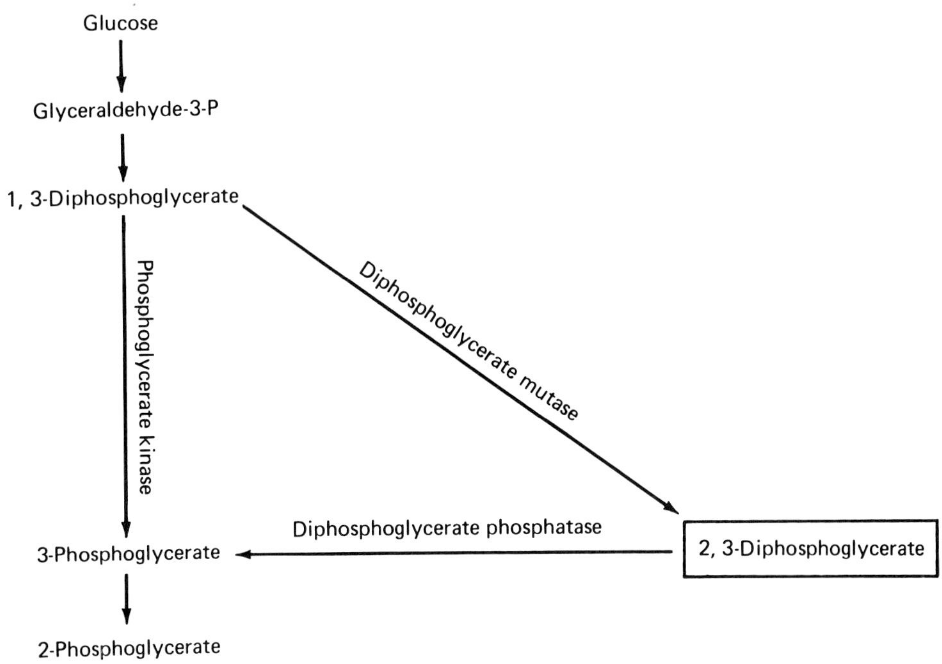

FIG. 5-9. Chemical pathway involved in the production of erythrocyte 2,3-diphosphoglycerate.

finity for oxygen. 2,3-DPG is predominantly, if not solely, produced in erythrocytes (Fig. 5-9), and numerous factors affect the production of intraerythrocytic 2,3-DPG, as listed in Table 5-4. Several clinical situations are associated with marked changes in 2,3-DPG. Uremia, characteristically associated with elevated circulating phosphate levels, is associated with high levels of 2,3-DPG and reduced affinity of hemoglobin for oxygen.[84,85] This may be an advantage in terms of tissue oxygen delivery, because these patients are generally severely anemic. Chronic hypoxemia is associated with increased 2,3-DPG and reduced affinity of hemoglobin for oxygen.[86] In other situations, the effects on oxygen delivery to tissues may, in fact, be detrimental. For example, in sustained metabolic acidosis seen during the development of diabetic acidosis, the hemoglobin affinity for oxygen is reduced (with improved tissue release of oxygen) as a result of the decreased *p*H. Subsequently, as the acidosis inhibits production of 2,3-DPG, the hemoglobin affinity for oxygen is increased, resulting in reduced unloading of oxygen at the tissue level.[66] Similarly, massive transfusions of stored blood with high oxygen affinity may measurably impair oxygen transport.[87–90]

Many variants of the hemoglobin molecule have been described with different binding characteristics for oxygen.[70–72,74] Fetal hemoglobin, the most common, has a left-shifted curve with apparent advantages for the fetus whose arterial Po_2 approximates maternal venous Po_2. Hemoglobin A_{1c}, a variant of normal adult hemoglobin, is present in high concentrations in diabetes. It has increased affinity for oxygen,[90a90b] but its significance in oxygen transport is not yet established. Methemoglobin and carboxyhemoglobin have an increased oxygen affinity.

Hemoglobinopathies with a left-shifted curve are commonly associated with polycythemia. It has been suggested that all polycythemic patients should have evaluation of their oxyhemoglobin affinity.[70,91] Hemoglobinopathies with a right-shifted curve are less common and several patients have been reported with comparatively low hemoglobin levels, suggesting more efficient oxygen transport.

Some medications are associated with changes in hemoglobin affinity for oxygen. The shift of the curve to the right, associated with propranolol, has been credited with improved oxygen transport to the ischemic heart.[91a]

The physiological advantages and disadvantages of shifts in the oxyhemoglobin dissociation curve have not been clarified. It is likely that the body's requirements need to be understood better.[91b] Reduced arterial Po_2, anemia, altered hemoglobin affinity for oxygen, reduced cardiac output, or regional ischemia undoubtedly have unique effects on tissue oxygen delivery which may be even more complex because of organ-specific tissue differences. The experimental work in this field leaves great uncertainty as to the benefits or liabilities of changing the hemoglobin affinity for oxygen.[63]

Cardiac Output and Tissue Perfusion

Normally, the cardiac output is regulated at least in part by the tissue oxygen requirements. Exercise, fever, hyperthyroidism, and anxiety are all associated with elevated cardiac output. This increase in blood flow is generally distributed to the most metabolically active tissue. There is no easy way to assess the cardiac output at the bedside. Clinical clues include warm, well-perfused skin; good urinary output; a normal pulse pressure suggestive of normal stroke volume and heart rate; and normal sensorium. Laboratory techniques for measuring cardiac output include indicator dilution techniques (which involve intravascular injections and blood sampling), assessment of ventricular stroke volume by ultrasound, radioisotope angiography with measurement of stroke volume, and the Fick method.

Direct sampling of arteriovenous differences, use of flow meters, or isotope angiography may be used to assess the regional distribution of blood flow to various organs.

The distribution of blood within the microcirculation of various organs is more elusive, and no clinically available technique provides an accurate assessment of tissue oxygenation or blood flow. Research techniques involving isotope angiography or tissue diffusion of isotopes can be utilized to identify the regions of decreased or increased tissue blood flow. Recently, attempts have been made to assess tissue oxygenation by oxygen electrodes or tissue sampling probes. Although these techniques now have limited clinical applicability, they may eventually be refined to provide additional information regarding distribution of oxygen in the body tissues.[92,92a,93]

Tissue Oxygen Transport

Metabolic requirements by tissues, and the factors affecting cellular respiration, are now of considerable interest.[94–96] Thyrotoxicosis, salicylate poisoning, malignant hyperthermia and many other conditions result in increased mitochondrial oxygen requirements. Hypothyroidism and cyanide poisoning are among those conditions that result in decreased mitochondrial oxygen consumption.[95,96] Mitochondrial edema and dehydration both reduce the oxygen consumption of cells. Further clarification of these changes in mitochondrial function may be of great importance in understanding adaptation to diseases involving reduced oxygen availability to tissues. Adaptive responses are now known to include changes in intracellular enzyme concentration.[96]

Various organs have specific requirements for nutrients and oxygen availability. Consequently, reduced oxygen delivery as a result of severe hypoxemia may have less severe effects than will ischemia. Ischemia adds the insult of accumulated CO_2, metabolic acids, and reduced *p*H as a result of inadequate tissue washout. When arterial hypoxemia is severe, it produces similar tissue effects to those seen with ischemia.

At present the tissue factors that determine oxygen transport are poorly defined. Distribution of perfusion, rate of diffusion, and local disease (*e.g.*, edema) can all be predicted to have importance.

Polycythemia, a Response to Hypoxia

Increased red cell and hemoglobin production is a normal response to arterial hypoxemia. This bone marrow response is generally viewed as an adaptive mechanism through which oxygen transport to tissue is maintained by an increase in the oxygen-carrying capacity of the blood. The response is mediated by a humoral substance, principally released or activated by the kidney. It is believed that renal erythropoietic factor acts upon a plasma precursor to produce active erythropoietin.[97–100] The renal stimulus to release the erythropoietic factor is apparently related to tissue hypoxia which may result from reduced arterial P_{O_2}, reduced oxygen transport due to anemia[98] or carboxyhemoglobin,[101] reduced oxygen release due to high-oxygen affinity hemoglobins,[91] or local factors causing tissue hypoxia. It is not blocked by cyanide and therefore not dependent on mitochondrial enzymes. The renal sensor has not been established. The effect of erythropoietin on bone marrow includes increased incorporation of iron into hemoglobin and increased maturation of red cell precursors. Laboratory measurement of erythropoietin levels may permit diagnosis of primary (reduced erythropoietin) and secondary (increased erythropoietin) polycythemia.[99]

Hypoxemia is implicated as a cause of polycythemia when the arterial P_{O_2} is less than 65 mm Hg and the oxygen saturation less than 92%. Chronic severe arterial hypoxemia may cause dramatic increases in hematocrit; values as high as 80% are not uncommon in cyanotic congenital heart disease.[102] With increasing altitude there is a predictable increase in hemoglobin with reduced arterial P_{O_2} in otherwise normal people. Other causes of secondary polycythemia are much less predictable in terms of quantitative increases in hemoglobin concentration. Physical activity, nocturnal hypoxemia, cardiovascular status, cigarette smoking, iron stores, and other factors probably account for this variability.

The precise level of hemoglobin or hematocrit above which the diagnosis of polycythemia should be made is not established. Measurement of the red-cell mass is usually necessary to establish the diagnosis of true polycythemia.[103] Values greater than 36 ml per kg in males or 32 ml per kg in females are considered elevated. In general a hematocrit greater than 53% should provoke consideration of the accompanying list, Mechanisms of Polycythemia. Relative polycythemia should be considered, particularly in patients taking diuretics or who may be dehydrated. The thoughtful physician recognizes that arterial hypoxemia is frequently present owing to other lung disease, even when the cause of polycythemia is not hypoxia. Generally such patients, particularly those with polycythemia vera, have mild hypoxemia,[104] which in itself does not explain the severity of polycythemia.

Mechanisms of Polycythemia

- Polycythemia vera (reduced erythropoietin)
- Secondary polycythemia (increased erythropoietin)
  - Physiologically appropriate (hypoxemia)
    - High altitude
    - Abnormal gas exchange in lungs
      - Disorders of the respiratory pump
      - Airways or parenchymal disease
    - Intracardiac or pulmonary right-to-left shunts
    - Abnormal hemoglobin-oxygen binding
      - Carboxyhemoglobin
      - High oxygen affinity
  - Physiologically inappropriate
    - Tumors
      - Renal carcinoma, cerebellar hemangioblastoma, hepatoma, uterine fibroid, adrenal cortical adenoma, ovrian carcinoma
    - Renal disease
      - Carcinoma, cysts, hydronephrosis, Bartter's syndrome, transplantation
    - Cobalt, testosterone administration
  - Familial polycythemia
- Relative polycythemia (reduced plasma volume, normal red cell mass)

The optimal circulating hemoglobin and hematocrit level has not been established. Early studies suggested that cardiac output and oxygen delivery to tissues were improved to hematocrit levels as high as 60%, with gradual decreases at higher hematocrits, due to increasing viscosity. More recent and perhaps more discriminating studies suggest that certain tissues, notably the brain, develop reduced perfusion above hematocrit levels of 46%, more than negating the benefits of increased carrying capacity for oxygen.[105,105a] The optimal hematocrit level for a specific patient will depend on many poorly understood and interdependent factors. These include the range of tissue requirements, short-term and long-term cardiovascular and tissue adaption, and special needs for times of stress (*e.g.*, nocturnal hypoxemia). At present it is not entirely clear whether polycythemia is adaptive or maladaptive. While these matters remain a subject for clinical research, a general therapeutic guideline is to maintain the hematocrit at levels below 55%, and this may soon require revision to lower levels. (See also Chap. 1, Altitude; Chap. 14, Obstructive Disease.)

Critical Levels of Tissue Oxygenation

At the present time, the minimum oxygen delivery to tissues without producing adverse effects has not been established. Furthermore, no precise information regarding the most critical vascular beds is available.[77,106] Studies carried out to establish the critical level of jugular venous Po_2, below which manifestations of abnormal cerebral function would occur, have generally indicated potential danger below a Po_2 of 20, but this has not been uniformly confirmed.[107,108] Evidence of anaerobic metabolism and metabolic acidosis may occur in some conditions, with a mixed venous Po_2 as high as 30; whereas, in other circumstances, in normal persons, the arterial Po_2 may be below that level, with no evidence of major tissue dysfunction. Presumably, these differences reflect alterations in regional blood flow to critical tissues.

The importance of oxygen delivery must be considered in the light of specific organ requirements. It has been calculated[77] that the kidney extracts oxygen under normal circumstances to produce an average arteriovenous difference of 1.7 vol %. The heart, on the other hand, extracts 13 vol %. Therefore, a decrease in arterial oxygen content (as a result of a reduced Po_2 or severe anemia) to half of the normal value would mean that the heart would not be able to extract sufficient oxygen, even though the kidney would still have reserves. The heart, therefore, would have to either increase its blood flow or decrease the oxygen consumption. In normal persons, blood flow is readily increased. Furthermore, the effects of tissue CO_2 and metabolic acids within the heart capillaries would promote oxygen release through reduced hemoglobin affinity for oxygen (to a greater degree than would occur in the kidney capillaries). Differential distribution of blood flow, favoring brain over skeletal muscles, has been well demonstrated.[108] Diseased persons may not have normal ability to redistribute blood flow or increase cardiac output, and simple extrapolations of known arterial oxygen transport mechanisms may be misleading.

When hypoxia is severe, clinical evidence of decreased tissue oxygenation may become important. Some organs, such as the brain, may demonstrate loss of function. A decrease in aerobic glycolysis results in reduced oxygen consumption, increased production of lactic acid, and measurable metabolic acidosis.[106,109–111] This is reviewed in Chapter 1, in relation to the effects of high altitude.

The earliest manifestations of cellular hypoxia relate to synthetic processes in the cell, including the neurotransmitters. It is not surprising, then, that measures of impaired energy metabolism, such as evidence of anaerobic glycolysis, may occur later than the subtle changes in organ function.[96] Alterations of substrate utilization, biosynthesis, intracellular electrolytes, and high-energy phosphates are well-known; changes are characteristic of specific tissues. In advanced hypoxia, damaged cell membranes may leak, with increased flow of enzymes into the extracellular fluid and the blood stream. This is the basis for the well-known elevations of creatine phosphokinase in myocardial ischemia. The factors that determine reversibility of hypoxic or ischemic tissues are not well established, but clearly vary from tissue to tissue.[106]

It is appropriate, then, to make every effort to ensure adequate oxygen delivery by the known transport mechanisms until a clearer assessment of the critical levels of oxygenation of specific tissue dysfunction becomes possible.

Methods of Assessing the Oxygen Transport System

Table 5-5 lists the methods in common clinical use for estimating oxygen delivery to the tissues. Clinical methods are notoriously unreliable except when hypoxia is severe. Dyspnea is generally mild in conditions resulting in hypoxia, when compared with conditions that increase the work of breathing. Hyperventilation may be

TABLE 5-5. Methods of Assessing the Oxygen Transport System

Clinical Features

Dyspnea
Abnormal organ function (e.g., mental function)
Hyperventilation
Cyanosis

Laboratory Analysis

Component	*Method of Assessing*
Dissolved oxygen	Po_2 (blood gas electrodes)
Oxygen-carrying capacity	Oxygen content of fully saturated blood
Hemoglobin	Hb (clinical laboratory)
Hemoglobin affinity for oxygen	P_{50} (blood gas electrodes, tonometer, spectrophotometer, for assessing oxyhemoglobin)
Oxygen content, oxygen capacity	Van Slyke chemical analysis, Lexington instruments polarographic technique
Oxyhemoglobin saturation	Spectrophotometer Ear oximetry
Carboxyhemoglobin	Spectrophotometer
Meth- or sulfhemoglobin	Spectrophotometer
Cardiac output	Fick method, indicator dilution technique
Regional perfusion	Difficult Individual organ blood flow
Tissue oxygen levels	Tissue Po_2 electrode Mixed venous Po_2
Tissue oxygenation	Cytochrome a, a_3 NAD/NADH

Causes of Cyanosis

- Increased unoxygenated hemoglobin in capillaries
  - Decreased arterial Po_2 (generally less than 55 mm Hg)
  - Mildly reduced arterial Po_2 with polycythemia
  - Normal arterial Po_2 with severe reduction in blood flow (shock)
  - Hemoglobinopathy (e.g., Kansas)
- Abnormal hemoglobin pigment
  - Methemoglobin
  - Sulfhemoglobin
- Other pigmentation
  - Argyria
  - Hemochromatosis

present but is also nonspecific. When abnormal organ function occurs, it is a late manifestation of hypoxia. Cyanosis can be helpful for diagnosis when present, but is frequently misleading whether present or absent.[112] This bluish discoloration is best sought for in vascular capillary beds of nails, conjunctivae, lips, and tongue.

Cyanosis has been described to occur when the capillary content of reduced hemoglobin exceeds 5 g/100 ml. This may occur when arterial hemoglobin is unsaturated or when tissue extraction is high. When the extremities demonstrate cyanosis but central tissues such as the tongue and conjunctiva do not (peripheral cyanosis), the cause may be reduced peripheral perfusion with increased tissue oxygen extraction. When central and peripheral tissues are cyanosed (central cyanosis), it generally indicates unsaturated arterial hemoglobin (see list above). Hemoglobinopathies with severely reduced oxygen affinity have been reported as a rare cause of cyanosis with a normal Po_2. More commonly, the altered color characteristics of sulfhemoglobin or methemoglobin result in central cyanosis. These generally result from reactions to drugs or chemicals, although congenital methemoglobinemia has been reported.[72]

Equally important are the conditions associated with severe hypoxemia in which cyanosis may not be present (see list below). With anemia, as is now commonly seen in patients in chronic renal dialysis programs, total hemoglobin values of 3 to 5 g/100 ml of blood are not uncommon. In spite of severely reduced arterial blood oxygen saturation resulting from a low arterial Po_2, these persons are rarely, if ever, cyanosed. Carboxyhemoglobin is red, similar to oxyhemoglobin, and, therefore, fatal carbon monoxide poisoning does not produce cyanosis. In patients with fever and peripheral vasodilatation, the high capillary blood flow may reduce oxygen extraction and minimize otherwise apparent cyanosis. Finally, cosmetics have frequently masked the underlying cyanosis of the lips and nail beds. The examination for cyanosis is not complete until several vascular beds have been examined.

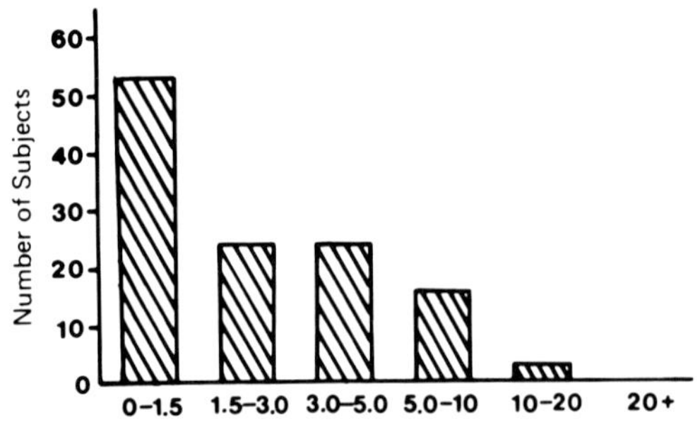

FIG. 5-10. Carboxyhemoglobin levels in patients during routine pulmonary function tests. One hundred and twenty-one consecutive patients who were evaluated in the clinical pulmonary-function laboratory in the Foothills Hospital in Calgary, Alberta, had carboxyhemoglobin determinations. Note the large number who had carboxyhemoglobin levels greater than 3%. Such levels are considered to have a significant affect on patients with cardiopulmonary disease. Most of these elevated values could be directly attributed to tobacco smoking; several nonsmokers had been exposed to urban environmental pollution.

Conditions with Severe Hypoxemia Without Cyanosis
Reduced circulating hemoglobin (anemia)
Abnormal hemoglobin (carboxyhemoglobin)
Systemic vasodilation with rapid blood flow
Abnormal pigmentation

Of the laboratory techniques available, measurement of arterial Po_2, hemoglobin, arterial oxyhemoglobin saturation, and, in some hospitals, an estimate of the oxyhemoglobin dissociation curve are in most common use. For special studies, use of the noninvasive ear oximeter, which assesses oxyhemoglobin spectrophotometrically through the capillary bed of the ear is now being applied more widely.[113] Most clinicians must make an assessment of cardiac output and regional distribution of perfusion on clinical grounds. Mixed venous Po_2 may be helpful in following a specific patient. Although no fixed level has been established to be helpful, levels below 30 mm Hg Po_2 are considered ominous.[114,115] Additional information about oxygen delivery can be obtained by knowing the patient's temperature, blood *p*H, amount of carboxyhemoglobin, and evidence of other factors affecting the oxyhemoglobin dissociation curve. The common exposure to carbon monoxide and increased concern about the adverse effects of moderate amounts of carboxyhemoglobin have resulted in more common use of this analysis (Fig. 5-10).

Methods of assessing cardiac output, regional blood flow and tissue oxygen levels are generally only available in tertiary care teaching hospitals with research interests. The place of the tissue Po_2 electrodes in clinical medicine remains to be defined.[92,115] Recent advances in measurement of tissue cytochrome a, a_3, NAD, NADH and flavoproteins show promise for more definite assessment of intracellular oxidation-reduction states.[116]

CARBON DIOXIDE TRANSPORT

Approximately 200 ml of carbon dioxide are removed per min from the tissues at rest, and 2000 ml are removed per min during exhaustive exercise. As is true for oxygen, the solubility of carbon dioxide in plasma provides a negligible amount of transport. Carbon dioxide produced in the mitochondria is diffused through the cytoplasm to interstitial spaces and then into the blood (Fig. 5-11). In the blood, the carbon dioxide diffuses through the plasma, where some is dissolved or is bound to plasma proteins as carbamino groups. Most of it, however, diffuses into the erythrocyte, where the enzyme carbonic anhydrase facilitates hydration of the carbon dioxide to form carbonic acid:

$$CO_2 + H_2O \underset{\text{carbonic anhydrase}}{\rightleftarrows} H_2CO_3$$

The carbonic acid then dissociates to some degree, producing free hydrogen ions and bicarbonate. Some bicarbonate then diffuses out of the erythrocyte into the plasma, thereby reducing the concentration in the erythrocyte. This takes place according to standard laws of concentration gradients. Because this results in a net

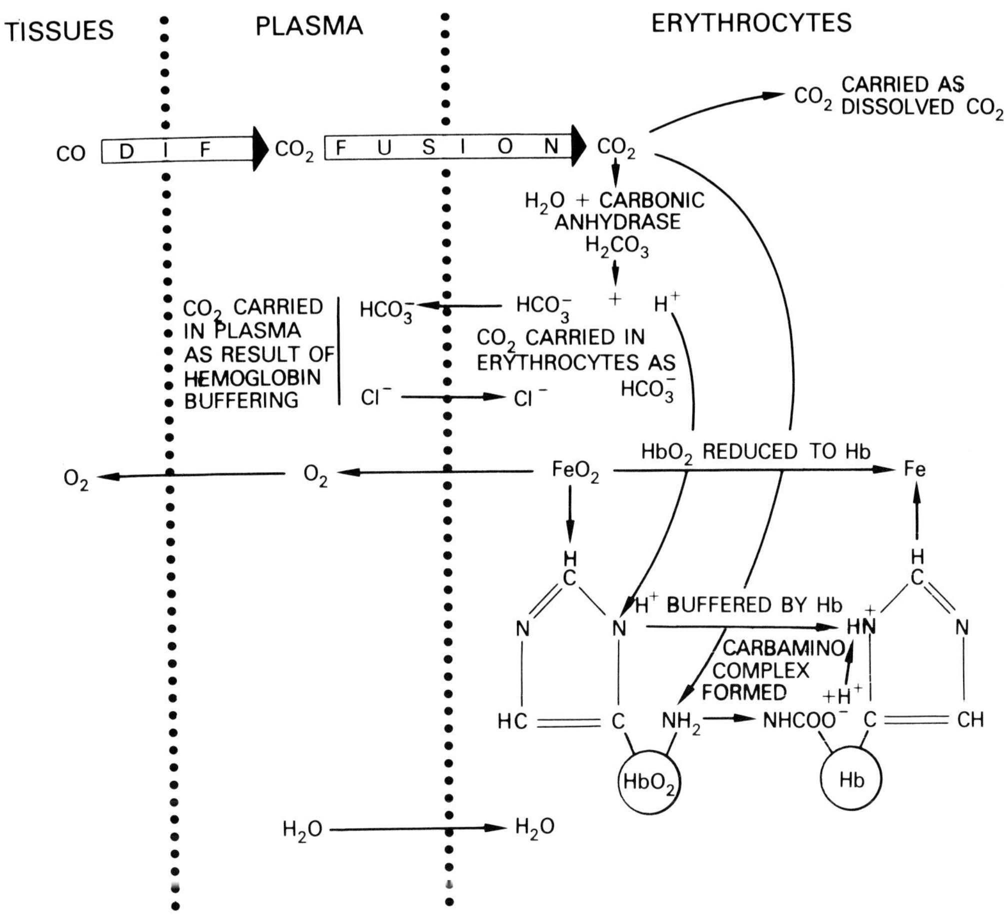

FIG. 5-11. Carbon dioxide transport. Note that carbon dioxide diffuses from cells and tissues through plasma into erythrocytes. Here it is dissolved, bound to reduced hemoglobin as carbamino groups, or hydrated to carbonic acid. This dissociates to produce bicarbonate, which may diffuse into the plasma. When the blood reaches the alveolar level, the entire process is reversed, and the diffusion is in the direction of the alveolus rather than the tissues. (Davenport H W: The ABC of Acid–Base Chemistry, 6th ed. Chicago, University of Chicago Press, 1974)

increase in negatively charged ions in the plasma, an additional transfer of negatively charged ions must take place into the cell; and chloride generally moves intracellularly.[117,118] In addition, the carbon dioxide may combine with the protein of reduced hemoblogin to form carbamino groups.

The majority of carbon dioxide, then, is transported from the tissues to the lungs in the form of bicarbonate in the plasma or as carbamino groups in the erythrocytes.[118,119] When the blood reaches the lungs, carbon dioxide is diffused from the plasma into the alveolar air, along diffusion gradients. In the lungs the entire process that occurred in the tissues is reversed; in the presence of carbonic anhydrase the carbon dioxide is quickly released from carbonic acid, and plasma and erythrocyte bicarbonate levels are decreased. Furthermore, in the presence of oxygen, hemoglobin binds to oxygen, eliminating carbamino groups. The cyclic unloading of carbon dioxide at the alveolar level is therefore facilitated by the loading of oxygen, and the uptake of carbon dioxide at the tissue level is facilitated by the release of oxygen.

As with oxygen, the carbon dioxide blood transport mechanisms normally function with substantial reserves, so that in circumstances of decreased rate of blood flow or increased metabolic activity, adequate transport is available. Abnormalities of the carbon dioxide transport system have not been incriminated as a mechanism of symptoms. Most studies have concentrated on the role of oxygenation in regional tissue metabolism rather than on the role of carbon dioxide removal. Consequently, at the present time, metabolic effects of regional tissue hypercapnia are not considered to be clinically significant. This entire area, however, has not been investigated adequately and, as recently emphasized, the chapters on this subject "belong to the future."[120] It is quite clear that major acidosis in the systemic venous bed, as seen in shock, can be partly attributed to increased carbon dioxide in venous blood, caused by low circulatory rates. When regional perfusion is strikingly impaired, severe tissue acidosis might be expected, even though the arterial blood may have a normal or nearly normal *p*H and P_{CO_2}. Tissue perfusion is therefore recognized as a major determinant of CO_2 removal from the tissues. It has also been demonstrated that regional ventilation–perfusion relationships in the lung may determine the removal of CO_2 from the blood.

The 20-fold range of P_{CO_2} apparently tolerated by different vertebrate species suggests that CO_2 *per se* is not of major importance in regulating metabolism.[118] The evidence now supports hydrogen ion concentration, directly influenced by CO_2, as the important factor.

RESPIRATORY ASPECTS OF ACID–BASE BALANCE

Hydrogen ion metabolism is important for many aspects of cellular function. Mitochondrial hydrogen ions are maintained at a low level, with a definite cytoplasm–mitochondrial gradient. Transfer of sodium, chloride, calcium, and other cations is intimately related to hydrogen ion distribution. The spatial configuration of various proteins and activity of certain enzymes are modulated by hydrogen ion concentration. In spite of these many recognized functions, clinical medicine is unable to assess tissue or cellular concentrations of hydrogen ions. The clinical applications remain at the level of measurement of acid–base balance in the blood, with crude extrapolations and speculation regarding organ function.

Relationship of Respiratory Gases to Acid–Base Balance in Blood

In body fluids, as in classical chemistry, a fluid with increased hydrogen ion concentration is acidic; one with decreased hydrogen ion concentration is basic. The major respiratory factor controlling hydrogen ion concentration in the blood is the amount of carbonic acid, which is directly proportional to the dissolved carbon dioxide, which is proportional to the P_{CO_2}. The following formula describes the relationships:

$$H_2O + CO_2 \rightleftarrows H_2CO_3 \rightleftarrows H^+ + HCO_3^-$$

An increase in carbon dioxide results in a shift of the equation to the right, forming more carbonic acid that will dissociate and form more hydrogen ions. Because bicarbonate is a weak base, this results in increased acidosis. Unfortunately, the practice of clinical medicine has been complicated by the concept of *p*H. This concept, apparently well founded in the laws of physics,[121–123] requires use of the inverse logarithm (log) of the hydrogen ion concentration. This complex relationship is described in the Henderson-Hasselbach equation:

$$pH = pK + \log \frac{[HCO_3]}{[H_2CO_3]}$$

or

$$pH = 6.10 + \log \frac{[HCO_3^-]}{0.03\ P_{CO_2}}$$

Normally, the ratio of bicarbonate to carbonic acid is approximately 20 to 1; when P_{CO_2} is introduced into the equation, it is apparent that an increase in P_{CO_2} reduces the ratio of bicarbonate to carbonic acid and thereby reduces the *p*H.

The concentration of bicarbonate is controlled by metabolic processes, and the P_{CO_2} by alveolar ventilation. Therefore, metabolic acid–base disturbances affect the numerator, and the respiratory acid–base disturbances affect the denominator.

Acute or severe changes in hydrogen ion concentration (and *p*H) are generally detrimental to the body. Because the process of cellular metabolism produces thousands of milliequivalents (mEq) of hydrogen each day, elaborate mechanisms are available to control the concentration. Buffer systems in the body act immediately to modify the hydrogen ion concentration. These include phosphates, sulfates, reduced hemoglobin, and proteins. Respiratory responses are early, increasing or decreasing the ventilation to blow off or retain carbon dioxide as required. Finally, the control of bicarbonate levels through renal excretion or conservation takes hours or days to become effective.

Changes in *p*H that result from changes in P_{CO_2} can be predicted with reliability.[118,119,124–128a] The precise quantitative interrelationship of hydrogen ion concentration and dissolved CO_2 observed in blood *in vitro* is somewhat modified *in vivo*. Consequently, recent studies have attempted to quantitate the *p*H–P_{CO_2} relationships *in vivo* in a variety of acid–base disorders.[126,128a]

It is now common practice to diagnose acid–base disturbances after measurement of *p*H and P_{CO_2} in arterial blood.[127] This permits calculation of the bicarbonate concentration and the hydrogen ion concentration.[128] Venous carbon dioxide is measured by widely differing techniques in clinical laboratories, adds no new information, and tends to be somewhat less reliable.[127] This may, however, be helpful in assessing the anion gap as described below. The hydrogen ion concentration has been widely discussed and is considered preferable to *p*H by many authors.[121–123,129] This has a particular advantage over *p*H by demonstrating change in milliequivalents, thus facilitating therapeutic decisions. The following table illustrates the *p*H-hydrogen ion relationships:

***p*H**	**H^+ concentration m moles/L**
7.00	100
7.10	80
7.22	60
7.30	50
7.40	40
7.52	30
7.70	20
8.00	10

Figure 5-12 is a composite drawing in which *in vivo* titration curves were utilized to establish normal ranges. This emphasizes the nonlinear relationships of bicarbonate and *p*H with increasing or decreasing P_{CO_2}.[126] Similar displays have been prepared by Davenport[117] and Sigaard-Andersen[125] and are in popular use. Each of the nomograms makes certain assumptions which limit the applications in complex acid–base disturbances.

When interpreting acid–base data, an arterial *p*H of less than 7.35 is generally considered to document acidemia; a *p*H of greater than 7.45 documents alkalemia. If the P_{CO_2} is normal or near-normal the mechanism is considered nonrespiratory or metabolic. If the P_{CO_2} is markedly abnormal, the mechanism is respiratory or includes a respiratory component.

If the bicarbonate is elevated or reduced beyond the range demonstrated in Figure 5-12 for acute respiratory acidosis or alkalosis, a metabolic contribution must be present. Use of the bicarbonate can be further refined by calculation of the anion gap,[130,131] a calculation which assumes electrical neutrality of the blood. All measurable cations are added up and expressed in mEq/L. Then all measurable anions are added up and expressed in mEq/L. The anions are then subtracted from the cations:

$$\text{Anion gap} = [Na^+ + K^+ + Ca^{++} + Mg^{++}] - [HCO_3^+ + Cl^- + PO_4^= + SO_4^=]$$

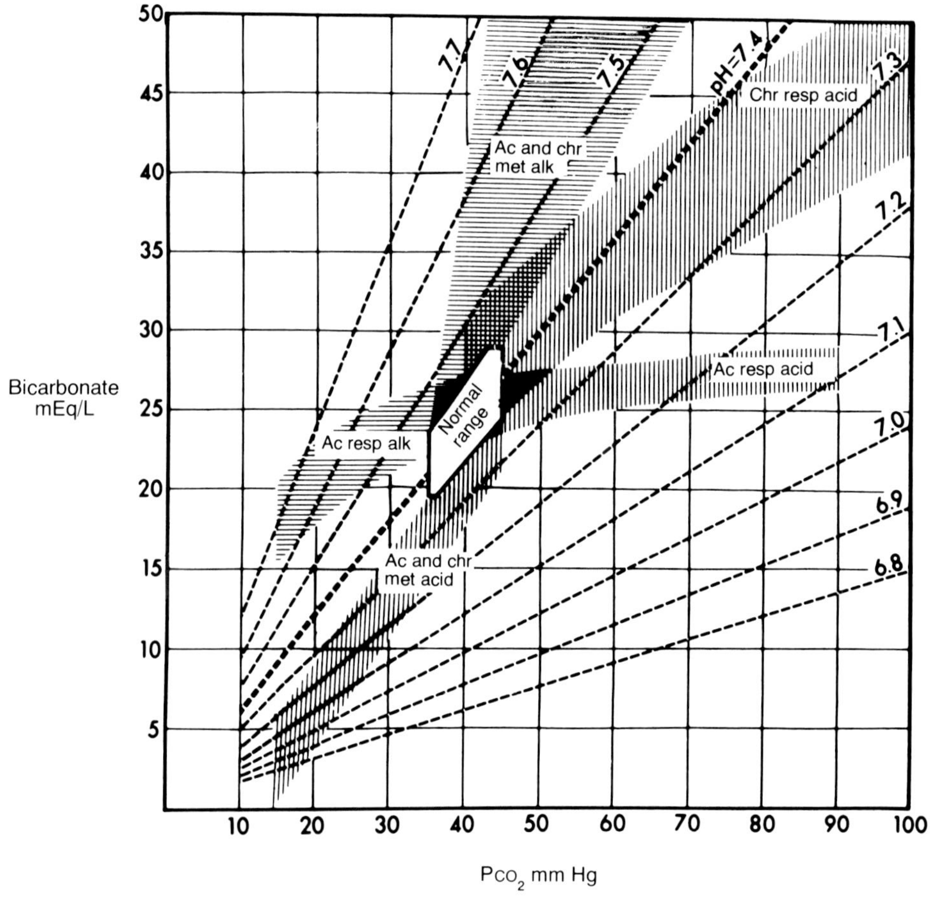

FIG. 5-12. Nomogram for acid-base disturbances *in vivo.* This graph displays the quantity and direction of changes in *p*H, Pco_2, and bicarbonate in a variety of metabolic and respiratory acid–base disorders. The shaded areas represent the range of variability observed in selected populations with pure acid–base disorders as designated. In general, patients whose values lie outside of the "significance bands" have mixed acid–base disturbances. *Ac* indicates acute; *Chr* indicates chronic; *Alk,* alkalosis; *Met,* metabolic. (Arbus GS: An in vivo acid–base nomogram for clinical use. Can Med Assoc J 109:291, 1973)

This equation can be simplified for clinical use, since the calcium, magnesium, phosphates and sulfates approximately cancel out. The following is a more suitable formula and permits an estimate to be made on the basis of readily available serum electrolytes:

$$\text{Anion gap} = [Na^+ + K^+] - [HCO_3^- + Cl^-]$$

Because the potassium concentration is relatively stable, it can be further simplified to:

$$\text{Anion gap} = Na^+ - [HCO_3^- + Cl^-]$$

The normal value, using this simplified formula, is 8 to 16 mEq/L.

Patients with metabolic acidosis who have increased circulating organic acids will have abnormally high anion gaps because these acids have not been measured. Some causes of metabolic acidosis, such as ingestion of ammonium chloride or renal tubular acidosis, have a normal anion gap, because the anion is routinely measured. In general, an elevated anion gap indicates that metabolic acidosis is contributing to the acid–base disturbance. Small increases in anion gap have been reported in metabolic alkalosis as a result of hemoconcentration causing an increased concentration of the normally negatively-charged blood proteins.[131]

Respiratory Alkalosis

Hyperventilation results in a decrease in the level of dissolved carbon dioxide (and consequently carbonic acid) in the blood, a reduced hydrogen ion concentration, and an increase in *p*H. Values of *p*H that are above 7.45 may be accepted as indicating clinically significant alkalemia. When the hyperventilation persists, as occurs at high altitude or with chronic hypoxemia, there is compensatory excretion of bicarbonate by the kidneys, which results in maintenance of the *p*H near normal. Under these circumstances, the *p*H generally ranges from 7.40 to 7.45. This is called a *compensated respiratory alkalosis.*

Respiratory alkalosis may be symptomatic when there is a substantial elevation in *p*H (alkalemia). In general, this requires *p*H levels greater than 7.50 to 7.55. Blood *p*H values greater than 7.70 are rarely tolerated for prolonged periods. The physiological effects and clinical manifestations of respiratory alkalosis are summarized in Table 5-6 (see also Chap. 6).

TABLE 5-6. Respiratory Alkalosis

Physiological Effects	Clinical Manifestations
Nervous System	
Decreased cerebral blood flow	Anxiety, numbness and tingling, seizures, light-headedness
Increased excitability	
Increased neuromuscular irritability	
Renal and Metabolic	
Chloride retention and bicarbonate excretion	Carpopedal spasm
	Increased reflexes
Decreased ionized serum calcium and magnesium	Chvostek's and Trousseau's signs
Increased glycolysis and metabolic rate	
Increased production of lactic acid	
Increased catecholamine release	
Cardiovascular	
Systemic vasoconstriction	Palpitations
	Arrhythmias
Tachycardia	
Increased myocardial irritability	
Respiratory	
Bronchoconstriction	Dyspnea

Respiratory Acidosis

Hypoventilation leads to elevated dissolved carbon dioxide (and consequently carbonic acid) in the blood. If this occurs acutely, there is a dramatic decrease in *p*H. A small increase in bicarbonate occurs acutely in response to the elevated carbon dioxide (about 3 mEq of bicarbonate per liter when the arterial P_{CO_2} is increased to 90 mm Hg). Therefore, the *p*H change *in vivo* is approximately equal to that predicted in blood *in vitro.*[133] With chronic hyperventilation, bicarbonate is retained and thereby buffers the effects of CO_2 on *p*H. Therefore, dramatic increases in blood bicarbonate may be expected in chronic hypercapnia (Fig. 5-12).

Symptoms in respiratory acidosis are also related to the change in *p*H more than the change in P_{CO_2}.[134] The physiological effects and clinical manifestations of respiratory acidosis are summarized in Table 5-7. They are minor at a *p*H of about 7.30, increasing at *p*H values below 7.25, and marked at *p*H values as low as 7.10. With rare exceptions, *p*H values below 6.90 in arterial blood are sustained for only short periods of life.

Interpretation of Acid–Base Disturbances

As listed in Table 5-8, simple acid–base disturbances are readily understood. Increased *p*H indicates alkalemia; decreased indicates acidemia. Alkalosis or acidosis refer to the acid–base de-

TABLE 5-7. Respiratory Acidosis

Physiological Effects	Clinical Manifestations
Central Nervous System	
Dilated cerebral vessels → increased cerebrospinal fluid pressure	Headache, dyspnea, somnolence, psychosis, papilledema, focal neurological signs, neuromuscular irritability (asterixis) may progress to frank coma
Depressed cortical function	
Respiratory center stimulation (medulla and carotid bodies)	Hyperventilation
Renal and Metabolic	
Transfer of H^+ into cells and K^+ out. Thus, early increased serum K^+, subsequent increased excretion of K^+	None significant
Excretion of Cl^- and reabsorption of bicarbonate	
Depressed glycolysis and cellular metabolism	
Reduced hemoglobin affinity for oxygen	
Cardiovascular	
Decreased myocardial contractility	Heart Failure
Increased or decreased irritability	Arrhythmias
Decreased responsiveness to catecholamines	
Systemic vascular dilatation	Systemic hypotension
Pulmonary vascular and bronchial smooth muscle contraction	Pulmonary hypertension

TABLE 5-8. Acute and Chronic Acid–Base Disturbances

	P_{CO_2}	*p*H Acute	*p*H Chronic	HCO_3^- Acute	HCO_3^- Chronic
Respiratory alkalosis (hyperventilation)	↓	↑	↑⟷	⟷	↓
Respiratory acidosis (hypoventilation)	↑	↓	↓⟷	⟷	↑
Metabolic acidosis	⟷↓	↓	↓⟷	↓	↓
Metabolic alkalosis	⟷↑	↑	↑⟷	↑	↑

rangement, even if the H^+ has been buffered or compensated for. When acidosis is caused by respiratory mechanisms, the P_{CO_2} is elevated. When acidosis is caused by metabolic mechanisms, the bicarbonate is reduced. When alkalosis is caused by respiratory mechanisms, the P_{CO_2} is reduced; when metabolic, the bicarbonate is increased.

After the primary derangement has been established, compensatory mechanisms become active. The mechanisms of compensation for respiratory acid–base disturbances are metabolic. Therefore, the patient with chronic hyperventilation developes a reduced bicarbonate; the patient with chronic hypoventilation, increased bicarbonate. Chronic or compensated acid–base disturbances always represent mixed mechanisms.[124–126]

TABLE 5-9. Mechanisms of Metabolic Acidosis

Mechanisms	Clinical Conditions
Increased production of acids	
Ketones, beta hydroxybutyric	Diabetes mellitus
	Starvation
Lactic acid	Severe hypoxia (shock, severe anemia, arterial hypoxemia, severe exercise)
	Drugs (phenformin, INH overdose, salicylate overdose, alcohol, ethylene glycol, methanol)
	Idiopathic
Decreased excretion of acids	
Reduced tubular hydrogen ion excretion	Pyelonephritis, multiple renal diseases, drugs (carbonic anhydrase inhibitors)
Reduced glomerular filtration	Acute renal failure
Exogenous acids	NH_4Cl infusions, ethylene glycol, methanol

Many laboratories report various computed values reflecting bicarbonate concentration. Base excess, the most popular of these, reflects the total available buffer base in the blood and is expressed in mEq per liter. This takes into account alterations in bicarbonate that are directly related to increased or decreased P_{CO_2}, as well as varying hemoglobin concentrations. The clinician can generally utilize base excess or bicarbonate equally well if a nomogram such as Figure 5-12 is understood.

Difficulties in the interpretation of acid–base disturbances arise when (as occurs so commonly in very ill patients) mixed factors are active.[135] Under these circumstances, clinical information that documents loss of hydrogen ions, loss of bicarbonate, or recent dramatic change in status may permit the conclusion that metabolic and respiratory factors are present. A common example in respiratory medicine is the patient with chronic obstructive pulmonary disease and chronic hypercapnia who presents with a nearly normal *p*H (*e.g.*, 7.43) and increased P_{CO_2} (*e.g.*, 58). This patient has an alkalosis that at first glance is not respiratory. Closer observation and historical information may permit the conclusion that, in fact, he chronically has an even greater P_{CO_2} (*e.g.*, 65), but he transiently hyperventilated at the time of sampling of the arterial blood, thus changing the *p*H from 7.38 to 7.43. Nomograms are not helpful in coming to a specific diagnostic conclusion; however, Figure 5-12, which incorporates the broad range of changes in *p*H, P_{CO_2}, and bicarbonate in pure acid–base disturbances, permits a judgment regarding the presence of multiple factors.

Metabolic acidosis frequently presents as a primary respiratory problem because of the obvious hyperventilation. Blood gas analysis may provide the important clue; when the *p*H is low, the P_{CO_2} normal or low (due to compensatory hyperventilation), and the bicarbonate low, the causes of metabolic acidosis listed in Table 5-9 should be considered.

Primary acid-base disturbances are readily diagnosed. Complex disturbances require a sophisticated analysis of the history, factors contributing to electrolyte shifts, and use of drugs or ingestion of toxins. No formula permits identification of specific cause.

REFERENCES

1. PETTY TL, BIGELOW DB, LEVINE BE: The simplicity and safety of arterial puncture. JAMA 195:693, 1966
2. MORTENSEN JD: Clinical sequelae from arterial needle puncture, cannulation and incision. Circulation 35:1118, 1967
3. MORGAN EJ, et al: The effects of unanesthetized arterial puncture on PCO_2 and *p*H. Am Rev Respir Dis 120:795, 1979

3a. SHAPIRO BA: Clinical Application of Blood Gases, 2nd ed. Chicago, Year Book Medical Publishers, 1977
4. GARDNER RM, et al: Percutaneous indwelling radial artery catheters: Risk of thrombosis and infection. N Engl J Med 290:1227, 1974
5. LUCE EA, et al: Compression neuropathy following brachial arterial puncture in anticoagulated patients. J Trauma 16:717, 1976
6. BEDFORD RF, WOLLMANN H: Complication of percutaneous radial artery cannulation: An objective prospective study in man. Anesthesiology 38:228, 1973
7. BEDFORD RF: Radial artery function following percutaneous cannulation with 18 and 20 gauge catheters. Anesthesiology 47:37, 1977
8. FALOR WH, HANSEL JR, WILLIAMS GB: Gangrene of the hand: A complication of radial artery cannulation. J Trauma 16:713, 1976
9. GREENHOW DE: Incorrect performance of Allen's test: Ulnar–artery flow erroneously presumed inadequate. Anesthesiology 37:356, 1972
10. MATTHEWS JI, GIBBONS RB: Embolization complicating radial artery puncture. Ann Intern Med 75:87, 1971
11. MICHAELSON ED, WALSH RE: Osler's node: A complication of prolonged arterial cannulation. N Engl J Med 283:472, 1970
12. LOWENSTEIN E, LITTLE JW, HING HL: Prevention of cerebral embolization from flushing radial artery cannulas. N Engl J Med 285:1414, 1971
13. BAND JD, MAKI DG: Infections caused by arterial catheters used for hemodynamic monitoring. Am J Med 67:735, 1979
14. LINDESMITH LA, et al: Arterial punctures by inhalation therapy personnel. Chest 61:83, 1972
15. SACKNER MA, AVERY WG, SOLOLOWSKI J: Arterial punctures by nurses. Chest 59:97, 1971
16. KELMAN GR, NUNN JR: Nomograms for correction of blood Po_2, Pco_2, pH, and base excess for time and temperature. J Appl Physiol 21:1484, 1966
17. SEVERINGHAUS JW: Blood gas calculator. J Appl Physiol 21:1108, 1966
18. FOX MJ, BRODY JS, WEINTRAUB LR: Leucocyte larceny: A cause of spurious hypoxemia. Am J Med 67:742, 1979
19. COMROE JH: A sea of air. Am Rev Respir Dis 111:355, 1975
20. GUENTER CA: The effects of acute severe arterial hypoxemia on the electrocardiogram during exercise. Chest 68:149, 1975
21. BRISTOW GK, KIRK BW: Venous admixture and lung water in healthy subjects over 50 years of age. J Appl Physiol 50:552, 1971
22. LENFANT C: Measurement of ventilation/perfusion distribution with alveolar–arterial differences. J Appl Physiol 18:1090, 1963
23. RAINE JM, BISHOP JM: A-a difference in oxygen tension and physiological dead space in normal man. J Appl Physiol 18:284, 1963
24. MELLEMGAARD K: The alveolar–arterial oxygen difference: Its size and components in normal man. Acta Physiol Scand 67:10, 1966
25. COLE RB, BISHOP JM: Effect of varying inspired oxygen tension on alveolar-arterial oxygen tension difference in man. J Appl Physiol 18:1043, 1963
26. WEST JB: Ventilation–perfusion relationships. Am Rev Respir Dis 116:919, 1977
27. CARDUS D: Oxygen alveolar–arterial tension difference after ten days recumbency in man. J Appl Physiol 23:934, 1967
28. TRIMBLE C, et al: The effect of supine bed-rest upon alveolar–arterial oxygen gradients and intrapulmonary shunting in normal man. J Thorac Cardiovasc Surg 63:873, 1972
29. HOLLAND J, et al: Regional distribution of pulmonary ventilation and perfusion in elderly subjects. J Clin Invest 47:81, 1968
30. NUNN JF: Measurement of pulmonary shunt. Acta Anaesthiol Scand (Suppl) 70:144, 1978
31. BALL WC, et al: Regional pulmonary function studied with xenon[133]. J Clin Invest 41:519, 1962
32. WEST JB, DOLLERY CT, NAIMARK A: Distribution of blood flow in isolated lung: Relation to vascular and alveolar pressures. J Appl Physiol 19:713, 1964
33. ANTHONISEN NR, MILIC-EMILI J: Distribution of pulmonary perfusion in erect man. J Appl Physiol 21:760, 1966
34. HUGHES JMB, et al: Effect of interstitial pressure on pulmonary blood flow. Lancet 1:192, 1967
35. HUGHES JMB, et al: Factors determining the distribution of pulmonary blood flow in patients with raised pulmonary venous pressure. Clin Sci 37:847, 1969
36. RITCHIE BC, SCHAUBERGER G, STAUB N: Inadequacy of perivascular edema hypothesis to account for distribution of pulmonary blood flow in lung edema. Circ Res 24:807, 1969
37. BERGLUND E, MALMBERG R, SIMONSSON BG: Effect of body position on regional lung perfusion at normal and elevated pulmonary pressures. Scand J Respir Dis 48:208, 1967
38. SWYER PR, JAMES GCW: A case of unilateral pulmonary emphysema. Thorax 8:133, 1953
39. MACLEOD WM: Abnormal transradiancy of one lung. Thorax 9:147, 1954
40. WELCH MH, et al: The lung scan in alpha$_1$ antitrypsin deficiency. J Nucl Med 10: 687, 1969
41. HOLLAND J, et al: Regional distribution of pulmonary ventilation and perfusion in elderly subjects. J Clin Invest 47:81, 1968
42. WAGNER HN JR: The use of radioisotope techniques for the evaluation of patients with pulmonary disease. Am Rev Respir Dis 113:203, 1976

43. BERGOFSKY EH: Active control of the normal pulmonary circulation. Moser KM (ed): In Pulmonary Vascular Diseases, Chap. 3. New York, Marcel-Dekker, 1979
44. COURNAND AF: Pulmonary circulation. Its control in man, with some remarks on methodology. Am Heart J 54:172, 1957
45. FISHMAN AP, HECHT HH (eds): The Pulmonary Circulation and Interstitial Space. Chicago, University of Chicago Press, 1969
46. HARRIS P, HEATH D: The Human Pulmonary Circulation: Its Form and Function in Health and Disease. Edinburgh, Churchill Livingstone, 1977
47. BRODY JS, STEMMLER EJ, DUBOIS AB: Longitudinal distribution of vascular resistance in the pulmonary arteries, capillaries and veins. J Clin Invest 47:783, 1968
48. LOPEZ-MAJANO V, et al: Effect of regional hypoxia on the distribution of pulmonary blood flow in man. Circ Res 18:550, 1966
49. HAUGE A: Hypoxia and pulmonary vascular resistance. The relative effects of pulmonary arterial and alveolar P_{O_2}. Acta Physiol Scand 76:121, 1969
50. ABRAHAM AS, et al: Factors contributing to the reversible pulmonary hypertension of patients with acute respiratory failure studied by serial observations during recovery. Circ Res 24:51, 1969
51. KILBURN KH, et al: Effects of breathing 10 per cent carbon dioxide on the pulmonary circulation of human subjects. Circulation 39:639, 1969
52. FERRER MI: Disturbances in the circulation in patients with cor pulmonale. Bull NY Acad Med 41:942, 1965
53. HOUSELY E, et al: Effect of acute and chronic acidemia and associated hypoxia on the pulmonary circulation of patients with chronic bronchitis. Cardiovasc Res 4:482, 1970
54. MOSER KM (ed): Pulmonary Vascular Diseases. New York, Marcel-Dekker, 1979
55. BRODY JS, STEMMLER EJ: Differential reactivity in the pulmonary circulation. J Clin Invest 47:800, 1968
56. BERGOFSKY EH: Mechanisms underlying vasomotor regulation of regional pulmonary blood flow in normal and disease states. Am J Med 57:378, 1974
57. MURRAY JF, KARP RB, NADEL JA: Viscosity effects on pressure–flow relations and vascular resistance in dogs' lungs. J Appl Physiol 27:336, 1969
58. AGARWAL JB, PALTOO R, PALMER WH: Relative viscosity of blood at varying hematocrits in pulmonary circulation. J Appl Physiol 29: 866, 1970
59. COMROE JH, et al: The Lung: Clinical Physiology and Pulmonary Function Tests, 2nd ed. Chicago, Year Book Medical Publishers, 1962
60. PONTOPPIDAN H, GEFFIN B, LOWENSTEIN E: Acute respiratory failure in the adult. N Engl J Med 287:743, 1972
61. WHIPP BJ, WASSERMAN K: Alveolar–arterial gas tension differences during graded exercise. J Appl Physiol 27:361, 1969
61a. WEST JB, WAGNER PD: Pulmonary gas exchange at high altitude. Prog Resp Res 16:287, 1981
62. BATES DV, MACKLEM PT, CHRISTIE RV: Respiratory Function in Disease: An Introduction to the Integrated Study of the Lung. 2nd ed. Philadelphia, WB Saunders, 1971
63. BROMBERG PA, BALCERZAK SP: Blood oxygen transport in humans. In Robins ED (ed): Extrapulmonary Manifestations of Respiratory Disease, Chap. 1. New York, Marcel-Dekker, 1978
64. PERUTZ MF: Hemoglobin structure and respiratory transport. Scientific American 239:92, 1978
65. EDWARDS MJ, MARTIN RJ: Mixing techniques for oxygen hemoglobin equilibrium and Bohr effect. J Appl Physiol 21:1898, 1966
66. BELLINGHAM AJ, DEHER JC, LENFANT C: Regulatory mechanisms of hemoglobin oxygen affinity in acidosis and alkalosis. J Clin Invest 50:700, 1971
67. BELLINGHAM AJ, LENFANT C: Hemoglobin affinity for oxygen determined by oxygen–hemoglobin dissociation analyzer and mixing technique. J Appl Physiol 30:903, 1971
68a. SCHEID P, MEYER M: Mixing technique for study of oxygen–hemoglobin equilibrium: A critical evaluation. J Appl Physiol 45:818, 1978
68. LEDWITH JW: Determining P_{50} in the presence of carboxyhemoglobin. J Appl Physiol 44:317, 1978
69. WINSLOW RM, et al: Variability of oxygen affinity of normal blood: The automated method of measurement. J Appl Physiol 45:289, 1978
70. BELLINGHAM AJ: Hemoglobins with altered oxygen affinity. Brit Med Bull 32:234, 1976
71. BUNN HF, FORGET BG, RANNEY HM: Human hemoglobins. Philadelphia, WB Saunders, 1977
72. BUNN HF, FORGET BG, RANNEY HM: Hemoglobinopathies in Major Problems in Internal Medicine, Vol XII. Philadelphia, WB Saunders, 1977
73. ROSA R, et al: The first case of a complete deficiency of diphosphoglycerate mutase in human erythrocytes. J Clin Invest 62:907, 1978
74. POYART C, et al: Hemoglobin Creteil: Oxygen transport by erythrocytes.. Ann Int Med 88:758, 1978
75. RAND PW, et al: Responses to graded hypoxia at high and low 2,3-diphosphoglycerate concentrations. J Appl Physiol 34:287, 1973
76. LENFANT C, TORRANCE JD, REYNAFARJE C: Shift of the O_2-Hb dissociation curve at altitudes: Mechanism and effect. J Appl Physiol 30: 625, 1971

77. KLOCKE RA: Oxygen transport and 2,3-diphosphoglycerate (DPG). Chest 62: 79S, 1972
78. HEBBEL RP, et al: Human llamas. Adaptation to altitude in subjects with high hemoglobin oxygen affinity. J Clin Invest 62:593, 1978
79. WRANNE B, NORDGREN L, WOODSON RD: Increased blood oxygen affinity and physical work capacity in man. Scan J Clin Lab Invest 33:347, 1974
80. MALMBERG PO, HLASTZLA MP, WOODSON RD: Effect of increased blood oxygen affinity on oxygen transport in hemorrhagic shock. J Appl Physiol 47:889, 1979
81. RIGGS TE, SHAFER AW, GUENTER CA: Acute changes in oxyhemoglobin affinity: effects on oxygen transport and utilization. J Clin Invest 52:2660, 1973
81a. KRALL MA, et al: Physiological effects of lowered blood oxygen affinity in dogs. Resp Physiol 33:362, 1978
82. BENESCH R, BENESCH RE: Intracellular organic phosphates as regulators of oxygen release by hemoglobin. Nature 221:618, 1967
83. BREWER GJ, EATON JW: Erythrocyte metabolism: Interaction with oxygen transport. Science 171:1205, 1971
84. RAICH PC, et al: Effect of hemodialysis on erythrocyte 2,3-diphosphoglycerate in patients with uremia. Am J Med Sci 265:147, 1973
85. SZWED JJ, et al: Effect of hemodialysis on oxygen–hemoglobin affinity in chronic uremics. Chest 66:278, 1974
86. BREWER GJ: 2,3-DPG and erythrocyte oxygen affinity. Annu Rev Med 25:29, 1974
87. MCCONN R, DERRICK JB: The respiratory function of blood: Transfusion and blood storage. Anesthesiology 36:119, 1972
88. HERMAN CM, et al. Changes in the oxyhemoglobin dissociation curve and peripheral blood after acute red cell mass depletion and subsequent red cell mass restoration in baboons. Ann Surg 174:734, 1971
89. SHAFER AW, et al: 2,3-diphosphoglycerate in red cells stored in acid-citrate-dextrose and citrate-phosphate-dextrose: Implications regarding delivery of oxygen. J Lab Clin Invest 77:430, 1971
90. PAPADOPOULOS MD, MORROW G, OSKI FA: Exchange transfusion in the newborn infant with fresh and "old" blood: The role of storage on 2,3-diphosphoglycerate, hemoglobin–oxygen affinity, and oxygen release. J Pediatr 79:898, 1971
90a. DITZL J: Changes in red cell oxygen release capacity in diabetes mellitus. Fed Proc 38:2484, 1979
90b. KOENIG RJ, CERAMI A: Hemoglobin A_{Ic} and Diabetes Mellitus. Annu Rev Med 31:29, 1980
91. EDITORIAL: High affinity hemoglobins. Br Med J 2:1040, 1977
91a. SCHRUMPF JD, et al: Altered hemoglobin affinity with long term propranolol therapy in patients with coronary artery disease. Am J Cardiol 40:76, 1977
91b. DANIEL A: The relationships among arterial oxygen flow rate, oxygen binding by hemoglobin, and oxygen utilization in chronic cardiac decompensation. J Lab Clin Med 91:635, 1978
92. BRANTIGAN JW, GOTT VL, MARTZ MN: A teflon membrane for measurement of blood and intramyocardial gas tensions by mass spectroscopy. J Appl Physiol 32:276, 1972
92a. GUENTER CA: Respiratory monitoring in acute multiple organ system failure. Adv Shock Res (in press)
93. WILSON GJ, et al: Mass spectrometry for measuring changes in intramyocardial P_{O_2} and P_{CO_2}. In Bicher HI, Duane FB (eds): Oxygen Transport to Tissue: Instrumentation, Methods, and Physiology. New York, Plenum, 1973
94. SIMON LE: Regulation of biosynthesis/biodegradation of oxygen related enzymes by molecular oxygen. In Robin ED (ed): Extrapulmonary Manifestations of Respiratory Disease, Chapt 5 New York, Marcel-Dekker, 1978
95. ROBIN ED: Dysoxia and intrinsic mitochondrial diseases. In Robin ED (ed): Extrapulmonary Manifestations of Respiratory Disease, Chapt 6 New York, Marcel-Dekker, 1978
96. ROBIN ED: Of men and mitrochondria: Coping with hypoxic dysoxia. Am Rev Respir Dis 122: 517, 1980
97. BERLIN NI: Diagnosis and classification of the polycythemias. Semin Hematol 12:339, 1975
98. BALCERZAK SP, BROMBERG PA: Secondary polycythemia. Semin Hematol 12:353, 1975
99. ERSLEV AJ, et al: Plasma erythropoietin in polycythemia. Am J Med 66:243, 1979
100. SPIVAK, JL, AND GRABER, SE: Erythropoietin and the regulation of erythropoiesis. Johns Hopkins Med J 146:311, 1980
101. FOSTER LJ, CORRIGAN K, GOLDMAN AL: Effectiveness of oxygen therapy in hypoxic polycythemic smokers. Chest 73:572, 1978
102. ROSENTHAL A, et al: Blood volume changes in cyanotic congenital heart disease. Am J Cardiol 27:162, 1971
103. ERSLEV AJ: Polycythemia. In Beeson PB, McDermott W, Wyngaarden JB (eds): Cecil, Textbook of Medicine, Section 5. Philadelphia, WB Saunders, 1979
104. LERTZMAN M, et al: Hypoxia in polycythemia vera. Ann Intern Med 60:409, 1964
105. HUMPHREY PRD, et al: Cerebral bloodflow and viscosity in relative polycythemia. Lancet 873, 1979
105a. WILLISON JR, et al: Effect of high hematocrit on alertness. Lancet 846, 1980

106. MAKER HS, NICKLAS WJ: Biochemical responses of body organs to hypoxia and ischemia. In Robin ED (ed): Extrapulmonary Manifestations of Respiratory Disease, Chapt 4. New York, Marcel-Dekker, 1978
107. BOYSEN G, et al: On a critical lower level of cerebral blood flow in man with particular reference to carotid surgery. Circulation 49:1023, 1974
108. LARSON CP JR, et al: Jugular venous oxygen saturation as an index of adequacy of cerebral oxygenation. Surgery 62:31, 1967
109. EDELMAN NH, et al: The effect of impairment of O_2 delivery on the aerobic metabolism of brain and skeletal muscle. Chest 61:49S, 1972
110. PERETZ DI, et al: The significance of lactic acidemia in the shock syndrome. Ann NY Acad Sci 119:1133, 1965
111. CAIN SM: Relative rates of arterial lactate and oxygen-deficit accumulation in hypoxic dogs. Am J Physiol 224:1190, 1973
112. COMROE JH JR, BOTHELLO S: The unreliability of cyanosis in the recognition of arterial anoxemia. Am J Med Sci 214:1, 1974
113. SAUNDERS NA, POWLES ACP, REBUCK AS: Ear oximetry: Accuracy and practicability in the assessment of arterial oxygenation. Am Rev Respir Dis 113:745, 1976
114. KASNITZ P, et al: Mixed venous oxygen tension and hyperlactatemia. JAMA 236:570, 1976
115. HILLER C, BONE R, WILSON F: Comparison of tissue and mixed venous oxygen tension in endotoxic shock. Am Rev Respir Dis (Suppl) 119:127, 1979
116. JOBSIS FF, LAMANNA JC: Kinetic aspects of intracellular redox reactions. In Robin ED (ed): Extrapulmonary Manifestations of Respiratory Disease, Chapt 3. New York, Marcel-Dekker, 1978
117. DAVENPORT HW: The ABC of Acid–Base Chemistry 6th ed. Chicago, University of Chicago Press, 1974
118. KLOCKE RA. Carbon dioxide transport. In Robin ED (ed): Extrapulmonary Manifestations of Respiratory Disease, Chapt 9. New York, Marcel-Dekker, 1978
119. SIGGAARD-ANDERSEN O, GARBY L: The Bohr effect and the Haldane effect. Scand J Clin Lab Invest 31:1, 1973
120. ROBIN ED: Abnormal tissue metabolism related to alterations of carbon dioxide and *p*H. In Robin ED (ed): Overview in Extrapulmonary Manifestations of Respiratory Disease, Part 2. New York, Marcel-Dekker, 1978
121. DAVIS RP, LOG I, GIBBS A: Ion view of acid—base balance. Am J Med 42:159, 1967
122. LENNON EJ, LEMANN J JR: Defense of hydrogen ion concentration in chronic metabolic acidosis. A new evaluation of an old approach. Ann Intern Med 65:265, 1966
123. HILLS AG, REID EL: *p*H defended—is it defensible? Ann Intern Med 65:1150, 1966
124. SIGGAARD-ANDERSON O: Blood acid–base alignment nomogram. Scand J Clin Lab Invest 15:211, 1963
125. SIGGAARD-ANDERSON O: An acid–base chart for arterial blood with normal and pathophysiological reference areas. Scand J Clin Lab Invest 27:239, 1971
126. ARBUS GS: An in vivo acid–base nomogram for clinical use. Can Med Assoc J 109:291, 1973
127. BRASHEAR RE, et al: Relationship between arterial and venous bicarbonate values. Arch Intern Med 139:440, 1979
128. MASORO EJ, SIEGEL PD: Acid–base Regulation. Philadelphia, WB Saunders, 1977
128a. JONES NL: Blood Gases and Acid–Base Physiology. New York, Brian C Decker, 1980
129. STEWART PA: Independent and dependent variables of acid–base control. Respir Physiol 33:9, 1978
130. EMMETT M, NARINS RG: Clinical use of the anion gap. Medicine 56:38, 1977
130a. NEVINS RG, EMMITT M: Simple and mixed acid–base disorders: A practical approach. Medicine 59:161, 1980
131. MADIAS NE, AYUS JC, ANDROGUE HJ: Increased anion gap in metabolic alkalosis. N Engl J Med 300:1421, 1979
132. PARLIN EG, HORNBEIM TF: Organ and tissue disturbances produced by acid–base abnormalities. In Robin ED (ed): Extrapulmonary Manifestations of Respiratory Disease, Chapt 11. New York, Marcel-Dekker, 1978
133. BRACKETT NC, COHEN JJ, SCHWARTZ WB: Carbon dioxide titration curve of normal man: Effect of increasing degrees of acute hypercapnia on acid–base equilibrium. N Engl J Med 272:6, 1965
134. BRACKETT NC JR: Acid–base response to chronic hypercapnia in man. N Engl J Med 280:124, 1969
135. WELT LG: Acidosis and alkalosis. In Wintrobe MM, et al (eds): Principles of Internal Medicine, 8th ed. New York, McGraw-Hill, 1978

Part TWO

Respiratory Illness

Chapter 6

Disorders of the Respiratory Pump

WILLIAM A. WHITELAW

The function of the normal respiratory pump was outlined in Chapter 2. In order to analyze disorders of the pump, an understanding of the integrated mechanisms required to regulate breathing is essential. This chapter deals with clinical conditions that produce abnormal function. Patients with such conditions rarely present with a clinical problem whose symptoms direct the physician to the underlying disorder. They present with dyspnea, clinical manifestations of respiratory failure, respiratory infections, right heart failure, or thromboembolic disease. For this reason, this chapter precedes chapters dealing with those clinical problems. Disorders of the control systems, neuromuscular disease, and thoracic wall abnormalities are dealt with separately, but all have their primary respiratory effects on the respiratory pump.

DISORDERS OF THE NEURAL CONTROL SYSTEM

HYPERVENTILATION

Most patients with hyperventilation, indicated by a low arterial P_{CO_2}, have pulmonary disease such as pneumonia, asthma, or pulmonary edema. There is usually some hypoxemia, and the hyperventilation might be explained as the result of stimuli from carotid chemoreceptors. Clinical experience, however, shows that correction of the hypoxemia will restore the P_{CO_2} only partly towards normal. Some other stimulus must be responsible for much of the hyperventilation and tachypnea. The mechanism likely involves receptors within the lung, since much of the increase in ventilation in animals with experimental lung disease can be abolished by cutting the vagus nerve, which carries afferent nerves from pulmonary stretch, irritant, and "J" receptors.[1] A few patients with pulmonary fibrosis, tachypnea, overventilation, and severe dyspnea have had their vagus nerves sectioned with the result that minute ventilation, respiratory frequency, and dyspnea all decreased.[2]

For a classification of causes of hyperventilation, see the list on p. 195.

Central Neurogenic Hyperventilation. Patients with extensive neurologic damage, such as those with head injuries or intracranial bleeding, sometimes have persistent hyperventilation and chronic respiratory alkalosis. To be certain that the origin of the hyperventilation is within the brain one must exclude peripheral stimuli. Hypoxia and acidosis can be measured in arterial blood and the stimuli from them estimated, but it is not often possible to rule out stimuli from lung receptors.[3] A few cases have been described in which lung disease could be excluded with reasonable certainty, and autopsies showed lesions in the rostral pons.[4] Aside from local damage to centers or pathways involved in control of breathing, extensive ischemia or destruction of neural tissue might lead to accumulation of lactic acid in brain interstitial fluid, and thus to stimulation of central chemoreceptors. The mechanisms also seem to include a heightened sensitivity to hypoxemia, since administration of oxygen often brings about a substantial drop in ventilation.[5] Whatever the mechanism, hyperventilation of central origin is a poor prognostic sign in head-injured patients.[6]

Hyperventilation in Tense or Anxious Patients. This "hyperventilation syndrome" seems to be an exaggeration of the normal ventilatory re-

Causes of Hyperventilation

Alveolar ventilation increases in proportion to carbon dioxide production; arterial P_{CO_2} remains normal. (More correctly called hyperpnea.)

- Exercise
- Hyperthyroidism
- Hypermetabolism due to carbohydrate loading

Alveolar ventilation increases out of proportion to carbon dioxide production; arterial P_{CO_2} is below normal.

- Chemoreceptor stimulation
  - Arterial hypoxemia
  - Metabolic acidosis
  - Hypotension
  - Cyanide poisoning
- Stimulation of pulmonary receptors
  - Pneumonia
  - Pulmonary embolism
  - Asthma
  - Pulmonary edema
  - Pulmonary fibrosis
- Anxiety neurosis (hyperventilation syndrome)
- Drugs
  - Nikethamide, ethamivan, doxapram
  - Theophylline
  - Catecholamines
  - Salicylates
  - Progesterone
- "Central neurogenic hyperventilation" of head injury
- Associated with Cheyne-Stokes breathing
- Hepatic failure
- Fever

sponse to anxiety or a disorder in perception of breathing movements, since many patients are convinced that they are not breathing enough at a time when alveolar ventilation is two or three times normal. Patients may have short-lived attacks of extreme overventilation with a severe acute respiratory alkalosis, or may go on for days or weeks with a chronic, compensated alkalosis and have superimposed spells of more marked acute hyperventilation.[7,8] In the acute form transitory gross hyperventilation culminates in tetany or fainting. More commonly, a period of anxiety results in intermittent, variable episodes, with symptoms in various organ systems. Hypocapnia leads to constriction of cerebral vessels, causing faintness, dizziness, impaired concentration, or rarely, loss of consciousness.[9] Shifts in *p*H and in calcium and magnesium ion concentrations are thought to be responsible for changes in peripheral nerve and muscle.[10] Numbness and tingling is felt in the fingers and toes or around the mouth. Myalgia, twitching, carpopedal spasm, and generalized tetany occur. Palpitations, tachycardia, and sharp twinges of chest pain are common, but a sensation indistinguishable from angina pectoris may also occur and the electrocardiogram may show ST and T wave changes.[11,12] There may be a feeling of tightness in the chest, but patients sometimes deny feeling short of breath or describe their dyspnea in an unusual way. Characteristically, they say they are unable to take a big enough breath, or that air does not seem to be going into their lungs when they breathe. The pattern of breathing is slow and deep, using the intercostal muscles more than the diaphragm. If arterial blood gas measurements are obtained during symptoms, the P_{CO_2} is generally less than 25 mm Hg and the *p*H greater than 7.50.

Treatment consists of patient education, reassurance, and rebreathing from a reservoir, such as a paper bag, for several breaths during acute attacks. This maneuver returns arterial P_{CO_2} and *p*H toward normal and reduces symptoms. Most acute attacks of hyperventilation syndrome occur in normal but emotionally labile subjects under conditions of acute emotional stress, especially when hot weather and crowds of people induce an illusion of "suffocation." Other investigators have emphasized the importance of bereavement in setting the emotional stage. Such attacks respond promptly to treatment and typically do not recur. Occasionally, chronic anxiety states may be associated with chronic hyperventilation and respond poorly to treatment. Treatment of the underlying emotional disturbance is crucial to the management of these patients. The hyperventilation syndrome occasionally occurs in patients with underlying organic disease of the heart and lungs and complicates both diagnosis and management.

A disorder in which acute episodic dyspnea may mimic the hyperventilation syndrome is pulmonary embolism. Acutely, patients with this disorder often become severely dyspneic and hypoxemic without an apparent mechanical hindrance to ventilation; respiratory alkalosis is usual.

CHEYNE-STOKES AND RELATED PERIODIC BREATHING

Cheyne in 1818 described a patient with apoplexy who displayed a peculiar pattern of breathing in which he would become apneic for a period of 30 sec, then begin making very small respiratory efforts which would slowly increase in amplitude and slowly die away again, the period of the whole cycle being about 1 min.[13] Such breathing, in a more or less exaggerated form, is very frequently seen among patients on any general medical ward, although it often goes unrecognized or is reported as "apneic spells." The spectrum of periodic breathing ranges from minor waxing and waning of the amplitude of respiratory movements to a pattern of long apneic spells interrupted by brief bursts of a few large breaths.[14,15] Whereas slow oscillation in tidal volumes is the most prominent feature of Cheyne-Stokes breathing, it is but one manifestation of a general oscillation of central nervous system activity and autonomic function. In a typical case the patient appears to be asleep while apneic. Near the beginning of the phase of hyperpnea, he makes a few restless movements, then opens his eyes as he takes his first breaths, seems aware of his surroundings and may answer questions, only to lapse again into stupor or sleep with the next apneic phase. The first, feeble attempts to breathe at the beginning of the hyperpnea are often prevented by obstruction of the upper airway and the first breath is often a snore indicating that the upper airway muscles are inactive during apnea and may remain so a bit longer than the other inspiratory muscles. Some patients have neurologic abnormalities (a squint, unequal pupils, or a Babinski sign) that come and go with the apnea. Blood pressure, pulse rate, and tone of cerebral and peripheral vascular beds also oscillate.[16] Blood gases vary, but in a way that is surprising at first glance: P_{CO_2} is usually lowest and P_{O_2} highest during the apneic phase. Although the patient may seem to be underventilating with only two or three sizeable breaths per minute, the usual finding is a chronic respiratory alkalosis.

Periodic breathing is commonly found among patients with diffuse loss of cerebral cortical function or with chronic heart failure. It is also found in normal subjects during the early stages of slow-wave sleep, more often in older people and at high altitude.[17] By itself, it seldom has any significance beyond that of the neurologic or cardiac disorder which underlies it. A few patients have been reported to get dangerous cardiac arrhythmias during periodic breathing; in comatose patients with severe head injury, this breathing pattern implies a poor prognosis.[18] Surprisingly, patients are seldom aware of Cheyne-Stokes breathing, and if it is reported at all, it is by their spouses who notice either apnea or gasping during the night. Occasionally a patient himself may take notice of the breathing of the hyperpneic phase while he is on the verge between waking and sleep. Such patients usually describe this as shortness of breath, so that awareness of Cheyne-Stokes breathing is an uncommon cause of nocturnal dyspnea.[19] The periodic breathing can often be abolished by administration of oxygen or aminophylline.

The mechanism usually proposed to explain this sort of regular periodic breathing comes from the theory of negative-feedback control systems. It is easily understood by analogy with the system that controls the temperature of water in a shower bath. Here, the man in the shower detects the temperature of water on his skin and adjusts it by turning a tap. If there is a long pipe between the tap and spout and thus a delay between turning the tap and detecting the effect of the adjustment, the man always tends to overcorrect, making the water run alternately too hot and too cold. The amplitude of the temperature oscillation depends on both the length of the pipe and the sensitivity of the subject. An oversensitive person will reach for the tap quickly and turn it violently to try to correct the too-hot or too-cold water, whereas a phlegmatic person will react slowly, suiting his motions to the sluggish response of the plumbing. The respiratory system controls arterial P_{O_2} and P_{CO_2}

by measuring these and feeding back the information to the respiratory centers, increasing or decreasing ventilation to restore gas tensions toward normal. Ventilation would be expected to oscillate if there were a long delay between lungs (the tap) and chemoreceptors (the skin) or if the chemoreceptors were oversensitive. The first could occur when circulation is slowed, as in heart failure, and the second when the ventilatory response to carbon dioxide is increased, as it is in diffuse cerebral disease.[20] Animal models for both these disturbances do produce periodic breathing.[21,22] An interesting recent modification of this theory suggests that with the breathing cycle the patient may also oscillate between waking and sleep and in so doing may continuously change the sensitivity of his chemoreceptor system.[23] A quite different theory says that the oscillation is a manifestation of a cycle of activity that is intrinsic to the central nervous system and is only exaggerated by heart failure or disinhibition arising from loss of cerebral function. Such a central rhythm in breathing and blood pressure has been demonstrated in an animal model in which the chemoreceptor and other feedback loops were interrupted.[24] In patients it is impossible to prove which mechanism is important and either could equally well explain most of the observations.

ATAXIC BREATHING (BIOT'S BREATHING)

Ataxic, or Biot's, breathing is an irregular pattern in which deep and shallow breaths occur at random, interspersed with long and short pauses. In spite of its name it is not associated with disorders of balance or damage to the cerebellum. It results from damage to the medulla caused by compression, trauma, hemorrhage, demyelination, meningitis, or poliomyelitis.[25] The ventilatory response to carbon dioxide is depressed. Apnea frequently occurs, often with sleep or small amounts of sedative, so that careful monitoring of ventilation and preparations for mechanical support may be indicated.[18] Patients with medullary lesions, when able to report their symptoms, are usually free of dyspnea.[26]

APNEUSTIC BREATHING

A few patients with apneustic breathing have been described.[27] They had extensive lesions of the pons, causing nearly complete transsection above the level of the trigeminal nerve roots, similar to the experimental lesion that produces the same breathing pattern in cats. They had pauses of from 30 to 60 sec in both inspiration and in active expiration. These patients were able to swallow, cough in response to stimulation of the tracheal mucosa, and respond with bradycardia to carotid sinus massage. Their apneusis was inconstant, alternating with other irregular rhythms. Similar breathing patterns are occasionally observed in metabolic brain disease and meningitis.[18]

MISCELLANEOUS NEURAL DISORDERS

Respiratory Apraxia. A disorder of elderly people with signs of diffuse extrapyramidal disease, respiratory apraxia is an inability to perform voluntary respiratory acts such as deep breathing or breath holding. It is associated with generalized increase in muscle tone, suck, grasp, and rooting reflexes, and decreased mental acuity. Metabolic respiratory function is preserved and normal blood gases are maintained.[28]

Posthyperventilation Apnea. Normal subjects continue to breathe regularly after a period of voluntary or mechanical hyperventilation, allowing their low P_{CO_2} to correct itself gradually in the course of approximately ten minutes.[29] Patients who stop breathing after hyperventilation are found to have diffuse cerebral disease and presumably depend more than do normal people on simple direct chemical feedback to control their breathing.[28]

Hiccough. Hiccough is a spasmodic inspiratory movement involving both diaphragm and intercostal muscles combined with transient closure of the glottis, so that the resulting airflow is negligible.[30] Persistent hiccough is a distressing and tiring symptom which is strangely confined mainly to male patients. Central nervous system diseases causing hiccough always involve the medulla. The more frequent cases of hiccoughs associated with disease in the upper abdomen, diaphragm, mediastinum, or heart are presumed to be due to irritation of the phrenic or vagus nerves. Uremia is also a common cause. Successful symptomatic treatments include stimulation of the pharynx with a nasal catheter or cold water, drugs such as chlorpromazine and methylphenidate, and maneuvers such as breath holding and inhaling carbon dioxide.

Diaphragmatic Flutter (Respiratory Myoclonus). This is a disorder in which the diaphragm, and in some cases intercostal muscles as well, make rapid rhythmic contractions with a frequency of from 30 to 500 per min. It may be associated with disease of the thorax or abdomen (in which case irritation of the phrenic nerve has been suggested) and has followed encephalitis lethargica in a few cases. Often, however, no underlying disease can be found. Attacks seem to be precipitated by coughing, sneezing, deep breathing, emotion, and exercise and are of varying duration.[31,32]

PRIMARY ALVEOLAR HYPOVENTILATION

Clinical Features. Primary alveolar hypoventilation, an uncommon primary disorder of control of ventilation, was first noticed in patients with polycythemia and cyanosis.[33,34] Unlike ordinary cases of secondary polycythemia, these had no demonstrable lung disease and had originally been classified as polycythemia vera. After cyanosis was noticed, arterial oxygen tension was found to be low while carbon dioxide tension was high. It was quickly shown that most of the patients failed to increase their ventilation in the normal way during exercise, or when stimulated with carbon dioxide.[35] Although it was considered possible that primary polycythemia might cause local damage to respiratory centers through thrombosis of brain stem vessels, a primary disorder of ventilation was seen as the most reasonable explanation for these findings.[34]

Numerous patients in this category have been reported over the past two decades.[36,37] The syndrome occurs in infants, children, and adults. These patients usually come to the attention of the physician because of mental symptoms due to chronic hypoxemia and hypercapnia (drowsiness, difficulty concentrating, or irritability) or because of edema and high venous pressure due to cor pulmonale. Many report an incident in the distant past that can be interpreted as a transient encephalitis, but often the time and manner of onset of the disease remain obscure. At autopsy there is cor pulmonale and signs of chronic pulmonary hypertension due to hypoxia. The few reports of brain histology have shown a range of lesions from nothing at all through minor nonspecific cell damage to cell destruction spread throughout the brainstem.[38,39] There is no clear correlation between the physiological derangement and damage to identifible groups of respiratory neurons. A few cases in infants have shown loss of serotonergic cells in the brainstem.[40]

Owing to the dissemination of new ideas about respiratory control, these patients are now being more extensively tested, and new classifications can be expected. Many turn out to have sleep apnea of the central or obstructive type,[41] but this may be a nonspecific result of damage to respiratory centers. Similarly, the blunted ventilatory response to carbon dioxide found in many of them may indicate selective damage to medullary chemoreceptors, but could also arise from nonspecific damage to respiratory neurons. The increase in ventilation seen with exercise is often impaired, as is the response to hypoxia.[37]

Chronic hypercapnia by itself seems to blunt responsiveness to carbon dioxide, and it is possible that episodes of nocturnal hypoxemia and hypercapnia may cause further deterioration.[42] These patients are peculiarly susceptible to respiratory depression induced by sedatives and narcotics.

It is remarkable that even quite severe airways obstruction and neuromuscular disease do not often cause carbon dioxide retention. If respiratory acidosis is found in a patient with moderate myopathy, moderate emphysema, or extreme obesity, it is reasonable to wonder whether he does not also have some problem of the neural control system.[43]

Diagnosis and Assessment. Because there are no specific signs or symptoms of respiratory acidosis and because clinical assessment of alveolar ventilation is grossly inaccurate, this condition is diagnosed only after arterial blood gases are measured in the course of searching for the explanation of polycythemia, pulmonary hypertension, or cor pulmonale. Arterial P_{CO_2} often varies widely through the day, and a single specimen may show normal or alkaline *p*H. An otherwise unexplained increase in bicarbonate may suggest chronic respiratory acidosis and gives an estimate of the average level of carbon dioxide through the day.

In order to treat a patient with chronic carbon dioxide retention, the physician must first exclude recognizable diseases which can be expected to depress ventilation (see list at right). Thus, pulmonary function tests, tests of muscle function, careful neurologic examination, assessment of acid–base status, and a drug history are primary requirements. Special tests necessary to characterize the defect include those for ventilatory responses to hypoxia, hypercapnia, and exercise; polygraphic sleep recordings; and assessment of response to mechanical loads. Specific tests of diaphragm function may be required in order to exclude major dysfunction of this muscle.

Causes of Alveolar Hypoventilation

- Lack of usual stimulus
  - Metabolic alkalosis
  - Hyperoxia
  - Sleep
- Reduced "respiratory center" activity
  - Drugs, e.g., sedatives, hypnotics, narcotics
  - Local CNS damage, e.g., head injury, poliomyelitis
  - Myxedema
  - Idiopathic alveolar hypoventilation
- Damage to descending tracts or peripheral nerves
  - High spinal cord injury
  - Bilateral phrenic nerve palsy
- Neuromuscular junction disease
  - Myasthenia gravis
  - Drug overdose—succinyl choline, aminoglycoside antibiotics
  - Botulism
- Muscle disease
  - Myositis, dystrophy or myopathy
  - Muscle weakness due to hypokalemia or hypophosphatemia
  - Muscle fatigue
- Fixed chest wall
  - Kyphoscoliosis
- Uncoupling between chest wall and lungs
  - Flail chest
  - Pneumothorax
- Increased impedance to ventilation in the lungs
  - Acute obstruction of trachea, larynx, or bronchi
  - Chronic diffuse airways obstruction
- Inefficiency of gas exchange
  - Increased dead space
  - Decreased tidal volume

Treatment. Treatment is not always satisfactory. Any secondary contributing causes must be removed. Bronchodilators, cessation of smoking, and weight reduction may all help. Sedatives are definitely contraindicated. Drugs (theophylline, ASA, progesterone, acetazolamide, amphetamines) are seldom helpful, although thiamine was useful in one reported case,[44] and doxapram infusion is helpful in acute situations.[45] Mechanical ventilation during the night by cuirass, tank respirator,[46] or rocking bed will return blood gases toward normal; for some as yet unexplained reason P_{CO_2} often takes many hours to drift back up during the day. Electrophrenic respiration can be used for those for whom simpler measures are ineffective.[47] If obstructive sleep apnea is present, other special measures may be indicated.

BREATHING DURING SLEEP, SLEEP APNEA, AND HYPOXEMIA OF SLEEP

There is a great deal yet to be learned about the pathogenesis of nocturnal disorders of breathing, and the classification is likely to change in the next few years. In any case, the physician must be aware that alterations in respiration during sleep make patients vulnerable to pulmonary disease, aggravate many cardiorespiratory problems, and can be responsible for significant daytime symptoms.

Physiology of Respiration in Sleep

During an ordinary good night's sleep, normal subjects pass in and out of several different clearly defined sleep states.[23] After first dozing off, they show electroencephalographic changes of increasing slow-wave activity and loss of alpha rhythm, progressing through four stages of sleep. The first hours of repose are spent mainly in slow-wave sleep (SWS), but as the night goes on these are interrupted by intervals of rapid-eye-movement (REM) sleep, during which electroencephalograms show bursts of fast alpha rhythm, there are rapid movements of the eyes, dreams occur, skeletal muscle tone falls markedly with loss of deep tendon reflexes, and heart rate and breathing become irregular. The intervals of rapid eye movement become longer and more frequent toward morning. SWS and REM sleep are physiologically as different from one another as each is different from the waking state.

During wakefulness breathing is controlled by a complex interlocking set of neural structures responsive to a wide range of sensory stimuli. This sytem coordinates breathing with many other activities that share the breathing muscles, including exercise, change in posture, speech, eating, and expression of emotion. Through the course of all these activities ventilation is maintained, perhaps with infrequent reference to the chemical control system, but the basic respiratory pattern generator in the brain stem responds briskly to changes in chemical stimuli, so long as there is no overriding behavioral influence on breathing. Respiratory activity is widespread through many nuclei of the medulla, and respiratory drive is plentifully supplied to the diaphragm, intercostals, and upper airways. The metabolic and behavioral systems support each other to regulate carbon dioxide and oxygen tensions very closely. Definite changes in the respiratory control system occur in both kinds of sleep, tending in general to make it more vulnerable to disturbance and less effective at regulating blood gases.

During SWS the behavioral system becomes much less active, and responsibility for maintaining ventilation devolves largely upon the metabolic system alone. The ability to recognize and respond to mechanical loads is reduced, as is the conscious ability to anticipate demands on or threats to the respiratory system. Breathing is no longer being coordinated with so many other activities, and becomes slow and regular. The metabolic system is also less active than in the awake state. Response to carbon dioxide is somewhat reduced and respiratory drive is not so fully and widely supplied to all respiratory muscle groups.

In REM sleep, behavioral activity seems to reappear, and the breathing pattern again becomes irregular although now inexplicable, except perhaps to someone who knows the content of the subject's dreams. The activity of the diaphragm is maintained, but now other muscle groups are severely depressed and response to carbon dioxide is markedly reduced.

Two major changes in the use of respiratory muscles occur. First, there is a decrease in activity of the intercostal muscles. In REM sleep the diaphragm is almost completely unsupported by intercostal muscles. Without the stiffening effect of intercostal muscle contraction, the rib cage allows itself to be partly collapsed by the contracting diaphragm and inspiration becomes mechanically less efficient. (Fortunately, the supine posture which many people assume during sleep puts the diaphragm into a mechanically advantageous position). Second, activity decreases in a set of muscles in the pharynx and larynx that ordinarily contract with every inspiration in order to hold the upper airway open.[48] These include the posterior muscles of the pharynx, the genioglossus (which causes the tongue to protrude), and the posterior cricoarytenoid (the major abductor of the vocal cords). Without contraction of these muscles the soft tissues of the upper airway tend to be sucked together with each inspiration, partly or completely obstructing the passage of air. When this occurs to a major degree, snoring is the result. In an extreme form it is recognized as "obstructive sleep apnea." Relaxation of the upper airway muscles occurs to a slight degree in SWS and to a much greater degree in REM sleep.

TABLE 6-1. Respiratory Protective Mechanisms in Sleep

Mechanism	Effectiveness in Sleep
Cough reflex	Depressed
Gag reflex	Depressed
Loading response	Depressed
Mucociliary clearance	Slowed
Response to hypercapnia	Depressed
Response to hypoxia	Normal
Arousal response to:	
Hypercapnia	Decreased
Hypoxia	Decreased
Mechanical loading	Decreased
Airway irritation	Decreased

Table 6-1 lists mechanisms which the respiratory system uses to defend itself and which can be impaired in sleep. The cough reflex is depressed, as anyone knows who has had a viral bronchitis. Patients who are troubled incessantly through the day with an irritative cough often sleep comfortably through the night. Not only the threshold for cough, but also the threshold for arousal from sleep by bronchial irritation is raised.[49] Deprived of the most effective means of clearing secretions or aspirated material, the airways are prone to local obstruction with deteriorating regional ventilation–perfusion relationships and arterial hypoxemia. The gag reflex is similarly depressed, making the airways more vulnerable to aspiration. The ventilatory response to carbon dioxide is diminished, so that this chemical-feedback loop is less capable of finely controlling P_{CO_2}. The response to mechanical loading is reduced, so that increases in resistance and compliance do not elicit the increase of respiratory effort needed to prevent a fall in ventilation. Only the response to hypoxia seems to remain intact. To some extent in SWS and to a much greater degree in REM sleep, therefore, the basic controller of ventilation, sensitive to changes in P_{O_2} and P_{CO_2} and using the diaphragm as the main muscle of respiration, is stripped of the support of many accessory stabilizing mechanisms and becomes more vulnerable to disturbance of any kind.

The supine posture applies several stresses to stability. The fall in functional residual capacity (FRC) tends to worsen gas exchange, in part because some small airways remain closed throughout the whole breathing cycle. Regurgitation of stomach contents is more likely. Gravity draws the tongue back into the pharynx, so that more vigorous contraction of the upper airway muscles is necessary to keep the airway open.[50] In disease many of these problems may become exaggerated, particularly in asthma and in left ventricular failure. The recognition of these physiological changes in the respiratory system during sleep is recent, and the practice of monitoring patients during the night is only beginning. The trouble occurs mainly when the patient is unaware and the doctor is absent.

Sleep Apnea

The discovery that some patients have frequent apneic spells during sleep was made by Gastaut and associates in 1965, while making nocturnal polygraphic records in patients with the "Pickwickian syndrome."[51,52] Since then pathological sleep apnea has been observed in a wide variety of patients, and appears to be relatively common. Understanding of this area is rapidly developing in scientific circles and is becoming popularized in the lay press. It is possible that sleep apnea and related disorders may be involved in the pathogenesis of diseases ranging from psychosis to sudden death, and it can be expected that patients in increasing numbers will come to their physicians with direct questions or unspoken worries about observations of the breathing during sleep of their spouses or children. Clinical syndromes caused by sleep apnea usually center on neurologic, psychiatric, cardiac, hematological, or other systems and seldom point directly to a disorder of respiratory control. Recognition of these syndromes and their association with respiratory problems is therefore of great importance.

Normal men frequently have one or two spells of apnea (defined as lack of air flow for more than 10 sec) just after falling asleep, and again during REM sleep, when failure to breathe coincides with bursts of rapid eye movements. In addition many adult males, especially older ones, and especially at high altitudes, develop Cheyne-Stokes breathing in the early stages of sleep, and may have apnea associated with this.[17] In all, normal adult males average about two apneic episodes per hour during a night's sleep (the frequency tending to increase with age and obesity), and many have associated periods of arterial desaturation. An exaggerated sinus arrhythmia occurs in conjunction with the variable breathing pattern. These features of breathing in sleep are found in women about one-twentieth as often as in men. Snoring is, of course, very common. Although it has been suggested that snoring without apneic spells may be associated with mild pulmonary and systemic hypertension,[51] the evidence so far is not compelling.

Apneic spells, mild transient hypoxemia, and minor cardiac arrhythmias in sleep probably affect a large part of the normal population, and should not be a cause for alarm. They become clinically significant and warrant investigation if apnea is frequent enough to produce a "sleep apnea syndrome," or if a minor sleep abnormality interacts with underlying pulmonary or cardiac disease to produce severe nocturnal hypoxemia or dangerous cardiac arrhythmias.

After a patient with sleep apnea falls asleep, his breathing is interrupted by numerous episodes of apnea. In patients who suffer from daytime somnolence, more than thirty, usually hundreds of episodes occur in a night. Three types of apnea are described: *central*, *obstructive*, and *mixed*. In central apnea, all signs of respiratory activity stop. In obstructive apnea, the upper airway closes off, so that there is no flow of air, but inspiratory muscles continue to contract, generating large negative intrathoracic pressures and distorting the chest wall. "Mixed" apnea begins like central apnea, but turns into obstructive apnea as the first resuming inspiratory efforts are frustrated by upper airway closure. One patient may have predominantly central or obstructive apnea, but many show all three types in the course of a night's sleep.

The different types of apnea are best understood in terms of activity of two groups of muscles, namely the inspiratory muscles (diaphragm and intercostals) and the upper airway muscles (cricoarytenoids, genioglossus and pharyngeal). If the inspiratory muscles do not contract, there is no air flow, and no intrathoracic pressure is generated. This is a central apnea. If the inspiratory muscles contract, but the upper airway muscles fail to do so, the pharynx is sucked closed,[53] no air flow occurs, and negative pressure is generated in the thorax. This is an obstructive apnea and is clearly shown by electromyography to be caused by a temporary failure of neural drive to the upper airway muscles.[48,50] The terminology is confusing, since both types of apnea result from failure of respiratory center output: in one case to the diaphragm, in the other case to the pharynx. In mixed apnea there is clearly failure of neural drive to both groups of muscles. In central apnea the state of the upper airway is usually not known. In a few cases it is found to be open, but often it is closed, as shown when apnea was treated by electrophrenic respiration. When the phrenic nerves are electrically stimulated during an episode of central apnea, the result is often an obstructed inspiration or obstructive apnea. These findings suggest that in central apnea there is waning or disappearance of neural drive to both sets of muscles. Similarly, in obstructive apnea, where loss of upper airway patency is the main factor, neural drive to inspiratory muscles often wanes as well. Although large pressure swings are generated in the thorax by the frustrated efforts of inspiratory muscles, these efforts when measured correctly are found to be feebler than the efforts made in breaths preceding the apnea.[54] The ma-

Sleep Apnea Syndromes

- Obstructive
  - Symptomatic, obstructive, often associated with obesity
  - Asymptomatic, obstructive
  - Obstructive, associated with a deformity of the upper airway
- Central
  - Predominantly central, with insomnia
  - Associated with narcolepsy
  - Associated with known damage to respiratory centers
  - "Ondine's Curse"
- Mixed

jority of apneas—central, obstructive, and mixed—thus seem to be variations on a theme, a general waxing and waning of respiratory center activity and neural drive to all muscle groups.

Sleep apnea occurs in association with many other conditions, but the cause-and-effect relationships are not clear. In some cases a primary neurologic disorder can be postulated, for example when it occurs in conjunction with narcolepsy, but in others a peripheral defect seems more likely, as in obesity. Several groups of patients with sleep apnea have been identified, as listed and described below. There is considerable overlap between the groups, in symptoms, conceptions of pathogenesis, and treatment.

TABLE 6-2. Prevalence of Symptoms in Patients With Severe Obstructive Sleep Apnea

Symptom	Percentage of Patients With Symptom
Loud snoring	100
Abnormal motor activity in sleep	100
Intellectual deterioration	82
Excessive daytime sleepiness	78
Hypertension	52
Personality change	48
Impotence	42
Morning headache	36
Nocturnal enuresis	30
Morning nausea	8

Guilleminault C, Dement WC (eds): Sleep Apnea Syndromes. New York, A R Liss, 1978

Obstructive Apnea

Symptomatic Obstructive Sleep Apnea Often Associated With Obesity. This appears to be the most common clinical problem. It occurs much more commonly in men, the male/female ratio being about 8:1. Although it is certainly found in people of normal weight, the incidence is correlated with degree of obesity. For example, in a series of fifty patients, ten were of normal weight, ten were 5 to 15%, fifteen were 16 to 30%, and twenty were 40 to 100% overweight.[51] Onset of symptoms may occur in the second decade, but most patients are older (mean age of diagnosis approximately 45 yr). Few of the patients' complaints point to problems with sleep or respiratory control, and in most cases the patients are referred first to neurologists or psychiatrists. The list of complaints in Table 2 are ones which do not appear in the usual functional inquiry and would puzzle most physicians without suggesting any diagnosis or line of investigation. The disease is of very gradual, insidious onset, causing trouble for many years. Patients become used to the symptoms, have persuaded themselves that they are normal, or nearly so, and imagine they would be regarded as complainers or crazy if they made an issue of them.

Snoring is too common for most people to complain of it to a doctor, but these patients often snore loudly and persistently enough to be embarrassed about it. Most can recollect being told they were snorers before the age of 21. Spouses of course can give the best information, and may note that the noisy breathing stops from time to time for periods of 20 sec or so. In some cases, the noise actually drives the spouse to sleep in a separate room. Snoring is the symptom that points clearly to upper airway obstruction. Sometimes the patient has been observed to struggle to breathe while completely obstructed, but this is often interpreted initially as a seizure.

Another hazard of the conjugal bed is abnormal motor activity during sleep. Patients fling their limbs about, frequently kicking or slapping their bed partner, or falling out of bed. Somnambulism occurs commonly.

Daytime somnolence is the most widely known feature of this condition, and is the most common reason for referral of such patients to the major centers of sleep research. To be significant it must go beyond a habit of dozing off during boring lectures. Affected subjects have uncontrollable periods of drowsiness, perhaps most common in the early afternoon, but usually occurring as well in the mornings not long after waking up, and in many unusual circumstances, such as while driving a car, attending an exciting sports event, or in the middle of a conversation. They may drop off to sleep while being examined, and have a short interval (about 3 min, compared to a norm of 10 min) between settling down to rest and actually falling asleep. They often describe periods of drifting between wakefulness and sleep, with hypnagogic hallucinations and merging of real perceptions with imagination. During these periods the power of concentration decreases, intellectual performance may fall off to the point where only simple, semiautomatic tasks can be performed, and memory for events of that part of the day may be impaired. Episodes of automatic behavior resembling temporal lobe epilepsy are found in a few patients, and automobile accidents occur frequently.[55]

These problems are persistent, occur on most days, get steadily worse over the years, and are not surprisingly associated with long-term changes in intellectual capacity, personality, and behavior. Many patients become jealous, suspicious and hostile, given to outbursts of anger. They may lose their jobs or get divorced as a consequence.

Impotence and decreased libido are reported by about half the patients. About one-third have nocturnal enuresis and as many have morning headaches, both symptoms being more common in the obese. Morning nausea is the main complaint of a minority. Moderate systemic hypertension occurs in about one-half.

Nocturnal polygraphic recordings show numerous apneic spells, predominantly of the obstructive type. The patients reported have had more than 300 apneic spells per night, usually averaging about 80 per hr. The duration of each episode averages more than 20 sec, so that 40% of the night is spent with no airflow. Apnea occurs in all phases of sleep, but may be found predominately in either SWS or REM. Marked sinus arrhythmia occurs in synchrony with apnea. In one series of 15 patients,[56] six had periods with heart rates less than 30, including asystoles of up to 6 sec, and two had second-degree A-V block. Ten had multifocal premature ventricular contractions and two had transient ventricular tachycardia. Marked arterial hypoxemia may occur, leading in turn to cycles of pulmonary hypertension. Systemic blood pressure rises, as high as 250/145 mm Hg, but falls again as breathing resumes.[57] There may be mild sustained overall hypoventilation during sleep, with P_aCO_2 in the range of 40 to 50 mm Hg, but most of these patients seem to have normal alveolar ventilation during wakefulness.

The underlying pathogenetic mechanism of obstruction is obscure. In many ways it could be regarded as an exaggeration of a normal mechanism. The normal reduction in tone of upper-airway muscle activity during sleep may be accentuated in some subjects. In obesity, and particularly in those patients with short necks, accumulation of fat in the pharynx may increase the tendency for the upper airway to close, so that normal pharyngeal muscle effort is no longer sufficient to overcome it. The hypoxia and large swings in negative pressure may contribute to the genesis of cardiac arrhythmias, but arrhythmias also occur in pure central apnea, indicating that centrally generated fluctuations in vagal or sympathetic tone are partly responsible.

It has been assumed that a cycle of sleep–apnea–hypoxemia–partial arousal results in chronic sleep deprivation, and that lack of sleep causes the hypersomnolence and other neuropsychiatric problems. This fits very well with the dramatic reversal in neurologic symptoms that follows tracheostomy, and with the finding that oxygen prolongs the episodes of apnea. It must be the case, however, that some people are more susceptible to this mechanism than others since many with severe apnea are free of symptoms.[58] The physiological and biochemical processes of sleep and sleep deprivation are very poorly understood. The association of obesity and sleep apnea might also be explained by postulating a basic disorder of autonomic control that affects both breathing and the mechanism that regulates hunger and satiety.

There is some suggestion that once obstructive apnea begins, there is a vicious cycle in which apnea, through hypoxia, hypercapnia, or sleep deprivation, leads to more apnea.

With obese patients treatment usually begins with attempts to lose weight. Patients with apparently milder obstructive problems, with apnea occurring intermittently rather than continuously through the night, may improve considerably after drastic weight reduction. Patients who have episodes of apnea continually through the night tend not to improve after weight reduction. At any rate, treatment of obesity is no easier in these cases than usual, and is generally unsuccessful. Tonsillectomy and adenoidectomy sometimes help considerably by relieving part of the tendency to obstruct the upper airway. Medroxyprogesterone can be tried, but often is not helpful.[59,59a] Strychnine has been very successful in two patients.[60] Protryptyline, one of the tricyclic antidepressants, also shows promise.[60a]

The most drastic and most successful treatment is to place a permanent tracheostomy to bypass the obstruction. A fenestrated tube is used to permit normal laryngeal function during waking hours.[51] The operation is unusually difficult and risky because of obesity and the tendency for these patients to have very short thick necks.

Following tracheostomy most patients have a dramatic improvement in neuropsychiatric symptoms and in signs of cardiopulmonary disease. Needless to say, the idea of such surgery does not meet with ready acceptance by most patients, and there are obvious complications to be expected from long-term tracheostomy. This drastic step is generally recommended only when such symptoms as somnolence and intellectual deterioration are severe. Conceivably, it might be done to prevent life-threatening cardiac arrythmias, if these could not be controlled by other means.

Cardiac arrythmias disappear after tracheostomy, but recur immediately if the stoma is temporarily closed. Interestingly, the number of apneic episodes also tends to decrease, although nothing has apparently been done to alter CNS function except to restore the normal sleep pattern.

Prognosis is not very well defined. Without treatment some go on to chronic cardiac–pulmonary failure. Some die suddenly in their sleep, and there is a risk of automobile or other accidents. Knowledge of the probability of these events is limited, and it is not yet clear where the balance lies between the risks and benefits of surgery. The longest follow-up of chronic tracheostomy for obstructive apnea is about seven years.

Asymptomatic Obstructive Sleep Apnea. A number of asymptomatic patients—referred to sleep laboratories because their spouses observed curious patterns of breathing in sleep, and others studied with nocturnal recordings as part of a general study of obese patients—have been found to have intermittent or continuous obstructive sleep apnea indistinguishable in type and quantity from that of symptomatic patients.[58] It is not known whether such patients are at increased risk of sudden death in the night, and no treatment beyond weight loss can be recommended at present.

Obstructive Sleep Apnea Associated With a Deformity of the Upper Airway. It is easy to imagine that an anatomical abnormality that tends to constrict the upper airway would bring out any latent tendency to have obstructive apnea in sleep. Some of the conditions reported to do this are listed below. Many of them occur in children, where diagnosis is frequently delayed because neither the child nor the parents appreciate that the neurologic or psychological symptoms are abnormal or might have a correctable organic basis. Patients may be hypersomnolent, and some have very frightening hypnagogic hallucinations. Others develop severe cardiorespiratory failure. Surgical correction of the deformity is often possible and the prognosis is then excellent.

Anatomical Lesions Giving Rise to Obstructive Sleep Apnea

Micrognathia
Laryngeal stenosis
Laryngeal web
Enlarged tonsils or adenoids
Deviated nasal septum
Acromegaly
Lymphoma of hypopharynx

Central Apneas

Predominantly Central Apnea, Cause Unknown. A number of cases have been found with frequent central apneas not explained by recognized neurologic disease. Most of these patients complain of insomnia, rather than somnolence. They fall asleep readily but may wake up several times during the night, gasping for breath. Chronic fatigue and depression occur, together with loss of libido. They usually snore, but not loudly.

Sleep Apnea Associated With Narcolepsy. Many typical patients with the narcolepsy–cataplexy complex of symptoms also have sleep apneas. These are usually central, but may be obstructive or mixed. They are relatively infrequent, in the range of 6 to 9 per hr.[51]

Sleep Apnea Associated With Known Damage to Repiratory Centers. It should be possible for a degenerative or destructive disease of neural tissue to produce apnea that is predominantly obstructive (by affecting the nucleus ambiguus) or predominantly central (by damaging the basic rhythm generator, or the nuclei that supply neural drive to inspiratory motoneurons). Patients with previous bulbar poliomyelitis and hypersomnolence have been found to have severe sleep apnea, predominantly central, but with numerous obstructive and mixed episodes. The Shy-Dräger syndrome is a rare combination of autonomic insufficiency and parkinsonism associated with apnea which is predominantly obstructive.[60] Presumably because of failure of sympathetic or parasympathetic control of the heart, these patients are protected from nocturnal cardiac arrhythmias.

"Ondine's Curse" or "Failure of Automatic Ventilation." This colorful term, along with the "Pickwickian syndrome," has lent a pleasant atmosphere of erudition to the study of respiratory control, but regrettably has done little to improve the classification or understanding of cases of underventilation.[62,63] The details of the legend of the jilted nymph vary from source to source and the name has been applied to a variety of disorders of breathing. In the version of the story used by Giradoux in his play *Ondine*, the problem appears to be complete failure of automatic respiration, with intact voluntary control. A patient who had to breathe every breath deliberately has not been described, but the ones alluded to in the abstract[64] that christened the syndrome did have some apneas while awake and prolonged apnea as soon as they slept, and come close to resembling the character in the legend. These patients and others like them have had bilateral cervical cordotomies for relief of intractable pain. During the weeks immediately following the operation they have frequent apneas and are at great risk of dying suddenly in the night, but this problem seems to resolve with time. The most reasonable explanation is that the descending metabolic pathway in the ventrolateral cord has been severed on both sides, leaving only the "behavioral" pathway connecting the respirator centers to their motor neurons. "Failure of automatic ventilation" is an inaccurate description of the problem, since the behavioral system is as automatic as the metabolic one in most circumstances, even if its pathway also subserves voluntary control.

The term has been applied to infants with central alveolar hypoventilation who often have more severe acidosis during sleep[65] and may have sleep apnea. These patients have nothing in common with the first group.

Pathogenesis and Treatment of Central Apneas. The exact nature of the CNS damage is unknown. Many patients with central apnea have absent or severely depressed responses to CO_2 and hypoxemia. In central apnea the hemodynamic and blood gas consequences are similar to those of obstructive apnea.

If severe carbon dioxide retention or other serious complications occur, respiration must be supported by mechanical means or by repeated stimulation of the phrenic nerves through implanted electrodes. Cuirass respirators can be fitted for night-time use. Electrophrenic stimulators are available in a few specialized centers. Interestingly, once inspiratory pressure is artificially generated during apnea, it is often found that the upper airway muscles are also failing to contract, the central apnea being converted into an obstructive one.[41] It is then necessary to do a tracheostomy as well. Drugs have been generally ineffective in these patients, but are worth trying, and are summarized further on.

Hypoventilation During Sleep, Not Associated With Apnea

Normal subjects have a small drop in alveolar ventilation and rise in arterial P_{CO_2} during sleep, amounting to a few millimeters of mercury. More important decreases in ventilation during sleep occur in some cases of idiopathic alveolar hypoventilation, and in association with other pulmonary and chest wall diseases.

"Pickwickian Syndrome." The association of extreme obesity with hypersomnolence noted by Charles Dickens and later introduced to the medical literature[66] was once explained by postulating that increased work of breathing led to reduced ventilation in patients with a poor ventilatory response to carbon dioxide. Carbon dioxide retention was then thought to have a narcotic influence, inducing sleep. Many of these patients have since been found to have obstructive sleep apnea as the cause of their hypersomnolence, with only mild elevations of P_{CO_2} at night, and usually normal values during the day. Another group of obese somnolent patients do not have sleep apnea, and the reason for their somnolence is not entirely clear. They tend to be extremely obese with more marked changes in chest wall mechanics than those with only obstructive sleep apnea. Chest-wall compliance is lower and work of breathing higher, vital capacity is usually low, and ventilatory response to carbon dioxide is reduced.[67] They have a chronic respiratory acidosis during the day that worsens during sleep but do not suffer the sharp drops in P_{O_2} associated with apneic spells, keeping more steady and higher levels through the night. It is not clear what proportion of "Pickwickians" will turn out to have obstructive apnea *versus* the syndrome of chronic hypoventilation. The tendency of extremely obese patients to underventilate may result from the huge mechanical load on their chest wall eventually becoming too great to be fully compensated for by the available reflex and other mechanisms. Partial upper airway closure with marked increase in flow resistance during sleep may be important in many of them. Since sleep impairs many of the compensatory mechanisms, it is not surprising that ventilation is lower during sleep. The respiratory effects of obesity are discussed in greater detail further on in relation to chest wall abnormalities.

Hypoxemia During Sleep

Normal men and women may have changes in gas exchange as well as intermittent apnea during sleep.[68,69] The slight fall in alveolar ventilation is accompanied by a predictable fall in arterial P_{O_2}, but there is also some widening of the alveolar–arterial gradient for oxygen, and thus a more marked drop in oxygen tension than can be accounted for by hypoventilation alone. Continuous monitoring of arterial oxygen saturation by ear oximetry has recently pointed to hitherto unsuspected episodes of severe hypoxemia in several groups of patients. People living at high altitude who had severe polycythemia, out of proportion to the degree of arterial unsaturation found during the day, were monitored at night and found to have prolonged spells of severe hypoxemia.[70] Patients with chronic obstructive pulmonary disease (COPD) associated with pulmonary hypertension and cor pulmonale ("blue bloaters") had major drops in saturation while asleep, whereas "pink puffers" did not.[71] Marked drops in saturation were also found to occur in patients with asthma,[72] cystic fibrosis,[69] and obstructive sleep apnea.

Hypoxemia is usually more severe in REM sleep. While there are dips in oxygen saturation that coincide with apneic spells, hypoxemia also occurs in patients without apnea. Even in patients with chronic carbon dioxide retention, most of the drop in P_{O_2} is due to widening of the alveolar-arterial oxygen gradient.[73–75] The principal mechanism seems to be a fall in FRC that occurs in sleep, particularly REM sleep, and causes worsening ventilation–perfusion relationships.

Nocturnal hypoxemia has been associated with chronic polycythemia and can also be responsible for sustained pulmonary hypertension. In experimental animals, intermittent hypoxia is as effective as sustained hypoxia in causing pulmonary hypertension.[76] Low P_{aO_2} at night interferes with comfortable sleep[73] and may play a role in precipitating cardiac arrhythmias or angina.

Administration of oxygen through the night is effective in preventing severe hypoxemia,[77] but increases the duration of apneic spells and may lead to severe respiratory acidosis in sleep.[73] Patients who are given oxygen to prevent arrhythmias, improve polycythemia, lower pulmonary artery pressure, or help primary alveolar hypoventilation should have blood gases monitored in the night if there is any reason to be concerned about hypoventilation. Both medroxyprogesterone[70] and acetazolamide[78] have been found to improve nocturnal oxygen saturation in polycythemic patients at altitude. The efficacy of these drugs in other conditions remains to be established, and both have significant side-effects.

Assessment of Disorders of Breathing During Sleep

When sleep apnea or sleep hypoxemia is suspected, some form of continuous nocturnal polygraphic recording must be done to quantify the frequency and severity of the disorder and to determine if there are associated dangerous complications, such as cardiac arrhythmias.[79,80] Casual observation of the patient during the night may identify some episodes of obstruction, apneas, or arrhythmia, but these might also be found in normal people, and certainly would not justify serious consideration of long-term administration of stimulant drugs or surgery.

Nocturnal bronchospasm and left ventricular failure must always be excluded. Full assessment of pulmonary function and respiratory muscle strength, careful inspection of the upper airway, detailed neurologic examination with attention to respiratory nerves and muscles, and electroencephalography are important in excluding specific causes or associated diseases.

Full-scale sleep monitoring includes electroencephalography to establish sleep state[80] and correlate it with whatever abnormalities are discovered. This helps in classification and understanding of pathogenesis, but is not necessary in order to diagnose and quantify apneas. Cardiac rhythm is monitored by electrocardiography. Ear oximetry allows fairly accurate, continuous monitoring of oxygen saturation. With patients in whom hypercapnia during sleep may be a clinical problem (obese hypersomnolent, COPD), it is necessary to install an arterial cannula for intermittent checks of blood gases. Noninvasive monitoring of ventilation is more difficult. Flow can be monitored by strapping on a tight-fitting mask connected to a pneumotachograph, but this is usually very bothersome to the patient. Presence or lack of flow can be established by attaching small thermistors in front of the nose and mouth, and these can be made cheaply from discarded thermodilution-cardiac-output Swan-Ganz catheters.[81] Impedance pneumographs around the thorax and abdomen give continuous semiquantitative tracings of tidal volumes. More precise tidal volume data can be acquired from magnetometers or a vest that incorporates two magnetic coils, but sophisticated computerized calculations are needed to translate the electrical signals into volume measurements. With magnetometers, absolute lung volume can be followed. For most clinical purposes it is mainly important to identify apneas and separate obstructive from central ones. Obstructive apnea is most reliably detected by measuring intrathoracic pressure with an esophageal balloon. This technique also permits identification of partial obstruction due to upper airway narrowing, and some quantitation of respiratory muscle effort. If the patient cannot comfortably swallow a balloon, obstructive apneas can be recognized by the occurrence of paradoxical motion of rib cage and abdomen in tracings from pneumographs or magnetometers.[82] In some cases it may be desirable to monitor pulmonary or systemic arterial pressures, but this is seldom necessary for diagnosis or management.

DISORDERS OF CHEMICAL CONTROL

FAILURE OF CHEMORECEPTOR FUNCTION

To demonstrate the function of chemoreceptors the P_{CO_2} or P_{O_2} of arterial blood is artificially changed by making the patient inhale a gas mixture which is either high in carbon dioxide or low in oxygen; the response to this stimulus is assessed by measuring minute ventilation. In practice, the carbon dioxide level is usually raised by having the patient rebreathe gas from a small bag which is initially filled with a mixture of 7% carbon dioxide and 93% oxygen.[83] P_{CO_2} rises steadily at a rate of about 6 mm Hg per min and the test is completed in about 5 min. The most useful method for producing a hypoxic stimulus is the *progressive isocapnic hypoxia* method.[84] The range of normal values for both these tests is extremely wide,[85] (*e.g.*, from 2 to 10 liters/min/mm Hg for CO_2 response).

By changing carbon dioxide or oxygen and measuring ventilation, these tests assess not just the function of the chemoreceptor but of chemoreceptor plus respiratory centers, spinal connections, the muscular pump, and its interaction with resistance and compliance of the respiratory system (see chap. 2). A defect anywhere along this chain can reduce the ventilatory response. The effect of lung mechanics on the response can be separated from the rest of the chain by measuring the output of the respiratory centers as occlusion pressure rather than as ventilation. This measurement is relatively independent of lung compliance and resistance. If the electromyogram of the diaphragm is measured, the output of the respiratory centers may be seen to be normal even when ventilatory response is decreased because of muscle weakness or some other chest wall disorder. Still, disease or damage anywhere in the neuraxis may affect response. It is also true that carbon dioxide and oxygen responses interact, the slope of one being altered by changes in steady stimulus from the other. For practical purposes carbon dioxide stimulation tests central nervous system receptors, and hypoxic stimulation tests carotid bodies.

Isolated failure of oxygen sensitivity can be presumed in those patients who have had bilateral resection of the carotid bodies. Such patients have been studied and found to have no response to hypoxia, although they increase ventilation normally on exercise.[86,87] Unfortunately, there is little useful clinical data available about how these patients function in daily life. They appear to be normal in most respects although they could be predicted to be at particular risk in those situations where carotid bodies are thought to play a role: at high altitude, in airplanes, during hypoxic respiratory failure, in sleep apnea, and in metabolic acidosis.

Reduction in sensitivity to hypoxemia is found in patients with severe chronic hypoxemia in cyanotic congenital heart disease, and in people who dwell for years at very high altitude.[88] The wide variation in sensitivity through the normal population is partly explained by heredity. Insensitivity to hypoxemia has been found in association with the obesity–sleep–apnea syndrome, central sleep apnea, and idiopathic alveolar hypoventilation, but it is not certain to what extent it plays an important pathophysiological role.

In most cases where ventilatory response to carbon dioxide is reduced, it is unlikely that the dysfunction is confined to chemoreceptors. Usually the reduction in ventilation can be ascribed to impaired activity of many parts of the neural respiratory control system (as in the effects of sedatives, for example). Isolated dysfunction of central chemoreceptors could be suspected if ventilation responded normally to the stimuli of hypoxemia and exercise, but not to inhaled carbon dioxide. This combination of findings has rarely been reported, however. Reduced ventilatory response to carbon dioxide, probably indicative of general impairment of the metabolic control system, is found in association with idiopathic alveolar hypoventilation, sleep apnea, myxedema, neuromuscular disease, sedative or narcotic drug intake, and many other conditions.

METABOLIC ACIDOSIS AND ALKALOSIS

It is well recognized that primary metabolic acidosis brings about an increase in ventilation through stimulation of chemoreceptors, so-called respiratory compensation. It must be remembered, however, that two sets of chemoreceptors respond to changes in hydrogen ion concentration, namely the carotid bodies in arterial blood and the central chemoreceptors sampling brain interstitial fluid. Since neither hydrogen nor bicarbonate ions readily cross the blood–

brain barrier, the two sets of chemoreceptors may be temporarily exposed to environments of different acidity during an illness in which blood *p*H is changing rapidly.

In metabolic acidosis,[89–91] arterial *p*H depends on the rate at which acid is being generated and added to the circulation, and on alveolar ventilation. As acidosis develops, ventilation increases, and P_{CO_2} falls. The decrease in arterial P_{CO_2} constitutes a reduction in normal chemical stimulus to the carotid body and limits the degree of ventilatory compensation. If the metabolic process responsible for generating acid does not involve brain tissue, brain interstitial fluid *p*H begins by being normal. CO_2 equilibrates very rapidly with CSF, but the equilibration of arterial H^+ and HCO_3^- with CSF takes many hours, so at first brain interstitial fluid *p*H is governed mainly by the decreasing level of P_{CO_2}, and therefore rises. The central chemoreceptors' drive to breathe is thus reduced, further limiting ventilatory compensation. As acidosis persists, CSF bicarbonate falls gradually, CSF becomes more acid, and ventilation increases, making compensation of arterial *p*H more complete. If the cause of acidosis is corrected or venous infusion of bicarbonate is now given, the reverse process occurs. Arterial *p*H rises, stimulation of the carotid body by acidemia is less, and ventilation decreases. As P_{CO_2} rises but CSF bicarbonate stays low, CSF *p*H fails to improve, and may actually get worse. Since CSF and brain interstitial fluid acidosis adversely affect brain function,[92] the patient may remain stuporous or become more so as blood bicarbonate returns to normal. CSF *p*H remains low and stimulates ventilation so that prolonged hyperventilation unexplained by arterial gases is seen.

In metabolic alkalosis, ventilation can be depressed. (On the average, arterial P_{CO_2} rises 0.6 mm Hg/m Eq rise in bicarbonate).[90] In rapidly changing situations, discrepancies between arterial and CSF *p*H could occur.

GENERALIZED DISEASES OF MUSCLE AND NERVE

Respiratory muscles can be involved in general diseases of muscle, neuromuscular junction, or peripheral nerves. It is usually assumed that all the muscles are affected symmetrically, although damage to the major respiratory muscle groups is seldom assessed separately. In some cases the diaphragm is probably affected more or less than the intercostal or abdominal muscles, and this could be expected to make subtle differences in function. When axial muscles are involved, kyphoscoliosis may complicate the picture. When the primary disease is neurologic, as in poliomyelitis, there may also be damage to respiratory centers. Primary muscle diseases may also affect the heart, leading to left ventricular failure. Neuromuscular diseases that can produce significant damage to the respiratory pump are listed below.

GENERALIZED NEUROMUSCULAR DISEASE AFFECTING RESPIRATORY MUSCLES

- Neural
  - Acute
    - Guillain-Barré syndrome
    - Poliomyelitis
    - Porphyria
    - Tetanus
    - Strychnine poisoning
  - Chronic
    - Motor neuron disease
    - Multiple sclerosis
    - Parkinson's disease
    - Poliomyelitis
- Neuromuscular junction
  - Myasthenia gravis
  - Curare or succinyl choline
  - Anticholinesterase poisoning
  - Botulism
  - Aminoglycoside antibiotics
  - Tick paralysis
- Muscle
  - Myotonic muscular dystrophy
  - Other dystrophies
  - Polymyositis
  - Lupus erythematosis
  - Familial paralytic paralysis
  - Hypophosphatemia
  - Hypokalemia
  - Central core disease and other myopathies

CHRONIC NEUROMUSCULAR DISEASE

Pathophysiological Principles

The common clinical experience is that patients with respiratory muscle weakness go along for years without any suspicion of respiratory problems. Exercise limitation is attributable to weakness of other muscles, blood gases remain normal, and routine pulmonary function tests, if done at all, show signs interpreted as "restriction" or "poor effort." Respiratory failure is usually precipitated by pulmonary infection or an abdominal operation, and comes as a surprise.

The effect of uncomplicated, symmetrical muscle weakness on pulmonary function can be predicted from normal physiology. As inspiratory muscles weaken, they can no longer maximally distend the lungs and total lung capacity falls. This may be noted on routine pulmonary function testing and be misinterpreted as restrictive disease of the lung. Because the pressure–volume curve of the respiratory system is relatively flat near total lung capacity, it can be predicted that a major portion of inspiratory muscle strength must be lost before there is an appreciable reduction in total lung capacity or vital capacity. This is true to some degree, but in many patients total lung capacity is reduced more than would be predicted on the basis of measurements of muscle strength alone.[93] There is apparently also a decrease in pulmonary compliance, perhaps owing to a lack of deep breaths or sighs. The loss in compliance may be explained by areas of microatelectasis, or by an overall increase in surface tension.[94] A minor reduction in diffusing capacity can occur, and is best explained by the loss of lung volume. Expiratory muscle weakness interferes with the ability to breathe out below the resting volume and results in a rise in residual volume. Functional residual capacity may remain normal or be slightly decreased, either because of decreased lung compliance or because of a change in end-expiratory muscle tone.

In these diseases extensive damage occurs before symptoms develop. Much of the reserve capacity is used up and compensated for without the patient being aware, and even chronic underventilation, hypoxemia, pulmonary hypertension, and cor pulmonale may occur before the problem comes to the attention of the physician. As nerve or muscle cells degenerate and become less effective at generating pressure, the respiratory control system apparently detects the problem and overcomes it by increasing its output to remaining functioning motor units. It somehow does this without permitting a fall in alveolar ventilation or rise in P_{CO_2}. As this process goes on, however, it reaches a point where, to maintain normal CO_2 and O_2 transport at rest, the control system must be sending near-maximal signals to the remaining functional units. In this state the muscles are receiving great stimulation and working at close to their maximum capacity. If they are required to work even harder, as in exercise or pneumonia, or if they are hampered by a mechanical load (such as the increased resistance of bronchospasm, or severe obesity), they may be unable to maintain normal ventilation or may do so only at the expense of becoming fatigued. The mechanism by which patients with weak muscles detect the weakness and make compensatory efforts to maintain ventilation is not known. Since they maintain normal blood gases until the final stages, some neural mechanism other than the chemoreceptor is likely responsible. Sensitivity of such a neural mechanism to drugs might explain the peculiar susceptibility these patients have to respiratory depression by sedatives.

Patients with generalized neuromuscular disease may have dysphagia or a poorly functioning larynx, making them prone to aspiration. They frequently have an ineffective cough. Cough begins with a deep inspiration, after which the glottis is tightly closed. Expiratory muscles are then activated to make high positive pressures which suddenly expel air at high velocity when the glottis opens. Weakness or inefficiency of in spiratory, expiratory, or laryngeal muscles can impair this mechanism, leading to accumulation of secretions and infection.

Inactivity dictated by weakness of the limbs makes these patients prone to thrombosis and embolism. Myocardial failure complicates many kinds of dystrophy and myositis. Sleep apnea is also found in some cases.

When weakness becomes severe, other constraints apply stress to the control system. As inspiratory capacity approaches normal tidal volume these patients adopt a pattern of smaller-than-normal tidal volume and may have high dead-space-to-tidal-volume ratio.[95] The effort to make each breath becomes a large percentage of the maximal effort, and this introduces the possibility that the muscles will become fatigued with ordinary or slightly increased ventilation. The abnormally large effort by the weakened muscles produces only normal tension and normal deformation of the chest wall, so that those mechanisms for dyspnea that rely on perception of effort through tension and deformation are not triggered and dyspnea is a minor feature. Without this useful warning signal patients may fail to avoid stressful situations. Small tidal volumes and lack of effective sighs may increase the tendency to close small airways at end-expiration and lead to worse ventilation–perfusion distribution. In cases where functional residual capacity falls, this problem is exaggerated, and hypoxemia becomes an important factor.

Poliomyelitis

Poliomyelitis, caused by an enterovirus, is now a rare disease in the developed countries. The acute infection may be associated with potentially reversible paralytic disease which ranges from mild to severe, symmetrical or asymmetrical, rapid or gradual in onset, and is associated with an acute febrile illness.[96] The paralysis results from predominant infection of large motor neurons. Widespread use of immunization has provided a high level of prophylaxis. In its bulbar form this disease was frequently fatal, but some patients, after being kept alive for weeks or months on a tank respirator, have recovered enough function of respiratory muscles to return to fairly active lives. Many of these develop chronic, hypercapnic respiratory failure later in life,[97] usually in their fifth or sixth decades. Late deterioration may be attributed to loss of pulmonary reserve with aging, to progressively developing kyphoscoliosis, to pulmonary embolism, to recurrent infection, or to late degeneration of motor neurons. It is more likely if the original attack occurred after the age of ten. Since poliomyelitis affects both bulbar and anterior horn cells, complex mixed defects can occur. There may be failure of one or other or both hemidiaphragms, failure of intercostal muscles, or central damage leading to overall hypoventilation or sleep apnea.[98] Careful evaluation of each patient is necessary before the best treatment can be planned.[98a]

Kyphoscoliosis is a common and major complication, bringing with it all of the problems described in the section below.

Motor Neuron Disease

Motor neuron disease is the name applied to a family of disorders that share the pathological feature of progressive degeneration of neurons in the motor pathway, including Betz cells in the motor cortex, motor cells in cranial nerve nuclei, and motor neurons in the anterior horns of the spinal cord. Subgroups are distinguished by peculiar distributions of lesions. In *amyotrophic lateral sclerosis* upper motor neurons are preferentially affected, muscle weakness being associated with active deep tendon reflexes, but there is also loss of anterior horn cells, especially in the cervical, lower thoracic and lumbar regions, with relative sparing of the upper and mid-thorax. In *progressive muscular atrophy* spinal motor neurons supplying distal muscles are the first to degenerate, whereas in *progressive bulbar palsy* it is cranial nerve nuclei. Respiratory failure is a common mode of death in amyotrophic lateral sclerosis, which tends to affect expiratory muscles and the diaphragm. Diaphragm paralysis occurs in the Kugelberg-Welander syndrome[99] (which differs from progressive muscular atrophy in that proximal muscles are affected early in the course), whereas a normal diaphragm but impaired intercostal function is the rule in a related disease of infants, the Werdnig-Hoffman syndrome.[100] Pulmonary function testing should be part of the routine evaluation of patients with any of these diseases. Dyspnea on exertion is seldom a major complaint even when respiratory failure is imminent, although the characteristic orthopnea of diaphragm paralysis may be present, and a syndrome of hypersomnolence and periodic breathing has been reported.[101]

Amyotrophic lateral sclerosis characteristically produces a reduction in vital capacity, total lung capacity, and maximum inspiratory pressures by weakening the diaphragm, plus a rise in residual volume and fall in maximum expiratory pressure through weakness of abdominal muscles.[102] An early sign of expiratory muscle weakness that does not require special testing is a peculiar distortion of the flow–volume loop.[103,104] Maximum flow is reduced at the effort-dependent peak, is normal in the mid-range of vital capacity (where much less than normal maximum expiratory effort is required to collapse airways and reach flow limitation), but falls below the predicted curve again at residual volume. In some patients, however, involvement of bulbar neurons causes dysfunction of the larynx and gross distortion of the expiratory flow–volume loop.[104] The severity of respiratory abnormalities correlates only roughly with other manifestations of the disease. Occasionally severe hypercapnic respiratory failure develops before any abnormality can be detected by general neurologic examination, but the diagnosis can still be established by electromyography of peripheral muscles.[95,100]

Once the first respiratory abnormalities have appeared, pulmonary function tests offer one of the few simple quantitative ways of following the progress of the disease. There is usually a steady downhill course of one or two years. As in similar conditions, respiratory failure is usually precipitated by pneumonia, aspiration, or some other pulmonary complication. In spite of the grim long-term prognosis, many patients have survived a spell of hypercapnia with ventilator support, been successfully weaned, and returned home.[105]

The Muscular Dystrophies

The several types of muscular dystrophy have different effects on respiratory muscles. *Limb-girdle dystrophy* can cause diaphragm failure.[99] In *Duchenne's dystrophy*,[106] respiratory muscle weakness is a feature of advanced disease, the earliest detectable abnormalities occuring when the patient can no longer walk upstairs or get up from a chair. Inspiratory and expiratory muscles are affected symmetrically, but diaphragm function seems to be well preserved until near the end.

Myotonic dystrophy is distinguished by much more prominent respiratory disturbances than predicted by assessment of muscle strength alone.[107] Total lung capacity may be reduced, and residual volume increased, but more striking changes are seen in maximum inspiratory pressure. These changes are detectable fairly early in the course, when weakness of other muscles first becomes apparent. Many features point to an associated disorder of the central or reflex control system.[108] Daytime somnolence[109] occurs in patients with mild muscle disease and some shift into REM sleep at the onset of sleep, as in narcoleptics. In sleep some have frequent apneas, and many have severe hypoxemia. Upon stimulation with high carbon dioxide or low oxygen they breathe rapidly, but fail to increase tidal volume. Occlusion pressure and inspiratory flow rates rise normally, but minute ventilation does not,[110] which implies that expiration becomes unduly prolonged and suggests a central problem in rhythm generation. Cor pulmonale is a frequent problem, and patients are notably sensitive to respiratory depression by sedatives.

Other Muscle Diseases

Several rare diseases of muscle can end in respiratory failure. It is important to recognize that in some of them, as in myotonic dystrophy, the disorder of breathing may be out of proportion to measurable weakness of respiratory or other muscles.[111] Polymyositis can cause weakness of respiratory muscles, and this possibility must be considered in diseases such as systemic lupus erythematosis, where a "restrictive" picture in pulmonary function tests may be incorrectly blamed on interstitial pulmonary fibrosis.[112]

ACUTE NEUROMUSCULAR DISEASE

Some diseases that cause respiratory failure that comes on rapidly (over hours or days) and are self limited are listed on page 210. Survival is possible if adequate life support can be provided for days, weeks, or occasionally months.[113] In all cases the challenge for the physician is to recognize the problem, to anticipate when ventilator support is required, and to avoid complications of long-term respirator management.

The indications for ventilator support are the same as for other conditions (see Chap. 7). Weakness of muscles can be monitored by repeated measurement of the vital capacity and maximal inspiratory pressures, or simply by seeing how far the patient can count in one breath. The last test has the advantage that it requires no equipment and is easily calibrated, using the performance of the physician as normal. When the patient can count only one-third or one-fourth as far as normal, imminent respiratory failure can be predicted.[114]

Meticulous attention to detail is necessary in order to avoid the many complications of long-term intensive care. Optimal airway care; prevention of thromboembolism, aspiration, gastrointestinal bleeding and infection; good nutrition; careful fluid management; and physiotherapy to maintain mobility of joints are essential. Being paralyzed, these patients are helpless if the respirator stops; deaths have resulted from failure of alarm systems following disconnection of tubing or power failure.

Guillain Barré Syndrome, Acute Polyneuritis

These, and similar syndromes associated with acute intermittent porphyria, infectious mononucleosis, and hepatitis are characterized by fairly rapid development of flaccid paralysis of many muscles. In the most common form, paralysis begins in the legs and spreads upwards, but it may also begin in pharyngeal, facial, and respiratory muscles. The progress of weakness is quite unpredictable. Some patients have remained stable, with mild weakness for a week, only to lapse into respiratory failure in a day or two. For this reason it is recommended that even mildly affected patients be kept in hospital until recovery begins.[114] Ventilator support may be required for many weeks, but most patients recover completely in the end. Dysfunction of the autonomic nervous system complicates management by causing wild fluctuations in pulse and blood pressure, together with loss of sphincter control and lack of sweating.[113]

Myasthenia Gravis

This is an uncommon disorder in which the number of available acetylcholine receptors at skeletal neuromuscular junctions is decreased.[115–117] The resulting weakness is made worse by repeated efforts and is improved by rest. The extraocular, bulbar, neck, limb girdle, distal limb, and trunk muscles are involved, in that order. The degree of weakness fluctuates, so that episodes of transient respiratory failure can occur frequently. Anticholinesterase drugs, which favor the accumulation of acetylcholine at the receptor site, are used in initial diagnosis and treatment. Edrophonium is given intravenously to patients suspected of having myasthenia, as a diagnostic test. Improvement in strength within minutes supports the diagnosis, but a negative test does not exclude it. For long-term treatment, neostigimine or pyridostigmine are given orally, the dose and interval being adjusted to maintain strength throughout the day. An overdose of these drugs causes severe muscle weakness or "cholinergic crisis," and may be brought on by infection or surgery, which decrease the requirement for drugs, but this is indistinguishable from a "myasthenic crisis" in which the disease has worsened to the point where the usual dose of anticholinesterase is no longer sufficient. Separation of two types of crisis can be made by giving 10 mg of edrophonium, which will increase strength in a myasthenic crisis, but reduce it in a cholinergic one, as well as cause a great increase in tracheobronchial secretions.

Corticosteroids often make a dramatic improvement, but a transient exacerbation, reaching its nadir in about ten days, is commonly seen at the commencement of treatment. Ephedrine, thymectomy, thoracic duct drainage, and plasmapheresis help in some patients. Hypokalemia and drugs that interfere with neuromuscular transmission or muscle function (curare, quinidine, quinine, procaine, propranolol, aminoglycoside antibiotics) must be avoided, as well as narcotics and sedatives.

During myasthenic and cholinergic crisis, respiratory failure often develops, and ventilator support is required until strength returns. The problems peculiar to this disease are the high incidence of aspiration due to laryngeal muscle weakness; the management of a crisis that threatens to lead to respiratory failure; and the need to make ongoing assessments of variable strength of respiratory muscles.

When weakness first begins to affect respiratory muscles, vital capacity and inspiratory flow rates are reduced. When edrophonium is given in a mild case, FEV_1 may actually worsen because the anticholinesterase has the effect of increasing vagal tone, causing bronchoconstriction and hypersecretion of mucus. In more severe cases, FEV_1 rises with edrophonium in spite of increased airways resistance because vital capacity increases. Inspiratory flow rates increase in both situations. In a crisis, when it is necessary to determine whether the dose of anticholinesterase is too great or too little, it is essential to prepare for ventilatory support before administering edrophonium, because the test dose may precipitate severe hypoventilation. Furthermore, it is necessary to test respiratory muscle strength directly, because the effect of the drug varies unpredictably from one muscle group to the next, and a decrease in diaphragm strength may occur simultaneously with an improvement in handgrip.

Once the patient is intubated, repeated measurements of inspiratory muscle pressure or vital capacity are necessary to monitor drug doses and progress of the disease. Most patients recover from the acute crisis, but life expectancy in those who have had respiratory failure is sharply reduced. Special problems of management come up in anesthesia, surgery, pregnancy, and neonatal myasthenia.[113]

Tetanus

Tetanus is a major cause of mortality at all ages in underdeveloped countries, but in North America widespread prophylaxis has rendered it very uncommon.[118–120] It occurs mainly in young infants and in the elderly rural population who have escaped active immunization. The anaerobic soil bacterium *Clostridium tetani* infects deep penetrating wounds and secretes a toxin, tetanospasmin, into the blood, from where it is taken up by nerve endings and transmitted along axons to the central nervous system. At motor endplates it interferes with release of acetylcholine; in the spinal cord it interferes with release of inhibitory neurotransmitters. There is a marked increase in tone and overexcitability of skeletal muscle. A similar disinhibition apparently involves the autonomic nervous system, leading to unstable increases in sympathetic tone. The clinical features of trismus and severe spasms in response to slight stimuli are well known, but tetanus may at first be mistaken for seizures, meningitis, tetany, or strychnine poisoning.

The usual mode of death is respiratory, although cardiovascular complications become the main problem when good ventilator support and muscle relaxants are used. Mild cases usually have a reduced vital capacity,[121] which may be due to muscle weakness or to spasm of antagonist muscles; untreated severe cases die of asphyxia from spasm of inspiratory and expiratory muscles or of the larynx. Metabolic rate is greatly increased because of muscle plus sympathetic nerve activity, and ventilation increases to match carbon dioxide production,[122] unless spasms interfere. Altered autonomic activity shows itself as labile hypertension, tachycardia, profuse sweating, high temperature unresponsive to antipyretics, and constipation or ileus.[123] In part, the cardiovascular abnormalities are secondary to muscle spasms, increased metabolic rate, fear, hypoxemia, and the effects of drugs, but many of them persist after the patient is completely paralyzed and artificially ventilated, suggesting that they arise from a primary disturbance of autonomic control.[123]

Specific treatment consists of wound debridement, pencillin, passive immunization with human tetanus immune globulin, and the beginning of active immunization. Immune globulin is effective only against circulating toxin; the disease progresses after treatment is begun because toxin already taken up by motor nerves continues to be transported to the nervous system. Intrathecal injections of immune globulin may forestall some of this progression, but clinical trials to demonstrate its usefulness are not completed and available preparations are unsafe for this use.

Supportive treatment of the mild-to-moderate case consists of sedation, and protection from stimuli. At the first sign of laryngospasm or dysphagia threatening aspiration a tracheostomy or endotracheal tube must be placed to protect the airway.

There are several approaches to the treatment of muscle spasms. The older standard treatment consisted of barbiturates, chlorpromazine, paraldehyde, mephenesin, and occasionally morphine in various mixtures designed to achieve relaxation without respiratory depression. Recently diazepam alone has proven more satisfactory.[124] Huge doses may be required (300 to 400 mg/day), but respiratory depression is relatively uncommon and mortality rates have been reduced. Where mechanical ventilators and modern intensive care staff are available, another option is to paralyze the patient completely with a neuromuscular blocking agent, using small doses of sedative to keep the patient comfortable.

The second major problem in severe cases is to manage autonomic instability. The main threat is from sympathetic overactivity, both alpha and beta, which produces extreme elevations of heart rate and blood pressure and arrhythmias, and which has been blamed for myocardial infarction, pulmonary edema, and shock. Part of this problem, particularly the transient changes associated with spasm, goes away with muscle relaxation alone, but the primary autonomic disturbance does not seem to be improved by diazepam or d-tubocurarine, and may actually be aggravated by pancuronium. When the cardiovascular changes are a threat, they can be controlled by appropriate mixtures of alpha- and beta-adrenergic blockers, or in many cases by morphine, which may have a central effect.[125,126] These drugs themselves are dangerous, and deaths have occurred with their use in tetanus. Even with optimal treatment some patients still die of progressive hypotension or unexpected cardiac arrest.

Clearly, excellent nursing care and continuous monitoring of respiration, cardiac rhythm, and blood pressure are essential. The high metabolic rate is diminished by relaxants, but demands good nutritional support, usually by nasogastric tube. The risk of pulmonary embolism is high, and preventive measures are indicated. The planning of a pharmacological approach to muscle relaxation and autonomic control is difficult, but the choice of drugs is probably less important than the skill with which they are used.[127]

Botulism

Botulism is caused by a deadly neurotoxin secreted by the anaerobic, spore-forming bacillus *Clostridium botulinum.*[128] The toxin blocks release of acetylcholine from unmyelinated nerve fibrils proximal to the myoneural junction or synapse, and thus paralyzes skeletal muscle and interferes with the autonomic nervous system. The several types (A to G) elaborate toxins which are serologically distinct but have the same effect. All of them inhabit soil or sediments containing organic matter at the bottom of lakes or the sea.

Illness due to types A and B is most commonly associated with improper domestic canning, in which vegetables or fruits are not cooked long enough to destroy the spores, and the airtight seal produces the anaerobic condition necessary for the bacteria to proliferate. Although industrial canning procedures are designed to eliminate the hazard, outbreaks due to commercial products have occurred. Fish products as well as vegetables have been involved. Among Eskimos and northern Indians, poisoning (usually type E) sometimes arises from eating dried salmon or other uncooked fish products. A rare cause of botulism is wound infection.[129] *Clostridium botulinum* spores may contaminate a dirty wound, grow under anaerobic conditions, and produce toxic signs many days after the injury. Although a few epidemics have made news and provided the basis of important clinical reports, the great majority of cases are isolated ones. When a single case appears, the initial symptoms may be confusing, and rapid progression to respiratory paralysis can ensue. It is therefore useful to keep the clinical features in mind.

Blockade of both neuromuscular and autonomic cholinergic nerves occurs but initial symptoms usually refer to the latter. In mild cases, blurred vision, decreased accommodation and lacrimal secretion, constipation, nausea, and difficulty with micturition and sexual function may be the only symptoms.[130] With more severe intoxication, diplopia, dysphagia, and corresponding physical signs attest to blockade of cranial nerves III, IV, VI, IX, X, XI, and XII; palsy of nerve VI, IX, and X are most frequent.[131] Respiratory muscles are affected early on and severe involvement of the oculomotor nerve (ptosis plus dilated pupil and medial rectus weakness) correlates well with development of respiratory failure. Total paralysis of skeletal muscles occurs in severe poisoning, and this is associated with autonomic blockade. Parasympathetic functions are most evidently impaired, but sympathetic activity also appears to be blocked. There may be hypotension without tachycardia; failure of the pulse to respond to Valsalva maneuver, cold pressor test, tilting, or intravenous atropine; pupils fixed in midposition; ileus; urinary retention; and hypothermia.[132]

Diagnosis must be suspected from the history and physical findings. Botulism can be confused with myasthenia gravis, tick paralysis, Eaton-Lambert syndrome, Guillain Barré, or neomycin neuromuscular blockade. Rapid confirmation can be obtained with the help of electromyography and by injection of serum into laboratory animals. Electromyographic changes resemble those of Eaton-Lambert syndrome.[133] Specific treatment is of unproven value but is always given. Penicillin is given to remove any bacilli that might have been ingested and continue to secrete toxin (In the rare cases of wound infection, debridement and penicillin are essential). Specific equine antitoxin must be given early, since it is ineffective once toxin is fixed to neural tissue. Serum sickness, urticaria, or anaphylaxis may follow. Guanidine produces a definite increase in strength of the limbs but has almost no effect on respiratory muscles or autonomic function, and is therefore of little value in seriously ill patients.[134] Hypotension due to autonomic paralysis can be rectified by volume expansion. Because of denervation hypersensitivity, patients may have an exaggerated response to adrenergic pressor drugs. Prolonged paralysis increases the risk of complications of treatment, and mortality remains high in severe cases.

Infant botulism is a newly recognized problem. The bacteria enter the gut from an unknown source, establish themselves, and eventually cause a subacute illness consisting of constipation, cranial nerve deficits, generalized weakness, and hypotonia.[131]

Tick Paralysis

A rare but reversible form of progressive paralysis, with clinical features remarkably similar to botulism, tick paralysis may occur after establishment and engorgement of a tick. The Rocky Mountain tick and the American dog tick are usually responsible. Paralytic disease occurs days to weeks after the tick is attached, results from a toxin released by the engorged tick, and improves within hours to days of removal of the tick. Respiratory support and identification of the cause are generally life-saving.[135]

SPECIFIC RESPIRATORY MUSCLE WEAKNESS

Pathophysiological Principles

Many of the principles of chronic generalized weakness of respiratory muscles apply as well to cases of weakness or paralysis of individual muscles. The clinical manifestations are often subtle, although local muscle weakness more often gives rise to physical signs of asymmetrical or paradoxical chest movement. Except in cases where it is expected, as in spinal cord injury, local respiratory muscle weakness frequently goes undetected until respiratory failure has been precipitated by pneumonia. Dyspnea is usually a minor feature. Many diseases usually thought of as affecting muscles uniformly may in fact tend to weaken the diaphragm, intercostal, or abdominal muscles preferentially, but this information is not yet available because individual muscle function has so far been assessed in very few patients.

Some additional principles apply particularly to individual muscle weakness. When a major muscle is paralyzed, the remaining ones expand the chest in an abnormal way, and this changes the distribution of pleural pressure.[136] Ventilation is distributed differently, and normal ventilation–perfusion relationships are disturbed. The net effect on function of loss of one muscle is greater than would be predicted by merely subtracting from tidal volume the volume ordinarily displaced by that muscle. This is because loss of one muscle renders the others less efficient. When one muscle is paralyzed, the others must do more than their usual share of the work. There is less reserve, and the working muscles are more vulnerable to fatigue. Finally, loss of an individual muscle will be most noticeable in situations where the control system would ordinarily rely particularly on that muscle. All of these principles are most clearly understood at present with respect to the diaphragm, but most apply to some degree to all the other respiratory muscles.[137]

Unilateral Diaphragm Paralysis

It is much more common to find paralysis of one hemidiaphragm than of the whole muscle and there are many possible causes (see list at right).[138] Unilateral paralysis is recognized when one hemidiaphragm is elevated on physical examination or chest x-ray, but must be distinguished from elevation and fixation of the diaphragm by pleural or pulmonary disease, as well as subpulmonic effusion, eventration and rupture. At fluroscopy, the normal diaphragm descends but the paralyzed hemidiaphragm moves paradoxically upward when the patient sniffs, and the mediastinum may shift toward the affected side as the sharp inspiration against resistance generates a large negative intrathoracic pressure. A false positive "sniff test" may be found when there is subdiaphragmatic disease such as hepatic or splenic injury or subphrenic abscess and is seen in a few normal subjects, so that the test must be carefully performed.[139]

Patients seldom complain of dyspnea on exertion, but may be short of breath when lying on the affected side.[140] Vital capacity and total lung capacity are reduced about 20%, a bit more in the supine posture. Supine, there is less overall ventilation of the affected lung, and it is distributed more toward the apex than normal, but these changes are slight in upright patients.[141] In the supine posture, and even more so in the lateral decubitus with the affected side down, functional residual capacity of the affected lung is low, approaching residual volume, there may be airway closure, and since local blood flow is not reduced to match this, mild hypoxemia results. Abdominal wall displacement is not detectably different from normal.[142] Unilateral diaphragm paralysis may be particularly disabling in patients with associated pulmonary disease.

Causes of Unilateral Diaphragmatic Paralysis

- Surgical
- Tumor
  - Metastatic
  - Bronchogenic carcinoma
- Neurologic
  - Myelitis
  - Encephalitis
  - Herpes zoster
  - Poliomyelitis
  - Tetanus antitoxin
  - Diphtheria
  - Motor neuron disease
  - Brachial plexus neuritis
- Trauma
  - Wounds
  - Accidents
  - Brachial plexus block
  - Birth injury
- Mechanical
  - Substernal thyroid
  - Aortic aneurysm
- Infections
  - Tuberculosis
  - Pneumonia
  - ? Empyema
  - ? Adhesive pleurisy
  - ? Diaphragmitis
  - ? Subphrenic abscess
  - ? Hepatic abscess
- Miscellaneous
  - Syphilis
  - Pulmonary infarction
  - Congenital anomalies
  - Pott's disease

Bilateral Diaphragm Paralysis

Complete failure of the diaphragm, with more or less intact intercostal, abdominal, and accessory muscles, can be seen in a variety of clinical situations listed on p. 219. It is a subtle problem, frequently overlooked even in patients with an established diagnosis of neuromuscular disease and especially difficult when it is the sole manifestation of motor neuron disease or peripheral neuropathy. Patients may complain only of fatigue, disturbed sleep, or morning headache. Most have dyspnea that is worse in the supine posture, and this should strongly suggest the diagnosis. Paradoxical inward movement of the abdominal wall is seen in inspiration when the patient is supine, but when he is sitting or standing, it occurs only at the end of inspiration and is hard to detect by eye.[143] The accessory muscles of breathing are active and the lower border of the lungs as determined by percussion is too high and does not move, but there are no other useful clinical signs.

Causes of Bilateral Loss of Diaphragm Function

Anatomical
- Congenital absence
- Eventration
- Rupture

Myelopathies
- Motor neuron disease (amyotrophic lateral sclerosis)
- Poliomyelitis
- Carcinomatous encephalomyelitis
- Syringomyelia

Peripheral neuropathies (phrenic nerve)
- Guillain-Barré syndrome
- Diphtheria
- Beriberi
- Alcoholic neuropathy
- Brachial plexus neuropathy
- Lead neuropathy
- Surgery
- Closed chest trauma
- Idiopathic

Myopathies
- Myotonic dystrophy
- Duchenne dystrophy
- Systemic lupus erythematosis
- Polymyositis
- Acid maltase deficiency

Breathing is performed by intercostal, accessory, and abdominal muscles. The abdominals contract in expiration and relax in inspiration, raising and lowering the diaphragm. This normal-appearing excursion of the paralyzed muscle may deceive the fluoroscopist into believing there is no loss of function.[144] Total lung capacity and inspiratory capacity are sharply reduced. Upright vital capacity is about 50% predicted; supine, it is considerably less, and the difference between postures is a useful diagnostic point. Functional residual capacity is usually reduced, mainly because the end-expiratory level is set by expiratory muscle contraction, driving the chest wall below the relaxation volume that normally coincides with functional residual capacity. In addition, lung compliance is often below normal.

The normal gradient in pleural pressure is lost, so that when the patient lies on his side, ventilation is preferentially distributed to the uppermost lung, away from blood flow.[145] The alveolar–arterial gradient for oxygen is increased, more so in the supine posture, and severe hypoxemia and respiratory acidosis are often present. Since respiratory activity normally fades away from other respiratory muscles during sleep, patients with paralyzed diaphragms are particularly vulnerable to nocturnal worsening of respiratory acidosis and hypoxemia.[137,146]

The most reliable test of diaphragm function is to measure trans-diaphragmatic pressure, but electromyography may give additional information helping to distinguish neural from muscular disease.

These patients are in a perilous condition, on the edge of hypercapnic respiratory failure. Careful attention to details of supportive care is important. The upright posture improves muscle function and gas exchange to an important degree. Ventilation can be supported in the long-term patient by rocking bed, cuirass respirator, or electrophrenic respiration (diaphragm pacing) if the phrenic nerve is intact.[137]

Tetraplegia

Patients with high cervical cord lesions are deprived of intercostal and abdominal muscle function and may have involvement of the diaphragm as well. They have a poor prognosis in spite of good care, being vulnerable to both lung and kidney infections. When the lesion is below C5, diaphragm function is preserved, together with that of accessory muscles of the neck and upper thorax. The latter are capable of both inspiration (sternomastoids, levatores scapuli, scalenes, and others) and expiration (trapezius, serratus anterior). In chronic patients who are seated, inspiratory muscle weakness is shown by a low total lung capacity averaging 70% of predicted and low maximal inspiratory pressures. Marked expiratory muscle weakness results in a very low expiratory reserve volume (20% of predicted), high residual volume (170% of predicted), and very low maximal expiratory pressures. Vital capacity is reduced to about 40% of predicted, but is improved to about 60% when the patient is supine, as residual volume decreases, but total lung capacity is not changed.[147,147a] In the supine position the weight of abdominal contents aids expiration and puts the diaphragm into an advantageous position, helping it to generate more tidal volume for the same stimulus than it does in the sitting position.[148] These advantages of the supine posture may be outweighed by worsening in gas exchange owing to the fall in functional residual capacity that also occurs.[147] When the supine patient contracts his diaphragm, it draws the rib cage, with paralyzed intercostals, paradoxically inward, but this sign is often lacking when he is sitting up.[148,149] As spasticity develops in intercostal muscles, paradoxical inward movement of the rib cage lessens, and a small improvement in ventilatory function may occur. Interestingly, patients with complete spinal cord transection above C3 are unable to detect expansion of their thorax and lungs by a mechanical ventilator, though their pulmonary stretch receptors running in the vagus nerve are intact. They do get a tight feeling in the chest when the lungs are artificially deflated below functional residual capacity, suggesting that information from deflation receptors (these are the same as the irritant receptors) does reach consciousness.[150]

Normal alveolar ventilation appears to be maintained unless respiratory infection supervenes, but the diaphragm shows electromyographic signs of fatigue when called upon to do just a small amount more than its usual work. Respiratory muscle training can improve strength and endurance; it is not yet known whether it will affect longevity.[151]

If the lesion is above the phrenic nerve segments, only a few accessory muscles remain active. Significant ventilation can still be achieved by "glossopharyngeal breathing," in which the patient forces small volumes of air into the lungs with the muscles of mouth and pharynx.[152] Long-term ventilation can be achieved with electrophrenic stimultors.[153]

Tetraplegic patients have numerous other problems. Bladder dysfunction causes obstructive uropathy and recurrent pyelonephritis. An unstable vasomotor autonomic system can cause paroxysms of hypertension. Venous thrombosis and pulmonary embolism are major risks during the first 3 mon, but not thereafter. Muscle contractures and bed sores appear if not prevented. Spasms of pain and reactive depression present major difficulties. Nevertheless, with an excellent rehabilitation program, careful medical attention, and psychological support, many patients live useful lives and may even hold jobs.[154,155] About 30% die in the first few months after their injury, but after that the annual mortality rate in young patients is about 2%, not much different from that of paraplegics, and about twice that of the rest of the population. The long-term prognosis is better if the lesion is incomplete, but considerably worse for patients in older age groups.[156]

DISEASES OF PASSIVE ELEMENTS OF THE CHEST WALL

When the bony cage is deformed, the joints are immobilized, or the chest wall is made heavy by fat, respiratory muscles may be at a disadvantage when attempting to achieve normal tidal volumes and flows. Changes in geometry may put the muscles in positions where they are less effective, and fixation of part of the rib cage may make strong contractions of some muscles quite futile. Alterations in lung volume and shape lead to secondary disorders in gas exchange.

Obesity

Clinical Manifestations. Few patients consult a physician because of respiratory symptoms that obviously result from obesity. Many obese patients admit to exertional dyspnea upon questioning, however, and frequently the patient with obesity develops severe respiratory illness only when immobilized or bedridden owing to other illness. At such times (*e.g.*, postoperatively, during convalescence from a myocardial infarction, or other major systemic illness), pulmonary infection and atelectasis, resulting in clinically significant hypoxemia, become the major manifestations. Uncommonly, the patient

TABLE 6-3. Cardiorespiratory Effects of Obesity

Physiologic Parameters	Persons Without Hypoventilation	Persons With Hypoventilation
Total body O_2 consumption and CO_2 production	Increased	Increased
Cardiac output	Increased	Increased
Left ventricular work	Increased	Increased
Pulmonary artery pressure	Increased	Increased markedly
Right ventricular failure	Rare	Common
Arterial Po_2	Decreased, particularly when supine	Decreased severely, worse while supine and during sleep
Polycythemia	Occasional	Common
Arterial Pco_2	Normal or low	Increased, particularly while supine and during sleep
Ventilatory response to inhaled CO_2	Normal	Decreased
Oxygen cost of breathing	Increased	Increased
Vital capacity	Mildly decreased	Decreased
Functional residual capacity	Mildly decreased	Decreased
Lung compliance	Normal	Normal or decreased
Chest-wall compliance	Decreased	Decreased

presents with gradual spontaneous development of the obesity–hypoventilation syndrome.

As described previously, some obese patients develop obstructive sleep apnea, the result of interaction between increased upper-airway resistance probably due to fat and a defect in control of upper-airway muscles in sleep. Although this is common in the fattest persons, it also affects large numbers of those who are mildly or moderately overweight. Chronic alveolar hypoventilation, on the other hand, is found mainly in the extremely obese.[66] It may be partly due to chronically increased upper airway resistance, but the respiratory controller is probably overburdened by the combination of increased carbon dioxide production, requiring higher-than-normal alveolar ventilation, plus a chest wall too heavy to move easily.

Table 6-3 lists the effects of obesity on the cardiorespiratory system in those persons who do not develop hypoventilation, and contrasts them with the few persons who do.[157,158]

Oxygen consumption and carbon dioxide production are generally elevated at rest, presumably as a result of the increase in body mass. The cardiac output is generally elevated and, except during periods of frank heart failure, is increased approximately in proportion to the increase in resting oxygen consumption. As a result of the increase in cardiac output and the common presence of systemic hypertension, left ventricular work is generally increased, and some studies have indicated left ventricular failure that may be at least partly explained on this basis. Pulmonary artery pressure is commonly elevated in those who develop hypoxemia, but when hypoxemia is not present, the pulmonary artery pressure and pulmonary vascular resistance are normal. Right ventricular failure may occur in those who have increased pulmonary vascular resistance and is most striking in those with alveolar hypoventilation. The arterial Po_2 is generally reduced. This has been explained on the basis of mismatched ventilation–perfusion relationships in the lung. Studies of regional distribution of blood flow in the lungs demonstrated that obese subjects have approximately the same pattern of distribution of blood flow as do normal persons. However, those obese subjects with severely reduced functional residual capacity did not have a normal distribution of inspired air. Such patients, breathing at their normal resting level, inhaled most of their tidal volume into the upper lung zones rather than the lower lung zones. Thus, the lower lung zones continued to be perfused but were not ventilated.[159,160] This may be a result of closure of small airways in the dependent portions of the lungs.[161,162] Since these persons characteristically have a decrease in functional residual capacity, it is likely that the functional residual capacity is below the level at which some airways begin to close in the dependent lung zones.

In fact, severity of hypoxia should then be well correlated with the reduction of functional residual capacity, and hypoxia should improve as this increases toward normal with weight reduction. Polycythemia is commonly seen in those obese persons who have severe hypoxemia but occasionally is also seen in those persons who have nearly normal arterial blood gases, with tests performed on a casual basis. Such subjects may develop much more severe hypoxia when in the supine position, with elevated erythropoietin levels and secondary polycythemia.[163]

The adverse respiratory effects of obesity result predominantly from diaphragmatic elevation due to increased volume of the abdomen. Vital capacity is moderately reduced, but the most striking change is a drop in functional residual capacity.[164,165] Chest-wall compliance was found to be reduced in conscious subjects,[164] but under anesthesia, where the measurement is more reliable, it was normal.[166] Resistance is increased particularly in the upper airways[167,168] as is inertia.[169] Not only is the work of breathing increased,[170] but there is a loss in efficiency,[171] more oxygen being expended by the respiratory muscles per unit of work. Probably because of increased mechanical impedance, the ventilatory response to carbon dioxide is reduced, but occlusion pressure measurements show that most obese patients make normal or greater respiratory efforts in response to chemical stimuli.

Respiratory problems are magnified in the supine posture.[172,173] Functional residual capacity is even lower, there is increased venous admixture, and pulmonary artery pressure rises. General anesthesia produces further worsening of gas exchange.[174,175]

It is noteworthy that weight reduction is associated with dramatic improvement in respiratory function and complete reversal of all the cardiorespiratory effects of obesity. When this does not take place, underlying lung disease is generally present.[173,176–178]

Management. The management of the patient with respiratory effects of obesity must be tailored to the manifestations. In those persons whose only problems are related to hypoxia that is aggravated in the supine position, weight reduction is generally very effective. Persons presenting with respiratory complications in association with other illnesses may require vigorous therapy for atelectasis, pneumonia, or respiratory failure. In all these persons, the physiological effects of the supine position should be borne in mind. Maintenance of the upright or semirecumbent position may be effective in improving their respiratory failure. In the most severe forms of respiratory failure associated with alveolar hypoventilation, therapy must be instituted as for other types of ventilatory failure (see Chap. 7). Such persons are frequently best nursed in a chair during the 2 or 3 days during which critical hypoventilation is present. With adequate oxygenation, therapy for superimposed pulmonary complications (such as pulmonary embolism or pneumonia), management of heart failure, and occasionally the use of respiratory stimulants, patients with severe hypoventilation associated with obesity are generally significantly improved in 3 to 7 days of vigorous therapy. When weight reduction is achieved over several weeks of dietary restriction, the gas exchange in the lungs is dramatically improved. Although there is no defined relationship between the level of excess weight and the likelihood of developing alveolar hypoventilation, those persons who do develop this syndrome tend to do so at approximately the same weight on repetitive occasions.

Pregnancy and Ascites

It is commonly thought that in pregnancy the action of the diaphragm must be impaired by the presence in the abdomen of a greatly enlarged uterus, but this does not seem to be the case. In the third trimester small changes in lung volume occur, with functional residual capacity and residual volume being reduced by about 15%. The diaphragm dome moves upward about 4 cm, but tidal movements are normal. Alveolar ventilation increases out of proportion to metabolic rate, and arterial P_{CO_2} is reduced to about 25 mm Hg, but this is brought about by increasing tidal volume rather than frequency, suggesting that there is little hindrance to the effectiveness of inspiratory muscles. Although dyspnea is a very common complaint in pregnancy, its genesis is obscure.[179–181]

In ascites the diaphragm is pushed up, residual volume and functional residual capacity are reduced, and gas exchange may be impaired, generally in proportion to the increased abdominal pressure.

Ankylosing Spondylitis

Clinical Manifestations. Patients with this form of chest-wall disease rarely, if ever, develop respiratory failure, except when there is superimposed pulmonary disease.

Decreased movement of the thoracic cage as a result of rigidity of the bony thorax is the first respiratory manifestation of ankylosing spondylitis. Deformity of the chest wall frequently includes increased kyphosis, with marked rigidity of the thoracic spine. This is often first demonstrated by measurement of circumferential chest expansion.

Measurements of the change in anteroposterior and transverse diameters of the chest wall, or the circumferential distance around the thoracic cage (at the level of the fourth intercostal space anteriorly), demonstrate considerable individual variability in expansion. Mean circumferential expansion varies from 4 to 6 cm in the normal adult, approximately 20% lower in females than males, and decreases substantially with advancing age. Reduced expansion of the thoracic cage should be interpreted in the light of the effects of sex, age, and other associated respiratory disease. In general, persons who have less than 2.5 cm thoracic cage expansion on deep inspiration after a maximum exhalation should be evaluated for possible restrictive chest-wall disease.[182]

It must be emphasized that ankylosing spondylitis is a systemic disease that frequently involves multiple joints. Males are affected much more commonly than females. It begins predominantly in the third and fourth decades. Initially, most patients experience low back pain involving the sacroiliac joints; this gradually progresses to involve, in ascending fashion, lumbar intervertebral, thoracic intervertebral, and costovertebral joints.

Although marked changes in thoracic cage movement have been demonstrated in all studies, the effects on lung function appear to be minimal.[183–187] In general, vital capacity is slightly decreased, with the chest wall fixed in a relatively inspiratory position. Consequently, functional residual capacity and residual volume are increased. As a result, chest films appear to show hyperinflation. The rib cage is unable to expand, but normal tidal volumes are achieved even when ventilation is stimulated by carbon dioxide, by increased excursion of the diaphragm, partly due to increased abdominal muscle contraction in expiration. Intercostal muscles remain active and develop fatigue when ventilation is increased, as they strain against immobile ribs, but the diaphragm comfortably supports large increases in ventilation, and respiratory failure is rare.[188–191] Chest-wall compliance is severely reduced, but lung compliance is normal.[190] Although the distribution of ventilation in the lungs may be altered as a result of decreased mobility of the upper thoracic cage and increased activity of the diaphragm, only minor changes in pulmonary gas exchange are seen. Thus, mild hypoxemia and normal diffusion capacity are characteristic (see Table 6-4).[183]

The possibility that ankylosing spondylitis predisposes to respiratory infections has been debated.[191,192] Some evidence suggests that an increased incidence of tuberculosis may occur, and others have reported pulmonary aspergillomas, suggesting previous lung destruction. Since these persons frequently undergo a variety of therapies for the arthritis, the possibility of predisposition to infection resulting from iatrogenically altered immune mechanisms must be considered. In general, however, if there is a statistical predisposition to disease in the lungs, it appears to be of relatively minor importance.

Cor pulmonale, hypoventilation, or severe limitation of exercise as a result of the respiratory impairment occur uncommonly, except

TABLE 6-4. Cardiorespiratory Effects of Ankylosing Spondylitis

Cardiorespiratory Parameters	Changes Compared to Normal
Circumferential chest-wall expansion	< 2.5 cm
Vital capacity	Approximately 70% normal
Maximum expiratory flow rates	Normal
Residual volume and functional residual capacity	Commonly increased
Diaphragmatic movement	Increased
Arterial P_{O_2}	Normal or mildly reduced
Diffusing capacity	Normal
Lung compliance	Normal
Chest-wall compliance	Reduced markedly

where additional pulmonary parenchymal disease is present.

Some authors have suggested that these patients have an increased risk with abdominal surgery. This is a result of the impaired diaphragmatic function postoperatively (see also Chap. 11, Table 11-8).

A few patients with ankylosing spondylitis develop aortitis and aortic valvulitis with frank aortic insufficiency. This may occur in as high as 10% of those patients with severe, long-standing spondylitis with peripheral joint involvement. Occasionally, a prolonged PR interval heralds atrioventricular conduction problems. This is noteworthy because use of parasympathomimetics during anesthesia may precipitate complete heart block in these subjects.[193]

Apical fibrotic and cavitary disease, unexplained by infection, occurs more commonly than in patients without ankylosing spondylitis, and is thought to be an extra-articular manifestation of the basic process. It occurs in only about 1% of patients, however.[194] When such an x-ray abnormality is found, it cannot be assumed to be related to arthritis and must be investigated as it would in any other patient.

Kyphoscoliosis

Clinical Manifestations. The patient with respiratory symptoms related to kyphoscoliosis always has obvious, severe, chest-wall deformities. Kyphoscoliosis consists of lateral bending and rotation of the vertebral column. This results in marked distortion of the thoracic cage.[180,181] The lateral bending causes convexity of the vertebral column toward one side and concavity toward the other. Furthermore, rotation results in anterior displacement of the posterior ribs on one side, thus decreasing the volume in that hemithorax and producing posterior displacement of the ribs on the opposite side (generally the convex side), increasing the volume of that hemithorax. The patient with kyphoscoliosis, then, may be substantially shorter in stature, due to loss of length of the spine, and has marked asymmetrical alteration in the chest-wall configuration. Abnormalities of the lower portion of the thoracic spine tend to have more severe effects on ventilatory function than do abnormalities high in the thoracic spine. With thoracic lordosis, or loss of normal thoracic curvature in the sagittal plane, respiratory problems are particularly severe.[195–197] Physical examination of the chest may reveal marked displacement of the apex beat of the heart, the area of cardiac dullness, the area of mediastinal dullness, and marked variations in regional chest movement and breath sounds. Baseline physical findings recorded accurately at the time when the patients are clinically well are most helpful in subsequent evaluation during a severe respiratory complication. Thus, the careful physician will take more time in mapping out the details of the clinical findings for subsequent comparison.

Chest roentgenograms are frequently difficult to interpret, but if filmed in slight rotation, with the concave side of the chest rotated slightly anteriorly, the lung fields are generally visualized better.

Kyphoscoliosis may develop without identifiable cause (idiopathic); as a congenital abnormality, commonly associated with other congenital defects; following paralytic disease such as poliomyelitis; and less commonly in association with Marfan's syndrome, Hurler's syndrome, Morquio's disease, and Friedreich's ataxia. The respiratory effects and clinical manifestations of kyphoscoliosis depend, of course, on the severity of other associated disease, the severity of the kyphoscoliosis, and the time of onset.

Most commonly, scoliosis becomes more prominent during the rapid growth years, and the first respiratory symptoms relate to dyspnea on exertion. It is relatively uncommon for patients under age 20 to develop severe alterations in blood-gas exchange or evidence of cor pulmonale. However, in persons with severe kyphoscoliosis, life expectancy is markedly diminished. Patients do not suffer increased mortality as a result of a skeletal deformation *per se*, but rather as a result of respiratory complications.

Persons with severe spinal deformity generally present first with increasing dyspnea on exertion and exercise intolerance but eventually develop a deteriorating course punctuated with recurrent respiratory infections, hypoxia, and development of increased pulmonary vascular resistance, pulmonary hypertension, and right ventricular failure. This may be associated with polycythemia secondary to the hypoxemia. During this phase, severe exacerbations of the respiratory complications may occur as a result of infection, generalized systemic illness, or surgery. Towards the end, chronic alveolar hypoventilation supervenes and sleep apnea is found in some patients, perhaps related to reduced responsiveness of chemoreceptors.[198]

Abnormalities of cardiorespiratory function are summarized in Table 6-5. Nomograms predicting ventilatory parameters are not appropriate unless an estimated body height is used rather than the measured height. The body height may be estimated by measuring the armspan on full extension and, for most adults, multiplying times 1.03. The degree of scoliosis is usually expressed as the Cobb angle, measured from x-ray films of the spine.[202] In idiopathic kyphoscoliosis, vital capacity is generally reduced in proportion to the severity of the spinal deformity. In subjects with curvature of less than 60 degrees, there is seldom severe ventilatory impairment or significant alteration of gases. Individuals with 60 to 90-degree curvatures have an increasing frequency of severe ventilatory abnormalities, and with curvatures greater than 90 degrees, marked ventilatory abnormalities are predictable.[203–207] The residual volume and functional residual capacity are generally reduced.[208,209] Airway closure tends to occur at lung volumes above functional residual capacity in those persons with more than a 90-degree curvature of the thoracic spine.[210] In "paralytic" scoliosis, because of unpredictable associated abnormalities of respiratory muscles, ventilatory defect is more severe than in idiopathic cases, and correlates poorly with the measured angle.[211]

TABLE 6-5. Cardiorespiratory Effects of Kyphoscoliosis*

Vital capacity	Decreased
Functional residual capacity	Decreased
Residual volume	Decreased
Chest-wall compliance	Decreased markedly
Lung compliance	Decreased slightly
Regional ventilation	Decreased, particularly lower zones, concave side
Regional perfusion	Decreased, particularly lower zones, concave side
Arterial Po_2	Decreased
Pulmonary vascular resistance	Increased, proportional to hypoxemia
Respiratory infections	Increased

* Abnormalities approximately proportional to lateral curvature of thoracic spine: less than 60°, mild; 60° to 90°, moderately severe; greater than 90°, generally severe.

Detailed studies of regional lung function have been performed by several groups with varying results. In general, radioisotope scans of the lungs to assess regional ventilation indicate that the lung on the convex side has a larger volume, with a greater degree of ventilation in the upper lung zones; whereas the lung on the concave side tends to have a lower volume with less ventilation. Radioisotope scans of the lung to indicate pulmonary perfusion similarly reveal a greater blood flow through the lung on the convex side and a lesser blood flow through the lung on the concave side. In general, it would appear that the severity of distortion of pulmonary blood flow and ventilation is approximately proportional to the degree of angulation and is more marked in those persons with the primary curvature high in the thoracic spine than in those low in the thoracic spine.[212–214] These alterations in ventilation and perfusion probably result in mismatched ventilation and perfusion relationships, which, together with the reduced functional residual capacity, contribute to elevated alveoloarterial oxygen gradients and dead space characteristically seen with severe disease. Chest-wall compliance is generally reduced, although lung compliance may be normal or low. This results in an increased work of breathing and may contribute to the eventual development of alveolar hypoventilation.

The diffusion capacity is generally normal but may be reduced, particularly in those persons who have had recurrent respiratory infections.

Morphological studies suggest that lungs affected during the early growth period may actually have a reduced number of alveoli, hypoplastic bronchi, and pulmonary vessels. This would account for decreased ventilation, perfusion, and compliance and would make it unlikely that surgical correction of the skeletal deformity would improve lung function. Furthermore, there is evidence that progressive scoliosis, with altered thoracic cavity size, may result in atrophy and fibrosis of lung tissue.[215] These morphological changes may also explain the reduced maximum expiratory flow rates and elevated airways resistance, which are generally altered in proportion to reduction of lung volume.

Management. Vigorous efforts have been made to restore normal curvature to the spine by the use of external and internal splints. These have included plaster casts, spinal rods, and a variety of traction procedures, and spinal fusion. Several detailed analyses indicate only minimal improvement in ventilatory function.[203,204,207,216–218] In general, most patients do not change, 5 to 10% get a convincing increase in vital capacity but an equal number have substantial losses in function. The greatest improvement in function is seen 1 to 2 yr after surgery, when recovery from the effects of the operation is complete. The abnormal spinal curvature then tends to gradually increase again, in some studies returning to its original value after about 10 yr. Long-term follow-up of pulmonary function has not been reported, and there has not been a control study to show whether attempts to correct the scoliosis actually delay or prevent eventual respiratory dysfunction. The correctional procedures take months to years, and most casts and braces cause a temporary reduction in ventilatory function, by 15% or more. The few patients whose pulmonary function would benefit from surgery cannot be identified beforehand. Attempts to correct the deformity are often justified for cosmetic reasons, but cannot ordinarily be justified by an expectation that they will reduce the risk of cardiopulmonary disease.

Every effort should be made to avoid airways disease in these patients by encouraging them not to smoke, institution of early therapy of infections, and vigorous preoperative and postoperative chest care. Management of recurrent infections, hypoventilation, and cor pulmonale is undertaken as for other causes of respiratory failure. Recently, it has been suggested that positive-pressure ventilation increases the compliance of the lungs in these patients with decreased work of breathing for several hours. This form of therapy remains to be explored.[219]

Once respiratory failure develops, sleep apnea, nocturnal hypoventilation, and hypoxia are common features. Even before these disorders were recognized, it was found that such patients would do well if their ventilation was supported at night. Continuous or nocturnal ventilatory support can be provided in the long term by simple cuirass respirators, which must be tailor-made to fit each patient's deformed thorax.[220,221] Some patients treated in this way have survived for years and lived useful lives after their first episode of respiratory failure.[222,223]

Pectus Excavatum

Clinical Manifestations. Patients with a funnel-chest deformity generally develop this as a congenital abnormality. The lower portion of the sternum is displaced posteriorly, and when this is severe, there may be displacement of the intrathoracic structures laterally. On examination, there is marked bowing of the anterior ribs posteriorly, resulting in a depressed panel in the anterior chest wall. Most commonly, the child is presented to the physician because of concern regarding his appearance. Frequently, the child or the parent expresses concern regarding exercise intolerance, chest pain, and general anxiety regarding the ultimate potential for normal development. Occasionally, the first concern develops at the time of a chest roentgenogram, when the heart is considered to be enlarged as a result of its lateral displacement by the compression of the cardiac chambers.

The posteroanterior chest films commonly reveal a broadened cardiac silhouette, with some straightening of the left cardiac border. The posterior ribs tend to take off more horizontally from the vertebral spine, and the anterior ribs are angulated more inferiorly, thus causing an appearance of triangulation at the lateral chest wall. The cardiac displacement makes interpretation of heart size difficult, and the uninitiated may conclude that cardiomegaly is present. On the lateral view, the sternum can be seen coursing posteriorly towards the vertebral spine, and in the most severe instances, may be virtually apposed to the vertebral spine. In the normal adult, the distance between the posterior aspect of the sternum and the anterior portion of the vertebral bodies is about 8 cm. In most patients, posterior displacement of the sternum to within 2 cm of the vertebral spine is well tolerated.

No respiratory findings are noted on physical examination of the chest, and the only cardiovascular finding of note is a high incidence of systolic ejection murmurs heard along the left sternal border and generally of no hemodynamic significance. These have been attributed to distortion of the outflow tract of one or both ventricles.

Although some studies have suggested a mild (10 to 15%) reduction in ventilatory function, including vital capacity, total lung capacity, maximum voluntary ventilation, and flow rates,[224] most series have indicated normal ventilatory function and blood-gas exchange.[225] Furthermore, ventilatory function evaluated before and after surgical correction of the pectus deformity has not been associated with significant measurable changes in ventilatory function.[224,226]

Several individual patients have been reported with elevated right ventricular and right atrial pressures suggestive of cardiovascular effects of the chest-wall distortion. Most careful hemodynamic studies, performed at rest and during exercise, document a normal cardiac output response to increased demands. Reported differences in heart rate and stroke volume may be attributable to conditioning.

It is noteworthy that in a group of army recruits, emotional stability, acceptance of physical tasks, and ability to sustain employment were impaired in a group of young men with significant pectus deformity. What role this deformity may have played in their ultimate life adjustment is not established. Furthermore, a statistical increase in lower respiratory infection (pneumonia) was observed in those studied.[225] No mechanism for this predisposition to infection is established, and the observation has not been commented on in other series.

Management. Except for those rare instances of excessively severe funnel-chest deformity, in which careful analysis of cardiovascular and ventilatory status may be important, patients with this abnormality should be reassured and encouraged to accept the cosmetic defect in view of their normal function. In those rare instances where hemodynamic and ventilatory functions are definitely compromised, surgical correction may be undertaken.

Pectus Carinatum

The second commonest anomaly of the anterior chest wall has been referred to as "chicken breast" or "pigeon breast." The protrusion of the sternum may be general, forming a keel, localized to the manubrial portion, or the deformity may be unilateral. The pathogenesis is unclear.

Patients generally present for cosmetic reasons, but dyspnea, fatigue, and nondescript chest pain are common complaints. Pulmonary function is generally normal.

Physiotherapy, plaster casts, and other devices to compress the sternum have been tried and are ineffective. Surgical correction is frequently successful in improving the deformity, but there is no satisfactory information regarding the psychological or lung-function effects of this form of surgery.[227]

DIAGNOSIS OF THE PATIENT WITH DISEASE OF THE RESPIRATORY PUMP

Disorders of the nerves and muscles of respiration are seldom considered in the analysis of clinical problems. Especially if they occur alone, rather than as part of a general neurologic or muscular disease, they are usually not suspected until the patient develops full-blown respiratory failure. The first problem, therefore, is to remember that such problems can occur, and to include them in the lists of possible causes of respiratory failure, "restrictive" disease, and dyspnea.

The first and most important step is careful examination of the patient. Respiratory rate and rhythm may give indirect clues. If the patient happens to be asleep when the examiner arrives in the room, it is useful to watch him breathing for some time before awakening him, looking for Cheyne-Stokes rhythm, snoring, or obstructive apnea. If he is awake, it is important that he not be aware that his breathing is being observed, since all subjects tend to alter their pattern of breathing when they are made conscious of it.

Local muscle disease can be suspected by observing the motion of the chest wall. In bilateral diaphragm paralysis the abdomen is drawn in during inspiration. In intercostal paralysis the chest wall collapses somewhat when the diaphragm contracts; this is most noticeable at the lower end of the sternum. If there is severe generalized muscle weakness, the accessory muscles come into play. Contraction of the sternocleidomastoid and scalene muscles is best assessed by palpation. They often apear more prominent in inspiration, even if they are not active, because the overlying skin is drawn more tightly over them.

Observations of chest wall motion must be interpreted with great caution when the shape of the chest wall is abnormal, as in kyphoscoliosis or overinflation. In addition, the effects of lung mechanics must be considered. When the lungs are very stiff, as often occurs in the adult respiratory distress syndrome, intrathoracic pressure swings generated by inspiratory muscles are as much as ten times normal, and the pressure becomes the main factor determining chest-wall shape. Sternal indrawing or inward movement of the abdomen in inspiration may then be seen with normally functioning respiratory muscles. More refined quantitative analysis of chest-wall motion can be made with measurements of anteroposterior and lateral diameters of abdomen and rib cage by means of strain gauges or magnetometers, but this technique is as yet available only in a few specialized laboratories and much remains to be learned about interpretation of the data.

It is rare to have significant damage to brainstem respiratory centers without other definite neurologic signs. More subtle problems, such as respiratory apraxia and related disorders, are usually found in patients with diffuse cortical disease and can be demonstrated by asking the patient to hold his breath or do other voluntary respiratory maneuvers. These seldom have clinical significance independent of the underlying disorder.

Ordinary pulmonary function tests can be helpful if not often diagnostic. Most neuromuscular disorders give a "restrictive" picture with relatively little evidence of gas-exchange abnormality. Diffusing capacity is normal, and hypoxemia tends to be less prominent than in restrictive lung disease with an equivalent change in lung volume. If the inspiratory muscles are weak, total lung capacity is reduced; if expiratory muscles are weak, residual volume is increased. In both cases, the functional residual capacity is reduced owing to increased use of the abdominal muscles.

Near both total lung capacity and residual volume, the system is very stiff, so that large changes in pressure produce only small changes in volume. In many cases of neuromuscular disease there is, in fact, a significant loss of vital capacity greater than would be predicted from loss of muscle strength alone. This is explained by a fall in lung compliance that may result from failure to take deep breaths or sighs from time to time.

Respiratory muscle strength can be measured directly (see Chap. 2), and electromyography of the intercostal muscles and diaphragm can be performed.

Deformities and other abnormalities of the passive elements of the chest wall are best assessed by roentgenography and clinical examination. Chest-wall compliance is extremely difficult to measure, except in a paralyzed patient, because it is impossible to be sure the respiratory muscles are relaxed.

The importance of the respiratory pump,

demonstrated by the many and varied disorders outlined above, has only been fully appreciated in recent years. Careful clinical examination will undoubtedly reveal new clinical clues and suitable techniques for assessement of appropriate patients.

REFERENCES

1. PHILLIPSON EA et al: Role of vagal stimuli in exercise ventilation in dogs with experimental pneumonitis. J Appl Physiol 39:76, 1975
2. GUZ A et al: Experimental results of vagal block in cardiopulmonary disease. In Porter R (ed): Breathing, Ciba Symposium. London, J & A Churchill, 1970
3. PLUM F: Hyperpnea, hyperventilation and brain dysfunction. Ann Intern Med 76:328, 1972
4. PLUM F, SWANSON AG: Central neurogenic hyperventilation in man. Arch Neurol Psychiatry 81:535, 1959
5. LEITCH AG et al: Ventilatory response to transient hyperoxia in head injury hyperventilation. J Appl Physiol 49:52, 1980
6. VAPALAHTI M, TROUP H: Prognosis for patients with severe brain injuries. Br Med J 3:404, 1971
7. LEWIS BI: The hyperventilation syndrome. Ann Intern Med 38:918, 1953
8. YU PN, YIM BJB, STANFIELD A: Hyperventilation syndrome. Arch Intern Med 103:902, 1959
9. KETY SS, SCHMIDT CF: The effects of active and passive hyperventilation on cerebral blood flow, cerebral oxygen consumption, cardiac output and blood pressure of normal young men. J Clin Invest 25:107, 1946
10. BROWN EB JR: Physiological effects of hyperventilation. Physiol Rev 33:445, 1953
11. WHEATLEY CE: Hyperventilation syndrome: A frequent cause of chest pain. Chest 68:195, 1977
12. EVANS DW, LUM LC: Hyperventilation: An important cause of pseudoangina. Lancet 1:155, 1977
13. CHEYNE J: A case of apoplexy in which the fleshy parts of the heart was converted into fat. Dublin Hosp Rep 2:216, 1818
14. LANGE RL, HECHT HH: The mechanism of Cheyne–Stokes respiration. J Clin Invest 41:42, 1962
15. DOWELL AR, et al: Cheyne-Stokes respiration. Arch Intern Med 127:712, 1971
16. GOTOH F, MEYER JS, TAKAGI Y: Cerebral venous and arterial blood gases during Cheyne–Stokes respiration. Am J Med 47:534, 1969
17. WEBB P: Periodic breathing during sleep. J Appl Physiol 37:899, 1974
18. PLUM F, POSNER JB: Diagnosis of Stupor and Coma. Philadelphia, F.A. Davis, 1972
19. REES PJ, CLARK TJH: Paroxysmal nocturnal dyspnea and periodic respiration. Lancet 2:1315, 1979
20. CHERNIACK NS, LONGOBARDO GS: Cheyne–Stokes breathing. N Engl J Med 288:952, 1973
21. GUYTON AG, CROWELL JW, MOORE JW: Basic oscillating mechanism of Cheyne–Stokes breathing. Am J Physiol 187:395, 1956
22. CHERNIACK NS et al: Experimentally induced Cheyne–Stokes breathing. Respir Physiol 37:185, 1979
23. PHILLIPSON EA: Respiratory adaptations in sleep. Annu Rev Physiol 40:133, 1978
24. PREISS G, ISCOE S, POLOSA C: Analysis of a periodic breathing pattern associated with Mayer waves. Am J Physiol 228:768, 1975
25. NEWSOM DAVIS J: Diseases of the nervous system. In Campbell EJM. Agostoni E, Newsom Davis J (eds): The Respiratory Muscles. London, Lloyd-Luke, 1970
26. PLUM F, SWANSON AG: Abnormalities in the central regulation of respiration in acute and convalescent poliomyelitis. Arch Neurol Psychiatry 80:267, 1958
27. PLUM F, ALVORD EC JR: Apneustic breathing in man. Arch Neurol 10:101, 1964
28. PLUM F: Neurological integration of behavioural and metabolic control of breathing. In Porter R (ed): Breathing London, J & A Churchill, 1970
29. FINK BR: Influence of cerebral activity in wakefulness on regulation of breathing. J Appl Physiol 16:15, 1961
30. NEWSOM DAVIS J: An experimental study of hiccup. Brain 93:861, 1970
31. RIGATTO M, DE MEDEIROS NP: Diaphragmatic flutter. Am J Med 32:103, 1962
32. PHILLIPS JR, ELDRIDGE FL: Respiratory myoclonus. N Engl J Med 289:1390, 1973
33. RATTO O et al: Anoxemia secondary to polycythemia and polycythemia secondary to anoxemia. Am J Med 19:958, 1955
34. PARE P, LOWENSTEIN L: Polycythemia associated with disturbed function of the respiratory centre. Blood 11:1077, 1956
35. RICHTER T, WEST JR, FISHMAN AP: The syndrome of alveolar hypoventilation and diminished sensitivity of the respiratory centre. N Engl J Med 256:1165, 1957
36. MELLINS RB et al: Failure of automatic control of ventilation (Ondine's curse). Medicine 49:487, 1970
37. FARMER WC, GLENN WWL, GEE JBL: Alveolar hypoventilation syndrome: Studies of ventilatory control in patients selected for diaphragm pacing. Am J Med 64:39, 1978
38. NAEYE RL: Alveolar hypoventilation and cor pulmonale secondary to damage to the respiratory centre. Am J Cardiol 8:416, 1961
39. FINLEY KH: The neuroanatomy in respiratory

failure: Report of 2 cases. Arch Neurol Psychiatry 26:754, 1931

40. HADDAD GG et al: Congenital failure of automatic control of ventilation gastrointestinal motility and heart rate. Medicine 57:517, 1978
41. GLENN WWL et al: Combined central alveolar hypoventilation and upper airways obstruction. Am J Med 64:50, 1978
42. BARLOW PB et al: Idiopathic hypoventilation syndrome: Importance of preventing nocturnal hypoxemia and hypercapnia. Am Rev Respir Dis 121:141, 1980
43. RHOADS GG, BRODY JS: Idiopathic alveolar hypoventilation: clinical spectrum. Ann Intern Med 71:271, 1969
44. LONSDALE D, MERCER RD: Primary hypoventilation syndrome. Lancet 2:187, 1972
45. LUGLIANI R, WHIPP BJ, WASSERMAN K: Doxapram hydrochloride: a respiratory stimulant for patients with primary alveolar hypoventilation. Chest 76:414, 1979
46. MAN GCW et al: Primary alveolar hypoventilation managed by negative-pressure ventilators. Chest 76:219, 1979
47. GLEN WWL et al: Central hypoventilation; long term ventilatory assistance by radiofrequency electrophrenic respiration. Ann Surg 172:755, 1970
48. GUILLEMINAULT C et al: Obstructive sleep apnea: Electromyographic and fibreoptic studies. Exp Neurol 62:48, 1978
49. PHILLIPSON EA, SULLIVAN CE: Arousal: The forgotten response to respiratory stimuli. Am Rev Respir Dis 118:807, 1978
50. REMMERS JE, et al: Pathogenesis of upper airway occlusion during sleep. J Appl Physiol 44:931, 1978
51. GUILLEMINAULT C, DEMENT WC (eds): Sleep Apnea Syndromes. New York, A R Liss, 1978
52. GASTAUT M, TASSINARI CA, DURON B: Polygraphic study of the episodic diurnal and nocturnal (hypnic and respiratory) manifestations of the Pickwick syndrome. Brain Res 2:167, 1966
53. BOROWIECKI B et al: Fibreoptic study of pharyngeal airway during sleep in patient with hypersomnia obstructive sleep-apnea syndrome. Laryngoscope 88:1310, 1978
54. MARTIN RJ et al: Respiratory mechanics and timing during sleep in occlusive sleep apnea. J Appl Physiol 48:432, 1980
55. GUILLEMINAULT C et al: Altered states of consciousness in disorders of daytime sleepiness. J Neurol Sci 26:377, 1975
56. TILKIAN AG et al: Sleep-induced apnea syndrome: prevalence of cardiac arrhythmias and their reversal after tracheostomy. Am J Med 63:348, 1977
57. TILKIAN AG et al: Hemodynamics in sleep-induced apnea. Ann Intern Med 85:714, 1976
58. ORR WC et al: Hypersomnolent and nonhypersomnolent patients with upper airway obstruction. Chest 75:418, 1979
59. ORR WC, IMES NK, MARTIN RJ: Progesterone therapy in obese patients with sleep apnea. Arch Intern Med 139:109, 1979

59a. STROHL KP, HENSLEY MJ, SAUNDERS NA et al: Progesterone administration and progressive sleep apneas. JAMA 245:1230, 1981

60. DE GROOT WJ, ANCH AM, REMMERS JE: Acute and chronic effects of strychnine on upper airway obstruction in sleep. Am Rev Respir Dis 121:332, 1980

60a. CLARK RW et al: Sleep apnea. Treatment with protryptyline. Neurology (Minneap) 29:1287, 1979

61. LEHRMAN KL et al: Sleep apnea in a patient with Shy–Drager syndrome. Arch Intern Med 138:206, 1978
62. SUGAR O: In search of Ondine's curse. JAMA 240:236, 1978
63. COMROE JH JR et al: Frankenstein, Pickwick, and Ondine. Am Rev Respir Dis 111:689, 1975
64. SEVERINGHAUS JW, MITCHELL RA: Ondine's curse—failure of respiratory automaticity while awake. Clin Res 10:122, 1962
65. MELLINS RB et al: Failure of automatic control of ventilation (Ondine's Curse). Medicine 49:487, 1970
66. BURWELL CS et al: Extreme obesity associated with alveolar hypoventilation. A Pickwickian syndrome. Am J Med 21:811, 1956
67. ROCHESTER DF, ENSON Y: Current concepts in the pathogenesis of obesity hypoventilation syndrome. Am J Med 57:402, 1974
68. BLOCK AJ et al: Sleep apnea, hypopnea and oxygen desaturation in normal subjects. N Engl J Med 300:513, 1979
69. MULLER NL et al: Mechanisms of hemoglobin desaturation during REM sleep in normal subjects and in patients with cystic fibrosis. Am Rev Respir Dis 121:463, 1980
70. KRYGER M et al: Impaired oxygenation during sleep in excessive polycythemia of high altitude. Sleep 1:3, 1978
71. DOUGLAS NJ et al: Transient hypoxemia during sleep in chronic bronchitis and emphysema. Lancet 1:1, 1979
72. HUDGEL DW: Coexistence of sleep apnea and asthma resulting in severe sleep hypoxemia. JAMA 242:2789, 1979
73. KOO KW et al: Arterial blood gases and pH during sleep in chronic obstructive lung disease. Am J Med 58:663, 1975
74. LEITCH AG et al: Arterial blood gas tensions, hydrogen ion and electroencephalogram during sleep in patients with chronic ventilatory failure. Thorax 31:730, 1976
75. COCCAGNA G, LUGARESI E: Arterial blood gases

and pulmonary and systemic arterial pressure during sleep in chronic obstructive pulmonary disease. Sleep 1:117, 1978

76. NATTIE EE, BARTLETT D JR, JOHNSON K: Pulmonary hypertension and right ventricular hypertrophy caused by intermittent hypoxia and hypercapnia in the rat. Am Rev Respir Dis 118:653, 1978
77. FLICK MR, BLOCK AJ: Continuous in vivo monitoring of arterial oxygenation in chronic obstructive lung disease. Ann Intern Med 86:725, 1977
78. SUTTON JR et al: Sleep hypoxemia at altitude: Effect of acetazolamide. N Engl J Med 301, 1329, 1979
79. FLAGG WH, COBURN SC: Polygraphic aspects of sleep apnea. In Guilleminault C, Dement WC (eds): Sleep Apnea Syndromes. New York, A R Liss, 1978
80. RECHTSCHAFFEN A, KALES A: A manual of standardized terminology, techniques and scoring system for sleep stages of human subjects. National Institutes of Health, Publication No. 204. Washington, DC, 1968
81. RIEDY RM et al: Sleep apnea syndrome. Practical diagnostic method. Chest 75:81, 1979
82. SHARP JT et al: Use of the respiratory magnetometer in diagnosis and classification of sleep apnea. Chest 77:350, 1980
83. READ DJC: A clinical method for assessing the ventilatory response to carbon dioxide. Australas Ann Med 16:20, 1967
84. WEIL JV et al: Hypoxic ventilatory drive in normal man. J Clin Invest 49:1061, 1970
85. HIRSHMAN CA et al: Normal values for hypoxic and hypercapnic ventilatory drives in man. J Appl Physiol 38:1095, 1975
86. LUGLIANI R et al: Effect of bilateral carotid body resection on ventilatory control at rest and during exercise in man. N Engl J Med 285:1105, 1971
87. WHIPP BJ, WASSERMAN K: Carotid bodies and ventilatory control dynamics in man. Fed Proc 39:2668, 1980
88. BERGER AJ, MITCHELL RA, SEVERINGHAUS JW: Regulation of respiration (3). N Engl J Med 297:194, 1977
89. OHMAN JL et al: The cerebrospinal fluid in diabetic ketoacidosis. N Engl J Med 284:283, 1971
90. ARBUS GS: An in vivo acid–base nomogram for clinical use. Can Med Assoc J 109:291, 1973
91. BUREAU MA et al: Dynamics of the control of ventilation during metabolic acidosis and its correction. Am Rev Respir Dis 119:933, 1979
92. POSNER JB, PLUM F: Spinal fluid pH and neurologic symptoms in systemic acidosis. N Engl J Med 277:605, 1967
93. BRAUN NMT, ROCHESTER DF: Muscular weakness and respiratory failure. Am Rev Respir Dis [Suppl] 119:123, 1979
94. GIBSON GJ et al: Pulmonary mechanics in patients with respiratory muscle weakness. Am Rev Respir Dis 115:389, 1977
95. NEWSOM DAVIS J et al: The effects of respiratory muscle weakness on some features of the breathing pattern. Clin Sci Mol Med 50:10PP, 1976
96. PLUM F: Acute anterior poliomyelitis. In Cecil RF (ed): Textbook of Medicine, 15th ed, chap 307. Philadelphia, WB Saunders, 1979
97. LANE DJ, HAZLEMAN B, NICHOLS PJR: Late onset respiratory failure in patients with previous poliomyelitis. Q J Med 43:551, 1974
98. PLUM F, SWANSON AG: Abnormalities in central regulation of respiration in acute and convalescent poliomyelitis. Arch Neurol 80:267, 1958
98a. HILDES JA (ed): Respiratory polio rehabilitation in Manitoba. U of Man Med J 50:79, 1980
99. NEWSOM DAVIS J et al: Diaphragm function and alveolar hypoventilation. Q J Med 177:87, 1976
100. PARHAD IM et al. Diaphragmatic paralysis in motorneuron disease. Neurology 28:18, 1978
101. SERPICK AA, BAKER EI, WOODWARD TE: Motor system disease. Arch Intern Med 115:192, 1965
102. NAKANO K et al: Amyotrophic lateral sclerosis: a study of pulmonary function. Dis Nerv System 37:32, 1976
103. KREITZER SM et al: Respiratory muscle function in amyotrophic lateral sclerosis. Am Rev. Respir Dis 117:437, 1978
104. BRACH B: Expiratory flow patterns in amyotrophic lateral sclerosis. Chest 75:648, 1979
105. O'DONOHUE WJ et al: Respiratory failure in neuromuscular disease. JAMA 235:733, 1975
106. INKLEY SR, OLDENBURG FC, VIGNAR PJ: Pulmonary function in Duchenne muscular dystrophy related to stage of disease. Am J Med 56:297, 1974
107. KILBURN KH et al: Cardiopulmonary insufficiency in myotonic and progressive muscular dystrophy. N Engl J Med 261:1089, 1959
108. GUILLEMINAULT C et al: Respiratory and hemodynamic study during wakefulness and sleep in myotonic dystrophy. Sleep 1:19, 1978
109. COCCAGNA G et al: Alveolar hypoventilation and hypersomnia in myotonic dystrophy. J Neurol Neurosurg Psychiatry 38:977, 1975
110. BEGIN R et al: Control and modulation of respiration in Steinert's myotonic dystrophy. Am Rev Respir Dis 121:281, 1980
111. RILEY DJ et al: Blunted respiratory drive in congenital myopathy. Am J Med 63:459, 1977
112. GIBSON GH, EDMONDS JP, HUGHES GRV: Diaphragm function and lung involvement in systemic lupus erythematosis. Am J Med 63:926, 1977
113. HEDLEY-WHYTE J et al: Respiratory consequences of peripheral neurological disease, Applied Physiology of Respiratory Care. Boston, Little, Brown & Co, 1976. (Chapter 20)

114. HEWER RL et al: Acute polyneuritis requiring artificial respiration. Q J Med 33:479, 1967
115. DRACHMAN DB: Myasthenia gravis. N Engl J Med 289:136, 186, 1978
116. HARVARD CWH: Progress in myasthenia gravis. Br Med J 2:1008, 1977
117. ASHWORTH B, HUNTER AR: Respiratory failure in myasthenia gravis. Proc R Soc Med 64:489, 1971
118. KERR J: Current topics in tetanus. Intensive Care Med 5:105, 1979
119. EMONDSON RS, FLOWERS MW: Intensive care in tetanus complications and mortality in 100 cases. Br Med J 1:1401, 1979
120. STOLL BJ: Tetanus. Pediatr Clin North Am 26:415, 1979
121. FEMI-PEARSE D: Blood gas tensions, acid base status and spirometry in tetanus. Am Rev Respir Dis 110:390, 1974
122. FEMI-PEARSE D et al: Value of determination of oxygen consumption in tetanus. Br Med J 1:74, 1976
123. HÖRTNAGL H, BRUKE TH, NACKL JM: The involvement of the sympathetic nervous system in tetanus. Klin Wochenschr 57:383, 1979
124. JOSEPH A, PULIMOOD BM: Use of diazepam in tetanus—a comparative study. Indian J Med Res 68:489, 1978
125. RIE MA, WILSON RS: Morphine therapy controls autonomic hyperactivity in tetanus. Ann Intern Med 88:653, 1978
126. BUCHANAN N et al: Autonomic dysfunction in tetanus: the effects of a variety of therapeutic agents with special reference to morphine. Intensive Care Med 5:65, 1979
127. SAUNDERS RKM et al: Tetanus: Situational clinical trials and therapeutics. Prog Drug Res 19:367, 1975
128. BALL AP et al: Human botulism caused by Clostridium botulinum Type E: The Birmingham outbreak. Q J Med 48:473, 1979
129. LEWIS SW et al: Prolonged respiratory paralysis in wound botulism. Chest 75:59, 1979
130. TERRANOVA W et al: Ocular findings in botulism. Type B. JAMA 241:475, 1979
131. POLIN RA, BROWN LW: Infant botulism. Pediatri Clin NA 26:345, 1979
132. JENZER G et al: Autonomic dysfunction in Botulism B: A clinical report. Neurology 25:150, 1975
133. GUTTMANN L, PRATT L: Pathophysiologic aspects of human botulism. Arch Neurol 33:175, 1976
134. PUGGIARI M, CHERINGTON M: Botulism and guanidine, ten years later. JAMA 240:2276, 1978
135. Tick paralysis, pp 117, 118. In Cecil RF (ed): Textbook of Medicine, 15th ed. Philadelphia, WB Saunders, 1979
136. ROUSSOS CS et al: Voluntary factors influencing the distribution of inspired gas. Am Rev Respir Dis 116:457, 1977
137. GUENTER CA, WHITELAW WA: The role of diaphragm function in disease. Arch Intern Med 139:806, 1979
138. RILEY EA: Idiopathic diaphragmatic paralysis. Am J Med 32:404, 1962
139. ALEXANDER C: Diaphragm movements and the diagnosis of diaphragmatic paralysis. Clin Radiol 17:79, 1966
140. ARBORELUIS M, LILJA B, SENYK Y: Regional and total lung function in patients with hemidiaphragmatic paralysis. Respiration 32:253, 1975
141. AMIS TC et al: The effect of diaphragmatic paralysis on regional distribution of ventilation in the lung. Bull Eur Physiopathol Respir 15:89P, 1979
142. HIGENBOTTAM T et al: Abdominal wall movement in normals and patients with hemidiaphragmatic and bilateral diaphragmatic palsy. Thorax 32:589, 1977
143. KREITZER SM et al: Bilateral diaphragmatic paralysis with hypercapneic respiratory failure. Am J Med 65:89, 1978
144. LOH L, GOLDMAN M, NEWSOM DAVIS J: The assessment of diaphragm function. Medicine 56:165, 1977
145. LOH L, HUGHES JMB, NEWSOM DAVIS J: The regional distribution of ventilation and perfusion in paralysis of the diaphragm. Am Rev Respir Dis [Suppl] 119:121, 1979
146. SKATRUD J et al: Determinants of hypoventilation during wakefulness and sleep in diaphragmatic paralysis. Am Rev Respir Dis 121:587, 1980
147. FUGL-MEYER AR: Effects of respiratory muscle paralysis in tetraplegic and paraplegic patients. Scand J Rehab Med 3:141, 1971
147a. TROYER AD, HEILPORN A: Respiratory mechanics in quadriplegia. The respiratory function of the intercostal muscles. Am Rev Respir Dis 122: 591, 1980
148. MORTOLA JP, SANT AMBROGIO G: Motion of the rib cage and abdomen in tetraplegic patients. Clin Sci Mol Med 54:25, 1978
149. DANON J et al: Function of the isolated paced diaphragm and the cervical accessory muscles in C-1 paraplegics. Am Rev Respir Dis 119:909, 1979
150. NEWSOM DAVIS J: High cervical cord transection. Am Rev Respir Dis [Suppl] 119:69, 1979
151. GROSS D et al: The effect of training on strength and endurance of the diaphragm in quadriplegia. Am J Med 68:27, 1980
152. JAMES WS et al: Cervical accessory respiratory muscle function in a patient with a high cervical cord lesion. Chest 71:59, 1977
153. GLENN WWL et al: Total ventilatory support in a quadriplegic with radiofrequency electrophrenic respiration. N Engl J Med 286:513, 1972

154. YASHON D: Spinal Injury. New York, Appleton-Century Crofts, 1978
155. GUTTMANN L: Spinal Cord Injuries, 2nd ed. Oxford, Blackwell Scientific Publications, 1976
156. BERKE MH et al: Survival of patients with injuries of the spinal cord. JAMA 172:121, 1960
157. ROCHESTER DF, ENSON Y: Current concepts in the pathogenesis of the obesity hypoventilation syndrome. Am J Med 57:402, 1974
158. ALEXANDER JK, AMAD KH, COLE VW: Observations on some clinical features of extreme obesity, with particular reference to cardiorespiratory effects. Am J Med 32:512, 1962
159. HOLLEY HS et al: Regional distribution of pulmonary ventilation and perfusion in obesity. J Clin Invest 46:475, 1967
160. BARRERA F et al: Ventilation–perfusion relationships in the obese patient. J Appl Physiol 26:420, 1969
161. BATES DW, MACKLEM PT, CHRISTIE RV: Respiratory function in disease. Philadelphia, WB Saunders, 1971
162. DOUGLAS FG, CHONG PY: Infuence of obesity on peripheral airways patency. J Appl Physiol 33:559, 1972
163. WARD HP, BIGELOW DB, PETTY TL: Postural hypoxemia and erythrocytosis. Am J Med 45:880, 1968
164. NAIMARK A, CHERNIACK RM: Compliance of the respiratory system and its components in health and obesity. J Appl Physiol 15:377, 1960
165. TUCKER DH, SIEKER HO: The effect of change of body position on lung volumes and intrapulmonary gas mixing in patients with obesity, heart failure and emphysema. Am Rev Respir Dis 82:787, 1960
166. HEDENSTIERNA G, SANTESSON J: Breathing mechanics, deadspace and gas exchange in the extremely obese. Acta Anaesthesiol Scand 20:248, 1976
167. KAUFMAN BJ, FERGUSON MH, CHERNIACK RM: Hypoventilation in obesity. J Clin Invest 38:500, 1959
168. KRYGER M et al: The sleep deprivation pattern of the obese patient. Am J Med 56:530, 1974
169. SHARP JT et al: Total respiratory inertance and its gas and tissue components in normal and obese men. J Clin Invest 43:503, 1964
170. GILBERT R, SIPPLE JH, AUCHINCLOSS JH JR: Respiratory control and work of breathing in obese subjects. J Appl Physiol 16:21, 1961
171. CHERNIACK RM, GUENTER CA: The efficiency of the respiratory muscles in obesity. Can J Biochem Physiol 39:1215, 1961
172. PAUL DR, HOYT JL, BOUTROS AR: Cardiovascular and respiratory changes in response to change of posture in the very obese. Anesthesiology 45:73, 1976
173. BEDELL GN, WILSON WR, SEEBOHM PM: Pulmonary function in obese persons. J Clin Invest 37:1049, 1958
174. SANTESSON J: Oxygen transport and venous admixture in the extremely obese. Acta Anaesthesiol Scand 20:387, 1976
175. HEDENSTIERNA G, SANTESSON J, NORLANDER O: Airway closure and distribution of inspired gas in the extremely obese. Acta Anaesthesiol Scand 20:334, 1976
176. CHERNIACK RM: Respiratory effects of obesity. Can Med Assoc J 80:613, 1959
177. SANTESSON J, NORDENSTROM J: Pulmonary function in extreme obesity. Influence of weight loss following intestinal shunt operation. Acta Chir Scand [Suppl] 482:36, 1978
178. SODERBERG M, THOMPSON D, WHITE T: Respiration circulation and anesthetic management in obesity. Investigation before and after jejunoileal bypass. Acta Anaesthesiol Scand 21:55, 1977
179. HYTTEN FE, LEITCH I: The physiology of human pregnancy. London, Blackwell Scientific Publications, 1971
180. BADER RA, BADER ME, ROSE JD: The oxygen cost of breathing in dyspneic subjects as studied in normal pregnant women. Clin Sci 18:223, 1959
181. WEINBERG SE et al: Pregnancy and the lung. Am Rev Respir Dis 121:559, 1980
182. MOLL JMH, WRIGHT V: An objective clinical study of chest expansion. Ann Rheum Dis 31:1, 1972
183. FRASER RG, PARE JAP: Diagnosis of diseases of the chest, 2nd ed. Philadelphia, WB Saunders, 1979
184. HART FD et al: Ankylosing spondylitis. Q J Med 18:217, 1949
185. ZORAB PA: The lungs in ankylosing spondylitis. Q J Med 31:267, 1962
186. MILLER JM, SPROULE BJ: Pulmonary function in ankylosing spondylitis. Am Rev Respir Dis 90:376, 1964
187. GACAD G, HAMOSH P: The lung in ankylosing spondylitis. Am Rev Respir Dis 107:286, 1973
188. GRIMBY G, FUGL-MEYER AR, BLOMSTRAND A: Partitioning of the contributions of rib cage and abdomen to ventilation in ankylosing spondylitis. Thorax 29:179, 1974
189. TSANACLIS A, GRASSINO AE: Diaphragm and intercostal muscle behaviour in ankylosing spondylitis during CO_2 rebreathing. Am Rev Respir Dis [Suppl] 119:336, 1979
190. SHARP JT et al: Lung and thoracic compliances in ankylosing spondylitis. J Lab Clin Med 63:254, 1964
191. CROFTON J, DOUGLAS A: Respiratory diseases, 2nd ed. Oxford, Blackwell Scientific Publications, 1975
192. SCOBIE BA: Disturbed esophageal manometric responses in patients with ankylosing spondylitis

and pulmonary aspergilloma. Aust Ann Med 19:131, 1970
193. HURST JW: The Heart. New York, McGraw-Hill, 1979
194. ROSENOW EC et al: Pleuropulmonary manifestations of ankylosing spondylitis. Mayo Clin Proc 52:641, 1977
195. KAFER ER: Respiratory and cardiovascular functions in scoliosis. Bull Europ Physiopathol Respir 13:299, 1977
196. BERGOFSKY EH: Respiratory failure in disorders of the thoracic cage. Am Rev Respir Dis 119:643, 1979
197. WINTER RB, LOVELL WW, MOE JH: Excessive thoracic lordosis and loss of pulmonary function in patients with idiopathic scoliosis. J Bone Joint Surg 57A:972, 1975
198. MEZON B, WEST P, KRYGER M: Sleep stage and apnea in patients with blunted chemical drives to breathe. Am Rev Respir Dis [Suppl] 119:336, 1979
199. HEPPER NB, BLACK LF, FOWLER WS: Relationship of lung volume to height and arm span in normal subjects and in patients with spinal deformity. Am Rev Respir Dis 91:356, 1965
200. LINDH M, BJURE J: Lung volumes in scoliosis before and after correction by the Harrington instrumentation method. Acta Orthopo Scand 46:934, 1975
201. LINDERHOLM H, LINDGREN U: Prediction of spirometric values in patients with scoliosis. Acta Orthop Scand 49:469, 1978
202. MARKLUND T: Scoliosis angle. Acta Radiologica 19:78, 1978
203. WESTGATE HD: Pulmonary function in thoracic scoliosis before and after corrective surgery. Minn Med 53:839, 1970
204. HAMILTON F, THOMAS MP, PERALTA MM JR: Ventilation effects of the Harrington procedure for the treatment of scoliosis. Surg Gynecol Obstet 130:1067, 1970
205. KAFER ER: Idiopathic scoliosis. J Clin Invest 55:1153, 1975
206. WEBER B et al: Pulmonary function in asymptomatic adolescents with idiopathic scoliosis. Am Rev Respir Dis 111:389, 1975
207. SHANNON DC, RISEBOROUGH EJ, KAZEMI H: Ventilation perfusion relationships following correction of kyphoscoliosis. JAMA 217:579, 1971
208. TURINO GM, GOLDRING RM, FISHMAN AP: Cor pulmonale in musculoskeletal abnormalities of the thorax. Bull NY Acad Med 41:959, 1965
209. ZORAB P (ed): Scoliosis. London, William Heinemann, 1969
210. BJURE J et al: Respiratory impairment and airway closure in patients with untreated idiopathic scoliosis. Thorax 25:451, 1970
211. KAFER ER: Respiratory function in paralytic scoliosis. Am Rev Respir Dis 110:450, 1974
212. LITTLER WA, BROWN IK, ROAF R: Regional lung function in scoliosis. Thorax 27:420, 1972
213. BAKE B et al: Regional pulmonary ventilation and perfusion distribution in patients with untreated idiopathic scoliosis. Thorax 27:703, 1972
214. KAFER ER: Idiopathic scoliosis—gas exchange. J Clin Invest 58:825, 1976
215. DAVIES G, REID L: Effect of scoliosis on growth of alveoli and pulmonary arteries and on right ventricle. Arch Dis Child 46:623, 1971
216. GUCKER T: Changes in vital capacity in scoliosis. J Bone Joint Surg 44A:469, 1962
217. MAKLEY JT et al: Pulmonary function in paralytic and nonparalytic scoliosis before and after treatment. J Bone Joint Surg 50A:1379, 1968
218. MELLENCAMP DD, BLOUNT WP, ANDERSON AJ: Milwaukee brace treatment of idiopathic scoliosis. Clin Orthop 126:47, 1977
219. SHINHA R, BERGOFSKY EH: Prolonged alteration of lung mechanics in kyphoscoliosis by positive pressure hyperinflation. Am Rev Respir Dis 106:47, 1972
220. POWNER DJ, HOFFMAN LG: Bedside construction of a custom cuirass for respiratory failure in kyphoscoliosis. Chest 74:469, 1978
221. WIERS PWJ et al: Cuirass respiratory treatment of chronic respiratory failure in scoliotic patients. Thorax 32:221, 1977
222. ROBERT D et al: Long survival of patients with kyphoscoliosis end-stage respiratory failure treated at home by artificial ventilation. Am Rev Respir Dis 183:1215, 1980
223. ROM WN, MILLER A: Unexpected longevity in patients with severe kyphoscoliosis. Thorax 33:106, 1978
224. FINK A, RIVIN A, MURRAY JF: Pectus excavatum, an analysis of twenty-seven cases. Arch Intern Med 108:427, 1961
225. WEG JG, KRUMHOLZ RA, HARKLEROAD LE: Pulmonary dysfunction in pectus excavatum. Am Rev Respir Dis 96:936, 1967
226. KOOP CE: The management of pectus excavatum. Surg Clin North Am 36:1027, 1956
227. ROBICSEK R et al: Pectus carinatum. J Thorac Cardiovasc Surg 78:52, 1979

Chapter 7

Acute Respiratory Failure

ALAN K. PIERCE

Much of the treatment for patients with acute respiratory failure has been empirically derived and has not been substantiated by rigorous clinical investigations. This has allowed different medical centers to develop many variations in specific therapeutic modalities, although the underlying physiological and clinical considerations are similar. Because there are few definitive rules, this chapter emphasizes the principles of therapy.

Acute respiratory failure may be divided conveniently into three types (see list below). In some patients, the respiratory apparatus fails despite the presence of normal or nearly normal lungs. These patients develop a pure syndrome of alveolar hypoventilation in which the arterial oxygen tension (PaO_2) is depressed in proportion to the increase in arterial carbon dioxide tension ($PaCO_2$).[1] In such patients, an elevation of the alveolar–arterial oxygen tension difference ($A\text{-}aO_2$) above approximately 15 mm Hg while breathing room air indicates some type of superimposed pulmonary disease. This type of respiratory failure results from depressed respiratory center activity or from insufficient chest-wall bellows action.

Types of Acute Respiratory Failure

- Ventilatory failure with normal lungs
  - Insufficient respiratory center activity
  - Insufficient chest-wall function
    - Neuromuscular paralysis
    - Trauma with unstable chest wall
    - Kyphoscoliosis
  - Obesity
- Primarily failure of CO_2 excretion
  - Chronic obstructive lung disease
  - Severe asthma
- Primarily failure to oxygenate arterial blood
  - Adult respiratory distress syndrome
  - Cardiogenic pulmonary edema

The most frequent cause of respiratory center depression probably is an overdose of sedative drugs, commonly seen in an attempted suicide. Respiratory center depression, however, may result from cerebral trauma, vascular insufficiency, or tumors, and occasionally occurs as a primary syndrome.[2] Insufficient chest-wall function in the presence of normal lungs most commonly occurs because of neuromuscular disease such as the Guillain-Barré syndrome, myasthenia gravis, poliomyelitis, demyelinating diseases, or muscular dystrophies. Trauma to the chest wall, with multiple rib fractures resulting in an unstable thorax, most commonly is associated with pulmonary parenchymal contusion but may be associated with normal lungs. Kyphoscoliosis may result in alveolar hypoventilation if the angle of curvature of the spine is marked.[3]

Obesity may lead to hypoventilatory respiratory failure. Although the chest-wall abnormalities clearly lead to altered pulmonary function, the initiating mechanism of hypoventilation may be periodic upper airway obstruction during sleep, the sleep apnea syndrome.[4,5] These abnormalities are discussed in Chapter 6.

A second type of respiratory failure is manifested primarily by an inability to excrete carbon dioxide because of abnormal lungs. The pathophysiological mechanism is a marked imbalance of ventilation and blood flow throughout the lungs, with regional areas of hypoventilation predominating and resulting in an inability to excrete carbon dioxide.[1] The imbalance in ventilation and perfusion also causes hypoxemia, so that the PaO_2 is depressed out of proportion to the elevation in the $PaCO_2$. Thus, in addition to hypercapnia, hypoxemia may be severe. Chronic obstructive lung disease, a term used for coexisting chronic bronchitis and emphysema, is the most frequent cause of this type of respiratory failure. Additionally, patients with severe episodes of reversible airways disease (asthma) may develop respiratory failure as a near-terminal event.

A third type of respiratory failure is manifested by an inability to oxygenate arterial blood despite an ability to ventilate sufficiently to excrete carbon dioxide. This type of respiratory failure is due to excess pulmonary parenchymal liquid (*i.e.*, pulmonary edema). Although the term *pulmonary edema* frequently is considered to be synonymous with left ventricular failure, it has become apparent that a variety of insults lead to pulmonary edema, because of excessive pulmonary capillary permeability.[6] This diffuse alveolar injury syndrome, frequently termed the *adult respiratory distress syndrome* (ARDS), may be due to a variety of etiologic agents which will be discussed subsequently.

It is apparent that many patients will not fit into a single category of respiratory failure. Many of the principles of management apply to each type of patient. Nevertheless, these types of respiratory failure are sufficiently different that they can be considered separately.

VENTILATORY FAILURE

GUIDELINES FOR VENTILATORY SUPPORT

The most common disturbance that causes depression of the respiratory center and that necessitates ventilatory support is an overdose of sedative or narcotic drugs. The need for ventilatory support in such patients usually is apparent. The patient is comatose, and the level of coma usually is sufficiently deep that the patient does not respond to painful stimuli. With most sedative drugs, progressive depression of the respiratory center causes a progressive slowing of the respiratory rate. The major exception is glutethimide, which may cause sudden apnea despite a previously normal respiratory rate.[7] There is a tendency for hypotension to occur simultaneously, especially if the patient is hypovolemic from any cause. In such patients, it usually is clinically apparent that ventilation must be supported. It is not often possible to document hypoventilation by arterial blood gas analysis before resuscitative measures are undertaken. The results of arterial blood gas analysis performed when the patient is first observed usually are not available in time for assisting in a decision for intubation. Thus, these patients usually are intubated and ventilated because of their clinical appearance, and the subsequent information that the $PaCO_2$ was elevated merely confirms the clinical impression.

The need for intubation and mechanical assistance to ventilation is more difficult to assess in patients with neuromuscular disease that leads to insufficient chest-wall function. Guidelines that have been found to be helpful by one group of investigators are indicated below.[8] A similar value for vital capacity has been suggested by other physicians.[9]

Guidelines for Ventilatory Support in Patients with Ventilatory Failure

Respiratory rate	> 35/min
Vital capacity	< 15 ml/kg body weight
$FEV_{1.0}$	< 10 ml/kg body weight
Inspiratory force	< 25 cm H_2O

Data from Pontoppidan H, Geffin B, Lowenstein E: Acute respiratory failure in the adult. N Engl J Med 287:690, 743, 799, 1972

The important parameters that indicate a need for intubation in this type of respiratory failure relate to the mechanics of the chest wall; blood gas analysis is of marginal benefit. Despite progressive diminution in muscular force, as long as the patient is able to generate a tidal volume that is nearly normal, hyperventilation is common. With such diminished ventilatory reserve, however, it is not possible to periodically take the large tidal volumes necessary to inflate all lung units, and progressive atelectasis with a decrease in compliance and arterial oxygenation is likely to ensue.[10–12] Additionally, it is not possible for the patient to generate sufficient force for an effective cough, and airways obstruction from secretions may develop suddenly. If the neuromuscular weakness is relatively acute, hypoventilation with mounting hypercapnia tends to occur only as a terminal event. In this type of patient, it is safer to intubate early if there is any concern about the patient's ventilatory reserve than to wait until an emergency develops.

In patients with structural defects of the chest wall, such as kyphoscoliosis and obesity, respiratory failure is most likely to be in part chronic, and arterial gas analysis indicating hypercapnia is more reliable than in other patients with ventilatory failure and relatively normal lungs. These patients tend to be more similar to the patients in the category of primarily failure of carbon dioxide excretion, and initiation of ventilatory support is assessed by the criteria indicated in that section.

A complete discussion of the pathophysiologic mechanisms is included in Chapter 2, The Respiratory Pump, and Chapter 6, Disorders of the Respiratory Pump.

ARTIFICIAL AIRWAYS

A patient requiring ventilatory support must have some type of artificial airway. It is not possible by means of a mouthpiece or mask to successfully connect a ventilator to a patient for protracted intervals. If an artificial airway is required, the insertion of a cuffed endotracheal tube is the method of choice for initiating therapy. Such tubes may be inserted through the nose or the mouth. Nasotracheal tubes frequently are better tolerated than orotracheal tubes in alert or semicomatose patients; they are more easily secured, so that inadvertent slipping too far into or out of the trachea is less likely to occur. Nasotracheal intubation, however, has disadvantages, such as more difficult suctioning of secretions, owing to the smaller size of tube that can be inserted through the nose and to the angulation of the tube in the nasopharynx. Also, nasotracheal tubes may obstruct drainage from cranial sinuses, and some physicians find them more difficult to insert into the trachea, especially in emergency situations. In general, in patients with ventilatory failure without viscid tracheobronchial secretions, nasotracheal intubation is preferred at our hospital.

Inflatable cuffs are incorporated into both nasotracheal and orotracheal tubes, so that the trachea surrounding the tube may be occluded and the output from the ventilator delivered into the patient's lungs. Cuffs requiring high pressures for inflation (low compliance) are capable of occluding the trachea only by tracheal distortion, which may lead to pressure necrosis, with tracheal stenosis following extubation. Low-pressure (high compliance) cuffs that conform to the tracheal wall may occlude the tracheal opening around the endotracheal tube without producing as great a pressure on the tracheal wall, and tracheal damage is minimized.[13–17] Careful inflation of the cuff to allow an audible leak of air through the mouth during inflation of the lungs with a ventilator further minimizes tracheal injury.[18]

Before attempting intubation, all equipment should be checked to insure that it is functional: the light source of the laryngoscope, the inflatable cuff of the endotracheal tube, a syringe to inflate the cuff, an instrument to occlude the tube leading to the cuff, and adaptors to connect the endotracheal tube to a ventilator. Intubation of a comatose patient usually does not pose a problem, but the procedure may be very difficult in an agitated, dyspneic patient. In the latter type of patient, relaxation may be achieved by slow intravenous administration of morphine; the onset of action is rapid, and the dose may be adjusted until the desired state of relaxation is achieved. In the unusual case in which this method does not produce relaxation, an intravenous, short-acting, paralyzing drug, such as pancuronium bromide, 0.08 to 0.10 mg/kg body weight, may be used.[19] As soon as the patient is relaxed, an oral airway is inserted, the head hyperextended, and the patient ventilated by means of a self-inflating bag with a tightly fitting face mask. Additional oxygen is supplied to the bag in order to completely saturate the patient's blood with oxygen. An attempt to intubate the patient is made by the most experienced person immediately available. If the initial intubation is not successful within 1 min, the attempt should be discontinued and the patient again ventilated by mask and bag. Prolonged attempts at intubation may lead to hypoxemia, although prebreathing high concentrations of oxygen prolongs the time before such occurs.[20]

As soon as the tube has been inserted successfully, the cuff inflated, and the patient placed on a ventilator, the chest is auscultated carefully. If the endotracheal tube has been inserted too far, it most commonly passes down the right main bronchus, preventing ventilation of the entire left lung and the right upper lobe. Diminished breath sounds in these areas or lack of breath sounds indicate the necessity for withdrawing the tube until sounds are audible. When the tube position is apparently correct, the tube is securely fastened to the patient in such a way that it cannot slide up or down, and the oral airway is reinserted if the intubation has been by oral route. Subsequent radiographic examination of the chest should be obtained at the earliest convenient time, to verify the position of the tip of the endotracheal tube, since auscultation does not always reveal right main bronchial intubation.[21]

DETERMINATION OF VENTILATORY VOLUME

Patients with acute ventilatory failure with an intact respiratory center and sufficient inspiratory force to trigger a respirator usually are maintained on *assisted ventilation*. That is, the patient determines the respiratory rate while the physician determines the tidal volume by manipulation of the respirator controls. The effort necessary to initiate inspiration is maintained at a minimum by the sensitivity control of the respirator. With some respirators it is necessary to insure that the inspiratory effort control is not too sensitive, or it may inadvertently trigger the respirator without patient effort. The optimal tidal volume to be used has not been completely established. Similarly, the necessity for periodic hyperinflations in order to prevent atelectasis (and the optimal frequency of such hyperinflations) has not been resolved.[8] Clinical experience suggests that tidal volumes in the range of 10 to 15 ml per kg ideal body weight are reasonable. Indirect evidence suggests that hyperinflations of approximately 50% of the patient's predicted vital capacity reverse microatelectasis when present and prevent its occurrence if not yet established.[22] If the ventilator in use can be programmed for automatic hyperinflations, these are set at the most frequent interval possible for that ventilator. If the ventilator does not have the capability of automatic hyperinflations, they are administered by nursing or respiratory therapy personnel every 30 minutes.

Patients without an intact respiratory center or with insufficient inspiratory force to trigger a respirator are maintained on *controlled ventilation*. That is, the physician determines both the tidal volume and the rate at which the tidal volume is to be delivered. A convenient nomogram (Fig. 7-1) has been constructed as a guide to the appropriate respiratory rate for the tidal volume chosen.[23,24] This nomogram is appropriate only for persons with normal lungs.[25] Tidal volumes in the range of 10 to 15 ml per kg ideal body weight are determined, and the appropriate respiratory rate is determined from the nomogram. The largest tidal volume indicated on the nomogram, however, is 900 ml, which is not sufficient for larger patients. Moreover, the physician must understand more fully the determinants of successful ventilation in order to interpret individual patients' deviations from the expected results for a particular pattern of ventilation. Therefore, the determinants of alveolar ventilation will be described more completely.

Terms that frequently are used during controlled ventilation, the equations that are most helpful in understanding initial ventilatory management, and estimates of normal values useful in ventilatory management are shown on pages 242 and 243.

At the end of expiration, the patients' airways and a small fraction of the ventilator tubing are filled with alveolar gas, which is low in oxygen and high in carbon dioxide content. On the subsequent inhalation, this gas is rebreathed to an alveolar level but is not useful for further oxy-

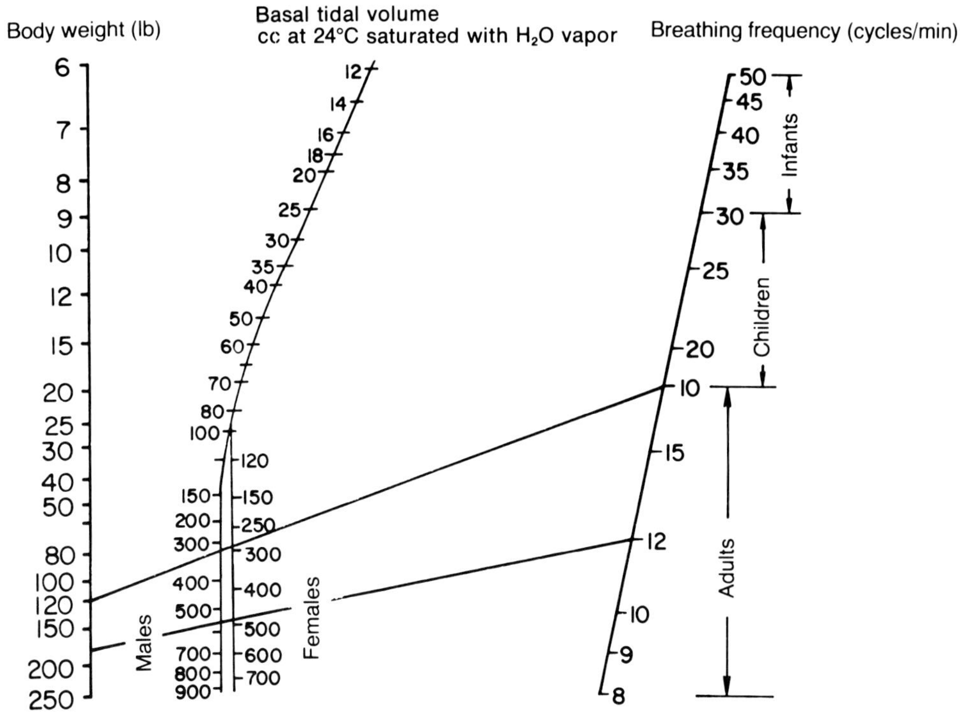

FIG. 7-1. The Radford nomogram[23,24] may be used to calculate the appropriate respiratory rate at the desired tidal volume for a patient on a ventilator. To use the nomogram, the patient's weight and desired tidal volume are connected with a straightedge, and the breathing frequency is read from the line to the right. Ventilation is underpredicted if conditions that increase metabolism are present, and the tidal volume should be increased: activity, add 10%; fever, add 5% for each degree above 37.2°C rectal; altitude, add 5% for each 610 m above sea level; metabolic acidosis, add 20%; artificial airway, subtract a volume equal to one-half the body weight if there is no apparatus dead space. If apparatus dead space exists, add an equal volume to the tidal volume. The nomogram is valid only for persons with normal lungs. (Radford EP Jr, Ferris BJ, Kirete BC: Clinical use of nomogram to estimate proper ventilation during artificial respiration. N Engl J Med 251:877, 1954. Reprinted by permission from the New England Journal of Medicine.)

genation of arterial blood or removal of carbon dioxide. The volume of this rebreathed gas is referred to as *dead space* (VD), anatomical and ventilator, respectively. In persons with normal lungs breathing at normal tidal volumes, the anatomical dead space is approximately equal to 1 ml per pound of ideal body weight (2.2 ml/kg). The volume of dead space in the ventilator tubing is dependent on the ventilator design (Fig. 7-2). If the ventilator is connected to the patient by a single tube, the apparatus dead space is that length of tubing between the patient and the exhalation valve (*i.e.*, the tubing filled with exhaled gas at the end of expiration). This volume most commonly is approximately 75 to 100 ml. If the tubing of the ventilator is designed so that inspiration is through one tube and exhalation through a separate tube, the only apparatus dead space is the small volume of the V where the inspiratory and expiratory tubes connect to the artificial airway. Because anatomical dead space is decreased by the artificial airway but ventilator dead space must be accounted for, an estimation of total dead space of 1 ml per pound of lean body weight (2.2 ml/kg) is reasonable in persons with normal lungs.

Definition of Terms Used During Controlled Ventilation

Alveolar ventilation ($\dot{V}_A$)	Total amount of fresh gas reaching the gas-exchange units of the lung per min*
Dead space ventilation ($\dot{V}_D$)	Total amount of gas ventilating the airways, the non-perfused lung units, and that part of ventilator tubing containing exhaled gas that is rebreathed by the patient per min*
Minute ventilation ($\dot{V}_E$)	Total amount of gas exhaled by the patient per min (includes $\dot{V}_A$ and $\dot{V}_D$)*
Carbon dioxide production ($\dot{V}_{CO_2}$)	Total amount of CO_2 exhaled by the patient per minute†
Tidal volume (V_T)	Volume of each breath*
Dead space (V_D)	Volume of dead space (non-gas-exchange) ventilation per breath*
Respiratory rate (f)	Number of tidal volumes per min
Dead space per tidal volume ratio (V_D/V_T)	Fraction of each tidal volume not taking part in gas exchange (normal ~0.3)

* Volumes commonly corrected from ambient temperature and pressure, saturated (ATPS) to body temperature and pressure, saturated (BTPS).
† Volumes commonly corrected from ambient temperature and pressure, saturated to standard temperature and pressure, dry (STPD).

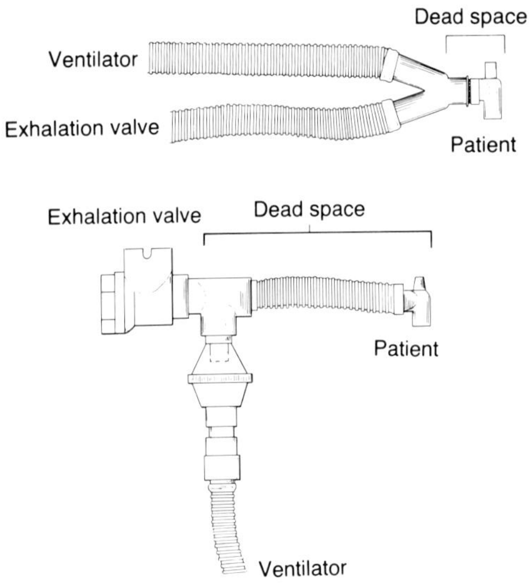

FIG. 7-2. Apparatus dead space is that volume of tubing which, at the end of expiration, is filled with exhaled gas that is rebreathed with the subsequent inspiration. If the tubing of the ventilator is designed so that inspiration is through one tube and exhalation through a separate tube, the only apparatus dead space is a small volume, where the inspiratory and expiratory tubes connect to the artificial airway. If the ventilator is connected to the patient by a single tube, the apparatus dead space is that length between the patient and the exhalation valve. In either system, if additional apparatus dead space is desired, additional lengths of tubing may be added between the patient and the tubing indicated in the diagram.

The volume of ventilation in excess of that necessary to fill the dead-space volume provides fresh gas to an alveolar level and is that volume of ventilation useful in gas exchange (alveolar ventilation). Thus, the total amount of gas breathed per minute (minute ventilation) is equal to the alveolar ventilation plus the dead space ventilation (Equation 1 in the list on p. 243). The minute ventilation is determined easily by measuring the averaged exhaled tidal volume and multiplying it by the respiratory rate (Equation 2). A number of measurement devices are available that may be placed on the exhalation valve of the ventilator. It is not possible, however, to measure alveolar ventilation or deadspace ventilation directly. Thus, each of these parameters must be estimated independently in order to determine the appropriate minute ventilation.

Alveolar ventilation may be estimated by Equation 3. A reasonable estimate of CO_2 production per minute in the basal state is 3.2 ml per kg body weight.[26] This estimate will be low if the patient is febrile or if there is excessive muscular activity. From the equation it can be seen that the alveolar ventilation of a 70-kg person approaches 5 liters per min in order to maintain a $PaCO_2$ of 40 mm Hg.

Equations 4a–i are a substitution and rear-

Equations Useful for Initial Ventilatory Management

1. Minute ventilation = Alveolar ventilation + dead-space ventilation

$$(\dot{V}_E) = (\dot{V}_A) + (\dot{V}_D)$$

2. Minute ventilation = Tidal volume × respiratory rate

$$(\dot{V}_E) = (V_T) \times (f)$$

3. Alveolar ventilation $(\dot{V}_A) = \dfrac{CO_2 \text{ production } (\dot{V}CO_2)}{PaCO_2} \times$ correction factor*

4. (a) $$\dot{V}_E = \frac{\dot{V}CO_2 \times 863}{PaCo_2} + \dot{V}_D$$

(b) $$\dot{V}_E - \dot{V}_D = \frac{\dot{V}CO_2 \times 863}{PaCO_2}$$

(c) $$\dot{V}_D = f\, V_D$$

(d) $$f\, V_T - f\, V_D = \frac{\dot{V}CO_2 \times 863}{PaCO_2}$$

(e) $$f\, (V_T - V_D) = \frac{\dot{V}CO_2 \times 863}{PaCo_2}$$

(f) $$f = \frac{\dfrac{\dot{V}CO_2 \times 863}{PaCO_2}}{V_T - V_D}$$

(g) $$f = \frac{\dfrac{3.2\text{ kg} \times 863}{PaCo_2}}{\text{kg}\, (V_T - 2.2)}$$

(h) $$f = \frac{\dfrac{3.2 \times 863}{PaCo_2}}{V_T - 2.2}$$

(i) $$f = \frac{69.04}{V_T - 2.2}$$

* The correction factor converts $\dot{V}CO_2$ from STPD to BTPS and the fractional concentration of alveolar CO_2 into $PaCO_2$. It is 863 if volumes are in ml and 0.863 if in liters.

Estimates Useful for Ventilatory Management

Volume of dead space (V_D)	1 ml/pound ideal body weight (2.2 ml/kg)
Carbon dioxide production ($\dot{V}CO_2$)	3.2 ml/kg body weight/min[26]
Initial respiratory rate if tidal volume (V_T) is:	
15 ml/kg ideal weight: 5 to 6/min	
10 ml/kg ideal weight: 8 to 9/min	

rangement of Equations 1 and 3, with algebraic manipulation to determine the appropriate respiratory rate (f) if the desired tidal volume (V_T) is known. Because all estimates, including tidal volume, are dependent on patient weight, Equation 4h indicates that patient weight may be eliminated from the calculation of respiratory rate. Because it is desirable to maintain the $PaCO_2$ at approximately 40 mm Hg, Equation 4i allows the respiratory rate to be determined knowing only the milliliters of tidal volume per kilogram of body weight desired. Thus, for initially establishing the pattern of artificial respiration, if a tidal volume of 15 ml per kg ideal weight is used, the respiratory rate should be approximately 5 to 6 breaths per minute. If the tidal volume is to be 10 ml per kg, the respiratory rate will be 8 to 9 per minute.

In determining the respiratory rate for initial ventilation, two assumptions have been made:

the carbon dioxide production per minute and the volume of dead space per breath. These, of course, may not be correct. After ventilating the patient for a brief interval (20 to 30 min), an analysis of arterial gases is obtained in order to correct the ventilatory volume. Then it may be assumed that the CO_2 production estimate is correct, and the measured $PaCO_2$ is used to determine the actual alveolar ventilation (Equation 1 in the list at right). This actual alveolar ventilation is subtracted from the measured minute ventilation that existed at the time of arterial gas analysis, and the true dead-space ventilation is thereby determined (Equation 2). When the dead-space ventilation per minute is divided by the respiratory rate (Equation 3), the dead space per tidal volume is obtained. This new estimate of dead space is divided by the patient's weight in kilograms (Equation 4), to obtain a better estimate of dead space in ml per kg patient weight. This new value is now substituted into Equation 4i in the list on page 243 in order to obtain the new, more appropriate respiratory rate at which to ventilate the patient for the tidal volume chosen.

If the respiratory rate is exceedingly slow, additional links of tubing between the ventilator exhalation valve (or V connector) and the patient may be added in order to increase the apparatus dead space, which will allow large tidal volumes at a faster respiratory rate. When the new settings have been used for ventilation for another 30 min, arterial gases are again obtained in order to assure the appropriateness of the ventilator settings.

Equations Useful for Correcting Ventilatory Management

1. Alveolar ventilation
$$= \frac{CO_2 \text{ production } (\dot{V}CO_2)\ (\text{ml}) \times 863}{PaCO_2}$$
2. $$\frac{\text{Minute ventilation}}{(\dot{V}E)\ (\text{ml/min})} - \frac{\text{Alveolar ventilation}}{(\dot{V}A)\ (\text{ml/min})} = \frac{\text{dead-space ventilation}}{(\dot{V}D)\ (\text{ml/min})}$$
3. $$\frac{\text{Dead-space ventilation}}{\text{Respiratory rate}}\ \frac{(\dot{V}D)}{(f)} = \text{dead space/breath } (V_D)$$
4. $$\frac{\text{Dead space/breath}}{\text{Patient weight (kg)}} = V_D/\text{kg}$$

VENTILATORS

Ventilators are classified by the mechanism that causes changeover from the inspiratory phase to the expiratory phase.[27,28] *Time-cycled machines* terminate inspiration after an interval set by the operator, no matter what volume of gas has been delivered or what mask pressure has been achieved. *Volume ventilators* cycle from inspiration to expiration when a predetermined volume of gas has been delivered, irrespective of the pressure necessary to deliver that volume. *Pressure-limited machines* cycle from inspiration to expiration when a predetermined pressure has been achieved, irrespective of the volume delivered to the patient. Any of the machines may be used for ventilating apneic patients as long as the physician and paramedical personnel are competent in manipulating the controls of the machine in use. It must be remembered, however, that the tidal volume actually received by the patient is the important parameter in ventilatory support, not the pressure necessary to generate the tidal volume. The exhaled tidal volume must be monitored. Because volume-limited ventilators tend to be more mechanically reliable, and because tidal volume is set directly by the ventilator controls, they are most frequently employed in the ventilation of apneic patients.

When utilizing a volume ventilator, the tidal volume is set directly by the appropriate ventilator control. In initiating ventilation with a pressure-limited ventilator, an estimate of the pressure necessary to deliver the desired tidal volume is made from the normal compliance of the lung and chest wall of ventilator patients without pulmonary disease (79.1 ± 14.7 ml/cm H_2O).[29] That is, one expects to deliver approximately 80 ml of gas into the patient's lungs for each centimeter of H_2O pressure generated by the machine. Thus, in patients with normal lungs, a tidal volume of approximately 800 ml will be delivered for 10 cm H_2O. With either type of machine, the velocity with which the tidal volume is delivered is determined by a flow control. This control is set so that the length of inspiration occupies no more than one-third of the total respiratory cycle. Applying positive pressure to the lung for protracted intervals tends to decrease venous return to the heart and the cardiac output.

The protracted breathing of a high concentration of inspired oxygen is toxic to the lungs, although the exact limits of human tolerance for oxygen have not been clearly defined.[30–32] Therefore, it is recommended that patients on prolonged ventilatory support be maintained at the lowest concentration of inspired oxygen that provides a nearly normal PaO_2.[33] In the patient with previously normal lungs, the fraction of inspired oxygen (F_IO_2) frequently need not exceed 0.21. Because volume-cycled respirators use room air for the ventilating gas, the F_IO_2 is 0.21, unless additional oxygen is added to the system. If higher concentrations are necessary, the oxygen concentration control is reasonably accurate.[33,34] Pressure-cycled machines that are powered by oxygen decrease the final concentration of inspired oxygen by means of a venturi air-mixing device. Pressure-limited ventilators powered by oxygen virtually always deliver a F_IO_2 in a potentially toxic range.[33–36] Thus, pressure-limited intermittent positive pressure breathing (IPPB) machines should be powered by compressed air. If additional oxygen is necessary, the machine should be powered by a mixture of oxygen and compressed air through a device that is able to deliver a known concentration of oxygen to the patient.[37] If supplemental oxygen is being administered with either a volume- or a pressure-limited machine, the F_IO_2 should be monitored periodically by an oxygen analyzer.

Inhaled gas is normally humidified by the nose or mouth. In patients with artificial airways, inspired gas is delivered directly to the trachea. If the gas is not saturated with water vapor at body temperature (44 mg H_2O/liter of gas), there is a tendency for drying of the mucosa and crusting of respiratory secretions in the artificial airway. Progressive obstruction of the airway may ensue. This must be prevented by completely saturating the gas from the ventilator at body temperature. This can be accomplished with either a heated humidifier or a heated nebulizer maintained at or slightly above body temperature. A thermometer should be incorporated into the ventilator tubing near the patient in order to insure that a proper temperature is maintained.

CONTINUING RESPIRATORY CARE

This chapter does not deal with the many facets of care necessary for bedfast patients, except those directly concerned with ventilation. One aspect of general care that differs in patients maintained on ventilators, as compared with other bedfast patients, however, is fluid administration. Insensible fluid loss through the respiratory tract is negligible as a result of the humidification. Numerous investigations have also indicated a relationship between positive-pressure ventilation and renal function.[38] Positive-pressure breathing at high pressures causes antidiuresis and sodium retention, partly owing to a diminished glomerular filtration rate. It is also debated whether artificial ventilation causes inappropriate secretion of antidiuretic hormone.[39] It has been suggested that positive water balance in ventilator patients may result in pulmonary edema in the absence of recognizable cardiac failure.[40] Although such a syndrome is not likely to be important in ventilator patients with normal lungs, fluid administration is usually limited to 20 to 25 ml per kg of body weight per 24 hr, unless other features of the patient's illness dictate a greater fluid administration.[8]

Patient Monitoring

It is necessary to periodically obtain arterial blood for gas analysis in patients on prolonged ventilatory assistance. After initially determining the proper volume of ventilation, this may not be necessary more often than once a day. The $PaCO_2$, *p*H, and PaO_2 should remain relatively constant as long as the ventilatory volume and F_IO_2 remain unchanged. Changes in $PaCO_2$ most likely indicate an inadvertent change in ventilator settings. A change in *p*H, if the $PaCO_2$ is constant, most likely represents a nonrespiratory complication. Acidosis may be seen if there is poor tissue perfusion, with tissue hypoxia leading to lactic acid accumulation, or acidosis may be observed in the course of renal failure. Alkalosis suggests insufficient potassium administration or insufficient electrolyte replacement for gastric acid suction. A fall in PaO_2 at the same F_IO_2 suggests that the patient is developing atelectasis, pulmonary emboli, pneumonia, or pulmonary edema. In the asymptomatic patient whose physical examination of the chest and chest roentgenogram prove normal, the most likely cause of the falling PaO_2 is microatelectasis, caused by insufficient tidal or sigh volumes. This can be confirmed by the return of the PaO_2 to its previous value after repeated inflation of the patient's lungs to approximately 50% of the vital capacity.

The pressure–volume relationships of the lung also should be followed and charted hourly. The peak ventilator pressure is not as useful as the ventilator pressure observed while the patient's lungs are briefly held inflated by keeping the exhalation valve shut after the ventilator has cycled to the exhalation phase. This is accomplished easily with volume ventilators that have an inflation-hold control. With pressure-limited ventilators, it is necessary to manually occlude the exhalation opening in order to observe static pressure. The peak ventilator pressure is necessary not only for distending the lungs and chest wall, but also for producing gas flow from the ventilator into the patient. Because the pressure necessary to produce gas flow depends on airway resistance, and because resistance varies the flow rate of gas, peak ventilator pressure in part reflects the flow with which the tidal volume is being administered. Static pressure measured without flow is an index of the pressure necessary to hold the patient's lungs and chest wall inflated, and it is always less than peak ventilator pressure.

If the exhaled tidal volume is divided by the static airway pressure, the *compliance* of the patient's lungs and thorax is obtained. In ventilator patients with normal lungs, static compliance is 97.3 ± 18.2 ml per cm H_2O.[29] Because the standard deviation is large, however, owing to patient size and to the weight of the chest wall, the measurement is most useful when followed serially in order to indicate change. Pressure measurements are not reliable if the patient makes respiratory efforts.

Changes in static compliance may be rapidly determined from the charting of ventilator settings. When a volume ventilator is being used and tidal volume held constant, a record indicating increasing static pressure indicates a fall in compliance. If a pressure-limited ventilator is in use and the inflation pressure held constant, a fall in the tidal volume achieved by that pressure indicates a fall in compliance. Falling compliance in a patient with a normal chest examination and a normal chest roentgenogram indicates the development of microatelectasis and suggests that tidal or sigh volumes have not been sufficient to prevent this complication.

Artificial Airway Care

The type of artificial airway to use for continued ventilatory support is controversial.[41–48] The prolonged use of both endotracheal and tracheostomy tubes is associated with postexubation complications. A prospective study comparing endotracheal and tracheostomy tubes in similar patients in the same hospital is not available. Thus, it is not clear which method is associated with fewer complications. In some institutions, when an artificial airway is necessary for longer than a few hours (commonly 72 hours), a tracheostomy is performed. In other institutions, endotracheal tubes are used for much more protracted intervals. At our hospital, at any time that it becomes apparent that an artificial airway will be necessary for an indefinite interval longer than a few days, a tracheostomy is performed.

Complications related to the artificial airway are common during the course of mechanical ventilation.[49] A frequent complication is accidental displacement of the tube, which may lead to complete extubation. Thus, the tube should be securely fastened, and it may be necessary to restrain the hands of an agitated or irrational patient. Tubes should be secured in such a way, however, that hard objects do not press firmly against soft tissues, because this may lead to tissue necrosis.[50] Endotracheal and tracheostomy tube cuffs may cause problems, such as herniation over the end of the tube, leading to sudden airway obstruction; the development of a leak, leading to deflation and causing difficulty in ventilation; incrustation with secretions while the cuff is deflated, preventing subsequent reinflation; and overinflation, leading to collapse of the endotracheal tube and airway obstruction.[51] Tracheostomy tubes have the additional potential of eroding into major blood vessels, leading to massive hemorrhage. Nasotracheal intubation has been reported to be associated with excessive gastrointestinal distention.[52] This was thought to occur because of the leak of gas around the endotracheal tube cuff into the oropharynx, with subsequent swallowing.

Intubated patients are not able to cough effectively, and suctioning must be performed to remove secretions that accumulate in the upper tracheobronchial tree. In patients with previously normal lungs, frequent suctioning usually is not necessary. Tracheal suctioning should be performed only when necessary to remove accumulated secretions, because mucosal hemorrhages and erosions are produced by the procedure,[53,54] although such may be minimized with proper catheter design.[55] The catheter should be inserted as far as possible, and suction should not be applied during insertion. The catheter is rotated while being removed slowly, and suction is applied only intermittently, to minimize mucosal damage. The entire suctioning procedure should last only a few seconds, because hypoxemia may occur during prolonged suctioning. If all secretions have not been removed, the patient may be resuctioned after being ventilated for a few minutes. Plastic suction catheters that have been packaged in a coiled position cannot be selectively directed into the major bronchi.[56] The use of catheters that have been packaged while straight may be more successful, especially if the tip has been slightly angled. Turning the patient's head markedly to the right may improve the ability to selectively catheterize the left mainstem bronchus.

Intensive-care-unit patients maintained on ventilators are at risk of developing nosocomial respiratory infections,[57] and suctioning of artificial airways may contribute to this potential. It has been demonstrated, however, that tracheal suctioning, using sterile catheters, sterile wash solutions, and sterile gloves, each opened at the time of suctioning, is no more successful in preventing bacterial colonization than the use of one sterile catheter per 8-hr shift maintained in benzalkonium chloride and passed with multiple packaged, disposable plastic gloves.[58]

EXTUBATION

A decision to discontinue ventilatory support and subsequently to extubate patients with a depressed respiratory center usually is not difficult. As the patient's state of consciousness improves and respiratory drive returns, controlled ventilation usually is replaced by assisted ventilation. As the patient rouses further, becomes aware of the environment, and is able to cough, assisted ventilation may be discontinued and the patient extubated shortly thereafter. In the case of glutethimide overdose, an artificial airway is continued until the patient is fully awake, because of the potential for sudden apnea.

In the case of patients with neuromuscular diseases, a decision to discontinue assisted ventilation may be more difficult. It has been suggested that the same criteria used for initiating ventilatory support may be used as an index to cease ventilatory support.[59,60] That is, when the parameters indicated on page 238 (Guidelines for Ventilatory Support in Patients with Ventilatory Failure) have returned towards normal, ventilatory support is no longer necessary.

When it is felt that the patient no longer needs assisted ventilation, weaning is begun. The patient is informed about the procedure to be carried out. The ventilator then is disconnected from the artificial airway. A T adaptor is attached to the airway, through which the patient is administered an aerosol from a heated nebulizer. The F_IO_2 should be the same or slightly greater than that that was being administered by the ventilator. The flow from the nebulizer should be sufficiently great that the entire minute ventilation is the desired F_1O_2; this is determined by observing mist escaping from the distal end of the T adaptor during inspiration. The patient is watched carefully during the early weaning process. Tachycardia, cardiac arrhythmias, a respiratory rate greatly different from normal, or obvious distress or dyspnea are indications that assisted ventilation should be reinstituted. If these abnormalities do not occur, arterial blood gases are obtained after 15 to 20 minutes to confirm that the patient is able to ventilate and oxygenate sufficiently.

Patients who show no abnormalities for 2 to 4 hours after stopping assisted ventilation may be extubated. Such will be the case for most patients recovering from respiratory-center depression. Patients with neuromuscular disease, however, may experience fatigue and dyspnea with progressive time off the ventilator. These patients are allowed to breathe spontaneously for some interval (such as 10 min), and assisted ventilation is reinstituted. The 10 minutes of spontaneous ventilation is repeated once an hour, and the time off the ventilator is progressively lengthened. When the patient is able to remain off the ventilator comfortably for 2 to 4 hours, extubation may be carried out.

Following extubation, many patients are hoarse and have difficulty in swallowing. Food and fluid by mouth are withheld for the first few hours postextubation; then bland liquids are given to determine the patient's ability to swallow. A few patients will have more marked upper airways obstruction, owing to edema of the vocal cords or larynx. Severe upper airways obstruction is indicated by respiratory stridor; these patients must be monitored especially carefully. Any progression of symptoms is an indication for reintubation. Such may be difficult through the obstructed upper airway, and it may be necessary to proceed with an emergency tracheostomy or cricothyroidotomy. Until an artificial airway is reestablished, administration of 80% helium and 20% oxygen, a mixture less dense than room air, may markedly alleviate symptoms. Adrenal cortical steroids usually are administered to patients with marked upper airways obstruction, although their efficacy is unproven.

FAILURE OF CO_2 EXCRETION

DESCRIPTION OF PATIENTS

Patients with severe asthma,[61] obesity,[4,5] severe kyphoscoliosis,[3] and neuromuscular disease[62,63] may develop hypercapnic respiratory failure. However, most episodes of acute respiratory failure in this category occur in patients with chronic bronchitis and emphysema. This section deals predominantly with patients who have chronic obstructive lung disease.

The differentiation of acute and chronic respiratory failure may be difficult. Although many authors define acute respiratory failure by an arbitrarily determined elevation of $PaCO_2$, marked hypercapnia may exist in such patients chronically, making such a definition unreliable.[64] Similarly, definitions of acute respiratory failure based on the degree of hypoxemia are not reliable. Although acutely worsening hypercapnia causes a fall in *p*H, values for patients with chronic hypercapnia overlap those for patients with acutely worsening hypercapnia to such a degree that this measurement does not separate the two groups.[65–67] The most useful index for determining acute respiratory failure in such patients is deterioration from steady-state blood gas values, if these are known. In many patients, a history of increasing dyspnea, increasing mental confusion, or coma in association with severely deranged blood gases is the best index of recent onset of the respiratory failure.

Patients with chronic obstructive lung disease presenting in acute respiratory failure usually have had symptoms of chronic cough, sputum production, and dyspnea on exertion for several years. Most commonly, airways obstuction has been persistently severe with the forced expiratory volume in 1 second ($FEV_{1.0}$) less than a liter, although carbon dioxide retention may occur at a much larger $FEV_{1.0}$.[68] There usually is marked mismatching of ventilation and blood flow, with lung regions that underventilate with respect to blood flow, leading to hypoxemia and a tendency to hypercapnia, and with lung regions that overventilate with respect to blood flow, leading to excess dead-space ventilation.[69] There usually is a change in the breathing pattern so that the inspiratory time is shorter, resulting in smaller tidal volumes; total minute ventilation tends to be normal owing to an increase in breathing frequency, but the small tidal volumes cause a large V_D/V_T, and alveolar ventilation tends to be low.[70,71] The abnormal pattern of breathing becomes more marked during episodes of acute respiratory failure.[72] Some chronically ill patients and many patients with acute respiratory failure have abnormalities in thoraco-abdominal motion, with inward abdominal motion coincident with outward rib-cage motion during inspiration.[73] This abnormality, which is often apparent by physical examination but may require instrumentation to detect, suggests that the diaphragm is not contributing to respiration. Additionally, the hyperinflated chest wall placing the muscles of respiration at a mechanical disadvantage and the excessive work load imposed by the lung disease are thought to potentiate respiratory muscle fatigue.[74,75]

In some patients, however, a respiratory infection is the precipitating factor. The infection need not be pneumonia; acute bronchitis may cause enough additional airways obstruction to precipitate respiratory failure. Lung infection is the precipitating event in less than half of the patients with chronic obstructive lung disease (COLD) in acute respiratory failure, when a diagnosis of infection is based on purulent sputum, leukocytosis, or pulmonary parenchymal infiltrates with fever. Systemic diseases accompanied by fever may cause deterioration, because the increased metabolic rate increases carbon dioxide production. Injudicious administration of sedative drugs or of high concentrations of inspired oxygen may depress ventilation to the degree that carbon dioxide retention occurs. However, even when such precipitating events are sought, most patients with severe lung disease deteriorate into acute respiratory failure without an obvious cause.[76]

Most patients are conscious at the time of admission.[65] The level of consciousness is related to the arterial gas concentrations. In one large series, semicoma or coma was not observed unless the $PaCO_2$ exceeded 75 mm Hg, the PaO_2 was less than 35 mm Hg, or the oxygen content was less than 11 ml/100 ml blood.[65] Coma occurred with increasing frequency at higher carbon dioxide and lower oxygen values. The arterial *p*H was maintained at relatively normal values despite severe hypercapnia, except in patients with coma, in whom the mean arterial *p*H was 7.26. These findings are consistent with data that demonstrate that the state of consciousness correlates well with the *p*H of the cerebrospinal fluid.[77] Cerebrospinal fluid *p*H falls proportionately to the blood *p*H during respiratory acidosis. Although conscious, many patients exhibit mental and neurologic dysfunctions, including disorientation, confusion, incoherence, somnolence, obstreperousness, combativeness, fine tremors, asterixis, myoclonic jerks, sustained myoclonus, or seizures.[78]

INITIATING THERAPY

The specific etiology leading to an episode of acute respiratory failure frequently is not determined.[76] When a patient with chronic obstructive lung disease with acute respiratory failure arrives at the hospital, the most immediate threat to life is tissue hypoxia.[79] The initial goal of therapy is to improve tissue oxygenation by partially correcting arterial hypoxemia. The successful regulation of therapy of patients with acute respiratory failure, however, is facilitated by the repeated analysis of arterial blood for *p*H, $PaCO_2$, PaO_2, and oxygen saturation. If the condition of the patient permits, these values should be obtained before the institution of oxygen therapy. This may be accomplished by a simple arterial puncture with a needle and heparinized syringe, but it is more efficient to place an indwelling needle in the radial artery so that repeated samples may be obtained. A radial artery is cannulized with a flexible plastic needle, and baseline arterial gas analysis is obtained. The needle is maintained patent by an inner cannula or by filling the dead space of the needle

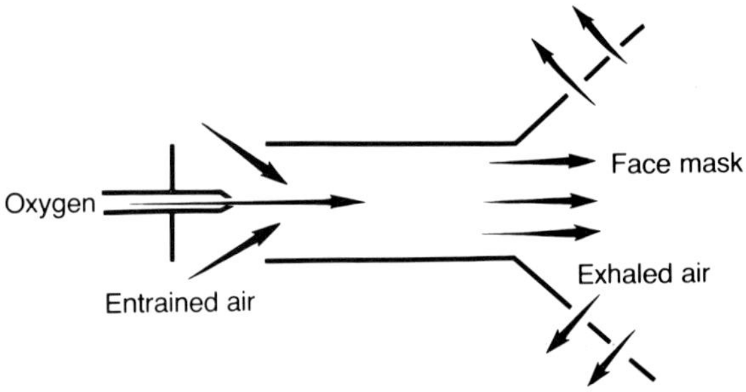

FIG. 7-3. This diagram depicts an oxygen mask incorporating the venturi principle. Oxygen at a flow of 4 L/min enters the mask through a jet. This flow creates a partial vacuum that entrains 80 additional liters of room air, causing a final concentration of oxygen to the patient of 24%, at a flow of 84 L/min. The inspired oxygen concentration cannot exceed 24%, and the environmental flow is great enough to minimize the likelihood of dilution below 24% by the inspiration of additional room air around the face mask. Some commercially available masks use less efficient jets, entrain less room air, and administer higher concentrations of oxygen (e.g., 28%, 35%, and 40%).

with a dilute heparin solution. If the patient is exceedingly ill, it may not be possible to devote time to an indwelling needle at the time of admission. Oxygen therapy is started as soon as the blood has been obtained and before results of gas analysis are known (see Chap. 5).

If pneumonia is not present, the major cause of hypoxemia is mismatching of ventilation and blood flow in the lungs; this type of defect may be significantly improved by a small increase in the inspired oxygen concentration. High concentrations of inspired oxygen must be avoided, because the primary drive to respiration may be hypoxemia, and too vigorous administration of oxygen may lead to further depression of ventilation or to apnea.

Administration of oxygen at a fixed low flow (1–3 liters/min) by means of a humidifier and nasal cannula or loose-fitting face mask may be successful, but this fixed-flow method has major disadvantages. The concentration of oxygen inspired by the patient cannot be accurately controlled, because it depends not only on the flow of oxygen but also on the total volume of ventilation. For example, a fixed flow of 2 or 3 liters/min may produce an inspired oxygen concentration of approximately 28% if the patient has a minute ventilation of 12 liters/min, but approximately 40% at a minute ventilation of 5 liters/min. The former inspired oxygen concentration would be satisfactory in most patients with respiratory failure, but the latter would aggravate respiratory depression in most patients, and the more the patient is depressed, the higher the inspired oxygen concentration rises. In addition, during the hurried activity generated by the care of an acutely ill patient, it is not uncommon for the oxygen flow to be increased by personnel not aware of the critical necessity of maintaining a low flow. Finally, commercially available flow meters are inaccurate at flows under 3 liters/min.

The safest technique by which to administer oxygen is a high flow of gas with a fixed oxygen concentration.[79] The area surrounding the patient's nose and mouth is flooded with gas of the desired oxygen concentration at such a high flow (over 50 L/min) that all of the patient's inspired gas is supplied by the system, with no additional dilution by room air. This is most easily carried out with commercially available, disposable oxygen masks that incorporate the venturi principle, an example of which is shown in Figure 7-3. At 4 liters/min of oxygen flow through the venturi jet built into the mask, 80 additional liters of room air are entrained, causing a final concentration of oxygen to the patient of 24% at a flow of 84 liter/min. The inspired oxygen concentation cannot exceed 24%, and the environmental flow is great enough to minimize the likelihood of dilution below 24% by the inspiration of additional room air around the face mask. This slight increase in inspired oxygen is enough to partially improve arterial hypoxemia and to minimize the risk of death from hypoxia, whereas it is not high enough to depress respiration in most patients.

Although almost all patients may be managed at this stage of therapy with only improved oxygenation, one of several factors may force the physician to use an artificial airway. The patient may arrive at the emergency room apneic or with such severe hypoventilation that gas exchange is not sufficient to maintain life. This situation may be produced by the injudicious administration of high concentrations of oxygen in an ambulance on the way to the hospital, or by sedatives administered to counteract the restlessness of increasing hypoxemia. In a severely debilitated patient, the large airways may be obstructed with tenacious secretions that cannot be cleared because of ineffectual cough. Hypoxemia and hypercapnia may have caused such manic behavior, with rapid, ineffectual respiration, that the situation is not ameliorated by better oxygenation, reassurance, or assisted respiration by means of a pressure-limited intermittent positive-pressure breathing machine.

In these circumstances an artificial airway is necessary. The airway of choice is a cuffed endotracheal tube. Oral endotracheal tubes are preferred at our hospital in this type of patient, because suctioning of the patient's viscid secretions is easier with this type of tube than with a nasotracheal tube. The same type of precautions concerning intubation indicated in the section on Ventilatory Failure are appropriate to these patients. Additionally, it should be remembered that these patients are severely hypoxemic, and adequate oxygenation should be assured before proceeding with endotracheal intubation. When the patient has been intubated, assisted ventilation is instituted by the most efficient means at hand. If the patient is capable of initiating respiration, a pressure-limited IPPB machine may be used at pressure settings that cause large tidal volumes. If the patient is not initiating respiration, the physician may continue to use the self-inflating bag, or any type of IPPB device capable of automatic ventilation. In such a circumstance, care must be taken not to allow marked overventilation, which would lead to alkalosis. It should be emphasized that very few patients will require intubation in the emergency room, and most patients can be managed by low levels of oxygen (e.g., through a venturi mask) (see Table 7-3).

The marked importance of respiratory rate in spontaneously breathing patients with obstructive airways disease cannot be overemphasized. Rapid inspirations cause a maldistribution of inspired gas to the areas of the lung that are least obstructed, causing overdistention of some lung units, with poor ventilation in other lung units. This results in an apparent stiffening of the lung (*i.e.*, frequency-dependence of compliance).[80] Forceful exhalation causes airway collapse, and expiratory flow is no greater than if lesser expiratory pressures were used.[81,82] These factors lead to a marked increase in the work of breathing, without improving minute ventilation. Additionally, forceful breathing causes a worse distribution of ventilation and blood flow than exists during quiet breathing, and hypoxemia and hypercapnia are worsened. By slowing the rate of respiration, these defects can be partially reversed, resulting in lessened dyspnea and improvement in arterial blood gases. Most patients with obstructive airways disease may be markedly relieved of dyspnea by simply slowing the respiratory rate, although their underlying airways obstruction is not thereby improved. Slowing of the respiratory rate is best accomplished by improving arterial oxygenation and by calm reassurance on the part of the physician

Initiating Therapy in Patients with Chronic Obstructive Lung Disease

1. Cannulate radial artery and obtain blood for gas analysis unless patient is in extremis
2. Begin 24% O_2 by venturi mask
3. Slow respiratory rate by calm reassurance of patient and oxygenation (may be achieved in some patients by successfully administered IPPB)
4. Meticulous evaluation by:
   a. History and physical
   b. Blood analysis of Hb/Hct, leukocyte count and differential, serum electrolytes, BUN
   c. PA—lateral chest roentgenograms
   d. Electrocardiogram
   e. Repeat arterial blood gas analysis
5. Begin intravenous fluids
   a. Normal saline if volume depleted
   b. D_5W if edematous
6. Aminophylline IV (if no arrhythmia)
   a. 6 mg/kg in 20 min
   b. O.5 mg/kg/hr infusion
   c. Reduce dose if heart failure, liver disease; or pneumonia exists
7. Oral endotracheal intubation only if patient:
   a. Is apneic on admission (usually from excessive oxygen or sedative drugs)
   b. Cannot cough and clear large airways
   c. Exhibits uncontrollable manic behavior

and all medical personnel coming in contact with the frightened, dyspneic patient. A pressure-limited IPPB machine may be useful in this regard if it can be administered in such a way that the patient's inspiration is assisted.

When the patient has been better oxygenated, usually by a venturi mask, and the respiratory rate has been slowed, the physician can proceed with a more meticulous evaluation, including a detailed history of recent events and a thorough physical examination. Blood is obtained for laboratory analysis, including hemoglobin and hematocrit, leukocyte count, serum electrolytes, and blood urea nitrogen. High-quality posteroanterior and lateral roentgenograms of the chest are obtained if possible. An electrocardiogram is performed. Repeated arterial blood gas analysis validates the partial relief of hypoxemia without significant worsening of hypercapnea.

An intravenous infusion is begun in most patients. If the patient is not edematous, and if there is historical or physical evidence for depletion of extracellular fluid volume, the patient is initially given normal saline at a rate appropriate for the clinical status. In edematous patients and patients without evidence of volume depletion, an intravenous infusion of 5% dextrose in water is begun. Unless hypotension or cardiac arrhythmias exist, aminophylline is administered with the intravenous fluids. A loading dose of 6 mg/kg given over approximately 20 min is reasonable unless the patient has recently taken oral theophylline, in which case the dose is reduced by one-half.[83] Since theophylline is metabolized primarily by the liver, alterations in hepatic function markedly influence blood levels.[84,85,86] Severe lung disease and pneumonia similarly decrease theophylline metabolism and cause increased serum concentrations for any dose.[87] A reasonable maintenance dose is 0.5 mg/kg/hr as a continuous IV infusion unless these conditions exist, in which case the maintenance dose should probably be decreased by one-half. A convenient nomogram has been published to help guide therapy,[88] but individual variability is so great that therapy should be directed by determination of serum theophylline concentrations, if possible. Levels of 10 μg/ml to 20 μg/ml are considered optimal.[89]

A summary of the intial steps of therapy is indicated above. The patient should now be sufficiently oxygenated to prevent the threat of immediate death, but hypercapnia is not likely to have increased significantly. Sufficient baseline data have been obtained to guide more definitive therapy, and the patient may now be transferred from the emergency room to the intensive care unit.

EARLY DEFINITIVE TREATMENT

The Spontaneously Ventilating Patient

The first goal of early definitive therapy is to increase the inspired oxygen concentration to a level that produces an adequate arterial oxygen content without causing such worsening of carbon dioxide retention that the patient becomes somnolent and unable to cooperate with therapy. Repeated analyses of arterial blood gas values are extremely helpful in this regard, and these determinations are facilitated by an indwelling arterial catheter. Thus, if an artery has not been cannulated in the emergency room, this should be accomplished shortly after arrival at the definitive treatment area. It should be emphasized, however, that decisions concerning the necessity for endotracheal intubation are not made from arterial gas values alone. The mental status of the patient and his ability to cooperate with therapy are more important in this regard. Every effort must be made to provide aggressive but conservative therapy directed at improving the ventilatory drive, reducing the work of breathing, and improving the distribution of gas in the airways of the lung. These measures, in addition to adequate oxygenation, generally prevent the need for intubation and respirator care.

An adequate PaO_2 does not insure adequate tissue oxygenation. Further components of oxygen transport include an adequate hemoglobin concentration, an adequate cardiac output, and efficient distribution of blood flow according to tissue needs. These considerations have led to widely varying suggestions for the therapeutic goal of PaO_2, from as low as 40 mm. Hg up to 80 mm Hg.[90] A better indicator of tissue hypoxia is the mixed venous Po_2,[90,91] but even this measurement may be an inaccurate indicator of hypoxia in an individual tissue or organ because of widely varying local perfusion rates. Thus, a reasonable goal of oxygen therapy is to provide an arterial oxygen content that is as high as possible without depressing ventilation.

As the PaO_2 is increased from very low values, the percentage saturation of hemoglobin increases almost linearly, until a PaO_2 of approximately 55 to 65 mm Hg is achieved (Fig. 7-4). As the PaO_2 increases above this level, the increase in hemoglobin saturation becomes proportionately less, and relatively little additional oxygen is added to the blood, despite large increases in PaO_2. Thus, when the PaO_2 is in a range of 55 to 65 mm Hg, causing an oxygen saturation of approximately 80 to 90%, a near-maximum amount of oxygen is transported by the blood. Additionally, it has been demonstrated that physiological responses to hypoxemia (such as an increased cardiac output, pulmonary hypertension,[92] augmentation of ventilation,[93–95] and an increase in erythrocyte mass[96]) begin to occur when the arterial oxygen saturation falls below approximately this range. These data suggest that a reasonable goal of oxygen therapy is an arterial oxygen saturation of 80 to 90%, corresponding to an arterial oxygen tension of approximately 55 to 65 mm Hg. These values refer to patients with a normal hemoglobin and, hence, a normal oxygen-carrying capacity. In patients who are seriously anemic (hemoglobin less than 10), transfusion of packed erythrocytes may be more important in maintaining tissue oxygenation than the administration of high concentrations of inspired oxygen. (See Chap. 5 for a detailed discussion of factors that affect oxygen transport.)

The patient arrives at the definitive treatment area on the 24% oxygen initiated in the emergency room. In the more comfortable ward environment, the same concentration of inspired oxygen that was tolerable in the emergency room may lead to mounting hypercapnia and CO_2 narcosis. The patient, therefore, is allowed to stabilize in this environment, and arterial gases are analyzed again. If the desired arterial oxygenation has not been achieved, if the patient has not become so somnolent as to be uncooperative with therapy, and if the $PaCO_2$ has not risen inordinately, the inspired oxygen concentration is increased to 28%. The patient is observed for signs of increasing somnolence on this new F_IO_2; if such does not occur over the next half hour, arterial gases are analyzed again. This procedure is repeated until the arterial oxygenation is in an acceptable range without serious worsening of hypercapnia, or until CO_2 narcosis supervenes. It will be found that most patients can be acceptably oxygenated without significantly worsening hypercapnia, and controlled oxygen administration may be continued. In patients in whom the arterial oxygen content cannot be raised to a satisfactory level without CO_2 narcosis, an artificial airway and assisted ventilation is indicated; these patients will be considered subsequently.

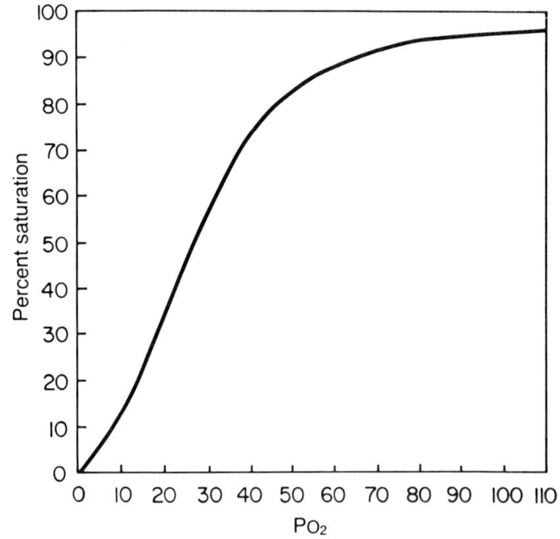

FIG. 7-4. The oxygen dissociation curve indicates that as the PaO_2 is increased from very low values, the percentage of saturation of hemoglobin increases almost linearly until a PaO_2 of approximately 55 to 65 mm Hg is achieved. As the PaO_2 increases above this level, the increase in hemoglobin saturation becomes proportionately less, and relatively little additional oxygen is added to the blood despite large increases in PaO_2. Thus, when the PaO_2 is in the range of 55 to 65 mm Hg, a nearly maximum amount of oxygen is transported by the blood.

As a guide to oxygen therapy, it is possible to roughly predict the PaO_2 that will be achieved by a given F_IO_2 (Fig. 7-5).[97] It also is possible to

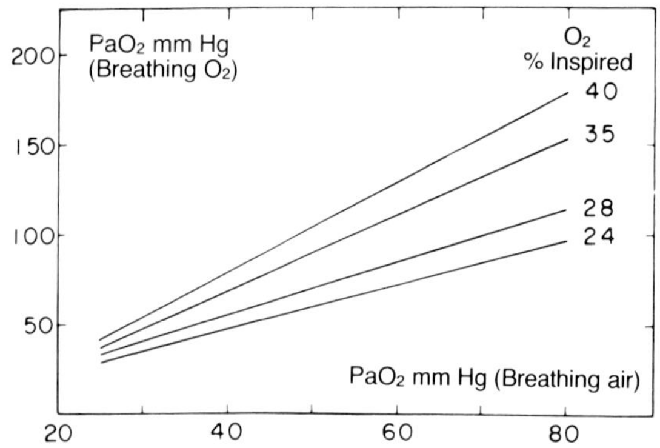

FIG. 7-5. This nomogram indicates the PaO_2 that is likely to be achieved by a given F_IO_2 in patients with acute respiratory failure due to chronic obstructive lung disease. The patient's PaO_2 while breathing room air is indicated on the horizontal axis. By reading vertically from this value to the isopleth indicating the percentage of inspired oxygen concentration, and horizontally from this point to the vertical axis, an estimate of the new PaO_2 may be obtained. (Mithoefer JC, Keighley JF, Karetzky MS: Response of the arterial PO_2 to oxygen administration in chronic pulmonary disease. Ann Intern Med 74:328, 1971)

suspect which patients are at greatest risk of developing CO_2 narcosis on oxygen administration. As would be expected, patients with the most severe hypercapnia at the outset are most likely to develop CO_2 narcosis. The state of oxygenation and the arterial *p*H before therapy, however, are also of help in predicting CO_2 narcosis.[79,98] Patients in whom somnolence develops during controlled oxygen therapy are, in general, severely hypoxemic or have moderate hypoxemia and acidosis on the initial blood gas determinations, and such patients are scrutinized especially carefully during manipulations of oxygen therapy. Using all of these criteria, it will be found that most patients can be successfully oxygenated on a 24-to-28% venti-mask.[98] Once oxygen has been begun, it is imperative that it be continuous. Arterial hypoxemia may be even more severe following oxygen administration and discontinuation than if oxygen had never been given at all.[99,100] This is particularly true immediately after cessation of oxygen therapy.

The Apneic Patient

Although most patients with acute respiratory failure may be managed by controlled oxygen therapy, approximately 15 to 25% will require more aggressive therapy with an artificial airway and assisted or controlled ventilation.[98,101,102] In addition to the indication for intubation included on page 251 (Initiating Therapy in Patients With Chronic Obstructive Lung Disease), some patients' ventilation is remarkably depressed even by controlled oxygen therapy. These tend to be the patients who had very elevated $PaCO_2$ and acidosis and very depressed PaO_2 on admission. In this type of patient, even partial correction of hypoxemia by controlled oxygen therapy may lead to CO_2 narcosis and inability to cooperate with therapy. Such usually does not occur immediately after the administration of low concentrations of oxygen, and the patient must be carefully observed for several hours after initiating therapy.

As described in the section on initiating therapy, the artificial airway of choice is an oral endotracheal tube. The maximum time an endotracheal tube may remain in place has not been established with certainty, but most patients tolerate intubation well for at least a week. Because this interval is sufficiently long for most patients to recover from acute respiratory failure, a tracheostomy may be obviated, and convalescence is thereby shortened. If at any time it becomes apparent that the artificial airway will be needed for a protracted interval, a tracheostomy may be done electively. The same precautions regarding the procedure of intubation that were discussed previously in this chapter pertain to these patients.

As soon as intubation has been accomplished, the patient is begun on assisted respiration. Although spontaneous ventilation may have been inadequate, many patients will be able to trigger an IPPB device at an appropriate rate to maintain or reduce the $PaCO_2$ with assisted respiration. If the patient is able to trigger the ventilator appropriately, this usually should be allowed. If the patient cannot trigger the respirator at a sufficient rate to maintain adequate ventilation while being relieved of hypoxemia, an automatic device must be used. A machine of either the pressure-limited or volume-limited principle may be used successfully. If the former is used, the exhaled tidal volume must be monitored either continuously or periodically, because the inflation pressure cannot be intelligently adjusted without knowledge of the tidal volume being achieved.

The principles of ventilator management in these patients are similar to those outlined in the section on ventilatory failure. Certain important differences, however, should be noted. First, the patient with chronic obstructive lung disease tends to have a large physiological dead space, and the dead space tends to remain a constant fraction of the tidal volume over a wide range of tidal volumes. Thus, in calculating ventilatory requirements, one estimates that approximately 50% of each tidal volume is wasted ventilation, which does not take part in gas exchange at the alveolar level. Second, it is not desirable to lower the $PaCO_2$ rapidly to a normal level. Most of these patients have chronic hypercapnia that has been at least partially compensated by bicarbonate retention. Rapid reduction in $PaCO_2$ results in a marked alkalosis. This has been demonstrated to lead to a central nervous system syndrome characterized by seizures, coma, and frequently death.[103,104] This syndrome evidently is due to a decrease in cerebral blood flow, causing cerebral hypoxia. Ventilation should be adjusted to create a sufficiently gradual reduction in $PaCO_2$ to avoid alkalosis by allowing time for renal bicarbonate excretion. Alternatively, more rapid reductions in $PaCO_2$ without alkalosis may be accomplished if the patient is simultaneously given carbonic anhydrase inhibitors intravenously to hasten bicarbonate excretion; 250 mg of acetazolamide IV administered on two or three occasions is usually sufficient.[105]

When using a pressure-limited ventilator to assist respiration in a patient spontaneously triggering the respiratory rate, it should be remembered that pressure-limited ventilators powered by a 100% oxygen source deliver high concentrations of inspired oxygen, despite air-mixing by the ventilator. The F_IO_2 delivered by such ventilators is likely to depress the respiratory center, and apnea may ensue despite the ventilator. The ventilator should be powered by an air- and oxygen-mixing device, so that a controlled F_IO_2 may be maintained. When ventilation is controlled with either a pressure- or a volume-limited ventilator, the F_IO_2 should be maintained sufficiently low to prevent oxygen toxicity.

During spontaneous respiration, inhaled gas is warmed to body temperature and saturated with water vapor by the nose or mouth. Because artificial airways bypass these structures, and because compressed air and oxygen contain virtually no water, patients on ventilators are at risk of having cold, dry gas delivered directly into the tracheobronchial tree, resulting in drying of the mucosa and further thickening of viscid secretions. The effluent gas from the ventilator must pass through some device that warms it to body temperature and saturates it with water vapor. Either a heated nebulizer or a heated humidifier can be used for this purpose.

Additional Therapy

Bronchodilators. The systemic infusion of aminophylline is continued during this phase of treatment. The previously suggested maintenance dose of 0.5 mg/kg/hr, or half of this amount if the patient has liver disease or congestive heart failure, is continued. Although this dose is satisfactory for most patients, occasional patients may experience toxic side-effects, most commonly nausea and vomiting. Theophylline-induced seizures and arrhythmias have been reported without antecedent symptoms of nausea and vomiting,[106] but such is not common. If serum theophylline concentrations can be obtained, the intravenous infusion is adjusted to give a serum concentration of between 10 and 20 μg/ml.[107]

Inhaled bronchodilators are administered periodically. The frequency of administration and the dosage depend on the particular preparation chosen, but on the average, inhaled bronchodilators are administered every 2 to 4 hr. It has been demonstrated that bronchodilators administered by proper use of a hand nebulizer are as effective as when delivered by IPPB to stable outpatients with chronic obstructive lung disease.[108] Many patients in acute respiratory failure, however, are not capable of the slow, deep inspirations that are thought necessary to maximize deposition of the inhaled bronchodilator. Thus, it may be beneficial to administer bronchodilators by IPPB to patients with acute respiratory failure who cannot or will not take deep breaths.[109] Pulmonary deposition of the bronchodilator may not be as great as with spontaneous large breaths, however.[110] Exhaled tidal volume should be monitored in order to insure that large tidal volumes are being inhaled.

Removal of Tracheobronchial Secretions. Patients with chronic obstructive lung disease and acute respiratory failure have thick, tenacious secretions within their airways. An important facet of therapy is the removal of these secretions. This is best performed by an effective cough.[111] Although it has not been conclusively demonstrated that physical therapeutic maneuvers are effective in facilitating removal of secretions, such measures are reasonable for patients who produce an appreciable amount (>30 ml) of sputum.[112,113,114]

Successfully administered IPPB, causing large tidal volumes, may stimulate and facilitate an effective cough. This is repeated as often as necessary and is followed by chest percussion or vibration and encouragement of the patient to cough. Modified postural drainage positions may be helpful, but many patients cannot tolerate a head-down position during this phase of therapy, because of dyspnea. If necessary, nasotracheal suctioning may be employed to stimulate cough and to remove secretions that have been raised to the trachea.[76] An experienced nursing and respiratory therapy staff may determine by trial and error the procedures most helpful in facilitating cough in a particular patient. These patients should generally be positioned with the chest elevated to a 30- to 60-degree angle, and they should be rolled from side to side at least once hourly. The elevation improves diaphragmatic effects on lung volumes. Side-to-side posturing provides systematic postural drainage to some areas.

In some patients with a depressed cough reflex, periodic stimulation of the trachea may lead to cough and production of secretions. This may be accomplished by placing a plastic catheter percutaneously into the trachea under local anesthesia.[115] A small volume of saline (2 ml) may be injected periodically in order to stimulate cough. This procedure may be helpful in patients with chronic obstructive lung disease, but is not recommended for patients with asthma, because tracheal stimulation may lead to bronchospasm.

Hydration. Even if patients are not clinically dehydrated at the time of admission, it is thought that the administration of large volumes of water, either orally or systemically, is useful in helping to thin viscid secretions. The administration of from 2.5 to 3.5 liters/day of water has been recommended and has been demonstrated to have no detrimental effect on right ventricular hemodynamics.[116] Salt-containing solutions may be necessary, depending on the extracellular fluid volume status of the patient.

The efficacy of inhaled water or saline aerosols in the treatment of patients with acute respiratory failure who do not have an artificial airway is controversial, but most studies indicate no benefit.[117,118] Advocates of bland aerosol therapy feel that the deposition of water in the tracheobronchial tree causes thinning and easier evacuation of respiratory secretions. Physicians not using bland aerosols note that only a small fraction of an inhaled aerosol is deposited in the tracheobronchial tree and that there is no evidence that such a volume of water enhances mucus clearance. In the absence of a well-controlled clinical study, such controversy will not be resolved. If water aerosol is to be used, it is administered by means of a heated nebulizer. In order to control the concentration of oxygen administered at less than 40%, it is necessary to drive the nebulizer from a separate flowmeter (Fig. 7-6). By varying the flow of compressed air and supplemental oxygen, it is possible to achieve any desired oxygen concentration. Table 7-1 indicates the final oxygen concentration achieved for varying flows of air and oxygen. If a nebulizer is used to administer water aerosols, it is important to ensure that the apparatus is decontaminated of bacteria at least once every 24 hr.[119] Nebulizers that are not carefully decontaminated become reservoirs of gram-neg-

TABLE 7-1. Oxygen Concentrations Achieved by Compressed-Air-Driven Nebulizers with Oxygen Enrichment

Oxygen Flowmeter Reading (L/min)	Nebulizer Flowmeter Reading (L/min)			
	8	10	12	14
1	23%	23%	23%	22%
2	26	25	24	24
3	28	26	26	25
4	30	28	27	26
5	32	30	28	27
6	33	31	30	29
7	35	33	31	30
8	37	34	32	31
9	38	35	33	32
10	40	37	35	33
11	41	38	36	34
12	42	39	37	35

The nebulizer is powered by compressed air, and the venturi on the nebulizer is set to 40% O_2. Oxygen is added from a separate flowmeter (Fig. 7-6).

ative bacilli, which may produce a hospital-acquired pneumonia.[120]

Bacterial Infection. A decision regarding the probable presence or absence of bacterial infection is made soon after admission. If historical or physical findings are suggestive of pneumonia or if a pulmonary parenchymal infiltrate is evident on a roentgenogram of the chest, it is assumed that a bacterial pneumonia is present. As in most adults, the most likely causative organism is *Streptococcus pneumoniae*, the pneumococcus, but these chronically debilitated patients are also at risk of developing pneumonia due to aerobic gram-negative bacilli.[121] A Gram stain of expectorated sputum is the only diagnostic technique available to the physician at the outset of therapy. Even when examined by experienced bacteriologists or bacteriology technicians, the Gram stain may not accurately predict the organisms subsequently recovered by culture, especially gram-negative bacilli.[122,123,124] Thus, one is usually unsure of the bacterial cause of the pneumonia at the outset. If the patient is only moderately ill, and if only gram-positive diplococci are observed in the sputum, it is reasonable

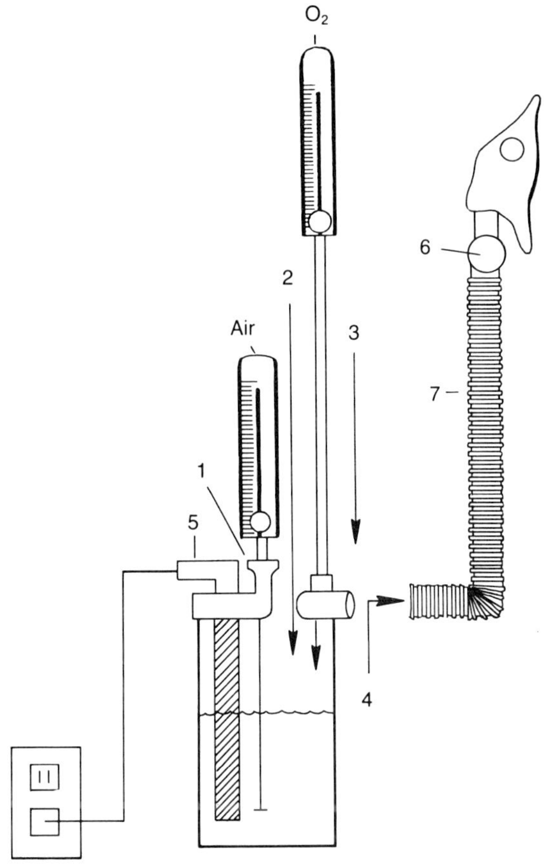

FIG. 7-6. It is possible to administer a heated water aerosol at any inspired oxygen concentration desired between 21 and 35% by use of the system illustrated in this diagram. The flow meter that powers a venturi-principle reservoir nebulizer is attached to a compressed air outlet. Air enters the nebulizer through a jet (1), causing a partial vacuum within the nebulizer cap. The air-mix control on the top of the nebulizer cap is set to the "40% oxygen" reading. This setting indicates that three times as much room air will be aspirated through the nebulizer cap (2) by the venturi jet as there is driving gas through the primary flow meter. A separate flow meter is attached to an oxygen outlet and to the nebulizer jar by plastic tubing (3). The total gas flow (4) will be four times the flow indicated on the primary flow meter (21% oxygen) plus the flow indicated on the oxygen flow meter (100% O_2). By manipulation of these flows, the desired oxygen concentration may be achieved (see Table 7-1). Additional features of the system are the variable heating element (5), a thermometer to determine the heat of the mist arriving at the face mask (6), and a 91-cm (36-inch) corrugated plastic tubing (7).

to administer only 600,000 units of procaine penicillin every 12 hr. However, if the patient is critically ill, or if gram-negative bacilli are observed in the sputum, it is wise to begin broad-spectrum antimicrobial coverage and to discontinue inappropriate drugs when the results of cultures become available. In addition to penicillin, gentamicin is reasonable, with a dose of 1.5 mg/kg at an interval in hours of eight times the serum creatinine value in mg/dl (*i.e.*, q.8hr for a normal creatinine).

It may be difficult to determine whether acute bacterial bronchitis is the cause of the respiratory failure in patients with no roentgenographic infiltrates. It is most commonly assumed that such is present if the patient's sputum is clearly purulent. The organisms most often associated with purulent sputum are *Streptococcus pneumoniae* and *Hemophilus influenzae*, although it is not clear that these bacteria are important in precipitating acute respiratory failure.[125] Because both organisms usually are sensitive to ampicillin, this antibiotic usually is given to patients with purulent sputum in a dosage of 250 mg to 500 mg four times a day. (See also Chap. 8, on Acute Respiratory Tract Infections.)

Other Treatment Modalities. The beneficial effects of adrenal cortical steroids in patients with asthma are well known, but studies of their efficacy in patients with stable COLD are conflicting.[126,127] In the only controlled study of steroid use in patients with COLD in acute respiratory failure, it was found that 0.5 mg/kg body weight of methylprednisolone IV every 6 hr for 72 hr resulted in a greater improvement in $FEV_{1.0}$ than that caused by a placebo when all other therapy was similar.[128] Whether such therapy results in improved survival is not known at present. Additionally, some patients thought to have fixed airways disease demonstrate marked reversibility of airways obstruction with steroid therapy.[129] Such therapy should not be continued, however, unless there is objective evidence of benefit.

Many patients who present with acute respiratory failure additionally manifest right ventricular failure from cor pulmonale. There is little evidence that digitalis is significantly beneficial in this clinical setting.[130] Conversely, digitalis is associated with a high incidence of cardiac arrhythmias in these patients.[76,79,131] Thus, it is wise to avoid digitalis administration in the early management of these patients unless there is evidence of left ventricular failure.

Careful attention must be paid to the electrolyte and acid–base balance of patients in acute respiratory failure. Hypokalemia and hypochloremia (and presumably, total body deficits of these ions) are common, and deficits may be magnified in patients who have been treated with diuretics.[132,133] In the nonedematous patient, intravenous fluid therapy should include saline, on the order of 1 liter daily. A total body deficit of potassium should be assumed to exist unless the patient has renal disease manifested by azotemia. Intravenous therapy should include potassium supplements on the order of 60 to 80 mEq daily.

CONTINUING TREATMENT

Discontinuing Assisted Ventilation

As patients improve, mechanical ventilation should be discontinued and extubation should be accomplished as early as possible, because serious complications frequently occur in bedfast patients. Unfortunately, the criteria used for extubation in patients with other types of respiratory failure (see Guidelines for Ventilatory Support in Patients with Ventilatory Failure) may not be applicable to patients with COLD. The ratio of dead space to tidal volume (V_D/V_T) may be helpful, because it has been observed that a patient with a V_D/V_T greater than 0.6 is less likely to be successfully weaned from a respirator.[134] Because such a measurement is inconvenient in most hospitals, weaning from ventilatory support is usually estimated by the clinical appearance of the patient and is performed by trial and error.

When it is felt that the patient no longer needs assisted ventilation, a procedure similar to that described previously in the section on extubation of the patient with ventilatory failure with normal lungs is carried out. The patient is observed carefully for tachycardia, cardiac arrhythmias, tachypnea, or obvious distress. If these abnormalities do not occur, arterial blood gases are obtained after 15 to 20 min to confirm that the patient is able to ventilate and oxygenate sufficiently. Because most patients have an increase in $PaCO_2$ when ventilatory support is discontinued,[135] moderate increases are not considered a contraindication to continue weaning, unless the *p*H falls to a low value.

It is rarely possible with this type of patient to discontinue ventilatory support abruptly. These patients tend to tire with time off the ventilator, and many lack coordination of their respiratory muscles. Repeated and progressively longer times off the ventilator are usually necessary, and the whole process may take several days in some patients.

A system of weaning, termed *intermittent mandatory ventilation* (IMV), has been suggested as a means of expediting the weaning process.[136] The patient is left attached to the ventilator, but the system is modified to allow the patient to breathe spontaneously between inhalations produced by the ventilator (Fig. 7-7). Weaning is accomplished by a gradual reduction in the number of breaths that the ventilator delivers, which allows the patient to slowly assume more responsibility for ventilation. No controlled series have been carried out to determine if IMV significantly accelerates the weaning process. Thus, the role of IMV in this regard has not been established.

When the patient is able to maintain spontaneous ventilation for a period of hours, extubation may be carried out. The patient must be observed carefully in the postextubation period, to make sure that he does not tire with time. If such occurs, reintubation and assisted ventilation may be necessary.

Additional Therapy

As the patient with acute respiratory failure superimposed on COLD improves, it is possible to discontinue intravenous fluids. The patient is encouraged, however, to continue a large oral fluid intake. At this juncture, the patient's regimen is changed from intravenous to oral aminophylline. With uncoated tablets of aminophylline, peak plasma concentrations are observed between 1 and 3 hr after administration, and the average plasma half-life of theophylline is 4 to 5 hr.[83] Thus, the drug is administered every 6 hr and should be administered in a fasting state. The suggested dose of uncoated oral aminophylline tablets is 3 mg/kg/6 hr for initial therapy and 6 mg/kg/6 hr for optimal dosage. Because plateau plasma concentrations are attained within 1 or 2 days following change of dosage, the dose can be increased every 2 or 3 days in an attempt to find the optimal dose for maximum benefit and minimum side effects. It has been demonstrated that the addition of ephedrine to aminophylline adds little to bronchodilation but increases toxicity.[137,138] However, the bronchodilating effects of aminophylline and terbutaline are additive.[139] Thus, the combined use of aminophylline with terbutaline (2.5 mg or 5 mg) three times a day, depending on side effects, may be useful in some patients. More commonly, oral aminophylline and inhaled sympathomimetics are used.

Prolonged bed rest has been demonstrated to be markedly detrimental to cardiac and musculoskeletal performance, even in normal young persons.[140] The defects in performance imposed by bed rest are overcome only after a protracted period of reconditioning. Patients with COLD in the stable state are already deconditioned in regard to their cardiovascular and musculoskeletal systems.[141] The additional deconditioning imposed by prolonged bed rest in elderly patients may cause even more severe debility on recovery from an episode of acute respiratory failure than had existed previously. These patients, therefore, should be encouraged from the outset of treatment of respiratory failure to be as physically active as possible under the circumstances. They should be mobilized as rapidly as possible and made to walk to the limits of their capacity. In some patients, such exercise should be supported with oxygen breathing.[142]

In this phase of therapy, the patient should be progressively transferred from the inhaled bronchodilator and the physical therapeutic regimen outlined previously to that which the patient will be expected to carry out after discharge from the hospital. The principles of home management are outlined in Chapter 14, Obstructive Airways Diseases. An important facet of

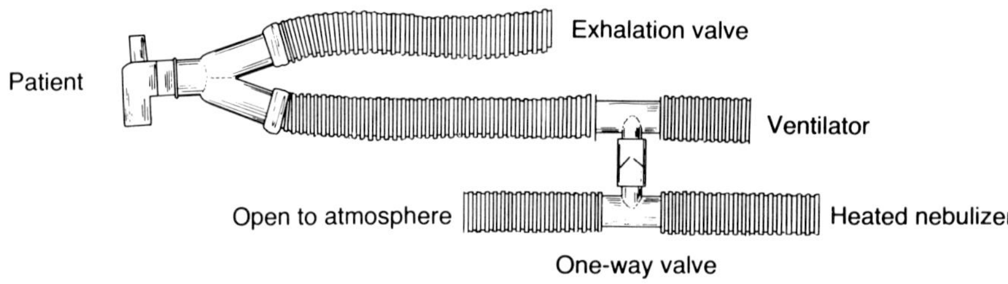

FIG. 7-7. This diagram depicts the principles of intermittent mandatory ventilation (IMV). An H connector containing a one-way valve is placed into the tubing connecting the ventilator to the patient. One additional arm of the H is connected to a heated nebulizer, and the final arm is left open to the atmosphere. When the ventilator cycles into the inspiratory mode, both the exhalation valve and the one-way valve are closed, and the patient's lungs are inflated by the ventilator. When the ventilator cycles to the expiratory mode, both valves are open, and the patient breathes in the mist generated by the nebulizer through the one-way valve and breathes out through the exhalation valve. During IMV, the patient's inspiratory efforts do not trigger the ventilator, and the patient breathes spontaneously, except during the automatically-cycled ventilator tidal volumes.

care is to devote sufficient time to the patient and the patient's family to ensure that the principles of outpatient care are understood and will be adhered to after discharge.

Prognosis

Approximately 70% of patients with COLD survive an episode of severe acute respiratory failure.[102,143–147] A fatal outcome usually does not relate to the respiratory failure directly, because an inability to ventilate and oxygenate the patient is unusual. Mortality more often results from superimposed complications.

As in other types of patients who require continued ventilatory support, complications related to the artificial airway are common during the course of mechanical ventilation.[49] The same types of precautions indicated in the section on artificial airway care for patients with ventilatory failure should be observed in patients with failure of CO_2 excretion.

The precipitating cause of acute respiratory failure in these patients may be pneumonia. Although the most frequent causative organism is the pneumococcus, chronically debilitated patients such as these may have oropharyngeal colonization and subsequent pneumonia from gram-negative bacilli.[148] In addition, severely ill, hospitalized patients tend to become colonized with such bacilli, which may then cause a hospital-acquired pneumonia. Because many gram-negative bacilli are resistant to antimicrobial therapy, this type of infection is a potential cause of death.[120]

Pulmonary embolization is a frequent event in intensive-care-unit patients.[121] Anticoagulant therapy, however, is not used prophylactically, because these patients also have a high incidence of peptic ulcer and gastrointestinal hemorrhage. Low-dose heparin prophylaxis has not been evaluated in this condition but shows great promise in most immobilized patients (see Chap. 10).

Severe cardiac arrhythmias are a potential cause of death.[76] Arrhythmias may be potentiated by digitalis toxicity, acid–base abnormalities and hypokalemia, catecholamine bronchodilators, or theophylline derivatives.

Although most patients survive the acute episode of respiratory failure, the long-term prognosis is guarded, owing to the progression of their underlying chronic obstructive lung disease. The 1-year survival rate following an episode of respiratory failure is approximately 50%,[147] and the 2-year survival rate is approximately 30%.[143,146,150] Nevertheless, many of the survivors are able to lead relatively comfortable lives following recovery from their first episode of acute respiratory failure.

FAILURE TO OXYGENATE ARTERIAL BLOOD

MECHANISMS OF PULMONARY EDEMA

A third type of respiratory failure is manifested by an inability to oxygenate arterial blood despite an ability to ventilate sufficiently to excrete carbon dioxide. The underlying pathophysiological mechanism is an excess of pulmonary parenchymal liquid (i.e., pulmonary edema). This type of respiratory failure may occur because of two types of derangement: an increase in the hydrostatic pressure or an increase in the permeability of the pulmonary capillaries. An understanding of these mechanisms requires a review of lung fluid formation and reabsorption and of the ultrastructure of the lung.[151,152,153,154,155]

A diagrammatic representation of an alveolar wall appears in Figure 7-8. The alveolar spaces are separated from the interstitium of the lung primarily by Type 1 alveolar epithelial cells which, under normal conditions, form a relatively impermeable barrier to fluid flow from the interstitium into air spaces. A large fraction of the interstitial space is made up of pulmonary capillaries, the walls of which are composed of a single layer of endothelial cells resting on a basement membrane. The remainder of the interstitial space contains connective tissue meshworks of collagen and elastic tissues, the fibroblasts that synthesize connective tissue, phagocytic cells, and a variety of other cell types. The important determinants of extravascular fluid formation are the hydrostatic and oncotic pressure differences between the lumens of the capillaries and the interstitial space, and the permeability of endothelial cells to water, solutes, and large molecules such as plasma proteins.

These determinants of transvascular movement of fluid are summarized in Starling's equation:

$$\dot{Q}f = K(PMv - Ppmv) - K\sigma(\pi mv - \pi pmv)$$

where $\dot{Q}f$ is the net transvascular flow of fluid, K is the capillary filtration coefficient, Pmv is the microvascular hydrostatic pressure, Ppmv is the perimicrovascular (interstitial)hydrostatic pressure, σ is the plasma-protein reflection coefficient (which determines the transvascular protein osmotic-pressure difference), πmv is the protein osmotic pressure in the plasma, and πpmv is the perimicrovascular (interstitial) protein osmotic pressure. In normal circumstances, pulmonary microvascular (capillary) hydrostatic pressure is approximately 10 mm Hg. The perimicrovascular pressure is not subject to direct measurement, but it is probably moderately subatmospheric.[156–158] The plasma-protein osmotic pressure is approximately 25 mm Hg. In experimental animals the interstitial protein osmotic pressure is between 12 and 20 mm Hg.[153] The endothelial cell has a high permeability to water, small ions, and uncharged metabolites such as urea and glucose,[159] but high-molecular-weight substances such as protein are markedly

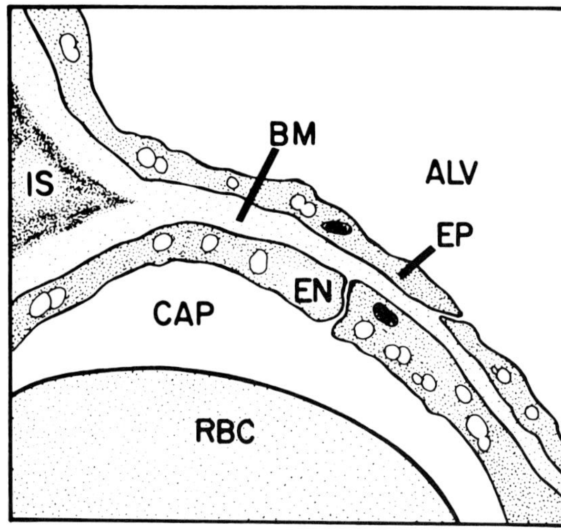

FIG. 7-8. In this diagrammatic representation of an alveolar wall, an alveolar space (ALV) is to the right, and a pulmonary capillary (CAP) is to the lower left. Separating the alveolar space from the capillary lumen are an alveolar epithelial Type 1 cell (EP) resting on a basement membrane (BM), and the capillary endothelial cell (EN) resting on a basement membrane (BM). Along a part of this interface, the basement membranes are fused. The interstitial space (IS) is represented to the left, and in some locations this space contains a variety of cell types as well as connective tissue meshworks of collagen and elastin.

limited in movement out of the vasculature.[159–161] The net balance of forces allows continuous filtration of fluid from the pulmonary capillary into the interstitial space. It is clear that a mechanism is necessary to continuously drain this fluid from the interstitial space of the lung; this mechanism is the lymphatic system.

The loose connective-tissue spaces of the lung are richly endowed with lymphatic vessels that end as anatomical structures at about the level of the terminal bronchioles. The alveolar interstitial spaces do not contain anatomically distinct lymphatics. The three-dimensional meshworks of alveolar interstitial spaces, however, act as conduits for fluid to flow to the lymphatics. The fluid is probably transported from the lung by rhythmic contraction of the lymphatic vessels and ultimately is returned to the venous system.[162] It is estimated that lung lymphatic flow is approximately 20 ml/hr in a normal 70 kg person.[152]

In diseases leading to increased pulmonary capillary pressure or to increased permeability, an excess of interstitial lung fluid is formed only when the capacity of the lymphatics to remove excess fluid is exceeded. It has been estimated that lymph flow can increase to approximately ten times the baseline level.[163] Following saturation of this system, an interstitial phase of edema exists for a variable period before alveolar flooding occurs. Initially, the edema is most marked in the loose interstitial connective-tissue spaces, but such is followed temporally by alveolar-wall edema.[164] If the excess lung fluid is more severe, a phase of alveolar flooding may begin abruptly and consists of rapid filling of individual alveoli with fluid. The exact route of fluid flow into alveoli is not clear,[165,166] but this phase results in more profound physiological derangements than had previously existed.

It is important to recognize that the chain of events described may be caused by either an increase in pulmonary capillary pressure or an increase in permeability. Thus, the physiological and clinical effects of either type of pulmonary edema are similar, at least at the outset. A differentiation of which type of pulmonary edema exists in an individual patient may be exceedingly difficult. In many instances the correct diagnosis may be made only by direct measurement of the pulmonary capillary wedge pressure. In the rare instance that pulmonary edema fluid may be collected from the patient's airways, measurement of the protein content may be helpful. It has been demonstrated that the protein concentration in edema fluid of patients suffering from excess capillary permeability is similar to that of the patient's serum,[167–170] whereas edema due to high pulmonary capillary pressure has considerably less protein than serum.[171] In many cases the diagnosis is not made with assurance and depends on associated clinical findings rather than on the nonspecific pulmonary findings of edema. Rapid resolution speaks for the etiology being increased capillary pressure, whereas a delayed resolution suggests increased permeability.

The Starling equation indicates that the protein osmotic-pressure difference across the pulmonary capillary endothelium is important in edema formation. In the case of high pulmonary capillary pressures in the presence of normal endothelial permeability, the excess fluid transuded into the interstitial space tends to have a low protein concentration.[172] This reduces the osmotic forces tending to favor pulmonary edema and is thought to minimize extravascular fluid formation. In patients with a variety of critical illnesses, however, it has been reported that exceedingly low plasma oncotic pressures are usually associated with pulmonary edema and with a high mortality rate.[173,174,175]

PATHOPHYSIOLOGY OF PULMONARY EDEMA

Correlation among anatomical, physiological, radiological, and clinical findings have not been reported in detail. Part of the following, therefore, is conjecture not supported by investigation and may prove to be inaccurate. However, this pathophysiological schema gives a frame work with which to approach the patient with pulmonary edema.

The earliest change of pulmonary edema is an increase in lymphatic flow. Pulmonary lymphatics are located predominately in the loose interstitial connective tissue surrounding pulmonary arterioles and small airways (Fig. 7-9). The engorged lymphatics impinge on these tubular structures and alter the pressure relationships between them and the surrounding lung parenchyma. This results in mild obstruction to small airways, which has been shown to be the earliest physiological change in patients with left ventricular failure that can be measured by noninvasive means.[176] This has not been measured in pulmonary edema due to excess capillary permeability. Since this is not a uniform lesion throughout the lung, changes in distribution of ventilation and perfusion result, leading to mild hypoxemia. Impingement on small arterioles also results in the earliest roentgenographic abnormality in left ventricular failure, a redistribution of blood flow from the base to the apex of the lung in the upright patient.[177] Clinically, this phase is not likely to be associated with serious signs or symptoms, and it may account for the latent interval observed following the initial insult in many patients with the adult respiratory distress syndrome.

If interstitial fluid formation exceeds the capacity of the lymphatic system, a period of alveolar-wall edema may ensue. During this phase, compliance is moderately decreased (*i.e.*, the lung becomes stiff).[178] This results in tachypnea, which is probably the earliest clinical finding in patients with pulmonary edema. Additional mismatching of ventilation and blood flow leads to worsening hypoxemia. However, carbon dioxide excretion is not impaired, and patients typically manifest hyperventilation with respiratory alkalosis. There may also be some contribution to hypoxemia by diffusion defects, and increased right-to-left shunting through unventilated alveoli probably occurs at this stage.[179] Roentgenographically, there is an interstitial or reticular infiltrate. If the patient is alert, dyspnea is present. Physical examination is likely to demonstrate, in addition to tachypnea, increased transmission of breath sounds and inspiratory rales on auscultation.

During the phase of alveolar flooding, all findings become more severe. Compliance decreases markedly, leading to rapid, shallow breathing and to the necessity of high inflation pressures if the patient is on a ventilator. Since alveoli are filled with fluid while blood flow to them continues, right-to-left shunting of blood becomes extreme, leading to hypoxemia that is resistant to increased inspired oxygen concentrations.[180] Unless the lesion is exceedingly severe, however, hyperventilation and respiratory alkalosis continue. Roentgenographically, the picture is that of an alveolar infiltrate spread throughout the lung, although the perihilar and basilar regions are typically the most involved. If the patient is alert, dyspnea is severe. The patient demonstrates tachypnea, tachycardia, and cyanosis if ventilation is unsupported. This condition has been referred to as the adult respiratory distress syndrome (ARDS).

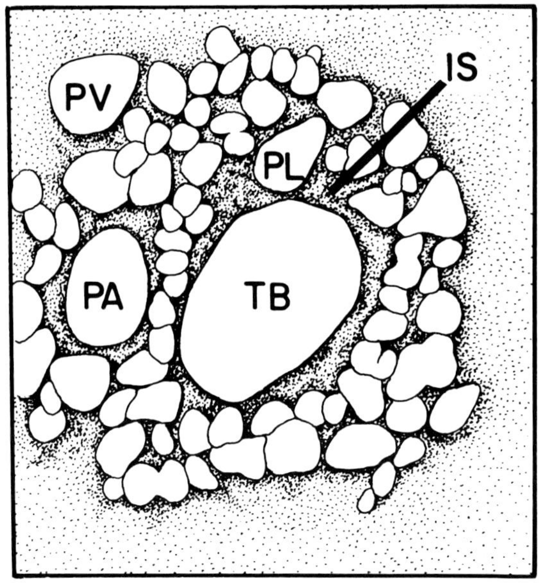

FIG. 7-9. This low-power view of the loose interstitial connective tissue space (IS) demonstrates the relationships among the terminal bronchiole (TB), pulmonary artery (PA), pulmonary lymphatic (PL), and pulmonary vein (PV). The unlabeled spaces are alveoli, which extend outward into the lightly stippled area.

Microatelectasis is a prominent feature of ARDS. These changes are thought to be due to surfactant abnormalities secondary to the primary lung insult.[181,182] The reduced surfactant activity may also lead to additional transudation of fluid from capillaries into the lung parenchyma by increasing alveolar-surface tension.[183]

DIFFERENTIAL DIAGNOSIS OF PULMONARY EDEMA

One approach to the differential diagnosis of a patient with pulmonary edema is to first determine which of the two pathophysiological mechanisms is likely to exist: increased pressure or increased permeability of the pulmonary capillaries (see list below). The possibilities indicated in the list below do not include all reported syndromes. The mechanism for some of the syndromes has not been elucidated, and in some syndromes both mechanisms may exist. However, this simplified differential diagnosis should suffice for most clinical purposes.

Differential Diagnosis of Acute Respiratory Failure Due to Pulmonary Edema

- Increased pulmonary capillary pressure
  - Cardiogenic pulmonary edema
    - Left ventricular failure
    - Mitral stenosis
  - Venous congestive syndrome
  - ? Neurogenic pulmonary edema
  - ? Altitude pulmonary edema
- Increased pulmonary capillary permeability
  - Post-traumatic pulmonary insufficiency
  - Aspiration of gastric contents
  - Sepsis
  - Pneumonia (any cause)
  - Heroin (narcotic) overdose
  - Smoke inhalation and respiratory burns
  - Inhalation of toxic chemicals
  - Oxygen toxicity
  - Near-drowning
  - Fat embolism
  - Uremia
  - Pancreatitis
  - Miscellaneous disorders

Increased Pulmonary Capillary Pressure

Cardiogenic Pulmonary Edema. The most common cause of pulmonary edema is left ventricular failure. A complete discussion of this important syndrome is beyond the scope of this chapter and is well covered in textbooks of cardiology. For the purposes of this chapter, it is important to recognize the difficulty in determining in an individual patient whether the cause of pulmonary edema is cardiogenic or is due to ARDS.[184,185] Clinical, laboratory, and roentgenographic findings may be similar in the two syndromes. Frequently, the correct diagnosis may be made only by measurements of the pulmonary capillary wedge pressure, a procedure that may be carried out at the bedside of critically ill patients by means of a flow-guided catheter.[186] In some patients, the presence or absence of cardiomegaly or pleural effusions may be helpful. It is unusual for left ventricular failure to occur in the presence of a normal-sized heart, unless the cause is an acute myocardial infarction. Pleural effusions are unusual in ARDS; when present, effusions suggest that the pulmonary edema is due to increased pulmonary capillary pressure.

Venous Congestive Syndrome. Patients with an overexpanded intravascular volume may develop increased pulmonary capillary pressure and pulmonary edema in the presence of a normal heart.[187] Expansion of the intravascular volume need not be marked for venous congestion to occur, since systemic vasoconstriction may cause a shift in the blood volume to the central circulation. This syndrome most commonly occurs in patients who have been given large amounts of intravenous crystalloids or blood, especially if renal function is impaired. Simultaneous administration of adrenal corticosteroids with sodium-retaining properties causes further venous congestion.

The venous congestive (fluid overload) syndrome is most likely to occur in patients with extensive trauma who have received large amounts of intravenous fluids to support the circulation. In the recovery phase, pulmonary edema may ensue, and the syndrome may be mistaken for left ventricular failure or for ARDS. Venous congestion and ARDS may be differentiated by the normal pulmonary capillary wedge pressure found in the latter syndrome. Venous congestion may be differentiated from left ventricular failure by the normal cardiac output and normal arteriovenous oxygen content difference found with venous congestion. The appropriate therapy for venous congestion is diuresis; digitalis is of no benefit.

Neurogenic Pulmonary Edema. Patients with lesions of the central nervous system and postictal patients may develop pulmonary edema.[188,189] In experimental animals, pulmonary edema has been shown to occur within minutes of the injury,[190] and it has been demonstrated that edema may be prevented by a blockade of the sympathetic nervous system.[191] The edema is caused by high pulmonary capillary pressures greatly in excess of those seen in left ventricular failure. The elevated pressure is present for only the brief interval of a few ventricular contractions, and subsequent measurements of cardiovascular pressure or performance are normal.[192] The mechanism is thought to be hypothalamic stimulation causing a massive discharge of the adrenergic nervous system, in turn resulting in a shift in blood from the systemic to the pulmonary circulation and in a decrease in the compliance of the left ventricle. Despite the transient nature of the cardiovascular disturbance, the pulmonary edema is long-lasting and has a high protein concentration similar to that found in ARDS.[193] This is discussed further in Chapter 11, Chest Trauma.

Neurogenic pulmonary edema is most common in persons with head trauma, but it may occur in association with intracranial diseases of many types. It is particularly common in younger patients. In persons with head injury or acute intracranial hemorrhage, pulmonary edema develops very rapidly; it is present even in patients who die instantaneously or within a few minutes of the injury.[188] A neurogenic mechanism may explain the early pulmonary edema in heroin users who are found dead with the injection apparatus still in their veins. Treatment is directed at correction of the nervous system lesion, oxygenation, and mechanical support to ventilation.

Altitude Pulmonary Edema. Normal persons ascending to altitudes greater than 2700 m (9000 ft) may develop pulmonary edema in the absence of demonstrable precipitating events. This serious but uncommon condition may occur during a person's first ascent to high altitudes,[194] but it is more commonly encountered in fully acclimatized persons who have been at much lower altitudes and then return to high altitude. At least a week at low altitude has been thought to be necessary;[195] however, shorter intervals have been reported.[196] Children and adolescents are at greater risk than adults, but even among this age group subsequent episodes of reascent from low altitude are usually not associated with recurrent pulmonary edema[195,196,197] (see Chap. 1, Altitude Illness).

The cause of high-altitude pulmonary edema is not known. Cardiac catheterization studies of affected persons reveal marked pulmonary hypertension with normal wedge pressures. This evidence indicates that left ventricular failure is not the mechanism.[198,199] It has been suggested that the mechanism is pulmonary hypertension caused by the hypoxia of altitude; this has been demonstrated to be more severe in persons who develop altitude pulmonary edema than in persons who do not.[200,201] According to this hypothesis, intense vasoconstriction of a large fraction (but not all) of the pulmonary arteries causes high pressures to be transmitted to the capillaries of the pulmonary arteries that remain patent.[202]

Symptoms of high-altitude pulmonary edema typically occur from 6 to 36 hr after arrival at high altitude.[203] Vigorous exercise during this interval makes edema more likely. Early symptoms include a dry cough, dyspnea, and a feeling of pain or pressure in the lower substernal area. Anorexia, nausea, and vomiting may occur. As the syndrome becomes more severe, the findings are typical of any form of pulmonary edema, with hemoptysis and orthopnea being particularly prominent. The temperature may be slightly elevated, and there may be a transient leukocytosis, but the role of infection is not established.

Treatment with bed rest and oxygen administration or removal to a lower altitude results in prompt improvement within 24 hr. The patient usually is entirely asymptomatic and has a normal chest roentgenogram within 3 days. Administration of digitalis does not hasten improvement, but diuretics may be helpful.[203]

Increased Pulmonary Capillary Permeability

Pulmonary edema due to increased capillary permeability, the adult respiratory distress syndrome, is estimated to occur in 150,000 persons per year in the United States.[204] Although many cases result from a direct pulmonary insult, many cases occur as a complication of extrapulmonary disease or injury. Unfortunately, many such patients are young, previously healthy persons who would otherwise recover from their primary injury or disease process. Considerable investigation has been directed at the mediators of the increased permeability.[204] Factors thought to be potentially important include lysosomal enzymes of polymorphonuclear leukocytes aggregated in pulmonary capillaries owing to complement activation or other stimuli,[205–208] lysosomal enzymes from platelets or plasma proteolytic enzymes,[209,210,211] release of mediators from mast cells,[212] other humoral substances,[172,213] oxygen toxicity,[214,215] and vascular obstruction causing flow damage to the endothelium of vessels which remain patent.[153] A review of these investigational studies is beyond the scope of this text, in which a more clinical approach will be used (see also Chapter 11, Chest Trauma).

Post-Traumatic Pulmonary Insufficiency. Although it had previously been recognized that traumatized patients may suffer pulmonary complications in the postresuscitative interval, specific reports of pulmonary edema in this circumstance first appeared during World War II.[216,217] Owing to improved management of other problems related to trauma and the more rapid evacuation of traumatized patients to sophisticated treatment centers, the syndrome apparently has increased in frequency in recent years. The incidence of post-traumatic pulmonary insufficiency among severely wounded persons has been estimated to be between 1 and 40%[218,219,220] (see Chap. 11).

Many injured patients, during resuscitation, develop significant hypoxemia that may last for several days.[221,222] The causes of hypoxemia in this circumstance are probably similar to those causing hypoxemia following laparotomy for any cause and are reviewed in the chapter on pulmonary complications of general surgery. Additional features of pulmonary edema are necessary in order to make the diagnosis of post-traumatic pulmonary insufficiency. Up to 25% of severely wounded patients may require ventilatory support for up to 3 days following trauma.[219] Some of these patients probably have pulmonary edema as a result of the previously described venous congestive syndrome. This transient respiratory failure is probably not best classified as post-traumatic pulmonary insufficiency, a more protracted syndrome.

The cause or causes of post-traumatic pulmonary insufficiency are not known,[223,224] although histological studies emphasize the presence of fibrin and platelet microthromboemboli in the pulmonary vasculature.[225,226] It may be that several of the syndromes indicated as "increased pulmonary capillary permeability" in the list on Differential Diagnosis of Acute Respiratory Failure due to Pulmonary Edema contribute to this form of pulmonary edema. Early laboratory and retrospective clinical investigations suggested that the etiology is hemorrhagic hypotension, leading to the term, *shock lung*. However, subsequent laboratory[227] and prospective clinical[219,228] investigations do not support the concept that hypotension alone is sufficient to lead to post-traumatic pulmonary insufficiency. Whatever the etiology, it is important to note that the patient's injuries need not involve the thoracic cage in order for this syndrome to develop.

Patients with post-traumatic pulmonary insufficiency frequently follow a predictable course.[229] In the early postresuscitation period, patients are frequently mildly alkalotic due to a combination of hyperventilation and administration of alkaline solutions during resuscitation. Most patients recover without incident, but those with more severe pulmonary derangements develop signs that suggest the onset of post-traumatic pulmonary insufficiency. These include cardiovascular instability, low urine output, persistent hyperventilation, and arterial hypoxemia. In the early phase of symptomatic respiratory distress, the patient continues to hyperventilate and develops refractory hypoxemia in spite of the administration of high concentrations of inspired oxygen, indicating that a large fraction of the cardiac output is traversing unventilated lungs, functioning as right-to-left shunts. The magnitude of these shunts has been estimated to be as high as 15 to 30% of the cardiac output. In the phase of obvious progressive pulmonary difficulty, the patient becomes more dyspneic, exhibits a very large minute ventilation with a large fraction of respiratory dead space, and increases the shunt fraction even more. Roentgenographic infiltrates occur, and rales may become evident on physical examination. In a terminal phase, it becomes impossible to prevent hypoxemia with very high levels of inspired oxygen, and increasing metabolic acidosis ensues. In this terminal phase, hypercapnia may occur. The evolution of the entire syndrome may require hours to days; although the mortality rate remains high, it has been suggested that early aggressive therapy with positive end-expiratory pressure may be beneficial.[230]

The aspiration of gastric contents may lead to ARDS. Animal experiments suggest that the severity of the syndrome relates to the acidity of the solution aspirated.[231] and to the volume of aspirate.[232] Acid with a *p*H of 2.5 or less instilled into the lungs causes a marked, long-lasting increase in alveolar–capillary permeability, while acid with a higher *p*H causes only transiently increased permeability similar to that of water or saline.[233,234,235] Gastric enzymes do not contribute to the injury, and the lesion is bacteriologically sterile.[231] The gastric juice spreads throughout the lungs within seconds,[236] and lung tissue is buffered to a normal pH in a matter of minutes.[237] With severe insults hypotension may ensue, which is thought to be due to a reflex decrease in cardiac output mediated by the vagus nerve.[238]

Disturbances of consciousness lead to the possibility of regurgitation and aspiration.[239,240] An overdosage of sedative drugs and general anesthesia are the most common predisposing conditions, and obstetrical or emergency surgical patients have been reported to have the highest incidence with anesthesia because of inadequate preoperative preparation.[241] A single oral dose of 300 mg of cimetidine, a specific competitive histamine H_2 antagonist that reduces basal gastric acid output, given at least 60 min preoperatively, has been demonstrated to be effective in raising gastric fluid *p*H to greater than 2.5 and thus may reduce the incidence of ARDS in patients undergoing general anesthesia.[242,243,244] Although symptoms begin immediately in most patients, a "latent period" of up to 5 hr between aspiration and the development of signs or symptoms may occur.[245] In addition to the usual findings in patients with pulmonary edema, fever and leukocytosis occur in the majority of cases. Shock or apnea in the early postaspiration interval suggests a poor prognosis. Roentgenographic manifestations are extremely variable, with no typical appearance.[246] The most common findings are small, irregular, bilateral infiltrates in perihilar or basal regions.

Approximately 15% of the patients sustain a massive injury and die within 24 hr.[241] Another 60% of the patients stabilize after the initial injury and demonstrate prompt clinical and roentgenographic improvement. Roentgenograms return to normal in this group of patients within 2 to 16 (mean, 4.5) days.[241] Approximately 30% of the patients demonstrate early improvement but then deteriorate clinically and roentgenographically, most commonly on the third to fifth day. These patients have a recrudescence of fever and leukocytosis, and sputum cultures reveal potential pathogens. These findings suggest a superimposed infection on a healing aspirational injury. The most common offending organisms are gram-negative bacilli. The mortality rate of patients with superinfections is approximately 60%.[241]

Sepsis. Septicemia by gram negative bacilli from extrapulmonary infection is an important cause of pulmonary edema due to increased pulmonary capillary permeability (see Septic Shock in Chapter 8). In experimental animals, infusion of *Escherichia coli* or *E. coli* endotoxin causes marked pulmonary functional abnormalities,[247] changes in ultrastructure of pulmonary vessels,[248] and pulmonary edema.[249] Infusion of *Pseudomonas aeruginosa* has been demonstrated to cause pulmonary edema by increasing pulmonary capillary permeability.[250] The pulmonary edema of sepsis has been demonstrated clinically to be due to increased capillary permeability by the careful exclusion of increased capillary pressure,[251,252] and by the finding of high-molecular-weight substances in the pulmonary edema fluid.[167] Indeed, these patients commonly manifest a high cardiac output.[253] It is not clear whether these changes are a direct effect of the organisms or whether they are mediated by some biologically active substance resulting from the organisms.[254] It is clear, however, that a diffuse pulmonary edema results without active multiplication of organisms within the lung; that is, these are not the changes of pneumonia.

Pulmonary edema is a common feature of septic shock, but it is apparently not related to hypotension *per se*, since patients with sepsis without shock may develop the lesion.[251] The syndrome has been reported most frequently in surgical patients with sepsis from traumatic wounds or from intra-abdominal catastrophes with peritonitis.[255] These critically ill patients usually have positive blood cultures in addition to fever, leukocytosis, and other manifestations of sepsis. If shock is associated with septicemia, the pulmonary edema commonly develops within 12 hr of the onset of hypotension. Despite therapy with appropriate antimicrobial agents and ventilatory support, the mortality rate may approach 90%.[254]

Sepsis is such a frequent finding in patients diagnosed as having post-traumatic pulmonary insufficiency that it is considered by some to be the most important causative factor, except in patients with burns, intracranial lesions, or pulmonary contusion.[219,223,228,254] (See also Chap. 8.)

Pneumonia. Infections of the lung are reported as causes of diffuse pulmonary edema with increasing frequency. Mycobacterial, pyogenic bacterial, mycoplasma, Legionella, rickettsial and fungal infections have all produced this clinical picture. The most common etiology, however, is viral pneumonia.

Viral infections produce pulmonary edema by direct pulmonary infection. The histological and electron-microscopic picture is similar to that of other types of pulmonary edema due to increased capillary permeability.[256] The only viruses that regularly produce respiratory failure from diffuse pulmonary edema are influenza and varicella viruses (see also Chap. 8).

Patients with primary influenza virus pneumonia present during the course of an influenza epidemic with a relatively uniform clinical picture.[257] The onset is characteristic of influenza, with chilly sensations or overt shaking chills, high fever, sore throat, a dry nonproductive cough, headache, myalgias, and prostration. Over the first 24 to 48 hr, the patient develops increasingly severe respiratory distress. There may be production of bloody, nonpurulent sputum. On physical examination the patient appears acutely and seriously ill, with high fever and marked respiratory distress. The physical and roentgenographic findings in the chest are typical of pulmonary edema. In the acute phase, the only abnormal laboratory finding is a moderate leukocytosis of polymorphonuclear leukocytes, with an increase in immature forms.

Influenzal pneumonia was originally reported in patients with preexisting cardiac disease, especially mitral stenosis. It may be that the prevalence among such patients is increased, but influenza pneumonia may also occur in previously well persons. The mortality rate continues to be high.

Although varicella is typically a disease of childhood, most cases of varicella pneumonia occur in persons over age 20.[258] The incidence of pneumonia in adults with varicella is approximately 15%. The disease occurs primarily from January through May.

After an incubation period averaging 14 days, the disease begins with mild to moderate fever, followed by a generalized papulovesicular skin eruption. Symptoms of pneumonia develop from within 1 to 6 days after the onset of rash and consist of cough, dyspnea, tachypnea, hemoptysis, and pleuritic pain. The physical findings of the chest are minimal in relation to the extent of the disease revealed roentgenographically. The chest roentgenogram demonstrates the nonspecific findings of pulmonary edema, but many patients have a more nodular infiltrate than is characteristic of other forms of edema. The nodules are rarely greater than 0.5 cm. in diameter and tend to have ill-defined margins. Additionally, there may be pleural effusions or hilar adenopathy. The roentgenographic findings correlate with the severity of the skin rash; as cutaneous lesions disappear, the roentgenogram clears rapidly. The leukocyte count is usually normal, but approximately one-third of the patients have a mild leukocytosis.

Varicella pneumonia continues to be a serious disease that may lead to death from respiratory insufficiency. Among all adults, the mortality rate is approximately 12%. However, among pregnant women, the mortality rate has been reported to be 41%.[259] (See Chap. 8).

Heroin (Narcotic) Overdose. Narcotic pulmonary edema is most commonly associated with heroin, since most addicts in the United States use this drug,[260] but it has also been described with intoxication due to morphine, methadone, propoxyphene, and ethchlorvynol.[261] The cause of pulmonary edema is not known, and there may be more than one mechanism. In some patients, the pulmonary edema occurs so rapidly that the patient dies while the injecting needle is still in the vein.[260] In such patients, it may be that heroin pulmonary edema represents a form of neurogenic pulmonary edema that also may occur instantaneously. If this mechanism exists, altered hemodynamics are transient, since cardiac catheterization within 24 hr of formation of pulmonary edema reveals normal wedge and nearly-normal pulmonary artery pressures.[263] In most patients, respiratory distress does not occur for some interval,[264] and a neurogenic mechanism is less attractive. In these patients, increased pulmonary capillary permeability seems more likely, and it has been demonstrated that the edema fluid contains the same concentration of protein as does serum from the same patient.[168] The mediator of increased capillary permeability is not known. Measurements of blood and tissue concentrations of morphine at the time of death support the concept that toxic reactions are dose-related.[265]

The illicit drug user has no way of predicting the concentration of heroin that has been purchased. In studies from different metropolitan areas it has been found that street-obtained consumer packages may have from 0 to 33.3 mg of heroin per package.[266,267] Thus, the possibility of overdose is always present. Additionally, addicts who have been incarcerated and thereby kept drug-free may return to drug abuse with the amount of heroin used previously, disregarding the abstinence-related loss of tolerance for the drug. Once overdose has occurred, the user experiences the usual torpor, but this rapidly progresses to stupor, which usually is accompanied by irregular, slow respiration. Coma and respiratory arrest may occur, and in some cases, death occurs rapidly.

Although the method of reporting patients is variable, it is possible to gain a relatively clear impression of the clinical spectrum with which the patient presents to an emergency room.[264,268–271] Most patients are young, and over 90% are men. Approximately 25% have a mixed overdose, with the most common additional drug being alcohol. Data are not available to indicate the percentage of patients with overdose that develop pulmonary edema, but of those who are hospitalized, approximately 50% develop pulmonary edema. At the time of presentation, almost all patients are comatose or semicomatose. Approximately 70% have a markedly depressed respiratory rate, but, paradoxically, approximately 20% demonstrate tachypnea. Ninety percent of the patients have a tachycardia greater than 100 beats per min, but only 10% are hypotensive at the time of admission. Ninety percent of patients have constricted pupils; but in approximately 5% the pupils are normal, and in 5% the pupils are dilated. The latter is thought to be due to cerebral anoxia in some patients and mixed drug overdose in others. Fever that cannot be attributed to infection is present in 15% of patients at the time of admission. In approximately 50% of the patients, the examiner is able to find evidence of repeated intravenous injections, most commonly in the antecubital fossae. Of those patients who ultimately develop pulmonary edema, 75% have rales in the lung bases and 90% demonstrate pulmonary edema roentgenographically on presentation to the hospital. The electrocardiogram frequently demonstrates nonspecific changes of the ST-T waves.

A small number of tracings have evidence suggesting pulmonary hypertension, including peaked P waves or a right-bundle-branch-block pattern. Approximately 10% of the patients have some abnormality of rhythm or conduction. Approximately 60% of the patients demonstrate a leukocytosis, not uncommonly greater than 20,000 cells/mm^3. An additional 20% of patients have less than 5000 cells/mm^3. On urinalysis, 40% of the patients have been reported to have glycosuria, and 45%, proteinuria. On the average, arterial oxygenation is markedly depressed at the time of admission, with the PaO_2 characteristically less than 50 mm Hg while breathing room air and less than 200 mm Hg breathing 100% oxygen. Most patients demonstrate hypoventilation, but some are hyperventilating. The *p*H is reduced out of proportion to the increase in $PaCO_2$, indicating a combined respiratory and metabolic acidosis, with an average *p*H less than 7.20.

Patients suspected of narcotic overdose should be given a narcotic antagonist, N-allyl-nor-oxymorphone (Narcan), intravenously. The initial adult dose is 0.4 mg (1 ml), and if improvement in respiratory function is not obtained within 2 minutes, it may be repeated at 2- to 3-minute intervals. Failure to obtain significant improvement after 2 or 3 doses suggests that the cause of coma is not a narcotic. If the patient responds, additional drug may be necessary minutes to hours later if a recrudescence of symptoms occurs.

When the patients are treated with a narcotic antagonist, with oxygenation, and with ventilatory support when necessary, their clinical, roentgenographic, and arterial-blood-gas improvement is usually dramatic. The patients frequently become alert within 2 hr. The physical findings of pulmonary edema characteristically clear during the course of 24 hr. Roentgenographic clearing is usually marked within 2 days, but complete clearing takes, on the average, 4 days and may take as long as 4 weeks.[272,273] Patients whose roentgenograms demonstrate a progressive worsening, especially in localized areas, should be assumed to have superimposed bacterial pneumonia. Assessment of lung function indicates that abnormalities persist longer than indicated by clinical or roentgenographic response.[271] The physiological dead-space-to-tidal-volume ratio is larger than normal for at least 5 days. The vital capacity and total lung capacity are reduced for at least 10 days, and lung compliance parallels the changes in lung volumes. The diffusing capacity tends to be markedly decreased and does not tend to improve over a 10-day period following the pulmonary edema. Two patients studied 10 and 12 wk, after initial insult still had functional abnormalities.[274] Longer follow-up has not been reported.

Smoke Inhalation and Respiratory Burns. It has long been recognized that respiratory tract damage is a major cause of mortality in burn victims,[275] and it is now apparent that inhalation of smoke in the absence of thermal burns is also a major cause of death.[276,277] Respiratory burns have been reported to occur in approximately 15% of hospitalized burned patients[278] and have been reported to be the major cause of death in up to 70% of burned patients who do not survive.[279] Smoke inhalation or asphyxia was reported to be the primary cause of death in 30% of all fire fatalities in New York City during the years 1966 and 1967.[280]

A respiratory burn is thought to be caused by thermal energy. The amount of coexisting body-surface burn is extremely variable, and the presence or absence of facial burns does not correlate well with respiratory tract involvement.[281] The respiratory lesion tends to involve the pharynx, larynx, trachea, and major bronchi, with a severe inflammatory and necrotizing lesion. Smoke inhalation may involve persons without significant body surface burns and is apparently a chemical injury. The type of respiratory damage probably relates to the type of burning material and the chemicals contained in the resulting smoke.[282] Smoke may produce tracheobronchitis, bronchiolitis, and pulmonary edema. Many patients have a combined thermal and chemical injury, and clinically it is wise to consider these lesions together.[263]

The incidence of respiratory complications after thermal injury is related to the severity of surface burn and the presence or absence of smoke inhalation.[284–286] The compromise in pulmonary function after smoke inhalation is usually an early event.[286,287] The diagnosis of potentially serious smoke inhalation may be made in approximately 85% of patients by the finding of greater than 15% carboxyhemoglobin,[277] and serious airways obstruction may be demonstrated by spirometry within a few hours of the exposure.[286] Airways obstruction progresses for approximately 24 hr, and ARDS may supervene during this interval. During the next 24 hr airways obstruction tends to improve, but resolution may require many weeks in survivors. Patients with only large surface burns develop primarily a restrictive lung defect and hypoxemia, which is maximal on the third day after injury.[286] The severity of changes correlates with the percentage of chest burn and with the net fluid intake. Patients with both smoke inhalation and large body-surface burns develop a combined pulmonary lesion that is more severe than when the injuries occur independently.

Patients with severe airways involvement demonstrate physical findings similar to those of asthmatic patients: wheezing, a cough producing sputum that is characteristically thick and may be black, and quiet breath sounds if airway obstruction is severe. The chest roentgenogram may reveal hyperinflated lung fields. Patients with an alveolar injury demonstrate the physical and roentenographic findings of pulmonary edema. There may be a combination of these findings in some patients. During the course of resolution, a superimposed bacterial pneumonia very commonly occurs, especially in patients who have had bronchiolitis.[279] One defect thought to lead to pneumonia is an impairment of alveolar macrophage chemotaxis induced by smoke inhalation.[288] The most common bacterial pathogens are *Staphylococcus aureus* and *Pseudomonas aeruginosa*.

The mortality rate for this syndrome varies from 10 to 50%. Long-term studies of a significant number of patients who survive are not available; presumably, most survivors have normal lung function. However, cases of delayed onset of tracheal stenosis, bronchiectasis, and bronchiolitis obliterans have been reported.[289,290]

The inhalation of toxic chemicals may produce a lung lesion very similar to that of smoke inhalation. Pulmonary edema has been reported as a result of exposure to phosgene,[291] chlorine,[292,293] the oxides of nitrogen,[294] ozone,[295] sulfur dioxide,[296] metallic oxides,[297] acid fumes,[298] and more complex chemical fumes.[298] The term *silo filler's disease* has been applied to pulmonary edema secondary to the oxides of nitrogen, since grains stored in closed spaces may spontaneously generate these chemicals. Gases that are extremely soluble in water, such as sulfur dioxide, may produce serious ocular, nasal, and tracheobronchial inflammation as well as cause pulmonary edema.[296] The pulmonary edema has been demonstrated to result from diffuse damage to alveolar epithelial and endothelial cells, resulting in increased capillary permeability.[299,300]

Industrial accidents or mishaps in the transport of chemicals cause most of the incidents of toxic fume inhalation. Most commonly, the patient and witnesses are aware of the exposure because of the color or smell of the fumes and the immediate onset of symptoms, such as lacrimation, rhinorrhea, or cough. However, in some instances, the exposure may not have been appreciated, and the correct diagnosis can only be made by taking a meticulous history of work conditions.

The clinical presentation is similar to that for patients with smoke inhalation. It is important to note that the onset of symptoms may be delayed for several hours; asymptomatic patients with chemical fume exposure should be observed for at least 24 hr following the event. Symptoms, physical abnormalities, and roentgenographic findings depend on the presence or absence of involvement of the tracheobronchial tree, in addition to pulmonary edema. In surviving patients, resolution most commonly requires several days. The incidence of secondary bacterial pneumonia evidently is not as high as with smoke inhalation. The mortality rate depends on the intensity of the exposure. Long-term follow-up has been performed best in patients with chlorine intoxication and has suggested permanent pulmonary fibrosis in some patients.[292] Chronic bronchiolitis obliterans following exposure to the oxides of nitrogen,[301] and fixed airways obstruction following sulfur dioxide[296] have been reported.

Oxygen Toxicity. Unfortunately, toxic chemicals and smoke are not the only inhalants that produce pulmonary edema; prolonged breathing of high concentrations of oxygen is toxic to the lungs. The adverse effects of oxygen were described in animals as long ago as 1899.[302] The mortality and pathological findings associated with oxygen toxicity subsequently have been studied extensively in a variety of laboratory animals. There is marked variability in the time of onset of pulmonary alterations, with a latent period averaging between 24 and 72 hr of exposure to 100% oxygen. When lesions appear, the histological picture is similar to that of pulmonary edema due to increased pulmonary capillary permeability. Similar lesions have been described in humans who have been treated with prolonged courses of high concentrations of inspired oxygen.[303-306] The earliest change observed by electron microscopy is thickening of interstitial spaces by edema fluid containing fibrin strands, leukocytes, thrombocytes, and macrophages.[307] This occurs before demonstrable damage to endothelial cells, but with more severe injury, these cells are seen in various stages of destruction. Alveolar epithelial cells degenerate only late in the course. Animals surviving prolonged oxygen exposure may show resolution of these changes or may have permanent changes of fibrosis and emphysema.[308,309]

Normal persons experience symptoms from 6 to 30 hr after breathing 100% oxygen at atmospheric pressure, and symptoms become severe enough to limit further exposure in 53 to 75 hr.[310] Symptoms include substernal distress, paresthesias, nausea and vomiting, general malaise, fatigue, and dyspnea if exposure continues. Pulmonary function analysis reveals a progressive decrease in lung volumes and diffusing capacity, with no indication of airways obstruction.[311-318] Mucociliary clearance of the tracheobronchial tree is impaired by high concentrations of inhaled oxygen.

Clinically, it is rarely necessary to administer 100% oxygen. An important question, therefore, is the length of administration of lesser concentrations of oxygen that produces pulmonary damage. Normal humans have been found to withstand an inspired oxygen concentration equivalent to 55% for 7 days.[314] However, each subject experienced substernal pain from the second day onward, suggesting early oxygen toxicity. In a separate experiment, normal subjects were able to withstand the equivalent of 35% oxygen for 30 days without demonstrable effects.[315] It seems reasonable to believe that the normal person's tolerance for oxygen for protracted intervals lies between these two values. However, experimental evidence suggests that pre-existing injuries to the alveolar epithelium and capillary endothelium increase susceptibility to the toxic effects of oxygen.[316] Thus, no definitive dose–time relationship for oxygen can be given for oxygen therapy.

The only patients who require protracted administration of high concentrations of oxygen are those with pulmonary edema due to increased capillary permeability. It may be impossible to differentiate among a worsening of the underlying disease, left ventricular failure, the onset of bacterial pneumonia, or oxygen toxicity. In these circumstances, the patient develops a progressively stiffer lung, requiring greater inflation pressures by the ventilator, and worsening hypoxemia due to additional right-to-left shunting. Physical examination and chest roentgenogram demonstrate a worsening of the diffuse pulmonary infiltrates.

In most clinical reports, it is not possible to determine the course of oxygen toxicity *per se*, separate from the underlying lung disease. In a report of patients with respiratory insufficiency secondary to muscular weakness who developed oxygen toxicity, most patients improved markedly within 2 to 5 days after reduction of the inspired oxygen concentration from 87 to 40%.[317] Roentgenographic infiltrates decreased in 1 to 4 wk and disappeared in from 3 to 7 wk. One patient studied 11 wk later had normal pulmonary functions.

At present the free-radical theory of oxygen toxicity indicates that the highly reactive metabolites of molecular oxygen cause the pulmonary damage observed with hyperoxia.[215,318,318a] Normal cellular oxidation–reduction processes lead to the formation of a highly reactive cytotoxic free-radical, superoxide anion (O_2^-). Subsequent intracellular reactions of O_2^- lead to the formation of hydrogen peroxide, hydroxyl radicals, and singlet oxygen. These short-lived species, the formation of which are greatly increased during hyperoxia, are capable of various toxic activities. This theory has led to attempts to augment the normal antioxidant protective systems by exogenous administration of various substances. Vitamin E has been used in premature infants, who are normally deficient in this vitamin, to reduce the incidence of retrolental fibroplasia,[319,320] hemolytic anemia,[321] and perhaps bronchopulmonary dysplasia[322] caused by therapy with high concentrations of inspired oxygen. The administration of superoxide dismutase, an intrinsic antioxidant enzyme, has not lead to consistent results in animal studies.[323,324] However, animal investigations to test the protective effect of small doses of bacterial endotoxin have been more encouraging.[325,326] Thus, clinical measures to protect against the deleterious effects of oxygen therapy may be available within a few years.

Near-Drowning. Persons who survive immersion in fresh water or seawater may develop pulmonary edema.[327] Autopsies on persons who do not survive reveal the same pulmonary pathological changes described for other causes of pulmonary edema. Drowning victims also frequently aspirate foreign materials other than water, including vomitus, mud or sand, and fragments of aquatic vegetation.[328] Electron microscopic studies in animals reveal that the changes in freshwater drowning are predominantly osmotic in nature, as indicated by severe cellular disruption, mitochondrial swelling, and endothelial destruction.[329] In seawater drowning, the lung structure is preserved, but formation of vacuoles, discontinuity of alveolar lining cells, and swelling of cells occur.[329]

While drowning, the victim usually aspirates some volume of water. Fresh water is hypotonic, and seawater is hypertonic, relative to the blood, causing movement of fluid across the alveolar–capillary membranes into the blood or into the lungs, respectively. The resultant changes in electrolyte concentrations in blood are proportional to the volume of fluid aspirated.[330,331] In experimental animals that survive near-drowning, electrolyte values return to normal with 1 hr of aspiration,[332] and serum electrolyte values in patients who survive are usually normal at the time the patient arrives at a medical treatment facility.[328,333] It is likely that patients who aspirate large quantities of fresh water succumb at poolside to ventricular fibrillation due to profound electrolyte changes and to hypoxemia. In the case of drowning in seawater, fibrillation is unlikely, and it is probably hypoxemia that leads to the patient's death. In either case, if the patient survives long enough to reach a medical treatment facility, the primary problem is the management of pulmonary edema.

Following an episode of near-drowning, most patients are apneic and require mouth-to-mouth resuscitation.[333,334] When admitted to the emergency room, most patients are unconscious, and many develop additional signs referable to the central nervous system, such as convulsions. Most patients demonstrate tachypnea, tachycardia, and the findings of pulmonary edema. Some, however, may appear normal at the time of admission but develop the signs of pulmonary edema a few hours later, a syndrome sometimes referred to as *secondary drowning*.[330,334] Cardiac arrhythmias, excepting for premature ventricular contractions, are unusual. The chest roentgenogram is typical of pulmonary edema.[335] Fever and a polymorphonuclear leukocytosis up to 38,000 cells per mm^3 are present in over half of the patients. Serum electrolyte values are normal or nearly normal. Victims of freshwater drowning may demonstrate evidence of hemolysis.

With early therapy of pulmonary edema, most patients survive. The course of resolution of the pulmonary edema has not been carefully recorded, but apparently it is similar to that for aspiration of gastric contents (*i.e.*, on the average, 4 to 5 days). It is assumed that pulmonary function returns to normal following an episode of near-drowning, but no long-term studies are available.

Fat Embolism. Some injured patients develop a distinctive form of respiratory failure in the postinjury period: fat embolism. (See also Chap. 11.) The causative mechanisms of fat embolization are still not entirely clear.[336] The neutral fat that embolizes the lung evidently is liberated from marrow fat by mechanical forces.[337] The triolein of neutral fats is probably in part hydrolyzed to free fatty acids by lipoprotein lipase within the lung,[338] and the major lung damage is due to the free fatty acids.[339] However, part of the lung damage may be mediated by pulmonary hypertension caused by the embolization,[340] thrombocytopenia induced by the circulating fat,[341] or fibrin coagulation and lysis in the lung.[342,343] Whatever the etiology, the lung responds with the same histological appearance that characterizes other causes of high-permeability pulmonary edema, with the additional feature of fat globules in small blood vessels and free in alveolar spaces.

Although fat globules have been demonstrated to be present in femoral vein samples following total hip replacement or fractures of the lower extremities,[344,345] most patients do not develop the fat-embolization syndrome. Many patients, however, develop transient hypoxemia following injury involving fractures.[346] More severe pulmonary damage correlates with thrombocytopenia,[347] suggesting associated disseminated intravascular coagulation; and patients who develop the fat-embolization syndrome may be constitutionally different from those who do not in regard to carbohydrate and lipid metabolism, coagulation, capillary fragility, and neurohumoral regulation in response to exercise.[348]

The syndrome most commonly occurs in patients with long bone fractures, especially of the femur or tibia. The diagnosis is established primarily on clinical grounds.[349–352] Major features include the symptoms and signs of pulmonary edema, central-nervous-system symptoms unrelated to head injury, and a petechial rash distributed to the upper part of the body.[353] Less important diagnostic features include tachycardia, fever, retinal petechiae, and oliguria or anuria. Useful laboratory findings include fat globules in the urine, a sudden drop in hemoglobin concentration, thrombocytopenia, an elevated sedimentation rate, and fat globules in the sputum. Serum lipase levels frequently are elevated late in the course. Fat globules may occasionally be demonstrated by microscopic examination of whole blood. Most of these findings are nonspecific, may occur without pulmonary manifestations, and are present in fewer than half of the patients suspected of having fat embolism. Consequently, this diagnosis is generally made on the basis of pulmonary edema and cerebral symptoms occurring in the clinical setting of a patient who has had bony fractures for from 4 hr to 5 days before the onset of symptoms.

Specific forms of therapy for fat embolism not suggested for other patients with ARDS have been proposed. Owing to a lack of understanding of the major cause of the pulmonary lesion, these therapies are mutually contradictory.[336,351] Intravenous infusion of alcohol has been suggested on the basis of its action as a lipoprotein lipase inhibitor, in order to retard the conversion of neutral fat to free fatty acids. Heparin has been suggested in order to activate lipoprotein lipase to accelerate conversion and decrease the amount of circulating neutral fat. Low-molecular-weight dextran has been suggested to reduce intravascular aggregations of erythrocytes. Due to a lack of proven efficacy and to the contradictory nature of these therapies, most attention now is directed at an early recognition of the syndrome and treatment of the pulmonary edema. The mortality rate reported in the literature as 10 to 40%, is probably much lower with modern management.

Uremia. Patients with renal failure frequently develop pulmonary edema. In many patients, left ventricular failure exists because of some combination of anemia, hypertension, atherosclerosis, and vascular calcification. In some patients, increased intravascular and plasma volumes may lead to a venous congestive syndrome in the absence of myocardial disease. However, pulmonary edema may exist in some patients with normal pulmonary capillary pressures,[354] and pulmonary edema may resolve following dialysis, despite a positive fluid balance.[355] These findings suggest that uremic pneumonitis exists in some patients because of increased pulmonary capillary permeability. The histological findings in the lung of such patients are similar to those found in other causes of pulmonary edema due to increased capillary permeability.

Patients with uremic pneumonitis develop progressive dyspnea over the course of days. Fibrinous pleuritis with pleural pain is not uncommon in patients with chronic uremia and may occur concomitantly with the pulmonary edema.[356] Physical findings of the chest are typical of pulmonary edema. The chest roentgenogram frequently demonstrates symmetrical alveolar infiltrates limited to the hilar areas, with clear peripheral zones, the so-called bat wing or butterfly wing pattern.[357] These changes revert toward normal rapidly after dialysis.

Pancreatitis. Up to 55% of patients with acute pancreatitis develop pulmonary complications, including elevated diaphragms, atelectasis, pneumonia, pulmonary infarcts, and pleural effusions.[358,358a] Pulmonary edema has been reported in approximately 40% of patients dying of pancreatitis.[359] Although there are many potential causes of pulmonary edema in these critically ill patients, 5 to 22% of all patients with pancreatitis are thought to have ARDS.[360–362a] The high protein concentration of the edema fluid supports this diagnosis.[361,363] Release of toxic substances such as trypsin, phospholipase A, and kallikrein during pancreatitis has been the suggested mechanism.[364–369]

Many patients with pancreatitis are seriously hypoxemic.[370,371] The full syndrome of ARDS, however, develops 2 to 7 days following hospitalization for acute pancreatitis, and in survivors resolves slowly over 1 to 3 wk. Physical, roentgenographic, and laboratory findings are similar to those of other forms of ARDS. In a single patient tested 3 mon after the episode, the diffusing capacity was found to be 50% of that predicted. The mortality rate, when the severe syndrome develops, may be as high as 80%.[362] Less severely ill patients frequently have reduced vital capacity and diffusing capacity as their only abnormalities of function.[362a]

Other Disorders. Pulmonary edema due to increased pulmonary capillary permeability has been reported to occur with disorders other than those listed on page 264 (Differential Diagnosis of Acute Respiratory Failure due to Pulmonary Edema) and discussed above. These include disseminated intravascular coagulation,[372–374,375] prolonged cardiopulmonary bypass using a disk oxygenator,[376,377] paraquat poisoning,[378] and injection of meglumine diatrizoate for intravenous pyelography,[379] among others. The clinical and pathological manifestations are similar to those described. (See also Chap. 11).

Various drugs may cause pulmonary edema in addition to the narcotics described previously. These are summarized in Chapter 13 under Drug-Induced Disease. Patients with salicylate intoxication may develop a severe illness with encephalopathy, proteinuria, and pulmonary edema.[379a]

It is clear that ARDS represents a limited response of the lung to a variety of toxic insults. It is not clear whether many of these insults damage the lung through a common mediator or mediators. The similar pathophysiology produced, however, suggests that the principles of therapy are similar in all of these syndromes.

THERAPY FOR THE ACUTE RESPIRATORY DISTRESS SYNDROME (ARDS)

The principles of ventilatory support indicated in other sections of this chapter pertain as well to patients with pulmonary edema due to increased pulmonary capillary permeability, especially those sections on artificial airways, determination of ventilatory volume, ventilators, continuing respiratory care, and extubation. These principles will not be reiterated in this section; only modifications of such therapy necessary for patients with pulmonary edema will be indicated.

Oxygen and Ventilatory Support

Patients with mild pulmonary edema and patients whose course can not be predicted may need only supplemental oxygen without ventilatory support. Humidified oxygen is administered by means of nasal cannulas (nasal prongs), a loose-fitting face mask, or a face tent. The delivery device is not critical and depends primarily on patient acceptance. Because nasal cannulas allow a free range of motion for the patient, this device usually is preferred. Although it is not possible to accurately predict the fraction of inspired oxygen (F_IO_2) when using these devices, it is not necessary to give a precisely controlled dose of oxygen to this type of patient. The range of F_IO_2 obtained for several devices is indicated in Table 7-2,[380] and suggested devices for a variety of conditions are listed in Table 7-3. The measurements in Table 7-2 were made in normal persons, and patients with ARDS usually hyperventilate; therefore, the F_IO_2 for patients is probably lower than indicated. It is not possible to continuously administer oxygen at 15 liters/min by means of nasal cannulas, because of patient discomfort. It is apparent that the inspired oxygen concentration achieved is not likely to be sufficiently high to lead to oxygen toxicity. The list below gives factors that affect the inhaled oxygen concentration in patients. Clearly, if the inspiratory flow rate is 20 liters/min, and if inhalation takes only one-third of the time of the total respiratory cycle, 5 liters of oxygen per minute, flowing continually, will provide a very small supplement to the inhaled oxygen concentration.

The decision that endotracheal intubation and ventilatory support is necessary may be difficult. Experimental studies of ARDS in animals suggest that early ventilatory support decreases morbidity and mortality more than ventilatory support after the lesion has become fully developed.[381,382] Thus, it is probably wise to initiate assisted ventilation if there is any concern about the patient's status. Guidelines that have been found helpful by one group of investigators are indicated below.[8]

When a decision to initiate assisted ventilation has been made, the same precautions concerning endotracheal intubation indicated in a previous section must be observed (see p. 239). It is im-

TABLE 7-2. Concentration of Inspired Oxygen Using Various Modes of Delivery

Method	Flow (L/min)	Range (%)	Mean (%)
Nasal cannula			
Mouth closed	5	31–41	36
	10	38–53	45
	15	42–62	52
Mouth open	5	31–39	35
	10	36–48	42
	15	37–57	47
Face mask	5	27–41	34
	10	33–45	39
	15	33–53	43
Face tent	5	31–45	38
	10	37–57	47
	15	37–63	50

TABLE 7-3. Selection of Device for Oxygen Administration to Hypoxemic Patients

Method of Administration	Approximate Inhaled Oxygen Concentration (%)	Patient Best Suited
Room air	21	Normal
Low-range oxygen	25–30	Patients with chronic respiratory disease whose P_{CO_2} rises when given oxygen
Low-flow (1–2 L/min): mask or nasal cannula		
Venturi mask	24, 28, 32	
Medium-range oxygen	35–45	Most patients with moderate hypoxemia due to a variety of causes
Medium flow (4–6 L/min): mask or nasal cannula		
High-range oxygen	70–90	Patients with severe hypoxemia not corrected by medium range oxygen
High-flow (10–15 L/min): mask with reservoir bag		
Endotracheal tube	Any concentration to 100	
Endotracheal tube and respirator	Any concentration to 100	
Endotracheal tube and respirator with positive end-expiratory pressure	Any concentration, frequently permits reduction to safe levels of inhaled oxygen	Patients who require greater than 60% of inhaled oxygen

Factors Affecting Inhaled Oxygen Concentration

Oxygen flow rate, at mouth or nose
Minute ventilation of patient
Inhalation flow rate
Duration of inhalation

portant to recognize that patients with ARDS undergoing endotracheal intubation usually are seriously hypoxemic, and 100% oxygen should be administered before attempting intubation. Since tenacious secretions requiring frequent endotracheal suctioning are not common in most of these patients, nasotracheal intubation is preferred at our hospital.

Patients who relax while being ventilated and allow the ventilator to assume their work of breathing generally are maintained on assisted ventilation; that is, the patient is allowed to trigger the respiratory rate while the tidal volume is determined by the ventilator. Clinical experience suggests that initially, tidal volumes in the range of 10 to 15 ml per kg of ideal body weight are reasonable.[7]

Guidelines for Ventilatory Support in Patients with ARDS

Respiratory rate	> 35/min
PaO_2 on mask O_2	< 70 mm Hg
PAO_2-PaO_2 on 100% O_2	> 450 mm Hg
V_D/V_T	> 0.60

Patients who are agitated and cannot allow the machine to assume their work of breathing are sedated by the slow, intravenous administration of morphine or diazepam, and the patient is begun on controlled ventilation. In some cases, it may be necessary to produce relaxation by paralyzing drugs such as pancuronium bromide. In these patients, the principles of determination of ventilatory volume, already enumerated in the section on ventilatory failure, apply, with certain modifications. Patients with ARDS tend to have large dead-space-to-tidal-volume ratios (V_D/V_T), which remain constant despite increasing tidal volumes.[383] In initiating controlled ventilation, it is reasonable to assume a V_D/V_T ratio of 0.5, irrespective of the tidal volume to be administered. The equation to determine respiratory rate (f), modified from the list on page 243, (Equations Useful for Initial Ventilatory Management), then becomes

$$f = \frac{69}{0.5 \times V_T \text{ (per kg)}}$$

Since the V_D/V_T ratio may be considerably different from that estimated, arterial blood gases are obtained after a brief interval to determine the corrections necessary to normalize the $PaCO_2$. If the slow respiratory rate appears to agitate the patient, additional links of tubing between the ventilator exhalation valve or V connector and the patient may be added in order to increase the apparatus dead space and allow large tidal volumes at a faster respiratory rate.

Continuous assisted or controlled ventilation in these patients should improve arterial oxygenation, as well as carbon dioxide retention or metabolic acidosis, should these exist.[384–387] Oxygenation is improved because of the reopening of lung units that had not been ventilated, decreasing the amount of right-to-left shunt. Metabolic acidosis is improved because of the decreased work of breathing. To maximally improve oxygenation, large tidal volumes should be used. Excessively large tidal volumes, however, require inflation pressures that may result in a decreased cardiac output and less oxygen delivery to the tissues[388] and may potentiate lung rupture with pneumothorax.[389] Excessive tidal volumes also may be deleterious to the conservation of surfactant.[390] Thus, tidal volumes may be either too small or too large for optimal patients care.

Measurements of static compliance may be of help in determining the optimal tidal volume (see p. 246). The static compliance (exhaled tidal volume divided by static airway pressure) is obtained at several different tidal volumes, allowing the construction of a pressure volume

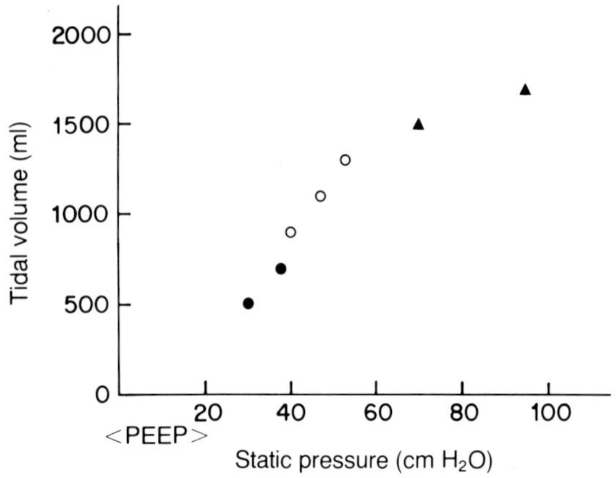

FIG. 7-10. This graph represents the static pressure–volume relationship of the lungs and thorax in a patient with ARDS. Each observation represents the inflation-hold manometer pressure obtained on the ventilator (horizontal axis) for the tidal volume indicated on the vertical axis. The static compliance equals tidal volume divided by inflation-hold pressure minus PEEP pressure. In this example, in which PEEP pressure is 10 cm H_2O, compliance for tidal volumes indicated by the closed circles is 25 ml/cm H_2O; open circles, 30 ml/cm H_2O; and triangles, 25 and 20 ml/cm H_2O.

curve over the entire lung volume above functional residual capacity (Fig. 7-10). At low tidal volumes, the compliance may be less than at tidal volumes in a mid-lung range; this suggests opening of atelectatic lung units when sufficiently large tidal volumes are delivered. At high lung volumes, compliance also is worse than in then mid-lung range; this suggests that some lung units are being distended beyond their total capacity. Patients with tidal ventilation in the range of lung volume with the highest compliance are less likely to experience pneumothorax[389] and are most likely to have the best possible oxygen delivery to tissues (cardiac output times arterial oxygen content).[391] Since compliance changes with improvement or worsening of the pulmonary parenchymal disease, measurements of compliance over the entire lung volume should be performed at least once a day, to direct selection of the appropriate tidal volume.

Patients with very severe pulmonary edema due to increased pulmonary capillary permeability may remain hypoxemic despite successful ventilatory support, unless very high concentrations of inspired oxygen are administered, and some remain hypoxemic even with a F_IO_2 of 1.0. In patients requiring an F_IO_2 greater than 0.40 to 0.60, the use of positive end-expiratory pressure (PEEP) may improve arterial oxygenation and allow a reduction of the F_IO_2 into a less toxic range.[392–394] With this technique, the patient's lungs are inflated during the inspiration with whatever positive pressure is necessary to cause the desired tidal volume, and during expiration the patient is made to breathe out against a lesser positive pressure. The positive end-expiratory pressure causes an increase in the functional residual capacity (*i.e.*, the patient's lung remains at a greater degree of inflation during expiration).[395] The larger lung volume may improve arterial oxygenation by preventing the collapse of small airways and alveoli during expiration. However, in some patients hypoxemia is worsened by PEEP; if the lung injury is not relatively uniform, there may be a shift in regional perfusion away from the better-ventilated lung.[396,397] PEEP does not cause a decrease in the magnitude of the pulmonary edema in syndromes due to excess pulmonary capillary permeability.[398,399] Further, although the arterial oxygen content may be improved, the delivery of oxygen to tissues may be decreased because of a decrease in cardiac output. Although the cause of the decreased cardiac output is not entirely defined, it is evidently due to a decrease in venous return and a decrease in myocardial contractility due to the increased intrathoracic pressure and to reflexes mediated in the vagus nerve due to lung inflation.[400–406]

Positive end expiratory pressure should be considered if a patient with severe pulmonary edema due to increased capillary permeability does not have acceptable arterial oxygenation on standard ventilator therapy with an inspired oxygen concentration that may be toxic to the lungs. Therefore, if the PaO_2 is approximately 60 mm Hg or less, the F_IO_2 0.5 or more, and usual measures to improve ventilation have been instituted, positive and expiratory pressure may be indicated. All commercially available volume ventilators have PEEP controls. Approximately 5 cm H_2O PEEP is applied, and the patient is observed for adverse cardiovascular effects, such as marked tachycardia, bradycardia, arrhythmia, or hypotension. If such does not occur, arterial blood gases are obtained after 30 to 60 minutes of equilibration, to determine if the desired improvement in PaO_2 has been achieved. If possible, measurements of cardiac output are desirable in order to calculate net tissue oxygen delivery; alternatively, mixed venous Po_2 may be used for the same purpose, although some evidence suggests that mixed venous PO_2 may not accurately reflect adequacy of tissue oxygenation in these circumstances.[407] If no apparent deleterious effects have occurred, but the PaO_2 or net oxygen delivery has not improved, PEEP is increased by 3 to 5 cm H_2O. This procedure is repeated until deleterious cardiovascular effects or the desired improvement in oxygen transport is achieved. The latter allows a decrease in the F_IO_2 to a nontoxic range. It should be noted that PEEP causes an increase in the functional residual capacity, which may dictate a decrease in tidal volume to prevent overdistention of the lungs. To measure effective compliance of a patient on PEEP in order to ventilate the patient in the lung volume range of the best compliance, PEEP pressure should be subtracted from static inflation pressure before dividing into tidal volume. On the average, the level of PEEP and tidal volume that results in the best static compliance allows the best cardiac output.[391]

Patients being treated with PEEP evidently are more liable to lung rupture and pneumothorax than are patients treated with IPPB alone. This may be because more severely damaged patients are treated with PEEP, or it may be caused by ventilating patients at too high a lung volume. In any event, sudden deterioration of a patient during this form of therapy suggests a tension pneumothorax, which in many instances is bilateral. Emergency chest-tube therapy may be necessary, based only on the physical examination without the benefit of a chest roentgenogram. Such patients generally have a rapid deterioration of the cardiovascular status.

When patients with ARDS improve, PEEP is progressively reduced in the same stepwise manner in which it was applied. A decision to discontinue ventilatory support may be based on the criteria used for initiating ventilatory support (see Guidelines for Ventilatory Support). That is, when these parameters have returned toward normal, ventilatory support may no longer be necessary. The weaning of these patients from ventilatory support is similar to that described in the previous section on extubation.

A ventilatory technique used successfully in infants with the neonatal respiratory distress syndrome is the application of continuous positive airway pressure (CPAP).[408] The airway is connected to a system which is continuously pressurized by the controlled inflow and outflow of gas. The patient inspires voluntarily by muscular force with some assistance from the positive airway pressure and expires, preferably with lung and chest-wall elastic recoil, against the positive airway pressure. Variations of this technique have been used in adult patients who are able to ventilate with their own muscular effort; such techniques may be associated with fewer cardiovascular and barotrauma side-effects than standard ventilator therapy with PEEP.[409–412]

Flow-guided catheters frequently are used to measure both pulmonary vascular and wedge pressures, as a guide to fluid or diuretic therapy in patients with ARDS. The transducers used for pressure measurement are referenced to atmospheric pressure, as is done in standard cardiac catheterizations while patients are spontaneously breathing. However, during spontaneous breathing the pressure surrounding the heart (pleural pressure) is subatmospheric and alveolar pressure is approximately atmospheric, whereas such pressures are above atmospheric pressure in patients on ventilatory support with PEEP. Thus, net ventricular-filling pressure and the pulmonary capillary pressure measured in patients on PEEP may not be directly comparable to normal values obtained in spontaneously breathing persons.[413,414] Directional changes in pressure over time may be more valuable than a single set of measurements. Further, while the serious complication rate of such catheters is low,[415] invasive procedures must always be used with caution.

Although it is clear that various ventilatory techniques may result in improvement in physiological parameters and survival of some seriously ill patients with ARDS, there have been no prospective studies randomizing adult patients to differing ventilator treatment regimens to determine which yield the greatest reduction in mortality. Indeed, an uncontrolled, retrospective study has suggested that ventilatory therapy with PEEP yields no more survivors than ventilator therapy without PEEP among patients with very severe hypoxemia.[416] Until appropriate studies are available, vigorous advocacy of one form of mechanical therapy over another seems unwise.

Additional Therapy

Adrenal corticosteroids have been recommended for treating most types of pulmonary edema due to increased capillary permeability. Some authors recommend pharmacologic doses.[334,417–419] Experimental studies in animals have been contradictory, with some studies supporting the use of steroids,[232,236,418–426] and some studies finding no benefit.[237,427–433] Similarly, uncontrolled clinical studies have suggested beneficial effects,[239,245,434–436] or no demonstrable effect[241,257,351,389,437] from corticosteroid therapy. A prospective, double-blind randomized control study of any of these disorders evidently is not available. Thus, the correct role of corticosteroids in the treatment of these disorders is not known at present.

Diuresis and Plasma Expanders. The use of diuretic agents in patients with pulmonary edema due to left ventricular failure is well established. Several clinical studies report improvement in post-traumatic or postoperative hypoxemic patients with the intravenous administration of the potent diuretics furosemide or ethacrynic acid.[438–440] In many of the patients reported, it is clear that pulmonary edema was associated with the administration of excessive amounts of intravenous fluids, and, hence, the diuretics were used in patients with a venous congestive syndrome rather than a true increased pulmonary capillary permeability syndrome. In some patients who apparently had true ARDS, however, there was improvement in oxygenation. These data are consistent with the demonstration in experimental animals that small increases in pulmonary capillary pressure cause marked increases in extravascular lung water in animals with excessive pulmonary capillary permeability.[152] In addition, diuretics have an extrarenal effect that is thought to reduce the vascular surface area for exchange of fluid in the lung and thereby decrease pulmonary edema.[441] Thus, diuretic-induced hypovolemia may improve arterial oxygenation in patients with ARDS; however, cardiac output may be reduced simultaneously, resulting in poor tissue perfusion or even shock.

In clinical practice, it may not be possible to correctly estimate the relative importance of these factors in an individual patient. When possible, fluid and diuretic therapy should be guided by direct measurement of pulmonary capillary wedge pressure, which should be maintained in a low-normal range. When this measurement is not available, mild diuresis may be attempted, with careful monitoring of the patient's pulse, blood pressure, urine output, and blood gas values.

High-molecular-weight substances such as dextran and salt-poor human albumin have been administered in order to increase intravascular osmotic pressure, in an attempt to cause reabsorption of pulmonary extravascular lung water.[167,438] Although transient improvement may be observed, these substances traverse the excessively permeable pulmonary capillaries rapidly and cease to exert the desired effect.[442]

Antimicrobials. Although bacterial infection is the cause of ARDS only in patients with sepsis, and perhaps patients with post-traumatic pulmonary insufficiency, it is clear that these critically ill patients are at increased risk of developing a superimposed bacterial infection.[57,121,148] Because prophylactic antibiotics are of no benefit in this circumstance,[443] antimicrobials are not administered unless evidence suggesting bacterial pneumonia develops. The roentgenographic appearance of a new or progressive pulmonary infiltrate in association with fever, leukocytosis, and purulent tracheobronchial secretions suggests that superinfection has occurred. Although gram-negative bacilli are the most frequent cause of nosocomial pneumonia, gram-positive cocci or anaerobic bacteria may be the cause.

Thus, broad antimicrobial therapy, such as penicillin and gentamicin, is used. Details regarding the precise diagnosis of lung infections and selection of antibiotics are discussed in Chapter 8, Acute Respiratory Tract Infections.

Prognosis

Patients with all of the manifestations of ARDS are at high risk of dying. Of all patients between the ages of 12 and 65 yr who require endotracheal intubation for 24 hr or more with inspired oxygen concentrations of 50% or greater, the mortality rate is approximately 66%; and for patients with arterial oxygen tensions of 50 mm Hg or less while breathing 60 to 100% oxygen at 5 cm H_2O or more PEEP, the mortality rate exceeds 90%.[444] For patients over 65 years with ARDS, mortality exceeds 80%. Death is frequently not due to an inability to support ventilation. The mortality risk for respiratory failure only is 40%. However, failure of other vital organ systems during the course of therapy is common and greatly increases the probability of an unfavorable outcome.

REFERENCES

1. WEST JB: Causes of carbon dioxide retention in lung disease. N Engl J Med 284:1232, 1971
2. RICHTER T, WEST JR, FISHMAN AP: The syndrome of alveolar hypoventilation and diminished sensitivity of the respiratory center. N Engl J Med 256:1165, 1957
3. BERGOFSKY EH: Respiratory failure in disorders of the thoracic cage. Am Rev Respir Dis 119:643, 1979
4. LUCE JM: Respiratory complications of obesity. Chest 78:626, 1980
5. GUILLEMINAULT C, TILKIAN A, DEMENT WC: The sleep apnea syndromes. Annu Rev Med 27:465, 1976
6. ROBIN ED, CROSS CE, ZELIS R: Pulmonary edema. N Engl J Med 288:239, 1973
7. MAHER JF, SCHREINER GE, WESTERVELT FB, JR: Acute glutethimide intoxication. Am J Med 33:70, 1962
8. PONTOPPIDAN H, GEFFIN B, LOWENSTEIN E: Acute respiratory failure in the adult. N Engl J Med 287:690, 743, 799, 1972
9. WILLIAMS MH, JR, SHIM CS: Ventilatory failure. Etiology and clinical forms. Am J Med 48:477, 1970
10. MEAD J, COLLIER C: Relation of volume history of lungs to respiratory mechanics in anesthetized dogs. J Appl Physiol 14:669, 1959
11. FERRIS BG, POLLARD DS: Effect of deep and quiet breathing on pulmonary compliance in man. J Clin Invest 39:143, 1960
12. BENDIXEN HH, SMITH GM, MEAD J: Pattern of ventilation in young adults. J Appl Physiol 19:195, 1964
13. COOPER JD, GRILLO HC: The evolution of tracheal injury due to ventilatory assistance through cuffed tubes. Ann Surg 169:334, 1969
14. COOPER JD, GRILLO HC: Experimental production and prevention of injury due to cuffed tracheal tubes. Surg Gynecol Obstet 129:1235, 1969
15. SHELLY WM, DAWSON RB, MAY IA: Cuffed tubes as a cause of tracheal stenosis. J Thorac Cardiovasc Surg 57:623, 1969
16. GRILLO HC, COOPER JD, GEFFIN B et al: A low-pressure cuff for tracheostomy tubes to minimize tracheal injury. J Thorac Cardiovasc Surg 62:898, 1971
17. DUNN CR, DUNN DL, MOSER KM: Determinants of tracheal injury by cuffed tracheostomy tubes. Chest 65:128, 1974
18. BRYANT LR, TRINKLE JK, DUBILIER L: Reappraisal of tracheal injury from cuffed tracheostomy tubes. JAMA 215:625, 1971
19. Drug Commentary: Evaluation of a muscle relaxant, pancuronium bromide (Pavulon). JAMA 225:745, 1973
20. HELLER ML, WATSON TR, JR: Polarographic study of arterial oxygenation during apnea in man. N Engl J Med 264:326, 1961
21. JAY SJ, JOHANSON WG, JR, PIERCE AK: Respiratory complications of overdose with sedative drugs. Am Rev Respir Dis 112:591, 1975
22. WILSON JE, III, et al: Hypoxemia in pulmonary embolism, a clinical study. J Clin Invest 50:481, 1971
23. RADFORD EP, JR, FERRIS BJ, KRIETE BC: Clinical use of nomogram to estimate proper ventilation during artificial respiration. N Engl J Med 251:877, 1954
24. RADFORD EP, JR: Ventilation standards for use in artificial respiration. J Appl Physiol 7:451, 1955
25. PONTOPPIDAN H, et al: Ventilation and oxygen requirements during prolonged artificial ventilation in patients with respiratory failure. N Engl J Med 273:401, 1965
26. RUCH T, PATTON H (eds): Physiology and Biophysics. Philadelphia, WB Saunders, 1966
27. PIERCE AK: Assisted respiration. Annu Rev Med 20:431, 1969
28. MCPHERSON SP: Respiratory therapy equipment. St. Louis, C. V. Mosby 1969
29. ROBERTSON J, JOHANSON WG, PIERCE AK: Measure-

ment of compliance in ventilator patients (abstr.) Am Rev Respir Dis 105:979, 1972
30. CLARK JM, LAMBERTSEN CJ: Pulmonary oxygen toxicity: A Review. Pharmacol Rev 23:37, 1971
31. NORTHWAY WH, JR, ROSAN RC, PORTER DY: Pulmonary disease following respirator therapy of hyaline-membrane disease. N Engl J Med 276:357, 1967
32. NASH G, BLENNERHASSETT JB, PONTOPPIDAN H: Pulmonary lesions associated with oxygen therapy and artificial ventilation. N Engl J Med 276:368, 1967
33. PONTOPPIDAN H, BERRY PR: Regulation of the inspired oxygen concentration during artificial ventilation. JAMA 201:11, 1967
34. BOSOMWORTH PP, SPENCER FC: Prolonged mechanical ventilation. I. Factors affecting delivered oxygen concentrations and relative humidity. Am Surg 31:377, 1965
35. KOTHEIMER TG, JR, DICKIE KJ, DEGROOT WJ: Mechanical determinants of inspired oxygen concentration in a pressure-cycled ventilator. Am Rev Respir Dis 103:679, 1971
36. SELLERY GR, FAIRLEY HB: Inspired oxygen concentration delivered by the Bird ventilator. Anesthesiology 28:453, 1967
37. DRINKER PA et al: A constant ratio air-oxygen mixer. JAMA 202:531, 1967
38. GAUER O, HENRY JP: Circulatory basis of fluid volume control. Physiol Rev 43:423, 1963
39. PHILBIN DM, BARATZ RA, PATTERSON RW: The effect of carbon dioxide on plasma antidiuretic hormone levels during intermittent positive-pressure breathing. Anesthesiology 33:345, 1970
40. SLADEN A, LAVER MB, PONTOPPIDAN H: Pulmonary complications and water retention in prolonged mechanical ventilation. N Engl J Med 279:448, 1968
41. TONKIN JP, HARRISON GA: The effect on the larynx of prolonged endotracheal intubation. Med J Aust 2:581, 1966
42. PILCHER J: Prolonged orotracheal intubation without tracheostomy for respiratory failure. Br J Dis Chest 61:95, 1967
43. WEG JG: Prolonged endotracheal intubation in respiratory failure. Arch Intern Med 120:679, 1967
44. DIXON TC, SANDO MJW, BOLTON JM et al: A report of 342 cases of prolonged endotracheal intubation. Med J Aust 2:529, 1968
45. HEDDEN J, ERSOZ CJ, DONNELLY MH et al: Laryngotracheal damage after prolonged use of orotracheal tubes in adults. JAMA 207:703, 1969
46. LINDHOL CE: Prolonged endotracheal intubation. Acta Anaesthesiol Scand (Suppl) 33:1, 1969
47. MEAD JW: Tracheotomy—its complications and their management. A study of 212 cases. N Engl J Med 265:519, 1961
48. GEFFIN BG, GRILLO HC, COOPER JD et al: Stenosis following tracheostomy for respiratory care. JAMA 216:1984, 1971
49. ZWILLICH CW et al: Complications of assisted ventilation. A prospective study of 354 consecutive episodes. Am J Med 57:161, 1974
50. ZWILLICH CW, PIERSON DJ: Nasal necrosis: A complication of nasotracheal intubation. Chest 64:376, 1973
51. DIETZ GW, PIERCE AK, CHRISTENSEN EE: Endotracheal tube compression demonstrated by roentgenogram. JAMA 206:2512, 1968
52. COOPER JD, MALT RA: Meteorism produced by nasotracheal intubation and ventilatory assistance. N Engl J Med 287:652, 1972
53. PLUM F, DUNNING MF: Technics for minimizing trauma to the tracheobronchial tree after tracheostomy. N Engl J Med 254:193, 1956
54. AMIKAN B, LANDA J, WEST J et al: Bronchofiberscopic observations of the tracheobronchial tree during intubation. Am Rev Respir Dis 105:747, 1972
55. SACKNER MA, LANDA JF, GREENELTCH N et al: Pathogenesis and prevention of tracheobronchial damage with suction procedures. Chest 64:284, 1973
56. HABERMAN PB et al: Determinants of successful selective tracheobronchial suctioning. N Engl J Med 289:1060, 1973
57. JOHANSON WG, JR, PIERCE AK, SANFORD JP et al: Nosocomial respiratory infections with gram-negative bacilli. Ann Intern Med 77:701, 1972
58. REINARZ JA, WELLS DE, MURPHY TE: An evaluation of tracheostomy care in control of pseudomonas colonization—a Trojan horse! Clin Res 16:56, 1968
59. PONTOPPIDAN H, LAVER MB, GEFFIN B: Acute respiratory failure in the surgical patient. Adv Surg 4:163, 1970
60. FEELEY TW, HEDLEY-WHYTE J: Weaning from controlled ventilation and supplemental oxygen. N Engl J Med 292:903, 1975
61. MCFADDEN ER, JR, LYONS HA: Arterial-blood gas tension in asthma. N Engl J Med 278:1027, 1968
62. KREITZER S, FELDMAN N, SAUNDERS N et al: Bilateral diaphragmatic paralysis with hypercapnic respiratory failure. Am J Med 65:89, 1978
63. SKATRUD J, IBER C, MCHUGH W et al. Determinants of hypoventilation during wakefulness and sleep in diaphragmatic paralysis. Am Rev Respir Dis 121:587, 1980
64. REFSUM HE: Acid–base status in patients with chronic hypercapnia and hypoxemia. Clin Sci 27:407, 1964
65. REFSUM HE: Relationship between state of consciousness and arterial hypoxemia and hypercapnia in patients with pulmonary insufficiency, breathing air. Clin Sci 25:361, 1963
66. MCNICOL MW, CAMPBELL EJM: Severity of respira-

tory failure, arterial blood gases in untreated patients. Lancet 1:336, 1965

67. LAL S: Blood gases in respiratory failure, state on admission to hospital and management. Lancet 1:339, 1965
68. PAROT S, SAUNIER C, GAUTIER H et al: Breathing pattern and hypercapnia in patients with obstructive pulmonary disease. Am Rev Respir Dis 121:985, 1980
69. WAGNER PD, DANTZKER DR, DUECK R et al: Ventilation–perfusion inequality in chronic obstructive pulmonary disease. J Clin Invest 59:203, 1977
70. SORLI J, GRASSINO A, LORANGE G et al: Control of breathing in patients with chronic obstructive lung disease. Clin Sci Mol Med 54:295, 1978
71. BRADLEY CA, FLEETHAM JA, ANTHONISEN NR: Ventilatory control in patients with hypoxemia due to obstructive lung disease. Am Rev Respir Dis 120:21, 1979
72. AUBIER M et al: Central respiratory drive in acute respiratory failure of patients with chronic obstructive pulmonary disease. Am Rev Respir Dis 122:191, 1980
73. SHARP JT et al: Thoracoabdominal motion in chronic obstructive pulmonary disease. Am Rev Respir Dis 115:47, 1977
74. DERENNE J-PH, MACKLEM PT, ROUSSOS CH: The respiratory muscles: Mechanics, control, and pathophysiology. Am Rev Respir Dis 118:119, 373, 581, 1978
75. MACKLEM PT: Respiratory muscles: The vital pump. Chest 78:753, 1980
76. WILLIAMS MH, JR: Ventilatory failure. Medicine 45:317, 1966
77. POSNER JB, PLUM F: Spinal-fluid pH and neurologic symptoms in systemic acidosis. N Engl J Med 277:605, 1967
78. KILBURN KH: Neurologic manifestations of respiratory failure. Arch Intern Med 116:409, 1965
79. CAMPBELL EJM: The J. Burns Amberson lecture: The management of acute respiratory failure in chronic bronchitis and emphysema. Am Rev Respir Dis 96:626, 1967
80. WOOLCOCK AJ, VINCENT HJ, MACKLEM PT: Frequency dependence of compliance as a test for obstruction in the small airways. J Clin Invest 48:1097, 1969
81. MEAD J, TURNER JM, MACKLEM PT et al: Significance of the relationship between lung recoil and maximum expiratory flow. J Appl Physiol 22:95, 1967
82. PRIDE NB, PERMUTT S, RILEY RL et al: Determinants of maximal expiratory flow from the lungs. J Appl Physiol 23:646, 1967
83. PIAFSKY KM, OGLIVIE RI: Drug therapy: Dosage of theophylline in bronchial asthma. N Engl J Med 292:1218, 1975
84. PIAFSKY KM et al: Theophylline kinetics in acute pulmonary edema. Clin Pharmacol Ther 21:310, 1977
85. PIAFSKY KM et al: Theophylline disposition in patients with hepatic cirrhosis. N Engl J Med 296:1495, 1977
86. JENNE JW et al: Apparent theophylline half life fluctuation during treatment of acute left ventricular failure. Am J Hosp Pharma 34:408, 1977
87. POWELL JR et al: The influence of cigarette smoking and sex on theophylline disposition. Am Rev Respir Dis 116:17, 1977
88. JUSKO WJ et al: Intravenous theophylline therapy: Nomogram guidelines. Ann Intern Med 86:400, 1977
89. EATON ML et al: Efficacy of theophylline in "irreversible" airflow obstruction. Ann Intern Med 92:758, 1980
90. MITHOEFER JC: Indications for oxygen therapy in chronic obstructive pulmonary disease. Am Rev Respir Dis (Suppl) 110:35, 1974
91. MITHOEFER JC, HOLFORD FD, KEIGHLEY JFH: The effect of oxygen administration on mixed venous oxygenation in chronic obstructive pulmonary disease. Chest 62:112, 1974
92. FISHMAN AP, FRITTS HW, JR, COURNAND A: Effects fects of acute hypoxia and exercise on the pulmonary circulation. Circulation 22:204, 1960
93. KELLOG RH: Central chemical regulation of respiration. In Fenn WO, Rahn H (eds): Handbook of Physiology. Section 3, Vol 2, p. 507. Baltimore, Waverly Press, 1965
94. LAMBERTSEN CJ: Effects of oxygen at high partial pressure. In Fenn WO, Rahn H (eds): Handbook of Physiology, Section 3, Vol 2, p. 1027. Baltimore, Waverly Press, 1965
95. WEIL JV et al: Hypoxic ventilatory drive in normal man. J Clin Invest 49:1061, 1970
96. WEIL JV, JAMIESON G, BROWN DW et al: The red cell mass arterial oxygen relationship in normal man. J Clin Invest 47:1627, 1968
97. MITHOEFER JC, KEIGHLEY JF, KARETZKY MS: Response of the arterial P_{O_2} to oxygen administration in chronic pulmonary disease. Ann Intern Med 74:328, 1971
98. BONE RC, PIERCE AK, JOHNSON RL, JR: Controlled oxygen administration in acute respiratory failure in chronic obstructive pulmonary disease. Am J Med 65:896, 1978
99. CAMPBELL EJM: Respiratory failure, the relation between oxygen concentration of inspired air and arterial blood. Lancet 2:10, 1960
100. MASSARO DJ, KATZ S, LUCHSINGER PC: Effect of various modes of oxygen administration on the arterial gas values in patients with respiratory acidosis. Br Med J 2:627, 1962
101. SMITH JP, STONE RW, MUSCHENHEIM C: Acute respiratory failure in chronic lung disease. Am Rev Respir Dis 97:791, 1968
102. KETTEL LJ et al: Treatment of acute respiratory

acidosis in chronic obstructive lung disease. JAMA 217:1503, 1971
103. ROTHERAM EB, JR, SAFAR P, ROBIN ED: CNS disorders during mechanical ventilation in chronic pulmonary disease. JAMA 189:993, 1964
104. KILBURN KH: Shock, seizures, and coma with alkalosis during mechanical ventilation. Ann Intern Med 65:977, 1966
105. BEAR R et al: Effect of metabolic alkalosis on respiratory function in patients with chronic obstructive lung disease. CMA Journal, 117:900, 1977
106. ZWILLICH CW et al: Theophylline-induced seizures in adults. Ann Intern Med 82:784, 1975
107. WEINBERGER MM, RIEGELMAN S: Rational use of theophylline for bronchodilation. N Engl J Med 291:151, 1974
108. GOLDBERG I, CHERNIACK RM: The effect of nebulized broncho-dilator delivered with and without IPPB on ventilatory function in chronic obstructive emphysema. Am Rev Respir Dis 91:13, 1965
109. MURRAY JF: Indications for mechanical aids to assist lung inflation in medical patients. Am Rev Respir Dis (Suppl) 122:121, 1980
110. DOLOVICH MB et al: Pulmonary aerosol deposition in chronic bronchitis: intermittent positive pressure breathing versus quiet breathing. Am Rev Respir Dis 115:397, 1977
111. OLDENBURG FA, JR, DOLOVICH MB, MONTGOMERY JM et al: Effects of postural drainage, exercise, and cough on mucus clearance in chronic bronchitis. Am Rev Respir Dis 120:739, 1979
112. MURRAY JB: The ketchup-bottle method. N Engl J Med 300:1155, 1979
113. ROCHESTER DF, GOLDBERG SK: Techniques of respiratory physical therapy. Am Rev Respir Dis (Suppl) 122:133, 1980
114. DARROW G, ANTHONISEN NR: Physiotherapy in hospitalized medical patients. Am Rev Respir Dis (Suppl) 122:155, 1980
115. RADIGAN LR, KING RD: A technique for the prevention of postoperative atelectasis. Surgery 47:184, 1960
116. FARBER MO, RUSK BJ, WINTER LW: Right heart hemodynamics during acute respiratory failure from chronic obstructive lung disease (COLD). Clin Res 20:806, 1972
117. GIBSON LE: Use of water vapor in the treatment of lower respiratory disease. Am Rev Respir Dis (Suppl) 110:100, 1974
118. WANNER A, RAO A: Clinical indications for and effects of bland, mucolytic, and antimicrobial aerosols. Am Rev Respir Dis (Suppl) 122:79, 1980
119. PIERCE AK, SANFORD JP: Bacterial contamination of aerosols. Arch Intern Med 131:156, 1973
120. PIERCE AK, SANFORD JP, THOMAS GD et al: Long-term evaluation of decontamination of inhalation therapy equipment and the occurrence of necrotizing pneumonia. N Engl J Med 282:528, 1970
121. PIERCE AK, SANFORD JP: Aerobic gram-negative bacillary pneumonias. Am Rev Respir Dis 110:647, 1974
122. LEPOW ML et al: Interrelationships of viral, mycoplasmal, and bacterial agents in uncomplicated pneumonia. Am Rev Respir Dis 97:533, 1968
123. MERRILL CW, GWALTNEY JM, JR, HENDLEY JO et al: Rapid identification of pneumococci. N Engl J Med 288:510, 1973
124. DIPOALA JA: Prognosis of pneumonia. NY State J Med 77:1259, 1977
125. TAGER I, SPEIZER FE: Role of infection in chronic bronchitis. N Engl J Med 292:563, 1975
126. SAHN SA: Corticosteroids in chronic bronchitis and pulmonary emphysema. Chest 73:389, 1978
127. SHIM C, STOVER DE, WILLIAMS MH, JR: Response to corticosteroids in chronic bronchitis. J Allergy Clin Immunol 62:363, 1978
128. ALBERT RK, MARTIN TR, LEWIS SW: Controlled clinical trial of methylprednisolone in patients with chronic bronchitis and acute respiratory insufficiency. Ann Intern Med 92:753, 1980
129. PETTY TL, BRINK GA, MILLER MW et al: Objective functional improvement in chronic airway obstruction. Chest 57:216, 1970.
130. FISHMAN AP: Chronic cor pulmonale. Am Rev Respir Dis 114:775, 1976
131. HUNTER CC, JR: Errors in management of patients dying of chronic obstructive lung disease. JAMA 199:488, 1967
132. COCHRAN RT, JR: Pulmonary insufficiency and hypercapnia complicated by potassium-responsive alkalosis. N Engl J Med 268:521, 1963
133. ROBIN ED: Abnormalities of acid–base regulation in chronic pulmonary disease, with special reference to hypercapnia and extracellular alkalosis. N Engl J Med 268:917, 1963
134. SKILLMAN JJ, MALKOTRA IV, PALLOTTA JA et al: Determinants of weaning from controlled ventilation. Surg Forum 22:198, 1971
135. BERRY PR, PONTOPPIDAN H: Oxygen consumption and blood gas exchange during controlled and spontaneous ventilation in patients with respiratory failure. Anesthesiology 29:177, 1968
136. DOWNS JB et al: Intermittent mandatory ventilation: A new approach to weaning patients from mechanical ventilation. Chest 64:331, 1973
137. WEINBERGER MM, BRONSKY EA: Evaluation of oral bronchodilator therapy in asthmatic children. J Pediatr 84:421, 1974
138. WEINBERGER MM, BRONSKY EA: Oral bronchodilator therapy. J Allergy Clin Immunol 53:78, 1974
139. WOLFE JD, TASHKIN DP, CALVARESE B et al: Bronchodilator effects of terbutaline and aminophylline alone and in combination in asthmatic patients. N Engl J Med 298:363, 1978
140. SALTIN B et al: Response to exercise after bed rest

and after training. Circulation [Suppl VII] 38:1, 1968
141. PIERCE AK, TAYLOR HF, ARCHER RK et al: Responses to exercise training in patients with emphysema. Arch Intern Med 113:28, 1964
142. PIERCE AK, PAEZ PN, MILLER WF: Exercise training with the aid of a portable oxygen supply in patients with emphysema. Am Rev Respir Dis 91:653, 1965
143. ASMUNDSSON T, KILBURN KH: Survival of acute respiratory failure: A study of 239 episodes. Ann Intern Med 70:471, 1969
144. O'DONOHUE WJ, JR et al: The management of acute respiratory failure in a respiratory intensive care unit. Chest 58:603, 1970
145. ROGERS RM, WEILER C, RUPPENTHAL B: Impact of the respiratory care unit on survival of patients with acute respiratory failure. Chest 62:94, 1972
146. MOSER KM, SHIBEL EM, BEAMON AJ: Acute respiratory failure in obstructive lung disease. Long-term survival after treatment in an intensive care unit. JAMA 225:705, 1973
147. BURK RH, GEORGE RB: Acute respiratory failure in chronic obstructive pulmonary disease, immediate and long-term prognosis. Arch Intern Med 132:865, 1973
148. JOHANSON WG, PIERCE AK, SANFORD JP: Changing pharyngeal bacterial flora of hospitalized patients: emergence of gram-negative bacilli. N Engl J Med 281:1137, 1969
149. BAUM CL, FISHER SD: The relationship of fatal pulmonary insufficiency with cor pulmonale, right sided mural thrombi and pulmonary emboli: a preliminary report. Am J Med Sci 240:609, 1960
150. SUKUMALCHANTRA Y, DINAKARA P, WILLIAMS MH, JR: Prognosis of patients with chronic obstructive pulmonary disease after hospitalization for acute ventilatory failure: A 3-year follow-up study. Am Rev Respir Dis 93:215, 1966
151. STAUB NC: Pulmonary edema. Physiol Rev 54:678, 1974
152. STAUB NC: Pathogenesis of pulmonary edema. Am Rev Respir Dis 109:358, 1974
153. STAUB NC: Pulmonary edema due to increased microvascular permeability to fluid and protein. Circ Res 43:143, 1978
154. HURLEY JV: Current views on the mechanisms of pulmonary oedema. J Pathol 125:59, 1978
155. PIETRA GG: The basis of pulmonary edema, with emphasis on ultrastructure. Monogr Pathol 19:215, 1978
156. LEVINE OR, MELLINS RB, SENIOR RM et al: The application of Starling's law of capillary exchange to the lungs. J Clin Invest 46:934, 1967
157. MEYER BJ, MEYER A, GUYTON AC: Interstitial fluid pressure. V. Negative pressure in the lungs. Clin Res 22:263, 1968
158. MELLINS RB, LEVINE OR, SKALAK R et al: Interstitial pressure of the lung. Circ Res 24:197, 1969
159. MEYER EC, DOMINGUEZ EAM, BENSCH KG: Pulmonary lymphatic and blood absorption of albumin from alveoli: A quantitative comparison. Lab Invest 20:1, 1969
160. WANGENSTEEN OD, WITTMERS LE, JR, JOHNSON JA: Permeability of the mammalian blood–gas barrier and its components. Am J Physiol 216:719, 1969
161. TAYLOR AE, GAAR KA, JR: Estimation of equivalent pore radii of pulmonary capillary and alveolar membranes. Am J Physiol 218:1133, 1970
162. HALL JG, MORRIS B, WOOLEY G: Intrinsic rhythmic propulsion of lymph in the unanesthetized sheep. J Physiol (Lond) 180:336, 1965
163. BRINGHAM KL, WOOLVERTON WC, BLAKE LH et al: Increased sheep lung vascular permeability caused by pseudomonas bacteremia. J Clin Invest 54:792, 1974
164. STAUB NC, MAGANO H, PEARCE ML: Pulmonary edema in dogs, especially the sequence of fluid accumulation in lungs. J Appl Physiol 22:227, 1967
165. EAGAN EA, NELSON RM, GESSNER IH: Solute permeability of the alveolar epithelium in acute hemodynamic pulmonary edema in dogs. Am J Physiol 1:H80, 1977
166. NELSON RM, MCINTYRE BR, EGAN EA: Solute permeability of the alveolar epithelium in alloxan edema in dogs. J Appl Physiol 44:353, 1978
167. ROBIN ED et al: Capillary leak syndrome with pulmonary edema. Arch Intern Med 130:66, 1971
168. KATZ S et al: Heroin pulmonary edema: Evidence for increased pulmonary capillary permeability. Am Rev Respir Dis 106:472, 1972
169. GELB AF, KLEIN E: Hemodynamic and alveolar protein studies in noncardiac pulmonary edema. Am Rev Respir Dis 114:831, 1976
170. ANDERSON RR et al: Documentation of pulmonary capillary permeability in the adult respiratory distress syndrome accompanying human sepsis. Am Rev Respir Dis 119:869, 1979
171. VREIM CE, SNASHALL PD, STAUB NC: Protein composition of lung fluids in anesthetized dogs with acute cardiogenic edema. Am J Physiol 231:1466, 1976
172. BRIGHAM KL, OWEN PJ: Increased sheep lung vascular permeability caused by histamine. Circ Res 37:647, 1975
173. WEIL MH et al: Routine plasma colloid osmotic pressure measurements. Crit Care Med 2:229, 1974
174. STEIN L et al: Pulmonary edema during volume infusion. Circulation 52:483, 1975
175. RACKOW EC, FEIN IA, LEPPO J: Colloid osmotic pressure as a prognostic indicator of pulmonary edema and mortality in the critically ill. Chest 72:709, 1977

176. HALES CA, KAZEMI H: Small-airways function in myocardial infarction. N Engl J Med 290:761, 1974
177. MCHUGH TJ et al: Pulmonary vascular congestion in acute myocardial infarction: Hemodynamic and radiologic correlations. Ann Intern Med 76:29, 1972
178. SHIMADA Y et al: Evaluation of the progress and prognosis of adult respiratory distress syndrome. Chest 76:180, 1979
179. LAMY M et al: Pathologic features and mechanisms of hypoxemia in adult respiratory distress syndrome. Am Rev Respir Dis 114:267, 1976
180. DANTZKER DR et al: Ventilation–perfusion distributions in the adult respiratory distress syndrome. Am Rev Respir Dis 120:1039, 1979
181. PETTY TL et al: Characteristics of pulmonary surfactant in adult respiratory distress syndrome associated with trauma and shock. Am Rev Respir Dis 115:531, 1977
182. PETTY TL, SILVERS GW, PAUL GW et al: Abnormalities in lung elastic properties and surfactant function in adult respiratory distress syndrome. Chest 75:571, 1979
183. PATTLE RE: Surface lining of lung alveoli. Physiol Rev 45:48, 1965
184. ROSENOW EC, HARRISON CE: Congestive heart failure masquerading as primary pulmonary disease. Chest 58:28, 1970
185. UNGER KM, SHIBEL EM, MOSER KM: Detection of left ventricular failure in patients with adult respiratory distress syndrome. Chest 67:8, 1975
186. STEVENS PM, FRIEDMAN GK, NICOTRA MB: The value of flow directed intravascular catheters in cardiorespiratory failure. Am Rev Respir Dis 107:1111, 1973
187. EICHNA LW: The George E. Brown memorial lecture: Circulatory congestion and heart failure. Circulation 22:864, 1960
188. SIMMONS RL, MARTIN AM, JR, HEISTERKAMP CA, III et al: Respiratory insufficiency in combat casualties. II. Pulmonary edema following head injury. Ann Surg 170:39, 1969
189. HUFF RW, FRED HL: Postictal pulmonary edema. Arch Intern Med 117:824, 1966
190. BEAN JW, BECKMAN DL: Centrogenic pulmonary pathology in mechanical head injury. J Appl Physiol 27:807, 1969
191. SARNOFF SJ, SARNOFF LC: Neurohemodynamics of pulmonary edema. II. The role of sympathetic pathways in the elevation of pulmonary and systemic vascular pressures following the intracisternal injection of fibrin. Circulation 6:51, 1952
192. WRAY NP, NICOTRA MB: Pathogenesis of neurogenic pulmonary edema. Am Rev Respir Dis 118:783, 1978
193. THEODORE J, ROBIN ED: Speculations on neurogenic pulmonary edema (NPE). Am Rev Respir Dis 113:405, 1976
194. MENON ND: High-altitude pulmonary edema. N Engl J Med 276:66, 1965
195. HULTGREN HN, MARTICORENA EA: High altitude pulmonary edema. Chest 74:372, 1978
196. SCOGGIN CH, HYERS TM, REEVES JT et al: High-altitude pulmonary edema in the children and young adults of Leadville, Colorado. N Engl J Med 297:1269, 1977
197. HOUSTON CS: High altitude illness. JAMA 236:2193, 1976
198. FRED HL, SCHMIDT AM, BATES T et al: Acute pulmonary edema of altitude, clinical and physiologic observations. Circulation 25:929, 1962
199. HULTGREN HN, LOPEZ CE, LUNDBERG E et al: Physiologic studies of pulmonary edema at high altitude. Circulation 29:393, 1964
200. GROVER RF, HARTLEY LH, MILLER H et al: Latent pulmonary circulatory abnormalities in men with a past history of pulmonary edema at high altitude. J Clin Invest 46:1064, 1967
201. HULTGREN HN, GROVER RF, HARTLEY LH: Abnormal circulatory responses to high altitude in subjects with a previous history of high-altitude pulmonary edema. Circulation 44:759, 1971
202. OHKUDA Ket al: Lung fluid exchange after uneven pulmonary artery obstruction in sheep. Circ Res 43:152, 1978
203. SINGH I et al: Acute mountain sickness. N Engl J Med 280:175, 1969
204. MURRAY JF: Mechanisms of acute respiratory failure. Am Rev Respir Dis 115:1071, 1977
205. CRADDOCK PR et al: Complement and leukocyte-mediated pulmonary dysfunction in hemodialysis. N Engl J Med 296:769, 1977
206. CRADDOCK PR et al: Hemodialysis leukopenia. J Clin Invest 59:879, 1977
207. CRADDOCK PR et al: Complement (C5a)-induced granulocyte aggregation in vitro. J Clin Invest 60:260, 1977
208. JACOB HS: Granulocyte-complement interaction. Arch Intern Med 138:461, 1978
209. BONE RC, FRANCIS PB, PIERCE AK: Intravascular coagulation associated with the adult respiratory distress syndrome. Am J Med 61:585, 1976
210. HECHTMAN HB et al: Pulmonary entrapment of platelets during acute respiratory failure. Surgery 83:277, 1978
211. SCHNEIDER RC, ZAPOL WM, CARVALHO AC: Platelet consumption and sequestration in severe acute respiratory failure. Am Rev Respir Dis 122:145, 1980
212. AUSTEN KF, ORANGE RP: Bronchial asthma: The possible role of the chemical mediators of immune hypersensitivity in the pathogenesis of subacute chronic disease. Am Rev Respir Dis 112:423, 1975
213. NAKAHARA K, OHKUDA K, STAUB NC: Effect of infusing histamine into pulmonary or bronchial artery on sheep pulmonary fluid balance. Am Rev Respir Dis 120:875, 1979

214. SACKS T et al: Oxygen radicals mediate endothelial damage by complement-stimulated granulocytes. J Clin Invest 61:1161, 1978
215. FRANK L, MASSARO D: Oxygen toxicity. Am J Med 69:117, 1980
216. BUFORD TH, BURBANK B: Traumatic wet lung. Observations of certain physiologic fundamentals of thoracic trauma. J Thorac Surg 14:415, 1945
217. BREWER LA III, BURBANK B, SAMSON PC et al: The "wet lung" in war casualties. Ann Surg 123:343, 1946
218. EISEMAN B, ASHBAUGH DG (eds): Pulmonary effects of nonthoracic trauma. Proceedings of a conference conducted by the Committee on Trauma, Division of Medical Sciences, National Academy of Science–National Research Council. J Trauma 8:623, 1968
219. FULTON RL, JONES CE: The cause of post-traumatic pulmonary insufficiency in man. Surg Gynecol Obstet 140:179, 1975
220. LEWIS FR, BLAISDELL W, SCHLOBOH RM: Incidence and outcome of post-traumatic respiratory failure. Arch Surg 112:436, 1977
221. SIMMONS RL et al: Respiratory insufficiency in combat casualties: III. Arterial hypoxemia after wounding. Ann Surg 170:45, 1969
222. SIMMONS RL et al: Respiratory insufficiency in combat casualties: IV. Hypoxemia during convalescence. Ann Surg 170:53, 1969
223. AMATO JJ, RHEINLANDER HF, CLEVELAND RJ: Post-traumatic adult respiratory distress syndrome. Orthop Clin North Am 9:693, 1978
224. PARDY BJ, DUDLEY HAF: Post-traumatic pulmonary insufficiency. Surg Gynecol Obstet 114:259, 1977
225. BLAISDELL FW: Pathophysiology of the respiratory distress syndrome. Arch Surg 108:44, 1974
226. HILL JD et al: Pulmonary pathology in acute respiratory insufficiency: Lung biopsy as a diagnostic tool. J Thorac Cardiovasc Surg 71:64, 1976
227. DEMLING RH, SELINGER SL, BLAND RD et al: Effect of acute hemorrhagic shock on pulmonary microvascular fluid filtration and protein permeability in sheep. Surgery 77:512, 1975
228. HOROVITZ JH, CARRICO CJ, SHIRES T: Pulmonary response to major injury. Arch Surg 108:349, 1974
229. MOORE FD et al: Post Traumatic Pulmonary Insufficiency. Philadelphia, WB Saunders, 1969
230. WEIGELT JA, MITCHELL RA, SNYDER WH: Early positive end-expiratory pressure in the adult respiratory distress syndrome. Arch Surg 114:497, 1979
231. TEABEAUT JR: Aspiration of gastric contents. An experimental study. Am J Pathol 28:51, 1952
232. WAMBERG K, ZESKOV B: Experimental studies on the course and treatment of aspiration pneumonia. Anesth Analg (Cleve) 45:230, 1966
233. JONES JG, BERRY M, HULANDS GH et al: The time course and degree of change in alveolar–capillary membrane permeability induced by aspiration of hydrochloric acid and hypotonic saline. Am Rev Respir Dis 118:1007, 1978
234. GLAUSER FL, MILLEN JE, FALLS R: Effects of acid aspiration on pulmonary alveolar epithelial membrane permeability. Chest 76:201, 1979
235. JONES JG et al: Alveolar–capillary membrane permeability. Am Rev Respir Dis 120:399, 1979
236. HAMELBERG W, BOSOMWORTH PP: Aspiration Pneumonitis. Springfield, Charles C Thomas, 1968
237. AWE WC, FLETCHER WS, JACOB SW: The pathophysiology of aspiration pneumonitis. Surgery 60:232, 1966
238. PAMINTUAN R, BRASHEAR RE, ROSS JC et al: Cardiovascular effects of experimental aspiration pneumonia in dogs. Am Rev Respir Dis 103:516, 1971
239. ARMS RA, DINES DE, TINSTMAN TC: Aspiration pneumonia. Chest 65:136, 1974
240. LEFROCK JL, CLARK TS, DAVIES B et al: Aspiration pneumonia: A ten-year review. Am Surg 45:305, 1979
241. BYNUM LJ, PIERCE AK: Pulmonary aspiration of gastric contents. Am Rev Respir Dis 114:1129, 1976
242. HUSEMEYER RP, DAVENPORT HT, RAJASEKARAN T: Cimetidine as a single oral dose for prophylaxis against Mendelson's syndrome. Anaesthesia 33:775, 1978
243. DETMER MD, PANDIT SK, COHEN PJ: Prophylactic single-dose oral antacid therapy in the preoperative period—comparison of cimetidine and maalox. Anesthesiology 51:270, 1979
244. COOMBS DW, HOOPER D, COLTON T: Acid-aspiration prophylaxis by use of preoperative oral administration of cimetidine. Anesthesiology 51:352, 1979
245. BERRIS B, KASLER D: Pulmonary aspiration of gastric acid—Mendelson's syndrome. Can Med Assoc J 92:905, 1965
246. LANDAY MJ, CHRISTENSEN EW, BYNUM LJ: Pulmonary manifestations of acute aspiration of gastric contents. Am J Roentgenol 131:587, 1978
247. GUENTER CA, FIORICA V, HINSHAW LB: Cardiorespiratory and metabolic responses to live E. coli and endotoxin in the monkey. J Appl Physiol 26:780, 1969
248. COALSON JJ, HINSHAW LB, GUENTER CA: The pulmonary ultrastructure in septic shock. Exp Mol Pathol 12:84, 1970
249. SNELL JD, RAMSEY LH: Pulmonary edema as a result of endotoxemia. Am J Physiol 217:170, 1969
250. BRIGHAM KL, WOOLVERTON WC, BLAKE LH et al: Increased sheep lung vascular permeability caused by pseudomonas bacteremia. J Clin Invest 54:792, 1974
251. MCLEAN APH, DUFF JH, MACLEAN L: Lung lesions

associated with septic shock. J Trauma 8:891, 1968

252. RIORDAN JF, WALTERS G: Pulmonary edema in bacterial shock. Lancet 1:719, 1968

253. HIRSCH EF, FLETCHER R, LUCAS S: Hemodynamic and respiratory changes associated with sepsis following combat trauma. Ann Surg 174:210, 1971

254. KAPLAN RL, SAHN SA, PETTY TL: Incidence and outcome of the respiratory distress syndrome in gram-negative sepsis. Arch Intern Med 139:867, 1979

255. CLOWES GHA, JR: Pulmonary abnormalities in sepsis. Surg Clin North Am 54:993, 1974

256. GREENBERG SD et al: Pulmonary disease studied by electron microscopy: Pathogenesis and pathophysiology. Tex Med 68:87, 1972

257. LOURIA DB et al: Studies on influenza in the pandemic of 1957–1958. II. Pulmonary complications of influenza. J Clin Invest 38:213, 1959

258. TRIEBWASSER JH, HARRIS RE, BRYANT RE et al: Varicella pneumonia in adults. Medicine 46:409, 1967

259. HARRIS RE, RHOADES ER: Varicella pneumonia complicating pregnancy: Report of a case and review of the literature. Obstet Gynecol 25:734, 1965

260. HELPERN M, RHOA YM: Deaths from narcotism in New York City. NY State J Med 66:2391, 1966

261. WILEN SB, ULREICH S, RABINOWITZ JG: Roentgenographic manifestations of methadone-induced pulmonary edema. Radiology 114:51, 1975

262. FISCHER P et al: The effects of ethchlorvynol on pulmonary alveolar membrane permeability. Am Rev Respir Dis 116:901, 1977

263. GOPINATHAN K et al: Hemodynamic studies in heroin-induced acute pulmonary edema. Circulation (Suppl III) 41:44, 1970

264. STEINBERG AD, KARLINER JS: The clinical spectrum of heroin pulmonary edema. Arch Intern Med 122:122, 1968

265. GARRIOTT JC, STURNER WQ: Morphine concentrations and survival periods in acute heroin fatalities. N Engl J Med 289:1276, 1973

266. LOURIA DB, HENSLE T, ROSE J: The major medical complications of heroin addiction. Ann Intern Med 67:1, 1967

267. HUBER DH, STIVERS RR, HOWARD LB: Heroin-overdose deaths in Atlanta. JAMA 228:319, 1974

268. STERN WZ, SPEAR PW, JACOBSON HG: The roentgen findings in acute heroin intoxication. Am J Roentgenol Radium Ther Nucl Med 103:522, 1968

269. SILBER R, CLERKIN EP: Pulmonary edema in acute heroin poisoning. Am J Med 27:187, 1959

270. DUBERSTEIN JC, KAUFMAN DM: A clinical study of an epidemic of heroin intoxication and heroin-induced pulmonary edema. Am J Med 51:704, 1971

271. FRAND U, SHIM CS, WILLIAMS MH, JR: Heroin-induced pulmonary edema. Sequential studies of pulmonary function. Ann Intern Med 77:29, 1972

272. SABA GP et al: Pulmonary complications of narcotic abuse. Am J Roentgenol 122:733, 1974

273. LIGHT RW, DUNHAM TR: Severe slowly resolving heroin-induced pulmonary edema. Chest 67:61, 1975

274. KARLINER JS, STEINBERG AD, WILLIAMS MH, JR: Lung function after pulmonary edema associated with heroin overdose. Arch Intern Med 124:350, 1969

275. PHILLIPS A, COPE O: Burn therapy III: The revelation of respiratory tract damage as a principal killer of the burned patient. Ann Surg 155:1, 1962

276. WEBSTER JR, MCCABE MM, KARP M: Recognition and management of smoke inhalation. JAMA 201:287, 1967

277. ZIKRIA BA, BUDD DC, FLOCK F et al: What is clinical smoke poisoning? Ann Surg 181,151, 1975

278. STONE HH, MARTIN JD, JR: Pulmonary injury associated with thermal burns. Surg Gynecol Obstet 129:1242, 1969

279. SOCHOR FM, MALLORY GK: Lung lesions in patients dying of burns. Arch Pathol 75:303, 1963

280. ZIKRIA BA, WESTON GC, CHODOFF M: Smoke and carbon monoxide poisoning in fire victims. J Trauma 12:641, 1972

281. MOYLAN JA, ADIB K, BIRNBAUM MM: Fiberoptic bronchoscopy following thermal injury. Surg Gynecol Obstet 140:541, 1975

282. ZIKRIA BA, FERRER JM, FLOCK HF: The chemical factors contributing to pulmonary damage in "smoke poisoning." Surgery 71:704, 1972

283. MELLINS RB, PARK S: Respiratory complications of smoke inhalation in victims of fires. J Pediatr 87:1, 1975

284. ACHAUER BM, ALLYN PA, FURNAS DW et al: Pulmonary complications of burns: The major threat to the burn patient. Ann Surg 117:311, 1973

285. AGEE RN et al: Use of xenon in early diagnosis of inhalation injury. J Trauma 16:218, 1976

286. WHITENER DR et al: Pulmonary function measurements in patients with thermal injury and smoke inhalation. Am Rev Respir Dis 122:731, 1980

287. STEPHENSON SF, ESRIG BC, POLK HC, JR et al: The pathophysiology of smoke injury. Ann Surg 182:652, 1975

288. DEMAREST GB, HUDSON LD, ALTMAN LC: Impaired alveolar macrophage chemotaxis in patients with acute smoke inhalation. Am Rev Respir Dis 119:279, 1979

289. DONNELLAN WL, PITICHA SM, HOLINGER PH: Management and complications of severe pulmonary burn. JAMA 194:155, 1965

290. PEREZ-GUERRA F, WALSH RE, SAGEL SS: Bronchio-

litis obliterans and tracheal stenosis. Late complications of inhalation burn. JAMA 213:1568, 1971

291. CAMERON GR, CORTICE FC: The production and removal of oedema fluid in the lungs after exposure to carbonylchloride (phosgene). J Physiol (Lond), 105:175, 1946
292. KOWITZ TA, REBA RC, PARKER RT et al: Effects of chlorine gas upon respiratory function. Arch Environ Health 14:545, 1967
293. HEDGES JR, MORRISSEY WL: Acute chlorine gas exposure. J Am Coll Emer Phys 8:59, 1979
294. GRAYSON RR: Silage gas poisoning: Nitrogen dioxide pneumonia, a new disease in agricultural workers. Ann Intern Med 45:393, 1956
295. BILS RF: Ultrastructural alterations of alveolar tissue of mice: III ozone. Arch Environ Health 20:468, 1970
296. CHARAN NB, MEYERS CG, LAKSHMINARAYAN S et al: Pulmonary injuries associated with acute sulfur dioxide inhalation. Am Rev Respir Dis 119:555, 1979
297. KLEINFELD M: Acute pulmonary edema of chemical origin. Arch Environ Health 10:942, 1965
298. CONNER EH, DUBOIS AB, COMROE JH, JR: Acute chemical injury of the airways and lungs. Anesthesiology, 23:538, 1962
299. SHERWIN RP, RICHTERS V: Lung capillary permeability. Nitrogen dioxide exposure and leakage of tritiated serum. Arch Intern Med 128:61, 1971
300. YUEN TGH, SHERWIN RP: Hyperplasia of type 2 pneumocytes and nitrogen dioxide (10 ppm) exposure. Arch Environ Health 22:178, 1971
301. LEIB GMP, DAVIS WM, BROWN T et al: Chronic pulmonary insufficiency secondary to silo-filler's disease. Am J Med 24:471, 1958
302. SMITH JL: Pathological effects due to increase of oxygen tension in air breathed. J Physiol (Lond) 24:19, 1899
303. FRANK L, MASSARO D: The lung and oxygen toxicity. Arch Int Med 139:347, 1979
304. NORTHWAY WH, JR, ROSEN RC, PORTER DY: Pulmonary disease following respiratory therapy of hyaline-membrane disease. N Engl J Med 276:368, 1967
305. NASH G, BLENNERHASSETT JB, PONTOPPIDAN H: Pulmonary lesions associated with oxygen therapy and artificial ventilation. N Engl J Med 276:368, 1967
306. GOULD VE et al: Oxygen pneumonitis in man. Ultrastructural observations on the development of alveolar lesions. Lab Invest 26:499, 1972
307. KISTLER GS, CALDWELL PRB, WEIBEL ER: Development of fine structural damage to alveolar and capillary lining cells in oxygen-poisoned rat lungs. J Cell Biol 32:605, 1967
308. KAPANCIY et al: Pathogenesis and reversibility of the pulmonary lesions of oxygen toxicity in monkeys. II. Ultrastructural and morphometric studies. Lab Invest 20:101, 1969
309. TIERNEY DF, AYERS L, KASUYAMA RS: Altered sensitivity to oxygen toxicity. Am Rev Respir Dis 115:59, 1977
310. WELCH BE, MORGAN TE, JR, CLAMANN HG: Time-concentration effects in relation to oxygen toxicity in man. Fed Proc 22:1053, 1962
311. CALDWELL PRB, LEE WL, JR, SCHILDKRAUT HS et al: Changes in lung volume, diffusing capacity, and blood gases in men breathing oxygen. J Appl Physiol 21:1477, 1966
312. BURGER EJ, JR: Pulmonary mechanics associated with oxygen toxicity and a suggested physiological test for susceptibility to the effects of oxygen. Aerospace Med 38:507, 1967
313. BURGER EJ, JR, MEAD J: Static properties of lungs after oxygen exposure. J Appl Physiol 27:191, 1969
314. MICHEL EL, LANGEVIN RW, GELL CF: Effects of continuous exposure to oxygen tension of 418 mm Hg for 168 hours. Aerosp Med 31:138, 1960
315. ROBERTSON WG, HARGREAVES JJ, HERLOCHER JE et al: Physiologic response to increased oxygen partial pressure. II. Respiratory studies. Aerospace Med 35:618, 1964
316. AYERS LN, TIERNEY DF, IMAGAWA D: Shortened survival of mice with influenza when given oxygen at one atmosphere. Am Rev Respir Dis 107:955, 1973
317. HYDE RW, RAWSON AJ: Unintentional iatrogenic oxygen pneumonitis—response to therapy. Ann Intern Med 71:517, 1969
318. MUSTAFA MG, TIERNEY DF: Biochemical and metabolic changes in the lung with oxygen, ozone, and nitrogen dioxide toxicity. Am Rev Respir Dis 118:1061, 1978

318a. MCCORD JM, FRIEDOVICH I: The biology and pathology of oxygen radicals. Ann Intern Med 89:122, 1978

319. JOHNSON LH, SCHAFFER DB, BOGGS TR, JR: The premature infant, vitamin E deficiency and retrolental fibroplasia. Am J Clin Nutr 27:1158, 1974
320. CURRAN JS, CATOLINO SJ: Vitamin E (injectable) administration in the prevention of retinopathy of prematurity: Evaluation with fluorescein angiography and fundus photography. Pediatr Res 12:404, 1978
321. GROSS SJ, LANDAW SA, OSKI FA: Vitamin E and neonatal hemolysis. Pediatrics 59:995, 1977
322. EHRENKRANTZ RA et al: Amelioration of bronchopulmonary dysplasia after Vitamin E administration: A preliminary report. N Engl J Med 229:564, 1978
323. RHODES ML, PATTERSON CE: Effect of exogenous superoxide dismutase on paraquat toxicity (abstr). Am Rev Respir Dis 117:255, 1978

324. MCLENNAN G, AUTOR AP: Effects of continuous intraperitoneal infusion of superoxide dismutase on pulmonary oxygen toxicity in the rat (abstr). Am Rev Respir Dis 117:371, 1978
325. FRANK L, YAM J, ROBERTS RJ: The role of endotoxin in protection of adult rats from oxygen-induced lung toxicity. J Clin Invest 61:269, 1978
326. FRANK L, ROBERTS RJ: Endotoxin protection against oxygen-induced acute and chronic lung injury. J Appl Physiol 47:577, 1979
327. MODELL JH: The Pathophysiology and Treatment of Drowning and Near-Drowning. Springfield, Charles C Thomas, 1971
328. FULLER RH: The clinical pathology of human near-drowning. Proc R Soc Med 56:33, 1963
329. REIDBORD HE, SPITZ WU: Ultrastructural alterations in rat lungs. Changes after intratracheal perfusion with fresh-water and seawater. Arch Pathol 81:103, 1966
330. MODELL JH, MOYA F: Effects of volume of aspirated fluid during chlorinated fresh water drowning. Anesthesiology 27:662, 1966
331. MODELL JH et al: The effects of fluid volume in seawater drowning. Ann Intern Med 67:68, 1967
332. MODELL JH et al: Physiologic effects of near-drowning with chlorinated fresh water, distilled water and isotonic saline. Anesthesiology 27:33, 1966
333. MODELL JH et al: Blood gas and electrolyte changes in human near-drowning victims. JAMA 203:99, 1968
334. SLADEN A, ZANDER HL: Methylprednisolone therapy for pulmonary edema following near drowning. JAMA 215:1793, 1971
335. ROSENBAUM HT, THOMPSON WL, FULLER RH: Radiographic pulmonary changes in near-drowning. Radiology 83:306, 1964
336. GOSSLING HR, ELLISON LH, DEGRAFF AC, JR: Fat embolism. The role of respiratory failure and its treatment. J Bone Joint Surg 56A:1327, 1974
337. KERSTELL J: Pathogenesis of post-traumatic fat embolism. Am J Surg 121:712, 1971
338. DIMANT J, SHAFRIR E: Lipase activities in the lungs of rats subjected to experimental hypertriglyceridemia and fat embolism. Isr J Med Sci 10:1551, 1974
339. SZABO G, MAGYAR Z, REFFY A: The role of free fatty acids in pulmonary fat embolism. Injury 8:278, 1977
340. MCKEEN CR, BRIGHAM KL, BOWERS RE et al: Pulmonary vascular effects of fat emulsion infusion in unanesthetized sheep. J Clin Invest 61:1291, 1978
341. LAHNBORG G, MYLÉN S, SYLVÉN C: Induced fat embolism in rabbits: Effects of defibrinogenation and thrombocytopenia. Eur Surg Res 8:428, 1976
342. SALDEEN T: Fat embolism and signs of intravascular coagulation with post-traumatic autopsy material. J Trauma 10:273, 1970a
343. KUNZ F, HORTNAGL H, KROESEN G et al: Plasma lipids, coagulation factors and fibrin formation after severe multiple trauma, and in adult respiratory distress syndrome. J Trauma 18:115, 1978
344. HERNDON JH, BECHTOL CO, CRICKENBERGER DP: Fat embolism during total hip replacement. J Bone Joint Surg 56-A:1350, 1974
345. MEEK RN, WOODRUFF B, ALLARDYCE DB: Source of fat macroglobules in fractures of the lower extremities. J Trauma 12:432, 1972
346. RISEBOROUGH EJ, HERNDON JH: Alteration in pulmonary function, coagulation and fat metabolism in patients with fractures of the lower limbs. Clin Orthop 115:248, 1976
347. CURTIS AM et al: The three syndromes of fat embolism: Pulmonary manifestations. Yale J Biol Med 52:149, 1979
348. AVIKAINEN V, WILLMAN K, ROKKANEN P: Stress hormones, lipids, and factors of hemostasis in trauma patients with and without fat embolism syndrome: A comparative study at least one year after severe trauma. J Trauma 20:148, 1980
349. PELTIER LF: The diagnosis and treatment of fat embolism. J Trauma 11:661, 1971
350. GURD AR, WILSON RI: The fat embolism syndrome. J Bone Joint Surg 56-B:408, 1974
351. MURRAY DG, RACZ GB: Fat embolism syndrome (respiratory insufficiency syndrome). J Bone Joint Surg [Am] 56-A:1338, 1974
352. HERNDON JH, RISEBOROUGH EJ, FISCHER JE: Fat embolism: A review of current concepts. J Trauma 11:673, 1971
353. TACHAKRA SS: Distribution of skin petechiae in fat embolism rash. Lancet 1:284, 1976
354. GIBSON DG: Haemodynamic factors in the development of acute pulmonary oedema in renal failure. Lancet 2:1217, 1966
355. HENKIN RI, MAXWELL MH, MURRAY JF: Uremic pneumonitis. A clinical, physiological study. Ann Intern Med 57:1001, 1962
356. NIDUS BD, MATALON R, CANTACUZINO D et al: Uremic pleuritis—a clinicopathological entity. N Engl J Med 281:255, 1969
357. GOODRICH WA: Pulmonary edema. A correlation of x-ray appearance and physiological changes. Radiology 51:58, 1948
358. FINLEY FW: Respiratory complications of acute pancreatitis. Am Surg 35:591, 1969
358a. MURPHY D, PACK AI, IMRIE CW: The mechanism of arterial hypoxia occurring in acute pancreatitis. Q J Med 44:151, 1980
359. ROVNER AJ, WESTCOTT JL: Pulmonary edema and respiratory insufficiency in acute pancreatitis. Radiology 118:513, 1976
360. INTERIANO B, STUARD ID, HYDE RW: Acute respi-

ratory distress syndrome in pancreatitis. Ann Intern Med 77:923, 1972
361. WARSHAW AL, LESSER PB, RIE M et al: The pathogenesis of pulmonary edema in acute pancreatitis. Ann Surg 182:505, 1975
362. PALVIK R, LIIGENT A, SISSAK HM: Respiratory failure in acute pancreatitis. Intensive Care Med 3:97, 1977
362a. DETROYER A et al: Impairment of pulmonary function in acute pancreatitis. Chest 72:360, 1978
363. HAYES MF, JR, ROSENBAUM RW, ZIBELMAN M et al: Adult respiratory distress syndrome in association with acute pancreatitis. Evaluation of positive end-expiratory pressure ventilation and pharmacologic doses of steroids. Am J Surg 127:314, 1974
364. KELLERMEYER RW, GRAHAM RC, JR: Kinins—possible physiologic and pathologic roles in man. N Engl J Med 279:859, 1968
365. OFSTAD E: Kinins in acute hemorrhagic pancreatitis. Scand J Gastroenterol 5:9, 1970
366. EDITORIAL: Mechanism of pancreatic autodigestion. N Engl J Med 283:487, 1970
367. MORGAN AP, JENNY ME, HAESSLER H: phospholipids, acute pancreatitis, and the lungs: Effect of lecithinase infusion on pulmonary surface activity in dogs. Ann Surg 167:329, 1968
368. KELLUM JM, JR, DEMESSTER TR, ELKINS RC et al: Respiratory insufficiency secondary to acute pancreatitis. Ann Surg 175:657, 1972
369. KELLERMEYER RW, GRAHAM RC, JR: Kinins—possible physiologic and pathologic roles in man. N Engl J Med 279:754, 1968
370. IMRIE CW, FERGUSON JC, MURPHY D et al: Arterial hypoxia in acute pancreatitis. Br J Surg 64:185, 1977
371. MCWILLIAMS H, GROSS R: Pancreatitis and the lungs. Am Surg 40:448, 1974
372. BLAISDELL FW, LIM RC, JR, STALLONE RJ: The mechanism of pulmonary damage following traumatic shock. Surg Gynecol Obstet 130:15, 1970
373. PLEET AB: "Shock lung" syndrome following diabetic ketoacidosis: Treatment with heparin. Chest 63:434, 1973
374. GREIPP PR, BROWN JA, GRALNICK NR: Defibrination in acute pancreatitis. Ann Intern Med 76:73, 1972
375. BONE RC, FRANCIS PB, PIERCE AK: Intravascular coagulation associated with the adult respiratory distress syndrome. Am J Med 61:585, 1976
376. RITTENHOUSE EA, KERENDINO KA: Acute pulmonary edema in the absence of left ventricular failure. Circulation 40:873, 1969
377. LLAMAS R, FORTHMAN HJ: Respiratory distress syndrome in the adult after cardiopulmonary bypass. A successful therapeutic approach. JAMA 225:1183, 1973
378. THURLBECK WM, THURLBECK SM: Pulmonary effects of paraquat poisoning. Chest 69:276, 1976
379. CHAMBERLIN WH, STOCKMAN GD, WRAY NP: Shock and noncardiogenic pulmonary edema following meglumine diatrizoate for intravenous pyelography. Am J Med 67:684, 1979
379a. HEFFNER JE, SAHN SA: Clinical characteristics of salicylate-induced pulmonary edema. Am Rev Resp Dis 123:25–69, 1981
380. SHULMAN M, SCHMIDT G, SADOVE MS: Evaluation of oxygen tensions. Dis Chest 56:356, 1969
381. CAMERON JL, SEBOR J, ANDERSON R et al: Aspiration pneumonia. J Surg Res 8:447, 1968
382. FLINT L, GOSDIN G, CARRICO CJ: Evaluation of ventilatory therapy for acid aspiration. Surgery 78:492, 1975
383. HEDLEY-WHYTE J, PONTOPPIDAN H, MORRIS MJ: The response of patients with respiratory failure and cardiopulmonary disease to different levels of constant volume ventilation. J Clin Invest 45:1543, 1966
384. MILLER WF, SPROULE BJ: Studies of the role of intermittent inspiratory positive pressure oxygen breathing (IPPB/I-O_2) in the treatment of pulmonary edema. Dis Chest 35:469, 1959
385. DAMMANN JF, JR et al: The management of the severely ill patient after open heart surgery. J Thorac Cardiovasc Surg 45:80, 1963
386. THUNG N et al: The cost of respiratory effort in postoperative cardiac patients. Circulation 28:552, 1963
387. CLOWES GH, JR, COOK WA, VUJOVIC V et al: Patterns of circulation response to the use of respirators. Circulation (Suppl 1) 31:157, 1965
388. BURNHAM SC, MARTIN WE, CHENEY FW, JR: The effects of various tidal volumes on gas exchange in pulmonary edema. Anesthesiology 37:27, 1972
389. BONE RC, FRANCIS PB, PIERCE AK: Pulmonary barotrauma complicating positive end-expiratory pressure. Am Rev Respir Dis 111:921, 1975
390. CLEMENTS JA: Pulmonary surfactant. Am Rev Respir Dis 101:984, 1970
391. SUTER PM, FAIRLEY B, ISENBERG MD: Optimum end-expiratory airway pressure in patients with acute pulmonary failure. N Engl J Med 292:284, 1975
392. ASHBAUGH DG, PETTY TC, BIGELOW DB et al: Continuous positive pressure breathing (CPPB) in adult respiratory distress syndrome. J Thorac Cardiovasc Surg 57:31, 1969
393. UZAWA T, ASHBAUGH DG: Continuous positive pressure breathing in acute hemorrhagic pulmonary edema. J Appl Physiol 26:427, 1969
394. ASHBAUGH DG: Effect of ventilatory methods and patterns on physiologic shunt. Surgery 68:99, 1970
395. KUMAR A et al: Continuous positive pressure ventilation in acute respiratory failure. Effects on

hemodynamics and lung function. N Engl J Med 283:1430, 1970

396. KANAREK DJ, SHANNON DC: Adverse effect of positive end-expiratory pressure on pulmonary perfusion and arterial oxygenation. Am Rev Respir Dis 112:457, 1975
397. MURRAY JF: Effects of lung inflation on pulmonary arterial pressure in dogs with pulmonary edema. J Appl Physiol 45:442, 1978
398. KUDSK KA, PFLUG B, LOWERY BD: Value of positive end-expiratory pressure in aspiration pneumonitis. J Surg Res 24:321, 1978
399. HOPEWELL PC: Failure of positive end-expiratory pressure to decrease lung water content in alloxan-induced pulmonary edema. Am Rev Respir Dis 120:813, 1979
400. LUTCH JS, MURRAY JF: Continuous positive-pressure ventilation: Effects on systemic oxygen transport and tissue oxygenation. Ann Intern Med 76:193, 1972
401. SCARF SM, CALDINI P, INGRAM RH, JR: Cardiovascular effects of increasing airway pressure in the dog. Am J Physiol 232:H35, 1977
402. CASSIDY SS, ROBERTSON CH, PIERCE AK et al: Cardiovascular effects of positive end-expiratory pressure in dogs. J Appl Physiol 44:743, 1978
403. CASSIDY SS et al: Cardiovascular effects of positive-pressure ventilation in normal subjects. J Appl Physiol 47:453, 1979
404. PREWITT RM, WOOD LDH: Effect of positive end-expiratory pressure on ventricular function in dogs. Am J Physiol 236:H534, 1979
405. BUDA AJ et al: Effect of intrathoracic pressure on left ventricular performance. N Engl J Med 301:453, 1979
406. ROBOTHAM JL et al: The effects of positive end-expiratory pressure on right and left ventricular performance. Am Rev Respir Dis 121:677, 1980
407. DANEK SJ et al: The dependence of oxygen uptake on oxygen delivery in the adult respiratory distress syndrome. Am Rev Respir Dis 122:387, 1980
408. GREGORY GA et al: Treatment of the idiopathic respiratory distress syndrome with continuous positive airway pressure. N Engl J Med 284:1333, 1971
409. KIRBY RR et al: High level positive end expiratory pressure (PEEP) in acute respiratory insufficiency. Chest 67:156, 1975
410. GHERINI S, PETERS RM, VIRGILIO RW: Mechanical work on the lungs and work of breathing with positive end-expiratory pressure and continuous positive airway pressure. Chest 76:251, 1979
411. VENUS B, JACOBS HK, LIM L: Treatment of the adult respiratory distress syndrome with continuous positive airway pressure. Chest 76:257, 1979
412. PETERS RM: Lifesaving measures in acute respiratory distress syndrome. Am J Surg 138:368, 1979
413. LOSMAN J et al: Correlation of pulmonary wedge and left atrial pressures. Arch Surg 109:270, 1974
414. TOOKER J, HUSEBY J, BUTLER J: The effect of Swan–Ganz catheter height on the wedge pressure–left atrial pressure relationship in edema during positive-pressure ventilation. Am Rev Respir Dis 117:721, 1978
415. ELLIOTT CG, ZIMMERMAN GA, CLEMMER TP: Complications of pulmonary artery catheterization in the care of critically ill patients. Chest 76:647, 1979
416. SPRINGER RR, STEVENS PM: The influence of PEEP on survival of patients in respiratory failure. Am J Med 66:196, 1979
417. CHRISTY JH: Treatment of gram negative shock. Am J Med 50:77, 1971
418. WILSON JW: Treatment or prevention of pulmonary cellular damage with pharmacologic doses of corticosteroid. Surg Gynecol Obstet 134:675, 1972
419. SLADEN A: Methylprednisolone. Pharmacologic doses in shock lung syndrome. J Thorac Cardiovasc Surg 71:800, 1976
420. BANNISTER WK, SATTILARO AJ: Vomiting and aspiration during anesthesia. Anesthesiology 23:251, 1962
421. LAWSON DW et al: Corticosteroids as treatment for aspiration of gastric contents: An experimental study. Surgery 59:845, 1966
422. LEWINSKI A: Evaluation of methods employed in the treatment of the chemical pneumonitis of aspiration. Anesthesiology 26:37, 1965
423. THOMAS CS, BROCKMAN SK: The role of adrenal corticosteroid therapy in Escherichia coli Endoxin shock. Surg Gynecol Obstet 126:61, 1968
424. WERTZBERGER JJ, PELTIER LF: Fat embolism: The effect of corticosteroids on experimental fat embolism in the rat. Surgery 64:143, 1968
425. JONES RL, KING EG: The effects of methylprednisolone on oxygenation in experimental hypoxemic respiratory failure. J Trauma 15:297, 1975
426. CHENEY FW, JR, HUANG TH, GRONKA R: Effects of methylprednisolone on experimental pulmonary injury. Ann Surg 190:236, 1979
427. CHAPMAN RL et al: Effect of continuous positive-pressure ventilation and steroids on aspiration of hydrochloric acid (pH 1.8) in dogs. Anesth Analg (Cleve) 53:556, 1974
428. TAYLOR G, PRYSE-DAVIES J: Evaluation of endotracheal steroid therapy in acid pulmonary aspiration syndrome (Mendelson's syndrome). Anesthesiology 29:17, 1968
429. DOWNS JB, CHAPMAN RL, JR, MODELL JH: An evaluation of steroid therapy in aspiration pneumonitis. Anesthesiology 40:129, 1974

430. DUDLEY WR, MARSHALL BE: Steroid treatment for acid-aspiration pneumonitis. Anesthesiology 40:136, 1974
431. PARKER FB, JR, RACZ GB, WAX SD: The hemodynamics of experimental fat embolism and associated therapy. Chest 65:545, 1974
432. PINGLETON WW, COALSON JJ, HINSHAW LB et al: Effects of steroid pretreatment on development of shock lung. Lab Invest 27:445, 1972
433. WYNNE JW et al: Steroid therapy for pneumonitis induced in rabbits by aspiration of foodstuff. Anesthesiology 51:11, 1979
434. ASHBAUGH DG, PETTY TL: The use of corticosteroids in the treatment of respiratory failure associated with massive fat embolism. Surg Gynecol Obstet 123:493, 1966
435. FISCHER JE, TURNER RH, HERNDON JH et al: Massive steroid therapy in severe fat embolism. Surg Gynecol Obstet 132:667, 1971
436. PAZELL JA, PELTIER LF: Experience with sixty-three patients with fat embolism. Surg Gynecol Obstet 135:77, 1972
437. JOHNSON H: Pulmonary aspiration of gastric acid: Mendelson's syndrome. JAMA 179:900, 1962
438. SKILLMAN JJ, PARIKH BM, TANENBAUM BJ: Pulmonary arteriovenous admixture. Improvement with albumin and diuresis. Am J Surg 119:440, 1970
439. GEIGER JP, GEILCHINSKY I: Acute pulmonary insufficiency. Treatment in Vietnam casualties. Arch Surg 102:400, 1971
440. FLEMING WH, BOWEN JC: The use of diuretics in the treatment of early wet lung syndrome. Ann Surg 175:505, 1972
441. BLAND RD, MCMILLAN DD, BRESSACK MA: Decreased pulmonary transvascular fulid filtration in awake newborn lambs after intravenous furosemide. J Clin Invest 62:601, 1978
442. STAUB NC: Pulmonary edema. Physiologic approaches to management. Chest 74:559, 1978
443. PETERSDORF RG et al: A study of antibiotic prophylaxis in unconscious patients. N Engl J Med 257:1001, 1957
444. NATIONAL HEART, LUNG, AND BLOOD INSTITUTE COLLABORATIVE STUDY: Extracorporeal support for respiratory insufficiency. US Dept HEW, Dec, 1979

Chapter 8

Acute Respiratory Tract Infections

GARY D. HARRIS
WALDEMAR G. JOHANSON, JR.

INFECTIVITY AND RESPIRATORY DEFENSE MECHANISMS

ROUTES OF INFECTIVITY

Infective agents may establish themselves in the respiratory tract after arriving there by any of four major routes. Inhaled airborne organisms, spread of infective oropharyngeal organisms to the lower respiratory tract, spread from other septic foci by way of the blood stream, and spread from infected contiguous tissues all play a role under certain circumstances (Table 8-1).

In recent years our understanding of airborne infections has been greatly amplified. This is probably the major mode of transmission of most epidemic respiratory illness. Infectivity of oropharyngeal flora, particularly when aspirated into the lower respiratory tract in association with other organic materials, has long been recognized as a predisposing factor to the development of lung abscess. More recently, the possibility that pneumonia in debilitated patients may be preceded by changing flora in the oropharynx has lent credence to the suggestion that this route of transmission may be common. Spread of infection to the lungs from infected tissues, by way of the bloodstream, has long been recognized as an important factor in the development of septic emboli with infarction (see Chap. 10, Pulmonary Vascular Diseases). Furthermore, the pulmonary involvement in such diseases as Rocky Mountain spotted fever, leptospirosis, and several parasitic infections is brought about by vascular transmission from a distal infected site, generally with widespread systemic involvement. Infection from a contiguous focus, such as a subphrenic abscess, may spread through the diaphragm and involve the lung and pleural space. Rarely, esophageal rupture with mediastinitis may result in empyema and related pulmonary infection. Finally, pene-

TABLE 8-1. Routes of Respiratory Infection

	Organism	Illustrative Illnesses
Inhaled aerosols	Virus	Influenza, measles
	Rickettsia	Q fever
	Bacteria	Tuberculosis, Legionnaire's disease
	Fungus	Coccidioidomycosis, histoplasmosis
Aspirated oropharyngeal secretions	Bacteria	Lung abscess, pneumonia
Circulatory spread	Virus	Enteric viruses
	Rickettsia	Rocky Mountain spotted fever
	Bacteria	Septic phlebitis, endocarditis, septicemia
	Fungi	Candidiasis
	Parasites	Ascariasis
Contiguous spread	Bacteria	Mediastinitis, subphrenic abscess
	Protozoa	Amebiasis

trating chest injuries may be associated with direct extension of infection.

Inhaled Aerosols

Droplets, varying in size, are generated from the respiratory tract by coughs, sneezes, or even talking. Upon contact with air these droplets evaporate rapidly, leaving a residual core of material which may include microorganisms. Large droplets settle rapidly out of the air but, because several infectious particles may be contained within each large droplet, they may pose an infection hazard for individuals within a few feet of the source. Spread of microorganisms by large droplets is considered a form of direct contact, not airborne transmission. On the other hand, small particles called *droplet nuclei*, on the order of 1 to 3 μ in diameter, may contain only a single organism but, because of their small mass, remain suspended in the air for long periods. Thus, infection may be caused in persons who are remote from the source, and large numbers of people may be exposed rapidly.

Several respiratory tract infections are most frequently transmitted by droplet nuclei. These include tuberculosis, measles, influenza, and smallpox.[1] Demonstration of airborne contagion requires that several criteria be met. Obviously, the organisms must be present in host secretions and be able to withstand rather drastic environmental changes. In addition to temperature and humidity alterations, airborne organisms may be subjected to tremendous osmotic or chemical forces as the shell of water in which they are suspended evaporates in the air, thereby concentrating other constituents. Finally, the organisms must be able to survive exposure to the ultraviolet rays present in sunlight. Although organisms vary in susceptibility to ultraviolet rays, pathogenic viruses and bacteria are generally quite sensitive.

The second major determinant of airborne contagion is the ability of the organism to produce disease with only a small inoculum. Consider, for example, that if a sneeze caused the formation of 10,000 infectious airborne particles, the concentration of particles in the air of a 100 m^3 room would be only 1 per 10 liters of air. Bacteria do not commonly cause infection when introduced into human hosts in such small numbers. However, each of the organisms known to be commonly transmitted by way of the air produces infection with minimal inocula, perhaps as small as a single organism in a susceptible host.[2]

A disease can more confidently be attributed to airborne transmission if it is easily recognized and similar in all infected persons. Measles and influenza produce quite homogeneous patterns of illness and, since their incubation periods are short, cases occur in clusters or outbreaks of varying proportions. In diseases with longer incubation periods and varying clinical expressions, such as infections due to *Mycoplasma pneumoniae*, it is more difficult to determine the time and mode of transmission. Tuberculosis is a special case since, although clinical illness is uncommon after initial contact with *Mycobacterium tuberculosis*, the development of delayed hypersensitivity can be used to document infection.

Thus, clear evidence of airborne transmission exists for relatively few infections, all of which are characterized by distinctive clinical presentations and the occurrence of outbreaks of cases under appropriate conditions. It seems likely that many viral infections may be transmitted by the airborne route. The agents which cause bacterial infections, with a few notable exceptions, such as tuberculosis and "Legionnaire's disease," are ordinarily not transmitted in this way, presumably because of the considerations discussed. Of these, the required inoculum appears to be of prime importance, a finding which emphasizes the role of host defense mechanisms in prevention of bacterial infection of the respiratory tract. From the foregoing, the principles that govern the control of airborne infection can be understood. Reduction of the number of organisms released by the source can be achieved by rapid institution of effective chemotherapy and covering of the mouth during cough. Reduction of the number of organisms in the air can be achieved by adequate ventilation (dilution) or, in selected instances, by use of ultraviolet radiation.

Aspiration of Oropharyngeal Secretions

Transmission of infectious microorganisms by direct contact implies that regions of the respiratory tract in close proximity to the environment are involved initially. Such regions, including the mouth, nose, and pharynx, contain a rich microbial flora which is surprisingly constant in number and composition. However, because of the very large bacterial population in oropharyngeal secretions (10^8 to 10^{10} organisms per ml), aspiration of even small quantities of secretions into the tracheobronchial tree represents a significant risk of infection. Aspiration of small quantities of oropharyngeal secretions occurs commonly, certainly in all subjects with impaired consciousness and probably in everyone during sleep.[3]

Certain pleuropulmonary infections are known with certainty to be caused by aspiration of oropharyngeal secretions. The strongest case can be made for anaerobic infections, since they are caused by oropharyngeal anaerobes and occur principally in clinical situations in which aspiration obviously occurs. Hospital-acquired gram-negative bacillary pneumonias occur in patients whose upper respiratory tracts have been colonized by these organisms.[4] It is likely that most bacterial pneumonias are fundamentally caused by aspiration, since oropharyngeal carriage of the responsible organism is common and pneumonias are especially common among individuals who are predisposed to aspirate. However, proof of these relationships is incomplete at present.

Circulatory Spread

Perhaps the best-documented spread of infection through vascular channels is for those patients with septic pulmonary infarction due to tricuspid valve endocarditis. In the population of addicts who require repetitive self-administration of intravenous drugs, septicemia, septic thrombophlebitis, and endocarditis are seen with some frequency. Although a wide range of organisms have been reported, staphylococci and enteric gram-negative bacilli are the most common offenders. Many other systemic infections may have pulmonary manifestations which result from transmission of the organisms via the circulation. These may include enteric viruses such as the Coxsackie group, or rickettsia such as that responsible for Rocky Mountain spotted fever, which enters the body through a tick bite. Furthermore, gram-negative pneumonias have been reported following pyelonephritis,[5] and in association with skin infections in burned patients.[6] In most instances, the primary site is readily identified and blood cultures document invasion of the bloodstream. Fungi and parasites may be disseminated by hematogenous routes, but rarely produce acute respiratory illness.

Contiguous Infection

Pulmonary infections transmitted from the chest wall are rare. Occasionally, osteomyelitis involving a rib, or an infection of the soft tissues of the chest wall, may involve the pleural space. More commonly, however, the subdiaphragmatic space is a source of pleuropulmonary disease. Subdiaphragmatic infection may be a result of pancreatitis or cholecystitis. Anaerobic abscesses may occur, following contamination of the peritoneum by bowel perforation. Occasionally, hepatic abscesses, particularly due to protozoa (ameba) may perforate through the diaphragm into the pleural space. Under any of these circumstances, an empyema is generally the predominant respiratory involvement, with associated pulmonary parenchymal inflammation. These conditions are discussed in the section on pleural effusions. A less common problem occurs in association with mediastinitis, particularly following esophageal perforation. Recognition of this route of spread of infection is particularly important since the problem is never adequately treated without drainage of the mediastinum.

DEFENSE MECHANISMS OF THE RESPIRATORY TRACT

A variety of defense mechanisms are required to protect the lung against injury. Bacteria are only one of the many potential agents of injury, but we will center our discussion of defense mechanisms around antibacterial factors since they are reasonably well known.[7,8]

Bacterial Flora of the Respiratory Tract

It is common knowledge that the upper respiratory tract, including the nose, mouth, and pharynx, contains a massive population of resident bacteria and is exposed daily to a variety of new bacterial species. Less often appreciated is the fact that the population of resident organisms is closely controlled as to species, numbers, localization within the region, and prevention of spread to adjacent regions.[9] The terminology applied to the resident flora is sometimes inconsistent and therefore confusing. *Saprophytic* refers to organisms which are free-living in nature but which may exist in healthy human hosts. *Commensal* organisms exist only in animal hosts, human or other. Either may cause *colonization* of the respiratory tract, meaning persistence in the absence of *infection*. *Infection* is best reserved for those circumstances in which evidence of tissue invasion and local responses are present or might be reasonably inferred.

Neonates acquire a respiratory tract flora within hours of birth. Evidence suggests that the source of these organisms is the infant's attendants. During subsequent years, the composition of the respiratory tract flora remains remarkably stable, with occasional loss of one species and acquisition of another; family members tend to have similar flora. In healthy persons it is difficult to experimentally interrupt this state of balance. Potentially pathogenic bacteria, when inoculated into the respiratory tracts of healthy individuals, are rapidly removed and rarely achieve colonization.[10] Treatment with antimicrobial agents suppresses susceptible resident organisms but usually fails to eradicate them; drug-resistant strains multiply if treatment is continued, tending to restore the original population density.

However, people obviously do acquire new and potentially pathogenic organisms from time to time. On some occasions this acquisition follows a viral infection or other known insult but frequently no preceding event can be identified. Colonization of the respiratory tract with gram-negative bacilli has been studied in some detail. Despite the ubiquity of these organisms around humans, respiratory tract colonization is present in only 2 to 6% of healthy subjects.[11] Among persons who become acutely and seriously ill, the prevalence of colonization rises to nearly 50%. Neither hospital personnel nor patients hospitalized for non-medical or surgical reasons show this change, so that the predisposing factor promoting colonization is in some way related to illness. Colonization occurs in the absence of antimicrobial therapy, although such therapy may further promote colonization by suppressing the normal flora.

The factors that facilitate persistence of new bacteria in the respiratory tract are not well understood. Members of the resident flora may inhibit the growth of other bacterial species by production of bacteriocins, bacteriophages, or other toxic factors, or by utilization of needed nutrients. Attempts to modify infections by the implantation of "nonpathogenic" bacteria with inhibitory activity against the infecting organism have been made for nearly 100 years.[12] Only one has found a place in current medical practice, that is, the inoculation of selected neonates with the 502A strain of *Staphylococcus aureus*, which tends to inhibit subsequent acquisition of more virulent staphylococci.[13] The physiochemical milieu of certain regions of the upper respiratory tract may be too inhospitable for some organisms and thus may prevent them from achieving colonization; this consideration probably applies only to very localized microcosms such as the periodontal crevices, where anaerobic species abound, but is not likely to be the reason that relatively hardy organisms such as gram-negative bacilli are excluded from the entire region.

More likely, the composition of the normal flora is explained by selective adherence of only some species to the regional epithelium.[14] Alpha streptococci adhere to buccal epithelial cells obtained from neonates in far greater numbers than do *Escherichia coli*.[15] Similarly, *Pseudomonas* adhere *in vitro* to epithelial cells from critically ill patients, but not to cells from healthy patients.[16] Cells recovered from different regions of the oral cavity bind most avidly the bacterial species which are present in that region. Thus, one would predict that the predilection for hemolytic streptococci to colonize the tonsils or *Neisseria meningitidis* the nasopharynx will be explained by differences in epithelial-cell surfaces which render them susceptible to adherence of one species but not of another. If the organisms stimulate the production of local antibody, colonization tends to disappear since IgA-coated bacteria do not adhere to the epithelium.

It is probable that some organisms are particularly well adapted to the human respiratory tract and are more likely than others to be successfully transferred from one person to another. In the pre-antibiotic era, for example, it was common for family contacts and even hospital personnel to become colonized with the organism causing the patient's pneumonia. Hospital personnel who are persistently colonized with certain pathogens, particularly *Streptococcus pyogenes* or *Staphylococcus aureus*, tend to transmit their organisms to the patients under their care. Although these events suggest that the colonizing organisms possess unusual virulence, this is probably not true. A recent hospital outbreak of polyresistant pneumococcal infection revealed that patients were far more likely than hospital personnel to acquire the organism, and only already-ill patients developed infection.[17] These observations indicate that alterations in the resistance of the host play the predominant role in maintenance of the respiratory-tract flora.

Despite the enormous bacterial population of the oropharynx, contiguous surfaces, including the middle ears, paranasal sinuses, and airways distal to the larynx are virtually sterile. Proof of the sterility of the normal lung has come from several types of observations, including bronchoscopically obtained cultures with meticulous precautions being taken to avoid contamination by upper-airway secretions, and from cultures of lungs obtained at surgery.[18,19] However, if the bronchus to a normal lung is mechanically obstructed by a sterile plug, bacteria proliferate distal to the obstruction.[20] The species present are generally those of the upper tract. These findings are best interpreted as follows: while the lung normally contains few cultivatible bacteria, this state of near-sterility is critically dependent upon ongoing antibacterial defenses; even transient impairment of these defenses may allow bacteria to multiply.

In summary, the respiratory tract has a surprisingly constant bacterial flora which is confined to specific regions of the tract. Exclusion of organisms from some regions, and exclusion of new bacterial species, are the functions of antibacterial defense mechanisms. We will now consider these mechanisms in greater detail.

Defense Mechanisms of the Respiratory tract

- Defense of Airways
  - Anatomical arrangement
  - Mucociliary system
  - Chemical factors: lysozyme, immunoglobulins, interferon
  - Reflexes
  - Complex actions: cough, sneeze, swallow
- Defense of Alveoli
  - Phagocytes: alveolar macrophages, neutrophils
  - Mucociliary system
  - Lymphatic drainage
  - Surface-lining fluid
  - Immunologic factors: immunoglobulins, lymphocytes, monocytes, macrophages

Defense of Airways

Anatomical Arrangement. As air enters the nasal passages, it flows past the anterior nasal hairs and nasal turbinates, into the posterior pharynx. The combination of this tortuous course and the effect of anterior nasal hairs result in the distributing of this flow to provide a large surface exposure, favoring impaction of particles in the nose. Furthermore, the vascular mucosa raises inspired gas to body temperature and saturates it with water vapor before it reaches the subglottic area.[21,22] Hygroscopic droplet nuclei are thereby enlarged and therefore more likely to settle on impact. The particles impacted on the nasal mucosa are propelled by ciliary action along the mucous blanket through the posterior pharynx. The flow of mucus is from the anterior portion of the nasal passages posteriorly, draining eventually into the oropharynx, where the material is swallowed.[23] It has been estimated that the flow of mucus clears the main passages every 10 to 15 min. Very large particles are cleared from the anterior nasal passages by sneezing or nose blowing.

Mathematical models and studies of isotope-labelled particles demonstrate that particles measuring 10 to 20 μ in diameter generally settle in the nasopharyngeal regions.[24] Particles in the range of 2 to 4 μ are well-suspended and may pass through the nasopharynx into the lower tracheobronchial tree. Smaller particles (less than 0.5 μ) are so stable in the air that they are generally inhaled and exhaled with minimal deposition. Deposition of particles is determined, however, by gravity and impaction in the central airways, and to a greater extent, by sedimentation and diffusion in the peripheral airways. The latter processes become dominant as the rate of flow of inspired gas—and therefore of the particulates suspended in it—becomes slower and slower. Because of the branching arrangement of the airways, the total cross-sectional area progressively enlarges, and flow in any one airway is therefore slower. Cross-sectional area enlarges dramatically as terminal bronchioles become respiratory bronchioles and alveolar ducts, and it is likely that no bulk flow occurs beyond this level. Rather, gas exchange and movement of suspended particles occur by diffusion into more distal airspaces. This slowing and cessation of flow causes particles to settle on the airway surface.

Mucociliary System. The mucociliary system of the respiratory tract provides one of nature's most fascinating examples of interdependence between markedly differing elements, each of which is required for normal function of the system.[25] It is difficult to discuss the role of ciliary activity without consideration of the overlying mucus, without which ciliary activity ceases. Similarly, abnormal depth or visco-elastic properties of mucus may impair the function of the transport system while ciliary activity is normal. Thus, it is important to distinguish between effects on one element of the system and effects on the function of the system as a whole.

Respiratory mucus arises from submucosal glands and goblet cells, both of which are numerous in the upper airways but diminish in number in peripheral airways. Other secretory cells in the lungs (*e.g.*, Clara cells in terminal airways and alveolar type II cells) contribute to airway secretions, but their quantitative contribution is uncertain. Secretion by submucosal glands is under parasympathetic control; the control of goblet cell function is less clear.[26] The volume of secretions produced in the normal tracheobronchial tree is probably on the order of 10 to 100 ml per day; accurate estimates are obviously hampered by the likelihood that the intervention required to make the measurements may alter the processes under study.

Mucus in airways is stratified into two layers: the periciliary layer (sol phase) is less viscous than the outermost layer (gel phase). This arrangement allows the bulk of ciliary movement to occur in the less viscous sol layer, thus conserving energy. Recent evidence indicates that the gel layer is not continuous throughout the airways;[27] rather, it occurs in patches of varying size which have been likened to lily pads floating on the surface of a pond. The depth of the mucus layer appears to be closely regulated in normal airways. Whereas cilia are about 6 μ long, a sol layer of 10 μ would prevent ciliary contact with mucus in the gel phase and thereby inhibit transport. The mechanisms that sense and regulate the depth of mucus lining the airways are unknown, but the presence in airways of cells with microvilli suggests that an active resorbtive process may take place.

About 80% of cells lining the central airways contain cilia (Fig. 8-1); and the percentage of ciliated cells diminishes in peripheral airways. Each ciliated cell contains about 200 cilia which average 6 μ in length and 0.2 μ in diameter. Ultrastructural studies of cilia from humans and other mammals have revealed an interestingly consistent pattern of two central longitudinal fibrils surrounded by nine pairs of fibrils arranged around the periphery of the cilium (Fig. 8-2). Recently, several abnormalities in the ultra-

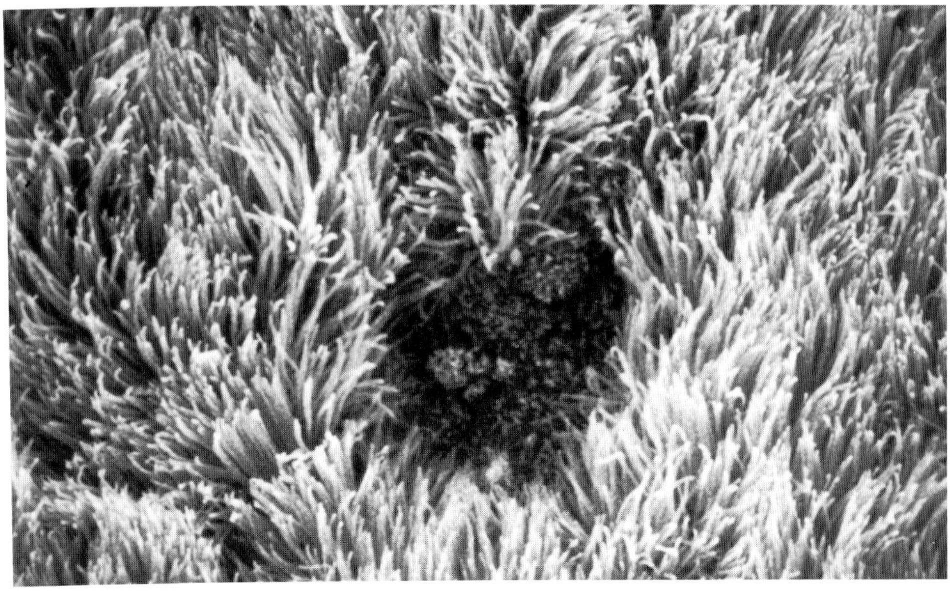

FIG. 8-1. A scanning electron micrograph of a normal human segmental bronchus. The central area devoid of cilia is a goblet cell that has recently discharged its contents. No mucus is visible owing to its removal during the process of fixation. Magnification ×4100. (Courtesy of J. J. Coalson, Ph.D.)

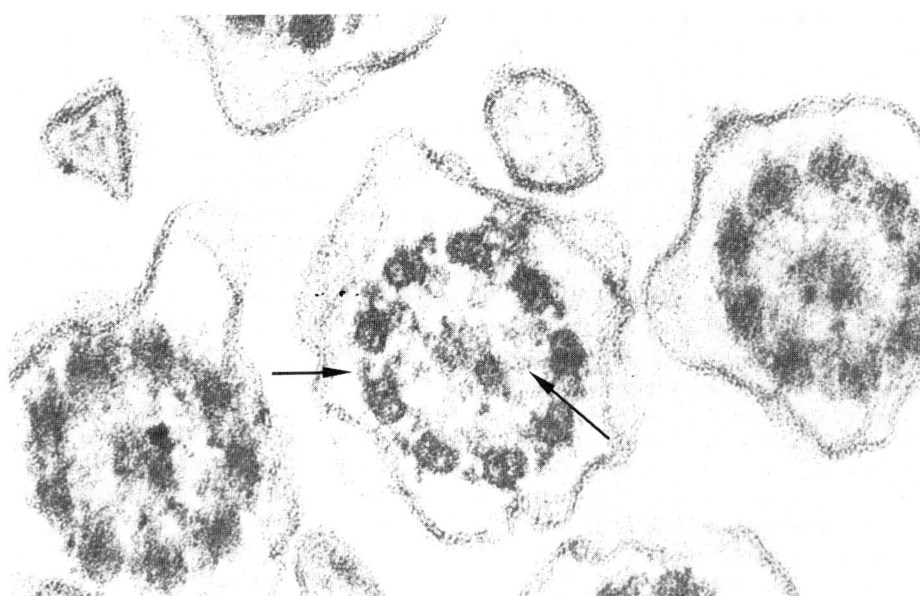

FIG. 8-2. A transmission electron micrograph of normal human bronchial cilia. Most of the structural features of cilia can be discerned, including the central pair of microtubules, the radial spokes leading to the periphery (*arrow*), and the nine peripheral microtubular doublets with dynein arms (*arrow*). The nexin links which connect adjacent doublets are not well seen. Magnification ×190,000. (Courtesy of J. J. Coalson, Ph.D.)

TABLE 8-2. Techniques For Assessing Mucociliary Function In Humans

Technique	Advantages	Limitations
Inhaled radiolabeled aerosol	Noninvasive	Marked variation of clearance rates with site of deposition
Deposition of tracheal particles	Rapid, useful for evaluating short-term changes	Limited to trachea, invasive
Deposition of contrast material (e.g., tantalum dust, barium)	Anatomic correlation possible	Invasive, limited range of observation, difficult to quantitate

structure of cilia have been described including a lack of appendages (*dynein arms*) to the doublet fibrils[28] and abnormalities in structures which radiate from the central fibrils to the periphery (*radial spokes*).[29] Each of these abnormalities has been associated with chronic airways disease, particularly bronchiectasis with onset early in life.[29a–b] Immotile cilia, a consequence of such abnormalities, appear to be a characteristic feature which involves all organ systems, including, for example, spermatozoa, which may provide a ready means of diagnosis in affected males.

The exact mechanisms of ciliary motion are not fully understood. However, cilia *in situ* beat about 1000 times per min, with a rapid effector or power stroke and a slower recovery stroke. Ciliary beating requires ATP, and the rate of beating is increased by digitalis glycosides. Ciliary beats tend to occur in waves (*metachronal waves*), in which the beats of adjacent cilia are coordinated so that a wave is propagated towards the pharynx. The mechanisms which coordinate the activity of cilia on adjacent cells are unknown but appear not to involve neuronal control.

Ciliary activity and mucociliary function have been studied in a variety of ways, including organ culture and direct observation through tracheal windows in living animals. Several techniques are now available which permit an assessment of overall mucociliary transport in humans (Table 8-2). Each technique has certain advantages, along with inherent limitations.

The first quantitative assessments of mucociliary transport in humans were made with inhaled radioactive particles;[30,31] the clearance of radioactivity from the lungs is followed with counters (collimators) placed over certain regions. A number of technical factors must be controlled, including the size and nature of the particles, the pattern of breathing during inhalation, and the positioning of the counting devices. This technique was instrumental in discovering that mucociliary transport from the respiratory tract occurs at differing rates as though differing compartments exist in terms of clearance. The exact anatomic correlates of these functional compartments are not known. However, it is apparent that half-times of clearance vary from 2 to 3 min for particles deposited in the trachea to several months or more for particles deposited in alveoli; mathematical models of such clearance data suggest that clearance zones exist with half-times of a few hr and 17 to 24 hr. Clearance slower than the latter may well represent mechanisms other than mucociliary.

The chief drawback to the aerosol technique is the uncertainty about the site of particle deposition. Patterns of deposition representing predominant deposition in either central or peripheral airways can be produced in normal subjects by altering the rate and depth of inhalation; similar differences may result from the presence of airways disease despite controlled inhalation. Since clearance is more rapid from central airways, deposition predominantly in these airways leads to an overestimation of the rate of lung clearance, and, for example, the finding of "normal" mucociliary clearance in subjects with cystic fibrosis.[32] A further disadvantage is the long period of monitoring required, which leads to the possibility that subject coughing will significantly alter overall clearance. Thus, this technique is best suited to investigation of subjects with little or no lung disease.

Placement of various markers on the tracheal mucosa of human subjects with minimal, if any, anesthesia of the larynx became possible with the advent of the bronchofiberscope.[33] Several types of markers have been used including small Teflon discs which are subsequently photographed by way of the bronchoscope, and radiopaque markers which can be followed fluoroscopically. These techniques provide a direct measure of movement of individual particles; because some may not move at all during the period of observation, usually only approximately 10 to 20 particles are deposited. These studies have shown that particle movement in the trachea spirals clockwise as viewed from the larynx and averages between 6 to 18 mm per minute. This technique provides a relatively rapid measurement of mucociliary transport and can be readily used therefore to determine the effect of drugs or other interventions on mucociliary transport. It provides information on a limited segment of the airways and does require bronchoscopy and sophisticated means of analysis of particle movement.

Deposition in the airways of radiopaque materials such as tantalum dust followed by fluoroscopy or serial radiographs, provides an opportunity to visualize the airway while observing its rate of clearance.[34] Mucociliary clearance is more difficult to quantitate with this approach.

It is generally agreed that the rate of mucus transport is on the order of 10 to 20 mm per min in the trachea and is less rapid in peripheral airways. Subjects with chronic bronchitis have impaired mucociliary transport. While the specific effects of smoking are less clear, some data suggest that impaired mucociliary clearance may precede other evidence of altered lung function.[27] Infection of the tracheobronchial tree is associated with decreased mucociliary transport. Adrenergic drugs, especially those with β-2 predominance, stimulate mucociliary transport, although the mechanism is not known. Cholinergic drugs also enhance mucociliary transport, but the accompanying bronchoconstriction induced by these agents limits their clinical application for this purpose.

Alterations of the chemical nature of mucus may influence overall transport.[27] Mucoid sputum from subjects with chronic bronchitis is chemically quite similar to secretions obtained from normal subjects, differing only slightly in fucose and neuraminic acid content. However, purulent sputum differs markedly from normal secretions chemically and in visco-elastic properties. Normal respiratory mucus has low viscosity and high elasticity, the latter presumably allowing mucus to remain intact as it is moved within the airways. Purulent sputum demonstrates high viscosity, apparently due to leukocyte-derived DNA, and reduced elasticity, probably the result of enzymatic action. Both asthma and cystic fibrosis are associated with changes in the biochemical composition of respiratory mucus. Whether these changes are major determinants in the reduced mucociliary transport associated with these diseases is not clear.

In summary, impaired mucociliary transport occurs in many acute and chronic lung diseases. When present, such impairment will tend to cause retention and inspissation of secretions, retention of foreign materials, and promote bacterial proliferation. Whether these changes are the initiating events in the pathophysiology of chronic disease, or occur as a consequence of other changes, is frequently unclear. However, the occurrence of chronic airways disease, especially bronchiectasis, in subjects with hereditarily deficient mucociliary transport suggests that impairment in this mechanism is fully capable of initiating a series of changes leading to permanent alterations in lung structure and function.

Chemical Factors. Respiratory tract secretions contain a variety of substances that may afford some measure of protection against microbes or other agents.[26] Lysozyme is present in respiratory secretions and in tears, but its antibacterial spectrum is limited to some gram-negative species. Properdin, complement proteins, and immunoglobulins, especially IgA and IgG, are present in the secretions of normal subjects. While IgG may serve as an opsonin, promoting phagocytosis, or may participate in immune lysis of organisms, IgA appears to exert its major antibacterial role in the prevention of bacterial adherence to respiratory epithelial cells. Interferon is produced by the respiratory tract as an early response to viral infection and has antiviral properties, in that viral replication is inhibited in its presence.[35] The spread of viral infection in the respiratory tract involves attachment and entry of virus into epithelial cells, viral replication within the cell, and finally, release of additional infective particles associated usually with cell death. Prevention of viral replication therefore limits the extension of the initial infection.

Reflexes and Complex Actions. Superficial *cough* or *irritant* receptors in the mucosa of the larynx and tracheobronchial tree are sensitive to mechanical deformation or chemical irritation. These stimuli are transmitted centrally by the afferent branches of the glossopharyngeal, vagus, and superior pharyngeal nerves. The efferent pathway involves the phrenic nerves to the diaphragm, intercostal nerves to the intercostal muscles, and the recurrent laryngeal nerves to the vocal cords.

Stimulation of the cough reflex results in an inspiratory phase, then adduction of the vocal cords, followed by a forceful contraction of the abdominal and expiratory intercostal muscles, generating an intrathoracic pressure in the range of 40 cm of water or more, and then a rapid opening of the glottis. At this point the high intrapulmonary pressures result in rapid expiratory flow of air, which carries mucus through the larger bronchi, the trachea, and the laryngeal structures. The membranous portion of the trachea is displaced anteriorly into the lumen, through the horse-shoe rings, narrowing the tracheal lumen. As the cross-sectional area of the trachea and main bronchi decreases to less than 40% of normal caliber during the compressive phase of the cough maneuver, the linear velocity of flow is greatly increased and, in fact, linear velocities have been measured as high as one-third the speed of sound.[36] This is a major defense mechanism in preventing the aspiration of particulate material into the lower respiratory tract. Together with the effect of the epiglottis on the distribution of materials during the swallowing process, it prevents contamination of the lower respiratory tract.

The cough mechanism may be modified by disease in several ways. If neurologic disease results in reduced sensitivity of the afferent pathways, the reflex may never be initiated. There is also clinical suspicion that prolonged stimulation, such as occurs with an indwelling nasogastric tube or an endotracheal tube, may result in decreased sensitivity of the cough receptors. Consequently, aspiration of particulate material may take place. Brain stem disease or injury to the vagus nerve supply of the larynx may prevent close apposition of the vocal cords, and high velocity of air flow through the larynx will not be achieved.

The velocity of expiratory flow during cough may also be reduced as a result of airways disease. Patients with emphysema commonly suffer severe dynamic compression of the peripheral airways, which reduces expiratory flow rates. At bronchoscopy, during the cough maneuver, it is commonly observed that bronchial collapse occurs in such patients, occasionally occluding the airway completely. Similarly, patients with bronchitis or asthma may have bronchospasm or produce secretions which reduce the maximal expiratory flow rates and impair the effectiveness of cough.

It appears that cough at high lung volumes is ineffective in emptying the peripheral portions of the lung; however, it is possible that cough at very low lung volumes might, in fact, help the drainage of the alveolar sacs and respiratory bronchioles.[36]

The laryngeal defense mechanism is apparently suppressed under a wide range of conditions which alter consciousness. Aspiration of foreign materials occurs in patients with transient unconsciousness from a drug overdose, epilepsy, alcohol ingestion, or head injury. In some patients this may occur during sleep, particularly when esophageal disease results in poor drainage of the oropharynx.

Stimulation of receptors located principally in central airways may produce other vagally-mediated effects, especially bronchoconstriction and mucus secretion. Even bronchoconstriction caused by inhalation of antigen in sensitized animals may be similarly mediated by means of the vagus.[26] Cough, bronchoconstriction, and mucus secretion may be viewed teleologically as responses which are beneficial for the individual, since they would tend to reduce entry and retention of foreign materials into the lung. However, such responses, if severe in intensity or active over prolonged periods of time, may be deleterious. The changes in the airways of persons with chronic bronchitis, consisting of hypertrophy of mucus glands, hyperplasia of goblet cells, and an increase in bronchial smooth muscle, could be the result of repetitive or continuing stimulation of these protective mechanisms. Once structural changes have occurred in the airways, the beneficial effects of these mechanisms are even less obvious. Although cough is dramatically effective in removing secretions from the airways of normal subjects, in the presence of chronic airway obstruction, coughing may impede movement of secretions due to complete airway closure by the coughing maneuver. Similarly, sudden mucus hypersecretion in a subject with impaired mucociliary transport and an ineffectual cough may lead to severe airway obstruction.

Defense of Alveoli

Phagocytic Cells. As discussed earlier, removal from the lung of inert particles deposited in alveolated regions occurs very slowly. Fortunately, defense of the lung against bacteria does not depend on these mechanisms of physical transport. Rather, the great majority of bacteria that enter the lung, whether by inhalation of droplet nuclei or aspiration of oropharyngeal secretions, are killed *in situ*. Nonphagocytic mechanisms, that is, physico-chemical agents, contribute little to this bactericidal activity of the lung. Under most circumstances bacteria in the lung are phagocytosed and killed by resident alveolar macrophages.[37] The alveolar macrophage is a descendant of precursor cells in the bone marrow, probably transported to the lung as a circulating blood monocyte. However, macrophages within the lung interstitium form a pool of cells which also maintain the number of alveolar macrophages, and which can be mobilized rapidly into the airspaces.[7] Alveolar macrophages differ from monocytes and from macrophages found in other body sites. In general, alveolar macrophages are more dependent on oxidative phosphorylation for cellular energy requirements and demonstrate properties associated with cell "activation" to an extent greater than other, similar cells.[38]

When experimental animals inhale staphylococci, about 90% of the deposited bacteria are phagocytosed by alveolar macrophages within 4 hr.[37] Bacterial killing lags only slightly behind ingestion, indicating that intracellular killing occurs rapidly for such organisms. Phagocytosis in the alveoli of normal animals is not influenced by the presence of specific antibody and represents "surface phagocytosis." Since polymorphonuclear leukocytes are rarely recovered by lavage from the lungs of healthy persons, it seems reasonable to conclude that neutrophils are not responsible for the absence of bacteria in normal lungs.

On the other hand, recent evidence has shown that not all bacterial species are handled in similar fashion. Certain pathogenic species, such as *Klebsiella pneumoniae*, cause a prompt recruitment of circulating PMNs when deposited in the lungs of normal animals.[39] Under these circumstances specific antibody, serum complement, and/or the number of PMNs may significantly influence how rapidly bacterial killing is accomplished;[40–42] for example, depletion of PMNs prior to bacterial inoculation markedly diminishes antibacterial defenses for these organisms.[40]

A number of environmental and host factors are known to impair lung antibacterial defenses.[8] Alveolar hypoxia, systemic acidosis, viral infection of the lung, and pulmonary edema are a few of a long list of conditions that have been studied. Environmental pollutants such as nitrogen dioxide and ozone also impair these defenses. Exactly how the antibacterial activity of the lung is impaired under these circumstances is not clear. Following ozone exposure reduced bacterial killing appears to result from defects in both bacterial ingestion by macrophages and in intracellular bacterial killing.[43] In mice, following Sendai viral infection, the overall antibacterial activity of the lung is markedly reduced, but the ability of macrophages isolated from these lungs to ingest and kill bacteria is normal.[44] These findings suggest that the principal defect following Sendai viral infection may relate to mobilization of phagocytes into regions where they are required.

Phagocytosis is an important aspect of alveolar defense against noninfectious agents as well. Most particles cleared from the lungs 12 to 24 hr after inhalation, as well as some fraction of particles cleared earlier, have been phagocytosed by alveolar macrophages; the rate of clearance of inhaled particles is more rapid in the presence of increased numbers of alveolar macrophages.[45] Whether clearance of these dusts is dependent upon prior phagocytosis or whether such phagocytosis is incidental to clearance is not firmly established. However, it is certain that processing of particulates by macrophages occurs for those dusts which remain in the lung for prolonged periods, and that such processing is an important aspect of the ultimate tissue response.[7] For example, materials that can be degraded by intracellular enzymes will be slowly solubilized and removed. Other particles such as asbestos or silica involve macrophages, lymphocytes, and fibroblasts in complicated interactions which lead to fibrosis of the lung, that is, to processes which permanently trap the foreign materials in the lung.

Mucociliary System. The mucociliary system and its probable role in alveolar clearance have been discussed previously.

Lymphatic Drainage. Pulmonary lymphatics begin as open-mouthed vessels in the region of the terminal bronchioles, that is the bronchoalveolar junction. Alveolar septae do not contain lymphatic vessels.[46] However, it is generally presumed that fluid is filtered from capillaries in these alveolar walls. It appears likely that such fluid moves through the interstitial spaces of the lung to the bronchoalveolar junction, where it enters lymph vessels. A number of observations suggest that particles deposited in alveoli may travel a similar route: (1) pneumococci appear in hilar lymph nodes within a few minutes of deposition in the lung, long before bacteremia occurs; (2) noninfectious particles such as those associated with pneumoconioses are regularly found in hilar nodes as well as in the lung parenchyma; and (3) inert dust particles instilled into the lungs of experimental animals can be traced through apparent steps of migration through the alveolar epithelium, transport through the interstitium, and entry into lymphatics at the bronchoalveolar junction.[47] Penetration of the alveolar epithelium probably occurs without prior phagocytosis of the particle. The presence of particles within macrophages in the lung's interstitium probably represents phagocytosis of particles which penetrated the epithelium alone.

Lymphatic drainage probably contributes little to the quantitative removal of foreign materials in the lung. However, because access to the lymphatic system requires internalization of the foreign particles, drainage by way of this system may play an important role in determining the host's response to the agent. In the case of bacterial infection, lymphatic invasion provides one mechanism of bacteremia.

Surface-Lining Fluid. Although the principal function of the alveolar surface-lining fluid is to lower surface tension, thereby promoting alveolar stability, some observations suggest that it may contribute to alveolar defense as well. Staphylococci which have had contact with this surface material *in vitro* are more readily killed by alveolar macrophages than organisms which have not.[48] The significance of this finding remains to be established.

Immunologic Factors. The role of immunologic factors in various diseases is discussed in Chapters 9, 13 and 14; only those aspects which may relate to general lung defense are discussed here. Bronchoalveolar lavage in normal subjects has revealed the presence of IgG, IgA, alpha-l-antitrypsin, and most of the complement proteins.[49] Obviously, the source of these proteins cannot be determined from such lavage specimens, but it seems reasonable to believe that they may be present on the surface of the normal alveolus. Although the immunoglobulins may represent transudation of serum proteins, there is ample evidence that they are synthesized by lymphoid tissue within the lung, especially around peripheral airways, the so-called bronchoalveolar lymphoid tissues, or BALT.[50] In the case of IgA, the moiety present in secretions contains secretory piece, a protein added by the respiratory epithelium. Experiments with differing sites of immunization have shown some compartmentalization of the immune response in that animals immunized by way of lung produce predominantly local antibody, whereas animals immunized systemically produce a generalized response with a lesser response in the lung.[51]

Cell-mediated immune responses show similar compartmentalization depending on the route of inoculation. These findings have two important implications. First, the lung contains a full complement of immunocompetent cells which are capable of a full range of immune responses. Second, systemic immune responses may underestimate the magnitude of response occurring in the lung, particularly if the antigenic challenge is presented principally to the lung.

As with other defenses, immunologic mechanisms may become the agents of lung injury under some circumstances. Such injury may represent an inadvertent side-effect of an immunologic attack on a foreign substance. Caseous necrosis resulting in cavitation of the lung in tuberculosis requires the presence of delayed hypersensitivity directed against mycobacterial antigens. Extensive pulmonary infiltrates may develop with measles infection in subjects who were previously immunized with the killed-virus vaccine.[52] In this situation, lung injury apparently occurs as a consequence of the interaction of measles virus and circulating antibody in the lung. In experimental animals, similar acute lung injury has been produced by intrabronchial administration of antigen to animals previously sensitized by parenteral injection.[53] Finally, immune mechanisms may be responsible for lung injury in the absence of a definable foreign antigen or stimulus. In Goodpasture's syndrome, diffuse hemorrhagic pneumonitis appears to be related to the presence of circulating anti-basement-membrane antibodies.[54] Under some conditions, the determinants of which are unknown, it appears that immune-mediated lung injury may lead to chronic interstitial pneumonitis, in that some patients with this disease have circulating immune complexes and deposits of complement and IgG in their lungs.[55]

ASSESSMENT OF PATIENTS WITH SUSPECTED RESPIRATORY TRACT INFECTION

Most patients with respiratory tract infection present with fever and varying combinations of nasal discharge, sore throat, cough, expectoration of sputum, chest discomfort, and shortness of breath. These symptoms serve to focus the physician's attention on the respiratory tract and to suggest the possibility of an infectious process. The ultimate aims of the physician are to establish that infection is present, identify the causative agent, and prescribe appropriate therapy. Accomplishment of these aims frequently requires that several types of data be obtained and interpreted in a skillful fashion.

HISTORY

The key items to be obtained from the patient's history are listed below. In addition to the exact symptoms the patient has experienced, the pace of the illness may provide valuable diagnostic information. For example, although both *K. pneumoniae* and anaerobic bacteria cause febrile illnesses with lung cavitation, the illness associated with the former is typically abrupt and fulminant, whereas that of the latter is quite indolent.

Key Historical Items

- Nature of symptoms
- Pace of illness
- Associated symptoms
- Previous episodes
- Illness in contacts
- Unusual exposures
- Treatment, if any
- Underlying disease

The presence of associated symptoms may provide useful information. Exacerbation of latent *Herpes labialis* infection ("fever blisters") usually indicates bacterial rather than viral infection. Other cutaneous eruptions are uncommon with bacterial respiratory infection but petechial rashes may occur with a variety of viral infections including rubeola (typical and atypical), ECHO, and adenovirus, as well as the rickettsial diseases. These infections must be differentiated from bacterial processes which produce petechial eruptions including bacterial endocarditis, gonococcemia, meningococcemia, and hemolytic streptococcal or staphylococcal infection.

Diarrhea may occur in any acute infection but is particularly common in Legionnaire's disease. Pulmonary involvement in primary enteric infection such as salmonellosis, when it occurs, usually presents as clinically insignificant bilateral interstitial infiltrates with cough and mild hypoxemia. Jaundice or chemical evidence of hepatocellular injury is a typical feature of some respiratory infections such as Q fever and infectious mononucleosis. Altered liver function may occur in overwhelming bacterial infections owing to hypoxemia and hypotension, although liver abscess should be considered.

An altered mental state is an ominous sign in the presence of acute respiratory infection. In aged patients, pneumonia commonly produces obtundation or disorientation in the absence of meningitis. Other infections, notably Legionnaire's disease, produce delerium or disorientation in patients of any age. Since bacterial invasion of the central nervous system can occur from any of several sites within or adjacent to the respiratory tract, including the nasopharynx, paranasal sinuses, or middle ears, as well as from the blood stream, the presence of an altered mental state requires thorough evaluation.

Recurring episodes of respiratory tract infection are rarely due to immunodeficiency states because the latter conditions are uncommon. Most often, recurrent pneumonia is due to underlying chronic bronchitis, bronchiectasis, or left ventricular failure.[56] Cancer of the lung uncommonly causes recurrent pneumonia; rather, bronchial obstruction tends to cause pneumonias which do not resolve radiographically. However, repetitive episodes of pneumonia in the same bronchopulmonary segments suggest a localized disease process such as bronchiectasis or sequestration, whereas recurrent pneumonias in differing sites suggest either diffuse airways disease or immunodeficiency. Hypersensitivity pneumonitis is an important consideration in patients with recurrent episodes of fever, cough, and pulmonary infiltrations; improvement attributed to therapy may simply reflect removal from exposure to the causative antigen. Patients whose symptoms return shortly after return home or to work should be particularly questioned about their exposures.

The presence of similar symptoms in close contacts and family members may be very useful. For proper interpretation one must keep the incubation period of the suspected disease in mind. Simultaneous appearance of fever, cough, and malaise in several family members may be due to an explosive outbreak of an illness with a short incubation period, such as influenza. Alternatively, such an occurrence could be due to simultaneous exposure to an agent such as *Legionella pneumophilia* or *Histoplasma capsulatum*. It is usually easy to sort out these possibilities, especially when the disease produces similar symptoms in all infected persons, as is the case with most viral agents. On the other hand, *mycoplasma pneumoniae* infections have a long incubation period (10 to 14 days), and the resultant illness may vary from bullous myringitis to pharyngitis to bronchitis to pneumonia, so that the transmission of the organism among family members may be obscured. It is uncommon for bacterial pneumonia to occur simultaneously in several family members. However, careful questioning commonly reveals the presence of a preceding viral infection in others who have recovered uneventfully.

Respiratory infection may be caused by organisms with which the general population has little contact; a history of possible exposure to such an agent may provide invaluable diagnostic clues. Birds, especially parrots or parakeets imported from Central or South America, may be carriers of the causative agents of psittacosis; contacts may become sick before the bird manifests illness, an occurrence sometimes due to the illegal practice of administering prophylactic tetracycline to the birds to prevent deaths during transportation. Other domestic birds, especially turkeys, may be infected with this agent, but most reported human causes of psittacosis resulting from such sources have occurred among workers at processing plants. Several fungal agents may be present in high concentrations in dust or soil and cause infection in persons who dig in or otherwise stir up the soil. Well-known examples include coccidioidomycosis from soil in the Southwestern United States, histoplasmosis in broad areas of the Ohio River Valley and Midwest, especially associated with pigeon or chicken roosts, and cryptococcal infection, also associated with pigeon roosts. A history of travel to areas in which certain infections are endemic also may be helpful. Coccidioidomycosis is the best known example, and deservedly so, since demonstrable infection is relatively common in exposed persons. Other infections to keep in mind include the subacute pneumonia caused by *Pseudomonas pseudomallei* in persons exposed in Southeast Asia, in which signs of infection may not appear for years after exposure; and pulmonary manifestations of various parasites, which also may not appear for prolonged periods after initial infection.

The patient's response or lack of response to therapy is important information to be obtained from the history. Little can be said about failure to respond within 24 hr of the initiation of treatment. On the other hand, failure of response to penicillin within 72 hr is strong evidence that a patient does not have pneumococcal pneumonia, or is suffering a complication of it. Lack of response to penicillin is characteristic of infections due to *M. pneumoniae*, gram-negative bacilli, and Legionnaire's disease.

Finally, the presence and the type of underlying disease may provide valuable insights into the pathophysiology of the infection, as well as leads toward diagnosis.

PHYSICAL EXAMINATION

This section is intended to highlight a few important aspects of the physical examination for patients with respiratory tract infections, and is not meant to be a comprehensive discussion. It is understood that a thorough, complete examination is necessary to detect underlying disease processes or extrathoracic complications.

Stridor, an inspiratory crowing sound, is an ominous finding which signifies obstruction of the upper airway usually at the laryngeal or epiglottic level. It occurs typically in infants with croup but may occur in adults with acute infections as well. *Wheezes* are high-pitched, whistling sounds heard during inspiration or expiration (either audible at the bedside or by auscultation), which signify partial obstruction of peripheral airways. The sounds produced by either central or peripheral airways obstruction are dependent on the degree of obstruction and the rate of gas flow through the obstruction. Hence, sounds may disappear as obstruction worsens and flow diminishes. Evidence of greater-than-normal respiratory effort may be shown by the presence of *retraction*, an inward sinking of intercostal spaces or supraclavicular tissues due to the negative pleural pressure caused by forceful diaphragmatic contraction in the presence of obstructed airways. Inspection of the skin and mucous membranes for *cyanosis* may be helpful if such is present, but this is a subtle finding and one which is imprecisely estimated at the bedside; suspicion of hypoxemia should lead to confirmation by blood gas analysis.

Palpation of the thorax may detect diminished or delayed excursion of all or part of one hemithorax. This finding has multiple causes including bronchial obstruction, acute or chronic pleural disease, and impaired diaphragmatic or chest wall motion. *Tactile fremitus* is elicited by having the patient speak loudly a phrase, like "ninety-nine," which resonates in the respiratory tract. Normally the vibrations produced by this maneuver can be readily felt over the main bronchi (interscapular regions) but are only weakly transmitted to more peripheral regions of the thorax. Decreased tactile fremitus, either absolutely or in comparison to the other side, is due to large airway obstruction or to pleural disease, the so-called "peripheral screen" effect. Increased tactile fremitus signifies greater-than-normal transmission of vibrations to the chest wall and occurs in the presence of consolidated lung served by a patent airway.

During auscultation the examiner should note the quality and intensity of breath sounds, as well as the presence of abnormal sounds. Increased transmission of sounds generated in large airways causes the normal bronchovesicular breath sounds to become "bronchial" or "tubular" in quality, meaning that they resemble sounds normally heard over the trachea or major bronchi. Such changes are due to increased transmission by consolidated or partially consolidated lung, and are usually accompanied by an increase in the intensity of the sounds. The change in quality is the more important finding. Intensity of breath sounds may be altered by partial airway obstruction or a peripheral screen effect, and thus may change in either direction in the presence of consolidation. Increased transmission of breath sounds in the chest wall is generally accompanied by increased transmission of the whispered voice (*pectoriloquy*) and distortion of some sounds such as the "E-to-A" sound (*egophony*).

Rales are short, discontinuous sounds which are probably produced by the opening of small airways during inspiration. Numerous fine rales heard near the end of inspiration are typically heard over areas of consolidation; as the consolidation progresses, rales may disappear only to return, usually with a coarser sound, as the process begins to resolve several days later. *Rhonchi* are similar to wheezes in timing but are low-pitched sounds which are generally due to excessive secretions in the airways.

RADIOGRAPHIC STUDIES

Most patients with suspected pneumonia should have posteroanterior and lateral roentgenograms of the chest. Valuable information may be gained from the type of pulmonary abnormalities demonstrated, their segmental location, and the presence or lack of associated changes.

Inspection of the film should identify whether areas of increased density are present, and if present, whether localized, diffuse, or multiple but discrete. Consolidative changes in dependent segments, including posterior segments of upper lobes, superior segments of lower lobes, or basilar–posterior segments suggest aspiration as a mechanism. Multiple areas of consolidation suggest a hematogenous mechanism; a classic variant is the multiple cavitating nodules associated with staphylococcal sepsis.

Cavitation occurs most often in the central positions of dense consolidation and is due to necrosis of lung parenchyma. Organisms which produce such necrosis include *M. tuberculosis*, fungal agents, anaerobic bacteria, enteric gram-negative bacilli, and *S. aureus*. *S. pneumoniae*, the most common cause of bacterial pneumonia, does not produce necrosis of lung tissue, with the rare exception of infection due to type 3 organisms.

Pleural effusion may be identified in PA and lateral films or may require lateral decubitus films for definition. Pleural effusion occurs in 10% of patients with pneumococcal pneumonia but is much more common with infections due to anaerobes, gram-negative bacilli, *S. aureus*, or *Str. hemolyticus*. Pleural effusion is very uncommon with viral infections, but may be present in small amounts in up to 20% of patients with *M. pneumoniae* pneumonia. These facts support the notion that identification of pleural effusion (or empyema) radiographically is of great significance in the initial evaluation of patients with respiratory tract infection and its cause should be aggressively pursued.

MICROBIOLOGIC TECHNIQUES

Swab Specimens From the Upper Respiratory Tract

Swab specimens have significance in few situations in adult patients. Attention must be paid to the site of collection. *Str. hemolyticus* is most often recovered from the tonsils, even in the presence of diffuse pharyngitis. *N. meningitidis* resides principally in the nasopharynx and cultures of other sites are usually negative. *S. aureus* may be recovered from any site in the oropharynx but is most commonly carried in the anterior nares. In infants and small children in whom sputum collection is not possible, cultures of the oropharynx may provide the only source of bacteriologic specimens.

As with materials discussed below, identification of specific organisms in swab specimens may require special precautions in collection, transport, and cultivation. Drying of the specimen is particularly deleterious to sensitive organisms like *N. meningitidis*, *Corynebacterium diphtheriae*, or *Hemophilus influenzae*. If direct plating at the bedside is not possible, the swab should be placed in a suitable transport medium which will preserve the specimen for some hours.

Most laboratories cultivate respiratory specimens on 5% sheep's blood agar; a media selective for enteric bacilli such as eosin methylene blue (EMB); MacConkey's agar; or chocolate agar. Special media are available and may be required for the isolation of uncommon pathogens; close cooperation between clinician and microbiologist is required for optimal results if unusual organisms are suspected.

Expectorated Sputum

To the uninitiated it would appear that the microbiologic evaluation of expectorated sputum should provide unimpeachable evidence of the etiology of respiratory infection. Unfortunately, this is not the case. The sensitivity and accuracy of sputum cultures has been carefully studied in bacteremic pneumococcal pneumonia in which the causative agent is known with certainty. Cultures of expectorated sputum fail to demonstrate pneumococci in about 45% of such cases (false negatives).[57] On the other hand, pathogenic bacteria other than pneumococci are isolated from sputum in about 30% of such patients (false positives). *S. pneumoniae* is present in the respiratory tracts of 15 to 30% of healthy persons and thus would be expected in sputum from at least a similar percentage of patients with pneumonia of any cause.

Several factors contribute to this frustrating situation. First and foremost is the enormous bacterial population of the oropharynx, which may contaminate lower respiratory tract secretions during passage through the region. In addition, studies of passively contaminated specimens have shown that recovery of a single species which is present in low concentration is inhibited by interference of microbial growth by other organisms. It is also possible that organisms causing infection in the distal portions of the lung are no longer present in more proximal regions, owing to more effective defenses in the latter.

Many approaches have been used to improve the reliability of the sputum culture. Quantitative cultures, in which the sputum is homogenized with a liquifying agent like N-acetylcysteine and plated at several dilutions on various media, have been useful in the hands of some investigators.[59–60] The presumptions behind this approach (neither of which is necessarily so) are that the organism causing pneumonia will be present in sputum, and present in greater concentration than other species. However, untreated acute bacterial pneumonia is reported to be associated with concentrations in sputum of the responsible species exceeding 10^6/ml in 70 to 90% of cases; about 20% of specimens from patients without acute infection contain one or more pathogens at concentrations exceeding 10^6/ml (false positives). Washing of the sputum sample with sterile saline prior to culture by either quantitative or only qualitative techniques removes some of the contaminants acquired in passage through the upper airways and tends to reduce the rate of false positivity. Because complete removal of organisms intentionally added to the specimen requires nine repetitions of this rinsing procedure, the technique is time-consuming and best applied in conjunction with quantitative cultures. Misleading false positives occur commonly in situations where secretions are retained for prolonged periods in the airways, permitting organisms to multiply and achieve high concentration; this is particularly likely in patients with bronchiectasis, or in the presence of artificial airways.

Liquefaction of the sputum specimen renders it relatively homogeneous; other investigators have handled the problem of nonuniformity simply by selecting the most purulent portions of the specimen for examination. This frequently requires excision of particularly tenacious portions with a sterile scissors. A further refinement of this approach is to verify microscopically the host cell population present in such areas before proceeding wih culture; cultures of specimens which contain fewer than 10 epithelial cells and more than 25 inflammatory cells per low-power field correlate well with cultures obtained from the lower respiratory tract by invasive techniques.[61]

These observations indicate that the "routine sputum culture" is a very imprecise tool in the investigation of respiratory infection. Several techniques, including quantitative cultures, rinsing of the specimen, or microscopic screening, can reduce the false positivity rate if applied by conscientious personnel. Each of these is time-consuming and expensive but failure to use one or another of these approaches in the culture of expectorated sputum renders the sputum culture essentially a waste of time and money.

Other Specimens

Bacteriologic results also can be improved by using specimens other than expectorated secretions. The most popular of these is the *transtracheal aspirate*, in which a small plastic catheter is inserted percutaneously into the trachea, usually through the cricothyroid membrane.[62,63] Care must be used to ensure that the catheter is threaded distally into the trachea and is not directed towards or coughed into the larynx or pharynx. Suction is applied by syringe or vacuum to obtain a small sample; if no material is obtained, a few millimeters of sterile saline may be injected through the catheter and the aspiration repeated. The catheter is then withdrawn and the specimen quickly processed for culture and microscopic examination. This technique substantially avoids contamination by the oropharyngeal flora and provides specimens in which both the number of bacterial species present and their concentrations are reduced as compared to expectorated sputum. However, false-positive samples occur in 20 to 30% of patients, without consideration of quantitation.[64] Most helpful is the fact that falsely negative results, that is, lack of a pathogenic species in a patient with bacterial pneumonia, occurs in less than 1% of patients if the aspirate is performed prior to antimicrobial therapy. Also helpful is the well-established observation that anaerobic bacterial species are present infrequently and in small numbers in transtracheal aspirates unless the patient has a large pool of such organisms seeding the airways from below, that is, a significant anaerobic infection. This probably occurs because oropharyngeal anaerobes are rapidly killed by ambient oxygen tensions so that aspirated anaerobic organisms survive only briefly in the tracheobronchial tree. In addition, transtracheal aspiration can be used to obtain specimens from patients who cannot cough and effectively clear secretions.

The chief complications of transtracheal aspiration are bleeding, and development of subcutaneous or mediastinal emphysema.[65,66] It is mandatory that bleeding and clotting parameters be normal or nearly so before attempting the procedure. Sudden patient movements while the needle is being passed into the trachea may be castastrophic, so the patient must understand what is to happen and be cooperative. Tracheal distortion by large masses in the neck, such as goiter, may pose an additional problem. Finally, the procedure should not be performed in subjects with a small trachea (children) or with partial tracheal obstruction, in which bleeding could likely result in complete obstruction. Subcutaneous emphysema results from vigorous coughing before the puncture of the tracheal wall has closed; although distressing to the patient, it requires no therapy and resorbs in a few days.

Specimens for examination may be obtained directly from the peripheral lung by bronchoscopy. The advent of *fiberoptic bronchoscopy* has made this approach a feasible bedside tool. However, bronchoscopic specimens are uniformly contaminated by upper respiratory secretions unless special precautions are taken. Because of upper airway contamination, specimens obtained by lavage following instillation of sterile saline through the bronchoscope are not useful in the evaluation of bacterial infections, but may provide valuable material for the demonstration of opportunistic fungi or parasites; bacterial cultures of such specimens should not be interpreted as evidence of the lung's flora. Such contamination can be largely avoided by passage of a "protected" swab through a bronchoscope positioned in a region of interest in the lung. The catheter containing the swab is sealed at the distal end and, once it is properly positioned, the swab is forced through the seal, specimens obtained, and the swab retracted into the catheter. Thus, the swab is exposed only at the site of specimen collection. Results obtained by such sampling indicate that a single pathogenic species is recovered most often, and that contamination by upper respiratory flora is infrequent.[67]

The most direct approach to specimen collection from the lung is *transthoracic aspiration* of an involved region with a sterile needle.[68–70] This approach obviously avoids upper airway contamination and the need for specialized equipment, but is appreciably more hazardous than the previous techniques. Fluoroscopic monitoring of the procedure is desirable but not mandatory in the hands of experienced operators, especially when the region of interest is clearly located, or if the lung lesion is diffuse. Transthoracic lung aspiration has been used by pediatricians for many years, and in previously healthy children its complications are few. In adults pneumothorax occurs in 5 to 25% of patients but only occasionally requires drainage. Empyema does not occur as a result of violating the pleural space, possibly because antimicrobial therapy is generally instituted promptly thereafter. Massive hemorrhage and air embolism are rare complications. Transthoracic lung aspiration should not be performed in patients receiving positive-pressure ventilation or in patients with severe obstructive lung disease unless a chest tube is placed before the aspiration. Falsely positive samples are obtained infrequently (0 to 10% in reported series) but falsely negative aspirations occur in 15 to 30% of cases. This latter finding may be due to the small area that is sampled by the technique. Use of a larger needle provides lung tissue for histologic examination, which may allow the detection of organisms as well as characterization of tissue responses. Complications are significantly more common after such procedures, however, and large needles should not be used routinely in the evaluation of suspected infections.

Routine bacteriologic cultures of respiratory tract specimens should always be supplemented by microscopic evaluation of a stained smear of the material. The information gained from a Gram stain (see below) of sputum may well be more useful than the results of cultures. Organisms contained within phagocytes are very likely pathogenic; in bacterial pneumonias one species of organism generally predominates in the smear, especially in association with inflammatory cells. On the other hand, a diverse population of many species suggests that the specimen under examination is principally saliva; the presence of squamous epithelial cells substantiates that suspicion and such specimens should be disregarded.

Gram Stain of Sputum: Rapid Method

1. Prepare thin smear of the most purulent sputum on glass slide with sterile loop or swab.
2. Air dry sputum smear.
3. Heat fix slide to a temperature just tolerable to the skin on back of hand.
4. Cover with crystal violet for 10 sec.
5. Rinse with water.
6. Cover with Lugol's iodine for 10 sec.
7. Rinse with water.
8. Cover with 95% ethyl alcohol.
9. Rinse with water.
10. Cover with Safranin for 10 sec.
11. Rinse with water.
12. Blot and dry.
13. Examine for bacterial organisms. Particularly note polymorphonuclear cells and intracellular organisms.

Thus, the physician faced with a patient who may have a bacterial infection of the lower respiratory tract has a complicated decision to weigh. Although innocuous to the patient, examination of expectorated sputum, even with the refinements of washing, carefully selecting the portion of the specimen for culture, or homogenization and quantitative culture, suffers from insensitivity and inaccuracy. More reliable microbiological data can be obtained by invasive procedures, all of which entail added risk, and to varying degrees, added expense. The choice of specimens for examination must be tailored to individual circumstances. In our opinion, clear indications for transtracheal aspiration are few. The procedure may be helpful in supporting a diagnosis of nonbacterial pneumonia if the clinical setting alone does not strongly suggest that possibility. Transthoracic lung aspiration is probably safer than generally believed in adults and, when the need for accurate microbiology is pressing, provides reliable specimens. However, fiberoptic bronchoscopy can be used to obtain several types of specimens including protected swabs, alveolar lavage, and transbronchial biopsy and, in our opinion, is usually the initial procedure of choice if any invasive technique is contemplated.

It should be remembered that bacteremia occurs in approximately one-third of patients with bacterial pneumonia. A positive *blood culture* is the single most useful finding in the evaluation of these patients, and should always be obtained before antimicrobial therapy is initiated in any patient who is sufficiently ill as to require hospitalization.

Pleural effusion is present on admission in 10% of patients with pneumococcal pneumonia, but is appreciably more common in pneumonias due to *Staphylococcus aureus*, hemolytic streptococci, gram-negative bacilli, or anaerobic species. Thus, presence of effusion on admission suggests a bacterial etiology other than pneumococcus, and the effusion should always be aspirated for examination prior to initiating antimicrobial therapy.

OTHER TECHNIQUES

Antibody Responses

The demonstration of specific antibody in blood or secretions of an ill patient against an agent known to cause a similar illness can be useful diagnostic information. Unfortunately, although a rising antibody titer provides the best evidence of recent infection, such rises require at least 7 to 10 days, so that the information is rarely helpful in clinical decision-making. Antibody may be directed at one or more components of the organism. In the case of *S. pneumoniae*, specific, protective antibody is directed against the polysaccharide capsule—which is also the basis of determination of capsular type. Cross-reactions occur among certain types, but demonstration of an antibody rise with pooled antisera against several types is sufficient for most diagnostic purposes. However, the diagnosis is rarely in doubt by the time serologic responses are demonstrable, and such titers are rarely used except as research tools. In *Str. hemolyticus* infections, antibody may be demonstrated against M-protein, technoic acid of the fimbriae, somatic antigens, or bacterial products such as streptolysin O. Antibody against the latter correlates best with recent infection. Gram-negative bacillary infections also evoke antibody responses against multiple components including somatic antigens, capsular antigens, and bacterial products such as proteases. Demonstration of the latter provides strong evidence of tissue invasion by the organism and assists in establishing a pathogenic role for the organism in contrast to merely establishing the fact of colonization; antibody against somatic antigens is common in healthy people, apparently owing to continuous exposure to these organisms by way of the gastrointestinal tract, and the fact that somatic antigens are similar among many enteric species.

A rising antibody titer may be the only means of confirming the diagnosis of infections due to organisms that are difficult to culture *in vitro*, such as those responsible for Q fever, psittacosis, and Legionnaire's disease. In general, antibody titers against such organisms are less common in the general population, so that a titer of any level is cause for suspicion; a significant titer rise is still required for confirmation, a factor which limits the usefulness of the findings in the acute situation.

Demonstration of Antigen

Although cultivation of the responsible organism allows confirmation of the diagnosis and permits further studies with the organism, such as determination of antimicrobial susceptibility, attempts at culture are not always successful. Recently, techniques that permit detection of microbial-associated antigens in body fluids or secretions have become available. Demonstration of microbial antigen in many circumstances has much the same significance as demonstration of the organism itself, and can be accomplished even more rapidly than cultural techniques. Demonstration of bacterial antigens by counterimmunoelectrophoresis (CIE) in pleural fluid or in blood confirms the presence of significant infection due to the organism, since false positives are rare.[71,72] Analysis of pleural fluid for such antigens may have particular significance in determining the etiology of parapneumonic effusions after treatment with antimicrobial agents. Such treatment markedly reduces the likelihood of recovery of the organism in culture.[73] Pneumococcal infections are characterized by local accumulation of capsular antigen at the site of infection, followed by antigenemia and antigenuria, and thus are particularly well suited to study by CIE. Antigen is present in blood in 20 to 40% of patients with pneumococcal pneumonia, many but not all of whom are bacteremic. Antigenemia persists for as long as 14 days despite antimicrobial therapy, and the titer of antigenemia appears to be directly related to the frequency and severity of complications. Antigenuria occurs in 60% of patients and also persists for days.[74]

More controversial is the significance of demonstration of pneumococcal capsular antigen in expectorated sputum.[75–78] Sputum from patients with pneumococcal pneumonia and positive sputum cultures is routinely antigen-positive. Some studies have found antigen in sputum in approximately twice as many pneumonia patients as has positive cultures. Others have reported that patients who were clinically well but had positive cultures were antigen-negative; these findings suggest that invasive pneumococcal infection of the lungs is associated with antigen accumulation and expectoration, whereas surface colonization is not.

Similar techniques of antigen demonstration have been used in the diagnosis of cryptococcal and meningococcal infections and in the demonstration of *L. pneumophilia* in respiratory secretions and lung tissue. Although the exact role of this relatively expensive procedure in clinical medicine is still uncertain, antigen demonstration does afford promise as an adjunct to respiratory culture techniques. In addition, it has unique advantages in the rapid demonstration of antigen in body fluids before cultures are completed, or when cultures are negative due to antimicrobial therapy or other reasons.

LABORATORY INVESTIGATION OF RESPIRATORY VIRUSES

Basically, a definitive viral diagnosis of respiratory infection can be made by virus isolation and identification, and serological techniques.[79]

Virus Isolation and Identification

As with bacteriological specimens, it is imperative that fresh, carefully collected specimens be obtained and dispatched immediately to the laboratory. Three types of specimens are generally considered suitable for the virus laboratory: throat swabs, nasal swabs, or tracheal suction specimens. It is important that they be taken early in the illness, because excretion of respiratory virus may be limited to two days following the onset of symptoms.

Rapid diagnostic techniques such as electron microscopy to identify viral particles and type-specific fluorescent antibody techniques can be employed directly on the submitted specimen. Although there are still difficulties and pitfalls in these techniques, they are sometimes useful in establishing the presence of a viral infection, especially in epidemic situations where the prevalent agent in the community is known.

Since viruses are obligatory intracellular parasites, they can only be isolated in living cells such as tissue cultures, embryonated eggs, or after animal inoculation. In most virus laboratories, tissue culture is the mainstay of isolation techniques.

Agents isolated in tissue culture are identified using a variety of immune-specific serological techniques such as neutralization of virus by homologous antisera, hemagglutination inhibition, fluorescent antibody, and hemadsorption techniques. Many laboratories have developed rapid techniques of identifying a virus before there are any changes suggestive of virus infection in tissue culture. Electron microscopic examination of the supernatant fluid from the tissue culture at regular intervals permits early recognition of virus particles. This depends on the identification of typical viral morphology, which only indicates which virus group one is dealing with. More refined techniques of immunoelectron microscopy are being developed for certain virus subgroups and may provide a definitive rapid identification.

Fluorescent antibody studies on infected tissue culture 48 hr after the cultures have been inoculated have been found useful in the hands of experienced workers. This technique allows a positive diagnosis to be made within three days of receipt of the specimen.

Serological Diagnosis

If a fourfold rise in antibody to one of the respiratory viruses is observed in convalescent serum, a serological diagnosis can be made. The time between sampling the acute and convalescent sera should be of the order of 10 to 14 days in adults. Infants under 6 mo may be slow to respond and convalescent sera should be submitted at 30- to 60-day intervals. In routine respiratory virus serology, the complement fixation test is preferred for most agents, although hemagglutination inhibition tests may be used for appropriate viruses. It is customary also for the virus serology laboratory to test sera for nonviral agents that present with syndromes similar to those caused by respiratory virus. An optimal viral screen includes serological tests for *Rickettsia burnetii* (Q fever), psittacosis group (*Chlamydia*) and *Mycoplasma pneumoniae*. In view of their high infectivity, it is extremely dangerous to laboratory personnel to attempt to isolate rickettsiae and psittacosis organisms unless special safety equipment is available, consequently most labs rely on serological methods to make the diagnosis.

VIRAL INFECTIONS OF THE RESPIRATORY TRACT

Acute respiratory infections account for a large proportion of all cases seen in general medical practice, and of all hospitalized patients with respiratory illness. As high as 30 or 35% of patients presenting in family practice have respiratory tract infection as their main complaint. These cases represent only the tip of the iceberg, as most people accept minor infections of the respiratory tract as inevitable, and do not seek medical advice. Those seeking help for minor ailments such as the common cold and flu often do so because of associated chronic disease, or concern that a more serious problem is developing. It is thus difficult to assess the true prevalence of infections of the respiratory tract in the total population.

The United States Public Health Services studied population samples and estimated that each person suffers an average of 1.4 respiratory infections per yr which require medical advice, or some alteration in routine, such as time off work or absence from school.[80] In more detailed family studies of mild disease, average figures of six respiratory infections per person per yr have been reported.[81] The number of infections and the severity of symptoms vary with the age of the patient. Children are afflicted more often and more severely than adults, with about 50% of clinically apparent upper respiratory tract infections occurring before age six. The frequency of these illnesses decreases with age.[82,83] Females have increased frequency of infections during childbearing years, and this has been ascribed to increased contact with infected preschool children. Infections occur more than twice as often during the winter months; although the reason for this has not been established, crowding, increased indoor social activity, and related factors promoting transmission of organisms are considered to play a greater role than cold air *per se*.[79,82]

In most surveys, viruses are incriminated as the causative initiating agent in 90% of cases of acute respiratory tract infection. The commonest nonviral agents are *Streptococcus pneumoniae*, and *Mycoplasma pneumoniae*.

The repetitive nature of viral respiratory illnesses is a result of the large variety of agents. It takes many years for a person to encounter the many variants, while the immunity developed is relatively specific. As a consequence, the viruses have the ability to cause periodic epidemics even in communities that are in constant contact with many parts of the world; only in isolated communities can one escape the nuisance of repeated respiratory infections. This was well illustrated by the Rev. MacAulay in the seventeenth century. He noted that, in the remote island of St. Kilda, off the west coast of Scotland, the inhabitants, whose only contact with the outside world was the annual visit of the rent collector's boat, all came down with colds and fever after its arrival. Similar experience has been noted in relation to other isolated islands and in the Antarctic expeditions.[84-86] Anecdotal evidence suggests that after a period of swapping viruses, the personnel transported to the polar stations were free from viral respiratory infections until visitors arrived or they left the Antarctic to return to civilization where they were again exposed to new strains of organisms.

The agents causing viral-like acute respiratory diseases are listed in Table 8-5.[79] It is customary to subdivide them into three groups; those viruses with predominant respiratory manifestations; viruses which involve other organ systems, but may have associated respiratory manifestations; and agents other than viruses which present in a manner similar to viruses (for example, mycoplasma, rickettsia). Table 8-3 lists the relative frequency of common viral agents in producing clinical illness.[79,83]

Transmission of Respiratory Viruses

Infected humans are the source and reservoir of the majority of the respiratory viruses. There is some evidence that animals such as horses and pigs may also serve as a reservoir for certain variants of influenza A.[79,87] In most instances, droplet transmission, as discussed earlier in this chapter, is undoubtedly the process by which inoculation of a susceptible host takes place. Certain viruses may be transmitted by direct contact with mucous membranes through close contact, such as kissing. In general, this is probably a less frequent mode of transmission. Some viruses may also affect the respiratory tract via fecal-oral contamination, and this has been postulated particularly for the enteroviruses.[79] Occasionally viruses such as that producing chicken pox may be transmitted from infected cutaneous secretions.

Recently, hand-to-hand contact was shown to be surprisingly effective in the transmission of rhinovirus among human subjects, actually demonstrating greater likelihood of producing infection than exposure to aerosolized virus.[88] The hands of the source case became contaminated by contact with his own secretions. Hand-to-hand contact with a susceptible host transfered the virus, which the new host subsequently autoinoculated into his respiratory tract.

The route of transmission is probably an important determinant of whether or not infection results from exposure to a given virus. The dose of rhinovirus or Coxsackie virus needed to establish respiratory tract infection is lowest when the virus is introduced into the nose; influenza and adenoviral infection is more likely to occur if the virus is delivered into the airways by small-particle aerosol.[79] The predilection of viruses to attack certain tissues is in part due to the necessity for cellular attachment to occur, a process which requires the availability of cell-surface receptors. Some tissue cells lack receptors for certain viruses and thus do not become infected. Binding of virus to the cell surface may be inhibited somewhat by nonspecific substances in secretions, and is markedly inhibited by specific antibody. Mucociliary transport aids in resisting respiratory infection by sweeping viral particles to the oropharynx for disposal by swallowing; most viruses are destroyed by acid in the stomach, although some such as the enteroviruses survive well in this environment.

Extensive studies to determine the factors which make a person more susceptible to respi-

TABLE 8-3. Viral Respiratory Illness in Older Children and Adults

Agent	Percent of All Viral Infections
Rhinovirus	40
Influenza A, B	10
Parainfluenza	8
Respiratory syncytial virus	6
Adenovirus	2
Coxsackie and echo virus	<1
Corona virus, herpes virus, and other	33

ratory virus infection have done little to increase our knowledge, but have done a lot to remove many of the commonly held myths of how "colds" are caught. Chilling has often been stated to be an important factor in making an individual more susceptible to viral infections. Attempts to reproduce this phenomenon experimentally have not met with success.[89,90]

Certain respiratory viruses such as influenza A are epidemic in nature, whereas other viruses tend to be endemic. This is probably related to differences in infectivity. Influenza A is a highly infectious agent, and thus when a variant of the virus appears in a community, susceptible subjects are rapidly infected and become immune, leaving the virus a limited substrate. It therefore disappears from the community.[91,92] This sequence is facilitated by short excretion periods. When a person is infected the excretion of the virus is limited to a period of a few days. Thus, even in large metropolitan centers such as New York, Tokyo and London, influenza A is unable to establish itself as an endemic agent. Adenoviruses 1, 3, 5, and 7 are commonly found in children during all seasons of the year. This is probably due to a lower infectivity and to prolonged excretion periods which may last for weeks. Adenoviruses may not require large populations to maintain themselves because of this prolonged excretion. Military training camps and mining centers often harbor what is known as a "place virus," usually an adenovirus, which infects new personnel entering the environment.[79]

Pathogenesis of Viral Illness

Once a virus has reached the respiratory tract mucosa, the principal site of infection appears to be the ciliated cells. Initially the ciliated epithelium degenerates and desquamates leaving a thin layer of basal replacement cells.[91] The replication of viruses takes place within the cells and spreads to adjacent cells; however, further inoculation up or down the tracheobronchial tree may also occur as a result of transmission of particles along the mucus blanket. These changes result in paralysis of cilia, frank necrosis of cells with desquamation, interference with function of the mucociliary blanket, and the attendant inflammatory responses, including exudation of fluid and erythrocytes. Pathological examination may reveal the entire range of findings. The mucosal insult and attendant changes in defense mechanisms along the respiratory epithelium probably account for the high incidence of secondary bacterial infection in patients with viral disease. The spectrum of severity is highly variable, and unpredictable in a given individual.

The general response to virus infection may be substantially modified according to the immunological history of the host. With increased knowledge of the immunological response of the host, it has been postulated that many of the clinical features of respiratory virus infection may be due to the injurious effect of the host's immune response to the foreign viral proteins and to the altered antigenicity of infected cells. Experience gained from the use of killed rubeola[93] and respiratory syncitial vaccines[94] has helped to elucidate some of these effects. Children who have received killed rubeola vaccine, instead of showing a diminished response when infected with wild rubeola, responded with a severe viral pneumonia, as if they had been somehow sensitized by their immunization. This led to the withdrawal of the killed vaccine from the market. In other attempts to control respiratory syncytial virus infection, a killed vaccine was used. Of the infants who received the control vaccine, only one required hospitalization, but of those who received the killed vaccine, approximately half required hospitalization for pneumonia and bronchiolitis. This raises the possibility that the presence of circulating antibody in the absence of cell immunity may lead not to protection, but to some form of hypersensitivity response.[95,96] Bellanti and coworkers suggested an Arthus type of reaction.[95]

Since many respiratory viruses share group antigens, a person who has had multiple previous infections, or vaccines (as for influenza A), will possess circulating antibody to components of new strains. These may not be sufficient to provide immunity. Consequently, the virus is able to multiply, and react with circulating antibody from previous infections, with the development of immune complexes and a hypersensitivity response. This might explain the strong

TABLE 8-4. Modification or Prevention of Respiratory Virus Infections

Virus*	Passive immunization† recommended for:	Active immunization‡ recommended for:
Influenza A and B		Chronically ill (see text)
Adenovirus		Military camps
Varicella zoster virus	(within 3 days) Contacts who are: Less than 2 yr old Immune suppressed Pregnant women (within 5 days)	
Rubeola	Contacts who are: Less than 3 yr old Pregnant women Tuberculous Immune-suppressed	Healthy children§

* See text for each specific organism.
† Hyperimmune human gammaglobulin administered parenterally.
‡ Contraindicated in individuals with hypersensitivity to egg protein.
§ Age, pregnancy, systemic disease or immune suppressing drugs may be contraindications.

similarity of clinical features between influenza and serum sickness. Until completion of more intensive studies of the immune response to respiratory viral infections, this fascinating aspect of pathogenesis must remain speculative.

Recovery From Virus Infection and Immunity to Specific Infections

The mechanism whereby patients infected by virus recover from their illness remains a mystery.[96] In the early days of virology, great emphasis was laid on the role of antibody production in eliminating the infecting virus; this has now been relegated to a more minor role. Many patients with abnormalities of circulating humoral antibody respond normally to viral infections. Quantitatively, the amount of specific antibody detectable in respiratory excretions is insufficient to explain the disappearance of the virus. Furthermore, antibody is usually first detectable after the clinical manifestations have subsided.[96] Interferons have been shown to protect susceptible cells against viral infection and they undoubtedly do play a role in the control of spread of virus, but this is unlikely the major mechanism of recovery from an infection. The cell-mediated immune mechanisms appear to be important in controlling the spread of certain types of viral infection. The devastating effect of the herpes and varicella group of viruses in patients in whom cell mediated immunity is artificially suppressed by drugs or disease processes, such as leukemia and Hodgkin's disease, supports this as an important immune mechanism. However, the same patients may respond in a normal fashion to other viral agents. The orchestration of these various contributions to the resistance of an individual to viral infection, or control of the disease remains to be defined.

Passive immunity may be developed by parenteral administration of human immune globulin, which thus has some place in the management of persons at high risk who have had contact with infectious patients. This is particularly true for varicella zoster infections, and rubeola (Table 8-4).

Active immunization for special groups may reduce the number of persons infected, and the severity of the disease. At present, this is most promising for influenza, adeno-, and rubeola virus infections. It should be noted that none of these measures provide complete protection, and each has an inherent risk.

Chemotherapy of viral infections continues to pose major problems, principally because of the toxicity of compounds with antiviral activity. The most promising approach involves the interferons, a group of proteins which are synthesized by virus-infected cells.[35] While many cells may produce interferon, human leukocytes and fibroblasts are the principal sources for *in vitro* production. Recombinant DNA technology affords the promise that bacteria may be caused to produce commercial quantities of human interferon. In concept, treatment may consist of administration of interferon or of an agent which induces its secretion by the host. A number of interferon inducers are known but their safety and efficacy for humans is not established.

In clinical trials, interferon has shown an effect in the treatment of herpetic keratitis, herpes zoster and cytomegalovirus infection. Topically applied interferon reduced clinical symptoms and nasal shedding of rhinovirus 4 in experimentally infected volunteers. In most trials, interferon has been most effective if given prophylactically. This is in keeping with its mode of action, which is to bind to cell-surface receptors and induce the formation of cellular enzymes that block viral replication. Its antiviral activity is nonspecific, being active against most human pathogens. Full exploration of its usefulness in antiviral chemotherapy awaits the availability of adequate supplies to permit clinical trials. Amantadine is an effective drug against influenza A and its use is described in the section on Influenza.

Lung Function Abnormalities Associated With Upper Respiratory Viral Infection

It has been generally considered that upper respiratory viral infections infrequently involve the lower respiratory tract. Recent studies have shown, to the contrary, that abnormalities in lung function commonly accompany "colds" in the absence of clinical evidence of lower tract disease, that is, in the absence of abnormal findings on physical examination or radiographic abnormalities.[97–102] Mild hypoxemia and airways dysfunction are the usual findings, suggesting that viral propagation has occurred throughout the respiratory tract. Of particular interest is the finding that individuals with acute upper respiratory viral infections transiently demonstrate bronchial hyperreactivity to inhaled aerosol.[103,104] This finding indicates that viral infection and environmental factors may act synergistically to impair lung function. Whether recurrent viral infection plays any role in the pathogenesis of chronic lung disease is unknown. The abnormalities of lung function that have been demonstrated during viral infection are generally transient, although several weeks may be required for full return of function.

Lung Function Abnormalities Associated With Lower Respiratory Tract Viral Infection

Viral pneumonias occur with varying severity; such variation appears to be due to the extent of disease, not to differing pathophysiologic processes. Affected patients demonstrate tachypnea, dyspnea, and cyanosis. When measured, lung volumes are reduced and lung compliance is low. Hypoxemia, if severe, responds poorly to increases in the concentration of oxygen inspired, indicating shunt physiology.[105–107] Radiographic changes tend to be diffuse, beginning as interstitial edema and progressing to frank alveolar flooding as the disease worsens. Early alveolar flooding consists of hemorrhage and edema fluid with a high protein content; later, the alveolar process becomes more cellular and fibrosis may occur within 7 to 10 days in patients maintained with mechanical ventilation.[108] Lung function tends to improve more rapidly than the chest radiograph as the alveolar process clears and/or organizes. Residual linear interstitial markings may persist for months. Lung function usually returns to normal, although such improvement may occur gradually over a protracted interval.[101]

However, recent observations suggest that bronchiolitis in infancy leads to persistent abnormalities in lung function and possibly in lung structure. Children who had bronchiolitis demonstrate increased airway reactivity, lower expired flow, and impaired gas exchange 8 to 10 yr later.[99,109] These findings raise the possibility that viral infection in childhood may predispose

TABLE 8-5. Common Respiratory Syndromes and Their Etiologic Agents

Pathogen	Child cold	Adult cold	Laryngo-tracheo-bron-chitis*	Flu	Adult pneumonia	Child pneumonia	Pleuritis, peri-carditis
Respiratory virus							
Influenza A	+	−	+	++	+	+	−
Influenza B	+	−	+	++	+	+	−
Influenza C	+	+	−	−	−	+	−
Parainfluenza	+	+	++	++	−	+	−
R. S. Virus	+	+	+	+	−	++	−
Adenovirus	++	+	+	++	+	+	−
Rhinovirus	+	++	+	+	−	−	−
Coronavirus	−	++	−	+	−	−	−
Non-respiratory viruses affecting respiratory tract							
Coxsackie virus	+	+	+	+	−	−	+
Echo virus	+	+	+	+	−	−	+
Rubeola	+	+	+	+	+	+	−
Varicella	+	+	+	+	+	−	−
Nonviral agents							
Psittacosis (*Chlamydia psittaci*)	−	−	−	+	++	+	−
Rickettsia (*Coxiella burnetii*)	−	−	−	+	++	−	−
Mycoplasma (*M. pneumoniae*)	−	−	+	+	++	+	±

* Presents as croup in the child.
− Rare, if ever
+ Occasional
++ Prominent feature

an individual to accelerated changes in lung function upon exposure to injurious agents such as cigarette smoke later in life.

COMMON VIRAL SYNDROMES

The viruses which may be responsible for each of the common viral syndromes are listed in Table 8-5.

The Common Cold: Coryza

Clinical Manifestations. The common cold is the commonest respiratory viral disease encountered by humans.[82] Although this upper respiratory tract syndrome is caused by many viruses, the presenting symptoms are remarkably similar from individual to individual. Variants peculiar to an individual also occur, and the same person tends to get the same combination of symptoms, whatever the causative agents. The disease usually starts with a feeling of dryness and stuffiness of the upper respiratory tract affecting mainly the nasopharynx. This is followed by hypersecretion of mucus and lacrymation. In the uncomplicated cases these fluids remain clear and mucoid. Generalized symptoms of headache and malaise may also be present. In more severe cases, fever and chills may be marked and mild prostration may occur. The disease process is usually over in 3 to 4 days.

Examination of the mucous membranes of the upper respiratory tract reveals them to be hyperemic, edematous, and bathed in mucous secretions. Biopsy of nasal mucosa shows a lymphocytic infiltration with edema and congestion of small capillaries. Recent studies suggest hyperreactivity of bronchial smooth muscle, which may account for exacerbations of asthma in some patients.[103,104]

Complications are rare, but in patients with a compromised respiratory tract, such as chronic bronchitics, the infection may descend to the trachea and the bronchial tree. Secondary bacterial infection, as evidenced by the respiratory secretions becoming purulent, and a bacterial bronchitis or pneumonia may develop. It is rare for a true viral pneumonia to ensue. In children otitis media is common, and in adults, sinusitis with secondary bacterial infection may follow.

Treatment of the uncomplicated case is symptomatic; there is no specific therapy. This knowledge is apparently not acceptable to the general public. In 1972 more than 600 million dollars were spent in the United States for nonprescription cold remedies.[110] Apparently, 94% of physicians' office visits for a cold resulted in prescriptions for the patient. About one-third of these were for antihistamines, which have not been shown to decrease severity or duration of the illness.[111] Salicylates, a time-honored symptomatic remedy, probably act by lowering the patient's temperature, increasing the pain threshold, and perhaps have an anti-inflammatory action. There is no evidence that they alter the duration of the illness, but they may actually increase viral shedding.[112] Recent enthusiasm for vitamin C for treatment or prevention of "colds" has some scientific support,[113] but is not generally accepted.[114] Osler's recommendation was: "There is just one way to treat a cold, and that is with contempt." The use of antibiotics should be avoided unless there is evidence of secondary bacterial infection, indicated by the presence of purulent discharge containing bacterial organisms. In patients such as chronic bronchitics, there may be an acute exacerbation of lower respiratory tract symptoms associated with each episode of the cold.

Many people develop the cold syndrome as a result of allergic rhinitis such as hay fever; this syndrome is generally improved by appropriate therapy for the allergy.

Pharyngitis

Clinical Manifestations. Sore throat, associated with difficulty in swallowing, is the hallmark of acute pharyngitis. Nasal stuffiness, cough, mild headache, and general malaise frequently characterize the illness if it is caused by a virus. Examination of the pharynx reveals erythema, swelling, lymphoid hyperplasia as in the tonsils, and occasionally exudative mucoid or purulent patches of secretions (particularly in association with the adenovirus). Submandibular lymph nodes may be enlarged, but are only mildly tender. Fever is generally mild, and the leukocyte count is normal or only slightly elevated.

Viral pharyngitis must be differentiated from other more severe and treatable causes of pharyngitis. The most common and most severe, streptococcal pharyngitis, is frequently clinically indistinguishable from viral pharyngitis. While the fever tends to be higher, the leukocyte count higher, and the illness generally more severe, cultures of the inflamed area may be the only practical method of differentiation. Diphtheria, now rare in countries with immunization programs, is associated with membranous lesions which have a creamy appearance, are tenacious, and difficult to remove. When the lesions are scraped off, the underlying mucosa tends to bleed. The patient appears inappropriately ill for the nasopharyngeal manifestations. Infectious mononucleosis is generally associated with generalized lymphadenopathy and, not infrequently, splenomegaly. The peripheral blood generally contains increased numbers of atypical lymphocytes and serology is positive for heterophile antibodies. Occasionally, fusospirochetal infections cause an ulcerative gingivitis and stomatitis (trench mouth); so-called Vincent's angina is readily recognized by the extensive lesions and foul odor.

Treatment. Viral pharyngitis requires no specific treatment. Symptomatic therapy may be appreciated by the patient. Exclusion of other nonviral causes of the disease is the most important aspect of the management. Streptococcal infections and diphtheritic infections, of course, require appropriate antibiotic therapy.

Acute Laryngotracheobronchitis

Clinical Manifestations. Adults with laryngitis develop hoarseness, loss of voice, and localized pain. This may be associated with a brassy cough which is generally productive of minimal sputum. Symptoms of associated tracheitis are common, consisting of a raw, burning, high retrosternal pain, accentuated by cough or deep breathing. In some patients a persistent, nonproductive cough, frequently occurring in paroxysms and aggravated by exercise or inhalation of cold, dry or dusty air, may be the only evidence of a viral bronchitis. The cough may last for a week, causing great concern as to other possible underlying causes. Chest-wall pain may develop as a result of the severe cough effort, and occasionally rib fractures occur (Chapter 11). If the condition is prolonged, increased mucus production takes place, occasionally becoming purulent. Mucopurulent sputum may result merely from increased cellularity due to inflammatory cells, or from secondary bacterial infection. In small children, respiratory distress may develop as indicated by dyspnea and stridor (croup). Prolonged inspiration and expiration, the use of accessory muscles of respiration, intercostal and supraclavicular indrawing of the chest wall, and cyanosis testify to the severity of an attack. Virtually all of these respond to inhalation of high humidity and oxygen within several hours, but may recur nightly for 3 to 5 days. Fever is minimal. Associated symptoms of a cold, otitis media, or in the older age groups sinusitis, are not uncommon.

Treatment. Symptomatic therapy, such as rest and salicylate administration, may be warranted in severe cases. High humidity in the environment and suppression of nonproductive cough by antitussive agents such as codeine may provide striking symptomatic relief. In some patients it appears that cough begets persistent cough, perhaps by providing recurrent mechanical trauma to the bronchial tubes and larynx. Complete cough suppression for 48 to 72 hr by use of drugs may terminate this aspect of the illness in the later stages, suggesting that the active infectious process has subsided.

Secondary bacterial infection must be diligently sought for, the organisms identified, and appropriate antibiotics considered. Persistent fever, purulent sputum, or pleuritic chest pain should arouse concern that a bacterial infection is in progress.

Bronchiolitis

Clinical Manifestations. Infants tend to develop severe obstruction at the bronchiolar level due to acute respiratory illness. Most often it is a result of respiratory syncytial virus, and occurs before age two.[115,116] As discussed in Chapter 3, the development of the lung is not complete at this stage, collateral ventilation is primitive, and the caliber of the distal airways remains relatively small, perhaps accounting for the severity of the obstructive manifestations. On examination, the child may have the clinical features of a cold, but dyspnea, cyanosis, and labored respiration are prominent. No tracheal stridor is heard, but examination of the chest demonstrates hyperinflation, poor air movement bilaterally, and generalized rhonchi or rales. Arterial blood gases demonstrate hypoxemia, and in severe attacks, increased arterial P_{CO_2}. Frequently a chest roentgenogram is required to demonstrate the absence of pneumonic infiltration convincingly, but bronchiolitis and pneumonia may co-exist. (See section on Respiratory Syncytial Infections.)

Although adults may develop bronchiolitis, due to several causes (Chap. 14) the symptoms are generally less severe.

Treatment. The major treatment is supportive, consisting of oxygen, increased humidity, bronchodilators, and diligent search for evidence of bacterial infection.

Viral Pneumonia

Clinical Manifestations. Some patients develop evidence of respiratory distress, with or without one of the preceding syndromes, where laryngitis, tracheobronchitis, or bronchiolitis are not likely to be the cause. They may have fever, dyspnea, and cyanosis on exertion; a nonproductive cough is a major clinical feature. Loss of

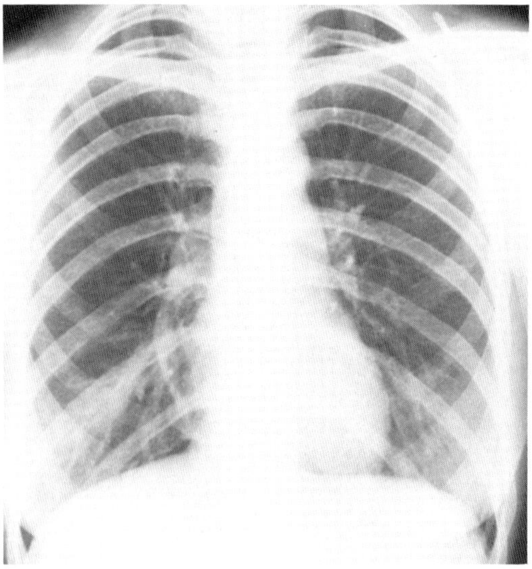

FIG. 8-3. Viral involvement of the lung is usually unrecognized roentgenographically. When it is demonstrable, it ranges through an entire spectrum of infiltrates. This patient with a right middle lobe infiltrate had minimal abnormality which completely cleared after 10 days without any form of therapy. Acute and convalescent sera demonstrated an eightfold rise in influenza A viral titers.

appetite is common. Examination of the chest reveals normal findings or minimal changes in breath sounds and resonance to percussion, with occasional scattered inspiratory rales. Roentgenographic examination of the chest may reveal minor infiltrates, or any degree of infiltrate up to severe bilateral infiltrates (see Figs. 8-3, 8-4, 8-5, 8-6). Frank lobar consolidation is uncommon, as are signs of pleural inflammation. In general, the physical findings in the chest are less dramatic than one would predict from the roentgenographic abnormalities. Viral pneumonia is discussed in detail under Influenza Viral Infections.

The differentiation of viral from bacterial pneumonias is discussed in detail in relation to the specific diseases (Table 8-6).

Treatment. The treatment of viral pneumonia is discussed in the section on Influenza Virus.

LESS COMMON VIRAL SYNDROMES

Herpangina

Some patients with Coxsackie virus infections characteristically develop small, rapidly ulcerating vesicles typically located on the anterior pillars of the tonsils and the soft palate. This finding may permit a clinical diagnosis of the cause of pharyngitis. It is also useful to the clinician when patients with other respiratory manifestations such as pleuritic pain are examined for further diagnostic clues. The acute illness is characterized by malaise, pharyngeal discomfort, and low grade fever. The patient presenting with an acute febrile illness, pleuritic pain, and the presence of herpangina should be considered to have a Coxsackie virus infection in the absence of other clinical features. Pleuritis, however, is generally the result of infection with the Coxsackie B types of virus, and herpangina generally the Coxsackie A group, so that the overlap is not great.

Pleurodynia

Patients with severe localized chest wall pain without apparent cause, or pleuritis with pleural friction rub, small pleural effusions, and pleuritic pain, may be victims of infectious virus illnesses generally of the Coxsackie variety, but occasionally other enteroviruses.[79] In most instances there is a clear-cut epidemic history, with other members of the family group affected, and the systemic manifestations are modest. Other features of enterovirus infection, including intestinal disturbances, are common.

The disease process is usually self-limited, with very severe pain lasting only for 2 to 4 days, fever decreasing within 2 to 5 days, and pleural effusions disappearing within a week. Thoracentesis reveals a straw-colored exudate (Fig. 8-7; see also Chap. 12, Pleural Disease). Although no reports are available, in the author's experience lung scans demonstrate diminished perfusion only in the region of the effusion. The major differential diagnosis includes other causes of acute onset of pleuritic pain. (See Chap. 12.)

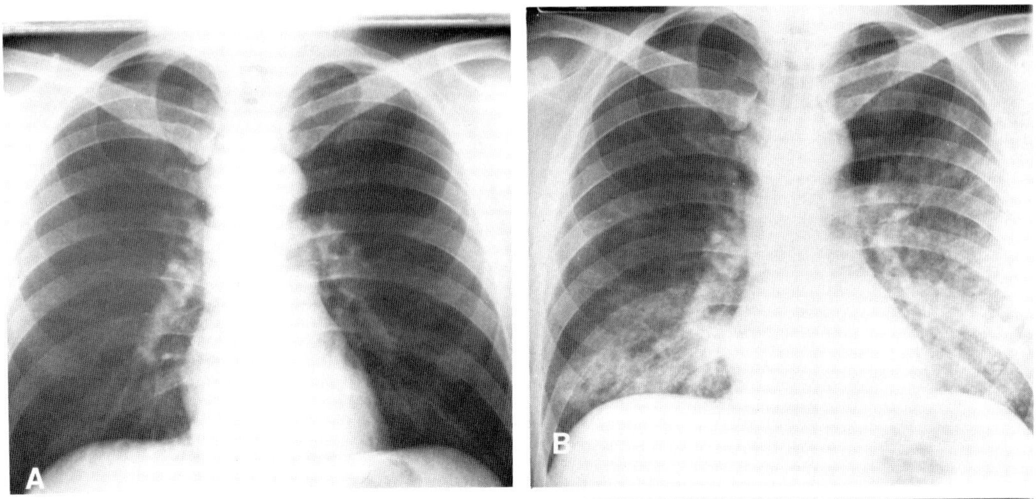

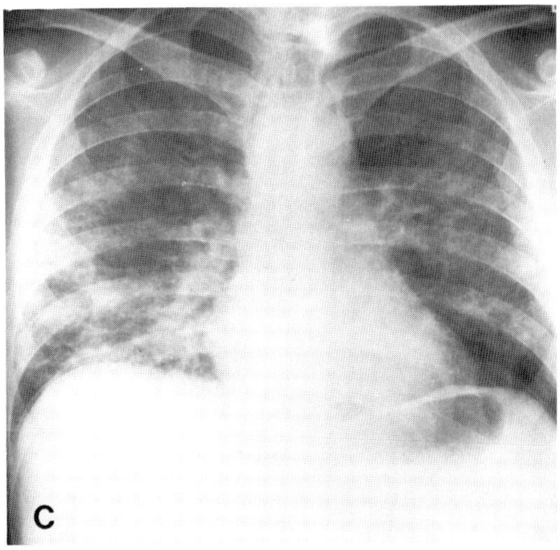

FIG. 8-4. The viral pneumonia shown here developed in a young male with acute myelogenous leukemia. A normal chest film taken six months prior to the viral infection (**A**) is contrasted with a film taken because of severe dyspnea (**B**), which demonstrates marked bilateral fluffy infiltrate with interstitial and alveolar components. At this time, there was a 20-fold rise in antibody titers to influenza A virus in convalescent as compared to acute serum. One month later, there was further loss of lung volume and a more reticular infiltrate. A lung biopsy at that time demonstrated interstitial fibrosis. A chest radiograph 6 months later (**C**) showed persistent infiltrate.

Treatment consists of analgesics and supportive care.

Pharyngoconjunctival Fever

Inflammation of the pharynx with conjunctivitis is a prominent manifestation seen commonly in relation to adenovirus infections. This is generally an acute and self-limited illness of childhood, associated with low-grade fever, and lasting 2 to 5 days.

Pericarditis

Viral pericarditis is occasionally associated with pleuritis as a result of Coxsackie infections. More commonly, however, the pericarditis appears as an isolated phenomenon, and follows the upper respiratory infection by 10 to 14 days. Pain is the major manifestation, but pericardial effusions may result in tamponade.

Differential Diagnosis of Common Syndromes

Recognition of the distinctive features of virus infections of the respiratory tract is of particular importance to the clinician and the patient since, for each syndrome, other important treatable causes of the clinical manifestations must be evaluated. When, for example, the young adult presents with acute onset of severe pleuritic chest pain, pulmonary embolism with infarction or an acute bacterial pneumonia with pleuritis

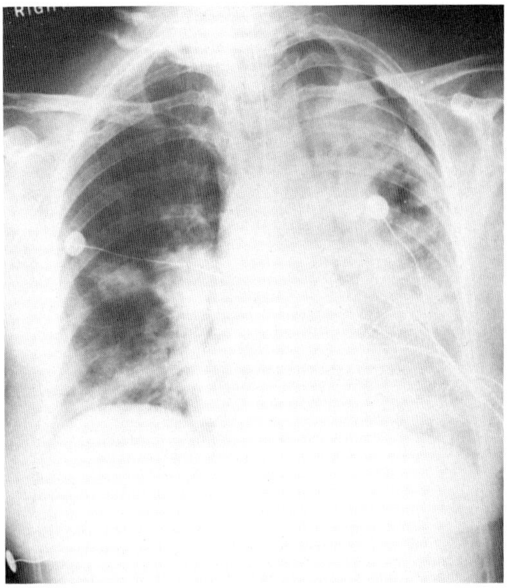

FIG. 8-5. This elderly woman was first seen with a dry hacking cough, and flu-like symptoms. She was treated with ampicillin but failed to improve. A chest roentgenograph demonstrated bilateral patchy infiltrates. On the seventh day of her illness she had a shaking chill, developed purulent sputum, and progressively deteriorated. *Staphylococcus aureus* was cultured from the sputum. This film demonstrates nodular infiltrates, an air bronchogram in the left upper lobe resulting from surrounding consolidation, a cavitary lesion in the left mid-lung field, and a pneumothorax on the left. Incidentally, note the superior vena cava catheter inserted from the right axillary vein, the thoracostomy tube on the left, the tracheostomy tube, the nasogastric tube, and the continuous ECG monitor electrodes.

are ominous diagnostic possibilities. The identification of an epidemic illness, associated with gastrointestinal symptoms, and occasional herpangina, provides firm clinical evidence that a viral process is accountable. Similarly, the patient presenting with a severe pharyngitis with a clearcut epidemic component, gastrointestinal disturbances, conjunctival irritation, or other distinguishing features, is more likely to have a viral than streptococcal infection. Since no definitive therapy is available in most instances, the precise identification of the type of virus is not at present necessary nor of any particular benefit. When definitive therapy does become available, identification of specific viral types may be critical in determining appropriate treatment. At the present time, this unfortunately remains an interesting but academic exercise.

INFLUENZA VIRUS INFECTIONS

The term *flu* is one of the most misused terms in lay medicine and is used to describe any respiratory infection (and some intestinal infections, *gastric flu*) with fever. The term *influenza* should be restricted to the acute viral respiratory tract infection, usually occurring in epidemics and characterized by a sudden onset of headache, myalgia, fever, and prostration, and often associated with pharyngitis, tracheitis, bronchitis and occasionally pneumonia.

Because of the epidemic nature of influenza, this disease has attracted the attention of many virologists, epidemiologists, and medical historians. The epidemiology has been characterized by pandemics followed by epidemics in the interpandemic periods. Thirty-four major pandemics have been identified between 1510 and 1979.[92] Certain of these pandemics were associated with extremely high mortalities with disastrous socio-economic effects. In the pandemic in 1918, the mortality world-wide was estimated at some 20 million, overshadowing the horrendous casualty figures of the First World War. Initially, after the association of *Hemophilus influenzae* with the 1889–92 pandemic, the disease was thought to be bacterial in origin. With the isolation of the causative myxovirus, influenza A in 1933 by Smith, Andrewes and Laidlaw in ferrets, the age of speculation ended.[117] The viral etiology now established, study of the epidemiology and pathogenesis could commence. Later, closely related viruses influenza B and influenza C were isolated from institutional outbreaks of influenzalike illness.

Characteristics of Influenza

The understanding of the epidemiology of influenza is dependent on a knowledge of the characteristics of the influenza viruses. Influenza C is, as far as is known, an antigenically stable virus. Infection with this virus tends to give a long-standing immunity, although there is some evidence to suggest that this immunity may de-

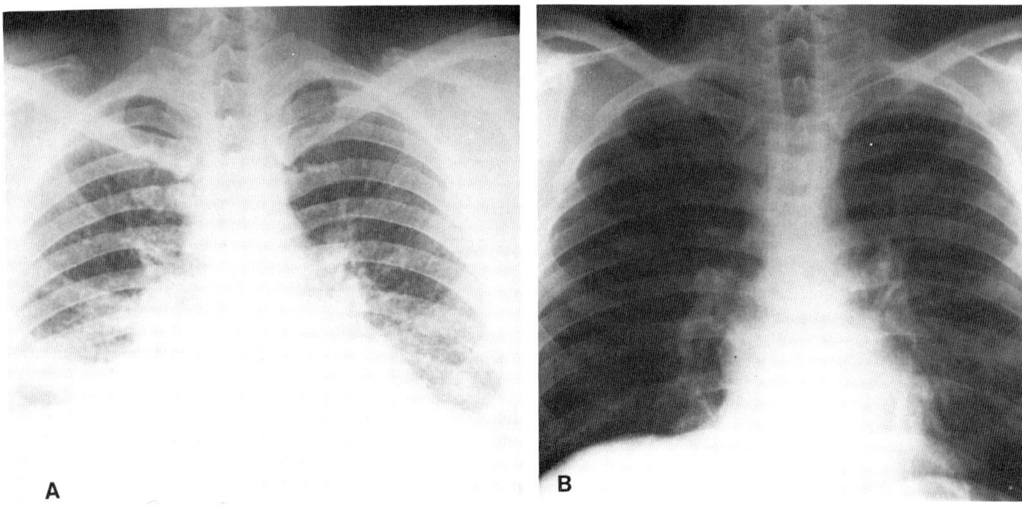

FIG. 8-6. A young man with chicken pox presented with severe dyspnea, tachypnea, and the bilateral finely nodular infiltrates noted on this radiograph (**A**). Marked clearing was apparent within three weeks (**B**).

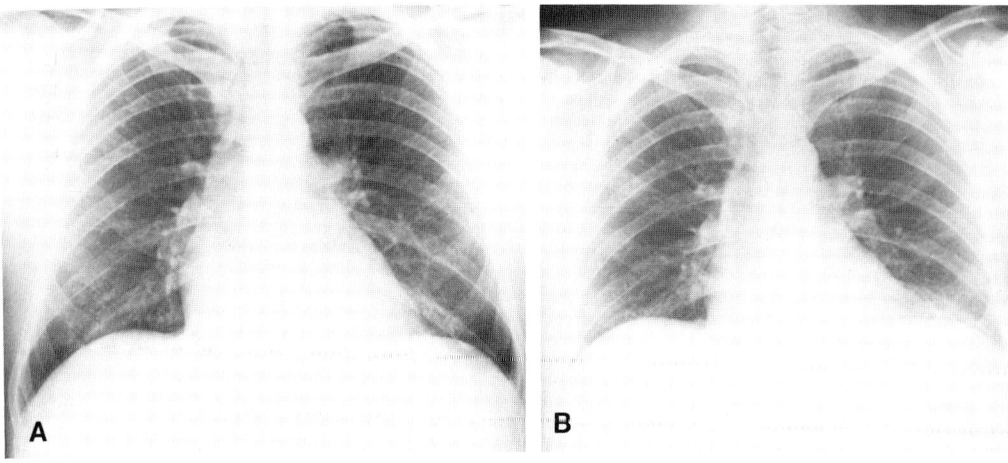

FIG. 8-7. This patient presented with severe pleuritic chest pain on the left. There was no hemoptysis, and no evidence of phlebitis. The initial chest film (**A**) was interpreted as being normal, but demonstrates minor blunting of the costophrenic angle on the left. A follow-up film taken three days later (**B**) demonstrates a definite pleural effusion on the left. A lateral decubitus film confirmed a significant effusion. This had entirely cleared ten days later. Acute and convalescent sera demonstrated a six-fold rise in antibodies to Coxsackie B virus.

cline in later life. It is usually a minor infection. Its high infectivity and prevalence in the general population is evident from the high frequency of antibody detected in surveys. Because of the difficulty in growing this virus in tissue culture, only limited information on its epidemiology is available. It causes outbreaks in institutions and is a frequent infecting agent in early childhood.

Influenza B is less antigenically stable, undergoing minor modifications. Hence, it is possible to undergo more than one infection in a lifetime. While epidemics are rare and pandemics as yet

TABLE 8-6. Differentiation of Pneumonia Resulting from Infectious Agents

Clinical Features	Organisms: Viral	Rickettsial	Mycoplasmal	Pyogenic Bacterial
Community history	Epidemic	Animal, bird contacts	Family illness	Not significant
Prodrome	Upper respiratory General malaise	General malaise	Upper respiratory General malaise	Occasional pharyngitis
Onset	Gradual	Gradual	Gradual	Sudden
Cough	Persistent Nonproductive	Persistent Nonproductive	Persistent Nonproductive	Persistent Purulent, bloody sputum
Chest Pain	Uncommon	Uncommon	Uncommon	Common, pleuritic
Physical findings on chest examination	Minimal	Minimal	Rales, rhonchi diffuse	Localized, well defined
Roentgenogram findings	Patchy, nonspecific	Patchy, nonspecific	Patchy, lower lobes, unilateral	Localized
Leucocyte count	Normal Leucopenic Mildly elevated	Normal Leucopenic Mildly elevated	Normal Leucopenic Mildly elevated	Polymorphonuclear Leucocytosis
Sputum smear	Few leucocytes Epithelial debris	Few leucocytes Epithelial debris	Few leucocytes Occasionally leucocytes without bacteria	Numerous leucocytes Intracellular bacteria
Pleural fluid	Rare	Rare	Rare	Occasional; with empyema
Blood cultures	Negative	Negative	Negative	+10 to 40%
Serology	Definitive	Definitive	Definitive	Not helpful
Response to antimicrobials	None	Good Tetracycline or chloramphenicol	Good Tetracycline or erythromycin	Good. Requires identification of organism
Secondary bacterial infection	Common	Uncommon	Uncommon	Uncommon

undescribed, quite large outbreaks have occurred in institutions, military camps and schools. In large community outbreaks, school children are most often affected.

Although influenza B is usually a milder illness than influenza A, it is associated with a greater incidence of post-infectious sequelae, especially Reye's syndrome. Reye's syndrome consists of an encephalopathy associated with acute fatty degeneration of the liver which afflicts children 1 to 14 years of age. Obtundation progressing to coma occurs as the child is recovering from the respiratory infection. The frequency of Reye's syndrome has been estimated to be 30 to 60: 100,000 cases of influenza B.[118]

Influenza A is antigenically unstable, appearing to be continuously changing. These antigenic changes are of two types: major antigenic "shifts" such as those which the virus underwent in 1947, 1957 and in 1968, and minor antigenic "drifts" that occur in the years between the major changes. The mechanisms of this antigenic variation are still debatable. When a major shift in antigenic type occurs, it is usually associated with a pandemic, indicating that the change in antigenicity has allowed the virus to infect persons who were immune to previous variants.

The markers of antigenic change are the surface proteins of the virus, namely the hemagglutinin (H) and the surface enzymatically-active protein neurominidase (N). These have been designated numbers H: 0–3 and N: 1–2. The influenza A viruses in several epidemics were classed as follows[91,92]:

Year	Old Nomenclature	New Nomenclature
1933	A_0	H_0N_1
1947	A_1	H_1N_1
1957	A_1 (Asian)	H_2N_2
1968	A_2 (Hong Kong)	H_3N_2

Strains that differ owing to antigenic drift are designated by the year and site of isolation. Recent major strains, all of which are H_3N_2 viruses, include influenza A/England/1973 and influenza A/Victoria/1975.

The major antigenic shifts and resulting pandemics of influenza appear to occur in repeating cycles of about 80 years. This suggestion is based on the observations that attack rates during pandemics are lowest among the elderly and that elderly persons appear to have pre-existing protective antibody. For example, persons alive in 1890 had antibody against the Hong Kong variant when it appeared in 1968. The appearance of "swine" influenza in sudden outbreak at Fort Dix, New Jersey, in 1976 was unexpected. This virus was antigenically similar to that which caused the pandemic of 1918–1919 and which was known to have occurred in sporadic human cases since. The Fort Dix outbreak spawned a massive compaign to prepare and administer influenza vaccine against the swine agent. However, epidemic disease did not occur and the major effect of the campaign was to publicize the fact that the Guillain-Barré syndrome is a rare complication of influenza vaccination.[119]

Pathogenesis and Pathology

General considerations of defense against viral infection have been discussed earlier (see Defenses Against Viral Infection). Influenza is spread from person to person by direct contact and by aerosol transmission. The very high attack rate among close contacts suggests that the necessary infecting dose is low; experimental studies suggest that fewer than 10 viral particles are required. Following implantation, viruses attach to and enter epithelial cells of the respiratory tract; to some degree the site of initial cell entry will be influenced by the route of inoculation, whether nasal, pharyngeal, or bronchial. However, intracellular multiplication is rapid, leading to cell death and expulsion of numerous newly-generated viral particles which then spread to adjacent cells and repeat the cycle. Available evidence indicates that with influenza this process is usually not limited to the upper respiratory tract. Experimental animals infected with influenza develop necrosis of respiratory epithelium from the nose to terminal bronchioles. Virus has been cultured from bronchial cells obtained at bronchoscopy from individuals with influenza but normal chest radiographs and no clinical evidence of lower respiratory involvement. Pulmonary function studies performed on previously healthy individuals with similarly "uncomplicated" influenza have shown abnormalities of small airways function in most infected persons. Thus, propagation of virus and spread throughout the respiratory tract is a regular feature of influenza.

Little is known of the pathology of this process except in experimental animals or persons who die, thereby introducing an obvious bias. These necropsy studies indicate that viral invasion is associated with hyperemia, edema, and cellular infiltration of the respiratory mucosa, followed by necrosis and sloughing of the epithelium.[120–123] Basement membranes remain intact. In fatal cases, alveolar inflammation is usually present, consisting of interstitial and alveolar edema and hemorrhage followed by Type II epithelial cell hyperplasia and an influx of mononuclear cells, chiefly macrophages. One of the early descriptions of alveolar hyaline membranes was in persons dying of influenza in the

1918 pandemic, long before oxygen, assisted ventilation, or other therapeutic modalities were available.[125] The presence of necrotizing bronchiolitis in such lungs is the pathologic clue to the etiology of the diffuse alveolar injury. A few survivors of complex treatment for influenza pneumonia have developed severe lung fibrosis.[107]

Although viremia and isolation of virus from other tissues has been reported, such findings are exceptional. Examination of tissues other than the respiratory tract, even in patients dying of influenza, usually reveals no lesions attributable to the infection.

Regeneration of the respiratory epithelium begins within 5 days and is complete within 10 to 14 days. The factors that diminish viral propagation in this short time period are not well understood.

Clinical Manifestations

These vary with different strains of the virus. During an outbreak, a typical pattern of disease emerges. One of the characteristic features is the suddenness of onset with little in the way of prodrome. The first symptoms are usually severe headache, chills, sometimes rigor, fatigue and muscle aches and pains. The patient feels weak. Respiratory symptoms are often lacking during this initial period. The eyes are often tender and watering, although photophobia is uncommon. Movement of the eyes often increases the intensity of the headache, and prostration usually ensues. It is only later that the respiratory elements of the disease become prominent. Nasopharyngeal irritation becomes evident with rhinorrhea and sneezing. The patient's body temperature rises during the first few hours of the illness, reaching 38 to 41°C. Fever is often a prognostic sign. In general, the higher the temperature, the more severe the disease. Heart rate is variable and the patient may have a slower heart rate than anticipated for the degree of hyperthermia. Certain patients show a drop in temperature within a few hours, but have a repeat of the pyrexial episode the next day. The majority of patients remain pyrexial for two to three days. The skin is usually hot and dry, but profuse sweating is sometimes observed. Upsets of the gastrointestinal tract are rare. Myalgia of the abdominal wall may mimic a surgical emergency. Anorexia, thirst, and constipation are usually present. The central nervous system is usually spared, although the mental state of the patient may vary from apathy to frank delirium.

Influenza encephalopathies do occur and may recur in certain individuals every time they contact influenza. Other uncommon manifestations of neurologic disease include polyneuritis, cranial nerve palsies, nerve deafness, hemiplegia, and psychosis. Of interest, but unexplained, is the often severe depression occurring in the recovery period. All of the nervous system manifestations are transient.

The respiratory manifestations occur some time after the onset of constitutional symptoms. A persistent, nonproductive cough, occasionally associated with other symptoms of tracheitis, is most common. The presence of purulent sputum should alert one to the possibility of secondary bacterial infection. Exertional cyanosis and dyspnea may be early indicators of pneumonia.

In the uncomplicated case, respiratory symptoms usually last 5 to 7 days; the constitutional upset generally subsides in 2 to 4 days. If, however, the fever has not subsided by the fifth day, one should reconsider the diagnosis or suspect a secondary bacterial infection (see Table 8-6).

Recovery tends to be slow, and patients having sustained a severe influenza infection frequently require 2 to 3 wk to regain their previous strength and activity.

Physical examination of the chest in most cases of influenza is unrevealing. Tachypnea and scattered rales may be the only findings, even when extensive pneumonia is present. Consolidation and pleural effusions are rare in uncomplicated influenza and are evidence of secondary bacterial infection.

The roentgenographic features are highly variable. Most commonly the lung parenchyma is not involved, and the chest roentgenogram is normal. Occasionally, even the patient with dyspnea and hypoxemia has a completely normal film. When abnormalities are observed, they may range from minimal infiltrates in any portion of the lung fields, to bilateral, fluffy infiltrates, to a completely consolidating bilateral process. Lung scans may demonstrate patchy perfusion defects, misleading the clinician to suspect pulmonary emboli.[125] Pleural effusions or localized consolidations should encourage the search for other organisms (Figs. 8-3, 8-4, 8-6). When bacterial infection becomes established, it takes on the clinical characteristics of the specific organism (Fig. 8-5).

Differential Diagnosis

Whereas flu-like illness is a common feature of many infectious and hypersensitivity diseases, the establishment of a diagnosis early in the course of influenza may be exceedingly difficult. In view of its epidemic character, the index of suspicion may be high as a result of information from worldwide epidemiological centers monitored by the World Health Organization, and published through the news media.[92]

Patients who were previously well can generally be observed by the physician at home or in the office for early signs of other serious and treatable disease. Patients with preceding underlying disease, such as chronic pulmonary disease, heart disease, or neoplastic disease, or who are pregnant, may require an exhaustive workup to establish that no other life-threatening illness has developed. Frequently, in such patients, the self-limiting "flu" will subside before a hospital workup is complete.

Laboratory Investigation

The peripheral blood leukocyte count is commonly reduced in uncomplicated cases. When the white cell count is above 12,000, serious concern should be raised regarding secondary bacterial infection. As indicated above, in the uncomplicated influenza infection, chest films are normal, but a wide range of abnormalities are present in severe lower respiratory infections.

Where facilities are available, the virus can readily be isolated. Myxoviruses are relatively unstable, so it is important that they be suitably transported to the virology laboratory as rapidly as possible. Specimens from tracheal suction, or throat swabs taken in the early stage of illness usually contain viable virus.

Complement fixing or hemagglutination inhibiting antibodies can be detected in acute and convalescent sera. A fourfold rise in titer is diagnostic of recent influenza infection. Serum specimens are usually obtained about 10 days apart, and therefore are of little use to the physician during the acute phase of the illness. Recent studies suggest that immunofluorescent staining of bronchial secretions may establish the diagnosis very early in the course of the illness, when necessary.[126]

Complications

The principal complications of influenza are listed in Table 8-7. Bronchiolitis and viral pneumonia represent either unusually severe infection or the usual course of the disease in a subject whose lungs were ill-prepared, by virtue of pre-existing disease, to handle this new insult. Bacterial pneumonia is due to suppression of normal antibacterial defenses.

Bronchiolitis presents as respiratory failure in a person with otherwise typical influenza. In infants the chest is quiet on examination, and the radiograph shows hyperinflation. Most adults with this complication have pre-existing chronic obstructive lung disease and present with in-

TABLE 8-7. Clinical Patterns of Influenza and Its Respiratory Complications

Presentation	Time of Onset	Groups at Special Risk	Prognosis
Bronchiolitis	Variable	Infants, COPD	Fair
Viral pneumonia			
Localized	Early	All	Good
Diffuse	Early	Underlying disease	Poor
Bacterial pneumonia			
Localized	Late	All	Good
Diffuse	Early	Underlying disease	Poor
Combined bacterial–viral pneumonia	Early	Underlying disease	Poor

creasing breathlessness. In these patients respiratory failure may occur at any time from shortly after onset of fever to 7 to 10 days later, an observation that probably relates to the variety of changes transpiring in their airways.

Viral pneumonia due to influenza was initially recognized only as a catastrophic, overwhelming process.[127] Affected patients typically sought hospitalization within 48 hr of the onset of influenza, with dyspnea their major complaint. Cyanosis refractory to oxygen therapy and diffuse alveolar infiltration radiographically were regularly present, and about 75% of such patients died. With aggressive management of acute respiratory failure the mortality may be slightly reduced, but survivors may develop diffuse lung fibrosis.[107]

It is now known that milder forms of influenza viral pneumonia also occur, and patients may present later in the course of infection (2 to 5 days) with localized interstitial or alveolar infiltrates due only to viral disease.[128] The prognosis of this localized form of viral pneumonia is much better than that of the diffuse form (Fig. 8-3).

Bacterial pneumonia has been a constant accompaniment of influenza in virtually all outbreaks. This process also occurs in two forms—localized and diffuse. Diffuse bacterial pneumonia with or without co-existing viral pneumonia is usually due to *S. aureus*, a predilection that is supported by animal studies but is still not fully explained. The frequency of *S. aureus* as a cause of pneumonia increases several-fold during influenza outbreaks, from 2 to 10% during nonepidemic periods to over 25% during outbreaks. However, as suggested by the latter figure, other bacterial species, especially the pneumococcus, are still the most common causes of bacterial pneumonia even in influenza epidemics. Diffuse bacterial pneumonia commonly represents a combined viral and bacterial process, although this may be difficult to prove in patients who survive.[129] The onset is rapid, typically requiring hospitalization within 48 hr of the onset of illness.

Localized pneumonia typically occurs 5 to 8 days after the onset of influenza; by this time the patients may have recovered sufficiently to have returned to their usual activities. Onset of pneumonia is heralded by recurrence of fever and onset of chest pain and sputum production. Physical examination and chest roentgenograms reveal localized alveolar consolidation. The prognosis of this type of post-influenza pneumonia is no different from that of pneumonia occurring independently of influenza.

Bacteriologic confirmation of the complicating process or demonstration of the absence of bacterial superinfection is an important aspect of the evaluation of these patients. In patients with diffuse infiltrates and severe illnesses, expectorated secretions may be misleading, both in suggesting the absence of bacterial pathogens when they are present and in demonstrating bacterial pathogens when the lung process is purely viral. Aggressive sampling techniques, such as transtracheal aspiration, bronchoscopic brushings, or transthoracic lung aspiration, may be indicated. All specimens obtained must be diligently examined for *S. aureus* microscopically, and the presence of large gram-positive cocci in clumps should always lead to treatment with agents resistant to penicillinase until culture results and microbial sensitivity tests are known.

Specific Chemotherapy

Amantadine hydrochloride is the only drug currently available with anti-influenza activity. Initially its use was restricted to Asian influenza (H_2N_2), but subsequent experience has shown the drug to be active against a variety of strains of influenza A; it is not effective against influenza B. The nature of its antiviral activity is not fully explained, but it appears to inhibit cellular penetration by the virus and the release of viral nucleic acid into the cell. Amantadine is most effective as a prophylactic agent, providing about 60% protection against clinical illness in exposed, susceptible populations.[130] If treatment of symptomatic influenza with amantadine is begun within 24 hr of the onset of symptoms, the course of illness is shortened and viral shedding is abbreviated. Unfortunately, amantadine does not appear to be efficacious in the treatment of influenza-viral pneumonia.

These observations indicate that amantadine has a definite role in the management of influenza.[131] It can be used chemoprophylactically if outbreaks occur before specific vaccines are available. Susceptible patients who have neglected immunization can be protected for several weeks until an antibody response to vaccination occurs. If the drug is administered as prophylaxis, it must be continued throughout the period of influenza activity; premature discontinuation renders the patient still susceptible to infection. With usual adult doses of 100 mg twice daily, 3 to 7% of people experience side effects of amantadine, predominantly insomnia, anxiety, and difficulty in thinking. Since the drug is excreted in the urine, the dose should be decreased in the presence of renal insufficiency.

Prevention

The great interest in world-wide studies concentrating on the control of epidemic influenza testifies to the inadequacy of our current methods of prevention. At present, investigation to develop virus-specific vaccines and interferons represents the major research thrust. Several forms of vaccination are currently available. Because of the changes in antigenicity of the influenza virus, the vaccine must be prepared with knowledge of the most likely characteristics of the current strain. As a consequence, formulation of a vaccine is generally determined a year in advance of its availability. The practice is to include single strains of Type A and B viruses that are the most representative. The effectiveness of these vaccines depends upon the recurrence of infections with the same or closely-related influenza strains.

Vaccination by Nasal or Aerosol Inoculation. Several studies have demonstrated the efficacy of vaccines administered nasally, or as an aerosol in adults or orally in children. The objective is to increase the level of secretory (IgA) antibodies, in order to provide a higher level of mucosal resistance. This route generally provides a lower level of serological antibody than subcutaneous injection.[132–136] The use of live attenuated vaccines in this fashion requires that the organism be appropriately antigenic, non-virulent, and yet infectious. Although early results have been promising, and this appears to be the method most widely practiced in the U.S.S.R., there remain some elements of doubt regarding its efficacy.

Subcutaneous and Intradermal Vaccines. At present measurable antibodies in serum can be developed in response to lower doses of intradermal than of subcutaneous vaccine. However, it would appear that the effect of a single dose is more protracted when given subcutaneously, and this is still the recommended method. Numerous studies have demonstrated that immediate immune response, as evidenced by rise in humoral antibodies, is greater with subcutaneous injections than inhalation.[132,134] This appears to be true for patients with chronic bronchopulmonary disease as well.[135,136] Complete protection however, has not been achieved. About 50% of individuals receiving the vaccine will develop minor local or systemic symptoms, predominantly related to the vehicle. Since the vaccine is prepared in embryonated eggs, and thus contains protein other than the virus antigens, individuals with a history of allergy to egg products should not be immunized. Complications of vaccination include anaphylactic reactions and febrile reactions; these are predominantly due to hypersensitivity to egg protein. Ascending paralysis (Guillain–Barré syndrome), though much publicized, is a rare complication.[119,136a]

Many new approaches are being actively explored, such as increasing the dose of antigen in the initial inoculation, in the hope that a higher level of antibodies will provide some cross-protection against changing antigenic strains. Furthermore, attempts to produce interferon-like substances which will be effective once an epidemic is already in progress are under active investigation.

At present there is substantial evidence that the severity of an influenza infection is reduced, and the rate of clinical infection decreased in a population which has been immunized with well-selected vaccine prior to an epidemic. In view of this limited effectiveness, the vaccine is currently recommended to those at greatest risk, should they become infected. These include patients with severe rheumatic valvular disease, chronic bronchopulmonary disorders, severe ischemic heart disease, advanced diabetes mellitus, the aged, and females in an advanced stage of pregnancy.

Supportive Therapy

In the uncomplicated case, bedrest, salycilates, high fluid intake, and antitussive agents if necessary, provide significant symptomatic improvement. Generally recovery occurs within 5 to 7 days.

Patients with viral pneumonia require observation for the onset of respiratory failure, which is managed as when due to other causes (see Chapter 7). There is no evidence at present that any definitive treatment modality changes the course of the disease but anecdotal evidence suggests that, in some patients, the administration of high-dose corticosteroids, equivalent to 40 or 60 mg of prednisone per day, may improve oxygenation and the rate of recovery.

A careful search for evidence of secondary bacterial infection must be made, so that this complication may be treated with appropriate antibiotics; antibiotic therapy should be given particularly when secondary infection is found in patients with underlying chronic disease. Patients with chronic bronchopulmonary disease may tolerate the superinfection very poorly. When antibiotics are selected empirically, the frequency of staphylococcal and gram-negative bacterial secondary invaders in influenza should be considered.

OTHER RESPIRATORY VIRUSES

Adenovirus

Pharyngitis, tracheitis, keratoconjunctivitis, and pneumonia may be caused by a variety of strains of adenoviruses.[79,83] Adenovirus pneumonia generally affects young adults, and major epidemics have been reported in military recruits. Types 4 and 7 have been the most common. In military recruits with adenoviral pneumonia, fever, cough, sore throat, rhinorrhea, nausea, retrosternal chest pain, and anorexia, were prominent symptoms.[137,138] Clinical evidence of pharyngitis, rhinitis, conjunctivitis, and adenopathy are common findings. Scattered rales and rhonchi may be present on auscultation of the chest. The white blood cell count and sputum characteristics are similar to other viral pneumonias (see influenza Pneumonia and Table 8-6). Epidemiological studies in children have found up to 12% of viral pneumonia resulting from adenovirus infection.[139]

Adenovirus infections have been implicated in the development of severe chronic lung changes including diffuse bronchitis, bronchiolitis, or bronchiectasis[140], and lobar or unilateral lung airways obstruction resulting in the unilateral hyperlucent lung (see Chap. 14). There is no specific therapy for adenovirus infection. Prevention with live viral vaccine given orally has been used successfully in populations of recruits.[79,137,141]

Parainfluenza Virus

Parainfluenza viruses cause less than 10% of respiratory infections, most commonly bronchitis, bronchiolitis, and occasionally pneumonia, in children.[99] Up to one-third of cases of croup have been documented as due to parainfluenza viruses. In the adult, parainfluenza viral infections generally cause mild respiratory illness with a mild influenza-like illness. Laryngitis is said to be more common than in influenza, and in a mild epidemic of flu-like illness, should lead one to suspect the presence of parainfluenza virus.

There is no specific treatment. There is no effective vaccine for parainfluenza virus at present, but considerable promise for aerosolized administration of attenuated vaccine.

Respiratory Syncytial Virus (RSV)

These viruses are most significant as pathogens during the first 6 months of life. During this period, bronchiolitis is a prominent potential problem.[83,94,95] In the older age groups (3–5 years) pneumonia is the more common.

Adults exposed to infants during an outbreak of RSV infection developed nasal discharge, cough, fever, and increased airways resistance demonstrating a previously underemphasized adult morbidity.[142]

Upper respiratory symptoms with cough, fever, and nasal discharge usually accompany other manifestations of RSV infection.

There is no specific treatment for respiratory

syncytial virus infections. No suitable RS virus vaccine is available at the present time.

Rhinovirus

Rhinoviruses are the most frequent cause of the typical common cold. Symptoms include nasal obstruction, nasal discharge, sneezing; on examination, there is swollen and boggy nasal mucosa. Sore throat and cough are frequent accompaniments, while only about one-fifth of persons have fever.

Exacerbations of respiratory symptoms in patients with chronic obstructive pulmonary disease and asthma have been attributed to rhinovirus infections in several studies.[99,103,143,144.]

There is no specific treatment and, because of the large number of antigenic types, immunoprophylaxis has proven unsatisfactory to date.

Enterovirus

The Coxsackie viruses and echo viruses have been discussed above in relation to pleurodynia, herpangina, and pericarditis. Coxsackie virus A_{21} is a common cause of febrile respiratory disease in military populations. The infection is prominently associated with nasal obstruction, discharge, headache, cough, and sore throat. Temperatures as high as 39° C have been reported, and the illness generally lasts about 5 to 10 days. Several studies have documented that the combined enterovirus infection rate in respiratory illnesses represents less than 1% of all cases.[79] Furthermore, the development of pleurodynia, pericarditis, or other major complications is rare considering the number of individuals infected.

Cultures of stool in addition to upper respiratory secretions are frequently useful in helping to establish the presence of the organism.

There is no specific treatment, and at present no satisfactory vaccine is in use. The large number of antigenic variants and the sporadic occurrence of cases make the widespread use of vaccine impractical.

Herpes Simplex Virus

Herpes simplex virus infections are apparently very common, as evidenced by the presence of neutralizing antibodies in 60 to 100% of individuals sampled in an adult population. The most common manifestation of infection is recurrent vesicles on the mucous membranes. In the newborn, primary infections may be severe, while in later infancy, gingivo-stomatitis accompanied by low-grade fever and cervical adenopathy is more common. In older children, pharyngitis may occur.

Several chemotherapeutic agents are effective against herpes simplex. Idoxuridine, vidarabine, and acyclovir are useful in treatment of herpetic keratitis.[35] Herpes encephalitis may respond to one of the former two agents. Unfortunately for the common man, neither labial or genital herpes responds well to topical agents.

Varicella-Zoster Virus

Clinical Manifestations. Varicella (chicken-pox) may occur at any age, but the highest attack rates are in the 2- to 8-year-old group. This is a highly infectious disease, and occurs in epidemics. In contrast, herpes zoster (shingles) frequently occurs in the absence of contact with any external source of virus. As a result it is considered an endogenous reactivation or reinfection. Varicella usually begins about 14 days after contact with a pre-existing case, but the incubation period may last up to 3 wk. In young children, the disease is generally mild, characterized by minimal systemic symptoms and red macular lesions which quickly progress to multilocular vesicles. The fluid is initially clear and then becomes turbid. The vesicles are easily broken by pressure. Concurrent pneumonia is rare in children. In adults, the entire disease is more severe. Temperatures tend to be higher, and 10 to 15% of patients develop pneumonia. Pneumonia occurs early in the course and is characterized by cough, dyspnea, diffuse bilateral nodular infiltrates, and a paucity of clinical findings, as is characteristic of other viral pneumonias (Fig. 8-6). The mortality has been reported to be as high as 20%, and is a result of respiratory failure or secondary bacterial infection. Females, particularly pregnant females, have more severe forms of varicella pneumonia[145] and should be followed especially closely.

The pulmonary lesions may be associated with effusions, hemoptysis, pleuritic chest pain, and findings indistinguishable from pulmonary infarction. In fact, the limited pathologic material which has been studied in such cases suggests an increased incidence of pulmonary embolism or *in situ* thrombosis.[145,146] Pulmonary function studies are similar to those in influenza pneumonia and remain abnormal for prolonged periods after symptomatic recovery, as evidenced by a high alveolar–arterial oxygen gradient and reduced diffusion capacity. In the late stages, diffuse pulmonary calcification has been demonstrated.[147]

Other complications of varicella infections, including encephalitis, myocarditis and corneal ulcers, are rare.

Herpes zoster generally presents with pain and paresthesiae in the distribution of a spinal nerve root. It may occur in the trigeminal distribution, but more commonly in a bandlike distribution in the lower thoracic or upper lumbar region. Following initial paresthesiae, which last 1 to 3 days, there is a papular rash, which is unilateral, and restricted to one or several dermatomes, followed by a vesicular eruption. The lesions generally appear first posteriorly and then anteriorly although the entire distribution of the intercostal nerve may not be uniformly involved. The major importance to the chest physician lies in the differential diagnosis of pleuritic pain, before the cutaneous eruption is apparent. This syndrome may be particularly prolonged, with chest-wall discomfort resulting in decreased respiratory excursion, in the older age groups. The incidence is strikingly increased in patients with lymphoproliferative disorders in whom the infection may disseminate, and in whom varicella pneumonia occurs with a much higher incidence.

Treatment. There is no specific treatment for either herpes zoster or varicella. Several agents such as adenine arabinoside,[35,130] idoxuride, and other antiviral agents have been used, but their effectiveness is not established. Passive immunization with human immune globulin may be of some benefit. Zoster immune globulin prepared from the plasma of patients recovering from herpes zoster is effective in prevention of varicella infections if administered within 72 hr of contact. Its use may be indicated in pregnant females and immune suppressed individuals.[148] Adrenocortical steroids may be of some benefit in reducing the duration of postherpetic neuralgia. In other patients, they appear to predispose to the development of the zoster syndrome and dissemination of infection, and are best avoided. The use of adrenocortical steroids in varicella pneumonia has no scientific basis at the present time.

Supportive therapy for patients with varicella pneumonia is similar to that for other causes of acute respiratory failure (see Chap. 7).

Picornavirus

These viruses appear to produce a mild form of the common cold. No distinctive features of clinical value are known at the present time.[79]

Rubeola

Clinical Manifestations. Rubeola (measles) is an acute febrile illness with marked cutaneous eruption. Widespread maculopapular rash is accompanied by conjunctivitis, photophobia, and a high spiking fever. This is a highly infectious illness, and is most common prior to the age of 6 yr. The incubation period is about 10 days. This is one of the severe infectious diseases, and may be complicated by encephalitis, myocarditis, or respiratory tract involvement. The respiratory illnesses include croup, bronchitis, bronchiolitis, or, rarely, interstitial pneumonia. The pneumonia is typical of viral pneumonias, in its roentgenographic and clinical features (Table 8-6). Secondary bacterial infection is a major concern.[149]

An atypical, severe form of measles is seen in some persons who have previously received inactivated measles vaccine.[52,93,150,151] These patients develop an atypical rash with maculopapules, vesicles, and petechiae. In contrast to natural measles, the rash frequently involves the feet and progresses proximally. Pneumonia is common, characterized by segmental or lobar consolidation, with hilar lymphadenopathy, and pleural effusions. Ill defined nodular shadows may persist in the periphery of the lungs for many months following the infection (Fig. 8-8). This is generally a self-limiting illness. The use of inactivated vaccine has been discontinued.

Treatment. There is no specific therapy for measles. In view of the potential severity of the ill-

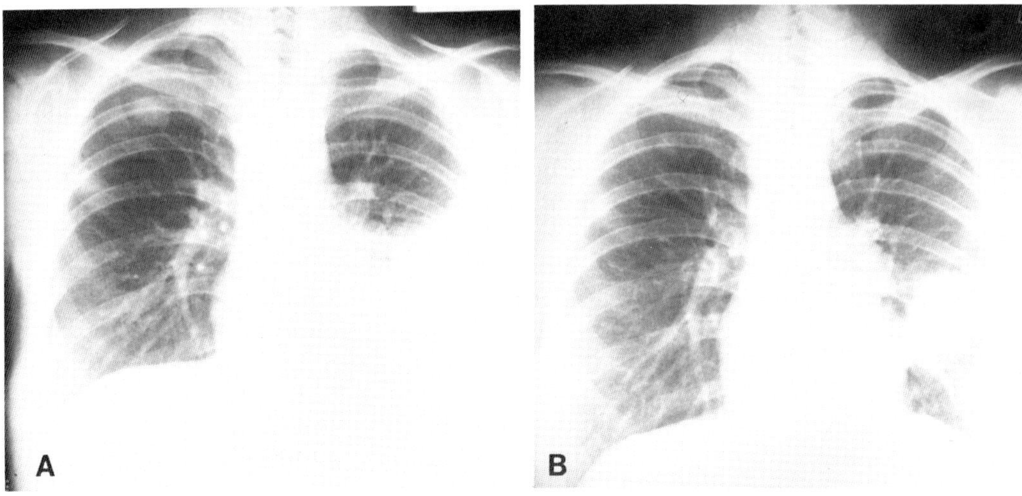

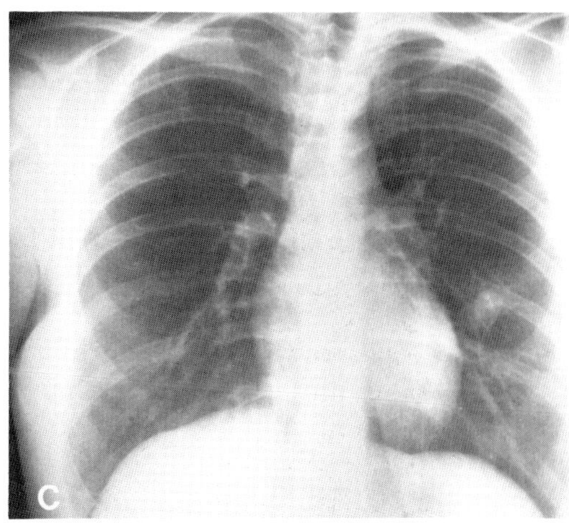

FIG. 8-8. This 14-year-old girl, previously immunized with killed measles vaccine, was exposed to a patient with rubeola. She developed a maculopapulo-hemorrhagic rash, cough, and fever. **A.** The chest roentgenograph reveals several nodular infiltrates in the right upper lung field, an extensive consolidating infiltrate in the left lower lung field, and a left pleural effusion. **B.** Follow-up film taken three days later demonstrates marked clearing with a residual rounded density in the left mid-lung field and tiny nodules in the right upper lung field. **C.** One month later, the nodule has almost completely cleared. This very unusual roentgenographic pattern is more consistent with a vasculitis or patchy pulmonary edema than with a frank infective process.

ness, passive immunization with gammaglobulin is justified following exposure, to prevent major manifestations of the disease. This is effective if given within 5 days of exposure, and is particularly important for children under age 3, for pregnant women, for patients with active and severe tuberculosis, and for those patients in whom immune mechanisms are impaired. Active immunity can be induced by the use of live attenuated measles virus vaccine. This results in a mild febrile illness, but is followed by a high level of prolonged immunity. Widespread immunization for children is now under way.[152,153] Live measles vaccine should not be given to pregnant women, to those sensitive to egg proteins, patients with disseminated lymphoproliferative disorders, or on immune suppressive drugs.

Once the disease is established, supportive therapy is the only available approach.

Cytomegalovirus (CMV)

Cytomegalovirus infections occur worldwide, are generally subclinical and their frequency is documented only by the high incidence of complement fixing antibodies (about 80% of the adult population).[154] Congenital cytomegalovirus infection may be very serious, with hepatitis, hemolytic anemia, splenomegaly, interstitial pneumonia and meningoencephalitis as prominent features. Adults tend to develop the CMV mononucleosis syndrome, which is much like

Epstein-Barr virus mononucleosis, but without pharyngitis or localized cervical adenopathy. Fever, atypical lymphocytes, and absence of heterophile antibodies should raise suspicion.

Immunosuppressed patients, particularly transplant recipients, frequently develop CMV pneumonia. This has all the clinical features of viral pneumonia. Electron microscopic examination of lung biopsies, bronchial washings, saliva, urine, or blood buffy coat may demonstrate the characteristic large nuclear inclusion bodies. Rising levels of complement-fixing antibodies are most helpful in establishing a diagnosis.

No specific therapy is available at the present time. A live vaccine is under trial.[154,155]

Infectious Mononucleosis: Epstein-Barr (EB) virus

Infectious mononucleosis is a systemic illness involving multiple organ systems. Skin rash, generalized lymphadenopathy, hepatosplenomegaly, fever, general malaise, and pharyngitis are common manifestations. Pneumonitis, pleural effusions, pericarditis, mild carditis, and encephalopathy are rare but serious complications. The diagnosis can be established on the basis of characteristic atypical lymphocytes in the peripheral blood and increased levels of heterophile antibodies in the serum. In most instances, this is a mild, transient, febrile illness in children and young adults. The incubation period is probably 2 to 6 wk, with low infectivity.

The major respiratory complication relates to upper airway obstruction as a result of tonsillitis and pharyngeal edema.

No specific therapy is available.

Rotavirus

This enteric virus commonly causes diarrheal disease in children. Recent studies have emphasized cough, otitis media, and nasal discharge preceding the gastrointestinal symptoms.

CHLAMYDIA INFECTIONS

Ornithosis (Psittacosis)

Chlamydia psittaci is a small, obligate intracellular parasite that produces infections in birds. Secondary spread to humans was first recognized from psittacine house pets but it is now known that a variety of birds may harbor the agent. Human infection results from inhalation of dried, contaminated bird feces or handling of infected viscera. Sporadic human cases virtually always are discovered to have had contact with birds.[156,157] Of the occasional outbreaks among humans, most have occurred in workers at turkey-processing plants.[158]

The incubation period ranges from 1 to 2 wk, and the illness then begins with fever, chills, anorexia, and severe headache, later followed by cough with scanty sputum. Physical examination of the chest is often unremarkable, even in the presence of patchy bronchopneumonia.

Patients with extensive pulmonary involvement develop severe arterial hypoxemia, tachypnea, and respiratory distress. Splenomegaly is common, and occasionally jaundice, albuminuria, and clinical evidence of meningitis or encephalitis may occur.

The leukocyte count is generally within normal limits, and laboratory diagnosis is dependent on growing the organism with specialized culture techniques or by documenting serological evidence of infection as evidenced by complement fixing, agglutinating and/or neutralizing antibodies.

Tetracycline is the antibiotic of choice, and results in a decreased severity and duration of illness.

Chlamydia trachomatis pneumonia

A pneumonia with distinctive clinical features among young infants has been recently attributed to natally-acquired *C. trachomatis*.[159,160] Affected infants become ill before age 3 mo, typically between age 2 to 6 wk, with tachypnea, congestion, and cough. All reported cases have been afebrile. Inclusion conjunctivitis precedes the development of respiratory symptoms in some infants; others may experience only conjunctivitis or lower respiratory tract infection. Chest radiographs reveal hyperinflation and a mixed alveolar and interstitial infiltrate. Common nonspecific laboratory abnormalities include eosinophilia and increased serum concentrations of IgM and IgG. The organism has been recovered from nasopharyngeal secretions of affected infants and from the genital tracts of their mothers. Elevated serum antibody titers against *C. trachomatis* are present in most patients.

The course of the illness is typically protracted with full recovery requiring 4 to 8 wk.

RICKETTSIA INFECTIONS

Coxiella burnetii is the etiologic agent of Q fever. The "Q" apparently was derived from "Query" rather than "Queensland," Australia, where the first described cases originated. This is one of several pulmonary-disease-producing rickettsia that often produce pneumonia.[161,162] Many domestic and wild animals, including cattle, sheep, goats, horses, pigs, swine, camels, and many species of birds are infected. The infection is generally acquired by inhalation. Person-to-person transfer is apparently unusual. The incubation period ranges from 2 to 4 wk, but the onset of illness is generally abrupt and is associated with chills, fever, malaise, severe myalgia, headache, confusion and disorientation.

The disease is commonly confused with mycoplasma pneumonia, influenza, and Chlamydia infections (Table 8-6). A dry cough and chest pain may arise within several days of onset. Physical findings related to lower respiratory tract infection are rare, but typical roentgenographic features of virus-like pneumonia are common. Fortunately, this is generally a relatively mild and self-limited illness. Rare fatal cases demonstrate extensive consolidation with fibrin and histiocytes, and focal necrosis.[163]

Hepatitis, associated with the development of granulomatous changes, may raise the entire spectrum of granulomatous diseases in the differential diagnosis. Endocarditis has also been reported.

Most laboratories do not attempt to culture the rickettsia because of the high incidence of transmission within the laboratory environment. However, urine and blood are generally good specimens from which to isolate the organism. Serological techniques permit identification of infected individuals during the convalescent phase. Complement-fixing and agglutinating antibodies appear in the second to third weeks. The proteus antibodies of the Weil-Felix reaction are absent.

Tetracycline and chloramphenicol are effective in modifying the course of the disease and constitute appropriate treatment.

Other rickettsiae including *R. tsutsugamushi* (scrub typhus) and *R. rickettsii* (Rocky Mountain spotted fever) may produce pulmonary involvement.

Most patients minimize the respiratory symptoms in the face of the more debilitating severe systemic illness. Careful examination demonstrates cough, auscultatory rales, pulmonary infiltrates, and hypoxemia in almost half of patients who are severely ill.[164] Pathology in fatal cases demonstrates interstitial infiltrates, hemorrhage, and edema.

The diagnosis is generally suspected on the basis of the petechial rash and a history of a tick bite in an endemic area. Serological confirmation of the diagnosis is specific, but too delayed to permit early treatment. Fluorescent antibody labelling of skin biopsies may be best and most specific early diagnostic tool.

Early treatment with antirickettsial drugs, tetracycline, or chloramphenicol is urgently advised and generally effective.

MYCOPLASMA INFECTIONS

Mycoplasma Pneumoniae

In the 1930s and 1940s, a number of patients were recognized with pneumonia that was not a result of identifiable etiological agents. These cases of pneumonia were called "atypical" and eventually Eaton defined an associated agent which was transmissible and the pneumonia became known as Eaton agent pneumonia. The particles were subsequently identified as virus-like particles, which are able to reproduce on cell free media. The organism was designated *Mycoplasma pneumoniae*.[165] Although a wide range of clinical conditions are attributed to this infection, the most severe manifestation is pneumonia.

Infections are worldwide, but occur in epidemic form, most prevalent in school-aged children and young adults. Attack rates within families are approximately 70% in children, and 20% among adults.[165a,166]

Mycoplasma pneumoniae is a primary respiratory pathogen, and infection is transmitted from person to person by means of infected secretions. The incubation period is about 3 wk.

Pathology and Pathogenesis. The organism establishes infection on the mucosal surfaces and epithelial lining. On gross examination, affected lungs exhibit patchy areas of infiltration. Microscopic sections reveal acute bronchiolitis with surrounding interstitial pneumonia consisting of thickening of the bronchiolar walls, edema, vascular congestion, necrotic epithelial debris, and infiltration with mononuclear cells.

There is increasing evidence that the pneumonia develops in subjects with partial immunity, with the major histopathology resulting from a hypersensitivity reaction.[166]

Clinical Manifestations. The vast majority of clinically apparent *Mycoplasma pneumoniae* infections are respiratory illnesses without pneumonia.[167,168a] These vary from a minor febrile upper respiratory illness with or without pharyngitis, to severe bronchitis. The airways component of the disease poses a particular problem in patients with chronic lung disease, and may be accountable for exacerbations of respiratory failure.[170] Furthermore, asthmatics may have exacerbations of bronchospasm and wheezing during mycoplasma infections.[171] Bullous and hemorrhagic myringitis has been reported in a small proportion of cases, but may raise the suspicion of this diagnosis when it occurs.

Clinically apparent pneumonia develops in only 3 to 10% of these infected with *Mycoplasma pneumoniae*, although in family studies, as many as 40% of infected persons have had evidence of pneumonia.[165a,172]

Patients with pneumonia present with fever, chills, cough that is generally nonproductive, headache, and generalized malaise. Hemoptysis and pleuritic pain are rare. Musculoskeletal and gastrointestinal symptoms are infrequent. Only occasionally is the disease so extensive as to cause dyspnea. Examination of the chest reveals occasional rhonchi and rales, but rarely evidence of consolidation. Conjunctivitis is generally mild, as are pharyngitis and cervical lymphadenopathy. Children with sickle-cell anemia may manifest unusually severe disease.[173]

Roentgenographic patterns of *Mycoplasma pneumoniae* infection range from minimal peripheral infiltrates, to extensive consolidating bronchopneumonia. Most commonly the infiltrates are unilateral, and involve the lower lobes. When pneumonia is present, the infiltrates are bilateral in 10 to 40% of cases[172] (Fig. 8-9). These findings are characteristically non-specific. In less than 10% of patients pleural effusions occur, and occasionally these may be bilateral.[168,168a,174] There is evidence that pleural effusions occur more commonly in childhood pneumonia than in adults. The effusion has the characteristics of an exudate. Although lung abscess has been reported, proof that this was a result of mycoplasma infection has not been well established.

Nonrespiratory manifestations of mycoplasmal infections include cold hemagglutinin-positive hemolytic anemia, aseptic meningitis, meningoencephalitis, peripheral neuropathy, cerebellar ataxia, generalized lymphadenopathy, splenomegaly, and a variety of skin lesions including erythema multiforme.[168a,172] Acute arthritis, myopericarditis, hepatitis, and gastroenteritis have all been reported occasionally.

Differential Diagnosis. Most patients presenting with mycoplasma infections have upper respiratory manifestations of pneumonia as their cardinal manifestations. The differential diagnosis generally includes viral and other bacterial causes. Table 8-6 identifies commonly useful criteria for differentiating these groups of infections. The presence of myringitis, family epidemic, and the absence of demonstrable bacteria in the sputum, are useful distinguishing features. *Mycoplasma pneumoniae* pneumonia is most likely to occur in persons 5 to 30 years of age, but as many as 15% of pneumonias in the older age groups may be caused by mycoplasma.

Laboratory Diagnosis. The peripheral blood leukocyte count is generally normal, although in severe cases of pneumonia, very high leukocyte

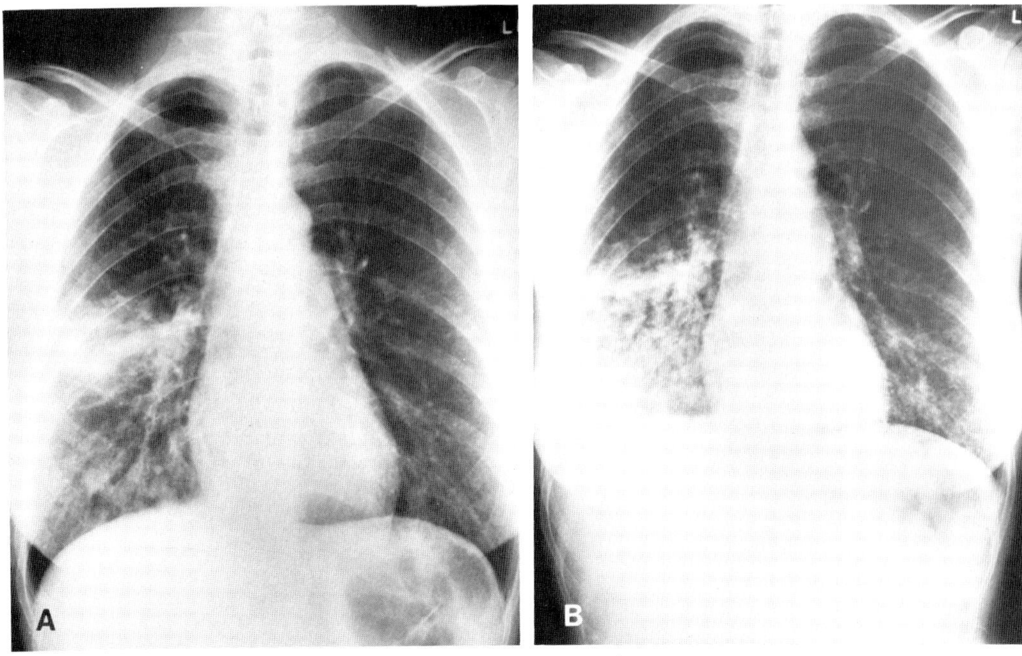

FIG. 8-9. A lower lobe infiltrate with areas of consolidation is characteristic of *Mycoplasma pneumoniae* infection. This patient had minimal sputum, no response to ampicillin therapy, and a dramatic improvement after the initiation of tetracycline orally. Chest roentgenogram **A,** taken ten days before **B,** demonstrates the gradual progression of the infiltrate while on ampicillin.

counts have also been recorded. Erythrocyte sedimentation rate is commonly elevated. Isolation of the organism is possible in many laboratories, after culture of throat swabs, sputum, or bronchial washings.

Serological confirmation of infection includes the demonstration of complement-fixing antibodies, metabolic inhibition, or neutralization tests. As with viral diseases, when a fourfold rise in titers occurs in paired acute and convalescent specimens, a recent or concomitant infection is generally considered established. When only convalescent specimens are available, a titer of 1 in 64 or greater is considered significant of infection. Titers remain elevated for 4 to 6 mo, after which there is a fall to minimal levels.

A nonspecific serological reaction, useful in the early diagnosis, is a test for cold hemagglutinins. These generally appear within 7 days, and rise sharply to reach their peak in 4 wk. Only 60 to 70% of patients will develop a positive cold agglutinin test, and other conditions such as infectious mononucleosis, rubella, influenza, adenovirus infections, dysproteinemias, and connective tissue disorders have been associated with cold agglutinins.

When serum antibodies are present, counter immunoelectrophoresis will detect them with a high sensitivity.[168a]

Treatment. This is generally a self-limiting disease of only modest severity. However, it has been shown that both tetracycline and erythromycin reduce the duration of fever, and hasten the roentgenographic clearing. Although 6 to 8 days of antimicrobial therapy appears effective, there is some evidence that more prolonged treatment (*e.g.*, for 2 to 3 wk) will improve results even further. Patients continue to shed organisms during antimicrobial therapy, and occasionally experience relapses when the antibiotics are discontinued early.[168a]

The choice between erythromycin and tetracycline may be made on the basis of related factors, since they provide similar therapeutic benefits.[175] If the major differential diagnosis includes Q fever and psittacosis, tetracycline is the drug of choice. On the other hand, if there is serious concern that the pneumococcus is the offending agent, and that, in fact, a bacterial pneumonia is present, erythromycin is the treatment of choice. In the adult, 2 to 3 g of tetracycline or erythromycin are the appropriate daily dose.

Prophylactic antimicrobial therapy has been effective in family studies where the risk of infection is high. Inactivated vaccines provide some protection against infection, but have not been widely used.

PYOGENIC BACTERIAL RESPIRATORY INFECTIONS

COMMON CLINICAL SYNDROMES

Understanding of the epidemiology and pathophysiology of bacterial respiratory infections coupled with development of specific antimicrobial therapy have provided the most significant advances in lung disease in this century. Acquisition of pathogenic bacteria and the respiratory defense mechanisms have been discussed above. This section will review common clinical syndromes associated with bacterial infection of the respiratory tract.

Acute Sinusitis

Infection of the paranasal sinuses is estimated to occur in up to 25% of adults.[176] The diagnosis is suspected in the presence of clinical features of pain and tenderness of structures overlying the involved sinuses. These are usually accompanied by fever, nasal discharge, and general malaise. Obstruction of drainage from the sinus is the usual cause of acute sinusitis. Documentation of fluid retention in the sinus can be obtained by transillumination or radiography.[177] Roentgenograms may also disclose mucosal thickening, which is evidence of recurring chronic sinusitis.

Fluid aspirated from infected sinuses is strongly acid and essentially devoid of oxygen, both of which are manifestations of the metabolic activity of bacteria and leukocytes.[178] These conditions favor the growth of strict anaerobes and bacterial species which are facultatively anaerobic such as *S. pneumoniae* and *H. influenzae*. Mycoplasma and Chlamydia species may be important pathogens in some cases. Smears and cultures of nasal discharge or of the oropharynx are unreliable indicators of the organisms responsible for acute sinusitis.

Treatment is with specific antibiotics and, where possible, relief of obstruction to promote drainage. The antibiotics advocated are doxycycline and minocycline, because of their activity against the usual pathogens and the levels of these drugs achieved in the mucosa of the paranasal sinuses. Ampicillin has also been widely used, although the increasing incidence of ampicillin resistance among *H. influenzae* has reduced its effectiveness.[179]

Systemic or topical decongestants aid in establishing drainage. When anatomical abnormalities such as nasal septal deviation or polyps are present, surgical correction may be required to promote drainage. Recurring or chronic sinusitis is a common complication of allergic rhinitis and immunodeficiency, which should be strongly suspected if symptoms persist.

Epiglottitis

Patients with epiglottitis present with a febrile illness, severe sore throat, and harsh, brassy cough. Examination of the hypopharynx reveals a beefy-red, swollen epiglottis, often with edema and erythema of the surrounding pharynx. Laboratory studies reveal a moderate leukocytosis and leftward shift. Cultures of the pharynx and epiglottis may reveal a variety of organisms, but *H. influenzae*, type B, is the usual cause.[180] When blood cultures have been reported, in excess of 90% of patients have had this organism in their blood.

Commonly thought of as a disease of children, epiglottitis also occurs in adults, where mortality rates are high. Treatment with humidity, antibiotics and, when necessary, endotracheal intubation or tracheostomy has reduced mortality to zero in at least two series.[181,182]

Pharyngitis

This syndrome is discussed under Viral Infections of the Respiratory Tract.

Purulent Bronchitis

Clinical Manifestations. Patients with acute bacterial infections of the tracheobronchial tree present with cough, sputum production, fever, and occasionally retrosternal pain aggravated by coughing. Findings on physical examination of the chest are frequently normal in previously healthy persons. Patients with underlying chronic bronchitis and an occasional previously well individual have abnormal auscultatory findings, usually consisting of rhonchi and coarse inspiratory rales, which are present bilaterally. Roentgenograms of the chest fail to demonstrate infiltrates.

Expectorated sputum is usually abundant and grossly purulent. The green-yellow color of purulent sputum is due to myeloperoxidase, an enzyme found in both neutrophils and eosinophils. Microscopic examination of sputum with either a wet-prep or staining technique is required to distinguish between these cell types. Gram stains of sputum usually reveal gram-positive cocci or small, pleomorphic gram-negative rods, *S. pneumoniae* or *H. influenzae*, respectively. Following influenza, *S. aureus* may be found, but this organism is otherwise an uncommon cause of bronchitis. Enteric gram-negative bacilli, especially *P. aeruginosa*, may be associated with purulent bronchitis in hospitalized patients or patients with bronchiectasis.

Purulent bronchitis due to primary bacterial infection is rare in previously healthy adults. In virtually all cases, a history of a preceding viral upper respiratory infection can be obtained and the bronchitic syndrome appears as a lingering sequel.

Patients with chronic bronchitis typically experience several episodes of purulent bronchitis each year. Several prospective studies have shown that 50% of such episodes are due to acute viral infection;[183] since only a small fraction of the many viruses that can cause this syndrome were sought in each of these studies, it seems likely that the true role of viral infection may be even greater. In contrast, the role of bacterial infection in purulent bronchitis is unclear despite decades of study. Early research in the United Kingdom suggested a strong association between purulent bronchitis and the presence of either *S. pneumoniae* or *H. influenzae* in sputum.[184] In other studies the presence of these organisms has been found to correlate poorly with sputum purulence and other evidence of active infection. Although antimicrobial therapy is used widely in treatment of purulent bronchitis, the few placebo-controlled studies available have failed to prove the superiority of antimicrobial therapy.[183] On the other hand, certain patients with chronic bronchitis suffer recurring episodes of purulent bronchitis related to *H. influenzae;* short-term antimicrobial therapy suppresses but does not eradicate the organism, and it reappears with increasing sputum volume and purulence shortly after discontinuance of treatment.[185]

Management. In previously healthy subjects, purulent bacterial bronchitis following viral respiratory infection should be treated with antimicrobial agents. In our experience, ampicillin, erythromycin, or tetracycline appears to be equally efficacious under most circumstances. We generally use similar drugs in the treatment of purulent exacerbations of chronic bronchitis, while recognizing the controversial aspects of such treatment. In selected patients in whom persistent *H. influenzae* appears to cause recurring episodes of purulent bronchitis prolonged therapy with ampicillin may lead to long-term eradication of the organism.

Since purulent sputum has markedly abnormal visco-elastic properties, bronchial clearance of secretions may be impaired during acute infection. This is usually not a significant problem in previously well patients but may lead to retention of secretions, atelectasis, and pneumonia in patients with previous airways disease. Postural drainage, perhaps with chest percussion, may assist in bronchial drainage in such patients. Bronchodilators may promote drainage by both dilating airways and stimulating mucociliary transport.[186] Although the use of inhaled bland aerosols is controversial, clinical experience suggests that this modality may be of value in some patients, if only by stimulating more vigorous coughing. Oral expectorants such as glycerol guaiacolate or potassium iodide are of limited value. Cough suppression should be considered when paroxysms of nonproductive coughing result from tracheobronchial irritation. Small doses of codeine effectively suppress cough with minimal sedation or other side-effects.

Acute Bacterial Pneumonia

The abrupt onset of a severe illness characterized by cough, productive of purulent or bloody sputum is the commonest presentation of bacterial pneumonia regardless of the causative organism (Table 8-6). Fever with temperatures up to 41 or 42° C is associated with tachypnea, dyspnea, and flaring of the nares. Young adults tend to have symptoms that can be well pinpointed to the respiratory tract, whereas infants and the elderly may have so few respiratory symptoms as to cause concern that the infection is, in fact, arising from another organ system. Not infrequently in the aged, the physician must initially systematically examine the urinary tract, the abdomen, and the chest, before it is clear which organ system harbors the infectious process. In infants, the elderly, and the severely ill, cough and sputum production may not be apparent, and clear evidence of bacterial infection may only be obtained in sputum from the tracheal aspirate. Pleuritic chest pain occurs in more than half of the patients, indicating pleural inflammation, and occasionally associated empyema.

Physical examination may reveal cyanosis, use of accessory muscles of respiration, tachypnea, tachycardia, and hyperthermia. The presence of clubbing should alert the physician to longstanding underlying disease. Physical examination of the chest demonstrates variable findings depending on the pattern of pneumonic involvement of the lungs.

Lobar pneumonia occurs as a result of infection of a discrete portion of the lung, generally a segment or lobe, with consolidation of the airspaces by edema, leukocytes, and erythrocytes, and ultimately a complete lack of aeration of that portion of the lung. This occurs most commonly in association with pneumococcal pneumonia, but occasionally also with *K. pneumoniae*, *S. aureus*, *H. influenzae*, or *Mycobacterium tuberculosis*. This distribution of infection generally represents an advanced stage, and has occurred less commonly with increasing early use of antibiotics in respiratory infections. Physical findings on examination of the chest may be restricted entirely to the lobe involved, and careful examination of the lungs in accordance with the anatomical knowledge of the lobes will generally permit the diagnosis to be established without roentgenography. The physical findings are those of consolidation, including decreased chest movement, dullness to percussion, bronchial breath sounds as a result of increased transmission of sound generated in the central airways, and occasionally high-pitched inspiratory rales in the region of the affected lung.

Bronchopneumonia tends to be patchy, may cross anatomical divisions between lobes, and is the common manifestation of bacterial pneumonia. The findings on physical examination are less discrete than those of lobar pneumonia. Owing to the patchy consolidation, there is again a reduction in air-entry, resulting in decreased chest movement, dullness to percussion, and either reduced or bronchial breath sounds over the affected region. As a result of accumulated tracheobronchial secretions, rhonchi and rales may occur. When the disease is limited to a segment or lobe, the physical findings are generally localized. On the other hand, if several lobes are involved, or there is bilateral involvement, definitive localization by physical diagnosis may be very difficult.

Hypoxemia is characteristic of pneumonia and, in the otherwise normal person, associated with marked hyperventilation. This results from a regional decrease in ventilation to some regions which remain perfused (at least initially), thereby producing a shunt-like effect. Compliance of the affected lung is diminished, with a reduction of the functional residual capacity. Regionally, there is a reduction in the surfactant levels, which may contribute to a loss of lung volume.[187–190] In patients with pre-existing respiratory disease, the additional work of breathing and impairment of regional ventilation may result in alveolar hypoventilation, with an elevation in P_{CO_2}.

During the febrile, septic phase of the illness, marked hemodynamic disturbances occur. Characteristically, there is profound peripheral vasodilatation, with a decrease in venous return and decreased cardiac output. Although the cardiac output may be normal for resting metabolic levels, it may be inappropriately low when the high metabolic demands associated with hyperthermia are taken into account.[191,192] This is discussed in greater detail further on under Septic Shock.

The prognosis is predictably worse with increasing age, with pre-existing debilitating disease, when the peripheral blood demonstrates leukopenia, in the presence of documented bacteremia, and in patients with immune deficiencies. Complications of pneumonia may be related to abnormalities of lung function, particularly hypoxemia; the course of the infection in the lungs; or distant spread of the infectious process.

Severe hypoxemia may result in altered levels of consciousness, arrhythmias, or death. These can all be avoided by management of the respiratory failure.

The infectious process in the lung may resolve completely; spread to contiguous areas such as the pleural space, with resultant empyema; or result in lung destruction. The production of single or multiple cavities within the lung is most characteristic of staphylococcal or gram-negative bacillary infections. When these occur, resolution is much slower and residual abnormalities of lung structure remain.

Bacteremia in association with pneumonia is relatively common (5 to 60%), but in most instances there is no spread of the infectious process. Meningitis, endocarditis, or abscesses of distant organs may occasionally result from hematological spread of the organisms. Delayed resolution of pneumonia should always alert the physician to the possibility of underlying disease. In the industrialized nations and in aging populations, the possibility of an underlying endobronchial neoplasm must always be considered as a cause of poor drainage and stasis. Occasionally, bronchostenosis, bronchiectasis, associated tuberculous or fungal infection in the lung, or other disease of the airways or lung parenchyma may impair the normal rate of resolution.

Bacterial pneumonia has been itemized as the fifth commonest cause of death.[193,194] It remains the commonest infective cause of death.[193] These figures may be somewhat misleading, since pneumonia is very commonly cited as the terminal illness in patients dying of other systemic disease. Furthermore, reported studies that indicate the incidence of various organisms as causative agents in pneumonia suffer from several shortcomings: (1) In most series, a significant fraction (up to 50%) of all patients with the clinical syndrome of bacterial pneumonia fail to demonstrate any pathogenic bacteria; (2) nonbacterial agents have not been extensively sought in many series; (3) patients are not thoroughly identified according to the presence of chronic illnesses; and (4) patients with milder illnesses, or lack of chronic diseases, are treated as outpatients and most reports only include hospitalized patients. However, certain generalizations can be made. Healthy young adults are much more likely to be infected by the pneumococcus, and in the pre-antibiotic era this was the case in 90 to 95% of bronchial pneumonias.[193,194,197,200] More recently, infections acquired while in hospital,[4] and among the debilitated and aging, have resulted in a much higher incidence of gram-negative bacillary pneumonias.[195,199] Anaerobic infections are not currently considered a common cause of primary bacterial pneumonia. These are more highly suspect in patients with necrotizing pneumonia, lung abscess, aspiration pneumonia, bronchiectasis, and empyema.[185] It is apparent that the offending organism varies with definable circumstances.

PATHOGENESIS OF BACTERIAL PNEUMONIA

There are three major steps in the pathogenesis of bacterial pneumonia, as outlined below.

Pathogenesis of Bacterial Pneumonia

1. Acquisition of causative agent
   a. Airborne organisms
   b. Direct contact
2. Entry into lungs
   a. Inhalation
   b. Aspiration
3. Interaction with host defenses
   a. Intrinsic lung defenses
   b. Systemic defenses

It is our view that only a few agents that cause bacterial pneumonia are transmitted by way of the air as droplet nuclei. The characteristics of such transmission, *e.g.*, simultaneous illness in many exposed persons, and transmission over some distance, are common with nonbacterial pneumonia but not with bacterial pneumonia. Notable exceptions occur, as with Legionnaire's disease, but ordinarily the organisms that cause bacterial pneumonia are acquired by direct contact. In fact, the organisms responsible for most bacterial pneumonias are commonly found in human hosts even in the absence of disease. However, multiple types or subgroups exist for each of these bacterial species, and the organisms with which a person has been chronically colonized may be different from those which produce acute infection. In the case of pneumococcus, which may account for up to 80% of community-acquired bacterial pneumonias, the majority of human infections are caused by only 12 of the 86 capsular types of the organism, but these 12 types are not prevalent among healthy pneumococcal carriers.[200,201] Only Type 3 is common both in carriers and in persons with infection.[195] These observations suggest that pneumococcal disease tends to occur shortly after acquisition of a virulent organism.

In hospitalized patients this sequence of events has been demonstrated prospectively. Gram-negative bacilli colonize the oropharynx in only 2% of healthy people.[11] However, sudden catastrophic illness or even elective surgical procedures cause the prevalence of colonization to increase to 30 to 50%. Nosocomial pneumonia is ten times more common among colonized patients than among noncolonized patients with similar illnesses, and is usually due to the organism which had earlier established colonization.[4] Airborne transmission of gram-negative bacilli does not appear to be a usual factor in nosocomial pneumonias. Rather, organisms are acquired directly from the patients by way of the hands of attendants.

Once established in the oropharynx, organisms probably enter the lungs principally through aspiration of small quantities of oropharyngeal secretions,[3] although aerosolization and inhalation of organisms from the upper respiratory tract cannot be excluded. Factors that promote aspiration, such as a depressed level of consciousness or impaired laryngeal reflexes, increase the risk of pneumonia; but aspiration probably occurs in all persons daily. Such aspiration is of such minute quantities of secretions as to be undetectable as a clinical event. However, owing to the enormous numbers of bacteria present, a small fluid bolus may contain 10^5 or more organisms. Because of the efficiency of the antibacterial defenses of the lung, bacterial pneumonia is not a daily occurrence.

Most persons who develop bacterial pneumonia have acute or chronic underlying diseases that might be expected to impair host defenses. When bacterial pneumonias occur in healthy persons, the history usually reveals a prodrome compatible with an acute viral respiratory illness, although proof of the causative virus is frequently lacking.[194,202,203] Both intrinsic lung defenses and the ability to rapidly mobilize systemic defenses are important. Persons with impaired mucociliary transport or pulmonary edema are at markedly increased risk of bacterial pneumonia, as are those who lack circulating antibodies or polymorphonuclear leukocytes.

If lung defenses are insufficient, bacterial proliferation occurs. Bacteria release substances which attract neutrophils from the blood and activate complement proteins. Bacterial products, neutrophil enzymes, and activated plasma proteins may each alter the permeability of the alveolar–capillary membrane, leading to the rapid development of protein-rich alveolar edema and hemorrhage accompanying intense accumulation of neutrophils. This stage of the process is called "red hepatization" because the consolidated lung is airless and of liver-like consistency. Lobar consolidation is in fact uncommon, probably because of early treatment with antimicrobial agents. Bronchopneumonia, in which many foci of inflammation are present around terminal bronchioles, is much more common. If untreated, such inflammation spreads through pores of Kohn and endobronchially to adjacent lung units until the pleural surfaces are reached, resulting in lobar consolidation.

At this stage the microbe has the advantage. While phagocytes can engulf nonopsonized bacteria enmeshed in fibrin strands or on surfaces, the milieu of the consolidated alveolus is unfavorable for the cell, being hypoxic, acidic, and filled with debris. Capsular polysaccharide accumulates as pneumococci die, and this material inhibits phagocytosis.[204]

Treatment with appropriate antimicrobial agents is more effective in eliminating organisms at the active, spreading edges of pneumonia than at the center.[205] Antimicrobial agents, with the exception of rifampin, do not cross cell membranes well, and thus exert their effect principally on extracellular bacteria. Additionally, bacterial multiplication is required for the antibacterial activity of most drugs. Therefore, in the central portions of a pneumonia, where bacteria may be quite inactive and may exist within phagocytes unable to kill them, the antimicrobial agents are least effective.

In the pre-antibiotic era, pneumococcal pneumonia persisted until the development of specific, opsonizing antibody.[206] This was heralded by prompt improvement in some patients ("crisis"), but more often by slower defervescence over several days ("lysis"). As the bacterial population is checked, either by antibody and phagocytes or by antibiotics, the neutrophilic exudate is gradually replaced by macrophages and the process begins to resolve. Interestingly, lung tissue does not necrose in pneumococcal pneumonia despite the presence of neutrophil and macrophage enzymes, which are known to be capable of digesting lung tissue. In contrast, lung necrosis is a common feature of pneumonias caused by gram-negative bacilli, staphylococci, or anaerobic organisms. Since these organisms secrete enzymes that can injure lung tissue, whereas the pneumococcus does not, it seems likely that lung necrosis results from the bacterial products and not host-cell enzymes. Presumably, this distinction reflects differing capabilities of serum- and tissue-protease inhibitors for enzymes derived from human virus or bacterial cells.

Antimicrobial therapy has reduced the mortality of community-acquired bacterial pneumonia from 20% to approximately 5% and markedly reduced the morbidity associated with these infections.[193,194] However, mortality from pneumococcal pneumonia for the first 4 to 5 days of treatment is still similar to that in the preantibiotic era[207] and the mortality of hospital-acquired *P. aeruginosa* pneumonia remains about 75% despite the use of antibiotics that are effective against organisms *in vitro*.[208] Clearly, prevention of bacterial pneumonia would be desirable. Prophylactic administration of antimicrobial agents to high-risk ambulatory or hospitalized patients has had only marginal success and leads to the emergence of drug-resistant strains. Immunization with polyvalent pneumococcal polysaccharide vaccine appears to be of benefit in certain high-risk populations.[201] Interestingly, such immunization leads both to a reduction in disease due to vaccine strains and a reduction in the prevalence of these strains in asymptomatic carriers. However, the impact of pneumococcal vaccinations on the overall incidence of bacterial pneumonia remains to be clearly demonstrated, especially among the aged, chronic bronchitic, and other groups at risk. The use of aerosolized or intratracheally-instilled antibiotics has no established place in the management of pneumonia. Recommended antibiotic treatment for bacterial pneumonias is outlined in Table 8-8; dosage adjustment for renal failure is outlined in Table 8-9.

STREPTOCOCCUS PNEUMONIAE PNEUMONIA

Incidence. The pneumococcus is responsible for the large majority of bacterial pneumonias acquired outside of the hospital. Although pneumococcal pneumonia occurs in young, healthy adults with no underlying illnesses, it is also the commonest cause of pneumonia in elderly patients and patients with various chronic diseases. From 15 to 30% of normal persons are pharyngeal carriers of the pneumococcus; however, the serotypes found most commonly among asymptomatic carriers are not those which most frequently cause pneumococcal pneumonia. Pneumonia occurs most commonly during the winter months, and the disease is less common in warm and dry climates. Nevertheless, it remains a

TABLE 8-8. Antimicrobial Agents in Respiratory Tract Infections

Causative Agent	First	Second	Third
Gram-positive cocci			
S. pneumoniae	Penicillin G	Erythromycin A cephalosporin	A tetracycline Chloramphenicol Clindamycin
Streptococci (anaerobic)	Penicillin G	Erythromycin	Chloramphenicol Clindamycin
Str. pyogenes	Penicillin G	Erythromycin	Clindamycin A cephalosporin
S. aureus			
Penicillin-sensitive	Penicillin G	A cephalosporin	Erythromycin Clindamycin
Penicillin-resistant	Penicillin G Nafcillin Methicillin	Vancomycin	Gentamicin
Methicillin-resistant	Vancomycin	A cephalosporin	Clindamycin
Gram-positive bacilli			
B. anthracis	Penicillin G Streptomycin	Erythromycin A tetracycline	A cephalosporin Chloramphenicol
C. diphtheriae	Penicillin G	Erythromycin	A cephalosporin
Gram-negative bacilli			
K. pneumoniae	Gentamicin Tobramycin	Amikacin A cephalosporin Chloramphenicol	Tetracycline Trimethoprim-sulfamethoxazole Kanamycin Polymyxin B Colistimethate
P. aeruginosa	Gentamicin/Tobramycin Carbenicillin/Ticarcillin		Colistimethate Polymyxin B
Proteus species (not *mirabilis*)	Gentamicin Tobramycin	Carbenicillin Amikacin	Chloramphenicol A tetracycline Trimethoprim-sulfamethoxazole Kanamycin Cefoxitin
E. coli	Gentamicin Tobramycin	Ampicillin A cephalosporin A tetracycline	Kanamycin Colistimethate Polymyxin B
Serratia	Gentamicin	Carbenicillin Ticarcillin Amikacin	Chloramphenicol Kanamycin Trimethoprim-sulfamethoxazole Cefoxitin
H. influenzae	Ampicillin	Chloramphenicol A tetracycline Streptomycin Sulfonamide	Cefaclor Cefamandole
Bacteroides (oral)	Penicillin G	Chloramphenicol	Tetracycline Clindamycin
Bacteroides (GI)	Clindamicin	Chloramphenicol	Tetracycline
P. pseudomallei	Tetracycline	Chloramphenicol	Trimethoprim-sulfamethoxazole Kanamycin

TABLE 8-8. Antimicrobial Agents in Respiratory Tract Infections (*Continued*)

Causative Agent	First	Second	Third
Non-gram-stained organisms			
L. pneumophilia	Erythromycin (IV)	Tetracycline	
M. pneumoniae	Erythromycin Tetracycline		

(Abramowicz M (ed.): The Medical Letter 22:2, New Rochelle, NY, 1980)

TABLE 8-9. Modification of Antimicrobial Management in the Presence of Impaired Renal Function

	Excretion or Inactivation	Maintenance Dosage Intervals for Varying Creatinine Clearance (ml/min)			
		80	50–80	10–50	<10
Aminoglycosides					
Gentamicin	Renal	8	12	12–26	48–72
Streptomycin	Renal	12	24	24–72	72–96
Kanamycin	Renal	18	24	24–72	72–96
Tobramycin	Renal	6–8	Need further evaluation		
Amikacin	Renal	8–12	12–18	24–36	36–48
Cephalosporins					
Cephazolin	Renal, hepatic	8	8	12	24–48
Cephalexin	Renal, nonrenal	6	6	6–12	6–12
Cephalothin	Renal, hepatic	6	6	6	8–12
Cefamandole	Renal	4–6	6	6–9	9
Penicillin					
Penicillin G	Renal, hepatic	8	8	8	8–12
Ampicillin	Renal, hepatic	6	6	9	12–15
Oxacillin	Renal, hepatic	6	6	6	6
Methicillin	Renal, hepatic	4	4	4	8–12
Carbenicillin	Renal, hepatic	4	4	6–12	12–16
Ticarcillin	Renal	4–6	4	8	12
Tetracyclines					
Tetracycline (NR)*	Renal, hepatic	6	8–12	12–24	24
Doxycycline	Renal, hepatic	12	12	12	12
Minocycline	Hepatic	12	12	18–24	24–36
Chloramphenicol	Hepatic, renal	6	6	6	6
Erythromycin	Hepatic	6	6	6	6
Clindamycin	Hepatic, renal	6	6	6	6
Lincomycin	Hepatic, renal	6	6	12	24
Trimethoprim-sulfamethoxazole	Renal	12	12	18	24
Vancomycin	Renal	24	24–72	72–240	240

(Adapted from Bennett WM et al: Guidelines for drug therapy in renal failure. Ann Int Med 86:754–783, 1977)
* NR—Not recommended

prominent worldwide problem, affecting also the warm African nations.

Clinical Manifestations. Patients present with general systemic manifestations of acute infectious illness including fever, tachycardia, and general malaise. The illness is generally abrupt in onset with cough productive of purulent or rust-colored sputum, pleuritic chest pain, and typically with a single, shaking chill. In many patients, symptoms of upper-respiratory viral infection precede the onset of pneumonia; despite this common apparent association between viral infection and pneumococcal pneumonia, efforts to document the former have been unsuccessful except for epidemic influenza. Hypotension is uncommon except in patients who have delayed seeking help for several days. Severe hypotension and dehydration may be the presenting features in elderly or debilitated patients. Jaundice and azotemia are present in some patients and are adverse prognostic signs. Azotemia is probably secondary to decreased renal perfusion due to hemodynamic changes. Jaundice is not well explained but has been ascribed to hemolysis, hepatic hypoxia with decreased bilirubin clearance, and red cell breakdown in the lung. The pneumonia in jaundiced patients is more frequently extensive, involving the right lower lobe, and may be associated with liver tenderness.[209]

Physical examination of the chest may be consistent with either bronchopneumonia or lobar consolidation. Pleural effusion occurs in 10% of patients and is typically small, thus causing minimal physical findings.

Laboratory Evaluation. Suspicion of pneumonia aroused by the patient's history and physical examination should be confirmed radiographically. Pneumococcal pneumonia has no characteristic pattern but typically results in one or more areas of alveolar consolidation. Complete lobar consolidation is uncommon. Hilar adenopathy, cavitation, or substantial pleural effusion should raise doubt about the diagnosis.

A Gram stain of lower respiratory secretions obtained by expectoration or other techniques should be examined to confirm presence of a distal inflammatory process, and to determine whether a specific organism predominates. This information is useful in guiding early empiric antibiotic therapy. Blood cultures should be obtained and incubated, both aerobically and anaerobically. If a pleural effusion is identified, the fluid should be aspirated for Gram stain, culture, and chemical characterization. The presence of organisms confirms existence of an empyema, which will require pleural drainage as part of the treatment. The pleural fluid *p*H may be useful in determining the need for drainage; an exudate with *p*H less than 7.2 usually requires drainage.[210] Pleural fluid as well as sputum may be assayed by CIE to identify the presence of pneumococcal antigens if the diagnosis is uncertain.[73]

Leukocytosis in the range of 15,000 to 20,000/mm^2 with a shift towards immature forms is usually present; either leukopenia or marked leukocytosis is an adverse prognostic sign. If jaundice is present, appropriate liver-function studies and hematological evaluation should be undertaken to establish the mechanism and to avoid missing co-existing disease. Arterial blood gas analysis should be performed for any patient sufficiently ill as to warrant hospitalization, since severe hypoxemia may be present without obvious clinical signs. In the presence of extensive lobar consolidation, hypoxemia is due in large part to shunting, and the arterial oxygen tension rises little with supplemental oxygen. However, as noted by Stadie in one of the pioneering applications of arterial blood gas analysis, the oxygen content of the blood is frequently lower in patients with scattered diffuse infiltrates than in patients with lobar consolidation.[211] It is now known that this is due to the effectiveness of hypoxic vasoconstriction, which reduces pulmonary blood flow to consolidated regions.[212]

Specific Treatment. Penicillin is the antibiotic of choice and is recommended in doses of 600,000 units of aqueous crystalline penicillin G, or procaine penicillin, administered at 12-hr intervals for 5 to 7 days, or at least 72 hr after the patient has been afebrile. Substantial evidence suggests that the minimum curative dose for infections with most strains of pneumococci is less than 60,000 units daily. Pneumococcal pneumonia can be treated orally with one of the well-absorbed penicillins, such as penicillin V, in doses of 1.0 g daily. Parenteral penicillin in doses exceeding 1.2 million units per day does not improve prospects of survival from severe pneumococcal infection[213] and does appear to be associated with a greater incidence of hospital-acquired superinfection.[214] Thus, the temptation to titer the given dose of penicillin against the severity of the patient's illness should be resisted. However, if extrapulmonary sites of infection are present, especially endocarditis or meningitis, penicillin should be administered intravenously in doses of 10 to 12 million units daily.

In patients who are allergic to penicillin, erythromycin or lincomycin is acceptable. Cephalosporins are effective, but should be given with caution in patients who are hypersensitive to penicillin because of the possibility of cross-sensitivity.

A truly alarming recent development is the report of disease caused by pneumococci which were highly resistant *in vitro* to multiple antimicrobial agents.[17] Occasional resistance has been known to occur for some time, especially to tetracycline, a fact which limits the usefulness of this drug in pneumococcal infections. However, with rare exceptions, resistance to penicillin has not been increasing despite years of exposure of the organism to this drug. In the recently described outbreaks, pneumococci resistant *in vitro* and *in vivo* to penicillin—as well as several other antimicrobial agents—were described. Refractory infections and nosocomial transmission of the organism to other ill patients were features of the outbreaks. Although *in vitro* susceptibility studies indicated that rifampin might be useful, therapy with this drug led to the emergence of resistant strains. Treatment ultimately required individualized regimens and the use of toxic agents such as vancomycin. Should similar organisms become common worldwide, the true ravaging nature of pneumococcal infections as witnessed in the pre-antibiotic era will once again become manifest.

Supportive Treatment. Death in early pneumococcal pneumonia is associated with hypotension, hypoxia, arrhythmias, and central nervous system depression. Confusion and disorientation, commonly reported in the older literature, are infrequent when management of these problems is pursued aggressively. Intravascular volume expansion with saline, or colloid-containing fluids, results in increased cardiac output and blood pressure, with improved renal perfusion and urine output. Treatment of hypoxemia by administration of supplemental oxygen is outlined in Chapter 7. Most patients are readily managed with intermediate flow rates of oxygen (*e.g.*, 4 to 6 liters per min by nasal cannula or mask), however, arterial blood gas analyses should be routinely repeated while the patient is on oxygen therapy, in order to establish that oxygenation is adequate.

Vigorous attempts to clear the airways of retained secretions will improve ventilation, and in the chronically debilitated patient or patients with pre-existing lung disease, nasotracheal suction, physiotherapy, and cough may provide striking benefit. Occasionally, tracheal intubation may be necessary to remove secretions and provide high oxygen concentrations.

Bronchodilators may improve regional ventilation and drainage of secretions. There are no studies available to clearly define their role for patients with pneumonia who do not have underlying airway disease. Inhalation of bland aerosols may relieve the patient's dry, irritated oropharynx, but there is little evidence to document improved drainage of bronchial secretions as a result of such therapy.

Supportive respiratory therapy must be tailored to individual patient needs. Most patients with pneumonia neither need nor benefit from such therapy, with the possible exception of oxygen.[215] However, an occasional patient with inadequate cough, markedly tenacious sputum, or bronchospasm may benefit from therapy directed towards these problems.

On effective therapy, the temperature generally returns to normal within 24 to 48 hr and the clinical manifestations of systemic toxicity are strikingly improved, but auscultatory and roentgenographic lung findings may actually progress for 24 hr while the patient is on antibiotics. Thereafter, the resolution is definite, but gradual. Once there is clear-cut evidence of response to antimicrobial therapy, the patient can generally be returned to his home environment, but there should be close follow-up of the case until resolution is complete.

Complications. Bacteremia can be demonstrated in about 30% of patients with pneumococcal pneumonia. Not surprisingly, the incidence of bacteremia increases with increasing extent of disease radiographically and the duration of the patient's symptoms. Overall, mortality rates are approximately 32% in patients with bacteremia and 6% in those without. Death usually occurs within the first 48 to 72 hr of hospitalization.

Delayed radiographic resolution is a common complication.[216] In young, previously healthy patients, the radiographic changes of pneumococcal pneumonia usually clear completely within 2 to 4 wk. Radiographic changes in elderly patients or patients with chronic lung disease usually also clear without permanent residue, although complete clearing may require as long as 18 wk. Volume loss, fibrotic stranding, and pleural thickening are common findings. Volume loss is a particularly worrisome finding since it suggests the presence of an obstructed bronchus. However, in the absence of continued clinical illness and with radiographic improvement, albeit slow, such obstruction is rarely found and bronchoscopy can be deferred. Persistent clinical illness and lack of radiographic improvement are indications for bronchoscopy.

Parapneumonic pleural effusions typically develop after 2 to 4 days of antimicrobial therapy.[217] The patient's temperature remains elevated and pleuritic chest pain is present. The pleural fluid is always exudative, typically containing 10,000 to 12,000 leukocytes per ml, with a mixture of neutrophils and lymphocytes. With effective antimicrobial therapy, organisms are neither seen on smears nor recovered in culture. If the patient's diagnosis is in doubt, the presence of pneumococcal antigen in pleural fluid by CIE confirms the presence of a parapneumonic, pneumococcal effusion. Treatment of these effusions is aspiration alone, because defervescence usually occurs promptly and reaccumulation of such sterile effusions is uncommon. Frank empyema is usually evident on the initial evaluation and it should be managed as outlined in Chapter 12, Pleural Disease.

Cavitation of the lung is rare in pneumococcal pneumonia, and is said to occur only with Type 3 infections. However, nonhomogeneous consolidation of an emphysematous lobe may give the radiographic appearance of necrotizing pneumonia.[218] Previous radiographs which demonstrate bullae or other changes of emphysema may be useful in making this distinction (Fig. 8-10). Extrapulmonary complications of pneumococcal pneumonia were common in the preantibiotic era and included endocarditis, meningitis, and arthritis. Antimicrobial therapy has largely eliminated these complications.

Prevention. The predominance of only 12 capsular types of pneumococci in serious human infections has made prevention by vaccination feasible. Studies in the pre-antibiotic era demonstrated the efficacy of vaccination in the reduction of pneumonia due to vaccinated types.[219] This approach was abandoned with the advent of antimicrobial therapy. However, the continued high mortality of pneumococcal disease in certain groups has rekindled interest in this approach.

The current vaccine contains 14 capsular type antigens (1, 2, 3, 4, 6, 8, 9, 12, 14, 23, 25, 51, and 56), which together account for nearly 80% of bacteremic infections in the United States.[201] This vaccine is acceptably immunogenic in normal subjects. Conflicting data on antibody responses in children with sickle-cell disease have been reported.[220,221] Minor local reactions occur in 30 to 40% and febrile reactions in about 3% of subjects. Field trials have shown the vaccine to be 82.3% effective in reducing bacteremic infections in South African gold miners.[201] However, serious pneumococcal infections have been documented in vaccinated subjects. At the present time, the reduction in incidence of serious pneumonias that might occur following widespread vaccination is unclear, and will depend on several factors, including the stability of the types of pneumococci which cause invasive disease; the antibody responses of persons with chronic illnesses; and the replacement of pneumococci by other, less virulent, but often less treatable bacterial species as the causative agents in pneumonia.

The vaccine is currently recommended for

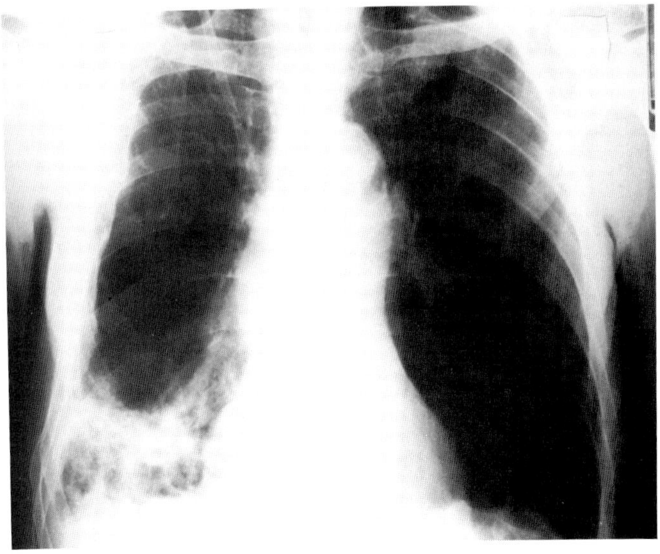

FIG. 8-10. Postero-anterior chest roentgenogram that demonstrates nonhomogeneous consolidation of the right lower lobe in a patient with a brief history of fever, right-sided chest pain, and purulent sputum. The thickened pleura resulted from thoracic trauma many years ago. Blood cultures grew *S. pneumoniae*. In this situation, the irregular consolidation of the lung is due to pre-existing abnormalities in the lung parenchyma, not to necrotizing infection.

persons age 2 yr or older with chronic diseases, those in chronic care facilities, persons convalescing from serious disease, and all persons over age 50 yr. Children under 2 yr of age do not respond satisfactorily and the vaccine is not recommended. It is not approved for use in pregnant women.

OTHER COMMON BACTERIAL PNEUMONIAS

Staphylococcal Pneumonia

Pneumonia due to *Staphylococcus aureus* occurs occasionally in children, but is unusual in adults except in certain specific instances. *S. aureus* remains a significant cause of nosocomial pneumonia among postsurgical patients. *S. aureaus* is responsible for about 1 to 5% of community-acquired bacterial pneumonias; however, its incidence rises to about 20% during outbreaks of influenza. Thus, community-acquired staphylococcal pneumonia is rare except in association with influenza.

In each of the above circumstances, pneumonia due to *S. aureus* shares most of the features of bacterial pneumonia discussed previously. Radiographic involvement tends to be patchy, not densely consolidated.

Pneumatoceles, thin-walled cystic structures, may arise within a few hours in children. These lesions have been variously ascribed to bronchiolar obstruction, lung necrosis, or subpleural emphysema.[222] Rupture of a pneumatocele through the pleura causes pyopneumothorax. Although pneumatoceles are uncommon in adults, cavitation of regions of consolidation is frequent, apparently owing to enzymes released from the organism. Pleural involvement is common in pneumonia due to *S. aureus* and the fluid loculates rapidly.

A distinctive syndrome consisting of chills, high fever, and prostration occurs in persons with *S. aureus* sepsis, usually from contaminated intravenous injections. The pulmonary manifestations may be slight with nonproductive cough and pleuritic chest pain being common symptoms. Roentgenograms of the chest reveal multiple, bilateral nodular lesions, 1-2 cm in diameter, which appear and enlarge rapidly. Some may show central cavitation (Fig. 8-11). Empyema occurs early in most patients. Some, but probably not all, patients with this syndrome have endocarditis; in most, the valvular process does not lead to major hemodynamic consequences.

Distant foci of infection may be established in patients with *S. aureus* bacteremia, including brain, liver, renal, and splenic abscesses. Diagnosis of these remote abscesses may pose a par-

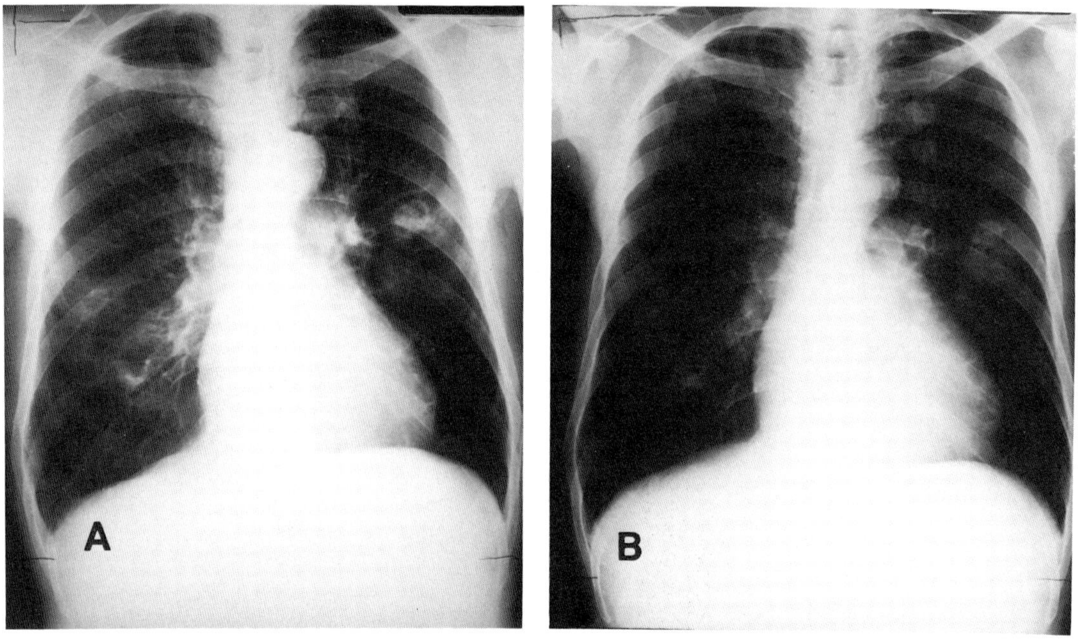

FIG. 8-11. **A.** Well-circumscribed cavity in left midlung field of patient with staphylococcal endocarditis. Similar lesions are seen in right lower lung field. **B.** One week after institution of antibiotic therapy.

ticularly vexing clinical problem because defervescence on treatment is frequently slow in *S. aureus* pneumonia, owing to the presence of pleural involvement.

Antimicrobial therapy should be instituted promptly when the diagnosis of *S. aureus* pneumonia is suspected on the basis of Gram stain of sputum or pleural fluid. Smears of the buffy coat or urine may be helpful in identifying septicemia. Initial therapy must include an agent that is resistant to penicillinase, such as methicillin or nafcillin, 2 g intravenously every 4 hr. Cephalothin, 1.5 g every 4 hr, or vancomycin, 0.5 gm every 6 hours, are suitable alternatives in patients with penicillin allergy.

Although *S. aureus* is generally susceptible to the aminoglycosides, these drugs are not considered the agents of choice. Recently, *S. aureus* "tolerance" to the penicillins has been described, in which the drug concentration required for a bactericidal effect is markedly greater than the minimum inhibitory concentration.[223] In such instances the addition of aminoglycosides may be helpful.

Treatment of empyema is discussed in Chapter 12, on Pleural Diseases.

Streptococcus pyogenes Pneumonia

Streptococcus pyogenes is an uncommon cause of pneumonia; it typically appears after influenza, measles, or pertussis in children, or in outbreaks in military populations. Silva and colleagues[224] reported a series of patients who developed *S. pyogenes* pneumonia following adenovirus infection. Studies of polymorphonuclear leukocytes from these patients suggested that the previous adenoviral infection had altered the neutrophils' capacity for killing the bacteria. Subjects in group settings where adenoviral infections are common might be expected to be at increased risk for *S. pyogenes* pneumonia, an expectation borne out by military experience as far back as the Civil War.

In such outbreaks the disease is characterized

by sudden onset of symptoms including severe chest pain. Empyema is commonly present on the initial examination. The diagnosis is most commonly based on a compatible clinical history, with positive sputum cultures, positive pleural fluid culture, and high ASO titers. Blood cultures are usually not positive. Treatment is with penicillin or a cephalosporin and, where necessary, drainage of empyema.

Klebsiella pneumoniae Pneumonia

This gram-negative encapsulated bacillus causes pneumonia in an older age group than the pneumococcus (mean age greater than 50), most commonly occurs in patients with underlying disease, particularly alcoholism, and has a predilection for the upper lobes. Chronic bronchopulmonary disease and diabetes mellitus also predispose patients to Klebsiella pneumonia.[194,199,225–229]

The clinical features and lung-function abnormalities found are similar to those of other acute bacterial pneumonias. The sputum has been described as nonputrid, thick, tenacious, and frequently brick red in color. However, its appearance is not at all consistently distinctive, and is therefore an unreliable sign.[199] Clinical examination of the chest generally reveals signs of consolidation and occasionally atelectasis in the region of the involved lobe. Involvement of more than one lobe is frequent. Roentgenographic examination demonstrates lobular or lobar consolidation, and lung abscess formation with multiple small thin-walled or large abscess cavities. Bulging of the fissure adjacent to the consolidation has been described as distinctive.[227,229] The rapid destruction of lung tissue has not been satisfactorily explained, but can occur within 24 to 48 hr, with frank abscess formation recognized within 4 days.[230] It is of utmost importance to recognize the nature of the infecting organism early, since extensive tissue destruction may be avoided. Carl Friedländer, in his initial description of eight cases of acute pneumonia, thought this to be the usual cause of lobar pneumonia, and the common eponym *Friedländer's pneumonia* resulted. Subsequent reevaluation through the years has demonstrated that only about 1% of primary pneumonias now occur as a result of Klebsiella infections.[199]

K. pneumoniae is a common cause of nosocomial pneumonia, especially among seriously ill patients.[4] In this setting radiographic changes are usually patchy and most common in the lower lobes. Classic signs of pneumonia, such as fever, cough, and rales, may be obscured by underlying disease processes. To further complicate the problem, most seriously ill patients become colonized with gram-negative bacilli, commonly *K. pneumoniae* in the absence of distal lung infection. Thus, the seriously ill patient may have signs and symptoms which are compatible with nosocomial pneumonia and have pathogenic organisms in his secretions in the absence of pneumonia. We have found the presence of new local consolidation radiographically and purulent tracheobronchial secretions to be helpful in determining the presence of pneumonia in such patients.

Prior to the antimicrobial era, mortality ranged from 50 to more than 90%. However, with the advent of drug therapy, the mortality has been reduced to 20 to 50%. Leucopenia, bacteremia, severe underlying disease, and increasing age are poor prognostic factors.

Aminoglycosides are the drugs of choice for infections due to *K. pneumoniae.* These drugs should be given in full doses for patients with normal renal function but must be adjusted downward according to the scheme in Table 8-8 when the creatinine clearance is impaired. In the critically ill patient, serum levels should be measured; the therapeutic range is 8 to 10 μg/ml. In infections due to organisms resistant to other aminoglycosides, amikacin may provide effective therapy. Cephaloporins have demonstrated *in vitro* activity against *K. pneumoniae* but clinical usage has lead to disappointing results; these agents are now second line drugs for this infection.

Pneumonia Due to Other Gram-Negative Bacteria

E. coli, *P. aeruginosa*, and Proteus species all occur most commonly in hospital-acquired infections, and result in a typical bacterial pneumonia syndrome, with characteristic necrotizing features. Pseudomonas bacteremia may produce a severe necrotizing vasculitis, which mimics a bland pulmonary infarct. Pseudomonas pneumonia may be difficult to distinquish from pneumonia or infiltrates due to other cause, with coincident colonization of the tracheobronchial tree. Clear evidence of infection due to the organism should be sought before undertaking aggressive, costly, and often futile chemotherapy.[231]

No diagnostic clinical features are demonstrable. Identification of the organism is of utmost importance. Antibiotics should be selected on the basis of the most likely infecting agent and treatment modified in accordance with information obtained from subsequent cultures.

Serratia marscesens infections are almost always nosocomial, and in recent years have been most commonly reported in association with the use of inhalation therapy equipment. Ultrasonic nebulizers, heated-mist nebulizers, and IPPB side-stream nebulizers have all been incriminated.[4,199] Identification of the organism is of some importance, since antimicrobial responses are at slight variance with those of other gram-negative bacteria.

Pneumonia due to *H. influenzae* is generally associated with chronic bronchopulmonary disease, but may occur rarely in adults as a primary infection. It generally presents as a bacterial pneumonia syndrome, with patchy bronchopneumonia radiographically. Occasionally, consolidating lobar pneumonia occurs.[232] Either ampicillin or chloramphenical have been effective against *H. influenzae*. However, both Type 6 and untypable strains of this organism have shown increasing resistance to ampicillin *in vitro*, so that in some localities ampicillin is no longer the drug of choice for severe infections. In addition to chloramphenical, suitable alternatives to ampicillin include cefaclor and the combination of trimethoprim–sulfamethoxazole.[233]

Bacterial Pneumonia Due to Uncommon Organisms

Bacillus anthracis is a gram-negative sporulating rod that causes anthrax. This uncommon infection generally results from contact with diseased animals, particularly sheep. The illness is generally diphasic, consisting of an initial chill, fever and myalgia, followed by some improvement, and then abrupt deterioration with clinical manifestations of acute bacterial pneumonia. The precise pathogenesis is not clear, but infection appears to depend on initial entry to the lung, followed by multiplication of the organisms in regional lymph nodes, followed by a toxic reaction with necrosis, hemorrhage, and edema in the lungs. Specific toxins and their precise role in the pathogenesis of the disease are not certain. If the organism is not cultured initially from blood or sputum, serological studies may permit identification of the organism. High-dose penicillin therapy and streptomycin are both effective against the organisms, and it is currently recommended that they be used in combination.[234,235]

Pasteurella species may produce pneumonia. These small gram-negative bacilli infect animals primarily, and transmission to man is generally by wood ticks, dog ticks, and a variety of wild animals including the rabbit. *Pasteurella multocida* causes occasional cases of severe pneumonia, and is best treated by penicillin.[236] *Pasteurella (Yersinia) pestis* is accountable for the disease known as bubonic plague. It is transmitted from wild animals or their fleas. It is associated with regional lymph node enlargement, but when lung involvement occurs, a fulminant septic course with profound prostration is characteristic.[236] Untreated bubonic plague has a mortality of 60 to 90%, but very early treatment of the pneumonic form may result in an improved prognosis. Tetracycline, chloramphenicol, sulfonamides, and streptomycin have all been effective in management. It has been recommended that streptomycin (20 to 30 mg per kg body weight per day, divided in three equal daily doses) and tetracycline (2 to 3 g divided in four equal doses) be given for at least 10 days. Because the disease is highly infectious, all contacts should also be treated with antibiotics, and observed for at least a 10-day period. Active immunization is possible in high-risk individuals.[237]

Bordetella pertussis is a gram-negative rod commonly responsible for whooping cough in children and occasionally in adults. Characteristically, this illness consists of a 1- to 2-week catarrhal stage with upper respiratory symptoms, followed by a paroxysmal stage lasting 1 to 6 weeks, during which a dry but persistent violent cough occurs; and a convalescent phase during which the patient gradually improves. This is an epidemic illness, characterized by minimal pulmonary signs, occasional roentgenographic evidence of mild pneumonitis, and a lymphocytosis during the paroxysmal stage of 60 to 80%. A cough specimen, or nasopharyngeal swab cultured on appropriate bacteriologic media will generally permit identification of the organism. The triad of an afebrile patient with lymphocytosis and typical paroxysms of cough generally permits a clinical diagnosis to be made. Active immunization in early life provides protection against the illness, and has strikingly reduced the incidence of this infection.[238] Antimicrobial agents including erythromycin and tetracycline are effective in eradicating the organism, though they do little to modify the course of the established disease.[239–241] The chief diagnostic confusion can occur with certain adenoviruses that cause upper respiratory symptoms with rhinorrhea, as well as paroxysms of cough.

Pseudomonas pseudomallei produces the condition melioidosis, which in its primary pneumonic form may result in chronic cavitary disease, occasionally with calcification. This gram-negative bacillus is endemic in rodents, cats and dogs in Southeast Asia, and most commonly has been recognized infecting Caucasian visitors to that area. The largest number of such cases occurred among military personnel during the Vietnam war. This is generally a chronic necrotizing pneumonia with no definitive characteristics. It is commonly confused with tuberculosis or fungal infection. The organism may be cultured, but a serological hemagglutination reaction and complement-fixing antibodies are helpful in identification of infected individuals.[242–244]

Treatment of meliodosis is with tetracycline, chloramphenicol, trimethoprim-sulfamethoxazole, or kanamycin.[245,246] Failure to become culture-negative in the presence of residual cavities is an indication for surgical resection in some centers.[245] Lobectomy has been advocated as the most useful procedure. Operation should be preceded by antibiotic therapy. In the limited number of cases reported, the sputum may remain positive for several weeks postoperatively. Therefore, antibiotics should be continued for 4 to 6 wk after resection.

Pleuropulmonary tularemia results from infection with *Francisella tularensis*. Ticks usually transmit the organism to humans from infected animals, although some individuals have developed infection after handling wild rabbits or squirrels, without evident tick bites.[247,248] Because of such cases, the possibility of infection by inhalation has been proposed.[249]

The most characteristic feature of tularemia is variability, with clinical presentations ranging from severe, overwhelming infection to asymptomatic radiographic abnormalities. Radiographic changes include bronchopneumonia, pleural effusion, localized consolidation, and hilar adenopathy. The "ovoid density" and cavitation are uncommon manifestations.[248]

The diagnosis is based on clinical suspicion and serologic changes. Isolation of the organism requires special media and may be hazardous to laboratory workers unaccustomed to this organism. Treatment consists of streptomycin for 10 to 14 days.

In 1976 a new organism, subsequently named *Legionella pneumophilia*, was identified as the causative agent of an epidemic of pneumonia with 15% mortality rate.[250] Retrospective serologic studies of unexplained outbreaks of acute respiratory illness, and ongoing studies of similar outbreaks have begun to define the epidemiology of this infection.[251,252] The organism appears to be widespread in nature. It is most likely spread by the airborne route from contaminated sources, usually air-handling systems, and there does not appear to be person-to-person spread. It appears more commonly in summer or early fall. Although the initial epidemics were characterized by a severe clinical syndrome, at least one epidemic in 1965 in Pontiac, Michigan, was characterized by a much milder illness with a short incubation period (1 to 2 days) and very high (95%) attack rate.

The usual clinical syndrome is that of a high, nonremitting fever with recurrent chills, relative bradycardia, early gastrointestinal symptoms, nonproductive cough, and lack of organisms on

Gram stain preparations of sputum or transtracheal aspirate.[252] Radiographs typically show poorly-marginated peripheral densities, which progress to bronchopneumonia and then to multilobar consolidation. Myalgia, hematuria, abnormal liver function tests, and toxic encephalopathy with an essentially normal cerebrospinal fluid are common associated findings.

The organism is extremely difficult to isolate in direct culture; diagnosis typically is made in retrospect by seroconversion. However, immunologic advances have made rapid diagnosis possible in some cases by demonstration of the organism in tracheal secretions and urine, using direct immunofluorescence or the enzyme-linked immunosorbent assay (ELISA) technique.[253] Infection in immunocompromised hosts may require lung biopsy to rule out the presence of other opportunistic organisms. Processing of such tissue must include Dieterle's silver stain, since *L. pneumophilia* is not visualized with the Gram stain. Direct immunofluorescence techniques can be used to demonstrate antigen in lung tissue.[254]

Because of the difficulty with isolation of the organism, and the progressive course of the disease, prompt treatment based on clinical features is warranted. To date, erythromycin, 4 g per day intravenously for 10 to 14 days, followed by an additional week of oral therapy, has been the most successful. Tetracycline has shown slightly less *in vitro* activity against the organism, and clinical results appear to be less satisfactory.

Additional new organisms are being identified as efforts have been intensified to explain previously undiagnosed pneumonias. Recent reports have identified acid-fast organisms with ultrastructures similar to *L. pneumophilia,* but with distinct serological differences, as the causative agents of opportunistic pneumonias in immunosuppressed patients.[255–257] These agents have been isolated by culture in embryonated eggs. These apparently new agents have been reported from widespread geographical areas, raising the spectre of a broad new category of bacterial, pneumonias that occur particularly in immunosuppressed hosts.

ANAEROBIC PLEUROPULMONARY INFECTIONS

Documentation of specific antimicrobial causes of pleuropulmonary infections is totally dependent on the selectivity and sensitivity of the specimens collected and the precision of the identification techniques. Several early studies of empyema noted a mixed flora on microscopic examination and the lack of microbial growth in culture. In the early 1900s, isolation of anaerobic bacteria from such specimens was shown, but the ascendency of interest in aerobic bacteria caused anaerobes to be overlooked as pathogens. In the late 1960s and the 1970s, there was a resurgence of interest in these organisms and the clinical syndromes they produce.

The most common clinical presentations of anaerobic infections are simple pneumonitis, necrotizing pneumonia, and lung abscess. Any of these may be complicated by empyema. The vast majority of such syndromes arise from aspiration of contaminated oropharyngeal contents; however, bacteremic spread or direct extension through the diaphragm from abdominal or genitourinary sites occurs occasionally.[258,259]

Patients typically present with a protracted illness consisting of cough, general malaise, and low-grade fever. Careful search will usually reveal an underlying disorder that might lead to aspiration, such as loss of consciousness, alcohol abuse, seizure disorder, disorders of swallowing, or neurologic defects. Physical examination usually reveals a chronically ill-appearing patient with fever. Examination of the chest may reveal localized signs of consolidation. Leukocytosis, sometimes in excess of 20,000 per mm^3, is present. Gram strain of sputum reveals mixed flora. Chest roentgenograms in simple pneumonitis reveal localized consolidation, usually within a lower lobe, and may be indistinquishable from pneumococcal infections. Necrotizing pneumonia appears as multiple cavities less than 1 cm in diameter.[258,259] Anaerobic lung abscesses are usually single cavities greater than 1 cm in diameter with an air–fluid level. The location of disease will be in the portion of lung most dependent at the time of aspiration; an-

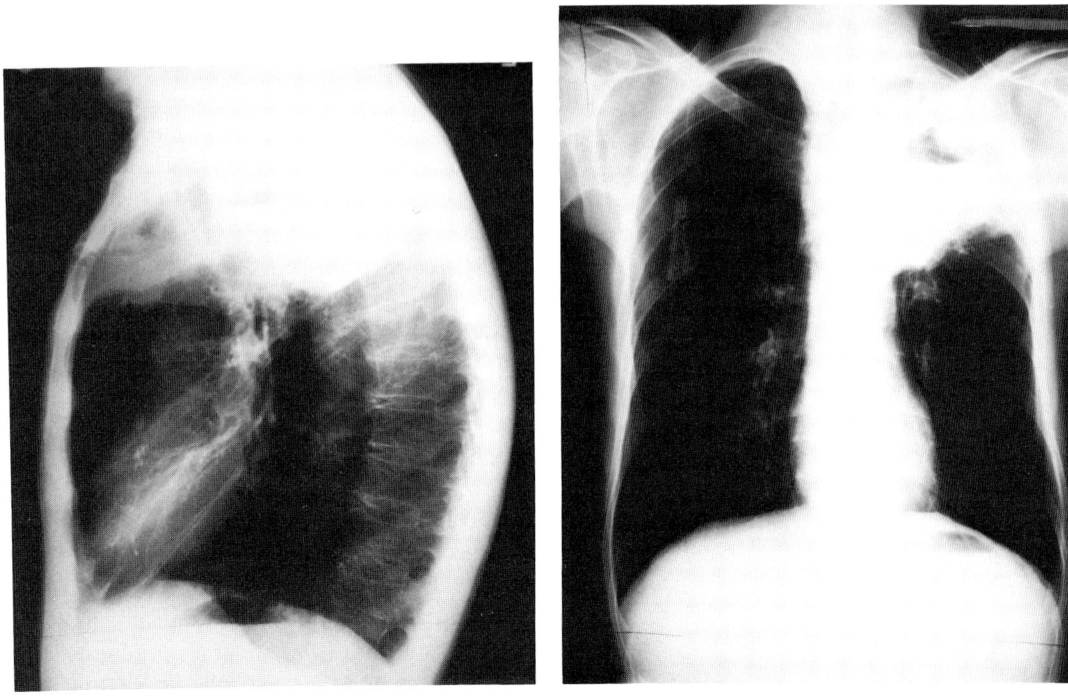

FIG. 8-12. Left upper lobe apical posterior segment abscesses due to mixed anaerobic and gram-negative infection.

aerobic infection with or without abscess formation rarely involves anterior lung segments. (Fig. 8-12)

A patient with lung abscess generally presents with a history of illness ranging from 1 to 3 wk in duration. The symptoms are variable, but are those of an acute febrile illness, with chills, fever, and at some point during the illness, the development of a productive cough. Commonly, a spiking fever will have been present and then decreased, concurrently with drainage of the abscess. On that day, copious foul-smelling sputum will have appeared, and generally the patient and other members of the household will be well aware that there has been a change in condition. The sputum will range from yellow-green to dark brown due to old blood, or be frankly bloody. Pleuritic chest pain may be present, depending on the location of the lesion.[259] Physical examination reveals a pale patient with temperature ranging from normal to 40°C. Unless there is associated pulmonary disease, the clinical findings are frequently remarkably localized. The specific segment of lung is most commonly identifiable because of its dullness to percussion, and decreased breath sounds, suggesting obstruction of the bronchus to that segment. However, if the bronchus is widely patent and drainage effective, the surrounding consolidated lung tissue will provide improved transmission of breath sounds to the periphery, and bronchial breath sounds and rales will be heard over the site of the lesion. When the pleura is involved, there may be signs of a pleural effusion, or a pleural rub.

Aerobic infections must be considered in differential diagnosis, particularly in patients with lung cavitation and empyema (see Table 8-10). These include gram-negative bacilli and *S. aureus*. Clinically these infections are usually abrupt, fulminant illnesses, whereas anaerobic infections are frequently subacute or even

TABLE 8-10. Causes of Cavitary Lesions in the Lung

Type of Cause	Manifestation
Infections	Primary lung abscess Necrotizing pneumonia Staphylococci Gram-negative bacilli Fungi Mycobacteria Septic emboli or infarction Parasitic infections *Entamoeba histolytica* *Paragonimus westermani* *Echinococcus granulosus* Infected cystic lesions of the lung Emphysematous bullae Bronchiectatic cysts Traumatic cysts Loculated hydropneumothorax in pleural space
Tumors	Primary or secondary
Developmental anomalies	Bronchogenic cyst Intralobular pulmonary sequestration
Vascular disease	Pulmonary infarction with cavitation Vasculitis (Wegener's granulomatosis)
Connective tissue disease	Necrotic rheumatoid nodule

(Adapted from Fraser RG, Pare JAP: Diagnosis of Diseases of the Chest. Philadelphia, WB Saunders, 1978)

chronic; nearly one-half of patients will report symptoms for over 4 wk. Mycobacterial and fungal infection must be excluded with care; air-fluid levels in cavities due to these organisms are uncommon. The stable acinar–nodose lesions characteristic of endobronchial spread of caseous material from tuberculous cavities does not occur with anaerobic infections. However, mycobacterial or fungal cavities may become secondarily infected with anaerobes, causing the initial presentation to be that of lung abscess.

Carcinoma of the lung produces cavitation by one of two mechanisms. Bronchial obstruction may lead to distal infection and cavitation, usually due to anaerobes. Alternatively, the tumor itself may undergo necrosis and cavitation. Bronchogenic carcinoma has been reported to underlie up to 30% of lung abscesses in men over age 45.[260]

Despite a voluminous literature reporting the presence of a variety of aerobic organisms in lung abscesses, it is quite clear that this process is an anaerobic infection. However, recent reports have suggested convincingly that hospital-acquired aspiration pneumonias may be due to both anaerobic and aerobic organisms, usually gram-negative bacilli. Such mixed infections are usually acute, rapidly developing pneumonias, not the indolent process associated with anerobic lung abscess.

Several controversies surround the bacteriologic evaluation of patients with suspected anaerobic infections. Expectorated sputum and bronchoscopically obtained lavage specimens always contain anaerobes and are therefore, of no value. There is universal agreement that pleural fluid, if present, should be aspirated for study. Transtracheal aspiration was critically important in defining the role of anaerobes in these syndromes, since contaminations by oropharyngeal anaerobes is generally avoided. However, the routine use of transtracheal aspiration in simple lung abscess is unnecessary, because proper empiric therapy is successful in the great majority of patients. Similarly, bronchoscopy is best reserved for patients with suspected cancer, patients with suspected foreign body aspiration, or patients in whom drainage of the cavity is delayed. Appropriate bacteriologic specimens for isolation of anaerobes can be obtained at bronchoscopy by the "protected brush" technique.[67]

Penicillin is the treatment of choice for anaerobic pleuropulmonary infection.[261–263] There is no good evidence that more than 2 to 4 million units per day are required. Oropharyngeal anaerobes are generally susceptible to penicillin. *Bacteroides fragilis* is resistant but is never the only anaerobe present in lung infections, as it may be in abdominal infections. Lung infections respond well to penicillin despite the presence of *B. fragilis*, a finding which attests to the synergistic nature of anaerobic infections. Individuals who are allergic to penicillin should be treated with clindamycin or chloramphenicol. Treatment should be continued until the process is clinically and radiographically stable, frequently 6 to 8 wk or more.

Bronchodilators, postural drainage, adequate hydration to improve liquification of secretions, chest physiotherapy, and supplemental oxygen may all be required during the early phase of management of the abscess. However, the clinical response is usually dramatic, with a marked decrease in sputum production, and these measures may only be necessary for 3 to 5 days.

When empyema complicates lung abscess, it is managed in the usual fashion, as discussed in Chapter 12, Pleural Diseases.

Surgical treatment for lung abscess should be deferred as long as possible. If the bronchus is patent, drainage is generally effective through the tracheobronchial tree. Under these circumstances, although clearing of the infiltrate and closure of the cavity may be very slow, surgery should be deferred until there is definitely no evidence of further healing on films taken every two weeks. Occasionally, surgery may be necessary because of reinfection of a large cavitary lesion, or to establish the diagnosis when a large infiltrate, thick-walled cavity, or persistent loss of lung volume suggest underlying neoplasm or chronic associated disease.

Patients with inflammatory lesions of the gingiva or oropharynx should have appropriate care. Most frequently, this requires dental extraction.

The outcome in a patient with a lung abscess is determined predominantly by associated disease. Where this is a complication of esophageal disease, bronchial obstruction, chronic debilitating disease, or alcoholism, the prognosis is less good than for an otherwise healthy, young individual. Mortality rates as high as 15 to 20% have been cited in patients with severe associated disease.[266,267]

Following management of lung abscess, there are characteristically residual roentgenographic abnormalities which include fibrotic strands, pleural thickening, residual cavitation, and atelectasis of the segment.

RESPIRATORY INFECTION IN THE COMPROMISED HOST

Throughout this chapter we have suggested that infections of the respiratory tract represent an adverse outcome to the interaction between invading microorganisms and the defense mechanisms of the host. Viral infections occur commonly with no predisposing cause, whereas bacterial infections most often follow other acute or chronic processes, many of which are known to impair host defenses. Thus, bacterial infections of the respiratory tract are closely linked to defects in host defense. In this section we will deal with patients who manifest recurrent respiratory infections by common pathogens or infections by organisms which rarely, if ever, cause disease in normal individuals (opportunistic infections). As a group, these patients are referred to as "compromised hosts," although the nature of their individual impairments varies widely.

These patients may present with no known compromise, but unexplained infection, recurrence, or unanticipated severity raise suspicion. Others with previously diagnosed disease or known immunosuppressive therapy may develop infections that can be anticipated to some extent. Cytomegalovirus has been particularly common in transplant recipients with iatrogenic immune suppression. Reactivation of tuberculosis and fungal disease occurs with administration of corticosteroids. Pyogenic infection is more common in patients with reduced humoral immunity or granulocytopenia. Malignant disease of the reticuloendothelial system produces greater immunodeficiency than solid tumors.[268] These factors may be useful in assessing a given patient.

The Compromised Host

The list on p. 364 presents an illustrative classification of various forms of host compromise. Certainly among adults, recurring bronchopulmonary infections are most often due to chronic pulmonary disease, usually the structural and functional changes associated with chronic bronchitis. In this disease, as in cystic fibrosis, asthma, and the immotile cilia syndrome, impaired mucocilliary transport appears to be a key factor in promoting bacterial infection.

Other conditions associated with recurrent infection lead to repetitive inoculation of the distal lung owing to aspiration of oropharyngeal or gastric contents, as is the case in alcoholism, or neuromuscular diseases, for example. Alcohol may also affect leukocyte function adversely.[268a,b] Splenectomy results in increased risk of pneumococcal infections.[269]

Acquired defects in host defenses have been demonstrated in many conditions associated with recurring infection (see Table 8-10). In some of these situations, the relationship between a demonstrated abnormality and infection is quite obvious. For example, the incidence of bacterial infection is clearly related to the number of circulating neutrophils, rising precipitiously when the neutrophil count falls below 1000 per m^3.[270,271] In other situations, such as diabetes mellitus, the role of abnormalities of leukocyte function is less certain, being but one facet of complex disorders of cellular metabolism.

That defects in immune defenses occur in the course of certain diseases is clear. Patients with multiple myeloma are remarkably predisposed to recurring episodes of pneumococcal pneumonia, occasionally with the same capsular type, owing to an inadequate humoral antibody response.[272] Conversely, the impaired T-cell function associated with Hodgkin's disease and other lymphomas is manifested by a unique susceptibility to intracellular microorganisms, particularly mycobacteria and fungi, which require intact delayed-hypersensitivity mechanisms for control.[273–275]

The Compromised Host: A Classification

- Nonimmune, nonmalignant diseases which predispose to recurrent respiratory infections
  - Lung diseases
    - Chronic bronchitis
    - Cystic fibrosis
    - Immotile cilia syndrome(s)
    - Asthma
  - Other cardiothoracic diseases
    - Pulmonary edema
    - Esophageal reflux and aspiration
  - Noncardiothoracic diseases
    - Alcoholism
    - Neuromuscular disease with aspiration
    - Splenectomy
- Primary deficiency states
  - Immunodeficiencies
    - B-cell functions—X-linked agammaglobulimenia, selective Ig deficiencies
    - T-cell functions—thymic hypoplasia
    - Both B- and T-cell functions—severe combined immunodeficiency, Wiskott–Aldrich syndrome
  - Abnormalities of inflammatory response
    - Humoral
      - Complement deficiency—C_3, C_5
      - Alternative pathway defects—sickle cell disease
    - Phagocytic function
      - Number—neutropenia
      - Chemotaxis–Job's syndrome, Chediak–Higashi syndrome
      - Phagocytosis and intracellular killing—chronic granulomatous disease
- Deficiency states associated with other diseases
  - Nonmalignant disease
    - Diabetes mellitus—impaired chemotaxis, phagocytosis
    - Uremia—impaired chemotaxis, T-cell function
    - Rheumatoid arthritis, SLE leukopenia, impaired chemotaxis
    - Viral infection—T-cell function transiently impaired
    - Postsurgical—impaired chemotaxia, T-cell function
    - Malnutrition—chemotaxis, T-cell function
  - Malignant disease
    - Leukemia—neutropenia, depressed B-cell function
    - Hodgkin's disease—depressed T-cell function, lymphopenia
    - Multiple myeloma—depressed B cell function
    - Cancer, many forms—impaired chemotaxis, T-cell function
- Drug-induced deficiency
  - Leukopenia
  - Impaired phagocyte function
  - Impaired B- and T-cell function

Understanding of the role of specific aspects of host defenses can be largely attributed to "experiments of nature," those uncommon congenital disorders of host defense (see list at left). The impairment of these hosts is generally apparent in early life. In the case of immunoglobulin deficiency, infections begin at 4 to 6 mo as maternal IgG disappears from the infant's circulation. Severely hypogammaglobulinemic infants experience recurring episodes of pyogenic bacterial infections, but handle viral infections quite normally. In contrast, abnormalities of T-cell function lead to overwhelming viral infection as well as infection with other intracellular organisms.

Basic principles of host defenses can be deduced from these observations (Table 8-11).

Laboratory Assessment for Immunodeficiency

Laboratory tests are readily available to screen for immunodeficiency and definitive tests are available in many referral centers (Table 8-12).

Clinical Features and Approach to Diagnosis

Acquired defects in host defenses due to chemotherapeutic agents and the diseases for which they are administered have assumed major significance in adult medicine, and are much more common than congenital defects. Patients with such defects often present difficult problems in differential diagnosis, for several reasons. The broad nature of their impaired defenses renders them susceptible to a wide spectrum of infectious agents, a fact which seriously limits the applicability of empiric therapy. Many chemotherapeutic agents cause lung injury leading to nonspecific inflammatory changes, which can mimic diffuse infectious processes clinically. Finally, the underlying disease for which the patient is being treated may manifest itself in the lungs and similarly mimic infection.

TABLE 8-11. Major Immune Defenses Against Infection

Organism	Major Immune Mechanism
Common gram-positive and gram-negative bacteria	Phagocytes, humoral factors (Ig, complement)
Mycobacteria, fungi	Cell-mediated
Viruses	Cell-mediated
Protozoa	Humoral- and cell-mediated

Most commonly, immunosuppressed patients with respiratory tract infection present with fever, radiographic infiltrates, and an array of nonspecific symptoms. The type of infiltrate may provide some clue as to the nature of the process (Table 8-13), but virtually all processes may appear as either diffuse or localized infiltrates, a fact which sharply reduces the specificity of the radiographic findings.

The microbiologic evaluation of such patients follows the general principles described in previous sections. All febrile immunosuppressed patients should have blood cultures drawn; pleural fluid, if present, should be aspirated for stain and culture. Expectorated sputum is frequently scanty and may be misleading; the organisms causing pneumonia may be present in the sputum in as few as 17% of patients.[276]

Immunologic techniques hold considerable promise for the future. Significant antibody rises are of no use in the acute situation, and single titers are rarely high enough to aid in diagnosis initially. However, identification of a variety of microbial antigens in respiratory secretions, blood, or pleural fluid is now possible with one or more techniques.[71–78] Influenza A, *L. pneumophilia*, and *Cryptococcus neoformans* are examples of widely differing organisms that can be rapidly and reliably identified by such means.[126,251] Up to the present time, however, these techniques have had limited application in the evaluation of groups of immunosuppressed patients with febrile illnesses.

In many patients the initial evaluation is inconclusive, and a decision must be made whether to proceed with empiric therapy or to obtain additional specimens to aid in diagnosis. One of the following three procedures is usually indicated: fiberoptic bronchoscopy with brushing, lavage, and transbronchial biopsy; transthoracic needle biopsy (aspiration); or lung biopsy by way of a small thoracotomy.[277,278] The advantages and disadvantages of each of these techniques are fairly obvious. Fiberoptic bronchoscopy is relatively safe. Peripheral brushing, especially with specially-constructed catheters

TABLE 8-12. Identification of Immunodeficiency

	Screening Tests	Definitive Tests
Peripheral leukocytes	Number Morphology	Rebuck window Chemotaxis Phagocytosis and killing Nitroblue tetrazolium dye reduction
B-cell function	Quantitation of IgG, IgA, IgM Presence of antibody to common viruses Antibody response to inoculation	Quantitation of IgG subclasses Antibody in secretions Quantitation of B cells in blood or tissue
T-cell function	Delayed hypersensitivity to common antigens (Candida, mumps, PPD) Chest radiograph to assess thymic size	Quantitation of T cells Induced hypersensitivity (dinitrochlorobenzene) Lymphocyte transformation Lymphokine production
Other	Complement (C_5, C_3)	Alternative pathway activation Complement components

TABLE 8-13. Causes of Roentgenographic Infiltrates in Compromised Hosts

Localized Infiltrates	Diffuse Infiltrates
Infection	Infection
Common bacterial agents	Common bacterial agents, especially in leukemia and severe neutropenia
L. pneumophilia and related organisms	Opportunistic fungi—Candida, Aspergillus
Pathogenic fungi	Viral—CMV, influenza, varicella-zoster
M. tuberculosis	Miliary tuberculosis
P. carinii	*P. carinii*
Other	Other
Pulmonary embolus	Malignancy—lymphangitic spread or multifocal
Lung hemorrhage	Leukoagglutinin reaction
Malignancy, especially cancer and lymphoma	Drug toxicity or hypersensitivity
Radiation pneumonitis	Sepsis

that avoid contamination by upper airway secretions, yields reliable bacteriologic information and may be useful in diagnosing pneumocystis infection.[279–281] A small-volume lavage may provide additional diagnostic material, although it is not useful for routine cultures. In the experience of many investigators, transbronchial biopsy adds significantly to the diagnostic yield, and appears to be particularly helpful in identifying malignant infiltrates, granulomatous processes, and pneumocystis. Transthoracic needle aspiration avoids upper airway contamination but samples a very small region of lung. Cytologic examination is frequently diagnostic in the case of solid nodules but is seldom helpful in diffuse disease. Positive cultures, when obtained, are easily interpreted. The small amount of tissue obtained and the frequency of complications (pneumothorax, 10 to 20%; bleeding, 10%) have limited the use of this procedure in this country.[282] With both transbronchial biopsy and transthoracic aspiration, bleeding is a major potential problem, and neither should be done until clotting parameters and platelet counts are known and major abnormalities corrected. Platelet counts less than 50,000 per mm^3 significantly increase the risk of hemorrhage.

Open-lung biopsy by way of small thoracotomy provides adequate tissue for a variety of studies, including special stains, cultures, and histologic evaluation. Bleeding sites and the pleural violation are controlled. The need for general anesthesia and postoperative thoracostomy tubes are obvious disadvantages.[278]

The relative diagnostic accuracy of these techniques has been examined by several investigators, with varying results.[278,279,283] Certain observations can be made from the available data. It is apparent that the incidence of particular infections varies from center to center. For example, *P. carinii* is the most common cause of diffuse lung disease in immunosuppressed hosts in some hospitals, while it is infrequently found in others. Pathogenic fungi, especially *Coccidioides imitis*, are fairly common causes of disease in endemic areas but not elsewhere. *L. pneumophilia* infections have occurred as a continuing nosocomial problem or in community outbreaks, which skews the findings in some series. The approximate frequency of infection among immunosuppressed hosts is shown in Table 8-14.

"Other tissue reactions" are common and a cause for concern when encountered. In some patients the lung injury is associated with epithelial-cell changes that are typical of certain drugs, notably bleomycin and busulfan, allowing a firm diagnosis of drug-induced lung damage. Most often, the histologic appearance is nonspecific, demonstrating varying degrees of edema, cellular infiltration, and fibrosis. These

TABLE 8-14. Lung Biopsy Findings In Immunocompromised Hosts with Infiltrates

	Nonmalignant Disease	Malignant Disease
Infection	40–60%	30–50%
Malignancy	—	10–15%
Other Tissue Reactions	40–60%	35–60%

TABLE 8-15. Chemotherapeutic Agents and Diffuse Alveolar Damage (DAD)

Known or Suspected Cause of DAD	Not Known to Cause DAD
Busulfan	Fluorouracil
Cyclophosphamide	Vinblastine–Vincristine
Bleomycin	Adriamycin
Nitrosoureas	Thiotepa
Chlorambucil	Azathioprine
Mitomycin	Corticosteroids
Hydroxyurea	
Methotrexate	
Procarbazine	

changes may be due to drugs, to the underlying disease, or to infection. Drugs known to cause such lung injury are listed in Table 8-15.[284]

Nonspecific findings are particularly troublesome if found in transbronchial biopsy specimens, owing to the small fragment of tissue available for study. However, in one series of 33 immunosuppressed patients, transbronchial biopsy yielded a specific diagnosis in 16 (48%) and only nonspecific findings in 15 (45%); 3 of the latter group were ultimately found to have other disease processes.[285] Thus, a diagnosis adequate to provide therapy was provided by transbronchial biopsy in 91% of patients. In other series, nonspecific findings on transbronchial biopsy have been shown to be due to specific causes in 44% of cases.[286] Overall, fiberoptic bronchoscopy with brushing, lavage, and transbronchial biopsy appears to provide a specific diagnosis in 30 to 50% of patients. Since nonspecific lung changes only account for the clinical syndrome in about one-half of patients, the rate of false negativity is about 10 to 20%.

Whether this failure rate is acceptable depends on the clinical situation. If the patient appears stable, the time lost with a negative bronchoscopy may not matter. However, in rapidly deteriorating patients, open-lung biopsy is the procedure of choice.

Treatment

Specific Treatment. Antimicrobial therapy for specific organisms is outlined in Tables 8-8 and

8-9. Certain principles should be kept in mind. Fever in patients with severe leukopenia (< 500 per mm^3) is due to infection in 95% of cases. Following collection of appropriate specimens, intravenous antibiotics with broad coverage of gram-positive and gram-negative organisms should be initiated without delay. Lung biopsy techniques are rarely indicated in such patients until blood cultures are known to be negative and the patient has not responded to therapy. Empiric treatment of suspected *P. carinii* with trimethoprim-sulfamethoxazole may be reasonable in institutions where infection is common and relative contraindications to biopsy exist. The toxicity of amphotericin B has generally precluded empiric therapy of suspected fungal infections with this agent. With newer, less toxic drugs such as ketaconazole, such may be possible.

Supportive Treatment. Principles of treatment for acute respiratory failure, as outlined in Chapter 7, should be followed. Survival from episodes of diffuse lung infiltration in immunosuppressed patients is approximately 50% and, since the etiology is usually potentially reversible, aggressive treatment is indicated.

The value of leukocyte transfusions in severely leukopenic patients is controversial. Such transfusions have reduced mortality in patients with proven infections when administered therapeutically.[287–292] They are of less certain value when given to patients with neutropenia and fever without proven infection, or when given prophylactically to patients with neutropenia only. If used, leukocyte transfusion must be continued for several days, usually 4 to 7, to provide benefit. The major drawback to the technique is the enormous expense involved. A recent report noted severe adult respiratory distress syndrome with diffuse pulmonary hemorrhage in patients with combined leucocyte transfusion and amphotericin B therapy.[292a]

Prevention. Hypogammaglobulinemia can be treated with intramuscular human gamma globulin in doses of 0.6 ml per kg of a 16% solution every 2 to 4 wk. Such replacement therapy is only effective for patients with IgG deficiency. Impaired T-cell function can be treated with infusion of transfer factor. Proven benefit has been shown in patients with mucocutaneous candidiasis, but the value of transfer factor in other settings is not established, despite occasional reports of its use in fungal infection, tuberculosis, leprosy, and congenital T-cell deficiency states.

Prevention of gram-negative bacillary infections among hospitalized, immunocompromised patients is largely ineffective. Protective isolation of severely neutropenic patients may limit their exposure to exogenous flora.[274] Intensive topical and oral antimicrobial therapy followed by complete isolation further reduces the likelihood of infection due to endogenous organisms during periods of severe neutropenia. Antimicrobial therapy with trimethoprim-sulfamethoxazole has been shown to reduce the number of febrile episodes and incidence of septicemia in granulocytopenic patients.[293] A similar regimen for patients with neoplastic disease on chemotherapy resulted in protection from pneumocystis carinii infections[294] and has been credited with similar effects in renal transplant patients.[295] Immunization with various *P. aeruginosa* antigens has proven to protect experimental animals from lethal infection and appears to offer similar protection in patients with burns. At the present time, this approach remains investigational.[296,297]

SEPTIC SHOCK

Patients with severe infections may develop hypotension, oliguria, and all the circulatory derangements of the shock syndrome. Typical manifestations of systemic infection are usual. Fever with temperatures as high as 42° C is common, although hypothermia occurs in a small percentage of cases. Leukocytosis with a marked polymorphonuclear response is characteristic, but the leukopenia with granulocytopenia may occur early in the bacteremic phase and, when sustained, suggests a poor prognosis. Warm, peripherally vasodilated extremities are common in spite of the hypotension,[298–304] but peripheral vasoconstriction may result in cold, clammy extremities. Confusion is common, perhaps a result of poor cerebral perfusion. As would be expected in hyperthermic states, the cardiac output is greater than normal in most patients, but tends to fall as the condition progresses. A low cardiac output generally signifies a poor prognosis.[298,305,306] Experimental evidence suggests that, initially, systemic vasodilation results in peripheral "pooling" of blood and reduced venous return. Depending on the extent of this "relative hypovolemia," the cardiac output may be decreased.[307–309] As the shock state persists, peripheral cyanosis, increased venous pressure, and evidence of myocardial failure become more prominent.[309] Although the heart appears to fail in the terminal stages of septic shock, experimental animals have normal myocardial contractility during the early phase of sepsis, and contractility is only impaired after many hours of profound hemodynamic derangement.[310–313]

The respiratory tract is the source of sepsis in a small portion of all patients with septic shock. Genitourinary tract infections, abdominal infections from the biliary tract, peritoneal infections, or post-surgical sepsis represent a much higher proportion.[299–303,305] Gram-negative sepsis is more frequent with increasing age, associated disease, use of antibiotics, immunosupression, surgery, and manipulation of the respiratory or urinary tract.[305] When the organism arises from the respiratory tract, *Pseudomonas* and *Klebsiella* species are most common. When the organism arises from the genitourinary tract, *E. coli* are most common. With gastrointestinal infections or peritonitis related to bowel perforation, *Bacterioides* becomes of increasing importance. Shock occurs in about 40% of hospitalized patients with documented gram-negative bacteremia.[305] The bulk of the literature stresses the importance of gram-negative bacteremia; however, gram-positive organisms have been shown experimentally to produce equally severe hemodynamic disturbances.[314] In patients it has been suggested that gram positive sepsis is more commonly associated with a high cardiac output, low peripheral resistance pattern of hemodynamic change.[315]

The respiratory effects of septic shock bear emphasizing. Most commonly, respiratory alkalosis occurs initially in association with high alveoloarterial oxygen gradients and arterial hypoxemia.[307,309,316,317] As the syndrome progresses, metabolic acidosis develops, and is frequently severe. A major cause of the acidemia is the accumulation of lactic acid. Oxygen transport to the tissues is also influenced by alterations in acid-base balance and modified distribution of peripheral blood flow. Shunting of blood past metabolizing tissues, through systemic vascular anastomoses, has been postulated.[318] There is little evidence for a direct effect of endotoxin on oxygen affinity for hemoglobin,[319] but 2,3-diphosphoglycerate may be reduced as a result of prolonged acidemia.

Numerous studies have implicated sepsis in the development of the "shock-lung" syndrome.[320–322] In this syndrome, widespread microatelectasis is associated with low functional residual capacity, decreased lung compliance, diffuse hazy pulmonary infiltrates, and impaired oxygen exchange. Some patients develop the pulmonary manifestations after successful resuscitation from the shock state. Patients and animals dying with septicemia commonly develop widespread patchy pulmonary edema with interstitial and intra-alveolar fluid. Electron microscopy demonstrates endothelial damage.[323] Unfortunately, the complexity of the illnesses in patients, and the wide variations in experimental models have made a clear understanding of a specific lung insult elusive.[324] Direct effects of circulating bacterial products such as endotoxin, deposition of antigen antibody complexes, intravascular coagulation, and intravascular disintegration of leukocytes or platelets have all been proposed as the mechanism of endothelial injury. The enormous intravascular leukocyte sequestration that occurs following the experimen tal injection of live organisms or endotoxin results in widespread pulmonary capillary deposition of leukocytes and platelets.[323–325] The possibility that the cellular components, by release of their lysosomal enzymes, might result in local tissue damage is under vigorous investigation.[324,326,327] At present no specific mechanism of lung injury is established in septic shock. (See also Chap. 7, under Differential Diagnosis of Pulmonary Edema due to Inceased Capillary Permeability).

The management of septic shock should be directed at appropriate fluid replacement. In most patients, administration of saline or colloid-containing solutions results in increased cardiac output. The rate of infusion must be adjusted in accordance with myocardial performance. In many patients, the use of a flow-directed catheter to measure left atrial filling pressures is important in gauging fluid replacement. Early institution of antibiotics should be carried out after specimens have been obtained for culture from sputum, urine, blood, or other appropriate body fluids. The antibiotics must be selected empirically, based on the most likely offending organism under the circumstances. Commonly, two or three antibiotics are instituted for wide-spectrum coverage until cultures provide definitive information, but multiple antibiotics may not improve survival more than a single well-chosen antibiotic.[304] Hypoxemia and respiratory failure is managed as outlined in Chapter 7.

A major therapeutic controversy relates to the use of adrenocortical steroids. Although numerous reports have suggested improved hemodynamics, pulmonary gas exchange, and life-expectancy associated with the use of corticosteroids,[328] these are difficult to evaluate critically. Controlled studies in primates failed to demonstrate any statistically significant improvement in hemodynamics, gas exchange, or morphologic abnormalities associated with the injection of endotoxin in steroid-pretreated animals.[329] Dogs with experimental Pseudomonas pneumonia deteriorated more rapidly and had a higher mortality when pretreated with corticosteroids.[330] In primates infused with live *E. coli*, neither methylprednisolone nor gentamicin alone prevented physiological deterioration and death, whereas the combination of these two agents did.[331] There is substantial reason to doubt that the widely divergent parameters reported to be improved by the administration of corticosteroids all have common mechanisms.[334–337]

A recent trial of digitalis early during the course of experimental shock suggests some cellular protection and improved myocardial contractility in animals given digoxin.[338]

The accumulated experience of Schumer and coworkers[337] gathered over several years in different institutions, demonstrated improved survival for septic patients given one injection of corticosteroids over that of patients given placebo, but another large series suggested reduced survival in steroid-treated patients.[304]

In the face of many unexplained pathophysiologic and biochemical phenomena, the mainstays of management of septic shock include appropriate fluid replacement, oxygenation, ventilation, and antibiotic therapy, and all other modalities assume less significance.

RESPIRATORY ASPECTS OF PARASITIC INFECTIONS

Clinical presentations of parasitic infections are highly variable.[339,340] Chest wall involvement of intercostal muscles by *Trichinella spiralis* may produce pain and limitation of respiratory excursion. Diffuse lung parenchymal infiltrations during the migratory phase of ascaris infestations, pleural effusions associated with *Entamoeba histolytica*, and discrete lung masses produced by hydatid cysts illustrate the spectrum of features. Occasionally, the manifestations will be incidental, as are most coin lesions produced by dirofilariae, or the healed cyst of the lung fluke (paragonimus).

The complex life cycles, morphology and distinguishing characteristics of these parasites are well described elsewhere.[341–342] Immunity to parasitic infections remains poorly understood.[348–352] Apparently, all parasites induce antibody production in humans (frequently to multiple antigens). There is little evidence, however, that measurable antibody titers correlate with protection against reinfection, or termination of established infection. Certain parasitic infections (*e.g.*, amebiasis) confer no protection against subsequent infections, whereas infection with leishmania and some malarial parasites induces lifelong immunity. IgA, IgG, IgM and IgE antibodies have been demonstrated under a variety of circumstances. The eosinophilia, bronchospasm, and tissue infiltrates that accompany certain parasitic infections probably result from hypersensitivity reactions to antigenic components of the organisms. The function of the eosinophilia has not been defined.[353]

Infection is established after inoculation of

immature parasitic forms into susceptible tissues. For helminths, this is most commonly the gastrointestinal tract. Spread through other tissues is determined by the specific characteristics of a given parasite. Although some infections are self limiting, others require chemotherapy, and a few are only cured by surgery. Generally useful drugs are itemized in Table 8-16. The physician planning therapy of a parasitic infection should consult detailed guides, since infections may be more susceptible to treatment at one stage than another. Severe hypersensitivity reactions may develop during chemotherapy.

The entire group of parasitic infections is distinctive in that specific geographic regions, socioeconomic factors, animal reservoirs, or definitive alterations in the host play a prominent role in determining infection. Consequently, the physician entertaining the diagnosis of parasitic infection frequently requires detailed information regarding travel, transient illness during travel, other organ system symptoms, or immune status of the patient.

In this section we will deal only with the predominant clinical manifestations of these infections as they present in the western world. This introduction does not deal with the highly varied presentations so common in endemic areas with high rates of infestation.

In the industrial nations, the patient will generally present to the respiratory physician with symptoms of cough, hemoptysis, chest pain, or dyspnea.[354,355] Because a chest radiograph is usually available, these infections will be discussed in relation to their major radiographic characteristics rather than the usual classification by class and genus (see list above right).

Chest Roentgenographic Patterns of Parasitic Infections

Infections with diffuse parenchymal infiltrates
- Pneumocystis carinii
- Toxoplasma gondii
- Schistosomes (bilharziasis)
- Paragonimus (lung fluke)
- Strongyloides
- Ancylostoma, Necator (hookworm)
- Dirofilaria (dog heartworm)
- Ascaris
- Toxicara (visceral larva migrans)

Infections with pleuro-pulmonary disease
- Entamoeba (amebiasis)
- Echinococcus (hydatid disease)

Infections with lung mass, cavity or cystic changes
- Entamoeba
- Paragonimus
- Echinococcus
- Dirofilaria

Normal chest radiograph with chest wall pain
- Trichinella (trichinosis)

INFECTIONS CAUSING DIFFUSE PARENCHYMAL INFILTRATES

Pneumocystis carinii

This protozoan organism is of world wide distribution, and endemic in some rodents. It produces a diffuse interstitial pneumonia, generally in patients who are immune suppressed. First documented in infants with agammaglobulinemia, it is now recognized most frequently in adults with iatrogenic immune suppression for a variety of diseases. Transmission is thought to occur by infected droplet, and normal people may be carriers.

Patients may present with insidious or abrupt onset of fever, tachypnea, hypoxemia, and typically bilateral diffuse alveolar and interstitial infiltrates on the chest roentgenogram. The chest roentgenogram may rarely be normal, or in about half the patients, will demonstrate patchy, assymetrical infiltrates, nodules, or pleural effusions. Leukocytosis and eosinophilia are seldom present.[270,275,293–295]

Lung aspirates, brushings, or transbronchial biopsies may demonstrate the organisms, particularly when examined with methenamine silver stains.[279–281] The pathological features typically consist of a foamy exudate filling the alveoli (when viewed with hematoxylin and eosin stains), but detailed study has demonstrated interstitial cellular infiltrates, fibrosis, increased alveolar macrophages, and lack of the typical foamy exudate in half the patients.[357]

When pneumocystosis is suspected, aggressive diagnostic measures should be undertaken

TABLE 8-16. Parasites that Affect the Respiratory System

Parasite	Major Presenting Features: Pulmonary	Major Presenting Features: Nonpulmonary	Drugs of Choice
Protozoa			
Entamoeba histolytica	Pleural effusion, lung abscess	Hepatic disease, diarrhea	Diiodohydroxyquin, metronidazole
Pneumocystis carinii	Diffuse pneumonia	None	Trimethoprim-sulfamethoxazole, Pentamidine
Toxoplasma gondii	Diffuse pneumonia	Cerebral, infectious mononucleosis-like syndrome	Pyrimethamine plus trisulfapyrimidines
Leishmania donovani	Minimal infiltrates	Leishmaniasis	Stibogluconate sodium, pentamidine
Plasmodium falciparum	Minimal infiltrates	Malaria	Quinine sulfate plus pyrimethamine plus sulfadiazine
Helminths			
Trematodes (flukes)			
Schistosoma hematobium, mansoni, japonicum	Patchy infiltrates, pulmonary hypertension	Hepatic, gastrointestinal, genitourinary disease	Niridazole, stibophen, antimony sodium domercapto-succinate
Paragonimus westermani, kellacotti	Cough, hemoptysis, cystic bronchiectasis	None	Bithionol, chloroquine sulfate
Cestodes (tapeworms)			
Echinococcus granulosis	Empyema, patchy infiltrates, hydatid cysts	Hepatic disease	Mebendazole
Nematodes (roundworms)			
Strongyloides stercoralis	Patchy infiltrates	Skin rash, pruritis, diarrhea, anemia, disseminated infestation	Thiobendazole
Ancylostoma duodenale; Necator americanus	Patchy infiltrates	Severe anemia, weight loss	Pyrantel pamoate, mebendazole
Ascaris lumbricoides	Migratory infiltrates, bronchospasm	Gastrointestinal, mild	Pyrantel pamoate, mebendazole
Toxicara canis, cati	Migratory infiltrates, bronchospasm	Splenomegaly, skin rash	Thiobendazole, corticosteroids for severe symptoms
Dirofilaria immitis	Infiltrates, coin lesions	None	Diethylcarbamazine
Trichinella spiralis	Chest pain, intercostal tenderness	Muscle pain, diarrhea	Corticosteroids for severe symptoms, thiobendazole

(Adapted from Definitions and classifications of infectious reactions of the lung. A.T.S. statement. Am Rev Respir Dis 101:116, 1970; Spencer H: Ch. 10, Pulmonary Parasitic Diseases. In Pathology of the Lung, 2nd ed. Oxford, Pergamon Press, 1976; Drugs for parasitic infection. Med Lett Drugs Ther, 20:4, 1978) as outlined under Diseases of the Compromised Host. Without treatment the mortality approaches 100%; with treatment the mortality is reduced to 15 to 30%. At present, high-dose tremethoprim-sulfoxazole in combination is the drug of choice, and has been demonstrated to provide protection when given in low doses to patients at risk for developing pneumocystosis.[294]

Toxoplasma gondii

This protozoal infection rarely produces pulmonary infiltrates in the adult. It more commonly causes congenital infection in infants, or very young children with abnormalities of the immune system. Adult infections have occasionally been reported. A pneumonic illness does occur but is generally associated with a syndrome resembling infectious mononucleosis.[342–344]

Schistosomes

The trematode flukes, *Schistosoma hematobium*, *mansoni*, and *japonicum* are endemic in Egypt and North Africa, East and Central Africa, and the Far East, respectively. *Schistosoma hematobium* causes predominantly genitourinary disease; mansoni, predominantly gastrointestinal disease, and *japonicum* more widespread disease with frequent central nervous system involvement. Most patients do not develop a clinically apparent pulmonary problem.

Snails are the natural reservoir for these organisms, and individuals develop percutaneous infection. Clinical disease follows a latent period of several months. The pulmonary lesions develop as a result of parasite emboli to the lungs. They may be grouped as follows: (a) those produced directly by the ovum (vascular obstruction); (b) those produced by an allergic response to the ovum and its products (bronchospasm, infiltrates); (c) chronic pulmonary hypertension due to (a) and (b).

Either the ova or adult flakes may be carried through the pulmonary circulation to the lungs. There they lodge in the pulmonary vessels. The majority lodge in branches of pulmonary vessels ranging from 100 to 50μ in diameter. There they produce an intravascular and perivascular granulomatous reaction. The ova may migrate through the bronchial wall, and produce bronchiectasis.[355] In endemic areas, schistosomal infections represent the commonest cause of cor pulmonale or heart failure.[359] Pulmonary function studies reveal restrictive and obstructive defects with reduced diffusing capacity and altered ventilation–perfusion relationships.[360]

The diagnosis of schistosomiasis may be very difficult. Roentgenographic abnormalities include miliary, nodular, or pneumonic infiltrates. The latter are probably on a hypersensitivity basis, and generally associated with definite leukocytosis and striking eosinophilia. The search for ova in urine, stool, and rectal biopsy may be diagnostic. However, the presence of a gastrointestinal infestation does not necessarily establish that disease of another organ is due to systemic infection. Serum antibodies are commonly used as diagnostic tools, but false negatives and false positives occur.[346,361]

The treatment is under active study, depends on the stage of the disease, and has been described in detail elsewhere.[345,346,362,363]

Strongyloides

Strongyloides infections occur throughout the world, but particularly in tropical and subtropical countries. The larvae of these roundworms are introduced through the intestinal mucosa, and migrate through venules or lymphatics to the lungs, where they produce pneumonitis. Hemorrhage and infiltration with leukocytes, particularly eosinophils, are common. Occasionally, bronchi may become blocked with areas of consolidation. A triad of cough, roentgenographic infiltrates, and eosinophilia is characteristic at this stage. However, the gastrointestinal symptoms of abdominal pain, indigestion, and diarrhea generally overshadow the pulmonary manifestations.[344,345,347]

In the Western Hemisphere, strongyloidiasis is not common. Recent reports emphasize that in immune-suppressed patients it may cause lethal disease.[364–367] Under these conditions, eosinopenia is commonly present and may indicate a poor prognosis. Widespread involvement of liver, lung, brain, and serous linings may develop. The diagnosis is best made by demonstration of larvae in the stools, optimally after concentration techniques. Serological assays for complement-fixing antibodies are frequently useful. The treatment of stongyloidiasis must include correction of the immune-suppressed state, if possible, and antihelminthic chemotherapy.

Ancylostoma and Necator (Hookworms)

These parasitic infections are particularly common in tropical countries, where they are associated with poverty, unsanitary habits, and close communal life. It has been estimated that more than 25% of the world population is infected. *Ancylostoma duodenale* and *Necator americanus* are the hookworms most commonly responsible and have widespread distribution. They may produce "creeping eruption" of the skin. They generally enter the unbroken skin of the feet after fecal contamination, bore their way to the bloodstream, and are carried to the heart and lungs.

Itch frequently occurs after the initial penetration, with dermatitis, followed shortly by bronchitis symptoms as the larvae pass through the lungs to the bronchi. The larvae then migrate through the bronchi and are swallowed, at which stage gastrointestinal symptoms begin. Severe iron-deficiency anemia is common.

A diagnosis is made by identification of the ova in the stool and therapy includes antihelminthics. In most instances, the pulmonary involvement with *Ancylostoma* and *Necator* is less severe and more short lived than with *Strongyloides.*[342–346]

Dirofilarae

Tropical eosinophilia or tropical eosinophilic lung[355] results in episodes of wheezing and cough. These commonly occur in attacks, worse at night. The leukocyte count is generally increased, with a striking eosinophilia. Pulmonary function studies reveal restrictive and obstructive changes.[368] Chest roentgenographs demonstrate bilateral patchy infiltrates, which are transient. The pathogenesis probably consists of filarii passing through the pulmonary circulation, with a hypersensitivity reaction. In the western world, *Dirofilaria immitis* is endemic in the right side of the heart in dogs, and intermediate hosts (see further on).

Ascaris lumbricoides

The roundworm, and the closely related *Toxicara canis* (dog roundworm), are transmitted by fecal–oral contamination. The larvae are released by digestion in the small intestine, and liberated into the blood stream where they pass through the portal circulation to the lungs. In the lungs, the parasites undergo changes that produce resistance to gastric digestion. The larvae then ascend the respiratory tract to the oropharynx, where they are swallowed and reach the intestine.

Pulmonary symptoms consist of dyspnea, wheezing, and cough. Occasionally, hemoptysis occurs. The injury to the lung occurs as a result of migration of the larvae through the alveolar wall into the airways. Ulceration, necrosis and hemorrhage result. A hypersensitivity reaction in the lung is suggested by the extensive edema, eosinophilia, and bronchospasm so commonly associated with the condition. The pulmonary manifestations are generally seen in children with severe infections, but are self-limiting.[345,355] Recently, a flurry of interest in the role of parasitic infections in the production of bronchial asthma in North America was reported:[369] a high incidence of ascaris, strongyloides, and necator infections were documented in a series of allergic patients. These findings were not confirmed by other investigators.[370]

The diagnosis is established by demonstration of the larvae in the sputum or the stool. Antihelminthic therapy is highly effective.

INFECTIONS WITH PLEURAL EFFUSIONS

Entamoeba histolytica

Amebiasis has a worldwide distribution, but clinical manifestations are common only in the underprivileged countries. This protozoal infection is transmitted by fecal–oral contamination.

After the cysts are swallowed, they become established in the colon and produce amebic dysentery. In the colon, an ulcer develops, with invasion of the wall and occasionally the blood stream. This may result in hepatic abscesses. Right-sided subphrenic abscesses result in penetration of the diaphragm with rupture into the thorax. This may be associated with an empyema, episodes of hemoptysis (currant-jelly material), and occasionally pericardial effusion. Abscesses may develop in brain, lungs, liver, and spleen, without direct extension from other organs.[371–377] Vague abdominal pain, intermittent diarrhea, indigestion, weight loss, and weakness are common accompanying symptoms.

The combination of hepatic infection, elevated right diaphragm with a pleural effusion, or right-lower-lobe lung abscess, associated with gastrointestinal symptoms, should suggest the diagnosis of amebiasis. Confirmation is dependent on identification of the cysts in sputum, pleural fluid, or stool.[345] Several serological tests have been useful, particularly a hemagglutination test.[378] This test remains positive for prolonged periods, and a high titer does not establish an active infection.

Antiamebic therapy is highly effective, though pleural drainage may occasionally be necessary.[373–377]

INFECTIONS WITH LUNG MASS, CAVITY, OR CYSTIC CHANGES

Most of the parasitic infections above may result in lung masses. Generally, these represent impaction of the parasite in a large vessel, death of parasitic forms in the tissues with surrounding granulomatous reaction, or localized abscesses as in the case of amebiasis. Several organisms, however, produce these changes more characteristically.

Amebiasis

When a lung abscess occurs without pleural involvement or hepatic involvement, spread is generally considered to have taken place through lymphatics or hematogenously. Occasionally, remote infection occurs without demonstrable hepatic lesions.[377]

Paragonimus

Infections due to *Paragonimus westermani* or *kellacotti* occur only in endemic areas. The lung fluke is confined to the Far East. The life cycle includes a water phase, and requires fecal contamination of water, with swallowing of immature forms while eating fresh-water crabs and crayfish. The larvae penetrate the wall of the intestine and migrate through the peritoneal cavity and the diaphragm into the pleural cavity, burrowing into the lungs.

The illness is gradual in onset, with chronic cough, hemoptysis, pleuritic chest pain, and frequently clubbing of fingers. In endemic areas, pulmonary tuberculosis very commonly is associated with paragonimiasis. Roentgenographic examination demonstrates clusters of cystlike spaces which eventually calcify. Occasionally, when the flukes are present in the spaces, multiple coin lesions are apparent.

The diagnosis is made by identification of ova in the sputum. Healed paragonimiasis may be manifested by calcified cystic lesions, apparent on the chest film.[379,380]

Echinococcus

The cestode *Echinococcus granulosa* produces hydatid disease. Most commonly, the unsuspecting physician interprets this discrete dense coin lesion in the lung as a tumor. This is an important condition in many sheep-raising areas of the world, including Australia, New Zealand, and the Middle East, and is also common in Iceland, Alaska, and Northern Canada.[381–386] The minute worms may inhabit the small intestine of dogs, wolves, caribou, moose, sheep, cattle, pigs, camels, or humans. Humans are nearly always infected through handling dogs. Fecal–oral contamination probably takes place. The embryo penetrates the intestinal wall, enters the portal circulation, and a small number pass through to the lungs. There the embryo gradually grows, but an adventitial layer forms a pulmonary cyst. There is minimal reaction, and the principal effects are compression and collapse of adjacent lung. The cyst may enlarge to erode bronchi, blood vessels, mediastinal structures, and even the chest wall. The cysts may be single or multiple, unilateral or bilateral (20%), and many (10 to 60%) pulmonary hydatids have coexisting hepatic cysts.[344,386] These cysts may gradually grow to a very large size, and calcification of the wall may develop. If the condition is unrecognized, the cysts may rupture into the pleural space, set up secondary cysts, and result in complete destruction of an entire hemithorax. Symptomatology depends on whether the cyst is small and well localized, or expanding with loss of functioning lung tissue, or ruptured. If a cyst is about to erode into a bronchus, hemoptysis is common and allergic reactions with severe episodes of bronchospasm may occur. Rarely, hepatic cysts rupture through the diaphragm and lung to form a hepatobronchial fistula, with cough productive of bile-stained sputum.[386a]

Roentgenographic evaluation most commonly demonstrates a well-circumscribed homogeneous density. If the adventitious laminated membrane has separated from the walls a free-floating calcified membrane, or "water lily" sign, may be apparent. If the cyst ruptures and the pleural fluid or bronchial fluid reveals the organism, the diagnosis is conclusive. A complement fixation test is the mainstay of hematological diagnosis. However, multiple antigens from cyst fluid have been used to develop hemagglutination, bentonite flocculation, and scoleo precipitation tests. A skin test for delayed hypersensitivity, the Casoni test, is generally positive.[386]

The management of hydatid cysts requires excellent judgment. Recent studies indicate a more severe clinical course in European (domestic animal) disease than in North American (wild animal) disease.[384] If there is active growth of the lesions, threatening effective lung function, evacuation of individual cysts may be curative.[387] If spread has occurred to the pleural space, a chronic empyema and obliterative pleuritis becomes established.

Patients with a positive Casoni test should probably receive corticosteroid therapy in high doses to protect against anaphylaxis at the time of surgery.

The indications for surgery have been (a) rapid growth of the cyst, (b) treatment of secondary infection after rupture of a cyst, (c) drainage of an empyema, (d) uncertain diagnosis.[384,386,388,389]

Recent reports of medical treatment with mebendazole are most encouraging. Whether drug treatment—alone or in combination with subsequent surgical resection—will be optimal, remains under active study.[390]

Dirofilarae

Dirofilaria immitis, the dog heartworm, normally infects the vena cava, heart, and pulmonary vasculature in dogs throughout the temperate zone. Well known to veterinary medicine, the first human case of disease due to this parasite was reported in 1941.[392] Since then, occasional case reports have appeared in the literature, generally representing pathological diagnosis of surgically-removed or autopsied lung masses. Characteristically, it presents as a coin lesion 1 to 4 cm in diameter, in the pulmonary parenchyma, with no distinctive features, only diagnosed after excision.[393–395] When symptoms are present, chest pain, cough, and hemoptysis are the most frequent. In almost all instances, the lesion is single and contains one worm, which is dead. No therapy is required and at present no preventive measures are generally recommended. It is thought that the larvae are transmitted to man by mosquitos.

INFECTIONS WITH CHEST WALL PAIN

Trichinella

Trichinosis is contracted in humans by ingestion of raw meat, generally pork, containing the encysted larvae of *Trichinella spiralis*.[396] Many other animals such as the bear, wolf, coyote, fox, horse, and cow have been noted to be infected or infective. After digestion in the gastrointestinal tract, the larvae migrate to the intestinal mucosa where reproduction begins, and from where they enter the vascular channels. They are then spread to muscles throughout the body, particularly the diaphragm, tongue, eye, deltoids, pectorals and intercostal muscles.

The first symptoms generally appear within a day or two of ingestion of uncooked meat. Diarrhea, abdominal pain, nausea, and fever may result. About the end of the first week, the patient may experience fever, edema of the eyelids, conjunctivitis, subconjunctival hemorrhages, muscle pain and tenderness, and often severe weakness. A wide range of neurologic symptoms may occur. Occasionally, myocarditis is present.

Eosinophilic leukocytosis is characteristic. A skin test for larval antigen becomes positive in the third week. Serological tests include precipitins, complement-fixing antibodies, indirect fluorescent antibodies, and bentonite flocculation tests. These all become positive in the third week and remain positive for several years. The most definitive test is a documented low level of antibodies initially, with a rise during the course of the disease. Muscle biopsy during the fourth week of infection is generally diagnostic, and myositis is a significant finding even in the absence of cysts or larvae.

The intercostal muscle pain and tenderness may result in compromised respiratory function, particularly in patients with underlying lung disease.[397]

The most important aspect of management is prevention, which is entirely the responsibility of the meat consumer. If all portions of meat are heated to 60°C, the larvae are destroyed. There is no adequate method of inspection which ensures that meat is free of Trichinella. In severe cases, chemotherapy may be used.

REFERENCES

1. RILEY RL: Airborne infection. Am J Med 57:466, 1974
2. KNIGHT V: Airborne transmission and pulmonary deposition of respiratory viruses. In Knight V (ed): Viral and Mycoplasmal Infections of the Respiratory Tract. Philadelphia, Lea and Febiger, 1973
3. HUXLEY EJ, et al: Pharyngeal aspiration in normal adults and patients with depressed consciousness. Am J Med 64:564, 1978
4. JOHANSON WG, et al: Nosocomial respiratory infections with Gram negative bacilli. Ann Intern Med 77:701, 1972
5. TILLOTSON JR, LERNER AM: Characteristics of pneumonias caused by Escherichia coli. N Engl J Med 277:115, 1967
6. RABIN ER, et al: Fatal pseudomonas infection in burned patients. A clinical bacteriologic and anatomic study. N Engl J Med 265:1225, 1961
7. GREEN GM, et al: Defense mechanisms of the respiratory membrane. Am Rev Respir Dis 115:479, 1977
8. HUBER GL, LAFORCE FM, JOHNANSON WG JR: Experimental models in pulmonary antimicrobial defenses. In Brain JD, Proctor DF, Reid L (eds): Respiratory Defense Mechanisms. New York, Marcel-Dekker, 1977
9. KRAUS FW, GASTON C: Individual constancy of numbers among the oral flora. J Bacteriol 71:703, 1956
10. BLOOMFIELD AL: The fate of bacteria introduced into the upper air passages. V. The Friedlander bacilli. Johns Hopkins Bull 31:203, 1920
11. JOHANSON WG, PIERCE AK, SANFORD JP: Changing pharyngeal bacterial flora of hospitalized patients. Emergence of Gram negative bacilli. N Engl J Med 281:1137, 1969
12. FLOREY HW: The use of micro-organisms for therapeutic purposes. Yale J Biol Med 19:101, 1946
13. SHINEFELD HR, et al: Interactions of staphylococcal colonization. Am J Dis Child 111:11, 1966
14. GIBBONS RJ, VAN HOUTE J: Bacterial adherence in oral microbial ecology. Ann Rev Microbiol 29:19, 1975
15. LONG SS, SWENSON RM: Determinants of the development of oral flora in normal newborns. Appl Environ Microbiol 32:494, 1976
16. JOHANSON WG JR, WOODS DE, CHAUDHURI T: Association of respiratory tract colonization with epithelial cell adherence of gram-negative bacilli. J Infect Dis 139:667, 1979
17. JACOBS MR, et al: Emergence of multiply resistant pneumococci. N Engl J Med 299:735, 1978
18. LEES AW, MCNAUGHT W: Bacteriology of lower respiratory tract secretions, sputum, and upper respiratory tract secretions in "normal" and chronic bronchitis. Lancet 2:1112, 1959
19. LAURENZI GA, POTTER RT, KASS EH: Bacteriologic flora of the respiratory tract. N Engl J Med 265:1273, 1961
20. LANSING AM, JAMIESON WG: Mechanisms of fever in pulmonary atelectasis. Arch Surg 87:168, 1963
21. INGELSTEDT S: Studies on the conditioning of air in the respiratory tract. Acta Otolaryngol [Suppl] 131:1, 1956
22. ANDERSEN I, LUNDQUIST GR, PROCTOR DF: Human nasal mucosal function in a controlled climate. Arch Environ Health 23:408, 1971
23. PROCTOR DF, ANDERSEN I, LUNDQUIST G: Clearance of inhaled particles from the human nose. Arch Intern Med 131:132, 1973

24. HATCH TF, GROSS P: Pulmonary Deposition and Retention of Inhaled Aerosols. New York, Academic Press, 1964
25. NEWHOUSE M, SANCHIZ J, BIENENSTOCK J: Lung defense mechanisms. N Engl J Med 295:990, 1045, 1976
26. COHEN AB, GOLD WM: Defense mechanisms of the lungs. Annu Rev Physiol 37:325, 1975
27. WANNER A: Clinical aspects of mucociliary transport. Am Rev Respir Dis 116:73, 1977
28. AFZELIUS VA: A human syndrome caused by immotile cilia. Science 93:317, 1976
29. STURGESS JM, et al: Cilia with defective radial spokes. N Engl J Med 300:53, 1979
29a. AFZELIUS BA, MOSSBERG B: Immotile cilia. Thorax 35:401, 1980
29b. STURGESS JM, CHAO J, TURNER JAP: Transposition of ciliary microtubules. N Eng J Med 303:318, 1980
30. MORROW PE, GIBB FR, GAZIOLU G: A study of particulate clearance from the human lung. Am Rev Respir Dis 96:1209, 1967
31. SANCHIZ J, et al: Quantitation of regional aerosol clearance in the normal human lung. J Appl Physiol 33:757, 1972
32. SANCHIZ J, et al: Pulmonary mucociliary clearance in cystic fibrosis. N Engl J Med 288:651, 1973
33. SACHNER MA, ROSEN MJ, WANNER A: Estimation of tracheal mucus velocity by bronchofiberoscopy. J Appl Physiol 34:495, 1973
34. GAMSA G, WEINTRAUB RM, NADEL JA: Clearance of tantalum from airways of different caliber in man, evaluated by a roentgenographic method. Am Rev Respir Dis 107:214, 1973
35. HIRSCH MS, SCHWARTZ MN: Antiviral agents. N Engl J Med 302:949, 1980
36. MACKLEM PT: Physiology of cough. Ann Otol 83:761, 1974
37. GOLDSTEIN E, LIPPERT W, WARSHAUER D: Pulmonary alveolar macrophage: Defender against bacterial infection of the lung. J Clin Invest 54:519, 1974
38. OREN R, et al: Metabolic patterns in three types of phagocytosing cells. J Cell Biol 17:487, 1963
39. PIERCE AK, REYNOLDS RC, HARRIS GD: Leukocytic response to inhaled bacteria. Am Rev Respir Dis 116:679, 1977
40. REHM SR, et al: Animal model of neutropenia suitable for the study of dual-phagocyte system. Infect Immun 25:299, 1979
41. GROSS GN, REHM SR, PIERCE AK: The effect of complement depletion on lung clearance of bacteria. J Clin Invest 62:373, 1978
42. LAFORCE FM: The effects of aerosol immunization with RE 595 Salmonella minnesota on lung bactericidal activity against Serratia marcescens, Enterobacter cloacae, and Pseudomonas aeruginosa. Am Rev Respir Dis 116:241, 1977
43. GOLDSTEIN E, et al: Ozone and the antibacterial defense mechanisms of the murine lung. Arch Intern Med 27:1099, 1971
44. MILLS J: Effects of Sendai virus infection on function of cultured mouse alveolar macrophages. Am Rev Respir Dis 120:1239, 1979
45. LABELLE CW, BRIEGER H: Patterns and mechanisms in the elimination of dust from the lungs. In Davies CN (ed): Inhaled Particles and Vapors. Vol II, Oxford/New York, Pergammon Press, 1967
46. LAUWERYNS JM, BAERT JH: Alveolar clearance and the role of the pulmonary lymphatics. Am Rev Respir Dis 115:625, 1977.
47. TUCKER ED, WYATT JH, UNDERY D: Clearance of inhaled particles from alveoli by normal interstitial drainage pathways. J Appl Physiol 35:719, 1973
48. LAFORCE FM, KELLEY WJ, HUBER GL: Inactivation of staphylococci by alveolar macrophages with preliminary observations on the importance of alveolar lining material. Am Rev Respir Dis 108:784, 1973
49. REYNOLDS HY, NEWBALL HH: Analysis of proteins in respiratory cells obtained from human lungs by bronchial lavage. J Lab Clin Med 84:559, 1974
50. BIENENSTOCK J, CLANCY RL, PERRY DYE: Bronchial associated lymphoid tissue: Its relationship to mucosal immunity. In Kirkpatrick HO, Reynolds Y (eds): Immunologic and Infectious Reactions in the Lung. New York, Marcel-Dekker, 1976
51. KALTREIDER HB, KYSELKA L, SALMON SE: Immunology of the lower respiratory tract. II. The plaque forming response of canine lymphoid tissue to sheep erythrocytes after intrapulmonary or intravenous immunization. J Clin Invest 54:263, 1974
52. MARTIN DB, et al: Atypical measles in adolescents and young adults. Ann Intern Med 90:877, 1979
53. JOHNSON KJ, WARD PA: Acute immunologic pulmonary alveolitis. J Clin Invest 54:349, 1974
54. WILSON CB, DIXON FJ: Renal response to immunologic injury. In Brenner BM, Rector FC (eds): The Kidney, Philadelphia, WB Saunders, 1976
55. DREISIN RB, et al: Circulating immune complexes in the idiopathic interstitial pneumonias. N Engl J Med 298:353, 1978
56. WINTERBAUER RH, BEDON GA, BALL WC: Recurrent pneumonia. Ann Intern Med 70:689, 1969
57. BARRETT-CONNOR E: The nonvalue of sputum culture in the diagnosis of pneumococcal pneumonia. Am Rev Respir Dis 103:845, 1971
58. KILBOURN JP, et al: Quantitative bacteriology of sputum. Am Rev Respir Dis 98:810, 1968
59. PIRTLE JK, et al: Diagnostic and therapeutic advantages of serial quantitative cultures of sputum in acute bacterial pneumonia. Am Rev Respir Dis 100:831, 1969

60. GUCKIAN JC, CHRISTENSEN WD: Quantitative culture and gram stain of sputum in pneumonia. Am Rev Respir Dis 118:997, 1978
61. MURRAY PR, WASHINGTON JA: Microscopic and bacteriologic analysis of expectorated sputum. Mayo Clinic Proc 50:339, 1975
62. KALINSKE RW, et al: Diagnostic usefulness and safety of transtracheal aspiration. N Engl J Med 276:604, 1967
63. RIES K, LEVISON ME, KAY D: Transtracheal aspiration in pulmonary infection. Arch Intern Med 133:453, 1974
64. BARTLETT JG: Diagnostic accuracy of transtracheal aspiration in bacteriologic studies. Am Rev Respir Dis 115:777, 1977
65. SPENCER CD, BEATTY HW: Complications of transtracheal aspiration. N Engl J Med 286:304, 1972
66. DERESINSKI SC, STEVENS DA: Anterior cervical infections: complications of transtracheal aspirations. Am Rev Respir Dis 110:354, 1974
67. EIMBERLEY N, FAILING LJ, BARTLETT JG: A fiberoptic bronchoscopy technique to obtain uncontaminated lower airway secretions for bacterial culture. Am Rev Respir Dis 119:337, 1979
68. DAVIDSON M, TEMPEST B, PALMER TL: Bacteriologic diagnosis of acute pneumonia. J Am Med Assoc 235:158, 1976
69. GEHRMAN CR, SIMON MJ: Pneumonia complicating severe underlying disease. A current appraisal of transthoracic lung puncture. Dis Chest 48:297, 1965
70. BRANDT PD, BLANK N, CASTELLINO RA: Needle diagnosis of pneumonitis: Value in high risk patients. J Am Med Assoc 220:1578, 1972
71. SIEGEL JD, GARTNER JC, MICHAELS RH: Pneumococcal empyema in childhood. Am J Dis Child 132:1094, 1978
72. COONROD JD, DRENHAN DP: Pneumococcal pneumonia: Capsular polysaccharide antigenemia and antibody responses. Ann Intern Med 84:254, 1976
73. COONROD JD, WILSON HD: Etiologic diagnosis of intrapleural empyema by counterimmunoelectrophoresis. Am Rev Respir Dis 113:637, 1976
74. TUGWELL P, GREENWOOD BM: Pneumococcal antigen in lobar pneumonia. J Clin Pathol 28:118, 1975
75. LEACH RP, COONROD JD: Detection of pneumococcal antigens in the sputum in pneumococcal pneumonia. Am Rev Respir Dis 116:847, 1977
76. TROLLFORS B, et al: Counterimmunoelectrophoresis of sputum and blood for the diagnosis of chest infection caused by pneumococci or *Hemophilus influenzae*. Scand J Infect Dis 11:31, 1979
77. MILLER J, et al: Diagnosis of pneumococcal pneumonia by antigen detection in sputum. J Clin Microbiol 7:459, 1978
78. SCHMID RE, et al: Sputum counterimmunoelectrophoresis in the diagnosis of pneumococcal pneumonia. Am Rev Respir Dis 119:345, 1979
79. KNIGHT V (ed): Viral and Mycoplasmal Infections of the Respiratory Tract. Philadelphia, Lea and Febiger, 1973
80. US Public Health Service: Acute conditions, incidence and associated disability. National Health Survey, US PHS Publ 1000 Ser IU, No 1, 1963
81. DINGLE JH, et al: A study of illness in a group of Cleveland families. Am J Hygiene 58:16, 1953
82. TYRRELL DAJ: Common Colds and Related Diseases. Baltimore, Williams and Wilkins, 1965
83. ASSAD F, COCKBURN WC: A seven-year study of WHO virus laboratory reports on respiratory viruses. Bull WHO 51:437, 1974
84. MUCHMORE HG, et al: Neutropenia in healthy men at the South Polar Plateau. Arch Intern Med 125:646, 1970
85. ALLEN TR: Common colds in Antarctica. J Hygiene 71:649, 1973
86. HOLMES MJ, ALLEN TR: Viral respiratory diseases in isolated communities. Br Antarctica Surv Bull 35:23, 1973
87. PERKINS FT, REGAMEY RH: International Symposium in Influenza Vaccines. Basel, S Karger, 1973
88. GWALTNEY JM JR, MOSKALSKI PB, HENDLEY JO: Hand-to-hand transmission of rhinovirus colds. Ann Intern Med 88:463, 1978
89. ANDREWES CH: Adventures among viruses. III. The puzzle of the common cold. N Engl J Med 242:235, 1950
90. JACKSON GG, et al: Susceptibility and immunity to common upper respiratory viral infections—The common cold. Ann Intern Med 53:719, 1960
91. KNIGHT V, KASEL JA: Influenza Viruses. In Knight V (ed): Viral and Mycoplasmal Infections of the Respiratory Tract. Philadelphia, Lea and Febiger, 1973
92. SCHILD GC: Influenza. Br Med Bull 35:1–92, 1979
93. SCOTT TFM, BONNANO DE: Reactions to live measles virus vaccine in children previously inoculated with killed virus vaccine. N Engl J Med 277:248, 1967
94. CHANOCK RM: Possible role of immunologic factors in pathogenesis of RS virus in lower respiratory tract disease. In Pollard M (ed): Virus Induced Immunopathology. New York, Academic Press, 1968
95. BELLANTI JA: Factors leading to the local production of respiratory antibody. The problems associated with immunologic imbalance. In Dayton DH Jr, et al (eds): The Secretory Immunoglobulin System. Washington, DC, US Government Printing Office, 1971

96. ROSSEN RD, BUTLER WT: Immunologic responses to infection at mucosal surfaces. In Knight V (ed): Viral and Mycoplasmal Infections of the Respiratory Tract. Philadelphia, Lea and Febiger, 1973
97. JOHANSON WG, PIERCE AK, SANFORD JP: Pulmonary function in uncomplicated influenza. Am Rev Respir Dis 100:141, 1969
98. PICKEN JJ, NIEWENHOWER DE, CHESTER EH: Prolonged effects of viral infection of the upper respiratory tract upon small airways. Am J Med 52:738, 1972
99. HALL WJ, HALL CB: Alterations in pulmonary function following respiratory viral infection. Chest 76:458, 1979
100. HORNER GJ, GRAY FD: Effect of uncomplicated presumptive influenza on the diffusing capacity of the lung. Am Rev Respir Dis 108:866, 1973
101. BERVEN H: Studies on the cardiopulmonary function in the post infectious phase of "atypical" pneumonia. Acta Med Scand [Suppl] 382:1721, 1962
102. ROSENZWEIG DY, et al: Changes in small airway function after live attenuated influenza vaccination. Am Rev Respir Dis 111:395, 1975
103. MINOR TE, et al: Rhinovirus and influenza type A infections as precipitants of asthma. Am Rev Respir Dis 113:149, 1976
104. EMPEY DW, et al: Mechanisms of bronchial hyperreactivity in normal subjects after upper respiratory tract infection. Am Rev Respir Dis 113:131, 1976
105. FERSTENFELD JE, et al: Recognition and treatment of adult respiratory distress syndrome secondary to viral interstitial pneumonia. Am J Med 58:709, 1975
106. FINUCANE KE, et al: The mechanism of respiratory failure in a patient with viral (varicella) pneumonia. Am Rev Respir Dis 101:949, 1970
107. WINTERBAUER RH, LUDWIG WR, HAMMAR SP: Clinical course, management, and long-term sequelae of respiratory failure due to influenza viral pneumonia. Johns Hopkins Med J 141:148, 1977
108. LAMY M, et al: Pathologic features and mechanisms of hypoxemia in adult respiratory distress syndrome. Am Rev Respir Dis 114:267, 1976
109. KATTAN M, et al: Pulmonary function abnormalities in symptom-free children after bronchiolitis. Pediatrics 59:683, 1977
110. SILVERMAN M, LEE P: Pills, Profits and Politics. Berkeley, University of California Press, 1974
111. WEST S, et al: A review of antihistamines and the common cold. Pediatrics 56:100, 1975
112. Oral Cold Remedies. Med Lett Drugs Ther 17:89, 1975
113. WILSON CWM: Colds, ascorbic acid metabolism and vitamin C. J Clin Pharmacol 15:570, 1975
114. Vitamin C and the common cold. Med Lett Drugs Ther 16:85, 1974
115. BRODIE HR, SPENCE LP: Respiratory syncytial virus infections in children in Montreal. Can Med Assoc J 109:1199, 1973
116. MCLEAN DM: Pediatric infections with respiratory syncytial virus. Can Med Assoc J 109:1181, 1973
117. SMITH W, ANDREWES CH, LAIDLAW PO: A virus obtained from the influenza patients. Lancet 2:66, 1933
118. COREY L, et al: Influenza B associated Reye's syndrome: incidence in Michigan and potention for prevention. J Infect Dis 135:398, 1977
119. CDC Bureau of Epidemiology, National Influenza Immunization Program, Viral Diseases Division, Influenza-Worldwide: Follow-up on Guillain-Barre syndrome, Vol 26, No. 1, p. 7. Morbidity and Mortality Weekly Report, US Dept of HEW, January 4, 1977
120. OSEASOHN R, ADELSON L, KAJI M: Clinical pathologic study of 33 fatal cases of Asian influenza. N Engl J Med 260:509, 1959
121. MULDER J, HERS JF: Influenza. Groningen, Wolters-Noerdhoff, 1972
122. HERS JF, MULDER J: Broad aspects of the pathology and pathogenesis of human influenza. Am Rev Respir Dis 83:84, 1961
123. BURK RF, SCHAEFFNER W, KOENIG MG: Severe influenza virus pneumonia in the pandemic of 1968 to 1969. Arch Intern Med 127:1122, 1971
124. WINTERNITZ MC, WASON IN, MCNAMERA FP: The Pathology of Influenza. New Haven, Yale University Press, 1920
125. LYNN DJ, WYMAN AC, VERMA VM: Influenza A infection simulating pulmonary embolism. JAMA 238:1166, 1977
126. BOGART DB, et al: Rapid diagnosis of primary influenza pneumonia. Chest 68:513, 1975
127. LOURIA DE, et al: Studies on influenza in the pandemic of 1957–58. 2 Pulmonary complications of influenza. J Clin Invest 38:213, 1959
128. LINDSAY MI, et al: Hong Kong influenza: Clinical microbiological and pathological features in 127 cases. JAMA 214:1825, 1970
129. PETERSDORF RG, et al: Pulmonary infections complicating Asian influenza. Arch Intern Med 103:262, 1959
130. HIRSCH MS, SCHWARTZ MN: Antiviral agents. N Engl J Med 302:903, 1980
131. AMANTIDINE: Does it have a role in the prevention and treatment of influenza? A National Institutes of Health Consensus Development Conference. Ann Intern Med 92:256, 1980
132. WALDMAN RH, MANN JJ, SMALL PA: Immunization against influenza: Prevention of illness in man by aerosolized inactivated vaccine. JAMA 207:520, 1969
133. LAUTERIA SF, et al: An attenuated influenza virus vaccine: Reactogenicity, transmissibility, im-

munogenicity and protective efficacy. J Infect Dis 130:380, 1974

134. EDMONDSON WP, et al: A comparison of subcutaneous nasal and combined influenza vaccination. Am J Epidemiol 93:472, 480, 1971

135. SHORE SL, POTTER CW, STUART-HARRIS CH: Antibody response to inactivated influenza vaccine given by different routes in patients with chronic bronchopulmonary disease. Thorax 28:721, 1973

136. PREVOST JM, et al: Live attenuated influenza virus vaccines in patients with chronic broncho-pulmonary diseases. Scand J Respir Dis 56:58, 1975

136a. GROUSE LD: Swine flu sequelae. JAMA 243: 2489, 1980

137. ROSE HM, et al: Adenoviral infection in military recruits. Arch Environ Heal 21:356, 1970

138. BRYANT RE, RHOADES ER: Clinical features of adenoviral pneumonia in Air Force recruits. Am Rev Respir Dis 96:717, 1967

139. BRANDT CD, et al: Infections in 18,000 infants and children in a controlled study of respiratory tract disease. I. Adenovirus pathogenicity in relation to serologic type and illness syndrome. Am J Epidemiol 90:484, 1969

140. HERBERT FA, et al: Adenovirus type 3 pneumonia causing lung damage in childhood. Can Med Assoc J 116:274, 1977

141. TOP FH JR: Control of adenovirus acute respiratory disease in US Army trainees. Yale J Biol Med 48:185, 1975

142. HALL WJ, HALL CB, SPEERS DM: Respiratory syncytial virus infection in adults. Ann Intern Med 88:203, 1978

143. STENHOUSE AC: Rhinovirus infections in acute exacerbations of chronic bronchitis: A controlled prospective study. Br Med J 3:461, 1967

144. STOTT EJ, GRIST NW, EADIE MB: Rhinovirus infections in chronic bronchitis, isolation of eight possibly new rhinovirus serotypes. J Med Microbiol 1.109, 1968

145. TREIBWASSER JH, et al: Varicella pneumonia in adults. Medicine 46:409, 1967

146. GLICK N, LEVIN S, NELSON K: Recurrent pulmonary infarction in adult chickenpox pneumonia. JAMA 222:173, 1972

147. BRANTON FJ, MOORE ME: A survery of pulmonary calcification following adult chickenpox. Br J Radiol 42:256, 1969

148. BRUNELL PA, et al: Prevention of varicella by zoster immune globulin. N Engl J Med 280:1191, 1969

149. DOVER AS, et al: Pneumonia associated with measles. JAMA 234:612, 1975

150. FULGINITI VA, et al: Altered reactivity to measles virus, atypical measles in children previously immunized with inactivated measles virus vaccines. JAMA 202:1075, 1967

151. HALL WJ, HALL CB: Atypical measles in adolescents: Evaluation of clinical features and pulmonary function. Ann Intern Med 90:873, 1979

152. KRUGMAN S: Present status of measles and rubella immunization in the United States. J Pediatrics 90:1, 1977

153. HINMAN AR, BRADLING-BENNET AD, NIEBURG PI: The opportunity and obligation to eliminate measles from the United States. JAMA 242:1157, 1979

154. NAKERVIS GA, KUMAR ML: Diseases produced by cytomegalo-viruses. Med Clin North Am 62:1021, 1978

155. GLAZER JP, et al: Live cytomegalovirus vaccination of renal transplant candidates. Ann Intern Med 91:676, 1979

156. SIEBERT RH, JORDAN WS, DINGLE JH: Clinical variations in the diagnosis of psittacosis. N Engl J Med 254:925, 1956

157. SCHAFFNER W, et al: The clinical spectrum of endemic psittacosis. Arch Intern Med 119:433, 1967

158. ANDERSON DC, STOESZ PA, KAUFMANN AF: Psittacosis outbreak in employees of a turkey processing plant. Am J Epidemiol 107:140, 1978

159. SCHACHTER J, et al: Pneumonitis following inclusion blennorrhea. J Pediatr 87:779, 1975

160. BEEM MO, SAXON EM: Respiratory tract colonization and a distinctive pneumonia syndrome in infants infected with Trachomatis. N Engl J Med 296:306, 1977

161. HUEBNER RJ, JELLISON WL, BECK MD: Q fever: A review of current knowledge. Ann Intern Med 30:495, 1949

162. DERRICK EH: The epidemiology of Q fever: A review. Med J Aust 1:245, 1953

163. URSO FP: The pathological findings in rickettsial pneumonia. Am J Clin Pathol 64:335, 1975

164. DONOHUE JF: Lower respiratory tract involvement in Rocky Mountain Spotted Fever. Arch Intern Med 140:223, 1980

165. COUCH RB: Mycoplasma pneumoniae. In Knight V (ed): Viral and Mycoplasmal Infections of the Respiratory Tract. Philadelphia, Lea and Febiger, 1973

165a. FOY HM, et al: Epidemiology of mycoplasma pneumoniae infection in families. JAMA 197:859, 1966

166. BALASSANIAN N, ROBBINS FC: Mycoplasma pneumoniae infection in families. N Engl J Med 277:719, 1967

167. FERNALD GW, CLYDE WA: Pulmonary immune mechanisms in mycoplasma pneumoniae disease. In Kirkpatrick CH, Reynolds HY (eds): Immunologic and Infectious Reactions in the Lung, Chapter 5. New York, Marcel-Dekker, 1976

168. FOY HM, et al: Mycoplasma pneumoniae pneumonia in an urban area. JAMA 214:1666, 1970

168a. LEVINE DP, LERNER AM: The clinical spectrum of

mycoplasma pneumoniae infections. Med Clin North Am 62:961, 1978
169. ALEXANDER ER, et al: Pneumonia due to Mycoplasma pneumoniae: Its incidence in the membership of a co-operative medical group. N Engl J Med 275:131, 1966
170. MCNAMARA MJ, PHILLIPS IA, WILLIAMS OB: Viral and mycoplasma pneumoniae infections in exacerbations of chronic lung disease. Am Rev Respir Dis 100:19, 1969
171. BERKOVICH S, MILLIAN SJ, SNYDER RD: The association of viral and mycoplasma infections with recurrence of wheezing in the asthmatic child. Ann Allergy 28:43, 1970
172. MURRAY HW, et al: The protean manifestations of mycoplasma pneumonia infection in adults. Am J Med 58:229, 1975
173. SHULMAN ST, et al: The unusual severity of mycoplasma pneumonia in children with sickle cell disease. N Engl J Med 287:164, 1972
174. CHESTER A, KANE J, GARAGUSI V: Mycoplasma pneumonia with bilateral pleural effusions. Am Rev Respir Dis, 112:451, 1975
175. SHAMES JM, et al: Comparison of antibiotics in the treatment of mycoplasmal pneumonia. Arch Intern Med 125:680, 1970
176. PANKEY GA: Sinusitis, bronchitis and mycoplasmal pneumonia. Bull NY Acad Med 54:156, 1978
177. GWALTNEY JM JR.: Early diagnosis and management of sinusitis and otitis. J Respir Dis 1:40, 1980
178. CARENFELT C, LUNDBERG C: The role of local gas composition and pathogenesis of maxillary sinus empyema. Acta Otolaryngol (Stockholm) 85:116, 1978
179. SCHWARTZ R, et al: The increasing incidence of ampicillin-resistant Hemophilus influenzae. A cause of otitis media. JAMA 339:320, 1978.
180. GORFINKEL HJ, BROWN R, KABINS SA: Acute infectious epiglottitis in adults. Ann Intern Med 70:289, 1969
181. HAWKINS DB, et al: Acute epiglottitis in adults. Laryngoscope 74:1211, 1973
182. BAXTER JD, PASHLEY NRT: Acute epiglottitis—twenty-five years experience in management in the Montreal Children's Hospital. J Otolaryngol 6:473, 1978
183. TAGER I, SPEIZER FE: Role of infection in chronic bronchitis. N Engl J Med 292:563, 1975
184. MAY JR: The bacteriology of chronic bronchitis. Lancet 2:534, 1953
185. JENNE JW, et al: The course of chronic Hemophilus bronchitis treated with massive doses of penicillin and penicillin combined with streptomycin. Am Rev Respir Dis 101:907, 1970
186. SANTA CRUZ R, et al: Tracheal mucus velocity in normal man and patients with obstructive lung disease: Effects of terbutaline. Am Rev Respir Dis 109:458, 1974
187. BATES DV, MACKLEM PT, CHRISTIE RV: Respiratory Function in Disease. Philadelphia, WB Saunders, 1972
188. MARSHALL R, CHRISTIE RV: The visco-elastic properties of the lungs in acute pneumonia. Clin Sci 13:403, 1954
189. KJELLMAN B: Regional lung function studied with Xe^{133} in children with pneumonia. Acta Paediatr Scand 56:467, 1967
190. COLP CR, PARK SS, WILLIAMS MH: Pulmonary function studies in pneumonia. Am Rev Respir Dis 85:808, 1962
191. BENSON H, et al: Hemodynamic effects of pneumonia. I. Normal and hypodynamic responses. J Clin Invest 49:791, 1970
192. KUMAR R, et al: Hemodynamic effects of pneumonia. II. Expansion of plasma volume. J Clin Invest 49:799, 1970
193. MOSTOW SR: Pneumonias acquired outside the hospital. Med Clin North Am 58:555, 1974
194. SULLIVAN RJ, et al: Adult pneumonia in a general hospital. Arch Intern Med 129:935, 1972
195. MCHENRY MC, et al: Hospital acquired pneumonia. Med Clin North Am 58:565, 1974
196. BARTLETT JG, FINEGOLD SM: Anaerobic infections of the lung and pleural space. Am Rev Respir Dis 110:56, 1974
197. CECIL RL, BALDWIN HS, LARSEN NP: Lobar pneumonia: A clinical and bacteriologic study of 2,000 typed cases. Arch Intern Med 40:253, 1927
198. BULLOWA JGM, WILCOX C: Incidence of bacteremia in the pneumonias and its relation to mortality. Arch Intern Med 55:558, 1935
199. PIERCE AK, SANFORD JP: Aerobic Gram negative bacillary pneumonias. Am Rev Respir Dis 110:647, 1974
200. AUSTRIAN R, GOLD J: Pneumococcal bacteremia with special reference to bacteremic pneumococcal pneumonia. Ann Intern Med 60:759, 1964
201. AUSTRIAN R, et al: Prevention of pneumococcal pneumonia by vaccination. Trans Assoc Am Physicians 89:184, 1976
202. FIALA M: A study of the combined role of viruses, mycoplasms and bacteria in adult pneumonia. Am J Med Sci 257:44, 1969
203. MUFSON MA, et al: The role of viruses, mycoplasmas, and bacteria in acute pneumonia in civilian adults. Am J Epidemiol 86:526, 1967
204. ANSFIELD MJ, WOODS DE, JOHANSON WG JR: Lung bacterial clearance in pneumococcal pneumonia. Infect Immun 17:195, 1977
205. WOOD WB, MCLEOD C, IRONS EN: Studies on the mechanisms of recovery in pneumococcal pneumonia. J Exp Med 84:377, 1946
206. WOOD WB: Studies on the mechanisms of recovery in pneumococcal pneumonia. J Exp Med 73:201, 1941
207. MUFSON MA, et al: Capsular types and outcome

of bacteremic pneumococcal disease in the antibiotic era. Arch Intern Med 134:505, 1974

208. STEVENS RM, et al: Pneumonia in an intensive care unit. Arch Intern Med 134:106, 1974
209. TUGWELL P, WILLIAMS AO: Jaundice associated with lobar pneumonia. Q J Med 46:97, 1977
210. LIGHT RW, et al: Diagnostic significance of pleural fluid pH and pCO_2. Chest 64:591, 1973
211. STADIE W: Oxygen of arterial and venous blood in pneumonia and its relation to cyanosis. J Exp Med 30:215, 1919
212. GOLDZIMER EL, KONOPKA RG, MOSER KM: Reversal of the perfusion defect in experimental canine lobar pneumococcal pneumonia. J Appl Physiol 37:85, 1974
213. BREWIN A, et al: High dose penicillin therapy in pneumococcal pneumonia. J Am Med Assoc 230:409, 1974
214. LOURIA DB, KAMINSKI T: The effects of four antimicrobial drug regimens on sputum superinfection in hospitalized patients. Am Rev Respir Dis 85:649, 1962
215. GRAHAM WGB, BRADLEY DA: Efficacy of chest physiotherapy and intermittent positive-pressure breathing in the resolution of pneumonia. N Engl J Med 299:624, 1978
216. JAY SJ, JOHANSON WG, PIERCE AK: The radiographic resolution of streptococcus pneumoniae pneumonia. N Engl J Med 293:798, 1975
217. TARYLE DA, POTTS DE, SAHN SA: The incidence and clinical correlation of parapneumonic effusions in pneumococcal pneumonia. Chest 74:170, 1978
218. ZISKIND MM, et al: Incomplete consolidation in pneumococcal pneumonia complicating pulmonary emphysema. Ann Intern Med 72:835, 1970
219. MACLEOD CM, et al: Prevention of pneumococcal pneumonia by immunization with specific capsular polysaccharides. J Exp Med 82:445, 1945
220. AHONKHAI VI, et al: Failure of pneumococcal vaccine in children with sickle cell disease. N Engl J Med 301:26, 1979
221. AMMANN AJ, et al: Polyvalent pneumococcal–polysaccharide immunization of patients with sickle cell anemia and patients with splenectomy. N Engl J Med 297:897, 1977
222. BOISSET GF: Subpleural emphysema complicating staphylococcal and other pneumonias. J Pediatr 81:359, 1972
223. SABATH LD, et al: A new type of penicillin resistance of Staphylococcus aureus. Lancet 1:443, 1977
224. SILVA JJ, NEALON TJ, REINARZ JA: A selective phagocytic defect for killing of N. meningitidus during adenoviral infections (abstr). Clin Res 20:55, 1972
225. LAMPE WT: Klebsiella pneumonia: A review of forty-five cases and re-evaluation of the incidence and antibiotic sensitivities. Dis Chest 46:499, 1964
226. REID JM, et al: Empyema due to *Klebsiella pneumoniae*. Thorax 22:170, 1967
227. HOLMES RB: Friedlander's pneumonia. Am J Roentgenol 75:728, 1956
228. LERNER AM: Primary Gram negative pneumonias. Med Times 97:118, 1969
229. JOFFE N: Acute fulminating Friedlander's pneumonia. Clin Radiol 12:286, 1961
230. KIRBY WMM, COLEMAN DH: Antibiotic therapy of Friedlander's pneumonia. Am J Med 11:179, 1951
231. DOGGETT RG (ed): Pseudomonas aeruginosa. New York, Academic Press, 1979
232. NORDEN CW: *Hemophilus influenzae* infection in adults. Med Clin North Am 62:1037, 1978
233. HIRSCHMANN JV, EVERETT ED: Haemophilus influenzae infections in adults: Report of nine cases and a review of the literature. Medicine 58:80, 1979
234. PLOTKIN SA, et al: An epidemic of anthrax, the first in the twentieth century. Am J Med 29:992, 1960
235. BRACHMAN PS, PAGANE JS, ALBRINK WS: Two cases of fatal inhalation anthrax, one associated with sarcoidosis. N Engl Med 265:203, 1961
236. BEYT E, et al: Human pulmonary pasteurellosis. JAMA 242:1647, 1979
237. FINEGOLD MJ: Pathogenesis of plague. AM J Med 45:549, 1968
238. KOPLAN JP, et al: Pertussis vaccine—an analysis of benefits, risks and costs. N Engl J Med 301:906, 1979
239. BASS JW, et al: Antimicrobial treatment of pertussis. J Pediatr 75:768, 1969
240. MORSE SI: Pertussis in adults. Ann Intern Med 68:953, 1968
241. PRESTON NW: Effectiveness of pertussis vaccine. Br Med J 2:11, 1965
242. HOWE C, SAMPATH A, SPOTNITZ M: The pseudomallei group: a review. J Infect Dis 124:598, 1971
243. SPOTNITZ M. RUDNITZKY J, ROMBAUD JJ: Melioidosis pneumonitis. JAMA 202:126, 1967
244. GILBERT DM: Potential medical problems in personnel returning from Vietnam. Ann Intern Med 68:662, 1968
245. EVERETT ED, NELSON RA: Pulmonary melioidosis: Observations in 39 cases. Am Rev Respir Dis 112:331, 1975
246. JOHN KF JR: Trimethoprim-sulfamethoxazole therapy of pulmonary melioidosis. Am Rev Respir Dis 114:1021, 1976
247. MORGAN HJ: Pleuropulmonary tularemia. Ann Intern Med 27:519, 1947
248. MILLER RP, BATES JH: Pleuropulmonary tularemia. Am Rev Respir Dis 99:31, 1969
249. PERMAN HH, MACLACHLAN WWG: Tularemic pneumonia. Ann Intern Med 5:687, 1931

250. FRASER DW, et al: Legionnaire's disease: Description of an epidemic of pneumonia. N Engl J Med 297:1189, 1977
251. BALOWS A, FRASER DW (eds): International Symposium On Legionnaire's Disease. Ann Intern Med 90:489, 1979
251a. ENGLAND AC¿ et al: Sporadic legionellosis in the United States: The first thousand cases. Ann Int Med 94:164, 1981
252. KIRBY DB, et al: Legionnaire's Disease: clinical features of 24 cases. Ann Intern Med 89:297, 1978
253. TILTON RC: Legionnaire's disease antigen detected by enzyme linked immunosorbent assay. Ann Intern Med 90:697, 1979
254. CHERRY WB, et al: Detection of Legionnaire's disease bacteria by direct immunofluorescent staining. J Clin Microbiol 8:329, 1978
255. MYEROWITZ RL, et al: Opportunistic lung infection due to "Pittsburgh pneumonia agent". N Engl J Med 301:953, 1979
256. ROGERS BH, et al: Opportunistic pneumonia: The clinical pathological study of five cases caused by an unidentified acid-fast bacterium. N Engl J Med 301:959, 1979
257. HERBERT GA, et al: The Ricksetta-like organisms TATLOCK (1943) and HEBA (1959): Bacteria phenotypically similar but genetically distinct from Legionella pneumophila and the WIGA bacterium. Ann Intern Med 92:45, 1980
258. BARTLETT JG: Anaerobic bacterial pneumonitis. Am Rev Respir Dis 119:19, 1979
259. BARTLETT JG, FINEGOLD SM: Anaerobic infections of the lung and pleural space. Am Rev Respir Dis 110:56, 1974
260. BROCK RC: Lung Abscess. Springfield, Charles C Thomas, 1952
261. ABERNATHY RS: Antibiotic therapy of lung abscess: Effectiveness of penicillin. Dis Chest 53:592, 1968
262. FINEGOLD SM, et al: Management of anaerobic infections. Ann Intern Med 83:375, 1975
263. BARTLETT JG, GORBACH SL: Treatment of aspiration pneumonia and primary lung abscess. Penicillin G vs Clindamycin. JAMA 234:935, 1975
264. ESTRERA AS, et al: Primary lung abscess. J Thorac Cardiovasc Surg 79:275, 1980
265. LAWRENCE GH, RUBIN SL: Management of giant lung abscess. Am J Surg 136:134, 1978
266. RUMBAUGH IF, PRIOR JA: Lung abscess: A review of 41 cases. Ann Intern Med 55:223, 1961
267. SHAFRON RD, TATE CF JR: Lung abscesses: A five-year evaluation. Dis Chest 53:12, 1968
268. SINGER C, KAPLAN MH, ARMSTRONG D: Bacteremia and fungemia complicating neoplastic disease. Am J Med 62:731, 1977
268a. HEINEMANN HO: Alcohol and the lung. Am J Med 63:81, 1977
268b. LEBOWITZ MD: Respiratory symptoms and disease related to alcohol consumption. Am Rev Respir Dis 123:16, 1981
269. PEARSON HA, et al: The born-again spleen: Return of splenic function after splenectomy for trauma. N Engl J Med 298:1389, 1978
270. CHANG H, et al: Causes of death in adults with acute leukemia. Medicine 55(3):259, 1976
271. GURWITH MJ, et al: Granulocytopenia in hospitalized patients. I. Prognostic factors and etiology of fever. Am J Med 64:121, 1978
272. ZINNEMAN HH, HALL WH: Recurrent pneumonia in multiple myeloma and some observations on immunologic response. Ann Intern Med 41:1152, 1954
273. BODE ER, PARE JAP, FRASER RG: Pulmonary diseases in the compromised host. Medicine 53:255, 1974
274. LEVINE AS, GRAW RG, YOUNG RC: Management of infection in patients with leukemia and lymphoma: Current concepts and experimental approaches. Semin Hematol 9:141, 1972
275. WILLIAMS DM, KRICK JA, REMINGTON JS: Pulmonary infection in the compromised host. Am Rev Respir Dis 114:359, 593, 1976
276. SICKLES EA, et al: Pneumonia in acute leukemia. Ann Intern Med 79:528, 1973
277. CUNNINGHAM JH, et al: Trephine air drill, bronchial brush, and fiberoptic transbronchial lung biopsies in immunosuppressed patients. Am Rev Respir Dis 115:213, 1977
278. ROSSITER SI, et al: Open lung biopsy in the immune suppressed patient. J Thorac Cardiovasc Surg 77:338, 1979
279. DREW WL, et al: Diagnosis of Pneumocystis carinii pneumonia by bronchopulmonary lavage. JAMA 230:713, 1974
280. KELLEY J, et al: Diagnosis of pneumonia due to pneumocystis by subsegmental pulmonary lavage via the fiberoptic bronchoscope. Chest 74:24, 1978
281. REPSHER LH, SCHROTER G, HAMMOND WS: Diagnosis of Pneumocystis carinii pneumonitis by means of endobronchial brush biopsy. N Engl J Med 287:340, 1972
282. ZAVALA DC: The diagnosis of pulmonary disease by nonthoracotomy techniques. Chest 64:100, 1973
283. HANSON RR, et al: Transbronchial biopsy via flexible fiberoptic bronchoscope: Results in 164 patients. Am Rev Respir Dis 114:67, 1976
284. WEISS RB, MUGGIA FM: Cytotoxic drug induced pulmonary disease: Update 1980. Am J Med 68:259, 1980
285. POE RH, et al: Sensitivity and specificity of the nonspecific transbronchial lung biopsy. Am Rev Respir Dis 119:25, 1979
286. NISHIO JN, LYNCH JP: Fiberoptic bronchoscopy in immunocompromised host: significance of a "nonspecific" transbronchial biopsy. Am Rev Respir Dis 121:307, 1980

287. ROSENSHEIN MS, et al: The cost effectiveness of therapeutic and prophylactic leukocyte transfusion. N Engl J Med 302:1058, 1980
288. HIGBY DJ, et al: Filtration leukaphoresis for granulocyte transfusion therapy: Clinical and laboratory studies. N Engl J Med 292:761, 1975
289. FORTUNY IE, et al: Granulocyte transfusion: A control study in patients with acute nonlymphocytic leukemia. J Transfus 15:548, 1975
290. VOGLER WR, WINTON EF: A control study of the efficacy of granulocyte transfusions in patients with neutropenia. Am J Med 63:548, 1977
291. ALAVI JB, et al: A randomized clinical trial of granulocyte transfusions for infection in acute leukemia. N Engl J Med 296:706, 1977
292. HERZIG R, et al: Successful granulocyte transfusion therapy for gram-negative septicemia: A prospectively randomized controlled study. N Engl J Med 296:701, 1977
292a. WRIGHT DG et al: Lethal pulmonary reactions associated with the combined use of amphotericin B and leucocyte transfusions. N Eng J Med 304: 1185, 1981
293. GURWITH MJ, et al: A prospective controlled investigation of prophylactic trimethoprim sulfamethoxazole in hospitalized granulocytopenic patients. Am J Med 66:248, 1979
294. HUGHES WT, et al: Successful chemoprophylaxis for pneumocystis carinii pneumonitis. N Engl J Med 297:1419, 1977
295. RAMSEY PG, et al: The renal transplant patient with fever and pulmonary infiltrates: Etiology, clinical manifestations and management. Medicine 59:206, 1980
296. PENNINGTON JE, et al: Use of a pseudomonas aeruginosa vaccine in patients with acute leukemia and cystic fibrosis. Am J Med 58:629, 1975
297. MARKELEY K. Vaccine prophylaxis for pseudomonas infections. Ann Intern Med 74:140, 1971
298. NISHIMIMA H, et al: Hemodynamic and metabolic studies on shock associated with Gram negative bacteremia. Medicine 52:287, 1973
299. WEIL MH, SHUBIN H, BIDDLE M: Shock caused by gram negative micro-organisms: Analysis of 169 cases. Ann Intern Med 60:384, 1964
300. WILSON RF, et al: Some observations on 132 patients with septic shock. Anesth Analg 46:751, 1967
301. MARTIN WJ: Bacteremia and bacteremic shock in surgical patients. Surg Clin North Am 49:1053, 1969
302. DUPONT HL, SPINK WW: Infections due to Gram negative organisms. An analysis of 860 patients with bacteremia at the University of Minnesota Medical Center, 1958–1966. Medicine 48:307, 1969
303. ALTMEIER WA, TODD JC, INGE WW: Gram negative septicemia: A growing threat. Ann Surg 166:530, 1967
304. KREGER BE, CRAVEN DE, MCCABE WR: Gram negative bacteremia. Re-evaluation of clinical features and treatment in 612 patients. Am J Med 68:344, 1980
305. KREGER BE, et al: Gram negative bacteremia. Reassessment of etiology, epidemiology and ecology in 612 patients. Am J Med 68:332, 1980
306. DIETZMAN RH, et al: High output, low resistance Gram negative septic shock in man. Angiology 20:691, 1969
307. GUENTER CA, FIORICA V, HINSHAW LB: Cardiorespiratory and metabolic responses to live E. coli and endotoxin in the monkey. J Appl Physiol 26:780, 1969
308. COALSON JJ, et al: Pathophysiologic responses of the subhuman primate in experimental septic shock. Lab Invest 32:561, 1975
309. CHRISTY JH: Pathophysiology of Gram negative shock. Am Heart J 81:694, 1971
310. HINSHAW LB, et al: Effects of endotoxin on myocardial hemodynamic, performance, and metabolism. Am J Physiol 221:504, 1971
311. HINSHAW LB, et al: Effect of endotoxin on myocardial performance. J Trauma 12:1056, 1972
312. HINSHAW LB, et al: Cardiac response to circulating factors in endotoxin shock. Am J Physiol 222:1047, 1972
313. HINSHAW LB, et al: Precipitation of cardiac failure in endotoxin shock. Surg Gynecol Obstet 135:39, 1972
314. GUENTER CA, HINSHAW LB: Comparison of septic shock due to Gram negative and Gram positive organisms. Proc Soc Exp Biol Med 134:780, 1970
315. KWAAN HM, WEIL MH: Differences in the mechanism of shock caused by bacterial infections. Surg Gynecol Obstet 128:37, 1969
316. MACLEAN LD, et al: Alkalosis in septic shock. Surgery 62:655, 1967
317. BLAIR E: Acid–base balance in bacteremic shock. Arch Intern Med 127:731, 1971
318. WRIGHT CJ, et al: Regional capillary blood flow and oxygen uptake in severe sepsis. Surg Gynecol Obstet 132:637, 1971
319. NAYLOR BA, et al: Blood affinity for oxygen in hemorrhagic and endotoxic shock. J Appl Physiol 32:829, 1972
320. CLOWES GHA JR, et al: Circulating factors in the etiology of pulmonary insufficiency and right heart failure accompanying severe sepsis (peritonitis). Ann Surg 171:663, 1970
321. RIGBY RA, CHRISTY JH: Recovery following prolonged gram negative shock and "shock lung." Am J Med 45:959, 1968
322. LEWIN I, et al. Pulmonary failure associated with clinical shock states. J Trauma 11:22, 1971
323. COALSON JJ, HINSHAW LB, GUENTER CA: The pulmonary ultrastructure in septic shock. Exp Mol Pathol 12:84, 1970
324. GUENTER CA: Role of Leukocytes in the Lung

After Endotoxin Administration: Fundamental Mechanisms of Shock, pp 77–80. New York, Plenum, 1972

325. WITTLES EH, et al: Pulmonary intravascular leukocyte sequestration: A potential mechanism of lung injury. Am Rev Respir Dis 190:502, 1974
326. KUX M, et al: Pulmonary effects of E. coli endotoxin: role of leukocytes and platelets. Ann Surg 175:26, 1972
327. PINGLETON WW, COALSON JJ, GUENTER CA: Significance of leukocytes in endotoxin shock. Exp Mol Pathol 22:183, 1975
328. CHRISTY JH: Treatment of Gram negative shock. Am J Med 50:77, 1971
329. PINGLETON WW, et al: Effects of steroid pretreatment on development of shock lung. Lab Invest 27:445, 1972
330. KATZ JD, et al: Pretreatment with methylprednisolone shortens survival on a canine model of pseudomonas pneumonia. J Surg Res 28:260, 1980
331. HINSHAW LB, et al: Is antibiotic/steroid post treatment capable of preventing death in Escherichia-coli L D_{100} shocked baboons. Surg Gynecol Obstet (in press)
332. MOTSAY GH, et al: Effects of corticosteroids on the circulation in shock: Experimental and clinical results. Fed Proc 29:1861, 1970
333. WILSON JW: Treatment or prevention of pulmonary cellular damage with pharmacologic doses of corticosteroid. Surg Gynecol Obstet 134:675, 1972
334. TECKLENBERG PL, et al: The effects of massive doses of methylprednisolone on myocardial contractility and peripheral vascular resistance. Am Heart J 85:216, 1973
335. SCHUMER W, ERVE PR, OBERNOLTE RP: Mechanisms of steroid protection in septic shock. Surgery 72:119, 1972
336. MASSION WH, ROSENBLUTH B, KUX M: Protective effect of methylprednisolone against lung complications in endotoxin shock. South Med J 65:941, 1972
337. SCHUMER W: Steroids in the treatment of clinical septic shock. Ann Surg 184:333, 1976
338. HINSHAW LB, et al: Prevention and reversal of myocardial failure in endotoxin shock. Surg Gynecol Obstet 136:1, 1973
339. Definitions and classifications of infectious reactions of the lung. A.T.S. statement. Am Rev Respir Dis 101:116, 1970
340. KATZ M: Parasitic infections. J Pediatr 87:165, 1975
341. WRIGHT FJ, BAIRD JP: Tropical Diseases, 4th ed. London, Churchill Livingstone, 1971
342. BROWN HW: Basic Clinical Parasitology, 4th ed. New York, Appleton-Century-Crofts, 1975
343. BECK JW, BARRETT-CONNOR E: Medical Parasitology. St Louis, C.V. Mosby, 1971
344. FAUST CE, RUSSEL PF, JUNG RC: Clinical Parasitology, 8th ed. Philadelphia, Lea and Febiger, 1970
345. WOODRUFF AW: Medicine in the Tropics. London, Churchill Livingstone, 1974
346. WILCOCKS C, MANSON-BAHR PEC: Manson's Tropical Diseases, 17th ed. Baltimore, Williams and Wilkins, 1972
347. DONALDSON RJ: Parasites and Western Man. Baltimore, University Park Press, 1979
348. COHN S: The immune response to parasites. In CIBA Symposium: Parasites in the Immunized Host, pp 3–18. Van Gorcum, Netherlands, 1974
349. Immunology of Schistosomiasis. Review Bull WHO 51:553, 1974
350. SADUN E: Soulsby EJL (ed): Immunity to Animal Parasites. New York, Academic Press, 1972
351. KAGAN IG: Diagnostic, epidemiologic, and experimental parasitology: Immunologic aspects. Am J Trop Med Hygiene 28:429, 1979
352. BLOOM BR: Games parasites play: How parasites evade immune surveillance. Nature 279:21, 1979
353. BASS DA, SZEJDA P: Eosinophils versus neutrophils in host defense, J Clin Invest 64:1415, 1979
354. CROFTON J, DOUGLAS A: Parasitic diseases of the lung. In: Respiratory Diseases, Chap, 24. Oxford, Blackwell Scientific Publishers, 1975
355. SPENCER H: Pulmonary parasitic diseases. In Spencer H: Pathology of the Lung, 2nd ed, Chap. 10. Oxford, Pergamon Press, 1968
356. Drugs for parasitic infections. Med Lett Drugs Ther 16:5, 1974
357. WEBER WR, ASKIN FB, DEHNER LP: Lung biopsy in *Pneumocystis carinii* pneumonia. Am J Clin Pathol 67:11, 1977
358. THEOLOGIDES A, KENNEDY BJ: Clinical manifestations of toxoplasmosis in the adult. Arch Intern Med 117:536, 1966
359. MOUSA AH, EL-GAREM A: Clinicopathological aspects of cardiopulmonary bilharziasis. J Egypt Med Assoc 47:270, 1964
360. FULEIHAN FJD, et al: Respiratory function in moderate schistosomal infection. Am Rev Respir Dis 100:651, 1969
361. MAHMOUD AA: Schistosomiasis. N Engl J Med 297:1329, 1977
362. MILLER MJ (ed): Proc Symposium on the Future of Schistosomiasis Control. New Orleans, Tulane University Press, 1972
363. GILLES HM: The search for new drugs for tropical diseases—"What the physician needs." Trans R Soc Trop Med Hygiene 73:144, 1979
364. NEEFE LI, et al: Disseminated strongyloidiasis with cerebral involvement: A complication of corticosteroid therapy. Am J Med 55:832, 1973
365. CRUZ T, ROCHALT RG: Fatal strongyloidiasis in pa-

tients receiving corticosteroids. N Engl J Med 275:1093, 1966

366. RIVERA E, MALDONADA N, GARCIA EV: Hyperinfection syndrome with *Strongyloides stercoralis*. Ann Intern Med 72:199, 1970
367. PORTILO DT, MEYERS WM, CONNOR DH: Fatal strongyloidiasis in immunosuppressed patients. Am J Med 56:488, 1974
368. NESARAJAH MS: Pulmonary function in tropical eosinophilia before and after treatment with diethylcarbamazine. Thorax 30:574, 1975
369. TULLIS DCH: Bronchial asthma associated with intestinal parasites. N Engl J Med 282:370, 1970
370. Letters to Editor. N Engl J Med 282:1045, 1970
371. IBARRO-PERES C SELMAN-LAMA M: Diagnosis and treatment of amebic "empyema." Am J Surg 134:283, 1977.
372. OCHSNER A, DEBAKEY M: Pleuropulmonary complications of amebiasis. J Thorac Surg 5:225, 1936
373. HERRERA-LLERONDI R: Thoracic repercussions of amebiasis. J Thorac Cardiovasc Surg 52:361, 1966
374. STEPHEN SJ, URAGODA CG: Pleuropulmonary amebiasis. Br J Dis Chest 64:96, 1970
375. VERGHESE M, et al: Management of thoracic amebiasis. J Thorac Cardiovasc Surg 78:757, 1979
376. CAMERON EWJ: The treatment of pleuropulmonary amebiasis with metronidazole. Chest 73:647, 1978
377. BLYTH DF, PIRIC D: Hematogenous amoebic lung abscess. S Afr Med J 53:147, 1978
378. KAGAN IG: Serologic diagnosis of parasitic diseases. N Engl J Med 282:685, 1970
379. GUTMAN RA, et al: Radiographic changes accompanying successful therapy of pulmonary paragonimiasis. Am Rev Respir Dis 99:255, 1969
380. BELAND JE, et al. Paragonomiasis (the lung fluke). Am Rev Respir Dis 99:261, 1969
381. LEROUX BT: Pulmonary hydatid disease. Thorax 27:365, 1972
382. HYDATIDOSIS: a global problem of increasing importance. Bull WHO 55:499, 1977
383. FINLAYSON DM, FERGUS A: Hydatid disease in Toronto. Can Med Assoc J 88:1004, 1963
384. MELTZER H, et al: Echinococcosis in North American Indians and Eskimos. Can Med Assoc J 75:121, 1956
385. AMIR-JAHED AK, et al: Clinical echinococcosis. Ann Surg 182:541, 1975
386. WILSON JF, DIDDAMS AC, RAUSCH RL: Cystic Hydatid disease in Alaska. Am Rev Respir Dis 98:1, 1968

386a. BORRIE J, SHAW JFH: Hepatobronchial fistula caused by hydatid disease. Thorax 36:25, 1981

387. BARRETT NR, THOMAS D: Pulmonary hydatid disease. Br J Surg 40:222, 1952
388. LICHTER I: Surgery of pulmonary hydatid cyst. Thorax 27:529, 1972
389. XANTHAKIS D, EFTHIMIADES M, et al: Hydatid disease of the chest: Report of 91 patients surgically treated Thorax 27:517, 1972
390. Editorial: Medical treatment for hydatid disease. B Med J 2:563, 1979
391. GERSHIN LH, GERSHWIN ME, KRITZMAN J: Human pulmonary dirofilariasis. Chest 66:92, 1974
392. FAUST EC, THOMAS EP, JONES J: Discovery of human heartworm infection in New Orleans. J parasitol 27:115, 1941
393. FELD H: Dirofilaria immitis as a cause of a pulmonary lesion in man. Radiology 108:311, 1973
394. DAYAL Y, NEAFIE RC: Human pulmonary dirofilariasis. Am Rev Respir Dis 112:437, 1975
395. AWE RJ, et al: Solitary and bilateral pulmonary nodules due to Dirofilaria immitis. Am Rev Respir Dis 112:445, 1975
396. PLORDE JJ, BENNETT IL, PETERSDORF RG: Trichinosis. In Thorn GW, et al: Harrison's Principles of Internal Medicine, 8th ed. New York, McGraw-Hill, 1978
397. ROBIN ED, CRUMP CH, WAGMAN RJ: Low sedimentation rate, hypofibrinogenemia and restrictive pseudoobstructive pulmonary disease associated with trichinosis. N Engl J Med 262:758, 1960

Chapter 9

Chronic Respiratory Tract Infections

JOHN G. WEG

PART ONE: TUBERCULOSIS

Tuberculosis is an infectious disease of worldwide importance. Prior to the development of specific chemotherapy, it carried a lifelong threat of exacerbation and a mortality rate exceeding many cancers. The experience of more than two decades documents that the completion of an appropriate course of drug therapy is virtually synonymous with cure. This remarkable ability to control a serious chronic disease is almost unprecedented. The term tuberculosis is generally reserved for infection with the organism *Mycobacterium tuberculosis* or *Mycobacterium bovis*. Infections by other mycobacteria are usually identified as mycobacterial disease caused by the specific organisms (*e.g.*, *Mycobacterium kansasii*).

MAGNITUDE OF THE PROBLEM

MORTALITY

Tuberculosis, the "White Plague" of the Middle Ages, has been estimated to be responsible for 30% of all deaths in 17th-century London. In Boston, New York, and Philadelphia in the early 19th century the tuberculosis death rate was about 400:100,000.[1] In 1900 the United States mortality rate was 202:100,000.[2] Since that time there has been a steady decrease in mortality. In 1953, shortly after truly effective chemotherapy came into widespread usage, the mortality rate had decreased to 12.4:100,000. Since that time this steady decline has continued to a rate of 1.3:100,000 in 1978, or 2,830 deaths.[3] The decrease prior to the chemotherapy era can be attributed to better living conditions, improved nutrition, and, perhaps, to the nonspecific therapeutic benefits attributed to sanitorium care and bed rest. The current death rate may be an overestimate since more people today die *with* tuberculosis than *of* tuberculosis. The unfortunate exceptions are the individuals in whom the diagnosis of tuberculosis is not made until postmortem examination, and the small but regular admission of patients with overwhelming disease who die before chemotherapy has had an opportunity to reverse the process.

MORBIDITY

Although death from tuberculosis in the United States has dramatically decreased, the number of people with disease has not declined quite so rapidly. Morbidity data have been reported as "new active cases" in the US through 1974. Cases were considered active if acid-fast organisms were identified microscopically or *M. tuberculosis* was grown in culture and in the presence of roentgenographic change or cavitation.[5] The new active case rate in the US was 76.7 per 100,000 in 1932; it had decreased to 55.4 per 100,000 in 1952, just prior to the chemotherapy era. A decade later the rate was 28.7 per 100,000; in 1972, 15.8 per 100,000 and in 1978, 13.1 per 100,000, or 28,251 cases[4] (see Fig. 9-1.)

INFECTION

An individual is identified as infected with *M. tuberculosis* when the reaction to a standard dose of tuberculin, 5 tuberculin units (TU), is significant (10 mm of induration or more in screening studies, and 5 mm or more when evaluating suspects or close contacts).[6] A good deal more will be said about the tuberculin skin test subsequently. It is a very sensitive indicator of the extent of the tuberculosis problem in a population. In 1968 it was estimated that 25 million people in the United States were infected on the basis of tuberculin skin testing of selected populations.[7,8] This figure was estimated at 15 million at the end of 1973.[9] In longitudinal studies of white Navy recruits, aged 17 to 21 yr, there has been a steady decline in infections from about 7% in 1949 to 2% in 1974.[10,11]

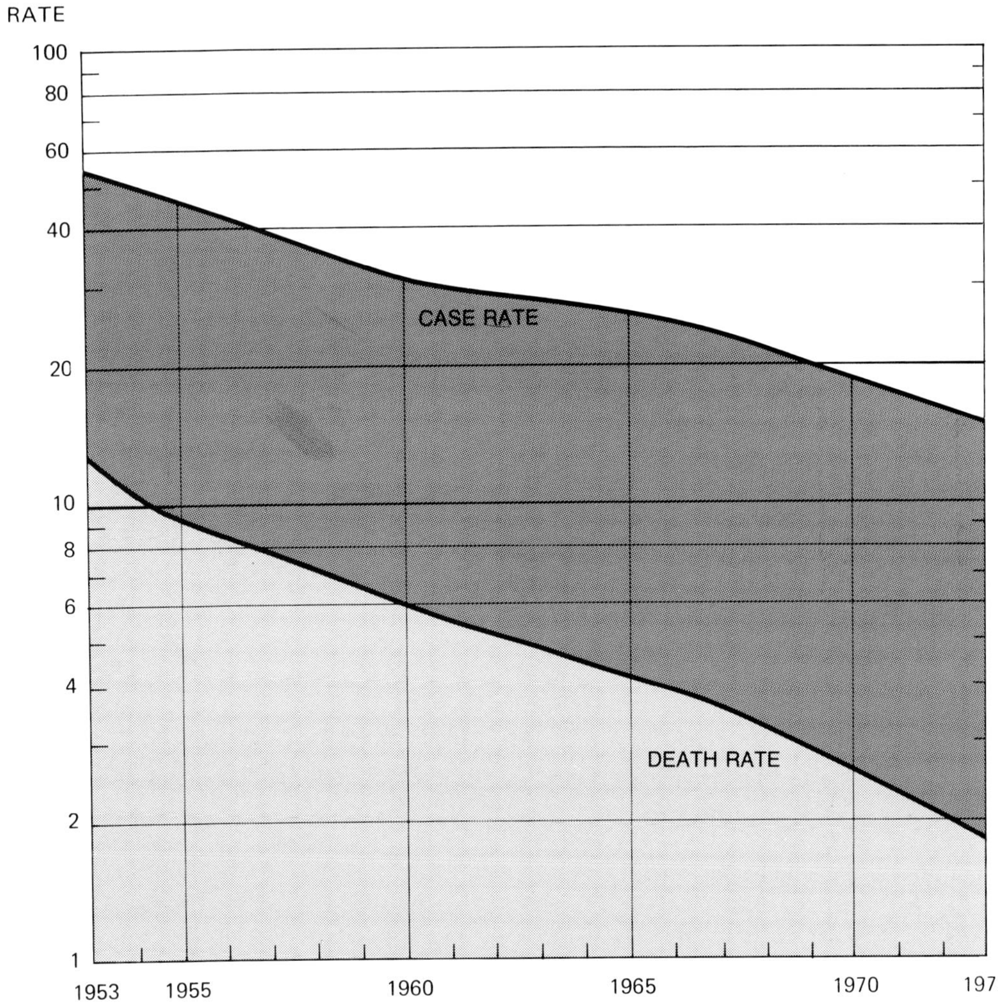

FIG. 9-1. Tuberculosis case and death rates in the United States, 1953–1973. Note that the death rates have declined more rapidly than the case rates. (US Department of Health, Education and Welfare: Reported Tuberculosis Data, 1973. Publication No. [CDC] 75-8201)

DISTRIBUTION OF THE PROBLEM

Although these nationwide figures for the United States indicate decreasing mortality, morbidity, and infection, they obscure the marked variation related to age, sex, race, geography, and most importantly, socioeconomic conditions. Most of the infected people in the US are over age 26 yr (see Fig. 9-2). The 1978 US figures indicate that 87% of the cases of tuberculosis develop in people over age 25 yr and 62% in those 45 and older.[10] There are approximately twice as many cases in men as in women. About 60% of the cases are in white and 40% in nonwhite patients; the case rate in nonwhites is about 4.5 times that in whites[12] (see Fig. 9-3).

The distribution of tuberculosis on a geographic basis is likewise quite variable. In 1978, the overall US case rate was 13.1 : 100,000, but the highest case rate by state was 32.3 : 100,000 in Hawaii (46.6 : 100,000 in the District of Columbia), while the lowest was 1.9 : 100,000 in Nebraska.[4] Table 9-1 lists the tuberculosis cases and deaths from 1953 to 1978. In 1978, 45% of cases came from cities with a population of 100,000 or more, and 34% from cities with

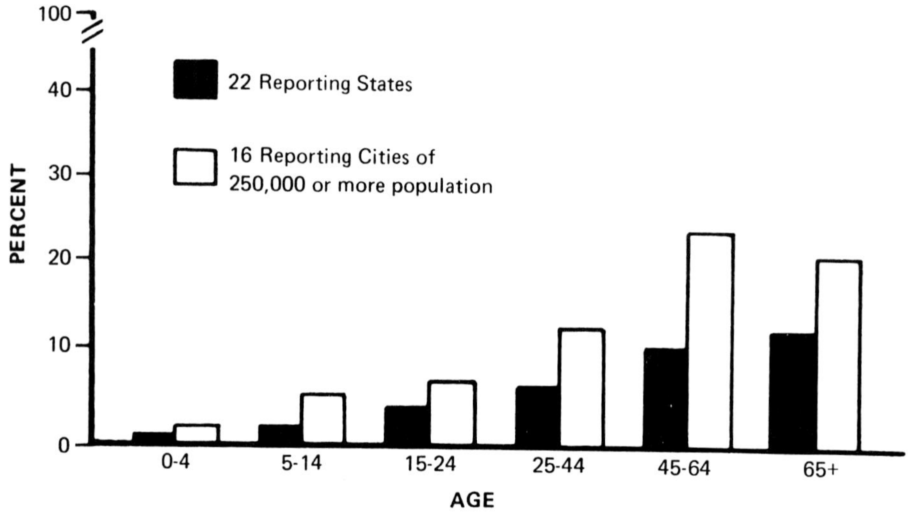

FIG. 9-2. Percent "positive" (10 mm or greater) tuberculosis reactors by age, selected areas, United States, 1978. Since data is based on selected areas of states and cities where reactor rates were expected to be high, they overestimate the infection rate. (US Department of Health and Human Services, Center for Disease Control: Tuberculosis in the United States. Publication No. [CDC] 80–8322, June, 1980)

FIG. 9-3. Tuberculosis case rates for whites and other races, males and females by age, United States, 1978. (US Department of Health and Human Services Center for Disease Control: Tuberculosis in the United States. Publication No. [CDC] 808322, June, 1980)

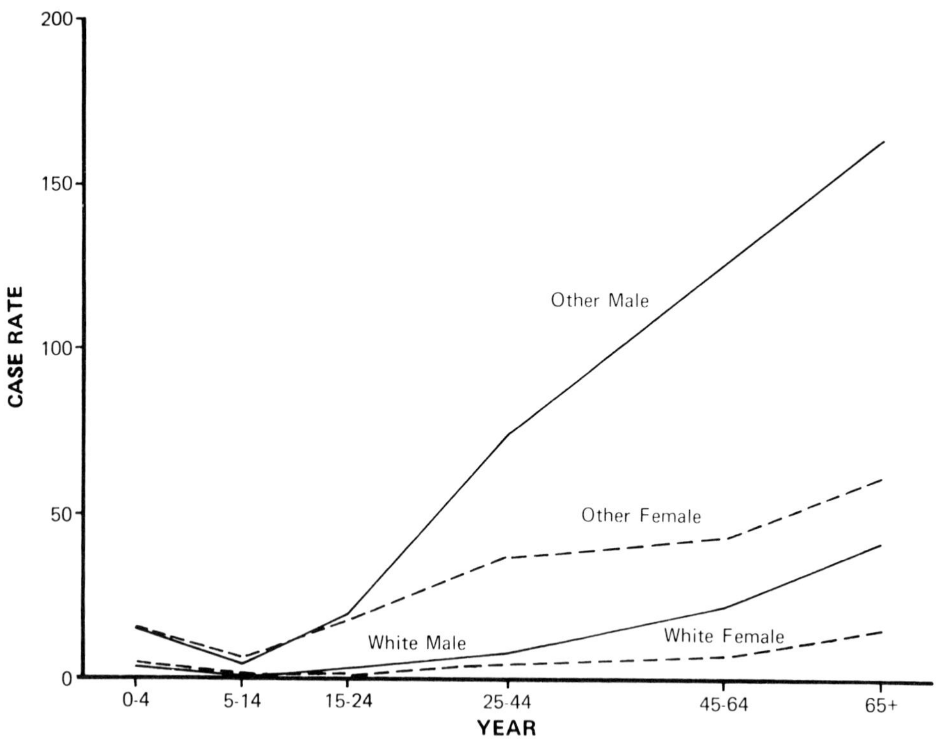

TABLE 9-1. Tuberculosis Cases and Case Rates, Deaths and Death Rates, United States, 1953–1978

	Tuberculosis Cases				Tuberculosis Deaths			
			Percent Change				Percent Change	
Year	Number	Rate	Number	Rate	Number	Rate	Number	Rate
1953	84,304	53.0	—	—	19,707	12.4	—	—
1954	79,775	49.3	−5.4	−7.0	16,527	10.2	−16.1	−17.7
1955	77,368	46.9	−3.0	−4.9	15,016	9.1	−9.1	−10.8
1956	69,895	41.6	−9.7	−11.3	14,137	8.4	−5.9	−7.7
1957	67,149	39.2	−3.9	−5.8	13,390	7.8	−5.3	−7.1
1958	63,534	36.5	−5.4	−6.9	12,417	7.1	−7.3	−9.0
1959	57,535	32.5	−9.4	−11.0	11,474	6.5	−7.6	−8.5
1960	55,494	30.8	−3.5	−5.2	10,866	6.0	−5.3	−7.7
1961	53,726	29.4	−3.2	−4.5	9,938	5.4	−8.5	−10.0
1962	53,315	28.7	−0.8	−2.4	9,506	5.1	−4.3	−5.6
1963	54,042	28.7	+1.4	0.0	9,311	4.9	−2.1	−3.9
1964	50,874	26.6	−5.9	−7.3	8,303	4.3	−10.8	−12.2
1965	49,016	25.3	−3.7	−4.9	7,934	4.1	−4.4	−4.7
1966	47,767	24.4	−2.5	−3.6	7,625	3.9	−3.9	−4.9
1967	45,647	23.1	−4.4	−5.3	6,901	3.5	−9.5	−10.3
1968	42,623	21.3	−6.6	−7.8	6,292	3.1	−8.8	−11.4
1969	39,120	19.4	−8.2	−8.9	5,567	2.8	−11.5	−9.7
1970	37,137	18.3	−5.1	−5.7	5,217	2.6	−6.3	−7.1
1971	35,217	17.1	−5.2	−6.6	4,501	2.2	−13.7	−15.4
1972	32,882	15.8	−6.6	−7.6	4,376	2.1	−2.8	−4.5
1973	30,998	14.8	−5.7	−6.3	3,875	1.8	−11.4	−14.3
1974	30,122	14.2	−2.8	−4.1	3,513	1.7	−9.3	−5.6
1975	33,989	15.9	—	—	3,333	1.6	−5.1	−5.9
1976	32,105	15.0	−5.5	−5.7	3,130	1.5	−6.1	−6.3
1977	30,145	13.9	−6.1	−7.3	2,968	1.4	−5.2	−6.7
1978	28,521	13.1	−5.4	−5.8	2,830*	1.3	−4.6	−7.1

* Provisional deaths for 1978 based on the NCHS ten-percent sample of death certificates. Note case data subsequent to 1974 are not comparable to prior years, owing to changes in reporting criteria which became effective in 1975. (US Department of Health, Education and Welfare, Public Health Service, Center for Disease Control: 1978 Tuberculosis Statistics, States and Cities. December, 1979).

250,000 or more people. During that year, 915 counties with 5.3% of the population reported no tuberculosis, while 7 counties each identified 400 or more cases[10] (see Fig. 9-4). It would appear that the major determinant of this marked variability in case rates relates to socioeconomic conditions. Prior to chemotherapy a regular decline in mortality and morbidity was documented as general living conditions improved. Most cases of tuberculosis in the US today arise in urban areas with crowding and substandard living conditions. Within these areas the highest rates correlate well with crowding and low income. Similar high rates do occur in non-urban areas with the same living conditions. This is most notable in migrant workers along the US-Mexican border, in Eskimos, and in American Indians.

Infection rates reflect this same variability. In Navy recruits at an average age of 19, the infection rate in whites was 4% and in nonwhites 12.9%, almost 3 times as great.[13] In studies of Air Force recruits the overall reaction rate was 4.2%. However, in white recruits the rate was 3.1%; in officer candidates, who generally came from a higher socioeconomic status, it was less than 1%; in blacks it was 10.7%; in those with Latin American surnames it was 20.2%; and in a

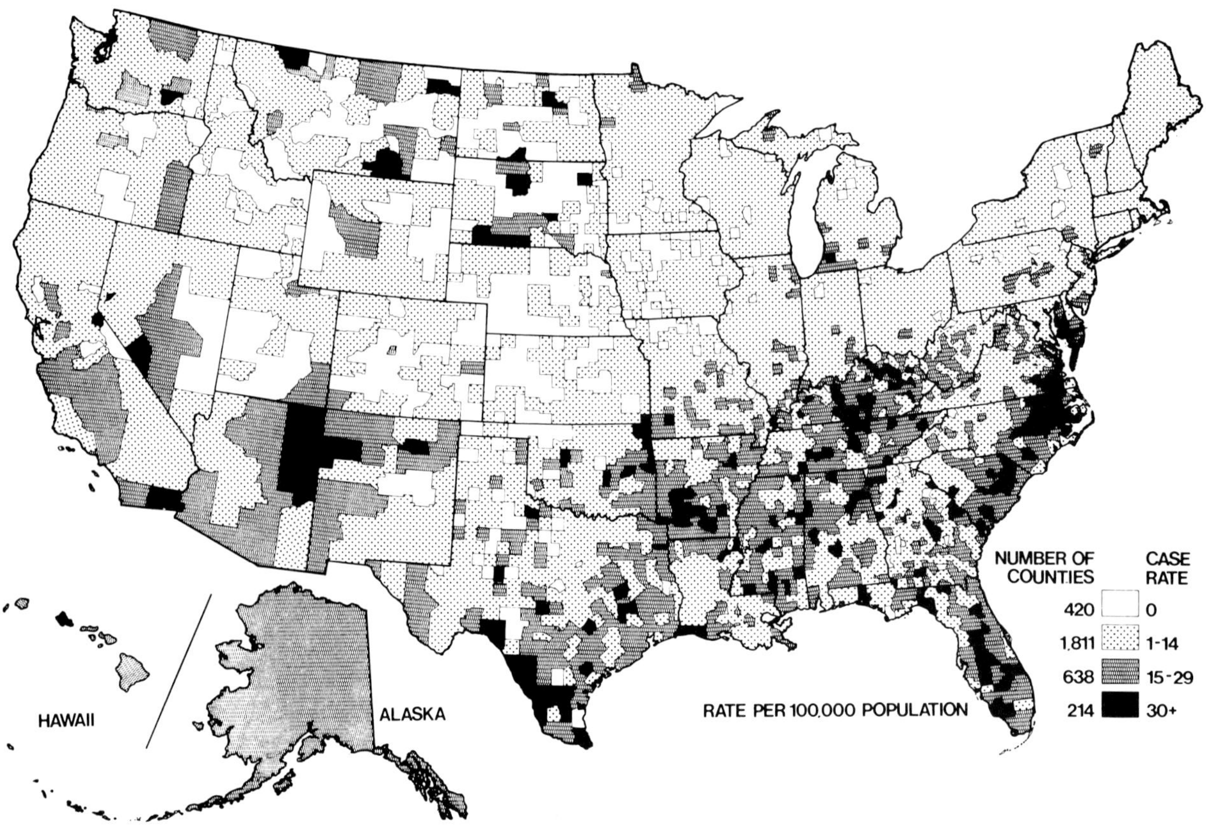

FIG. 9-4. Tuberculosis case rates by county, average 1976–78. (US Department of Health and Human Services, Center for Disease Control: Tuberculosis in the United States. Publication No. [CDC] 808322, June, 1980)

small group of American Indians it was 14.7%.[14]

In 1969 the incidence rate of tuberculosis in Indians and Alaskan natives was still eight times the US rate, although this represented a 94% decrease for the Alaskan natives.[15] On a Navaho reservation in 1973 the reactor rate was 29%.[16]

The probability of being infected in the general population in the United States is about 1 in 5000. The tuberculin-test reaction rate in US children under first grade was 0.32%; in first grade it was 0.37%, and from all other grades 1.07% in the 1972-1973 school year.[9]

It is estimated that 90% of the new active cases of tuberculosis will arise from people already infected. Figure 9-5 illustrates the relative risk of developing active disease in previously noninfected and infected populations in the United States.

The pattern of declining mortality, morbidity, and infection which is characteristic of highly developed countries is unfortunately not worldwide. In India in 1965, 27% of children under age 5 yr and 90% of the 40-year-olds had positive tuberculin skin tests. In Bolivia tuberculosis remains the leading specific infectious disease reported as the cause of death in adults, with an estimated mortality rate of 125:100,000, an estimated prevalence of active disease of 1.8%, and significant tuberculin skin test reactions in 50% of the population.[17] In 1971 the highest incidence of new cases was in Asia and Oceania with rates as high as 300 to 500:100,000. In some African countries, rates were as high as 250:100,000. This contrasts strikingly to rates of less than 20:100,000 in Denmark, the Netherlands, Canada, and the United States. A recent estimate of the worldwide annual incidence of tuberculosis in 1971 is over 3.5 million or

96:100,000.[18] The number of infectious cases of tuberculosis in the world is estimated at 15 to 20 million.[19]

It is important to appreciate the immense magnitude of the tuberculosis problem on a worldwide basis, since immigration may affect the incidence of tuberculosis quite appreciably.[20] The percentage of immigrants arriving from areas of high tuberculosis incidence is increasing in Canada and the United States.[21,22] A review of the effect of immigration on tuberculosis in Canada disclosed the following: (1) in 1971, 78% of the population was Canadian-born and 22% foreign-born, but they accounted for equal numbers of active new cases; (2) the morbidity in immigrants was comparable to that in their native country (*e.g.*, Asians 15 times greater than Canadians); (3) since immigrants were generally younger, the disease occurred in a younger age group than in Canadians; and (4) there was an increased incidence in the Canadian-born population of the same ethnic origin, since they generally interacted more with the newcomers.[22]

A more recent report emphasizes that the incidence is greater in recent immigrants and nonimmigrant long-term visitors such as students. It also reports bacillary resistance to isoniazid, streptomycin, or both in 3.3% of Canadian-born persons (excluding registered Indians) *vs.* 7.6% in Asian-born immigrants.[23]

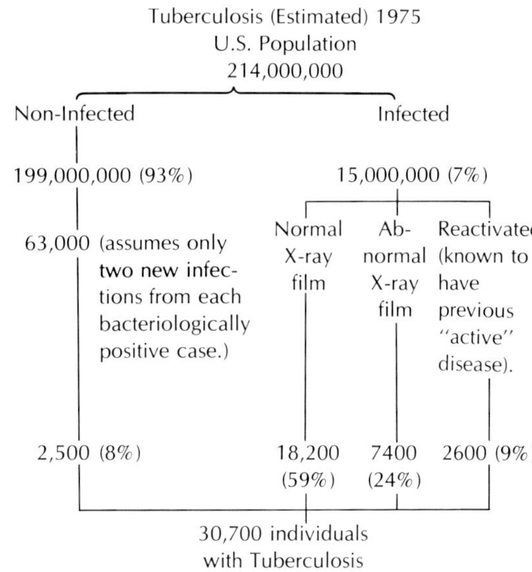

FIG. 9-5. A schematic representation of the epidemiologic picture of tuberculosis in the United States, 1975. (Sbarbaro, JA: Tuberculosis: the new challenge to the practicing clinician. Chest, 68:436 [Suppl.], 1975)

EPIDEMIOLOGY

TRANSMISSION

Tuberculosis is an airborne infection spread by droplet nuclei, which are invisible, minute particles suspended in the air and dispersed like cigarette smoke. Droplet nuclei are generated while one is talking, coughing, sneezing, and so forth. These 1μ to 10μ particles carrying the infectious agent, *M. tuberculosis*, will remain suspended in the air and are wafted about by normal air currents rather evenly throughout enclosed spaces such as a room. When inhaled, particles in this size range can reach an alveolar surface. One such particle is sufficient to establish a tuberculous infection.[6,24] Somewhat larger particles, if inhaled, impact in the nose, oropharynx, or trachea, where they are cleared by the mucociliary blanket. Organisms seldom invade intact mucosa or tissue. Still larger particles, such as those seen when someone sneezes or expectorates, settle almost immediately to a surface. On occasion, *M. tuberculosis* may be cultured from such material even after considerable periods of time, although most of the nonmotile tubercle bacilli are readily killed by heat, drying, sunshine, or ultraviolet light. These large particles which settle on a surface, however, play no role in the airborne transmission of tuberculosis. The immense amount of energy to resuspend them as droplet nuclei is generally not available. One must concede that the potential for infection through an open wound does exist, but, on the basis of experience, this risk appears to be uniquely reserved for mycobacterial laboratory technicians and pathologists. Therefore fomites such as books, clothes, bedding, and eating utensils are not involved in the spread of tuberculosis and require no special attention. Tubercle bacilli will not cause infection even when placed on unbroken skin. Ordinary handwashing removes these as well as other bacteria.[25]

Documentation that tuberculosis is spread by the airborne route rests on the initial studies of

Wells in 1934, with contributions by Perkins, which culminated in the studies of O'Grady and Riley[26–28] at the Baltimore Veterans Administration Hospital in association with the Johns Hopkins School of Hygiene. They vented all air from rooms of patients with active, infectious tuberculosis through a "T" system to animal chambers containing guinea pigs. Ultraviolet lighting was installed in one arm of the "T" system, which completely prevented tuberculosis infection in guinea pigs breathing this air. The guinea pigs breathing air through the other arm of the "T" were never in physical contact with the patients, but developed tuberculosis. Within 3 to 4 weeks, pearly white 3-mm tubercles were found on the surfaces of their lungs. Of the 130 guinea pigs exposed continuously, an average of 3 per mo became infected, and the characteristic lesion was a single tubercle. Riley estimated from these experiments that there was one infectious droplet nucleus per 12,000 to 14,000 cubic feet of air. He calculated that it would take a nurse 6 to 12 months, working on her ward 8 hours per day, to become infected. This was quite similar to the data on student nurses working at Bellevue Hospital in New York, where average time for skin-test conversion was 18 months in the pre-chemotherapy period of 1930 to 1948.[28] In contrast, Houk and associates detailed the characteristics of a mini-epidemic aboard a naval vessel with recirculating air conditioning where personnel were exposed for 24 hours each day.[29,30] Tuberculin skin-test conversion, the criterion of new infection, occurred in nearly 50% of the men at risk and in about one-tenth the time required for the student nurses. In this epidemic there was again solid evidence that exposure to air from the diseased sailor correlated strikingly with infection of previously uninfected individuals; there was no evidence of transmission of tuberculosis by direct contact.[24]

While tuberculosis is clearly an infectious disease spread by airborne droplet nuclei, it is not as highly infectious as some common viral illnesses such as measles and the common cold.[31] The household contacts of individuals with smear-positive tuberculosis have the greatest risk of being infected. However, most studies show that even those living in crowded, substandard conditions with repeated and intimate contact have an infection rate of 25 to 50%. In some studies the infection rate of household contacts of a person whose sputum culture is positive (while the sputum spear is negative prior to chemotherapy) is not different than in the surrounding community.[32] Others have found an increased rate of infection in household contacts of culture-positive, smear-negative index cases that was not as great as exposure to a smear-positive index case.[33]

On the basis of epidemiologic data, then, it would seem that exposure generally must be sustained and "close" (*i.e.*, breathing air containing droplet nuclei in an enclosed space). Subsequently, we will discuss the application of this concept in identifying potentially infected individuals who have been exposed to a person with untreated, bacteriologically positive tuberculous disease.

PREVENTION OF TRANSMISSION

Measures effective in preventing the spread of the tubercle bacillus can be considered under two major divisions: prevention of contamination, which requires cooperation by the individual with disease and the people exposed; and decontamination, which does not require individual cooperation.

Prevention of Contamination

Chemotherapy is the most effective definitive means of preventing the spread of infection. The effectiveness of chemotherapy in preventing new infection and subsequent disease was first clearly shown in the Madras studies in India under the auspices of the World Health Organization, the British Medical Research Council, and the Indian Medical Service. In 1956, with an estimated 1.5 million contagious patients and only 23,000 hospital beds for tuberculosis, a carefully controlled, randomized evaluation was initiated of hospital *vs.* home treatment of patients with extensive disease and positive bacteriology. All patients received isoniazid (INH) and para-aminosalicylic acid (PAS) daily for 1 yr. The hospital patients also observed bedrest and had an excellent diet. The patients treated at home were under careful supervision with home visits and, later in the study, surprise checks on urine samples to document drug ingestion. Seven (8.0%) of 87 tuberculin-negative contacts of the index cases who were treated in the hospital developed tuberculosis in the first year, while 7 (8.1%) of 86 contacts of the index cases treated at home developed disease. Tuberculin-positive contacts of hospitalized index cases had a 7.3% rate of disease, while contacts of the home-treated cases had a rate of 3.1%. Over a 5-year follow-up 10.5% of 86 contacts of the home-treated patients who were previously tuberculin-negative developed disease, while 11.5% of the tuberculin-negative contacts to index cases treated in hospitals developed disease. Of the initially positive tuberculin contacts 9.4% of 159 home-treated patients and 15.8% of 17 hospital-treated patients developed disease. There is no statistical difference in these infection or disease rates despite the extraordinarily substandard living conditions of these people. In the 5-year follow-up period, of 62 cases that developed tuberculosis, 32 were in the first year and 18 in the first 3 months. This strongly suggests that these contacts were already infected before the index case started treatment. Forty of these 62 cases were in people less than 15 years old, and 25 were in people less than 5 years old. The attack rate for the 5-year period was 25% in contacts under 5, 9% in those between 5 and 14, and 8% in those 15 years of age or older.[34]

More recent studies comparing hospital and home-treated patients in Arkansas clearly document the effectiveness of chemotherapy in preventing infection of household contacts of patients with tuberculosis who are receiving chemotherapy.[35] Chemotherapy reduces quite rapidly the number of organisms and the frequency of coughing.[33]

It is also recommended that persons with disease cover their nose and mouth with tissues while coughing and sneezing to reduce the number of droplet nuclei. In addition well-constructed "synthetic or glass fiber" masks that are well fitted have been shown to be 90 to 99% efficient in filtering 1 μm to 5 μm airborne particles.[36] These masks should be worn by the patient for short periods of time where others will be heavily exposed or by the person being exposed (*e.g.*, during bronchoscopy, attending to a disoriented patient who cannot cooperate, and so forth) until effective chemotherapy has been instituted. Gauze and paper masks are not effective. There is no need to wear gowns, gloves, boots, or caps, or to attempt to sterilize fomites such as bedding, dishes, and walls.[25]

Decontamination

Although not as desirable as prevention of contamination, decontamination has two major advantages: (1) it does not require individual cooperation, and (2) it provides protection even if the individual with tuberculosis is not identified. It is accomplished by adequate ventilation with fresh air; 20 or more room-air changes per hour are desirable. This requires a one-way or nonrecirculating air-control system. In its absence, however, even an open window with an exhaust fan is of some value. Alternatively, the use of ultraviolet irradiation of air in the upper parts of rooms and corridors will enhance the effectiveness of normal ventilation. Riley estimates that ultraviolet light can eliminate organisms at a rate equivalent to 50 air changes per hour.[31] While either or both of these methods should be used in areas where patients are admitted for the diagnosis and treatment of suspected or known tuberculosis, such protection is especially important in areas where an unidentified patient with tuberculosis is likely to visit (*e.g.*, emergency rooms and observation wards in areas where tuberculosis is regularly diagnosed).

PATHOGENESIS AND PATHOLOGY

When a tubercle bacillus carried on a droplet nucleus reaches a susceptible site such as the respiratory bronchiole or alveolus, it begins to multiply freely. In a host without prior tuberculosis exposure, macrophages migrate into the area and the organism is phagocytosed, but multiplication continues. There is edema formation and deposition of fibrin. A variable number of polymorphonuclear leukocytes can be found. This exudative response represents a rather nonspecific pneumonitis. At this point alveolar structures are still intact. Tubercle bacilli also enter lymphatic channels and reach regional lymph nodes. They also commonly spread hematogenously throughout the body. However, even though the bone marrow, liver and spleen are almost always seeded, they very seldom permit uncontrolled multiplication of the bacilli. In contrast, organisms deposited in regional lymph nodes, the upper lung zones, the renal parenchyma, epiphyseal lines, and the cerebral cortex may multiply before immunity is acquired. The fate of this initial lesion is dependent on the number of bacilli, the natural host resistance, and the development of acquired immunity. With the development of acquired immunity further multiplication of bacilli is controlled in the great majority of the initial lesions. The lesions resolve, leaving little or no residuum.[37] It has been estimated that 5 to 15% of patients initially infected with the tubercle bacillus will develop disease in the 5 years following infection and another 3 to 5% will develop disease during the remainder of their lifetime.[21]

Cellular or Type IV immunity develops 2 to 10 weeks after infection and results in inflammation and necrosis; this is manifested by a significant reaction to a tuberculin skin test. The inflammatory response consists of epithelioid cells and Langhans' giant cells. This is called *granulomatous inflammation.* It is usually surrounded by fibroblasts, lymphocytes, collagen deposition, and new capillaries. Within the center of this lesion, necrosis characteristic of tuberculosis generally develops. It is called *caseation necrosis.* Grossly it is a thick, grumous, white, cheeselike material. Within this material are many destroyed bacilli.[38] If the inflammatory response predominates, the lesion is called *proliferative.* If the necrosis predominates, it is called *exudative.* This granulomatous inflammation with or without caseation is the tubercle.

Subsequently, areas of caseation generally localize, undergo resorption, hyaline degeneration, and fibrosis. These necrotic areas may calcify. Less commonly, larger lesions may liquefy with the appearance of polymorphonuclear leukocytes and proteolytic enzymes; generally there is a concomitant increase in the number of organisms. This liquid material then empties into a bronchus, and the evacuated area becomes a cavity. Bacilli continue to proliferate in the necrotic cavity wall. The evacuated material leads to endobronchial spread of disease into new areas of lung; this can be a recurring process. The bacilli may also involve other mucous membranes by this route, resulting in laryngeal or middle-ear tuberculosis; swallowed organisms may lead to intestinal tuberculosis, including perirectal abscess and fistula. This material is also coughed up and tubercle bacilli are dispersed in the air in newly formed droplet nuclei capable of infecting other persons.

A lesion may also progress by direct extension if bacilli multiply rapidly and there is a marked exudative response. These lesions may extend through the pleura, resulting in a tuberculous pleural effusion with a small number of organisms. Similarly, pericardial effusions may occur. When large numbers of organisms enter the pleural space, usually with rupture of a cavity, a tuberculous empyema with a bronchopleural fistula may occur. The bacilli that initially travel through lung lymphatics to regional nodes may also multiply. The nodes develop granulomatous inflammation with caseation. Particularly in children these enlarged nodes may compress and obstruct bronchi; they may rupture into bronchi, producing a tuberculous endobronchitis. They may also rupture into the mediastinum or pleural space and lead to paraspinal or chest wall involvement.

In contrast to the small numbers of organisms that usually enter the blood stream during the initial infection, a large number of organisms may enter the blood stream under special circumstances such as rupture into a pulmonary vein of liquid caseous material from a cavity, from mediastinal nodes, or from other extrapulmonary foci.[37] This is disseminated disease, although it is commonly called "miliary tuberculosis." Strictly speaking, miliary tuberculosis is the roentgenographic manifestation of many tiny, discrete nodules scattered throughout the lung. With disseminated disease, similar bloodborne foci involve many organs, most notably, the brain, meninges, liver, kidney, and bone marrow. On occasion the chest roentgenogram is normal.

PATTERNS OF INFECTION

Initial infection is more commonly seen in the periphery of the middle or lower lung zones. Since these areas have greater ventilation than the upper zones, they are more exposed to droplet nuclei. The regional nodes, particularly the hilar and paratracheal nodes, are regularly involved. There is limited hematogenous seeding, more commonly to the kidneys, bone, brain, and mesenteric lymph nodes. In a small number of infections there may be direct progression to clinical illness, but usually there is an interval of months to years or even decades before disease is evident.[39–41]

In addition to the parenchymal disease in the middle and lower lung zones, tuberculous involvement of the hilar or paratracheal nodes may compress bronchi, resulting in atelectasis, pneumonia, and subsequently bronchiectasis. In infants and small children miliary and meningeal disease is a frequent complication.

This pattern has been called "primary tuberculosis" or "childhood tuberculosis." Today, however, it is not uncommon in adults, since the great majority of people in developed countries reach adulthood without previous tuberculous infections. Erythema nodosum may accompany the initial infection.

Usually there is an asymptomatic interval after initial infection that lasts for years or, less commonly, decades before clinical illness develops. The site most commonly involved is the upper lung zones, although extrapulmonary foci may exacerbate. This pattern has been termed "reinfection tuberculosis"; the term implies a new infection from an external source, which is most uncommon. Others have used the term "endogenous reinfection" for exacerbation to indicate that old foci of tubercle bacilli have begun to multiply and cause disease. This latter mechanism accounts for most of tuberculous disease in the western world today.[39–41]

HEALING

Tuberculous lesions may resolve entirely when small numbers of bacilli are adequately controlled by host defense mechanisms. Larger areas undergo hyalinization and collagen is formed. The resultant areas of fibrosis may shrink with time. These may become calcified, a process that usually takes years. With chemotherapy this process is hastened. Cavities commonly contract and close; however, some cavities may remain open. Their walls may be lined with fibrous tissue and occasional islands of granulation tissue, or the walls may be covered with bronchial epithelium.[42–45]

DIAGNOSIS AND CLASSIFICATION

The recent classification of tuberculosis (1981) is based on its pathogenesis. A person must first be exposed in order to be infected, and those who ultimately develop disease come from this infected population (usually at a time quite distant from the initial infection). The classification is applicable to all in whom the diagnosis of tuberculosis is, or should be, considered.[6] The new classification acknowledges as its mainstay the wisdom of Koch, who first identified the tubercle bacillus: "In the future it will not be difficult to decide what is tuberculosis and what is not . . . the demonstration of tubercle bacilli . . . will settle the question."[46] It reflects the unparalleled effectiveness of antituberculous chemotherapy in curing this once very chronic disease with its lifelong morbidity and high mortality. It streamlines older classifications without loss of necessary information, making it effective and functional for every practicing physician and other members of the health care team.

Tuberculosis usually presents with insidious symptoms. Many patients, even with extensive disease, have such slowly progressive symptoms that they are insensitive to them and only recognize them in retrospect when their disease has been treated; some may be truly asymptomatic. It is not uncommon to find extensive bilateral involvement with cavities demonstrated on the chest roentgenogram in an individual who volunteers no symptoms or only mild and nonspecific symptoms of not feeling well. These individuals can be recognized only through other measures such as a history of exposure to contagious tuberculosis, an abnormal chest roentgen-

Classification of Tuberculosis

0. *No tuberculosis exposure, not infected* (no history of exposure; reaction to tuberculin skin test not significant)
1. *Tuberculosis exposure, no evidence of infection* (history of exposure; reaction to tuberculin skin test not significant)
2. *Tuberculous infection, no disease* (significant reaction to tuberculin skin test; negative bacteriologic studies [if done], no clinical or roentgenographic evidence of tuberculosis)
   - *Chemotherapy status* (preventive)
     - None
     - On chemotherapy since (date)
     - Chemotherapy terminated (date)
       - Complete (prescribed course of therapy)
       - Incomplete
3. *Tuberculosis: current disease* (*M. tuberculosis* cultured [if done]; otherwise *both* a significant reaction to tuberculin skin test *and* clinical or roentgenographic evidence of current disease)
   - *Location of disease*
     - Pulmonary
     - Pleural
     - Lymphatic
     - Bone or joint
     - Genitourinary
     - Disseminated (miliary)
     - Meningeal
     - Peritoneal
     - Other

   The predominant site shall be listed. Other sites may also be listed. Anatomic sites may be specified more precisely.
   - *Bacteriologic status*
     - Positive by
       - Microscopy only (date)
       - Culture only (date)
       - Microscopy and culture (date)
     - Negative (date)
     - Not done
   - *Chemotherapy status*
     - On chemotherapy since (date)
     - Chemotherapy terminated, incomplete (date)

   The following data are necessary in certain circumstances:
   - *Roentgenogram findings*
     - Normal
     - Abnormal
       - Cavitary or noncavitary
       - Stable or worsening or improving
   - *Tuberculin skin-test reaction*
     - Significant
     - Not Significant
4. *Tuberculosis: no current disease* (history of previous episode[s] of tuberculosis, or abnormal stable roentgenographic findings in a person with a significant reaction to tuberculin skin test; negative bacteriologic studies [if done]; no clinical or roentgenographic evidence of current disease)
   - *Chemotherapy Status*
     - None
     - On chemotherapy since (date)
     - Chemotherapy terminated (date)
       - Complete
       - Incomplete
5. *Tuberculosis suspect* (Diagnosis Pending)
   - *Chemotherapy Status*
     - None
     - On chemotherapy since (date)

(Summarized from Diagnostic standards and classification of tuberculosis and other mycobacterial disease. Am Rev Resp Dis 123:343, 1981

ogram, a positive tuberculin skin test, or cultures which grow *M. tuberculosis*. To be practical, any system for recognition of tuberculosis must be incorporated into the routine daily pattern of medical practice. The clinical circumstances in which a diagnosis of tuberculosis should be actively pursued must be recognized and a practical diagnostic approach applied. This can be most logically approached by relating it to the host–parasite relationships that are the basis for the new diagnostic standards (see list at left).

0. NO TUBERCULOSIS EXPOSURE, NOT INFECTED

It is important to query each patient during initial evaluation as to exposure to persons with known tuberculosis (especially a close or prolonged exposure), even when they are asymptomatic. During an initial comprehensive evaluation a tuberculin skin test should be applied similar to other screening procedures, such as blood pressure measurement, blood count, blood urea nitrogen or creatinine, blood sugar, or urine analysis. This skin test is commonly applied during the first 2 years of life and before school entrance. It is reasonable to repeat it in early adulthood and at the time of hospitalization for an illness or surgical procedure in subsequent years. Exact guidelines for the frequency of tuberculin skin testing in persons without known exposure or other reasons to suspect tuberculosis are not available. The need for this evaluation also depends on the risk in a given population. Individuals with no history of exposure and a tuberculin reaction that is not significant generally require no further medical response concerning tuberculosis. However, if a patient has a compatible clinical picture, this lack of history of exposure and significant reaction does not exclude the diagnosis of tuberculosis. Such a patient requires further evaluation.

1. TUBERCULOSIS EXPOSURE, NO EVIDENCE OF INFECTION

If an individual relates a history of exposure to a person with tuberculosis, a tuberculin skin test should be applied. If the exposure was within the preceding 3 months, then a repeat tuberculin skin test about 3 months after exposure is essential. It generally takes about 6 weeks (2 to 10 weeks) for the development of delayed hypersensitivity to manifest as a positive tuberculin skin test. Careful evaluation of recently exposed individuals, especially household or other close contacts, is especially important since they represent a population who have an unacceptably high risk of progressing to disease. Even if the initial skin test is negative, the risk of developing disease in the first year has been estimated at 2.5% or 1 in 40.[47]

2. TUBERCULOSIS INFECTION, NO DISEASE

Infection has been defined as a significant reaction to a tuberculin skin test in a person with no evidence of mycobacterial disease. Thus, the chest roentgenogram should not have findings compatible with tuberculosis. There should be no symptoms due to tuberculosis and any bacteriologic studies for mycobacteria should be negative. While a significant tuberculin test indicates that tuberculous pathology exists somewhere in the body, the term *infection* is used since there are no symptoms or perceptible evidence of a morbid process that would warrant the term *disease*.

If a person has a significant tuberculin skin test, a chest roentgenogram should be obtained. If it is abnormal, further evaluation is necessary —specifically, retrieving old chest roentgenograms to identify change, if any; and studies for mycobacteria. Such studies will permit appropriate therapy and place the patient in Class 3 to 5. If the chest roentgenogram is negative, the individual belongs in Class 2 (unless extrapulmonary tuberculosis is identified). Calcified foci in lung parenchyma or lymph nodes are considered negative in this context. They could represent other granulomatous infections, and available evidence does not indicate that such individuals have a significantly increased risk of developing tuberculosis.

The risk of developing tuberculosis for an adult positive tuberculin reactor with a normal chest roentgenogram has been reported between 27:100,000 to 82:100,000 (0.03% to 0.08%) per year.[48,49] With various assumptions the risk to a person with a negative tuberculin in the US in 1975 has been estimated at 30:100,000 (0.03%).[21] This indicates that a person with a positive tuberculin without other risk factors has only a slightly greater chance of developing tuberculosis. However, when selected subsets of the populations are evaluated, a definite increased risk has been identified: in adolescents followed for two-and-a-half years the risk was 204:100,000 (0.2%);[50] in tuberculin converters it was 3.3% or 1:30; and in household contacts of new cases of tuberculosis it was 5% or 1:20.[47] An increased risk of progressing from infection to disease also exists in the following special clinical circumstances: (1) treatment with corticosteroids or other immunosuppressive drugs, including chemotherapy of tumors; (2) hematologic or reticuloendothelial diseases (*e.g.*, leukemia, lymphoma); (3) silicosis; (4) diabetes mellitus that is unstable, and (5) after gastrectomy.[47,51]

3. TUBERCULOSIS, CURRENT DISEASE

This category identifies individuals with or without symptoms who have evidence of current disease, such as an abnormal chest roentgenogram, and in whom the diagnosis is ideally confirmed by cultural proof of *M. tuberculosis.*

Class 3 includes all cases of current tuberculosis where diagnostic procedures are complete. If a diagnosis is pending, the individual is a tuberculosis suspect (Class 5). The predominant location of disease, bacteriologic and chemotherapeutic status, must be listed. Other sites involved, roentgenogram findings, and tuberculin reactions may be listed—for example, abnormal chest roentgenogram (unilateral hilar enlargement) with a parent with proven smear positive tuberculosis—would be diagnosed and treated as Tuberculosis, Current Disease (Class 3) without bacteriologic proof. With such a person the roentgenogram and skin test findings should be recorded. It must again be emphasized that those persons who fail to recognize symptoms or are asymptomatic can only be recognized through a history of exposure, an abnormal chest roentgenogram, a positive tuberculin skin test, or culture of *M. tuberculosis*. These people represent a sizable percentage of patients with tuberculosis; despite this knowledge the clinician is constantly surprised at the absence or scarcity of symptoms, even with extensive widespread disease. Excluding this group, patients with disease can be characterized as having generalized or systemic signs and symptoms, pulmonary signs and symptoms, signs and symptoms related to specific organ involvement (these will be discussed in relation to specific organ involvement), or a combination of these.[52]

Generalized or Systemic Signs and Symptoms

The usual onset of disease is characterized by the recognition of very slowly progressive fatigue, lethargy, anorexia, weight loss, irregular menses, ill-defined anxiety or low-grade fevers over weeks to months. The fevers classically occur in the afternoon and may be accompanied by defervescence and sweating at night (a nonspecific symptom). Often these vague symptoms are attributed to emotional stress or excessive work. Less commonly there is an acute onset with spiking temperatures, chills, myalgia, sweating, and generalized weakness not uncommonly attributed to an influenza-like illness. Even then medical attention may not be sought until the symptoms fail to clear over many days to weeks. These acute symptoms may be superimposed on the chronic pattern. Occasionally erythema nodosum signals the initial tuberculous infection.

Pulmonary Signs and Symptoms

Disease is heralded by the almost imperceptible onset of a cough which becomes more frequent over weeks to months. It is associated with the production of mucoid or mucopurulent sputum. Occasionally this is blood-streaked, but a large amount of blood (hemoptysis) is initially quite uncommon. There may be tightness or dull, aching pain in the chest. Dyspnea is also uncommon and may indicate other cardiopulmonary disease or a massive pleural effusion. However, patients do occasionally present in severe respiratory distress due to extensive parenchymal disease. They may be in severe respiratory failure requiring not only oxygen but total ventilatory support. Some patients acutely develop a productive cough, fever, chills, myalgia, and sweating, suggesting influenza, acute bronchitis, or pneumonia. This acute toxic febrile presentation is not so unusual as to warrant the exclusion of tuberculosis from diagnostic considerations. Children with pulmonary tuberculosis rarely cough. If there is pleural involvement the patient may have acute or recurrent pleuritic pain.

Physical examination of the chest, while usually abnormal, is in no way specific for tuberculosis. One may expect to find some dullness to percussion over involved parenchymal areas, associated bronchial breath sounds, rales, and increased transmission of spoken or whispered sounds. Rales may sometimes be recognized by having the patient let out almost all his breath, approaching residual volume, and then without taking in any air, gently coughing. Rales identified in this manner have been called "post tussive" rales; they are not specific for tuberculosis. Partial obstruction of a bronchus due to endobronchial disease or compression by lymph nodes may produce localized wheezing, particularly with a forced expiration. Extensive parenchymal necrosis may lead to volume loss, particularly of the upper lobes. This can frequently be identified by deviation of the trachea to one side or the other, detected by palpating deeply in the sternal notch. With pleural effusion there may be dullness, absence of breath sounds, and decreased-to-absent transmission of spoken or whispered sounds.

TUBERCULIN SKIN TESTS

The tuberculin skin test, first used by Robert Koch in the late 19th century, relies on the delayed hypersensitivity that develops in a person following mycobacterial infection. It is the most sensitive indicator of tuberculous infection. This cell-mediated or Type IV reaction is manifested by induration at the site of antigen injection in a sensitized person. Such a person is a "reactor." Reactor status is not synonymous with infection with *M. tuberculosis.* Infection with other mycobacteria, which are distributed worldwide, may result in a cross-reaction. In general, larger reactions with a given dose of antigen are more likely to be specific (*i.e.*, due to infection with the mycobacteria from which the antigen was derived).[6,53]

ANTIGENS

Two tuberculins are available. Old tuberculin (OT) is derived from heat-sterilized cultures of tubercle bacilli; the dead bacilli are filtered off and the filtrate is evaporated to one-tenth its original volume. Purified protein derivative (PPD) is a filtrate of heat-killed cultures of tubercle bacilli that have been grown on synthetic media and precipitated with trichloracetic acid or neutral ammonium sulfate. PPD-S was prepared by Dr. F. Seibert in 1939 from Batch No. 49608 and sent to the Division of Biologic Standards, National Institutes of Health, Bethesda, Maryland, as the US Standard; it was adopted by the World Health Organization as the International PPD-Tuberculin in 1952.[54] All other PPD-tuberculins should be designated by lot number and producer. Today, PPD-tuberculins are standardized as bioequivalent to PPD-S rather than by protein weight; 0.1 ml of PPD-tuberculin solution is equivalent to 5 tuberculin units (TU). This is commonly called the PPD-tuberculin intermediate. Since PPD is more specific and better standardized it is the preferable antigen. Currently available products have been stabilized by the addition of polysorbate 80 (Tween 80) to prevent the adsorption of the tuberculoprotein onto a glass or plastic surface. Prior to the addition of polysorbate 80 it had been shown that up to 25% of the tuberculin activity in a syringe could be lost in 20 min and more than 80% after 24 hr.[55] In addition, light will reduce potency of tuberculin stabilized with polysorbate stored in clear glass containers.[56]

At various times other strengths of tuberculin have been used (*e.g.*, 1 TU, 5 TU, 250 TU). The first strength (1 TU) was recommended to avoid untoward local or systemic reactions. Since even local untoward reactions of any severity are so uncommon and since very little epidemiologic information necessary for interpretation of reactions to 1 TU is available, its use is not recommended.[57] The second-strength tuberculin (PPD-2, 250 TU) is less specific; it has more cross-reactivity because of the larger amount of antigen. Therefore a positive reaction to PPD-2 adds little to the diagnostic evaluation. However, a negative response to a PPD-2 in an individual with intact delayed hypersensitivity does contribute to lessening the probability of a diagnosis of tuberculosis, since the larger dose of antigen elicits a positive response in a greater number of patients with tuberculosis than does a 5 TU dose. However, even the PPD-2 may not produce a significant reaction in up to 6% of patients with proven tuberculosis.[58] The PPD intermediate has been reported as not significant in from less than 1% to 15% of patients with proven tuberculosis in careful studies.[6,53,57–63]

Antigens have been prepared from other mycobacteria and have provided important epidemiological information about the distribution of these mycobacterial infections, particularly in the United States. In particular, PPD-Battey (PPD-B), prepared from a strain of *M. intracellulare* has been used extensively in dual skin testing with a PPD-tuberculin. In such surveys when the reaction to PPD-tuberculin has been between 6 and 9 mm and the reaction to PPD-B has been 5 mm or more larger, follow-up evaluations have indicated that the *infection* was with mycobacteria other than *M. tuberculosis.*[64] However, in an individual patient with disease, the lack of specificity of the other mycobacterial antigens is so great that they are of little or no value. In our experience and that of others with disease proven to be caused by other mycobacteria, the PPD-tuberculin reaction has commonly been larger, or conversely, with such frequency that we do not use them to differentiate the causative mycobacteria. At the present time this can only be done with cultures.[6,53,57,65]

TYPES OF TESTS

There are two basic types of tests in current use: the multiple-puncture techniques (Tine, Heaf, and Mono-vac), and the intracutaneous technique (jet injection or intracutaneous injection, Mantoux).

The multiple puncture (Tine, Heaf, Mono-vac) and the jet-injection techniques suffer from an inability to standardize the amount of concentrated tuberculin administered. Their advantages are better patient acceptance, particularly in children, and the ready-to-use nature of the Tine and Mono-vac. Induration without vesiculation should be confirmed with an intradermal Mantoux test with PPD-tuberculin (5 TU). Each of these techniques, because of their patient acceptance, rapidity, and ease of use, can be very effectively used in screening large population groups or in physicians' offices. However, they are not recommended for evaluation of an individual patient in whom the diagnosis of tuberculosis is suspected, in evaluations of close contacts of patients with tuberculosis, or in periodic surveillance programs to detect newly infected personnel.[6,57]

The intracutaneous (Mantoux) test is the standard test; it should be used whenever a diagnosis of tuberculosis or tuberculous infection is suspected, and to confirm reactions manifested by induration without vesiculation to screening tests. It is performed by the intracutaneous injection of 0.1 ml of PPD-tuberculin containing 5 TU (standardized by biologic activity), preferably into the skin of either the volar or dorsal area of the forearm. Other areas may be used, such as the suprascapular area in an elderly person with very thin and loose skin where difficulty is encountered in injecting within the dermis. A short (1 cm), bluntly beveled, platinum (26-gauge) or steel (27-gauge) needle with the needle bevel upward and a glass or plastic tuberculin syringe should be used. The injection of 0.1 ml should produce a discrete pale skin elevation, a wheal of 6 to 10 mm in diameter. However, the size may vary depending on skin conditions, and one should attempt to inject the entire 0.1 ml intracutaneously. If the tuberculin is injected subcutaneously, it is recommended that a second injection intracutaneously be made at least 5 cm away.

READING AND RECORDING

The reaction should be read 48 to 72 hr after the injection. However, little change in size occurs before the fifth day. *The reaction should be recorded as the diameter of induration in millimeters,* measured transversely to the long axis of the forearm; some also record the diameter of induration in millimeters parallel to the long axis of the forearm as a second measurement. Readings should be made in a good light; an oblique light often helps to identify the raised indurated area. Erythema is not measured since its relation to infection is not known. The indurated area should be carefully palpated; moistening the fingers or the area may help. A line drawn with a ballpoint pen toward the area may deviate when reaching induration. The diameter of induration must be measured with a ruler. A caliper with a millimeter ruler may be most accurate.[66]

This measurement of a biologic event has inherent variability. To this is added the unavoidable inter- and intra-observer variability. These can be minimized by careful measurement, preferably by an experienced observer.

INTERPRETATION

Our knowledge of the significance of the tuberculin reaction, the amount of induration, is based on large epidemiologic surveys of patients with documented tuberculosis, or with mycobacterial disease caused by other organisms, and individuals without known tuberculosis. People with disease due to *M. tuberculosis* generally have reactions between 15 and 20 mm induration, with few below 5 mm or over 30 mm. The distribution is unimodal; these are not two distinct populations of infected and not-infected.[53,66] The data does permit the development of statistical probabilities. The more sensitive the test is made (identifying individuals who have a given characteristic), the more likely the test is to be less specific (incorrectly identifying individuals who do not have the chosen characteristic). The selection of a given measurement as significant is therefore best determined by the intended use of the measurement. The available data indicate that 10 mm or more of induration identifies 90% or more of those truly infected with *M. tuberculosis* (sensitivity) with a low number of individuals identified falsely as infected (specificity). However, when evaluating high-risk groups such as suspects or close contacts of individuals with tuberculosis, a reaction of 5 mm induration or more is considered significant; this will identify more individuals as infected (greater sensitivity), but will include false positives more frequently (less specificity). Thus, the *interpretation* of the reaction is based appropriately on its *clinical use* rather than selecting a mm cut-off on a continuum. It must be emphasized that some patients with tuberculosis will have no reaction to tuberculin; *a negative tuberculin reaction cannot exclude the diagnosis of tuberculosis.*[6]

FACTORS AFFECTING REACTIONS

The problems of variable antigenicity and antigen adsorption are no longer significant in North America. However, the tuberculin must be protected from light exposure and should not be transferred from one container to another. It should be injected immediately after the syringe is filled. The reaction may be smaller if injected subcutaneously. The most common problem is careless measurement of reaction size, which is avoidable.

False-negative reactions may occur when cell-mediated reactions are decreased or absent. This may result from any severe or overwhelming febrile illness, including tuberculosis, measles, or probably other acute infectious diseases, live-virus vaccination, Hodgkin's disease, sarcoidosis, adrenal corticosteroid therapy, or other immunosuppressive drugs.[66] In patients who fail to react to PPD-tuberculin, the system of cellular immunity may be assessed by skin testing with a battery of other antigens to which almost all people have been sensitized: Candida; Trichophyton; mumps; dichloronitrobenzene (DCNB), which requires induction of sensitization; streptokinase-streptodornase (SKSD); or even lymphocyte transformation studies.[6] However, lack of reaction to tuberculin (even to 250 TU) in a patient with a reaction to one of the nonspecific markers of cellular immunity, does not exclude the possibility of tuberculosis.[67] There may be a decreased number or responsiveness *in vitro* of circulating T lymphocytes which may be specific for PPD. This may occur because of: (1) serum inhibitors such as serum immunoglobins, antibodies, or circulating antigen-antibody complexes; (2) a faulty inflammatory response, perhaps due to defective lymphokine production or serum inhibitors of polymorphonuclear leukocyte and monocyte chemotaxis; (3) compartmentalization of lymphocytes (in lymph nodes); (4) adherent suppressor cells; and (5) suppressor T lymphocytes.[68] A false-positive reaction may occur following a blood transfusion from a tuberculin-positive individual.[69] Tuberculin sensitivity tends to wane with age. This is particularly evident in those age 50 to 55 yr or older. In this age group a first tuberculin skin test, or one after many years, may give a small reaction or none at all. If a second skin test is applied within a week, a larger reaction in the positive range may appear and will last for at least 1 yr. This so-called booster effect is considered analogous to an anamnestic reaction in serology. This is not considered to be a sensitizing effect since repeated testing after the second test does not increase the response.[66] However, because of this booster effect which does occur even in young people, it is now recommended that if the reaction to 5 TU is less than 10 mm in periodic surveillance programs (*e.g.*, hospital personnel, mental institutions, prisons, old age homes), a second test be given within a week (two-stage testing) to avoid the incorrect identification of an individual as a converter when subsequently tested.[6,70,71]

ROENTGENOGRAPHIC EXAMINATION OF THE CHEST

While the tuberculin skin test is the most sensitive indicator of tuberculous infection, it does not document the presence of disease. Disease is most commonly recognized with the standard posterior–anterior (PA) and lateral chest roentgenograms. The PA film alone is inadequate since it fails to visualize approximately 25% of the lung fields. The apical lordotic view is of value in exposing lesions in the apical and subapical areas hidden by the bony thorax and in better defining middle-lobe collapse. Oblique views may aid in seeing lesions obscured by other structures, such as the heart.[72] Laminograms, planigrams, or body-section roentgenograms help in defining nodules, cavities or cysts, calcifications, contours of large bronchi, and vascular details. On occasion bronchography may be of value in identifying bronchiectasis or bronchostenosis, although the identification of the former seldom alters therapy and the latter can be seen at bronchoscopy. Because fluoroscopy exposes the patient and the examiner to larger amounts of radiation, its use should be limited to identifying localized lesions during diagnostic studies, such as bronchoscopy with peripheral biopsy or brushing, percutaneous lung biopsy, or during differential bronchospirometry, bronchography, and on occasion placement of catheters into the pulmonary vasculature.

FIG. 9-6. Posterior–anterior chest roentgenogram with enlargement of right hilum and slight infiltrate in apical segment of right upper lobe. This 25-year-old white male had a cough productive of small amounts of sputum for several weeks. PPD tuberculin intermediate measured 14 mm of induration. A biopsy of a narrowed right upper lobe orifice confirmed caseating granuloma. This was an initial tuberculous infection in an adult.

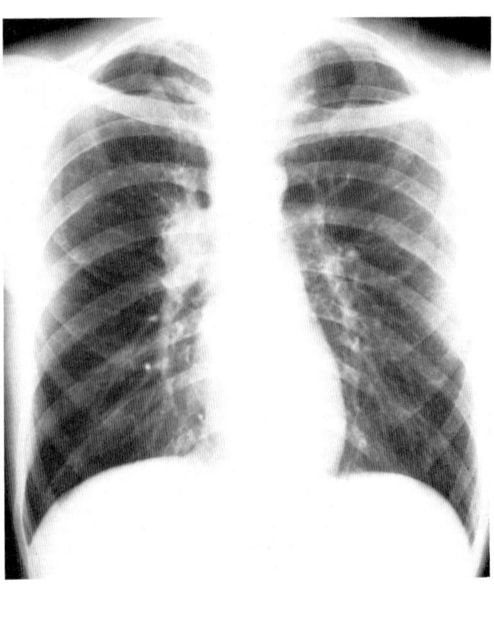

The initial manifestation of tuberculous involvement of the lung is usually a parenchyma–lymph node complex. The parenchymal lesion may be so small as not to be seen and initially is quite nonspecific. Characteristically in initial infection hilar or, somewhat less commonly, paratracheal lymph node involvement is seen (Fig. 9-6). In one series 80 of 83 children had hilar node enlargement and in the other three, central parenchymal involvement did not permit node assessment. In 13 of these children the hilar enlargement was equal bilaterally, and in the remaining 67 there was unilateral predominance.[73] In adults with initial infection, hilar node involvement was recognized in 43% of 37 patients.[74] At times hilar or paratracheal node involvement alone may be recognized.[75,76] Lymph node involvement tends to persist longer than parenchymal involvement. Parenchymal involvement even in the initial infection tends to be slightly more common in the upper than the lower lobes,[73] although some authors indicate it favors the superior segment of the lower lobe.[75] In children bronchial obstruction is considerably more common with resultant atelectasis (in 30% in one series); this is more common in the anterior segment of the upper lobe and the medial segment of the middle lobe. Cavitation and miliary disease are uncommon in children. Pleural involvement in initial infection in children approximates 10%. In one series parenchymal calcification was seen in 10% and lymph node calcification in 21%.[73] In children with initial infection about two-thirds completely resolve roentgenographic evidence of disease.[77]

In the characteristic presentation of tuberculosis in adults, most commonly due to exacerbation of an old initial infection, the lesions involve predominantly the apical and posterior segments of the upper lobes (85% in one series); and the superior segment of the lower lobes (9.5% in the same series; see Fig. 9-7).[72,78] *Isolated* involvement of an anterior segment of the upper lobe or the middle lobe is far less common, but it does occur. Therefore, tuberculosis should not be excluded from consideration under such circumstances.

While these non-specific initial nodular lesions of varying size are probably most common, tuberculosis also produces a necrotizing pneumonia. This characteristically leads to cavity formation and ultimately volume loss with associated elevation of the hilum and tracheal deviation (Figs. 9-8 and 9-10). Even this picture is not specific since it occurs in systemic fungal infections, sarcoidosis, lung carcinoma, Wegener's granulomatosis, and so forth. Lesions may also be lobar, segmental, or subsegmental, and simulate pyogenic bacterial pneumonia (Fig. 9-9). The characteristic pattern of hematogenous spread throughout the lungs results in small, 2-mm discrete nodules rather uniformly distributed throughout the lungs. They may appear larger in the upper lobes and may be seen more clearly behind the heart on the lateral roentgenogram. At times the lesions may appear considerably larger and coalesce (see Figs. 9-10 and 9-11). Although such a pattern may not be truly *miliary* (*i.e.*, the size of a millet seed), it can represent hematogenous dissemination. Thus the insistence on very small nodules serves little purpose.

Pleural effusion, usually unilateral, may be the only manifestation of tuberculosis. It is important to emphasize that tuberculosis may produce just about any chest roentgenographic abnormality and that no abnormality is specific for tuberculosis. Among the most common simulators of tuberculosis are the systemic mycoses, pulmonary fibrosis, neoplasm, sarcoidosis, lung abscess, and pneumonia.[79]

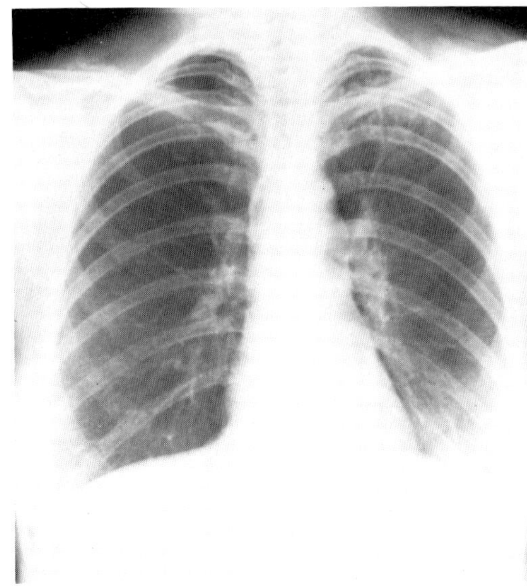

FIG. 9-7. Posterior–anterior chest roentgenogram with an infiltrate in the apical posterior segment of the left upper lobe. This 27-year-old female was asymptomatic except for a 5-pound weight loss and vague tiredness. The roentgenogram was obtained during preoperative evaluation for an elective surgical procedure. Auramine-rhodamine staining of a sputum smear was positive for mycobacteria. A culture grew *M. tuberculosis*.

PULMONARY PHYSIOLOGICAL CHANGES

No specific changes in pulmonary function occur with tuberculosis, although characteristically with extensive parenchymal disease a restrictive pattern is found. The vital capacity, total lung capacity, and other subunits of lung volume are reduced. Airways obstruction as manifested by a decreased FEV_1, FEV_1 percent, increased airways resistance, or an abnormal flow–volume curve may be seen with extensive fibrotic changes or endobronchial disease. However, these changes may well reflect concomitant chronic bronchitis and emphysema in older individuals, particularly smokers. Various studies of distribution of inhaled air, such as the single-breath nitrogen test, may be abnormal. There may be a widening of the alveolar–arterial oxygen gradient, but clinically significant hypoxemia even with extensive disease is

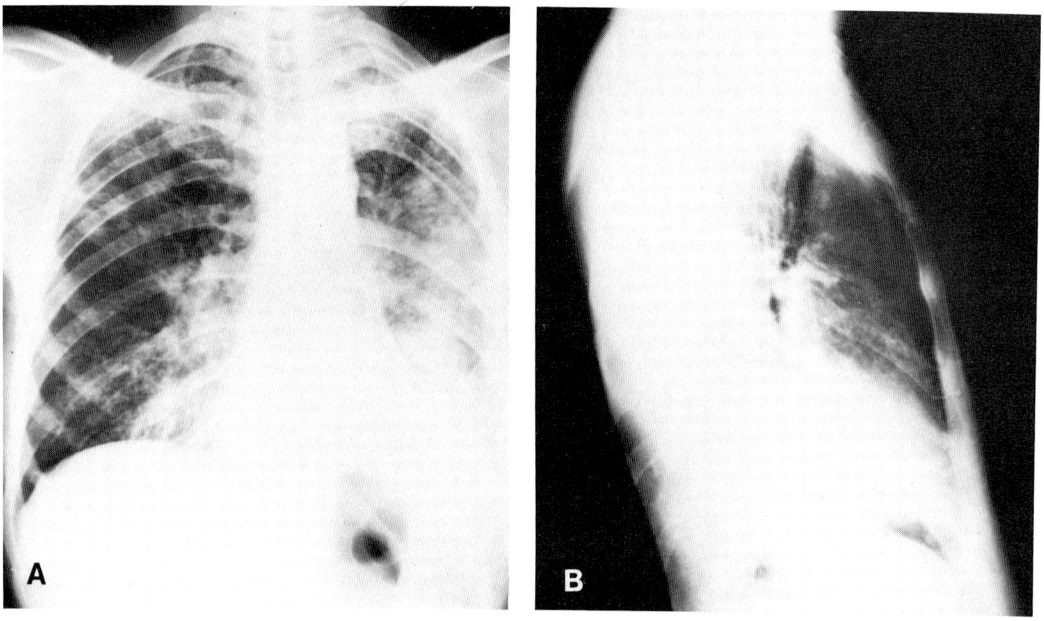

FIG. 9-8. Posterior–anterior (**A**) and lateral (**B**) chest roentgenograms wth extensive infiltrate and loss of volume throughout the left lung, which obscures the left heart border (lingula involved), but predominantly involves the left lower lobe. There are scattered infiltrates throughout the right lung. This 33-year-old inner-city male laborer had noticed fatigue, a productive cough, and malaise for 2 months. Two days before admission he became acutely ill, coughing up 4 to 5 ounces of purulent sputum each day, with progressive dyspnea even at rest and a temperature of 101°F.

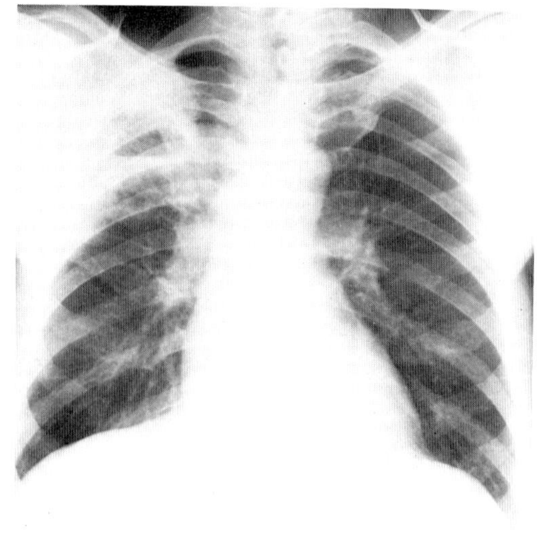

FIG. 9-9. Posterior–anterior chest roentgenogram with a 5 cm cavity in the right upper lobe and some elevation of the minor fissure. This 62-year-old lone alcoholic, sometime laborer was seen in the emergency room with a temperature of 103°F. He was toxic and coughing up large amounts of purulent sputum. Organisms seen on Gram stain were 90+% gram negative. Three blood cultures grew *E. coli.* Acid-fast smears of sputum were positive and cultures grew *M. tuberculosis.* In the presence of a temperature over 102°F, clinical signs of toxicity, advanced age, an elevated white blood cell count, and a roentgenographic picture compatible with cavitary tuberculosis, gram negative infections superimposed on tuberculosis should be considered.

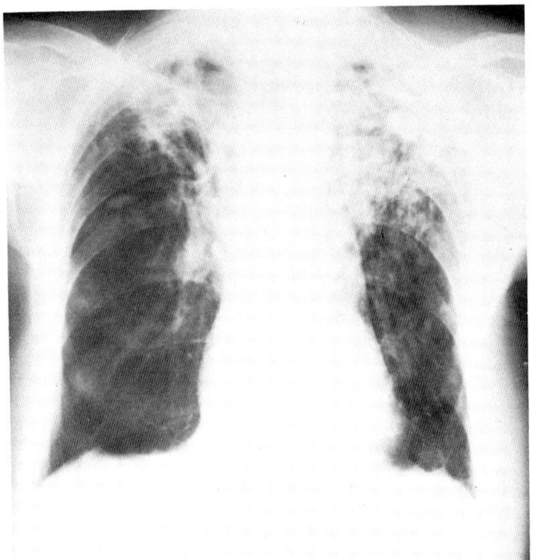

FIG. 9-10. Posterior–anterior chest roentgenogram with extensive bilateral disease. Both hilar areas are retracted upward, indicating volume loss. There are extensive bilateral infiltrates with multiple circular lucencies (cavities) and irregular, more linear lucencies (bronchiectasis). There are smaller nodular areas throughout both lung fields. The diaphragms are flattened. This 72-year-old man had his tuberculosis adequately treated 7 years ago and complained only of dyspnea. Cultures for tuberculosis were negative. Serial chest roentgenograms were unchanged. A single chest roentgenogram does not permit judgments concerning roentgenographic stability or mycobacteriologic status.

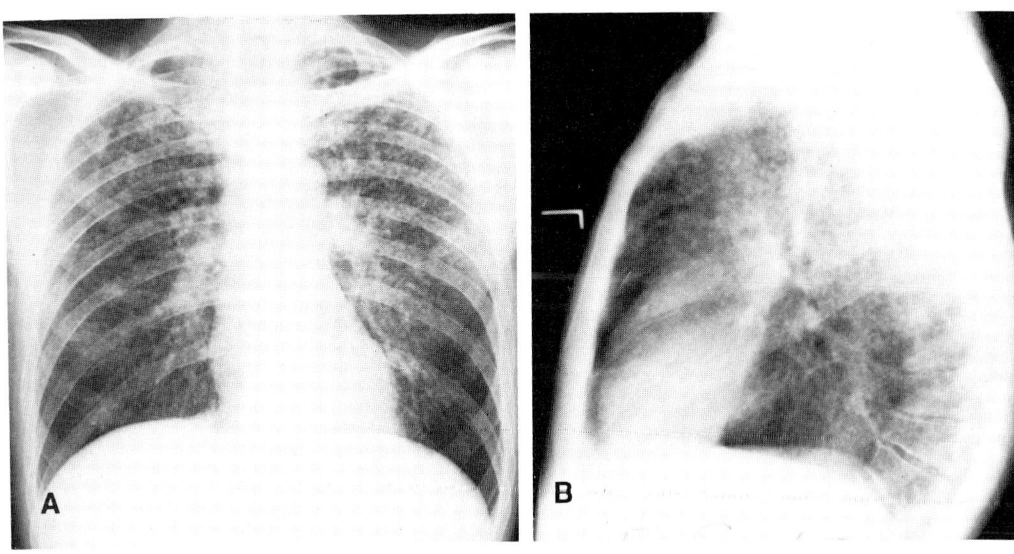

FIG. 9-11. Posterior–anterior **(A)** and lateral **(B)** chest roentgenograms with a myriad of bilateral nodules, 2 to 3 mm in diameter. The lateral view displays the nodules more clearly in the retrosternal and retrocardiac areas. This 39-year-old male had been chronically ill for 4 months with a weight loss of 10 pounds, a dry cough, anorexia, and almost daily sensation of fever. A PPD tuberculin intermediate skin test developed 11 mm of induration. Sputum for mycobacteria was negative on smear and culture. A percutaneous needle lung biopsy demonstrated caseating granuloma, and acid-fast bacilli were seen.

uncommon. This is probably a reflection of the necrotizing process which destroys pulmonary vessels as well as alveoli, resulting in what some have called an autopneumonectomy. During moderate exercise the arterial oxygen tension is generally quite well maintained. There may be some decrease in the diffusing capacity with extensive disease; this test appears to correlate fairly well with the degree of roentgenographic abnormality. When the disease is extensive, pulmonary hypertension and cor pulmonale may occur, related primarily to destruction of the vascular bed rather than hypoxemia. Extensive pleural or chest wall changes, such as occurred after pneumothorax therapy and thoracoplasty, may result in severe restrictive disease and cor pulmonale. Hypercarbia is seldom seen in the absence of concomitant chronic obstructive pulmonary disease.[80,81] In the sick and tachypneic individual with tuberculosis, arterial blood gases are recommended to identify, in particular, hypoxemia and to guide appropriate oxygen therapy; they will also identify hypoventilation. More extensive studies including the use of ventilation–perfusion scans and/or differential bronchospirometry may be of value in assessing regional lung function. These would be particularly helpful in considering the merits of pleural decortication, resectional surgery, plombage or thoracoplasty for mycobacterial disease, and the more common individual who may require surgical resection of a coexistent carcinoma. They may also be of value in documenting the extent of disability resulting from tuberculosis along with the entire clinical picture. However, disability due to lung destruction from tuberculosis without coexisting chronic obstructive pulmonary disease is uncommon.

Acute pneumonic tuberculosis such as may be seen with endobronchial spread may affect lung function like any other pneumonia, producing areas with decreased ventilation and intrapulmonic shunts manifested by severe hypoxemia. Similar changes may occur with extensive miliary or hematogenous dissemination. Either of these patterns may result in severe acute respiratory failure requiring not only oxygen, but total ventilatory support.[81–83] (see Chap. 7, Acute Respiratory Failure). While the number of patients with severe respiratory failure is not large, they are seen with unfortunate regularity in large city and county hospitals caring for the indigent with tuberculosis.

DEMONSTRATION OF TUBERCLE BACILLI

In order to make a definite diagnosis of tuberculosis, the organism *M. tuberculosis* must be cultured from clinical specimens. This demands vigorous and careful attention to collection of specimens and their prompt delivery to a laboratory qualified in mycobacteriology. It is essential that the clinician communicate with the laboratory to assure that specimens are submitted to the exact specifications of the laboratory. Although a diagnosis of tuberculosis on the basis of the total clinical picture, roentgenographic findings, tuberculin skin test and/or response to specific antituberculous chemotherapy may be warranted in special circumstances, every effort should be made to obtain adequate specimens for culture prior to the institution of specific antituberculous chemotherapy. Even the identification of acid-fast bacteria on smear or culture does not confirm the diagnosis of *M. tuberculosis.* Other mycobacteria are acid-fast and fluoresce. Nocardia, Actinomyces and the Pittsburgh Pneumonia Agent may take the acid-fast stain.[84]

SPECIMEN COLLECTION

In general, three 5- to 10-ml specimens of spontaneously produced sputum, collected over a short period, should be obtained. The patient must be instructed not to submit saliva or nasopharyngeal contents, but rather the material raised from the lungs after a cough. Early morning specimens are preferable. Pooled specimens collected over 12 to 24 hours may occasionally help; however, their increased contamination with other organisms over this period seriously limits their value.

If the patient cannot spontaneously produce sputum, it is induced with a 3 to 10% NaCl solution delivered through a heated aerosol generator or ultrasonic nebulizer. Since this produces vigorous coughing, this should be accomplished in a sputum induction booth equipped with an exhaust fan or in a portable hood with appropriate filters. A patient with asthma, chronic bronchitis, or emphysema, should be observed carefully since hypertonic solutions can produce severe bronchospasm. Bronchospasm may be ameliorated by pretreatment with a nebulized bronchodilator. Although induced sputum may appear quite thin and watery, it should be processed.

For the occasional patient who does not raise

sputum, gastric contents may be studied. After a fast of 8 to 10 hours and before arising from bed or brushing one's teeth, about 50 ml of gastric contents should be aspirated which may include tubercle bacilli swallowed overnight. Microscopic examinations of such specimens are of little value, although culture results are useful.[85]

Collection of material by tracheal suction after instilling 5 to 10 ml of saline without a bacteriostatic may be of value in patients who are too ill to cough effectively; the transtracheal technique is sometimes recommended. In a patient who cannot produce sputum, positive results may be obtained from washings obtained at bronchoscopy or in the sputum raised over the next several days. Recent experience indicates that brushing and/or biopsying through the flexible fiberoptic bronchoscope may increase the number of definite diagnoses with localized disease or with miliary disease.[86] In selected patients biopsy of lung tissue through the bronchoscope, via a percutaneous needle biopsy or open biopsy, continues to play an important role when routine studies fail to establish a diagnosis.[87,88] It should be emphasized that such invasive techniques are needed in only a small number of patients after other efforts have failed. Collection of other specimens will be discussed in relation to specific organ involvement. In certain clinical circumstances many physicians will eschew the need for bacteriological confirmation (*e.g.*, a small child with a positive PPD-tuberculin skin test and unilateral hilar node enlargement on chest roentgenogram who has been closely exposed to a parent with tuberculosis who has positive smears).

STAINING AND MICROSCOPY

Smears of sputum or other body fluids are generally stained with an acid-fast stain such as the Ziehl-Neelsen or a fluorochrome procedure which utilizes auramine and rhodamine for staining and examined either with ultraviolet or bright light illumination.[89–91] The fluorochrome technique is considerably more sensitive and less time-consuming for experienced technicians. The Center for Disease Control method provides an estimate of the number of acid-fast bacilli observed in 1,10, or 100 fields (F) when examined at 800–1000× (see Table 9-2).

TABLE 9-2. Standard Reporting of Smears With Acid-Fast Bacilli

Number AFB Observed	Reporting of Acid-Fast Bacilli on Smear, CDC Report	
0	Negative	(−)
1-2/300F	Number seen	(±)
1-9/100F	Average No./100F	(1+)
1-9/10F	Average No./10F	(2+)
1-9/F	Average No./F	(3+)
9/F	>9F	(4+)

Counts less than 3/300F are not considered positive; procedure should be repeated. (Smithwick RW: Laboratory manual for acid-fast microscopy, 2nd ed. Atlanta, Center for Disease Control, 1976).

DIGESTION AND DECONTAMINATION OF SPECIMENS

Since mycobacteria have an 18- to 24-hr generation time, other bacterial and fungal contaminants in most clinical specimens will overgrow the mycobacteria. The organic debris in the specimen is liquefied to permit a decontamination agent to reach unwanted microbes and to allow the mycobacteria access to the nutrient medium; N-acetyl cysteine and/or sodium hydroxide are generally used.[6,89–91]

CULTURE OF MYCOBACTERIA

Culture on appropriate media can detect as few as 10 mycobacteria per ml of digested concentrated material. Two general categories of media should be used: egg-potato base (Lowenstein-Jensen [L-J], American Trudeau Society [ATS]); and agar media (Middlebrook 7H-10, Middlebrook 7H-11, Dubos oleic albumin). An atmosphere with 5 to 10% carbon dioxide enhances growth. The following reporting system is recommended: no colonies—negative; fewer than 50 colonies—actual count; 50 to 100 colonies—1+; 100 to 200 colonies—2+; almost confluence (200 to 500 colonies)—3+; confluence (500 colonies)—4+.[6] Identification of mycobacteria should include culture characteristics, biochemical studies, and, on occasion, phage studies. *M. tuberculosis* grows as rough, nonpigmented, corded colonies on oleic-acid albumin agars. It produces a positive niacin test and a positive nitrate reduction test, and has weak catalase activity which is eliminated by heating to 68°C. Isoniazid-resistant organisms tend to grow more poorly or not at all and have a very weak or absent catalase activity. Growth and identification of the organisms generally require 2 to 8 wk.[6]

DRUG SUSCEPTIBILITY TESTING

Although all mycobacteria cultured should be identified, there is increasing agreement that susceptibility testing need not be routinely performed. *M. tuberculosis* organisms isolated from people never treated for tuberculosis have a very low and unchanging rate of drug resistance to the usual chemotherapeutic agents. This is particularly true in Canada, Western Europe, and the United States.[92–95] Routine drug-susceptibility studies on cultures from such people are very expensive and time-consuming. On the other hand, drug-susceptibility studies of cultures are clearly warranted for a previously treated individual, for a person in whom treatment is failing, for people from areas where drug resistance is quite common, such as Southeast Asia, or where the index case is known to have drug-resistant organisms.[95] They are necessary to intelligently manage treatment along with clinical and radiographic information. Additional details of laboratory methods, criteria for identification of mycobacteria, and drug-susceptibility testing are available.[6,93–99]

EXTRAPULMONARY TUBERCULOSIS

While the overall incidence of tuberculosis continues to decrease, the incidence of extrapulmonary tuberculosis in the US remains relatively unchanged. During the last 16 years the total number of extrapulmonary cases reported each year has remained constant at about 4000 per year while the number of pulmonary cases has decreased. Thus, the percentage of extrapulmonary cases has risen to 14.6% in 1978. In 1978, extrapulmonary tuberculosis was more common in the younger age groups, in nonwhites, and in females. Persons under age 45 accounted for 48% of extrapulmonary disease (*vs.* 36% of pulmonary); nonwhites about 49% of extrapulmonary (*vs.* 42% of pulmonary), and females 48% (*vs.* 32% of pulmonary.)[100] See Figure 9-12 for sites affected. This is an underestimate of the incidence of extrapulmonary tuberculosis, since extrapulmonary sites, with the exception of miliary tuberculosis, are commonly not reported if there is pulmonary involvement. Extrapulmonary tuberculosis represents a particularly difficult diagnostic problem when it affects older people who frequently have significant concomitant illness that may hinder the recognition of tuberculosis. Similarily, nonwhites from lower socioeconomic environments frequently have other diseases which may overshadow the recognition of tuberculosis. Patients requiring maintenance hemodialysis have increased risk of developing tuberculosis, particularly extrapulmonary; fever of unknown origin, anorexia, weight loss and/or hepatomegaly may be the signal findings.[101]

DISSEMINATED TUBERCULOSIS

The term *miliary* derives from the roentgenographic pattern of diffuse, uniform, discrete, nodular shadows about the size of a millet seed (about 2 mm), characteristically seen on the chest roentgenogram in hematogenously disseminated tuberculosis.[102,103] The roentgenographic pattern, however, is not always present and may appear considerably after the onset of symptoms.[104] This form of dissemination appears more commonly at the extremes of life, although it may occur at all ages. With decreased infection in infants, miliary disease is becoming less common in early life. Recent studies indicate a predominance of cases in individuals in their sixties and beyond.[105] Although patients may present acutely ill with fever, dyspnea, tachypnea, tachycardia, cyanosis, and, indeed, respiratory failure, a more chronic history is considerably more common. It is characterized by the insidi-

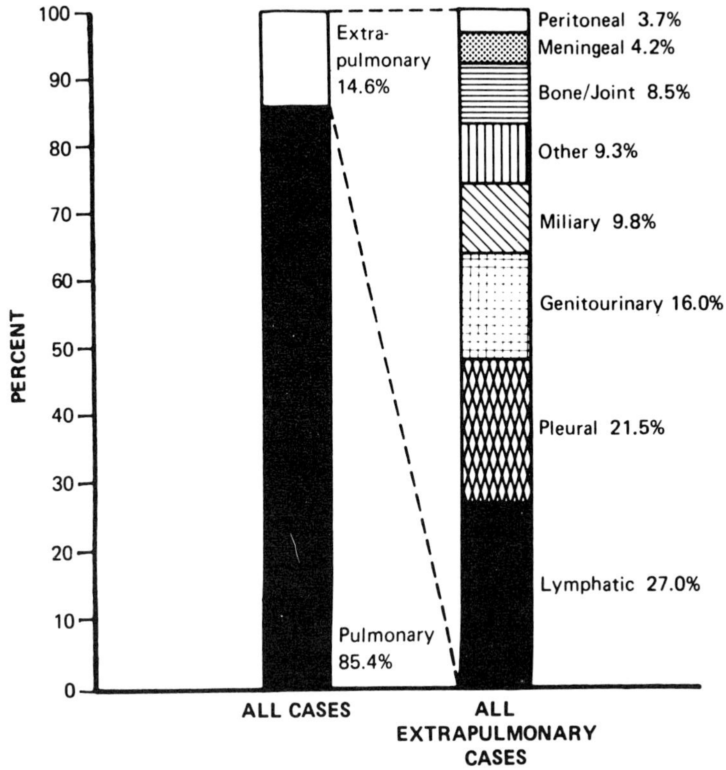

FIG. 9-12. Percent distribution of tuberculosis cases by form and site of disease, United States, 1978. (US Department of Health and Human Services, Public Health Service, Center for Disease Control, 1978: Tuberculosis in the United States, Publication No. [CDC] 808322, June, 1980)

ous onset of weight loss, fever, weakness, anorexia, fatigue, cough, dyspnea, headache, abdominal pain, and hemoptysis. In one recent series the mean duration of symptoms was almost 16 wk. Some patients had symptoms of 7 mo and one of two-and-a-half yr.[62] The complaint of headache is a strong indication of tuberculous meningitis, which occurs in about 30% of patients with miliary tuberculosis. Abdominal pain has been reported in about 10% of patients and correlates well with tuberculous enteritis or peritonitis. The initial signs that are most common are nonspecific: fever, inanition, tachycardia, tachypnea, and adventitious pulmonary signs (60 to 80%).[103] Less common signs include hepatomegaly (35%), lymphadenopathy (30%), nuchal rigidity (26%), and splenomegaly (12%).[62,103,105,106] Funduscopic examination may reveal choroidal tubercles. These are bilateral, grayish, oblong, indistinct lesions of about 1 mm in diameter with or without a central depression. Although they have been identified, with very careful examinations, in over 90% of children, in recent series of adults they have been observed in less than 10% of patients with miliary disease. Cutaneous lesions, including draining sinuses, abscesses, and ulcerations, are uncommon but important since smears and cultures of such lesions provide a high diagnostic yield.

Disseminated disease may present with only the previously described nonspecific systemic signs and symptoms and a protracted fever, without an obvious cause despite the usual diagnostic efforts. The chest roentgenogram may be normal or at least free of a miliary infiltrate. This presentation has been labeled as a "fever of unknown origin"[107] or "cryptic miliary tuberculosis."[108] Tuberculosis can quite frequently be confirmed by intensive, systematic, and often repetitive diagnostic studies including chest roentgenograms; tuberculin skin tests; studies of cerebrospinal, pleural, peritoneal, pericardial, and joint fluid; biopsy and culture of abnormal organs such as lung, pleura, liver and peritoneum; biopsy and culture of bone marrow; and even on occasion an exploratory laparotomy.[103,105,107] Miliary or disseminated tuberculosis is still quite commonly unrecognized.[105] This is especially true in older patients where concomitant disease obscures the clinical picture. In one series miliary disease was not recognized until autopsy in 15 of 21 patients, most over age 70.[109] More recently the diagnosis of miliary tuberculosis in a large teaching hospital was suspected in only 4 of 28 patients on admission; diagnosis was made in 14 of the 28 in an average of 14 days; and most strikingly, the lack of recognition and initiation of treatment was considered to be the major contributor to 10 deaths, only two of which received antituberculous therapy.[110] A variety of nonspecific laboratory abnormalities commonly accompany disseminated or miliary disease. They include mild-to-moderate anemia with hematocrits of 20 to 37% in 59% of one series[62] and usually a normal white blood cell count with a relative increase in polymorphonuclear leukocytes. Lymphocytosis is uncommon. Less commonly, severe leukopenia, pancytopenia, aplastic anemia, and leukemoid reactions have been reported.[103,108,111,112] Liver-function studies are commonly mildly abnormal: bromsulfalein retention is increased in about 50% of cases; alkaline phosphatase is elevated in 33%; and mild elevations in serum glutamic oxaloacetic transaminase appear in up to 90%. Low serum albumin and, rarely, bilirubin elevation are noted. There may be alterations in coagulation factors, but disseminated intravascular coagulation rarely has been reported.[113] Hyponatremia and hypochloremia may accompany disseminated or newly diagnosed tuberculosis in up to 10% of cases.[114] This has been attributed to an acquired excess release of antidiuretic hormone[115] or release of a similar principal from the tuberculous lung tissue.[116]

MENINGEAL TUBERCULOSIS

Meningeal involvement may occur at any age but is particularly common in infants and small children as a complication of initial infection. It is also a common complication of miliary disease.[105] There may be involvement of the cerebral cortex, cerebellum, or spinal cord with spread into the subarachnoid space. Tuberculomas, which are masslike lesions, may form in brain tissue. The granulomatous inflammation may proceed to dense fibrocollagenous changes most severe at the base of the brain. Arteritis and thrombotic vascular occlusion may produce cranial neuropathy, cerebral infarction, or obstructive hydrocephalus. With increased intracranial pressure, herniation of the brain stem may occur.[37,117,118]

The clinical presentation is usually insidious, with altered mental behavior, headaches, irritability, and vomiting. There may be seizures, disorientation, cranial nerve signs, paresis of one or more of the extremities, and ultimately coma and opisthotonos. Nuchal rigidity is usually present. Cerebrospinal fluid examination reveals increased protein, increased cells (usually mononuclear), and reduced sugar when compared with a concomitant blood sugar. Added confirmation is subsequently obtained when common bacterial pathogens fail to grow. Although a recent report from India found acid-fast mycobacteria in 30% of cerebrospinal fluid smears, this appears to be exceptional.[118] The yield of mycobacteria on culture is generally good. Other infectious meningitides, including fungi and viruses, may simulate tuberculosis. They can only be separated by culture and/or serologic studies. Tuberculous meningitis continues to have a high mortality of up to 20 to 25%,[119–122] and morbidity with persistent neurologic damage.[122] Thus antituberculous therapy must be started promptly with the suspicion of tuberculous meningitis long before cultural proof is available and without identification of mycobacteria on smears.

PLEURAL TUBERCULOSIS

Pleural involvement with tuberculosis is usually by direct extension from a subpleural focus. This focus may be so small that it cannot be seen even after the effusion clears. In a study prior to the chemotherapy era, when tuberculosis was more widespread, a serofibrinous effusion in a person with a positive tuberculin skin test, with or without cultural proof of *M. tuberculosis* and independent of initial clearing of the effusion, carried a 65% risk of developing some form of tuberculosis, usually a year or more later. This risk was even higher in those under age 25.[123]

The patient with tuberculous effusion may have nonspecific systemic symptoms that become gradually progressive with or without pleuritic pain. Some patients have an acute toxic febrile presentation. A person with a pleural effusion of unknown etiology should have a tuberculin skin test. If it is positive, this is strongly supportive of a diagnosis of tuberculosis, but further studies are required. The pleural fluid generally will be an exudate with a protein content of 3g/dl or greater; cells are generally lymphocytes, but occasionally an early effusion may have a predominance of polymorphonuclear cells. The pleural fluid glucose is usually less than 50% of a concurrent blood sugar.[124] However, the presence or absence of these findings does not make or exclude the diagnosis of tuberculosis. A needle biopsy of the pleura should be obtained; in various series granulomatous inflammation, with or without caseation, has been found in 65 to 75% of patients ultimately proven to have tuberculosis.[125] This yield is increased with a second or third attempt. If an adequate amount of pleural fluid (*e.g.* 1 liter) and a portion of tissue from the pleural biopsy are cultured for mycobacteria, the positive yield has exceeded 90%. The combination of histology and culture made the diagnosis in 20 of 21 patients in one series.[126] Pleuroscopy may be helpful in obtaining pleural biopsies from visualized areas of disease. While granulomatous inflammation of the pleura can result from other etiologies, such as sarcoidosis or fungal infections, its presence, especially in a tuberculin-positive individual, requires treatment for tuberculosis (see also Chapter 12, Pleural Disease).

GENITOURINARY TUBERCULOSIS

Urinary tract tuberculosis is usually of hematogenous origin. Prior to the chemotherapy era, in patients dying with extensive pulmonary tuberculosis, up to 73% had renal involvement and this was bilateral.[127] Spread is usually down the ureter to involve the bladder, prostate, seminal vesicle, and epididymis. However, clinically evident disease is commonly unilateral.[128,129]

The most common initial symptom in genitourinary tuberculosis has been reported as epididymitis (36%), followed by symptoms of urinary tract "irritation" such as frequency, burning, and dysuria (20%); gross painless hematuria (20%); mild dull aching flank pain; and less commonly, renal colic, hematuria with clots and pain, hematospermia, and absence of symptoms (10%).[130] A history of recurrent urinary tract infections or pyuria without growth of the usual bacterial pathogens should prompt the consideration of renal tuberculosis, particularly when any of the following symptoms are present: an acid urine; a beaded vas deferens; a draining sinus in the pelvic or scrotal area; epididymitis, especially with calcification; induration of the prostrate or seminal vesicles; and unexplained fever. Renal and skeletal tuberculosis frequently coexist. A history of previous tuberculous disease with current urinary tract abnormalities warrants evaluation for tuberculosis.

An excretory pyelogram may visualize abnormalities in the calices, pelves, ureters, or bladder. Tuberculosis tends to involve multiple areas. Dilatation of part or all of the pelvicalyceal system is the most common finding and poor definition of a minor calyx the earliest. Ureteral abnormalities occur in about one-half and vesical abnormalities in about one-third. Although renal cavitation, multiple ureteral strictures, and a shortened refluxing ureter are less common, they are more specific.[131]

Although considerably less common than urinary tract involvement, genital disease may appear in women. They may seek care for infertility, abdominal pain, profuse or irregular menses, or symptoms of pelvic inflammatory disease (salpingo-oophoritis or endometritis.). A history indicative of extragenital tuberculosis may be present in only about 50%; changes compatible with tuberculosis are seen on the chest roentgenogram in about 60%. A diagnosis requires a positive culture from the genital tract (occasionally urine) or microscopic identification of caseating granuloma with or without organisms.[132]

It is preferable to send multiple first-voided

morning midstream urine specimens for culture rather than 24-hour urine specimens, since the latter become excessively contaminated.[133] Broad-spectrum antibiotics may interfere with mycobacterial cultures. Smears for acid-fast bacteria are not done because of the false positives resulting from saprophytic mycobacteria (*M. smegmatis*).[6] Lack of urinary tract symptoms, a normal urinalysis, and even a normal pyelogram do not exclude genitourinary tract tuberculosis, since this may occur in up to 60% of patients with urine cultures positive for *M. tuberculosis* who have disease elsewhere. When urine from unselected, untreated patients with tuberculosis is cultured, 10% can be expected to grow *M. tuberculosis.* When people with evidence of only pulmonary disease are selected, the cultures will be positive in about 5%. However, in patients with extrapulmonary tuberculosis, positive cultures have been found in 21%. With extrapulmonary disease, urine is a good source of material for culture.[134] Positive urine cultures indicate genitourinary disease.[135]

BONE AND JOINT TUBERCULOSIS

Tuberculous involvement of the skeleton is most commonly of hematogenous origin. However, it may spread via the lymphatics to the spine when there is pleural or renal involvement.[136] While skeletal tuberculosis had been particularly prominent in children, it appears that it is now being seen more frequently in older persons;[100] the weight-bearing joints are most commonly involved. The spine is involved in about 50% of cases, the hips in 15%, and the knees in 15%.[137] However, any joint may be involved, including the ribs and the small joints of the hands and feet.[138,139]

The most common symptom of spinal involvement is pain followed by limitation of motion. Roentgenographically there is early disc-space narrowing with subsequent destruction and collapse of vertebral bodies. The pedicles are generally spared. There may be a paraspinous abscess, "the cold abscess."[140] With progression kyphoscoliosis may occur, the so-called gibbus deformity. About one-half of the patients will have no evidence of pulmonary tuberculosis, either remote or current. In comparison with osteomyelitis or tumor, the symptoms of tuberculosis of the spine tend to be of greater duration, not uncommonly exceeding a year (an indication of the delay in diagnosis). The lack of specificity of clinical and radiologic findings in separating osteomyelitis due to common bacteria or fungi from tuberculosis or tumor warrants aspiration or open biopsy for culture, cytology, and histology.[141,142]

Tuberculous arthritis of other joints is characteristically monarticular, but multiple areas may be involved.[137,140,143] Clinically there is the insidious onset of pain and swelling with limitation of motion; constitutional symptoms are usually present. The roentgenogram of the joint is usually abnormal with metaphyseal and subchondral erosion, joint space narrowing, or cysts. Roentgenographic evidence of pulmonary involvement varies from uncommon to about 50%. The presence of a destructive arthritis, particularly monarticular, warrants at least a tuberculin skin test since the PPD-tuberculin is usually positive in tuberculous arthritis. A definite diagnosis requires the identification and culture of *M. tuberculosis* from the synovial fluid or synovial biopsy, or histologic changes or tuberculosis in the biopsy.[137,144]

LYMPHATIC TUBERCULOSIS

Involvement of lymph nodes may be through direct extension or by hematogenous spread. Tuberculous lymphadenitis is commonly a delayed complication of initial infection, and is most prevalent in the young adult. The anterior and posterior cervical nodes are involved in more than half the patients, and the supraclavicular nodes in about 20%; submandibular, axillary, subauricular, and other nodes are involved less commonly. The patient usually seeks advice for painless swelling of the involved nodes with or without systemic symptoms. Occasionally the nodes may be painful or there is drainage of pus. Approximately half the patients have evidence of tuberculosis in other sites. The chest roentgenogram provides evidence of tuberculosis in up to 60% of patients; enlargement of mediastinal or hilar nodes has been found in 12 to 30%.

Diagnosis generally requires proof of *M. tuberculosis* on cultures of material from the nodes, usually obtained surgically. In adults, mycobacterial lymphadenitis is almost invariably due to *M. tuberculosis*.[60,145] However, in young children, infection with other mycobacteria is common (see further on).[146]

PERICARDIAL TUBERCULOSIS

Pericardial involvement most commonly results from lymphatic spread or direct extension from lung and mediastinal tissues. Pericardial tuberculosis is uncommon, amounting to 0.35% of tuberculosis admissions and 11% of autopsied cases. However, its mortality remains as high as 40%.[147] This can largely be attributed either to the lack of recognition of the tuberculous etiology of the pericarditis or the presence of pericarditis in patients with extensive tuberculosis. The former is most likely in patients who present with the signs and symptoms of pericarditis who have either normal pulmonary parenchyma on chest roentgenograms or only minor changes. All patients with pericarditis should be tuberculin tested; if the tuberculin test is positive, the etiology should be considered tuberculous until proven otherwise.[147] If a concomitant pleural effusion is present, it should be cultured for mycobacteria and a pleural biopsy obtained; the diagnostic yield is high and effusions have been reported in up to one-third of patients with tuberculous pericarditis. A negative tuberculin, especially in an older or debilitated patient, does not exclude a diagnosis of tuberculosis.[148–150]

In the presence of extensive tuberculosis involving the pulmonary parenchyma with or without pleural effusion, the recognition of pericardial disease may be quite difficult. Dyspnea, orthopnea, chest pain, and ankle swelling occur more frequently with pericarditis than would be expected with pulmonary or pleural tuberculosis alone. The more specific findings of a pericardial friction rub or pericardial tamponade evidenced by neck vein distention, decreased or muffled heart sounds, or a paradoxical pulse can be identified in less than one-half of patients. In a recent series 71% of patients had a concomitant pleural effusion, and 85% had cardiac enlargement roentgenographically. While the electrocardiogram was abnormal in all cases, the most common finding was nonspecific ST-T wave depression (84%), and "diagnostic" changes of acute pericarditis were present in only 9%.[147] A specific diagnosis can be made by culturing the pericardial fluid or with a pericardial biopsy. With documentation of parenchymal or pleural tuberculosis these procedures are generally not necessary. However, when the diagnosis cannot be otherwise substantiated and particularly in the individual with a positive tuberculin skin test, a pericardial biopsy is warranted.

TUBERCULOUS PERITONITIS AND ENTERITIS

Peritoneal involvement is usually of hematogenous origin.[105,151,152] Although direct extension or spread through the lymphatics, from intestinal lesions or the female genital tract, has been postulated,[153] involvement of these organs in patients with tuberculous peritonitis is quite rare.[151,152] Tuberculous peritonitis is characterized by the insidious onset of abdominal enlargement (ascites) and vague abdominal pain, usually of several months duration. Fever is almost invariably present, but may be intermittent with afebrile periods of a week or more. Ascitic fluid is moderate in amount. Small, single or multiple masses may be palpable; they represent a conglomerate of a thickened omentum, mesentery, and adherent bowel loops. The classic description of a "doughy abdomen" due to peritoneal, omental, and bowel inflammation with little ascites is most uncommon.

Evidence of parenchymal pulmonary involvement varies from 6 to 33% including residual scarring and calcification. A concomitant pleural effusion in recent series has occurred in about one-third of patients; this effusion has been exudative, and pleural biopsies have shown granulomas. The tuberculin skin test is usually positive. The ascitic fluid is exudative with a protein of 3 g/dl or more and an elevated specific gravity; cell counts are moderate (about 500), predominantly lymphocytes; bloody fluid is most unusual.

The diagnosis has been made on cultures in

83% when a liter or more of peritoneal fluid was submitted.[149] Documentation of granulomas, usually with caseation, is common in tissues obtained by needle biopsy, peritoneoscopy, culdoscopy or laporatomy; a portion of the tissue should be cultured.

The reported coexistence of tuberculous peritonitis and cirrhosis has been quite variable. In a series of Iranian patients with tuberculous peritonitis there were no cases of cirrhosis and in 100 cirrhotics only one case of tuberculous peritonitis,[152] in a series from India 8% of cirrhotics had tuberculous peritonitis[154]; and in an older series from the United States there was a 42% prevalence of alcoholic cirrhosis in patients with tuberculous peritonitis.[155] These variations probably reflect differing life styles. The presence of fever in a cirrhotic patient with ascites warrants aggressive study for concomitant tuberculosis or other bacterial peritonitis (*i.e.*, a tuberculin skin test, diagnostic paracentesis, and peritoneal biopsy).[151–158]

In a recent study, tuberculous enteritis and peritonitis occurred in 0.85% of patients admitted for tuberculosis; 21 had peritonitis, 11 enteritis, and 4 had both. The enteritis involved the ileum in 7, the colon in 2, both in 3 with isolated involvement of the rectum, stomach, and appendix. The tuberculin skin test was not significant in 28% and the chest roentgenogram was normal in about 20%. Culture-proven tuberculosis was present in 42%. Gastrointestinal tuberculosis was diagnosed unexpectedly in 12 patients at surgery. Complications included perforation of the ileum with peritonitis in 4, small bowel obstruction in 19, and bowel fistula in 5. Six patients died in the hospital related to the disease or its diagnosis. The enteritis usually develops because of swallowing infectious sputum.[158a]

UPPER RESPIRATORY TRACT TUBERCULOSIS

The upper respiratory tract (URT) is involved almost exclusively by tubercle bacilli carried in sputum with a high bacillary load. The larynx is most commonly involved and such patients are highly contagious. Other sites include the epiglottis, pharynx, tonsils, soft palate, tongue, and middle ear. In a recent survey, 1.8% of admissions had URT involvement. These patients had weight loss, change in cough pattern, hoarseness, and odynophagia for the preceding 4.6 mo. The vocal cord changes were variable. Erythema, edema, exudation, and exophytic or ulcerative changes were indistinguishable from carcinoma, fungal infections, or syphilis. However, chest roentgenographic changes of extensive or cavitary tuberculosis and positive sputum smears for mycobacteria were almost invariably present.[159]

TUBERCULOSIS IN OTHER ORGANS

Tuberculosis may involve any organ. Rarely it is the cause of superior vena cava obstruction with mediastinal involvement. The esophagus can develop diverticulae or strictures. It can produce adrenal insufficiency. Occasionally the chest wall is involved with a draining sinus or a "cold abscess." The mastoid sinuses may be involved. It may produce a rectal abscess or perianal fistula. Other sinus tracts from abdominal and pelvic tuberculosis may be found. In the intestinal tract, the ileocecal area is most commonly affected, particularly where *M. bovis* infections are prevalent and milk is not pasteurized. Chronic skin lesions with or without deep tissue penetration may occur. Tuberculosis is sometimes invoked, but seldom proven, as the etiology of chorioretinitis or iridocyclitis. Rarely direct infection of the conjunctiva is seen in physicians infected at bronchoscopy.

CHEMOTHERAPY AND MANAGEMENT

A logical approach to the treatment of tuberculosis follows the classification listed on page 400. Tuberculous infection has been defined as a significant reaction to a PPD-tuberculin skin test of an intermediate or 5 TU strength in a person without evidence of disease.[161] The following outline of therapy can be supplemented by specific details in three excellent recent reviews.[160–162]

The need for two or more drugs to treat tuberculosis is based on the estimate of the number of organisms in the host and thus the number of mutants with drug resistance that may develop. The largest number of tubercle bacilli may be found in cavities, approximately 1×10^7 to 10^8 as compared to a hard caseous focus where the number of bacilli are about 1×10^2 to 10^3. In a latent infection the number of organisms may be less than 1×10^2. Mutations producing resistance to a single drug occur in about 1×10^5 to 10^6 divisions. Thus a person with 1×10^8 to 10^9 bacilli might have 1×10^3 resistant organisms to a single drug. Resistance to two drugs resulting from mutation would require an exceptionally large number of organisms, since this can be expected to occur in about 1×10^{11} to 10^{12} divisions.[163]

0. NO TUBERCULOSIS EXPOSURE, NOT INFECTED

No medical action is required concerning tuberculosis unless the clinical picture of a patient warrants further investigation.

1. TUBERCULOSIS EXPOSURE, NO EVIDENCE OF INFECTION

If the exposure is remote, no further action is necessary. If the exposure is within 3 mo, a tuberculin skin test should be repeated about 3 mo after exposure is ended. This repeat testing is required since it may take this long for the development of delayed hypersensitivity.

INH Preventive Therapy

An important group of people are the initially skin-test-negative household contacts of persons with untreated infectious tuberculosis; they have a high risk of developing disease. This risk is even higher in young children. Children should receive isoniazid (INH) 10 mg/kg body weight once a day up to the adult dose of 300 mg once daily. The tuberculin skin test should be repeated 3 mo after exposure is terminated. INH can be discontinued if the reaction is negative; if it is now positive, INH is continued for a total of 1 yr. In young adults whose initial skin test is negative, the same course is followed. If the individual is older than 35, INH may be initially withheld; the skin test repeated at 3 mo, and if again negative, no further evaluation or therapy is given. If the skin test becomes positive, treat with INH 300 mg daily for 1 yr.[47,161]

BCG Vaccination

An alternative means of preventing tuberculous infection is vaccination of tuberculin-negative individuals with BCG (Bacillus of Calmette and Guèrin). The protection offered by vaccination has varied from 0 to 80%; the major determinant has most probably been the effectiveness of the individual lot of vaccine. Thus freeze-dried BCG vaccine administered intradermally with a preparation of documented efficacy is recommended only for (1) population groups who have a proven high rate of *new* infection (*e.g.*, a > 10-15% tuberculin-positive rate in school-age children [*vs.* US 0.2-0.7%] or a similar rate of tuberculin conversions in health workers repeatedly exposed to untreated sputum-positive tuberculosis); and (2) selected individuals, particularly very young children, who have had (or will have) repeated close exposures to sputum-positive, untreated tuberculosis, in whom follow-up investigation to determine new infection and INH preventive therapy cannot be reasonably assured.[164] The various aspects of the use of BCG vaccination have been summarized recently.[160,165–167]

2. TUBERCULOUS INFECTION, NO DISEASE

In the evaluation of a person with a significant tuberculin reaction, a chest roentgenogram should be obtained. It is considered negative for tuberculosis if there are no parenchymal infiltrates or hilar enlargement; calcified foci are also considered negative in this context.

High Disease Risk for Preventive Therapy

The people with the highest risk of developing tuberculosis are the tuberculin-positive household or other close contacts of a person with untreated, especially smear-positive, tuberculosis. Every effort should be made to treat each such child with INH 10 mg/kg body weight and each adult with 300 mg daily for 1 yr. Preventive therapy has been 60 to 80% effective despite variable drug ingestion, and the effect has persisted through 19 yr.[161,168–171] The physician must accept responsibility in cooperation with the health department to identify and treat every close contact. These contacts represent a most fruitful source in efforts to reduce the incidence of tuberculosis.[169]

Patients with tuberculous infection and the following conditions are also at great risk of progressing to disease; they should receive a year of INH, 300 mg daily:

1. The tuberculin convertor, with a tuberculin reaction that has increased by at least 6 mm within 24 mo from less than 10 mm in diameter.
2. Prolonged therapy with corticosteroids or immunosuppressive drugs (*e.g.*, cancer chemotherapy, renal transplant patients); we continue INH until 3 mo after such drugs are stopped.
3. Hematologic or reticuloendothelial diseases (*e.g.*, leukemia, lymphoma).
4. Silicosis.[172]
5. Diabetes mellitus that is unstable or difficult to control.
6. Gastrectomy.

Patients with a significant tuberculin reaction who are undergoing chronic dialysis or renal transplantation or intestinal bypass surgery should be considered for INH preventive therapy; however, the indications are not fully established.[173,173a]

In infected individuals age 35 or more, *without* the above increased risk factors, preventive therapy is not recommended. In individuals below age 35, INH preventive therapy is recommended by the American Thoracic Society and Center for Disease Control, Tuberculosis Branch, but others withhold preventive therapy in those over 20 without additional risk factors.[47,161,179]

INH-Associated Hepatitis

A mild, self-limited elevation in serum glutamic pyruvic transaminase (SGPT) occurs in 10 to 20% of people receiving INH. This usually occurs in the first 4 to 6 mo of therapy, and values generally return to normal while the drug is continued. However, true isoniazid-associated hepatitis does occur. It is age-related, occurring in 0.2% of those under age 20, up to 0.3% of those between 20 and 34, up to 1.2% of those between 35 and 49, 2.3% of those 50 to 64, and 0.8% of those age 64 and over; its risk appears greater in those who drink alcohol daily.[47,160,161,171,174–178]

The symptoms of INH-associated hepatitis are generally quite indolent and nonspecific, simulating a viral illness. Gastrointestinal symptoms include anorexia, nausea, vomiting, abdominal pain, dark urine, and jaundice. Systemic manifestations include fatigue, malaise, weight loss, fever, chills, arthralgia, myalgia, pruritus, and rash. Occasionally patients have developed acute abdominal symptoms which resulted in laparotomy for suspected acute cholecystitis.

With the indications cited above, the benefits of preventing tuberculosis outweigh the risk of hepatitis, which exists only during the year that INH is given.[178] Contraindications to INH preventive therapy are: (1) previous INH-associated liver disease; (2) severe adverse reactions to INH (*e.g.*, fever, chills, rash, and arthritis); and (3) *acute* liver disease of any etiology. An INH "challenge" is not recommended, if there is a history of a significant INH reaction. The risk of INH-associated hepatitis is minimized by ascertaining that preventive therapy has not been previously given; monitoring patients for the possible symptoms of INH-associated hepatitis monthly, utilizing a checklist administered by a nurse; thoroughly explaining the signs and symptoms of hepatitis to the patient, giving the patient a copy of the checklist; and advising him to stop the INH and "call in" if the listed symptoms persist for more than 3 days. Routine monitoring of liver function tests is not required. They are obtained in the presence of the listed signs and symptoms as part of a thorough medical evaluation. Monthly contact with patients receiving INH is essential not only to avoid serious side-effects, but to reinforce drug ingestion.

3. TUBERCULOSIS, CURRENT DISEASE

Conventional Chemotherapy

Every patient with tuberculous disease should receive adequate chemotherapy. Successful treatment is ultimately dependent on the medical care team's ability to persuade the individual or social unit (usually the family) to cooperate in the long-term self-administration or controlled administration of medications. Once an effective chemotherapeutic program is initiated, all other measures are secondary and should be altered as necessary to achieve completion of this primary requirement, long-term drug therapy.[179–185]

Initial Treatment

Every patient with tuberculosis should receive a minimum of two drugs to which the organisms are susceptible. In many countries the recommendations are directed at reduced duration of chemotherapy, as discussed under Short Course Chemotherapy further on. The most extensively studied regime consists of INH and EMB in a single daily dose.[180] Primary drug resistance (organisms resistant in a host never having received antituberculous drugs) should be anticipated if the index case has known drug-resistant organisms; initial therapy of such a person should be based on the index case's drug susceptibility.[184,185] In patients of Hispanic or Asian descent or those who have contracted their disease in Asia, primary drug resistance, especially to INH, may be very high. Primary resistance rates vary markedly in various regions of the US and Canada.[23,95] The clinician should know the local rates in the area of his practice. It is recommended that rifampin be substituted for INH in the initial treatment of such patients.[183] The recognition and prevention of INH-associated hepatitis has been discussed. In the usual dosage of INH (10 mg/kg in children and 5 mg/kg in adults) in an otherwise normal person, peripheral neuritis is rarely a problem. With higher doses of INH or in patients with alcoholism or poor diets, prophylactic use of pyridoxine is recommended. If patients requiring diphenylhydantoin are given INH, the dose of diphenylhydantoin should be reduced to 100 to 200 mg daily to avoid CNS side-effects as a result of the accumulation of diphenylhydantoin (diphenylhydantoin blood levels are useful in adjusting the dose).[186] Other side-effects, including skin rash, a rheumatic syndrome, and convulsions, occur rarely.[186,187] INH overdose may cause seizures, metabolic acidosis, coma, and death.[188] Ocular toxicity with EMB can be avoided by a careful ocular history and funduscopic examination along with determination of red–green color discrimination and visual acuity with a Snellen Eye Chart. During therapy red–green color discrimination and visual acuity should initially be monitored monthly. If color discrimination decreases or more than a one-line change in acuity occurs, the drug should be stopped. The patient is also instructed to report visual changes. The rare case of optic neuritis in humans has been reversible with discontinuation of medication and is extremely unusual at the 15 mg/kg daily dose. Ethambutol is contraindicated in the presence of optic neuritis. Its advantages must be weighed against possible risks in the presense of other serious ocular pathology. Although relatively little experience in pregnant women has been reported, there have been no teratogenic complications.[161,189,190]

The alternative initial oral drug is PAS. Although a drug of lesser effectiveness, its efficacy in two and three drug regimens is well established. However, the need to ingest 15 to 30 pills per day, the common gastrointestinal side effects, and the not-uncommon hepatotoxicity and hypersensitivity reactions (various dermatoses) seriously interfere with satisfactory therapy. The sodium salt of PAS should be avoided in patients over age 60 and in those with congestive heart failure or renal disease, in whom a salt load may contribute to edema formation. A combination without sodium may be substituted (see Table 9-3).

The alternative initial parenteral drug is streptomycin. The requirement for parenteral administration and the greater incidence of side-effects as compared with EMB make its use less common. When controlled therapy is necessary, parenteral administration assures delivery. With extensive or cavitary disease, where the number of organisms is great, streptomycin (1 g daily) is commonly given as a third drug, usually for the initial 60 days, or longer if sputum smears remain positive. However, recent studies indicate that a combination of INH and RIF is at least as effective.[160–162,191]

The "standard" length of therapy has been 2 yr. However, recent studies support treatment for as little as 12 to 18 mo, provided INH and

TABLE 9-3. Antituberculous Drugs and Their Side-Effects

Drug	Dosage (Adult Daily)	Side-Effects (Usual)	Monitoring*	Remarks
Most effective				
Isoniazid (INH)	5–10 mg/kg 300–600 mg	Peripheral neuritis, hepatitis, hypersensitivity, convulsions	SGOT/SGPT (not as a routine)	For neuritis, pyridoxine, 25–50 mg as prophylaxis; 50–100 mg as treatment
Streptomycin (SM)	0.75–1 g (frequently given for initial 60 days with extensive disease)	Otic and vestibular toxicity, decreased hearing, vertigo tinnitus; nephrotoxicity (rare)	Gross hearing (ticking of watch); if abnormal, audiograms; vertigo (if present, caloric testing); BUN and creatinine	More common in older patients (>60 yr); decrease dose or avoid drug if renal insufficiency
Rifampin	600 mg once daily (children 10–20 mg/kg to a maximym of 600 mg)	Hepatitis; hypersensitivity reactions	SGOT/SGPT	Extremely effective; drug interactions
Pyrazinamide	20–35 mg/kg; not over 3 g	Hyperuricemia, hepatotoxicity, arthralgia	Uric acid, SGOT/SGPT	Benemid or allopurinol to reduce serum uric acid
Supportive				
Ethambutol (EMB)	15 mg/kg†	Optic neuritis (reversible with discontinuation of drug; very rare at 15 mg/kg); skin rash	Visual acuity, red–green color discrimination (Snellen chart)	Ocular history and funduscopic exam before use; contraindicated with optic neuritis; use with caution if serious ocular problems
Para-aminosalicylic acid (aminosalicylic acid)	12–15 g	Gastrointestinal, sensitivity (rash), hepatotoxicity, sodium load	SGOT/SGPT	For GI irritation, temporarily reduce dose or use Ca, K, ascorbic acid, or resin combinations; avoid Na salt in elderly patients and patients with heart failure or renal disease
Ethionamide	750–1000 mg	Gastrointestinal, hepatotoxicity, hypersensitivity (rash)	SGOT/SGPT	Temporarily stop or reduce dose with GI irritation and hepatotoxicity
Cycloserine	750 mg	Psychosis, personality changes, convulsions, rash	Drug blood levels if poor renal function	Pyridoxine, 50–300 mg/day, may help; mental problems more common with predisposition

TABLE 9-3 (Continued)

Drug	Dosage (Adult Daily)	Side-Effects (Usual)	Monitoring*	Remarks
Capreomycin	1 g daily for 60–120 days, followed by 1 g 2 to 3 times weekly	Nephrotoxicity, ototoxicity, hepatotoxicity, hypersensitivity, hypokalemia	Same as streptomycin with SGOT/SGPT in addition	Effective, frequent cross-resistance with viomycin, also kanamycin; not for pediatric use; also as for streptomycin
Viomycin	1 g every 12 hr twice a week	Similar to streptomycin, but nephrotoxicity more common; hypokalemia, hypocalcemia	As for streptomycin, plus urinalysis	As for streptomycin; not currently available in US
Kanamycin	0.5–1 g—as for streptomycin	Similar to streptomycin	As for streptomycin	Rarely used; avoid concomitant ethacrynic acid, furosemide, or mercurial diuretics and mannitol

* The most important device is an informed patient having ready access to medical care, supplemented by a careful history and appropriate physical examination.

† For retreatment cases 25 mg/kg is recommended for the initial 60 days.

RIF are given for the first 5 mo. (INH and EMB may then be continued for the remaining required treatment.) This course should not be followed if there is extrapulmonary tuberculosis, drug resistance, or complicating medical conditions such as diabetes, silicosis, immunosuppressive drugs, or disease (see Short-Course Chemotherapy below.)[161,192]

Primary tuberculosis is usually treated with two drugs whether it occurs in the child or adult. However, in the young child INH is usually combined with PAS since EMB is not available in a pediatric form and children tolerate both INH and PAS surprisingly well. EMB can be used in the older child who is able to cooperate with eye testing. In children with tuberculosis INH is given in a dose of 10 to 20 mg/kg per day (not to exceed 300 mg). The 20-mg/kg dose is recommended in the acute phase of meningeal and miliary tuberculosis. The recommended dose of a PAS salt is 200 mg/kg.

The initial therapeutic intervention has the best chance of success (over 95%), since the physician has the most potent and least toxic drugs at his disposal. Therefore it is incumbent upon him to (1) have adequate specimens for identification and susceptibility studies, when appropriate, before therapy, and (2) seal the contract of firm commitment to completion of drug therapy with the patient and his family.

Rifampin (RIF) is bactericidal; extensive trials document its outstanding efficacy and relatively minimal side-effects. The combination of INH with RIF during the initial 16 to 26 wk, followed by INH-EMB, has been equal to or better than standard three-drug regimens.[160–162,191]

The usual adult dosage is 600 mg orally once daily, not with meals (children: 10-20 mg/kg to a maximum of 600 mg). The most frequent side-effect is relatively mild gastrointestinal complaints such as nausea, epigastric distress, and diarrhea, which usually do not require discontinuation of the drug. Liver dysfunction, including jaundice, occurs rarely, but about 10% of patients may develop slight SGOT elevations. The benefit of the drug in the presence of liver disease or pregnancy (on which information is inadequate) must be weighed against potential risks. Its hepatotoxicity appears to be somewhat greater than INH, and about the same as PAS.[162] Intermittent high-dosage programs cannot be recommended because of the association of significant hypersensitivity reactions and thrombocytopenia.[193] RIF interacts with warfarin and tolbutamide, requiring higher dosages of the latter drugs.[194] It decreases the effectiveness of the contraceptive pill.[195] It also accelerates the metabolism of corticosteroids, methadone, and digitoxin.[161] While altered immunologic responsiveness has been documented in patients taking RIF, the clinical implications of these changes are not clear.[162,196]

Its role as a potent agent in retreatment is clearly established. It offers an excellent alternative as a companion drug in initial therapy when isoniazid, ethambutol, or streptomycin are not tolerated, when the risks associated with these drugs, in an individual patient, are greater than those associated with rifampin, or when short-course chemotherapy is used.

Corticosteroids are of value in four instances: (1) in tuberculous meningitis, to prevent or ameliorate neurologic complications[118]; (2) in tuberculous pericarditis, to decrease the incidence of constrictive pericarditis[147]; (3) in tuberculous peritonitis, to prevent late intestinal obstruction[151]; and (4) in the very toxic patient, to "buy time" for specific chemotherapy and other measures to become effective. They should be used only under the cover of adequate chemotherapy: (1) in initial treatment, INH, EMB, and SM (or INH and RIF), or (2) in retreatment, INH along with at least two and probably three additional drugs that the patient has never received or to which the organisms are susceptible. Prednisone, 60 mg daily for the initial 2 to 3 wk, with a tapered dosage and discontinuation at 4 wk, is recommended.

Surgery. Since the advent of chemotherapy, therapeutic surgical intervention to control infection in the chest is rarely necessary. Occasional patients with cavitary disease who do not respond to drugs may require resectional surgery. Even more unusual is the patient with extremely limited pulmonary reserve whose sputum remains positive for *M. tuberculosis*. Such patients may require extraperiosteal plombage or thoracoplasty to attain negativity.[197] Surgery may be required for certain complications: (1) recurrent or massive hemoptysis,[198] (2) empyema with severe pleuritis requiring decortication, and (3) a bronchopleural fistula resulting from tuberculous empyema commonly with an associated bacterial infection. Since closure of a bronchopleural fistula—despite intensive drug therapy and tube thoracostomy—is uncommon, surgical intervention at a point some 4 to 8 wk after instituting therapy should be considered.

Extrapulmonary Tuberculosis is generally treated with three drugs: INH, EMB, and SM (or INH and RIF). The use of steroids in meningeal, pericardial, and peritoneal tuberculosis and in the toxic patient with or without disseminated disease has already been discussed. The other common areas for development of extrapulmonary tuberculosis, the genitourinary tract, bone and lymph nodes (scrofula in the neck), are generally amenable to triple drug therapy. Surgical intervention, such as nephrectomy, pericardiectomy, extirpation of nodes, and spinal fusion with debridement, is very rarely necessary,[130,137,144,147,199,200] although the opinion is not unanimous.[201,202]

Pregnancy. In pregnancy, INH and EMB are the drugs of choice; RIF also appears to be safe but less information is available. Ethionamide may be teratogenic. INH, RIF and SM are secreted in breast milk.[161,203]

Renal Failure. EMB is excreted almost entirely by the kidney. In renal failure, a dose of 9 mg/kg of body weight has been suggested, although we have not seen toxicity at 15 mg/kg. INH and RIF may be given in usual doses, as described above.[160–162,173]

Retreatment

The need for retreatment is usually the result of inadequate initial chemotherapy due most commonly to failure of the patient to complete the initial course of drugs. On occasion it results from idiosyncratic or allergic drug reactions, inadequate initial drug programs, or primary drug resistance. When reactivation occurs, as indicated by the finding of two or more positive cultures or a positive culture with roentgenographic progression, we generally treat the patient with INH, 8 to 10 mg/kg, and two additional drugs that the patient has never received before. Appropriate drug changes are subsequently made on the basis of drug susceptibility studies of the organisms. It is important to realize that patients occasionally have an isolated positive smear or culture with sparse growth while receiving successful treatment.[204] Therefore a single positive specimen in an asymptomatic patient with stable or improving chest roentgenograms may not indicate reactivation, but does indicate the need for careful reevaluation with multiple specimens submitted for culture. With retreatment, or if the initial treatment is failing, at least two new drugs should be given. If only one drug is added or substituted, the development of resistance to it is quite likely. In general, retreatment programs are best managed by physicians experienced in the use of the so-called second line drugs. A success rate of 80 to 90% or better is attainable.[160,162,179,205]

Drug Reactions

The approach to each drug reaction must be carefully individualized. If the reaction is severe, all drugs should be stopped. At least 10 to 14 days should elapse before reintroducing drugs. Earlier challenge may evoke a nonspecific response to almost any drug. Small doses of single drugs may be tried, the least suspect being started first. If a mild dermatitis develops, temporary discontinuation of the most likely offender may be all that is required. This drug can then be reintroduced in gradually increasing doses with careful observation. On occasion, if the drug is truly necessary, "desensitization" programs can be carried out under cover of corticosteroids.[206] In general, however, if the reaction is severe, alternative therapy should be used.

Short-Course Chemotherapy

Controlled clinical trials provide solid evidence that the duration of drug therapy may be radically reduced without loss of effectiveness.[192] The theory and basic bacteriologic mechanisms that underlie the major advances in intermittent and short-course chemotherapy have been recently reviewed.[208] Preventing the emergence of drug resistance and sterilizing the lesions remain the two major objectives. The use of INH, SM, and RIF for 6 mo had only a 2% relapse rate; INH and RIF for 6 mo had a 5% relapse rate; INH, SM, and PZA for 9 mo had a 4% relapse rate; and INH and RIF for 9 mo with either SM or EMB (better tolerated) for the first 2 mo resulted in no relapses. These results support such programs in efforts to improve patient compliance.[207,208]

Intermittent Therapy

Some people are unable to reliably take their drugs without close supervision (*e.g.*, the lone alcoholic). Several effective programs based on the controlled administration of drugs (direct observation of pill ingestion and drug injections) have been shown to be at least as effective as prolonged hospitalization, and certainly less costly. These have usually been provided by the public sector (health department or hospital), using public-health nurses to visit patients and/or a clinic that is readily available at convenient hours. Drugs are given daily in the hospital and then 5 days a week for the first 2 to 4 mo (usually until a negative culture is obtained). Thereafter, the following drugs are given twice weekly: either INH, 15 mg/kg orally and SM, 25 to 30 mg/kg intramuscularly, or INH, 15 mg/kg and EMB, 50 mg/kg orally. These programs are only recommended when regular treatment has not been or is unlikely to be satisfactory.[160–162,208,209]

Immunotherapy

Immunotherapy with transfer factor has been reported in a patient with progressive primary tuberculosis not responding to chemotherapy.[209a]

Patient Management

Hospitalization. The primary reasons for hospitalization are to provide care for the sick patient and to facilitate efficient, rapid diagnosis. Because many patients with tuberculosis are in the older age group, thorough evaluation for other diseases that may be more serious is necessary. Once the diagnosis is established, treatment can be started with close initial observation for drug side-effects. The patient and his family must be educated, stressing the requirement for long-term drug therapy even though whatever symptoms are present usually abate or disappear in a matter of days. Many well-controlled studies confirm that bed rest (beyond the brief symptomatic period), special diet, and climate control are not essential in the treatment of tuberculosis once an effective program of chemotherapy has been instituted.[21,25,34,35,160–162,179,181,182]

If the patient and his family understand the importance of taking medication faithfully and are committed to this, then the educational program has been successful. In hospitals treating large numbers of patients, this responsibility is shared by all personnel, including clerks, orderlies, nurses, medical social workers, and physicians. The least important reason for hospitalization today is the isolation of the patient. If the patient's illness does not require hospitalization and the diagnosis can be efficiently made while he is an outpatient, no hospitalization is necessary.

Isolation. Well-controlled experiments and clinical trials have clearly documented that tuberculosis is spread by droplet nuclei, aerosolized during coughing, laughing, singing, and speaking.[26–35] Since tuberculosis is not spread by fomites, only ordinary care of eating utensils, linens, books, and other articles is required.[25] When receiving effective chemotherapy, patients become rapidly noninfectious even before gross alterations in numbers of organisms in sputum smears or cultures are evident.[160,162,210,211] Therefore, from a strictly medical viewpoint, long-term hospitalization is unwarranted. Since long-term hospitalization is unnecessary for the average patient, with appropriate measures to control contagion, most patients can be treated economically and certainly with fewer personal social disadvantages in a general hospital.[210,212,213]

Discharge. The decision to discharge a patient from the hospital is based on several criteria: (1) the clinical well-being of the patient; (2) roentgenographic evidence of stability or improvement; (3) bacteriologic evidence of a reduction in the number of organisms being excreted*; and (4) most critically, the judgment on an individual basis that the patient, his home situation, and the outpatient health care delivery system will assure completion of the prescribed chemotherapy. Such an individual is encouraged to return to work immediately unless he works in a closed environment with highly susceptible contacts.[214,215]

Outpatient Care. It is of no medical importance whether the patient is treated for extended periods in a tuberculosis hospital, in a public clinic, or in the private physician's office. As already mentioned, some patients will require no hospitalization. However, it is incumbent upon the physician and the medical care team to assure effective chemotherapy with frequent roentgenographic and mycobacteriologic followup. Three months after beginning chemotherapy, 75% of patients should have negative cultures. At 6 mo, 95% should have negative cultures.[216] Early discharge without carefully defined plans and mechanisms to assure this continued treatment under close surveillance will almost surely be disastrous.[217] On the other hand, with such an early discharge program the patient can be quickly returned to his family and to a productive role in society.

Long-term Follow-up. The excellent success of chemotherapy over the last several decades has brought about a reevaluation of the need for lifelong follow-up examinations of patients who have taken an adequate course of chemotherapy. There is increasing agreement that annual (or more frequent) evaluations by chest roentgenogram and sputum cultures have a very low yield

* Currently we use as a *general* guideline two consecutive negative sputum smears, or a majority of negative smears with others containing only rare organisms. The patient who is well and can return to his home is often discharged in 2 wks or less once the number of organisms on smear is decreasing. An increasing number of patients who are not ill are being treated totally as outpatients, independent of their smear status.

in patients who have faithfully taken a prescribed course of effective therapy; the risk of reactivation in one study was 2.2 : 1000 cases per yr. However, with inadequate therapy, or none at all, the rate was 7.8 : 1000 and 6.7 : 1000 cases per yr, respectively.[218] Thus the major effort and necessary resources should be directed at completion of chemotherapy. In 1978, 84% of patients completed 12 mo of therapy and 75% completed therapy for 24 mo.[10] In addition, many of the patients who reactivate seek medical attention because of symptoms. Patients who have completed drug therapy are carefully instructed regarding symptoms that may indicate reactivation and advised to seek medical attention at that time. Their history of tuberculosis and its treatment is incorporated in their medical record to alert the physician(s) who will provide ongoing general medical care so that they will be aware of the need to consider possible reactivation of tuberculosis as a cause of future problems.

Reporting

Each case of tuberculosis should be reported to the local health department using the classification outlined in Table 9-2. Such reporting is not only essential for tuberculosis control programs, but more importantly, opens the door to the use of health department aid in: (1) investigation of contacts, (2) provision of laboratory and x-ray services, and (3) provision of drugs. These are generally provided without charge.

Education

The physician of today has an additional, extremely important role. He must educate not only the patient and his family but other medical and paramedical personnel concerning treatment and the remote dangers of tuberculosis to others, once effective chemotherapy has been established. Until the medical team is enlightened, it is difficult to expect the general community to accept these patients into their personal lives as they do people with other illnesses. Educational materials are available in North America at no cost from local Lung Associations. This need for education is secondary only to our paramount goal, the utilization of whatever resources are necessary to assure completion of a full course of effective chemotherapy as prescribed. This goal requires a highly individualized approach to each patient by the physician and the entire medical care team, one which will not only permit the patient to cooperate but will encourage and continually reinforce achievement of this end.

4. TUBERCULOSIS: NO CURRENT DISEASE

This category includes (1) people with a history of previous episode(s) of tuberculosis; and (2) people with abnormal stable roentgenogram findings, a significant tuberculin reaction, negative mycobacteriologic studies (if done), and no clinical or roentgenogram evidence of current disease. People in this class may never have had chemotherapy, may be receiving preventive chemotherapy, or may have completed chemotherapy, but do *not* have current disease. If current disease has not been excluded, the individual should be classified as a tuberculosis suspect until data permit classification as Class 3 or 4.

Preventive Treatment with Disease

A group of people can be identified with tuberculous disease who have a very small population of viable organisms. They are characterized by (1) a significant tuberculin skin test, (2) a parenchymal infiltrate on chest roentgenogram that is stable (old calcifications alone are excluded), (3) negative current smears and cultures for *M. Tuberculosis*, and (4) no symptoms referable to tuberculosis. Such patients are considered not to have current disease. They have a continuing risk of developing overt disease ranging between 0.8 and 1.0% for each year they live.[47,168] They should receive INH, 300 mg daily, for 1 yr. This is preventive therapy with a single drug because of the small number of organisms. The roentgenographic changes indicate disease; thus such persons are now placed in Class 4: Tuberculosis, no current disease.

5. TUBERCULOSIS SUSPECT

This class is for individuals in whom a diagnosis of tuberculosis is considered, whether or not treatment has been started. It is used until diagnostic procedures are completed. Persons should not remain in this class for more than 3 mo. When studies are completed, the sum total of information should be used by the clinician either to make a diagnosis of tuberculosis and appropriately classify the patient, or make a judgment that the patient does not have tuberculosis.

PART TWO: OTHER MYCOBACTERIAL DISEASES

Mycobacteria other than *M. tuberculosis* were recognized in the late 19th century. Their association with human disease was delayed another 30 to 40 years and it was not until the 1950s that this relationship was generally accepted. This delay probably reflects the limited techniques for cultural identification and the general lack of pathogenicity of these other mycobacteria for laboratory animals, particularly the guinea pig.

For many years these organisms were identified as *M. bovis* and the remainder placed in four groups (I-IV) by Runyan.

They were also called "unclassified," "anonymous," "atypical," or "nontuberculous" mycobacteria.[222–225] A recent book and exhaustive review provide detailed information on their bacteriologic and clinical presentations.[226,227]

MAGNITUDE OF THE PROBLEM

The overall incidence of pulmonary infections due to other mycobacteria is not well defined. Various estimates range from 1% or less to 10 to 15% of all patients with mycobacterial disease. There appears to be a considerable geographic variation (*i.e.*, Group I, *M. kansasii*, occurs more commonly in Dallas, New Orleans, Illinois, and Kansas; Group III, *M. avium-intracellulare* in Milwaukee, the southeastern US, Japan, and western Australia; about an equal number of both in Cleveland, Houston, and St. Louis; and *M. buruli* in the Nile Valley. However, these other mycobacteria have worldwide distribution.

EPIDEMIOLOGY

Human infection with *M. bovis* is almost nonexistent in areas where tuberculosis control has been achieved in cattle and where milk is pasteurized.[6] While *M. bovis* may be transmitted by the airborne route, it usually is transmitted by way of cow's milk and invades the intestines of infants and young children, involving the mesenteric nodes and other abdominal organs. Cervical node involvement may occur through extension from the pharynx or tonsils or may be a result of hematogenous dissemination, which can lead to bone and joint or pulmonary involvement.

The other mycobacteria can be generally found in the environment, in soil, water, food, plants, and animals.[225–228] Their mode of transmission is poorly understood. They may be isolated from sputum or gastric contents on occasion in healthy individuals.[229] Epidemiological surveys using antigens prepared from *M. kansasii*, *M. scrofulaceum*, and *M. intracellulare* indicate relatively high infection rates in the absence of disease.

This indicates a lower virulence for man. In addition, involvement of skin and joints is usually preceded by perforation skin. Disseminated disease is usually, but not always, found in the immunocompromised host. It has also been reported in sternal osteomyelitis with or without dissemination following coronary by-pass surgery and porcine valve replacement.[226,227]

Person-to-person transmission of infection with these mycobacteria has not been documented. Thus isolation of diseased individuals is not warranted.

PATHOGENESIS AND PATHOLOGY

The portals of entrance for these mycobacteria are considered to be (1) the respiratory tract (*e.g.*, pulmonary involvement with *M. kansasii*, *M. avium*, or *M. intracellulare*); (2) invasion through the oropharyngeal mucosa, producing cervical lymph node disease (scrofula) due most commonly to *M. scrofulaceum*, but also due to *M. kansasii* or *M. intracellulare;* (3) percutaneous inoculation (*e.g.*, *M. marinum* producing the so-called swimming pool granuloma; these organisms have been isolated from fish tanks and natural waters[230,231]). Disease due to *M. kansasii* and *M. avium* or *M. intracellulare* are usually localized to the lung; *M. scrofulaceum* usually involves the cervical lymph nodes in very young children and rarely the lung. Each of these may produce disseminated disease which usually occurs in the compromised host.[232]

TABLE 9-4. Mycobacteria Recovered from Vertebrates, Including Humans

	Potentially Clinically Significant		Usually Not Significant	
Group	**Species**	**Synonyms (Remarks)**	**Species**	**Synonyms**
	*M. tuberculosis** *M. bovis** *M. africanum**† *M. microti*		*M. bovis*, BCG*	
Photochromogen	*M. kansasii** *M. marinum** *M. simiae* *M. asiaticum**	(Yellow bacillus) *M. luciflavum* *M. balnei*, *M. platypoecilus* *M. habana*		
Scotochromogen	*M. scrofulaceum** *M. szulgai**	*M. marianum*, *M. paraffinicum*	*M. gordonae** *M. flavescens**	*M. aquae*, tap water scotochrome
Nonphoto chromogen	*M. avium** *M. intracellulare** *M. ulcerans** *M. xenopi** *M. malmoense** *M. haemophilum**	 (Battey bacillus) *M. brunense* *M. buruli* *M. littorale* (Needs hemin for growth)	*M. gastri** *M. nonchromogenicum** *M. terrae** *M. triviale**	
Rapid grower	*M. fortuitum** *M. chelonei** *M. chelonei* subsp. *abscessus**	*M. ranae*, *M. giae*, *M. minetti* *M. borstelense* *M. runyonii*, *M. abscessus*	*M. phlei** *M. smegmatis** *M. vaccae**	*M. moelleri*
Others	*M. paratuberculosis* *M. leprae** *M. lepraemurium*	*M. johnei* (needs mycobactin for growth) Hansen's bacillus (no growth on lab media) Stefansky's bacillus (no growth on lab media)		

* Indicates species found in humans.
† An organism intermediate between *M. tuberculosis* and *M. bovis;* status as distinct species being evaluated.
(Diagnostic standards and classification of tuberculosis and other mycobacterial diseases. Am Rev Resp Dis 123:343, 1981)

The pathology of these lesions is indistinguishable from that due to *M. tuberculosis*.

DIAGNOSIS AND CLASSIFICATION

The clinical, roentgenographic and pathologic patterns of pulmonary disease caused by these mycobacteria are indistinguishable from disease due to *M. tuberculosis*. A definite diagnosis requires (1) the presence of disease not attributable to another cause and (2) either the *repeated* growth of the same species of mycobacteria from sputum, usually in the absence of other pathogens, or isolation of the mycobacteria from a surgical specimen collected and processed by sterile techniques. Even with a surgical specimen one must assure that an isolate does not represent a contaminant from the laboratory or elsewhere. Rarely more than one mycobacterium can be *repeatedly* cultured from the sputum of a patient with compatible pulmonary disease, and appears to represent a double infection.[6]

Pulmonary infections with the other mycobacteria are more common in the presence of underlying pulmonary disease, such as chronic obstructive pulmonary disease, pneumoconiosis (silicosis, arc welding), previous tuberculosis, bronchiectasis, and chronic aspiration from esophageal disease.[226,227,233–235] (See below for a classification of the other mycobacterial diseases.)

SKIN TESTING

Differential skin testing with the most specific mycobacterial antigens currently available does not permit any reasonable separation of etiologic agents and therefore is not recommended. More specific antigens or *in vitro* testing techniques may resolve this problem in the future.

IDENTIFICATION OF OTHER MYCOBACTERIA

Microscopic evaluation of mycobacteria does not permit separation; however, certain cultural characteristics and biochemical studies do permit initial separation and identification of the organisms in many cases (see Tables 9-4 and 9-5).

M. bovis is both culturally and antigenically very similar to *M. tuberculosis*. It grows at 37°C. The niacin test is negative. *M. bovis* is more pathogenic for rabbits.

M. marinum (Group I) grows best at 22 to 33°C on initial isolation, and not at 37°C; it is usually niacin negative.

M. kansasii (Group I) grows at 37°C and is nonpigmented in the dark. With exposure to light for 12 to 24 hr it forms a bright yellow pigment and is thus a photochromogen. The niacin test is negative.

M. scrofulaceum Group II) grows at 37°C and produces an orange-yellow pigment both in the dark and the light, thus making it a scotochromogen. The niacin test is negative.

M. intracellulare or Battey bacillus (Group III) grows at 37°C.; the colonies range from off-

Classification of Other Mycobacterial Diseases

Mycobacterial disease caused by (Organism)

Location of disease
- Pulmonary
- Pleural
- Lymphatic
- Bone or joint
- Genitourinary
- Disseminated (miliary)
- Meningeal
- Peritoneal
- Other

Bacteriologic status
- Positive by
  - Culture only (date)
  - Microscopy and culture (date)
- Negative

Chemotherapy status
- None
- On chemotherapy since (date)
- Chemotherapy terminated (date)
  - Complete
  - Incomplete

Roentgenogram findings
- Normal
- Abnormal
  - Cavitary or noncavitary
  - Stable or worsening or improving

(Summarized from Diagnostic standards and classification of tuberculosis and other mycobacterial diseases. Am Rev Resp Dis 123:343, 1981

TABLE 9-5. Key Differential Features of Mycobacteria Recovered from Humans

Test or Property	*M. tuberculosis*	*M. bovis*	*M. kansasii*	*M. marinum*	*M. asiaticum*	*M. simiae*	*M. scrofulaceum*	*M. szulgai*	*M. gordonae*	*M. flavescens*	*M. xenopi*	*M. avium*	*M. intracellulare*	*M. malmoense*	*M. ulcerans*	*M. haemophilum*	*M. gastri*	*M. terrae complex*	*M. triviale*	*M. fortuitum*	*M. chelonei*	*M. phlei*	*M. smegmatis*	*M. vaccae*
Species of Mycobacteria →	TB Complex		Photochromogen				Scotochromogen				Nonphotochromogen									Rapid Grower				
Growth rate	S	S	S	S	S	S	S	S	S	S	S	S	S	S	S	S	S	S	S	R	R	R	R	R
Growth temperature: 22°–25° C	−	−	+	+			+	+	+	+	−	F	M	+	−	+	+	+	+	+	+	+	+	+
32°–33° C	+	+	+	+	+		+	+	+	+	F	+	+	+	+	5	+	+	+	+	+	+	+	+
35°–39° C	+	+	+	3	+	+	+	+	+	+	+	+	+	+	−	−	+	+	+	+	+	+	+	+
41°–43° C	−	−				−			−		+	+	M	−	−	−	M	M	F	M	M	+	+	F
Niacin production	+	−	−	F	−	+	−	−	−	−	−	−	−	−	−	−	−	−	−	−	V	−	−	−
Nitrate reduction	+	−	+	−	−	−	−	+	−	+	−	−	−	−	−	−	−	+	+	+	−	+	+	+
Catalase (>45 mm foam)	−	−	+	−	+	+	+		+	+	−	−	−	−	+	−	−	+	+	+	+	+	+	+
Catalase after 68° C 20 min	−	−	+	F	+	+	+		+	+	+	+	+	−	+	−	−	+	+	+	+	+	M	+
Pigmentation in dark	−	−	−	−	−	−	+	4	+	+	2	−	−	−	−	−	−	−	−	−	−	+	−	V
Pigment photoactivated	−	−	+	+	+	+	2	2,4	2	−	−	−	−	−	−	−	−	−	−	−	−	−	−	+
Tween hydrolysis (5 or 10 days)	F	−	+	+	+	−	−	F	+	+	−	−	−	+	−	−	+	+	+	M	−	+	+	+
Tellurite reduction (3 days)	−	−	−	−			−		−	F	−	M	M			−	−	−	−	M	F	M	+	M
Resistance 10μg TCH per ml	+	−	+	+	+	+	+		+	+	+	+	+		+		+	+	+	+	+	+	+	+
Growth in presence of 5% NaCl	−	−	−	−	−		−		−	+	−	−	−	−		−	−	−	+	+	M	+	+	+
Iron uptake (rusty colonies)	−	−	−	−			−		−	−	−	−	−		−		−	−	−	+	−	+	+	+
Arylsulfatase positive (3 days)	−	−	−	−	−		−	M	−	−	M	−	−		−		−	−	F	+	+	−	−	−
Growth on MacConkey agar	−	−	−	−			−		−	−	−	−	F				−	−	−	+	+	−	−	−
Urease activity	+	+	+				+		−	+	−	−	−	−		−	+	−		+	+			
Clinical significance	+	+	+	+		+	+	+	−	−	+	+	+	+	+	+	−	−	−	+	+	−	−	−

1. Key to symbols: S = slow; R = rapid; + = >84% of strains +; M = 50–84% of strains +; F = 16–49% of strains +; − = <16% of strains +;
 V = variable; blank spaces = few or no data available.
2. Pigment intensifies either with age or after prolonged (2 wk) exposure to light.
3. Strains adapt to growth at 37° C; on primary isolation, usually grow only at 31° to 33° C.
4. *M. szulgai* is scotochromogenic when grown at 37° C but photochromogenic at 25° C.
5. Grows from 25° to 30° C, no growth at 31° C. Requires hemin for growth.

(Diagnostic standards and classification of tuberculosis and other mycobacterial diseases. Am Rev Resp Dis 122:343, 1981) white to occasionally light yellow in color. The niacin test is negative.

MANAGEMENT

Disease due to *M. kansasii* responds to chemotherapy in the same manner as disease due to *M. tuberculosis*. The recommended initial treatment programs are: (1) INH, 8 to 10 mg per kg daily, and RIF, 600 mg daily, or (2) INH, 8 to 10 mg per kg daily, EMB, 15 mg per kg daily and SM, 1 g daily.[236] In vitro susceptibility studies may indicate some resistance, but drug therapy programs should be adjusted if there is a lack of clinical and/or bacteriologic response, rather than relying on susceptibility studies alone.

Cervical adenitis in young children generally requires extirpation of fluctuant or draining nodes. While this is considered localized disease resulting from invasion through the oropharynx, drug therapy in addition to surgery appears to be valid for *M. kansasii*, but questioned for *M. scrofulaceum* and *M. avium-intracellulare*.[226,227,237,238]

Disease due to *M. intracellulare* infection is notoriously refractory to chemotherapy. Some reports indicate that drugs alone have resulted in only a 20 to 25% conversion to negative sputum. Others have achieved 75% sputum conversion using four or five drug programs based on susceptibility studies.[205,225] Since the results of chemotherapy are so unpredictable, surgical resection of localized disease appears warranted.[239] Unfortunately, most patients have extensive and bilateral disease, precluding effective resectional surgery.[240] With extensive disease, one must evaluate the cost–benefit ratio. The use of four or more drugs may create more illness and threat to life than a roentgenogram abnormality. If there is roentgenogram stability with extensive disease and only slight symptoms, observation may be preferable to therapy.[241]

PART THREE: FUNGAL INFECTIONS OF THE LUNG

HISTOPLASMOSIS

Histoplasmosis is a systemic fungal infection caused by *Histoplasma capsulatum*. The organism is inhaled, invading the lung where it characteristically involves the body's reticuloendothelial system, producing a granulomatous reaction. The great majority of infections are benign and self-limited.

The organism was first identified by Darling in Panama in 1905 in three patients at autopsy.[242,243] Their illness had been characterized by fever, emaciation, hepatosplenomegaly, skin lesions, and lymph node and gastrointestinal involvement. It was not until 1932 that the organism was identified antemortem in a supravital blood smear of a child with an unusual and subsequently fatal anemia.[244] In 1933 it was cultured and animals were infected.[245] In the early 1940s, during United States Selective Service examinations, an increasing number of individuals with intrathoracic calcification on chest roentgenograms and negative tuberculin skin tests were recognized and a possible association with Histoplasma infection was suggested.[246] In 1944 skin testing of 180 children confirmed the association of intrathoracic calcification with histoplasmin reactivity.[247] However, as late as 1945 most reported cases represented a fatal systemic illness.[248,249] Histoplasmosis has been the subject of a recent extensive review.[250]

EPIDEMIOLOGY

Transmission

The spores of *H. capsulatum*, a soil saprophyte, are inhaled as "droplet nuclei" by man and animals and invade the alveolar walls. The respiratory tract is almost invariably the route of infection. Occasional cases may result from direct mucosal invasion of the oral pharynx or gastrointestinal tract, particularly in infants exposed to large numbers of organisms, but even such lesions may well reflect hematogenous dissemination. Rare cases of percutaneous inoculation have been reported.[251] Person-to-person or animal-to-human transmission generally does not occur. However, one case of direct inoculation into the perineal area from a penile lesion has been documented.[252] Thus while the route of infection is essentially identical to disease resulting from *M. tuberculosis*, the absence of person-to-person transmission is distinctly different.

Geographic Distribution

Histoplasmosis occurs worldwide. Infection, as identified by skin testing, has been found in more than 50 countries. Endemic areas have been identified throughout the western hemisphere. On the basis of skin test surveys 18 to 20% of the US population, some 50 million or more people, have been infected.[253,254] Areas with the highest infection rates in the US center about the Mississippi river valley and its major tributaries, the Ohio, Missouri, and Tennessee river valleys. In Canada the disease is endemic in the St. Lawrence river valley. Additional areas along the Atlantic seaboard (*e.g.*, Maryland and Virginia) have similar high-infection rates. Even within highly endemic areas infection rates may vary two- to tenfold within relatively short distances.[255] While the majority of cases of histoplasmosis arise in endemic areas, many cases occur in areas where the skin test reaction rate is as low as 2 to 3%. Thus the possibility of histoplasmosis should be considered in a patient with a clinically compatible history even when there has been no contact with an endemic area.

The histoplasma organism appears to thrive best in red-yellow podzolic soil with relatively high humidity and moderate temperatures. Its growth is enhanced in the presence of bird droppings, especially that of chickens and starlings, or bat guano mixed with soil, or in decaying matter such as wood. Starling roosts in urban areas have repeatedly been identified as a point source for epidemics.[256]

Epidemics occur from point sources or in groups who visit an endemic area. They have provided immensely valuable information about point sources, incubation time, and the spectrum of disease. The following point sources have been identified: chicken coops (particularly cleaning old ones); starling roosts; bats in both caves and buildings; dismantling old buildings (especially old schools); cleaning old buildings (barns, water towers, bridges, silos, church belfries); hollow trees; mycology laboratories; old storm cellars; building fires with old decaying wood; peat moss; digging for worms in woods; construction sites; major cleanup efforts (*e.g.*, Earth Day); and compost heaps.[257,258] Recently urban epidemics have been reported.[259] It has been recommended that known point sources, especially in urban areas, be "sterilized" with 2% formaldehyde, since such sources may harbor viable organisms and cause new epidemics for years.[260]

PATHOGENESIS AND PATHOLOGY

Experimental animal studies following the intranasal inoculation of histoplasma spores indicate that there is a polymorphonuclear response during the first 24 hr. At 36 hr epithelioid cells begin to replace the polymorphonuclear cells. Over the next several days the spore walls rupture, releasing their yeastlike contents to be phagocytosed by macrophages. Within a week granulomatous infiltrates involving alveoli and bronchioles appear. Dissemination of the yeast organisms to liver and spleen occurs; blood cultures may be positive. At 2 wk there is widespread involvement of the reticuloendothelial system. Within 4 to 8 mo caseating granulomas with giant cells appear in various organs.[261]

Studies in man indicate a striking similarity between the pathogenesis of histoplasmosis and tuberculosis. The incubation period is 5 to 18 days. The initial site of invasion is almost invariably the lung. This is followed by extension to adjacent lymphatics, lymph nodes, and the blood stream.[262] Hematogenous dissemination with the initial infection appears to be almost invariable. Mycobacteria and histoplasma grow relatively slowly. However, there are some apparent differences. Especially in the so-called epidemic form of histoplasmosis there are multiple airborne foci of pulmonary infection, manifested as multiple nodular densities, which is extraordinarily rare in tuberculosis. Histoplasmosis lesions in the lung and other organs, especially the spleen, calcify more frequently and to a greater extent. Histoplasmosis tends to have greater lymphatic involvement; mediastinal lymphatic involvement may produce fibrosing mediastinitis with obstruction of blood vessels leading to the superior vena cava syndrome and marked narrowing of the tracheobronchial tree. It also involves the adrenal glands, resulting in adrenal insufficiency more commonly than tuberculosis.[263]

Histoplasma capsulatum may be seen in tissues when present in large numbers with hematoxylin and eosin stains. However, they are more readily identified with periodic acid-Schiff, Gridley or Gomori methenamine-silver stains. The organism is usually 3 to 5μ, and almost always intracellular. However, there can be considerable variation in size, even as large as 15 to 20μ. They may appear to be growing by budding, and occasionally there is evidence of hyphae formation.[263] The organism is particularly difficult to identify in solitary pulmonary nodules, but careful study can be quite successful.[264]

A spectrum of disease has been proposed: severe clinical disseminated disease in an infant with marked susceptibility of macrophages to the organism and no tissue reaction or granuloma formation; an intermediate clinical and pathologic picture; and a milder more chronic form of disease characterized by more effective macrophage function and granuloma formation, as in an older male with an oropharyngeal ulcer.[250]

CLINICAL PATTERNS OF HISTOPLASMOSIS

Subclinical Infection

The most common form of infection by far is subclinical or unrecognized in the acute phase. Infection is documented subsequently by a positive histoplasmin skin test with or without other evidence of infection, such as parenchymal scarring, a pulmonary nodule, or mediastinal node enlargement, any of which may have calcification on chest roentgenograms. In endemic areas up to 80 to 95% of the population may have a positive histoplasmin skin test. A parenchymal lymph node complex has been identified in 67% of routine autopsies in an endemic area,[265] and postmortem roentgenographic studies of spleens have found 67% with calcifications and 44% with multiple calcifications characteristic of histoplasmosis.[266] In an evaluation of a small endemic focus in Milan, Michigan, 25% of 5-year-olds and 95% of 19-year-olds had positive histoplasmin skin tests as compared to an 8% rate for the rest of the county.[267] In evaluating 750 chest roentgenograms from this population, 185 were abnormal. Two-thirds of these had calcification, 40% unilateral hilar, 30% solitary parenchymal, and 30% both; other abnormalities were less common. Yet there was clinical evidence of disease in only two of these children.[268]

Acute Pulmonary (Benign) Infection

This form of the disease most often presents as a respiratory tract infection of varying severity or an influenza-like illness. The individual may have a cough with little or no sputum production, chest pain (perhaps related to the characteristic subpleural location of lesions), and systemic manifestions of fever, malaise, headache, anorexia, and myalgia. It is reasonable to assume that a large number of people with so-called inapparent infection may not have sought medical attention and are unable to subsequently recall these symptoms. Examination of the chest may be normal; there may be some localized rales or rarely an area of consolidation. If a chest roentgenogram is obtained, a localized infiltrate may be present, a picture similar to any number of pneumonias. There may also be hilar or mediastinal node enlargement. If a larger number of organisms has been inhaled there may be multiple nodular infiltrates. This latter pattern has been most commonly associated with point-source epidemics of histoplasmosis (Fig. 9-13). Over a period of time these nodules coalesce and may calcify, producing multiple tiny discrete calcifications (Fig. 9-14). Patients are seen with the latter who have not knowingly been exposed, and some cannot recall even a severe respiratory or influenza-like illness.

Acute Pulmonary (Severe) Infection

This presentation has also been characterized as fulminant or epidemic. It is due to inhalation of a large number of organisms, usually from a source that can be subsequently identified (*e.g.*, cleaning out an old feces-laden chicken coop, spelunking in a cave with bat guano). The individual appears acutely ill and quite toxic with a high fever, cough, commonly paroxysmal with little sputum production, marked tachypnea and dyspnea; cyanosis may be present. The chest roentgenogram discloses multiple nodular lesions varying from small and discrete to larger, fluffy lesions that tend to coalesce[270] (see Fig. 9-15).

Chronic Cavitary Infection

This presentation clinically and radiologically is indistinguishable from tuberculosis. It is more common in white males in their fifties who have lived in a non-urban environment. The patient has a productive cough and may have some hemoptysis. He may relate coughing up small bits of gravel or sandy, gritty material (*i.e.*, broncholithiasis) in reply to specific questioning. Nonspecific symptoms of anorexia, weight loss, and malaise are common. With extensive parenchymal involvement there may be dyspnea. There is fibronodular disease usually with cavities and volume loss, particularly in the upper lobes or the superior segment of the lower lobes on the chest roentgenogram (Fig. 9-16). Coexisting tuberculosis and histoplasmosis have been identified not infrequently, especially in tuberculosis sanitoria.[271–273]

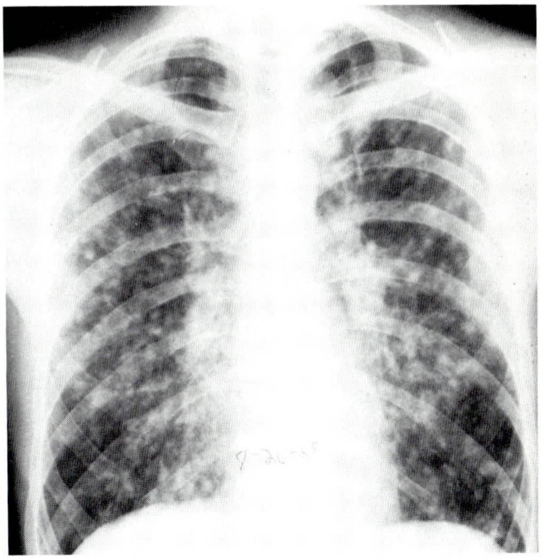

FIG. 9-13. Acute epidemic histoplasmosis with point-source exposure. Note the presence of multiple small nodules of varying size.

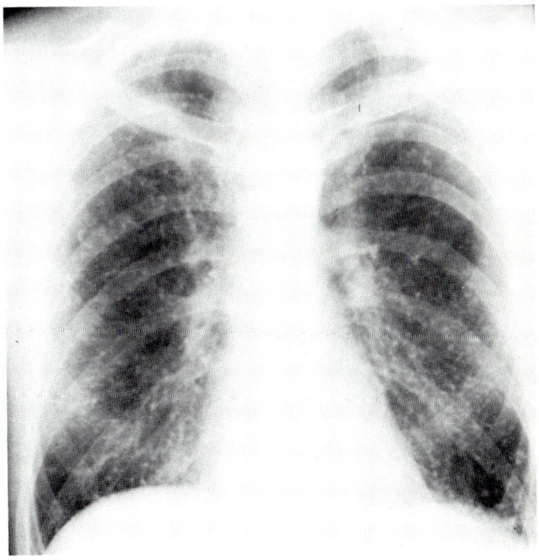

FIG. 9-14. Histoplasmosis with multiple punctate calcifications. This roentgenogram of the patient shown in Figure 9-13 was made 3 years later.

Thin-walled cavities may occur acutely and clear spontaneously. Cavitary disease is commonly found in association with centrilobular or bullous emphysema; some state that these

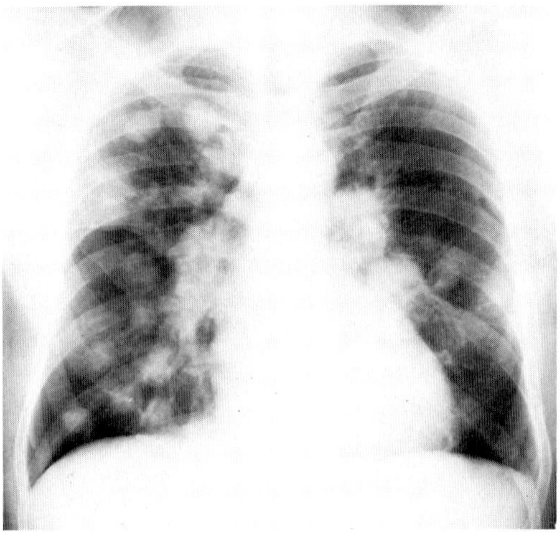

FIG. 9-15. Histoplasmosis with multiple large pulmonary nodules with hilar and mediastinal adenopathy simulating metastic malignancy.

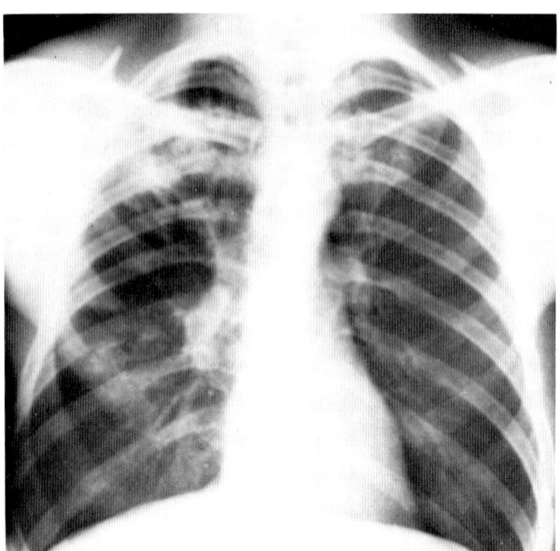

FIG. 9-16. Histoplasmosis with fibrocavitary disease in the right upper lobe, a pattern indistinguishable from other mycotic and mycobacterial diseases.

changes almost invariably precede cavitary disease.[250]

Histoplasmoma

Like other fungi and tuberculosis, histoplasmosis may cause a solitary pulmonary nodule—a histoplasmoma, on occasion, such a nodule may enlarge about 1 to 2 mm per yr. Calcification may occur centrally in 5 or more yr and concentric calcification is seen. While the stable calcified lesion is of no concern, enlarging lesions must be differentiated from carcinoma.[250]

Disseminated Infection

This form most commonly affects infants or older men.[274] Its presentation is reticuloendothelial or systemic rather than pulmonary. It is very rare; it probably occurs in less than 0.1% of acute infections. The individual has fever, malaise, weight loss, and anorexia. There may be generalized lymph node enlargement which is more prominent in adults. The individual may complain of pharyngeal pain, hoarseness or dysphagia; ulceration of the tongue, palate, epiglottis or larynx occurs in up to one-third of adults. Gastrointestinal involvement may be manifested by nausea, vomiting, diarrhea, and abdominal pain. Commonly there is hepatosplenomegaly. Frequently rather marked anemia, thrombocytopenia, and leukopenia are associated with bone marrow invasion. The most commonly involved organs are the adrenals, meninges, and brain; less commonly involved are the endocardium, pericardium, kidney, testes, prostate, esophagus, and pleura. Bone involvement is less frequent than in other systemic fungal infections. While pulmonary parenchymal or mediastinal involvement is common, it is not usually a prominent manifestation. Nodular or ulcerative skin lesions are also frequent. They are notable for their lack of specificity and commonly are not mentioned by the patient or recognized by the physician. This is most unfortunate since direct smears of the lesion using potassium hydroxide or one of the blue stains (*e.g.*, cotton methylphenyl blue) may immediately provide a diagnosis; a biopsy of the lesion wall for histology and culture should also be obtained.[275–278]

Specific Organ Involvement

Some patients with extrapulmonary disease present with primary manifestations related to a single organ. Thus a patient with meningeal involvement may relate slowly progressive symptoms of headache, altered mentation, and psychologic changes, and may have minimal meningismus. Others may present with lymphadenopathy, hepatosplenomegaly, jaundice, anemia, fever, or evidence of a coagulopathy simulating a primary reticuloendothelial disease. Some will present with chronic diarrhea, melena, or hematochezia. Rarely the presenting problem is that of pleural effusion, empyema or bronchopleural fistula.[279,280]

Pericardial involvement with histoplasmosis is another uncommon entity seen more often in children and young adults. In addition to respiratory symptoms, fever and tachycardia, chest pain and a pericardial friction rub are common. There may be neck vein distention and a paradoxical pulse. Mediastinal adenopathy, cardiac enlargement, and pleural effusion may be seen on the roentgenogram. Electrocardiographic evidence of pericarditis, S-T segment elevation, and T-wave flattening or depression are usually present. Identification or isolation of the organism in the pericardium or fluid is uncommon. Full recovery is often slow; there may be episodes of recurrent pericarditis. In a recent review overall mortality was 13%.[281]

The mediastinum may be involved with histoplasmosis in two forms that are of clinical importance: a lymph node may enlarge and impinge on a vital structure, or there may be extensive fibrosis extending throughout large areas of the mediastinum. Symptoms result from impingement on a vital structure. Thus a patient may present with (1) the superior vena cava syndrome: facial and upper extremity edema, facial flushing, headache, a choking sensation, increased venous pattern of the skin of the upper torso, neck vein distention, etc; (2) evidence of bronchial or even tracheal obstruction, with cough, often paroxysmal, recurrent pneumonia or atelectasis; (3) pulmonary venous obstruction simulating mitral stenosis; (4) pulmonary artery obstruction; and (5) esophageal obstruction. Mediastinal widening or a mass is seen on the chest roentgenogram. Histologic specimens may disclose organisms only with extensive searching. Clinical evidence of an active infection with histoplasmosis is almost always absent. The mechanisms for this response are not understood, but an abnormal host response to a residual Histoplasma antigen has been suggested.[282–284]

While it is useful to consider the presenting patterns of histoplasmosis individually, it is important to recognize that they often blend one into another. The data available would indicate that hematogenous dissemination at the time of initial infection occurs in essentially all individuals. Mild symptoms may or may not come to medical evaluation. Clinical judgment is required to separate a so-called benign acute pulmonary infection from a severe or fulminant infection. In individual disseminated cases the pulmonary involvement may be the major problem clinically, even though hepatosplenomegaly or skin lesions attest to the dissemination.

DIAGNOSIS

The absolute diagnosis of histoplasmosis requires cultural identification of the organism. Its identification in histologic preparation is often satisfactory. At times such proof may not be obtainable and a "clinical diagnosis" can be made on the basis of the clinical and roentgenographic picture, exclusion of other disease processes by careful study, and serologic evidence of infection.

Skin Test

Skin-testing material for histoplasmosis (histoplasmin) is made from a broth filtrate of the mycelial phase of *H. capsulatum*. The usual test dose is 0.1 ml of a 1:1000 solution. The reaction is read at 48 to 72 hr; a reaction of 5 mm of induration is considered significant. The actual measured induration should be recorded. A significant skin test reaction indicates infection with *H. capsulatum* at some time whether remote or recent. The reaction tends to wane over many years. There is frequent cross-reactivity with blastomycosis and on occasion with coccidioidomycosis. A false-negative reaction occurs in about 5% of patients with active pulmonary histoplasmosis and in one-third to two-thirds of patients with disseminated histoplasmosis. Most importantly a histoplasmin skin test may falsely elevate serologic studies to either the mycelial or yeast phase antigens in 25% or more of reactors.[285,286] This elevation is usually evident within 15 days and may remain for 3 or more mo. Even if a specimen for serologic study is obtained prior to skin testing, the clinical issue may be confused. The initial serological studies may be negative and a second set after a significant skin test, if elevated, may reflect a response to the skin test or the unknown disease process under study. Thus in an adult being evaluated for active disease which might be histoplasmosis, the histoplasmin skin test should not be used. The skin test may be quite helpful in an infant with possible active histoplasmosis, since a significant reaction even in an endemic area strongly supports the diagnosis. Histoplasmin skin testing has been and continues to be a very valuable epidemiologic tool in population surveys in identifying endemic areas. In a patient with a pulmonary nodule or parenchymal or lymph node calcification, a histoplasmin skin test result should not be considered as definitive of a specific etiology for the lesion. Often the local reaction may proceed to superficial ulceration.

Serologic Tests

The standard serologic study is the complement fixation technique using a mycelial phase antigen (MF), histoplasmin, and a yeast phase antigen (YF). The YF is usually elevated first after initial infection, while the MF rises later but tends to remain elevated with chronic disease for extended periods. After acute infection one or the other is elevated in 14% at 2 wk, 67% at 3 wk, 86% at 4 wk, and "almost all" after 4 wk.[287] Thus it is important to repeat serologic studies at 2- to 4-wk intervals to avoid "missing" a *titer* that has not yet risen. Even in chronic cavitary histoplasmosis the percentage of patients with elevated titers increased from 88% with a single specimen to 93% with multiple specimens.

In other studies, positive titers have occurred in 97% of culturally proven cases of pulmonary disease and up to 100% of cases with chronic progressive pulmonary disease. However, in cases where disease has only been documented by identifying the organism in tissue, positive results have been found less frequently. Unfortunately, in disseminated disease, false-negative results have occurred in 45 to 80%.[276,277] Thus a negative complement fixation study does not exclude histoplasmosis. False-positive reactions may occur particularly with blastomycosis and rarely with coccidioidomycosis, cryptococcosis, nonspecific uveitis, or carcinoma.[288]

The height of titers does not appear to correlate with the severity of disease or ultimate prognosis. Some authors consider the continued elevation of titers of 1:32 or greater, or titers that vary from zero to 1:8 or 1:16, as indications of continued activity and potential difficulty. We have seen initial titers in excess of 1:1024 which gradually decreased to 1:64 over 8 to 10 mo and ultimately became negative over several years with acute benign multinodular disease manifested as a mild, short-lived respiratory infection. Low-grade titers have been documented for many months without evidence of disease activity.

A histoplasmin latex agglutination test is frequently positive in acute infections but in only about 50% of chronic active infections. An agar-gel double-diffusion test with histoplasmin as antigen appears quite promising, although not generally available. The development of an H band is quite specific for active and progressive disease and usually is not influenced by skin testing. It may be found 1 to 2 yr after clinical recovery. An M band may be found with acute or chronic disease or following a positive skin test. It appears earlier than the H band and may persist much longer. An M band alone is of little diagnostic help; both bands are commonly found with active disease.[289] Cerebrospinal fluid serologies may be of value in diagnosing meningitis due to histoplasmosis.[290] The increased sensitivity of immunodiffusion and electroimmunodiffusion has been reviewed, but satisfactory clinical correlation is not yet available.[291]

A study comparing patients with active histoplasmosis to healthy people with a significant histoplasmin skin test found suppression of T cell function (lymphocyte transformation and skin-test reaction), which may be a result of circulating antibody or antigen-antibody complexes.[292]

Knowledge of the sensitivity and specificity of serologic studies as performed in the specific laboratory being used is essential. If reliability is at all questionable, state, federal government, or other reference laboratories should be used.

Identification and Culture

Specimen Source. Fresh single sputum specimens should be taken directly to the laboratory to minimize contamination with bacteria or saprophytic fungi. It may help to thoroughly rinse the mouth before coughing. If sputum cannot be raised spontaneously, induction with hypertonic saline (*e.g.*, 3–10% saline in a heated nebulizer or an ultrasonic nebulizer) should be attempted. When noninvasive techniques are unsuccessful, fiberoptic bronchoscopy for washings, brush specimens, and a transbronchoscopic biopsy are recommended. Rigid bronchoscopy is seldom helpful unless there is a quite central endobronchial lesion. Percutaneous needle or open lung biopsy may be necessary on occasion. When mediastinal nodes are involved they offer an alternative biopsy site. Scalene node biopsy has only rarely been helpful.

With acute disease and disseminated disease, blood and urine cultures are useful. A bone marrow biopsy is an excellent source of material for culture and histologic identification of the organism.[293] Any skin or mucous membrane lesion should have direct touch preparations and biopsy for culture and special staining for fungi. With evidence of other organ involvement (*e.g.*, meninges, pericardium, liver, pleura) appropriate specimens should be obtained.

Identification. Direct preparations of sputum or other material stained with Wright or Giemsa stain will demonstrate the organism as an oval 2 to 4μ body with a large vacuole; buds with a narrow attachment may be seen at the smaller end of the cell. Surrounding each organism is a pale capsule-like area (hence the name *capsulatum*) that represents an artifact due to protoplasmic shrinkage rather than a true capsule.

Culture. *Histoplasma capsulatum* has been most difficult to grow in many laboratories even when an appropriate specimen is provided. The organism will grown on brain–heart infusion glucose blood agar and Sabouraud's glucose agar at room temperature and 37°C with antibiotics added to prevent bacterial overgrowth. It can also be grown in laboratory animals such as mice.

MANAGEMENT

The vast majority of patients who develop histoplasmosis do not require treatment and with subclinical disease do not even seek medical attention. Patients with acute benign pulmonary histoplasmosis have a self-limited illness that requires nothing more than symptomatic and supportive therapy for a short period. This holds in the presence of a stable or regressive parenchymal infiltrate or mediastinal involvement even with slow resolution. In the presence of severe symptoms, clinical toxicity, and extensive, usually multinodular, infiltrate on chest roentgenogram one should seriously consider specific therapy, namely amphotericin B. Since this drug must be given intravenously over an extended period, its morbidity must be weighed against that of the primary illness. In an individual as just described, we generally initiate treatment with amphotericin B with a target total dose of a gram or less; the intent is to avoid the several weeks to 5 or 6 mo of morbidity manifested by severe fatigue, malaise, and possible recrudescence of acute illness with fever and prostration. Others are more restrictive in their use of amphotericin, requiring persistent and/or progressive symptoms for weeks before initiating treatment.

Chronic pulmonary histoplasmosis that is progressive or cavitary radiographically requires a full course of amphotericin B. In an evaluation of the course of 90 patients without chemotherapy, there were nine deaths due to the pulmonary disease (four others after pulmonary surgery) and roentgenographic progression in 79% of those followed for 3 yr.[269] In the United States Public Health Service Cooperative Mycoses Study 27 of 84 patients with untreated chronic pulmonary disease died at a fairly constant rate of 6 to 9% per yr: there was roentgenographic progression each year, increasing from 23% in the first to 64% in the sixth year. These patients had extensive bilateral, usually cavitary disease.[294] A subsequent study comparing treated *vs.* untreated patients clearly documented the efficacy of amphotericin B at a total dose of 25 mg/kg body weight or greater.[295] However, there is a report indicating that 16 of 20 patients with so-called early chronic pulmonary disease achieved stability or "inactivity" with prolonged hospitalization (average 3.6 mo), bed rest, and extended abstinence from usual activity or work (6 mo).[296] This approach, much like that for tuberculosis prior to chemotherapy, results in a formidable morbidity.

The usual current recommended total dose of amphotericin B is 2.0 to 2.5 g or a minimum of 35 mg/kg body weight. Since the drug must be given intravenously in a daily dose not to exceed 1 mg/kg, therapy is extended and difficult for patient and physician alike. Many physicians limit the daily dose to 50 mg and administer the drug every other day or three times a week to minimize toxicity. Administration of a dose which produces peak serum levels that are at least twice the *in vitro* inhibitory concentration daily over 10 wk is an effective alternative which reduces the total dose.[297] On occasion, doses in excess of 2 g may be necessary to control disease or treat recurrence.

Amphotericin routinely causes significant renal malfunction: elevation of the BUN and creatinine, fall in creatinine clearance, a potassium-wasting nephropathy, cylindruria, hyposthenuria, hyperuricemia, and renal tubular acidosis; other tubular dysfunctions and nephrocalcinosis may occur. Most of these disorders return toward normal after therapy is discontinued. A reduction in dose or temporary discontinuation of the drug is usually recommended when the BUN exceeds 50 mg/dl or the creatinine exceeds 3.5 mg/dl. Since about 25% of patients develop hypokalemia, it is useful to regularly give oral potassium chloride. Mild to moderate anemia occurs in about 75% and some patients develop thrombocytopenia. The nonspecific symptoms of fever, nausea, vomiting, and chills appear to respond to premedication with aspirin, a phenothiazine (chlorpromazine), and diphenhydramine. Local vein damage appears to be decreased by adding 20 to 30 mg of heparin and 25 to 50 mg of hydrocortisone to each IV bottle. The infusion of a small test dose on the initial day and then increasing this each day until the desired daily dose in achieved is recommended. At times, however, especially with doses in excess of 50 mg daily, the generalized debility and interference with alimentation caused by the drug may be so deleterious that temporary cessation of therapy is warranted.[298, 299] This polyene antibiotic preferentially increases fungal cell-wall permeability and has immunoadjuvant properties on humoral antibodies (IgG greater than IgM) and cell-mediated immunity. These effects are seen at lower than fungicidal levels and may represent an important component of the effectiveness of amphotericin B.[300]

Although resection of localized chronic, especially cavitary, disease has been a common practice, the response to amphotericin B has been so satisfactory that it is seldom if ever recommended to control infection. The resection of extensive residual disease or cavities does not appear to be warranted.

Disseminated histoplasmosis affects the very young as well as those beyond the fifth decade, and is often associated with other underlying severe disease. It has a mortality of over 80% if not treated. In one series 20 of 22 patients not treated died from 2 wk to 67 mo from the time of diagnosis, 16 within 4 mo. While in a group of 22 patients receiving an adequate course of therapy, all were alive at 3 mo; 13 died between 3 and 107 mo after starting treatment, but none died from active histoplasmosis. Relapses requiring treatment occur. Patients have been reported as cured with total doses as low as 460 mg, although most physicians recommend a total initial course of treatment consisting of 2 g or 35 to 40 mg/kg body weight.[301]

Effective therapy for generalized fibrosing mediastinitis has not been defined. On occasion a localized obstruction of a critical structure may be relieved by resection, although from a technical standpoint this is usually exceptionally difficult. There are no data indicating that amphotericin is of value; the histologic absence or scarcity of organisms support this. Although a potential benefit in interrupting a possible immunologic pathogenesis of this problem with corticosteroids is mentioned, documentation of a beneficial effect is not available. The potential of the corticosteroids to exacerbate or even cause dissemination of the initial infection may well contribute to the lack of reported clinical results with corticosteroids.

COCCIDIOIDOMYCOSIS

Coccidioidomycosis is a systemic fungal infection caused by *Coccidioides immitis.* The initial route of infection is almost invariably through the inhalation of arthrospores whose natural habitat is soil in fairly well-defined endemic areas. The great majority of infections are benign and self-limited. The disease has been called San Joaquin fever, valley fever, desert fever, desert rheumatism, valley bumps, coccidioidal granuloma, Posadas' disease, California disease, or simply "cocci."

The first patient with coccidioidomycosis, a soldier from the Argentine pampas, had disseminated disease with slowly progressing multiple skin lesions which were initially considered to be a form of neoplasia; an organism, thought to be a protozoan, was found in the lesions and inoculated material from the lesions produced disease in animals.[302] In 1896 the organism was named *Coccidioides immitis* in California.[303] The organism was isolated from soil in an area where four Filipinos contracted fatal disseminated disease in 1932.[304] Fairly common mild symptomatic disease with pneumonia and erythema nodosum was described in 1938.[305] Over the next 30 years Smith, Winn, and others made major contributions to the epidemiology, ecology, prevention, skin testing, and clinical course of the disease, and to the clinical correlation of serological studies.[302,306] A report on the Third International Coccidioidomycosis Symposium of 1976 and an extraordinarily comprehensive review have recently been published.[307,308]

EPIDEMIOLOGY

Transmission

Coccidioides immitis exists in the mycelial phase in soil. These spores are highly contagious for man and animals. Inhalation of spores is almost the invariable route of infection, although occasional cases of percutaneous inoculation have occurred.[309,310] Neither person-to-person nor animal-to-human transmission has been documented. However, infection carried by fomites does occur.[311] Organisms that reverted to the mycelial phase on a cast removed from a draining coccidioidomycosis sinus infected six hospital personnel.[312] Cases of coccidioidomycosis have occurred outside endemic areas with the individual never having visited such an area; these infections have been attributed to organisms carried by soil, food, cotton, wool, and the like from an endemic area. Since the organism is highly contagious in its mycelial form, accidental laboratory infection is a very real risk.[313]

Geographic Distribution

The endemic areas for coccidioidomycosis are relatively limited. The highest endemic areas are in the south-western United States and northern Mexico. The areas involved are generally semiarid (about 10 inches rainfall) with high summer temperatures (100°F) and mild winters (33°F or higher); these areas have been called the Lower Sonoran Life Zone. The soil is generally alkaline. The organism is quite resistant to high salt concentrations. It will grow readily in sterile soil, but less so in the presence of other microorganisms such as *B. subtilis.* Endemic areas are not limited to the Lower Sonoran Life Zone; some tropical areas, "Mediterranean Woodland areas" of northern California, and cool moist sandy areas are also involved.[308]

The most endemic areas recognized are Kern County in the southern San Joaquin valley, Maricopa County (Phoenix), and Pima County (Tucson) in Arizona and several southern counties in Texas bordering on the Rio Grande. In addition to these areas other parts of southern California, Nevada, Arizona, Texas, Utah, and New Mexico are also endemic. Outside the United States and northern Mexico endemic areas have been identified in Guatemala, Honduras, Venezuela, Paraguay, Argentina, and Colombia. The disease has been recognized in the Soviet Union, Pakistan, Algeria, and Australia. Cases outside the Western Hemisphere are questioned.[308]

It has been estimated that there are about 10 million people living who have been infected with coccidioidomycosis. Wild and domesticated animals including dogs and cattle also develop the disease. In some endemic areas 15 to 50% of newly arrived persons will be infected in 1 yr and 80% or more within 5 yr. The generally benign nature of the disease and the effectiveness of therapy are supported by the less than 100 deaths per yr in the United States. The infection rate is particularly high during the hot, dry periods when blowing dust increases.

Epidemics of coccidioidomycosis have been associated with digging at new sites of construction (*e.g.*, the California and Arizona airfields of World War II) and subsequently archeological diggings, rodent burrows, and mycology laboratory accidents.[313] Guidelines for protecting exposed persons are available.[308]

The names "San Joaquin fever" or "valley fever" tend to narrowly restrict diagnostic consideration of this disease. It deserves consideration in compatible clinical illness throughout the southwestern United States and other endemic areas. With the extent of modern travel and the possibility of transmission to unusual locations by fomites, it deserves consideration in any area in a patient with a compatible clinical picture in whom a specific diagnosis is wanting.

PATHOGENESIS AND PATHOLOGY

Spores settling on bronchial walls may cause endobronchitis. Those reaching alveoli evoke a macrophage response followed rapidly by polymorphonuclear invasion similar to a bacterial pneumonia; the sporangia with endospores may be identified in such lesions. These 30-to-60μ organisms are identifiable with hematoxylin and eosin stain. The 2-to-5μ endospores usually require periodic acid-Schiff, Gridley, or Gomori methenamine-silver stain for identification when released from the spherule. The pyogenic response is attributed to a chemotactic neutrophilic response evoked when the spherules rupture. The organism is phagocytized by macrophages. T lymphocytes exposed to antigen evoke cell-mediated immunity and activation of macrophages. B lymphocytes produce IgM and then IgG antibodies. Subsequently granuloma formation occurs about the spherule. The granulomata are indistinguishable from those of other infectious granulomatous disease with epithelial cells, caseation, and ultimately fibrosis and calcification. A third type of response that is quite common is a mixed pyogenic and granulomatous response in the same lesion. The pyogenic and mixed response is distinctly different than that seen in tuberculosis or histoplasmosis. As lesions become older and perhaps less active, a more typical granulomatous response is found. Hyphae have been found in over 70% of cavitary and 30% of granulomatous pulmonary surgical specimens.[314] Peribronchial and paratracheal nodes are routinely involved in the initial infection. The areas of caseation may shell out, producing cavities with varying amounts of surrounding granulomatous inflammation.

Initially the acute pyogenic and granulomatous reaction may produce little or no necrosis of alveolar septa; this type of lesion may heal without residua. More commonly healing occurs with residual fibrosis and hyalinization with or without central caseation or calcification. Organisms can commonly be cultured from resected nodules with central caseation.

In disseminated disease studied at autopsy the most commonly involved organs are lymph nodes, meninges, spleen, liver, kidney, skin, and adrenals. The involvement of the spleen, liver, kidney, and adrenals is believed to be late and rarely of clinical significance. There may also be a nonspecific myocarditis. The pericardium and peritoneum may be involved. The gastrointestinal tract is very rarely involved. Clinically significant disease involves primarily the lung, meninges, skin, and bone.[315]

Meningitis is one of the most common causes of death from coccidioidomycosis. A diffuse granulomatous meningitis surrounds the brain and often causes obstructive hydrocephalus. Cranial or spinal lesions may cause meningitis by direct extension. There may be pyogenic microabscesses. Significant brain invasion is rare.[316]

The pathogenesis of the initial coccidioidomycosis infection simulates tuberculosis with involvement of hilar or paratracheal nodes. Hematogenous dissemination of serious consequence likewise occurs in a small percentage of those infected. An initial benign hematogenous dissemination of organisms in coccidioidomycosis similar to that which occurs in histoplasmosis or tuberculosis is not as well documented. While granulomas are seen as often in pulmonary (localized) disease as in disseminated disease, the suppurative component may be more marked in disseminated disease. Clinical, immunologic, and pathologic correlations provide a framework to view coccidioidomycosis as a continuous spectrum of disease. The least serious disease with excellent host response is represented by acute pulmonary involvement, a high degree of cell-mediated immunity, spontaneous recovery, little or no antibody response (see Serology), excellent granuloma formation, and few intact organisms. The middle of this spectrum would be represented by increased extent and number of extrapulmonary areas involved. The most serious disease with least host response is represented by extensive dissemination involving the skin and the musculoskeletal system; minimal cellular immunity or none at all; a high probability of death without treatment; high antibody levels; prominent polymorphonuclear response; poor granuloma formation; and a large number of intact organisms. The response of the host is modulated by the number of organisms.

Initial infection appears to establish a very strong lifelong immunity to exogenous reinfection. However, such infection may occur with heavy exposure such as with laboratory accidents.[317]

CLINICAL PATTERNS OF COCCIDIOIDOMYCOSIS

Subclinical Infection

Various estimates indicate that 60 to 80% of persons infected with *Coccidioides immitis*, as defined by a positive skin test, are unable to recall any symptoms referable to the infection. Some of these may have had mild respiratory or influenza-like illness. There may be roentgenographic residua such as a nodule with or without calcification, hilar or paratracheal node enlargement or calcification, parenchymal scarring, or a cavity.[302]

Acute Pulmonary Infection

After an incubation period of 7 to 28 days, usually 10 to 16 days, the patient presents with the sudden onset of chest pain, cough that is usually dry, fever, malaise, anorexia, chills, sweating, headache, and streaks of hemoptysis. The most common symptom is chest pain (75–90% in various series). This pain is usually pleuritic and of short duration; it varies from mild to exceptionally severe. Some patients complain of substernal pain on swallowing. A fine erythematous macular or urticarial rash occurs during the first few days in about 10%. There may be clinical evidence of a pleural effusion or friction rub, episcleritis, conjunctivitis, or keratitis.[318] Although nonspecific, headache does occur. If there is any question of meningitis during early dissemination, the cerebral spinal fluid should be examined, and serologic studies performed.[308] Eosinophilia is common. Pleural biopsy is useful to identify the organisms.[308]

Erythema nodosum or erythema multiforme occurs between 3 and 21 days after symptoms begin. They are usually accompanied by arthralgias or arthritis without effusion, particularly in the ankles and knees. This occurs in 20 to 25% of adult white females and 5% of white male patients. Thus the terms "desert bumps" and "desert rheumatism." It is a good indication of strong host defense since dissemination is most unusual in such patients. On the chest roentgenogram there may be segmental or subsegmental parenchymal infiltrates usually in the lower lobes, single or multiple nodules, thin- or thick-walled cavities, hilar or mediastinal lymphadenopathy (unilateral or bilateral), or pleural effusion; these may occur alone or in various combinations. In one study of 59 patients admitted to a military hospital with acute coccidioidomycosis there was a segmental pneumonia in 46%, a minimal infiltrate in 27%, hilar lymphadenopathy in 19%, a pleural effusion in 19% (documented by lateral decubitus films), and a variety of the other findings mentioned in less than 10% each. In this series 22% showed progression, usually from an infiltrate to a nodule over extended time periods.[319] Nodules may excavate to form thin- or thick-walled cavities; these are usually in the upper lobes. A cavity is considered "thin" if the wall is 3 mm or less in thickness. Although uncommon, a diffuse multiple nodular presentation simulating that seen in epidemic histoplasmosis may occur without representing serious hematogenous dissemination. The resolution time for these initial roentgenographic findings averages 20 days. Small infiltrates may clear in 2 wk or less while larger infiltrates may require months to clear. About 1% of symptomatic patients will have a prolonged illness lasting weeks or months. Disease is considered to be persistent or chronic when symptoms or roentgenographic changes persist beyond 6 to 8 wk.[308]

Chronic Pulmonary Infection

Stable or Benign Form. It is estimated that 2 to 8% of symptomatic patients will have residual changes on chest roentgenogram. These may take the form of a nodule ("coin-lesion") which can be smooth or lobulated, or multiple nodules; they may calcify.

Chronic cavity formation may occur either with a thick or thin wall; there is usually a single cavity. Cavitation is estimated to occur in about 2% of hospitalized cases or 1 in 1000 patients with symptomatic coccidioidomycosis. Most patients are asymptomatic; reports vary from 24% in a civilian population to 58% in a military population, where chest roentgenograms are taken more frequently. The most common symptoms are small amounts of hemoptysis; cough; or vague chest pains or discomfort. It is stated that cavitary disease is more common in whites and males. Spontaneous closure is common; it occurred in 50% of 103 patients at a median of 2 yr after onset.[320]

Persistent Pneumonia. Some patients will have persistent infiltrates involving a considerable amount of lung and associated with fever, productive cough, chest pain, and prostration for many months if not treated.[308]

Progressive Form. The initial parenchymal lesions may progress over months to years and develop single or multiple cavities in association with respiratory and systemic symptoms that are indistinguishable from tuberculosis. Indeed, patients have commonly been hospitalized and treated for tuberculosis; concomitant infection with both organisms was not rare.[321] Diabetics appear to be predisposed to cavitation.[308]

Nodules may enlarge over a period of years, indicating activity and also raising concern over a possible malignancy. Nodules may excavate at some time remote from the initial infection ("abscessing coccidioma"). There may be spread of disease about the lesion. This may be associated with cough and sputum production or hemoptysis. Sputum cultures may grow *Coccidioides immitis.*

Cavitary lesions may gradually decrease or increase in size; enlargement may follow a previous decrease. They may fill with inspissated material ("blocked cavity") and subsequently empty. There may be bronchogenic spread of disease to other areas of lung. They may cross fissure lines (see Fig. 9-17). Those that are close to the visceral pleura or show variation in size have a greater propensity to rupture through the visceral pleura with a resultant empyema and bronchopleural fistula. Cavitary lesions may develop secondary bacterial infections with air–fluid levels or increased size. Dissemination is quite uncommon in patients with cavitary lesions.

Disseminated Infection

It is estimated that dissemination occurs in about 1 in 6000 infections or in 0.5% or less of symptomatic patients. The propensity for dissemination is highest in Filipinos, followed by blacks; in Kern County, California, in 1936 and 1937 the death rate for disseminated disease for Filipinos was 173 times, and for blacks 23 times, that of whites. It is estimated that dissemination occurs in 10 to 15% of dark-skinned people.[309] There also appears to be an increased risk in Native Americans (Indians) and Mexicans (Indians). However, when other factors are controlled such as underlying diseases, immunocompromised hosts, extent of exposure, and age, the extent of the influence of race may be revised.[322] In dark-skinned individuals dissemination usually follows closely on the initial infection and involves multiple systems. There is no known difference in infection rates or evidence for an effect of adverse socioeconomic conditions. Dissemination also occurs more frequently in pregnancy. The risk is greater in the second and third trimesters. Dissemination carries a very high maternal and fetal mortality, although congenital infection of the fetus is rare.[323,324] Recently, dissemination has been shown to be a significant problem in the compromised host (*e.g.*, Hodgkin's disease, lymphoma, other tumors, renal transplant, uremia, immunosuppressive therapy with associated granulocytopenia and lymphopenia, and corticosteroid therapy). This may occur even with remote infection with or without a significant skin test reaction. The underlying disease or the treatment may depress the skin-test reaction or serologic response. Thus, negative skin and serologic studies do not exclude the diagnosis. If there is a history of travel or residence in endemic areas, skin testing should be done before giving immunosuppressive therapy, if possible.[308] In this group of patients the dissemination may be explosive. The patients may present as acute respiratory failure (wet lung, adult respiratory distress syndrome).[325–327] (See also Chap. 7.)

Dissemination must be considered when there is persistent fever and toxicity beyond 4 wk after the onset of symptoms, supraclavicular or cervical lymphadenopathy (although this may be found without significant dissemination), evidence of skin, subcutaneous, or bone involvement, or meningitis. The chest roentgenogram may show slow resolution or extension of parenchymal disease; a miliary pattern may develop; there may be enlargement of hilar and paratracheal nodes (none of which assures the presence of dissemination). Untreated disseminated disease has a fatality rate in excess of 50% in 3 yr.[329]

In generalized dissemination osteomyelitis occurs in about half the cases. The ribs, vertebrae, and long bones are most commonly involved. Joint involvement with arthritis occurs in about one third of patients with dissemination. The bone lesions are usually osteolytic. There may be draining sinuses from bone lesions. With hematogenous dissemination blood and urine cultures may be positive.[327–329]

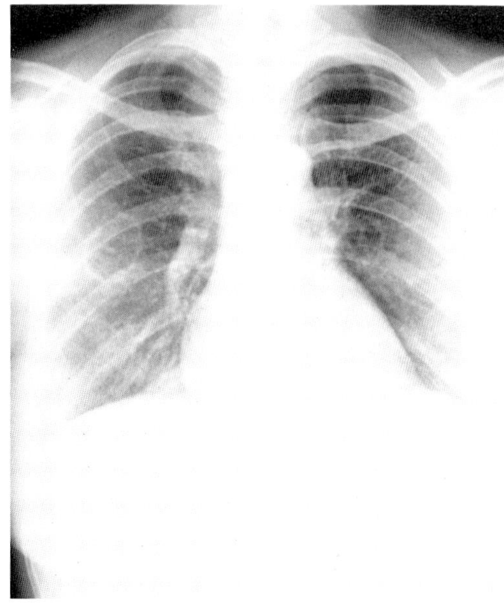

FIG. 9-17. Coccidioidomycosis with a thin-walled cavity in the superior segment of the right lower lobe of 4 × 5 cm. Rather than remaining stable, this disease process progressed over the next 9 years, crossing the fissure into the right upper lobe.

Specific Organ Involvement

Meningitis. The extrapulmonary site is limited to one organ in about 20% of patients with dissemination. There is a predilection for the meninges, and one-third to one-half of individuals with dissemination have meningeal involvement. Meningitis may lead to communicating or noncommunicating hydrocephalus. Meningeal involvement may be an acute and fulminant extension of the initial infection with headache, meningismus, and other neurologic signs. However, headache may accompany the initial infection without meningeal involvement. Examination of the cerebral spinal fluid will generally disclose increased lymphocytes, elevated protein, and a decreased sugar (compared to a concomitant blood sugar); however, a polymorphonuclear response can occur, as well as eosinophilia. Coccidioidomycosis complement-fixation titers of cerebral spinal fluid will be elevated in about 75 to 95% of patients.[330,331]

A chronic form of meningitis is more commonly found in whites. Symptoms may be limited to vague psychologic alterations, mild headache, or subtle neurologic signs over an extended period. There may be intermittent low-grade fever. In one series over 50% of the cases had no history of coccidioidomycosis, and all had a negative coccidioidin skin test; the diagnosis rested on complement-fixation studies of serum and cerebral spinal fluid.[332] Especially with this subtle presentation, the diagnosis is often only made at autopsy. Meningitis has a mortality approaching 100% without specific therapy.

Chronic Cutaneous Disease. Although this was the major feature of the originally described cases, it is quite rare as a sole manifestation of dissemination. It too is more common in dark-skinned individuals. Lesions commonly appear first as areas of induration about the face, head, and neck. They enlarge and grow into wartlike lesions, and may simulate epitheliomas or appear as indolent ulcers. The overall disease process may extend over many years, even without treatment, before multisystem involvement proves fatal. Skin lesions, far more commonly, are but one facet of multisystem dissemination.

DIAGNOSIS

Skin Test

The standard coccidioidin skin test is made from a filtrate of a broth culture of *Coccidioides immitis;* 0.1 ml of 1:100 solution is injected intradermally. A significant reaction is defined as 5 mm of induration or more in diameter when read both at 24 and 48 hr. If the reaction is not significant, testing with 0.1 ml of 1:10 solution is recommended; significant reactions in patients with histoplasmosis or blastomycosis have been reported with this strength. In a patient with erythema nodosum or erythema multiforme the initial test should be made with a 1:10,000 dilution to avoid exacerbating the skin lesions and developing systemic symptoms. The skin test reaction develops between 3 and 28 days after the onset of symptoms. Skin reactivity may persist for extended periods, even for life. However, reactivity does wane with age. In early reports skin test reactivity in acute pulmonary disease approached 100% contrasted to a figure of 30% or less with disseminated disease. More recent studies with coccidioidin 1:100 have shown an insignificant reaction in 55% of symptomatic archeology students after an exposure. One can only speculate whether current lots of coccidioidin (bioassayed to match Smith's original material) are less potent, or whether truly infected individuals were missed in the earlier studies, or both. When a significant skin-test reaction reduces or disappears, this is a strong indication of dissemination.[333] In 300 cases of chronic cavitary disease a significant reaction has been reported in 80% with 1:100 and an additional 12% with 1:10 coccidioidin;[334] in another series of 211 cases it was as low as 54% with 1:100.[320] The coccidioidin skin test does not affect coccidioides serology. Recently a more sensitive skin test antigen has been developed from the spherules of *Coccidioides immitis*, spherulin. In various studies it has identified 25 to 35% more reactors than coccidiodin and all those who reacted to the latter in the "usual skin test strengths" (equivalent to 1:100 coccidioidin). Probable cross-reaction to histoplasmosis occurred in about 1%. With the "high test strength" (equivalent to 1:10 coccidioidin) in persons who did not respond to the lower strengths, about 5% more reacted compared to 2.5% with coccidioidin 1:10; probable cross-reactions to Histoplasmosis occurred in 7%. Spherulin, "usual skin test strength," has also produced reactions in 74% of patients with active dissemination, compared with a 39% response to coccidioidin.

At present the use of spherulin to identify a greater number of truly infected persons (increased sensitivity) appears warranted in areas where histoplasmosis is not endemic. Its use in such areas will lower specificity. If one is attempting to identify occult or evolving dissemination, the problem is more difficult. The greater reactivity to spherulin may lower the number of disseminating individuals identified. A reasonable approach in evaluating a patient for this disease would be the initial use of coccidioidin; if a significant reaction occurs, infection has been identified and this antigen can subsequently be used to assist in indentifying dissemination. If it is not significant, spherulin, "usual" and then "high strength," if necessary, can be used to identify the infected. Subsequent changes in reactivity may indicate dissemination. In addition to the specific anergy to coccidioidal antigens with dissemination, depressed or absent reactions to other recall and sensitizing antigens occurs.[308,335] As with other skin tests, reaction indicates infection, whether remote or current; thus it may not aid in diagnosis of active disease. However, the conversion of a skin test during an illness is strong confirmatory diagnostic data.

Serologic Tests

The two standard tests are the tube-precipitin (TP) and the complement-fixation (CF) tests.[330] Precipitins become positive within 7 to 28 days of the onset of symptomatic initial infection in approximately 90% of patients, but are found in only about 10% of patients at 4 mo. Cross-reactions are extremely rare. The CF test usually is positive at 4 to 6 wk after the onset of symptoms and reaches a maximum response in acute pulmonary disease in 2 to 3 mo. CF is positive in approximately 90% of patients with uncomplicated acute disease and usually disappears in 6 to 8 mo; a titer of 1:8 or less may persist for years. This test is quite specific although weak cross-reactions may occur with disseminated histoplasmosis. It is extremely valuable in following the course of disease since a rising titer or one greater than 1:16 to 1:32 strongly suggests dissemination. With a single extrapulmonary lesion the serum titer may be less than 1:16. Persistently elevated titers correlate well with continued activity, and falling titers indicate improvement. An elevated titer is not a uniform finding with dissemination. The immunocompromised host may not be able to produce antibodies despite dissemination. In chronic cavitary disease positive complement-fixation tests, usually with titers of 1:8 or less, have been found in 74 to 82% of large series.[320,334] It must be emphasized that results will vary from laboratory to laboratory. Thus, these figures are guidelines. They are not a substitute for specific knowledge of results in the user's laboratory. Indeed, it is recommended that serial studies for comparison in an individual patient should be performed simultaneously on aliquots of each specimen.

Two screening procedures have been developed: the latex particle agglutination test, which correlates with the TP, and an immunodiffusion CF test, which correlates with the CF. Together they have been positive in 93% of patients ultimately proven to have coccidioidomycosis (any form) *vs.* 85% for the standard TP and CF tests. An immunodiffusion TP (tube precipition) that is more sensitve than the latex-particle agglutination test is also available.[308] Since the screening tests have some false positives, are not quantitative, and do not provide information about the course of the disease, positive tests should be verified with the standard techniques.[286]

Identification and Culture

The identification of the typical 30-to-60μ spherule filled with many 2-to-5μ endospores in pus from draining abscesses, biopsy tissue, or sputum is diagnostic. However, artifacts in sputum may be misleading. Sputum or pus should be placed in sodium hydroxide with or without ink or one of the blue stains. Identification in tissue has already been discussed. As with other systemic fungal infections, a careful search should be made for nonspecific, particularly indolent ulcers or sinus tracts from an underlying lesion that may be a cutaneous manifestation of dissemination. Direct preparation or biopsy may provide the diagnosis. For pulmonary lesions in patients without sputum production, sputum induction, fiberoptic bronchoscopy with brushings and transbronchial biopsy, and percutaneous or open lung biopsy should be considered in an orderly stepwise fashion.

The organism readily grows on Sabouraud's agar or similar media. Petri dishes or plate cultures should be avoided because of the great risk of accidental infection of personnel and all those sharing the laboratory's air. It is preferable to use slants or bottles that can be tightly sealed. Rigid hood protocol should be used if subculturing is to be done; formaldehyde may be poured over the slants prior to evaluation. Definitive diagnosis may require animal inoculation (using mice) to identify the spherules.

MANAGEMENT

The vast majority of patients who develop coccidioidomycosis do not require specific treatment and with subclinical disease do not seek medical attention. Most patients who develop acute pulmonary disease do well with symptomatic therapy and rest during the acute illness.

The standard of drug therapy is amphotericin B. A full course of intravenous therapy is recommended for (1) severe or progressive pulmonary disease; (2) impending or a high probability of dissemination as manifested by (a) clinical and roentgenographic evidence, (b) elevated or rising titers of 1:16 to 1:32 or greater, (c) a negative coccidioidin skin test, (d) the predisposition of Filipinos and blacks, (e) infection in the third trimester of pregnancy, (f) immunosuppression due to disease or the use of immunosuppressive drugs, or (g) diabetes mellitus; (3) disseminated disease as manifested by meningitis, lymph nodes in the neck, a destructive bone lesion, and so forth; and (4) chronic cavitary disease simulating tuberculosis or histoplasmosis. The latter has been associated with frequent superinfection.

Coccidioides meningitis requires not only an initial course of intravenous amphotericin B, but also intrathecal amphotericin B. This should be started as soon as meningitis is documented since early treatment appears to have a more favorable outcome. While this may be given through lumbar puncture sites, adhesive arachnoiditis occurs in a very high percentage of patients. Thus many authorities recommend intracisternal injections or the use of an Ommaya intraventricular catheter–subcutaneous reservoir. If obstructive hydrocephalus develops, a ventriculoatrial shunt is necessary. The CSF—CF titer is the most important criterion of the effectiveness of therapy. The development of a significant coccidioidin skin-test reaction also indicates a better prognosis. Intrathecal therapy may extend over weeks, months, or even indefinitely. In a series of 29 patients, 13 recovered fully, 6 require continued intrathecal therapy, 6 died of coccidioides meningitis, and 4 of unrelated causes.[336] In a comment 10 years after this report, only 3 of 23 alive at the time of the original report had died of their meningitis. Of 265 cases in the new report treated with amphotericin B, 130 died of their meningitis.[331]

The usual total dose of amphotericin required in coccidioidomycosis is considerably more variable than that recommended for histoplasmosis. A dose of less than 1 g may be adequate in acute severe pulmonary disease and in preoperative coverage.[337] In chronic cavitary disease the total dose of 30 mg/kg body weight or more is recommended (up to 2500 mg).[308,338] In disseminated coccidioidomycosis a goal is to keep the total dose below 5 g or even 3 g to minimize renal toxicity, although considerably higher doses are sometimes necessary. The appropriate dosage is best judged by following the clinical course of the patient and seeking a CF titer of less than 1:32 or a fourfold decrease. Administration of amphotericin B follows the same guidelines as described under histoplasmosis with the exception that the *in vitro* bioassay technique for assessing the organism's susceptibility has such appreciable hazards that it is generally not available.

Corticosteroids have been used effectively to ameliorate the symptoms of erythema nodosum or erythema multiforme despite a justifiable concern that they might facilitate dissemination. They have also been recommended for use in the severely ill patient who is receiving amphotericin B.[337]

The role of surgery in pulmonary coccidioidomycosis is still in the process of evolution. Surgery seems appropriate for (1) A rapidly enlarging cavity "with apparent imminent risk of rupture"; (2) bronchopleural fistula; (3) major hemorrhage (extremely rare); and (4) a bleeding mycetoma.[308] A cavity with secondary bacterial infection may require resection, but generally initial treatment should be medical management with antibiotics.

Other suggested indications for resection are an enlarging cavity, recurrent minor hemoptysis or blood streaking, a persistent cavity, a nodule that excavates, and a cavity with persistently positive cultures.[320,334,339] The use of preoperative amphotericin B for resectional surgery is controversial.[308,334,339] It appears that a trend away from aggressive surgical therapy, except for the clear-cut indications cited above, is developing much as it has for tuberculosis and histoplasmosis.

Miconazole, an imidazole, causes increased cell-wall permeability and interferes with purine transport. It must be given intravenously, intrathecally or by local instillation in bone and joint involvement.[340] A course of two to three months has been recommended. It produces hypovolemia, anemia, thrombocytosis, rouleau formation, phlebitis, hyperlipidemia; and interacts with the coumarin drugs. In 80 patients, almost all amphotericin B failures, about one-third with serious underlying disease and one-third dark-skinned, the following favorable responses to a course of treatment were reported: chronic pulmonary, 67%; skin and soft tissue, 50%; musculoskeletal, 41%; and meningitis, 35%. Relapses were common but treatment was not given for 2 to 3 mo.[308] More recently its use in musculoskeletal disease produced a 34% response rate.[340] Further studies to define its role are necessary.[300,308] Amphotericin B Methyl Ester, Econazole (R), R34000 (R), and Ambreticin (W 7783) are also under evaluation.[308] In addition promising results have been obtained with the use of transfer factor.[308,341,342] An experimental vaccine has been developed which may eventually be of value in individuals at high risk.[308,343]

BLASTOMYCOSIS

Blastomycosis is a systemic fungal infection caused by *Blastomyces dermatitidis.* The organism almost invariably is inhaled and invades the lung, resulting in a mixed pyogenic and granulomatous reaction. Information, although limited, appears to indicate that (1) many infections are benign and self-limited, and (2) the organism's natural habitat is the soil. Pulmonary symptoms or roentgenographic findings in association with chronic skin lesions are the most common presentation. Synonyms for the disease are North American blastomycosis, Gilchrist's disease, and Chicago disease.

In 1894 Gilchrist described the first case of skin involvement but thought the organism was *Saccharomyces homines* (cryptococcosis, torulosis, or European blastomycosis);[344] subsequently he and Stokes named the organism *Blastomyces dermatitidis.* Skin and systemic disease was reported from the Chicago area in 1908. Schwarz and Baum's report in 1951 established that initial infection occurred through the respiratory route.[345] Progressive pulmonary and systemic infection with a mortality of 92% without treatment was the recognized pattern.[346] In 1959 the first probable epidemic was reported, including symptomatic cases that resolved spontaneously.[347] In 1970 a report appeared of an accidentally infected laboratory worker who developed acute pulmonary disease which resolved spontaneously.[348] However, it was not until 1974 that a common-source epidemic demonstrated benign symptomatic and asymptomatic infection in 21 patients with a distribution similar to that reported for coccidioidomycosis and histoplasmosis.[349,350] A recent excellent review of blastomycosis reports two other epidemics with similar findings.[351]

EPIDEMIOLOGY

Transmission

It is believed that *B. dermatitidis* exists in the soil; its isolation from natural soil has been rare, although it will grow in sterile soil.[352] Person-to-person and animal-to-human transmissions have not been reported with the exception of conjugal transmission from an infected male.[353] The disease occurs in animals in endemic areas. Canine blastomycosis may be a harbinger of human disease.[354] It appears to occur more commonly in cool, wet periods. There are rare reports of primary percutaneous inoculation with the formation of an indurated ulcer, lymphangitis, and regional lymphadenopathy.[355]

Geographic Distribution

Adequate knowledge concerning the distribution of the disease is quite limited since the available antigens for skin testing and serologic studies are unsatisfactory. Such studies have been negative in more than 50% of patients with disease; there are also many false-positive reactions, particularly in patients with histoplasmosis. The best recognized endemic areas in the United States include the southeastern region (Mississippi, North Carolina, Kentucky, Tennessee, Louisiana, Virginia, and Georgia) and some midwestern states (Minnesota, Wisconsin, Illinois, and Arkansas). Endemic areas have been identified in Manitoba, southwestern Ontario and Quebec in Canada, and in Central America. Indigenous cases have also been reported from various areas throughout the African continent. Thus the term "North American" is best deleted.[356,357]

The majority of individuals with disease have an outdoor occupation, and males predominate 3 or more to 1. It is discovered most commonly in the 20- to 60-year-old group. In epidemics the disease is predominantly seen in the young, with no male predominance. Exposure while bird hunting in a wooded area, a suburban epidemic, and sporadic cases without significant outdoor exposure have been reported.[351]

PATHOGENESIS AND PATHOLOGY

The pathogenesis and pathology of blastomycosis are quite similar to those of coccidioidomycosis. The early pneumonia is an exudative purulent type with subsequent formation of a mixed purulent and granulomatous reaction with necrosis. The granulomas seldom caseate. Occasionally, "hard" noncaseating granulomas simulating sarcoidosis are found. In overwhelming infections, large numbers of organisms may occur without an inflammatory reaction.[351] There may be true abscess formation. Healing is characterized by fibrosis and hyalinization. The lung–regional-lymph-node complex so characteristic of histoplasmosis and tuberculosis is not a constant feature, and calcification is rare in blastomycosis.[358] The skin lesions are verrucous and hyperplastic, simulating carcinoma. Microabscesses under crusting, ulcerated lesions are common.

A specific diagnosis requires the identification of the organisms in tissue. They are usually between 8 and 15μ in diameter with a thick, doubly refractile wall; the cytoplasm usually shrinks from the wall. It has a single bud with a broad base and is commonly found extracellularly, unlike *Histoplasma capsulatum*. Blastomyces are generally well seen with hematoxylin and eosin stain. When organisms are scarce, such as in an old lesion, Gomori methenamine-silver or Gridley stains are of value.

The most common extrapulmonary location is skin, which has been involved in 38 to 80% of patients.[359] Although both pulmonary and skin lesions usually coexist, there may be no evidence of pulmonary disease. This is followed by bone with osteolytic lesions indistinguishable from other infections or neoplasm in 25 to 48%, and the male genitourinary tract (prostate, epididymis, testicle) in 5 to 33%. Meningitis, brain abscess, and spinal cord epidural abscess are uncommon. Gastrointestinal and renal involvement is rare. The female genital tract does not appear to be involved.

CLINICAL PATTERNS OF BLASTOMYCOSIS

Subclinical infection has been documented.[351,354] The incubation period has ranged from 33 to 44 days. In a point source epidemic in Big Fork, Minnesota, 11 of 21 patients without symptoms developed parenchymal infiltrates[349,350] which subsequently cleared without therapy, or had a positive blastomycin skin test. Acute pulmonary disease was also well documented in this epidemic. One group of patients presented with an abrupt onset of chills, fever, headache, photophobia, myalgia, and arthralgia. Initially there was a dry hacking cough which ultimately was productive of large amounts of purulent sputum. Some patients only had pleuritic chest pain, mild to quite severe, that lasted for only a few hours. In the 1955 epidemic, three children developed erythema nodosum, apparently a rarely reported finding in blastomycosis.[347] The roentgenographic changes varied from subsegmental or segmental consolidation to the multiple nodular pattern characteristic of epidemic histoplasmosis; pleural changes were not noted. Similar findings in six cases with symptoms for 3 wk have also been reported; chest pain occurred in most of these.[360] Pleural effusions with organisms identified in potassium hydroxide preparation and by culture have occurred.[351]

Chronic pulmonary disease presents with respiratory and systemic symptoms (although fever may be present in as few as 22%) that have been present for months or even years. The most common roentgenographic change is a fibronodular pattern with or without cavitation characteristic of tuberculosis or histoplasmosis.[361] This is followed by localized areas of consolidation, a hilar masslike density and diffuse disease. Pleural reaction was also noted in 30%.[360]

Disseminated disease is most commonly manifested by skin involvement and can be quite indolent. Skin lesions are verrucose or hyperplastic and tend to heal centrally. Ulcerative lesions may have multiple microabscesses. Involvement of subcutaneous tissues or bones may lead to draining sinuses. In some patients the skin lesions may be so indolent and inconspicuous that they are not recognized by the patient or the physician. The disease may appear in an extrapulmonary site with a normal chest roentgenogram and no identifiable antecedent acute respiratory illness.[351]

Genitourinary involvement in the male most commonly manifests as epididymitis; the testes may also be involved, and there may be draining scrotal lesions. The prostate may be enlarged and boggy; massage increases the number of positive urine cultures, and the organism may be seen in prostatic fluid.

Generalized multisystem dissemination may involve many organs and is similar to other disseminated systemic fungal infections.

Since the manifestations of this disease so commonly include extrapulmonary involvement that may be quite indolent, the separation into pulmonary and disseminated disease appears to be of less value in either recognizing the illness or estimating prognosis in comparison to histoplasmosis or coccidioidomycosis.

DIAGNOSIS

The commonly available skin-testing antigen and serologic studies are of no value in the diagnosis of blastomycosis.[286] Although an improved immunodiffusion test that identified 80% of 113 patients and appeared specific is available at the Center for Disease Control, serologic studies are still considered to be of little, if any, value.[351,354,362,363]

The organism may be identified in sputum, urine, prostatic secretions, and pus, by means of wet mounts, using potassium hydroxide. In pulmonary disease, evaluation of multiple sputum specimens enhances the direct identification; sputum cultures may be positive in up to 80%. If sputum is not rewarding, the use of escalating diagnostic studies to obtain tissue and material for culture, as described for tuberculosis and histoplasmosis, is recommended. The organism grows on Sabouraud's agar or blood agar at 25° C, usually in 14 to 18 days, although cultures should be observed for a month. Conversion of the mycelial forms to the yeast form by subculturing at 37° C is necessary for definite identification.

MANAGEMENT

Cases of acute pulmonary blastomycosis have been reported that have cleared spontaneously;[347–350,354] however, some authorities recommend treatment of acute pulmonary disease.[360] Those who eschew the treatment of acute disease recommend careful observation for 2 to 3 wk to be sure that the patient is improving clinically and roentgenographically. Symptoms clear in about a month, although roentgenographic abnormalities may persist. If the patient doesn't improve or worsens, there is consensus to use amphotericin B. While the data are too limited to firmly resolve the issue, withholding therapy from a patient who appears to be getting better and will be carefully followed does not seem unreasonable. One must accept the risk, however, of early deterioration or exacerbation at any time in the future either in the lung or in extrapulmonary sites.[300,351]

Fibrocaseous chronic pulmonary disease, with or without cavitation, should be treated. Amphotericin B is the drug of choice. The total dose recommended is 1.5 to 2.0 g or 20 to 30 mg/kg body weight.[364–366] Dosage in this range has resulted in a relapse rate of 4% *vs.* 29% with smaller doses. Similar doses are recommended for disseminated disease, although larger doses may be necessary. With meningitis intrathecal instillation has been recommended,[367] although more recently considered unnecessary.[351,368]

Prior to the advent of amphotericin, 2-hydroxystilbamidine in dosages of 8 g or greater given intravenously was reasonably successful.

Some authors still recommend its use for slowly progressive pulmonary or disseminated disease because its side-effects (hepatotoxicity) are less common and less serious than those of amphotericin B. An occasional patient has responded to 2-hydroxystilbamidine when amphotericin has failed. There are a few reports of successful treatment with both drugs, each given on alternating days.[369] In the series reported, over the last decade the mortality rate due to blastomycosis in patients receiving adequate therapy approximates 13%. Miconazole has been reported to be effective, although its role in therapy is yet to be defined.[300,368]

Surgical resection of pulmonary lesions other than for diagnosis does not appear to be warranted. Occasional successes with resection of localized cutaneous lesions without other evidence of disease have been reported.

ASPERGILLOSIS

EPIDEMIOLOGY

Members of the genus aspergillus cause a variety of diseases which have been termed aspergillosis. *Aspergillus fumigatus* and *Aspergillus niger* are the most common of the 300 species associated with disease in man. The genus aspergillus is ubiquitous. It is found in soil, decaying vegetation, organic debris, food, and as a common hospital contaminant, even in the laboratory.[370] It is often part of the normal oral and sputum flora. The common clinical presentations include (1) mycetoma, the aspergillus fungus ball; (2) bronchopulmonary allergic aspergillosis, the syndrome of asthma with pulmonary infiltrates and eosinophilia; (3) invasive pulmonary aspergillosis; (4) disseminated or systemic aspergillosis; and (5) as a colonizer of abnormal pulmonary tissues without invasion or other response.[371,372]

PATHOLOGY

Mycetoma

Fungus balls usually develop in cavities due to previous disease such as tuberculosis, histoplasmosis, bronchiectasis, sarcoidosis, lung abscess, cystic fibrosis, and within a cavitating carcinoma. The ball is composed of a mass of intertwined mycelia with fibrin, mucus, and cellular debris. Usually there is no invasion of the cavity or cyst wall. The organism may be identified with hematoxylin and eosin stain but is more clearly seen with Gridley, Gomori methenamine-silver, or periodic acid-Schiff stain. Fungus balls may be due to other organisms, such as *Candida albicans*, *Streptomyces*, *Coccidioides imitis*, *Allescheria boydii*, or *Nocardia asteroides*. They are more common in the upper lobes and may calcify. Tissue fragments of a cavitating carcinoma, necrotic lung tissue in a lung abscess, a disintegrating hydatid cyst or blood clot may simulate a fungus ball.[373,374]

Bronchopulmonary Allergic Aspergillosis

Superimposed on the pathologic picture of bronchial asthma, the more central segmental bronchi are blocked by mucous plugs containing aspergilli and eosinophiles. Bronchiectasis develops in these medium-sized bronchi.[371]

Invasive Aspergillosis

This is an acute necrotizing pyogenic pneumonia with abscess formation, and it has a predilection to invade blood vessels, causing thrombosis. A similar pattern is seen with dissemination throughout the body. The common organs involved in dissemination are brain, kidney, and myocardium.[375]

A chronic pneumonic form which may progress to abscess formation occurs rarely. Aspergillosis may cause endophthalmitis or sinus infections. Aspergillus organisms in the bronchi or a diseased area of the lung, without evidence of invasion, are commonly seen in postmortem examinations and are a reflection of colonization.

CLINICAL PATTERNS OF ASPERGILLOSIS

Aspergillus infections are often subtle, masked by the underlying lung disease or the associated manifestations. A wide spectrum of clinical manifestations makes early diagnosis more difficult.[376,378] In some patients sinusitis is the dominant feature.[377] The major pulmonary manifestations may present discrete patterns.

Mycetoma

Aspergillus fungus balls are usually asymptomatic. Patients may have recurrent pulmonary infections or hemoptysis. Recurrent hemoptysis is a serious sign presaging a massive pulmonary hemorrhage. The mycetoma is usually located within a cavity close to the pleura (see Fig. 9-18). Commonly there is pleural thickening; the development of pleural thickening may portend mycetoma formation. The fungus ball can be identified by a halo of air separating it from the cavity wall. Films obtained in various body positions will generally show movement of the ball within the cavitary lesion. If the cavity connects to an open bronchus, the organism may be cultured from the sputum. The aspergillus skin test is positive in approximately 20% of patients and precipitins are present in almost all patients.[379,380]

Bronchopulmonary Aspergillosis

Bronchopulmonary aspergillosis usually occurs in an individual with long-standing atopic bronchial asthma. There is a history of progressive recurrent exacerbations of the asthma—which becomes more difficult to treat—as well as sputum production, often with brownish bronchial casts which may contain the organism; fever; and eosinophilia. Roentgenographic findings include evidence of intermittent, often changing pulmonary infiltrates, particularly involving the upper lobes, with evidence of atelectasis which may spontaneously resolve; bronchiectasis or bronchial dilatation indicated by parallel dilated bronchial wall shadows; or mucoid impaction (*i.e.*, cylindrical shadows following the course

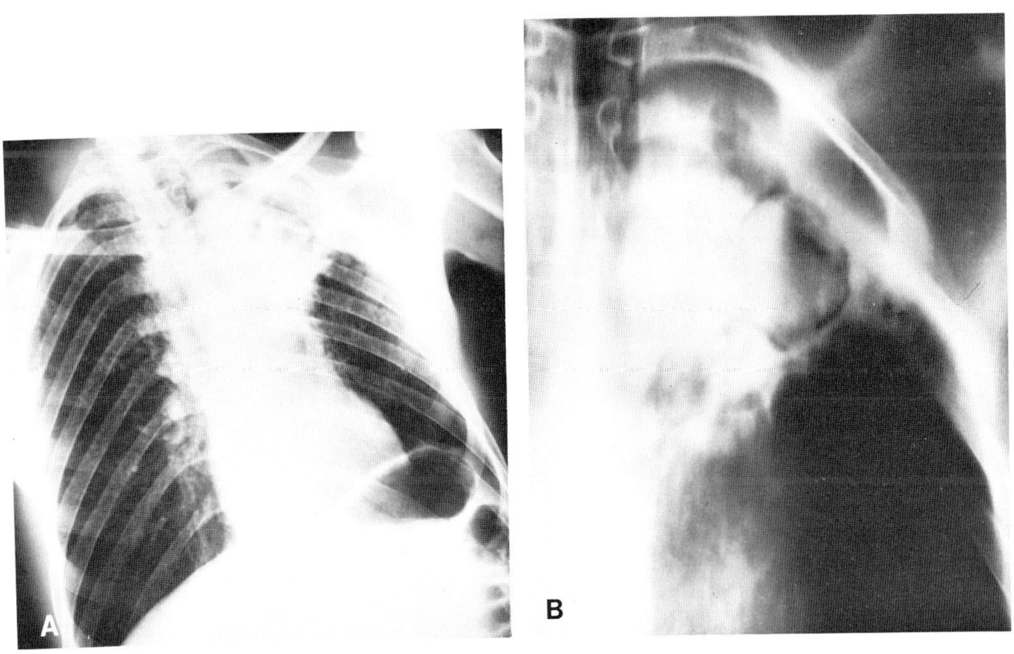

FIG. 9-18. **A.** Posterior–anterior chest roentgenogram obtained with the patient leaning to the right. There is marked pleural thickening surrounding a large left upper lobe (LUL) cavity. Within the cavity is an aspergillus fungus ball (mycetoma) resting on the lower medial cavity wall. The patient had been effectively treated for tuberculosis in the past and had a residual cavity. **B.** Laminogram (8.5 cm) of the LUL lesion shown in **A.** The mycetoma is now rather evenly surrounded by air. The patient is supine.

of medium-sized bronchi which are obstructed).[380–382] The roentgenographic pattern may simulate findings of tuberculosis, other fungal infections, or cystic fibrosis. The aspergillus skin test is positive in almost all cases producing both an immediate reaction and a delayed or Arthus reaction at 5 to 6 hr. The immediate reaction is considered diagnostic and is found in almost all cases. Aspergillus precipitins can be identified in approximately 70% of such patients.[383–385] Airways obstruction is an almost constant feature and a reduction of diffusing capacity occurs in most patients.

Invasive Aspergillosis

Invasive aspergillosis usually occurs in a patient who has serious underlying disease characterized by immunosuppression, such as leukemia or lymphoma, following the use of corticosteroids or other immunosuppressive drugs, such as in renal transplant patients and in patients following open-heart surgery.[375,378,386] The disease is usually a rapid, fatal, febrile illness characterized by toxicity and involvement of a wide variety of organs including lung, brain, kidney, and heart. There may be hematuria and symptoms of a space-occupying central nervous system lesion, such as coma or convulsions.

DIAGNOSIS

Identification of long-branching hyphal strands with conidiophores (expanded spore-bearing vesicles) in sputum, either by direct examination or with potassium hydroxide, is an indication of the presence of aspergilli. However, since the organism may be part of the normal flora, this does not definitely document the cause-and-effect relationship between the organism and pulmonary disease. Suspicion is strengthened by the repeated recognition of the organism on direct preparations or culture. A definite diagnosis requires the demonstration of tissue invasion by aspergilli; at postmortem examination colonization of no apparent significance may be seen in airways. With a mycetoma, sputum, especially when bloody, may contain intertwined masses of hyphae. This, along with a positive skin test and the appropriate clinical picture, are satisfactory for diagnosis.

In allergic bronchopulmonary aspergillosis the diagnosis is made in the setting of asthma, recurrent pulmonary infiltrates, and eosinophilia by the presence of an immediate reaction to the aspergillus skin test. Elevated IgE levels and the presence of organisms in the sputum are confirmatory.[384,385]

In invasive pulmonary aspergillosis the skin test and serologies are generally negative. The organism must be identified in tissue or from blood. Its presence in sputum along with a compatible clinical picture, while suggestive, does not permit a definite diagnosis.

MANAGEMENT

Aspergillomas generally require no therapy unless there is evidence of recurrent hemoptysis; this is considered to be a definite indication for resection of the fungus ball if this is possible.[387] However, some recommend surgery only with massive hemoptysis because complications are frequent.[388] Not uncommonly, individuals with widespread severe parenchymal diseases such as sarcoidosis or tuberculosis are not candidates for surgery. Systemic amphotericin or other antifungal agents have not been shown to be effective. On occasion, irrigation of the cavity with amphotericin B, introduced endobronchially or percutaneously, has been effective, but this is by no means a reliable response.[389,390]

In allergic bronchopulmonary aspergillosis there is usually a dramatic response to treatment with systemic corticosteroids. While some patients have done very well with corticosteroid therapy for periods of a few weeks to a month, many require continued low-dose corticosteroid therapy to maintain a satisfactory clinical status. There is some evidence that disodium cromoglycate may be of value as well.[391] Inhaled topical corticosteroids have also been used. Although the use of oral steroids for extended periods in low doses (*e.g.*, 7.5 to 10 mg prednisone or its equivalent) do control symptoms, long-term controlled studies documenting an alteration in the course of the disease are not available.[376,384]

Invasive pulmonary or disseminated disease

should be treated with amphotericin B. Since the disease is so rapidly progressive and the organism tends to be resistant, therapy is often unsuccessful. Treatment within the first four days may be more effective.[392]

CRYPTOCOCCOSIS

EPIDEMIOLOGY

Cryptococcosis is a systemic fungal infection caused by *Cryptococcus neoformans*. The organism has a worldwide distribution in soil; its growth is enhanced by pigeon droppings; it is found commonly in the dirt of urban areas. Infection is through the respiratory tract. Many infections are asymptomatic. In the healthy individual it invades primarily the lung, but in the compromised host it presents as disseminated disease involving particularly the meninges. Neither person-to-person nor animal-to human transmission is reported. Cryptococcosis is also called torulosis, European blastomycosis, and in Europe "signal malade" (a sign of serious underlying disease). For many years the disease was confused with blastomycosis.[393]

PATHOLOGY

C. neoformans causes little inflammatory reaction. Initially the lesion appears mucinous and later granulomatous. The gelatinous lesions contain many encapsulated budding organisms. They are about 5 to 10μ (but may be larger), usually with a thick capsule which is stained with mucicarmine but not hematoxylin and eosin stain; the former will stain the organism a faint purple. Identification of the capsule with mucicarmine permits a diagnosis. Periodic acid-Schiff or Gomori methenamine-silver also stains the organism. The organism is difficult to identify in pulmonary nodules or "coin lesions." The lung is commonly involved alone. With dissemination the meninges are most commonly involved; there is usually only minimal inflammation. The brain may be involved through embolization and develop mucoid cysts. Invasion of bone, skin, and the eye may also be evident.[394]

CLINICAL PATTERNS OF CRYPTOCOCCOSIS

Subclinical infections are probably the most common form of cryptococcosis. Such disease may only be recognized by resection of a nodule or identification of such a lesion at postmortem examination.

Pulmonary involvement may present with an acute onset of cough, fever, hemoptysis, pleuritic chest pain, and dyspnea or as a chronic illness with both respiratory and systemic manifestations. The chest roentgenographic changes are nonspecific: varying pneumonic infiltrates including a lobar distribution, diffuse bilateral involvement, solitary or multiple nodules or cavities. Nodular lesions may enlarge and cavitate.[395,396a]

Disseminated disease occurs more commonly in immune-compromised patients.[396a] Cryptococcal meningitis usually presents with the insidious onset of a progressive headache, fever, and meningismus. If the brain is involved there are symptoms of a mass lesion. Central nervous system disease may have a fulminant presentation and course.[397] The skin lesions are nonspecific papules, pustules or ulcers; bone lesions are osteolytic.[393]

DIAGNOSIS

Cryptococci may be identified on a wet mount, using a colloidal suspension such as India ink to outline them. Since India ink may agglutinate or contain other particles or organisms that may result in a false-positive identification, a control preparation with sterile saline is advised. The organism grows readily in a variety of non-antibiotic-containing media at 37°C. Although the organism may be identified in 24 to 48 hr, cultures should be observed for at least 4 wk. *C. neoformans* may be cultured from sputum in the absence of cryptococcal pulmonary disease. These are usually isolated cultures and may represent normal flora. Repeated positive cultures in the presence of chronic bronchopulmonary disease have been reported and attributed to colonization.[394,395,398]

Although not generally available, an indirect

fluorescent antibody test, a tube agglutination test, and a latex agglutination test for cryptococcal antigens appear to be quite useful.[399] When the three were used together in 66 cases of culturally proven cryptococcosis, a positive result was obtained in 95%. The latex agglutination test is most specific; false-positive reactions occurred only in sera with rheumatoid factor. The two antibody tests may cross- react in other fungal infections.[400]

MANAGEMENT

The role of specific treatment of pulmonary cryptococcal disease is not fully defined. The organism may be cultured from sputum in the absence of related disease. Individuals with an acute pneumonia or chronic localized disease have resolved without specific therapy. Specific therapy, amphotericin B, is recommended for acute pulmonary disease that is not localized, cavitation, and associated systemic disease. A total dose of 2 to 3 g is considered satisfactory. The role of surgery is confined to diagnostic procedures. Following such procedures amphotericin is usually not necessary unless there is dissemination.[394,395,398]

With disseminated disease a dose in excess of 2 g is recommended, and intrathecal therapy may be necessary. The mortality rate even with treatment is in excess of 40%.[401,402]

A new drug, 5-fluorocytosine, is effective *in vitro* against C. *neoformans* and at least initially in the treatment of cryptococcal meningitis. However, reports of rapidly developing resistance and relapse mitigate against its use.[402]

CANDIDIASIS

The common species of candida are a leading cause of deep mycotic infections in hospitalized and immunocompromised patients. The organisms are ubiquitous, frequently colonizing the upper respiratory tract without evidence of infection. *Candida albicans* is commonly cultured from the sputum or gastrointestinal tract in patients receiving antibiotics (particularly broad spectrum), or systemic or inhaled corticosteroids. Consequently there has been much confusion regarding the significance of this organism in the etiology of disease.[403–406]

Patients with immunodeficiency disease, particularly involving both the cellular and humoral components, are particularly prone to systemic infections by candida. (See Chapter 8, section on Diseases of the Compromised Host.) Systemic corticosteroid therapy, cytotoxic drugs, and hematologic malignancies are the most common predisposing conditions; diabetes and parenteral nutrition are frequently associated. Infection of the lungs may occur as a result of aspiration, or hematogenous spread from localized infection in mucosal sites.[405,406]

The lung-tissue response to Candida infection may include a polymorphonuclear exudative reaction with or without necrosis (abscess formation), or, less commonly, chronic changes including histiocytes and granuloma formation. The relatively large organisms can generally be identified on hematoxylin and eosin stains of the tissues. In the immunocompromised patient, multiple infections frequently occur. Cytomegalovirus or pyogenic infections may be associated and further confuse the clinical presentation.

The clinical picture may range from a minimal, localized pulmonary infiltrate to widespread bilateral consolidation with severe hypoxemia. Patients commonly develop fever, leukocytosis, hemorrhagic skin lesions, lesions in the fundi, and clinical evidence of septic emboli. In fatal cases endocarditis, renal failure, thrombocytopenia, and a bleeding diathesis are common.

The diagnosis is most reliable when organisms are identified on tissue (lung) biopsy. Positive blood cultures confirm fungemia, but cultures of sputum, stool, or urine may merely reflect colonization. Serology, identification of the species, and mycelial *vs* yeast phase of the organism are unreliable indicators of the relationship to disease.

In most patients the judgment to treat for candidiasis is based on persistent positive cultures from the appropriate tissue, and lack of evidence for an alternative pathogen. Evidence of associated persistant fungemia (after removal of indwelling lines) or systemic spread weigh heavily in favor of treatment.

Treatment is most reliable with amphotericin B although 5-fluorocytosine may be useful as well.[300]

OTHER FUNGAL INFECTIONS

SPOROTRICHOSIS

Sporotrichosis is usually a lymphocutaneous disease characterized by nodular suppurating and ulcerating cutaneous and subcutaneous lesions associated with ascending lymphangitis due to *Sporothrix schenckii.* It is usually implanted traumatically through the skin; individuals who work as farmers, gardeners (contact with sphagnum moss, thorns), and laborers (South African miners) are at greater risk. There may be mucous membrane or bone involvement; dissemination is rare. The lesions are mixed pyogenic and granulomatous. The organisms stain with periodic acid-Schiff or Gomori methenamine silver, but are extremely difficult to identify. A fluorescent antibody reagent is most helpful.[407]

Primary infection through the respiratory tract appears to be rare. The clinical picture is usually that of cough, sputum production, and constitutional symptoms of fever, gradual weight loss, and malaise. The roentgenographic picture is that of nonspecific chronic pneumonitis or fibronodular disease with or without cavitation that simulates tuberculosis.[408] Alternatively, cases have been reported with marked enlargement of hilar and mediastinal nodes.[409] Primary pulmonary infection with dissemination to a joint without skin lesions has been reported.[410] Direct examination of specimens from lymphocutaneous lesions or sputum rarely identify the organism. It grows readily on a variety of media. A skin test,[411] agglutination, and diffusion tests[412] appear quite specific and sensitive, but are not generally available.

Lymphocutaneous lesions usually respond to iodide therapy by mouth and topically. Amphotericin B is the drug of choice for pulmonary and disseminated disease.[413,414] It is also of value in lymphocutaneous disease that does not respond to iodides. Good response to a new antifungal agent, miconazole, after failure of amphotericin B, is reported.[415]

PHYCOMYCOSIS

The phycomycetes are an unusual cause of disease in man. Infection by organisms of the genus phycomycetes of the family mucoraceae is often called mucormycosis. The primary route of infection is through the respiratory tract. The organism is ubiquitous in the environment and may be part of the normal oral flora. It usually invades the compromised host.

The pathology is similar to that of aspergillosis with a particular predilection to invade blood vessels, producing major vascular occlusions. The organism appears as broad, usually nonseptate, hyphae readily seen with hematoxylin and eosin stain.

The usual presentation is that of rhinocerebral involvement with extension to the orbit, meninges, and brain; disseminated disease occurs. The most common predisposing diseases are diabetic ketoacidosis, lymphoma, leukemia, carcinoma, burns, and the use of corticosteroids.[416]

In the pulmonary form of the disease the patient usually presents with subacute or chronic cough and sputum with constitutional symptoms. The chest roentgenogram may disclose nonspecific infiltrates, multiple lung masses, abscess formation, or uncommonly a mycetoma. Leukemia or lymphoma is the most common predisposing factor.[417,418]

Diagnosis requires the identification of the organism microscopically or by culture. Organisms may be quite difficult to identify in sputum and may not grow even when recognized microscopically.

Amphotericin B therapy is recommended for pulmonary, rhinocerebral, and disseminated disease. On the basis of limited data indicating a high potential for massive fatal pulmonary hemorrhage, resection of mycetoma is suggested.[419]

PARACOCCIDOIDOMYCOSIS

This systemic fungal disease is caused by *Paracoccidioides brasiliensis.* It appears to be limited to South and Central America. Although the primary route of infection is believed to be the respiratory tract, the disease most commonly presents as mucocutaneous lesions of the oropharynx. Dissemination occurs. It causes a granulomatous and pyogenic reaction similar to blastomycosis. The organism appears as a 2-to-16μ chain of budding yeasts and grows on the usual fungal media. A highly specific and sensitive agar-gel double-diffusion precipitin test and a complement-fixation test are available; they are also useful in guiding therapy and prognosis. Prolonged treatment with sulfa drugs is the initial therapeutic choice. Amphotericin is highly effective and recommended when sulfa drugs fail.[420,421]

PATHOGENIC ACTINOMYCES

The actinomyces pathogenic for man are not fungi but so-called higher bacteria which belong to the order actinomycetales of the class Schizomycetes. Mycobacteria also belong in this classification. These organisms were thought to be transitional forms between bacteria and fungi since mycelial forms were noted in tissue. The two major systemic diseases related to this group of organisms are actinomycosis, usually due to *Actinomyces israelii*, and nocardiosis due to *Nocardia asteroides* or *Nocardia brasiliensis.*

ACTINOMYCOSIS

Actinomycosis is a chronic suppurative and granulomatous disease usually caused by *Actinomyces israelii.* The organism is part of the normal flora of the mouth and invades locally, usually in association with poor oral hygiene or trauma producing cervicofacial disease; it may be aspirated, causing thoracic disease, or it may present as an abdominal form, usually also in association with trauma. Actinomycosis is sometimes referred to as lumpy jaw, leptotricosis, or streptotricosis.

The disease was first recognized in the 1800s and was a fairly common clinical problem with significant mortality prior to the era of the sulfonamides and penicillin.[422] Recognition of the disease over the last 20 yr has appeared to decrease, whether due to improved oral hygiene or the more common use of antibiotics.[423]

Actinomyces organisms are normal inhabitants of the mouth, particularly the buccal mucosa and the tonsilar crypts; they are commonly found in sputum from individuals with chronic bronchopulmonary disease.[424] Person-to-person transmission of disease does not appear to occur, nor is there transmission of a similar disease from animals caused by *A. bovis.* The organism has not been cultured from environmental sources.

Pathology

A. israelii produces a chronic suppurative process which results ultimately in dense scarring. Grossly there are nodular lesions which have interconnecting sinus tracts with abscess formation that spread contiguously without regard to tissue planes. Sinus tracts may drain through the skin.

In lesions the "sulfur granules" can be seen with hematoxylin and eosin stains as round or oval bodies 100 to 300μ in diameter. They are composed of delicate filaments extending from a central core; the filaments commonly have clubbed peripheral ends. With a modified Gram stain, such as the Brown and Brenn or the MacCallum-Goodpasture, mycelia appear as an intertwined mass of gram-positive, delicate, occasionally branched filaments with or without occasional coccoid or bacillary bodies. Alternatively, Gomori methanamine-silver stain can be used to identify the filaments.

Actinomyces are usually not acid-fast, but with a modified Ziehl-Neelsen (Putt), they may be acid-fast.[425,426]

Clinical Patterns of Actinomycosis

Cervicofacial Actinomycosis. There is usually an antecedent history of oral or facial trauma, dental manipulation or dental infection preceding the development of a firm, indurated, "woody" mass on or near the mandible, with subsequent abscess formation and drainage. Multiple lumps usually connected by sinus tracts commonly develop. The serosanguinous or seropurulent material frequently contains sulfur granules which are highly suggestive but not diagnostic of actinomycosis. The lesions may extend into the maxilla and other cranial bones involving the eye and the meninges, the tongue and sublingual salivary glands, the neck, scapula, and upper extremities. Cervicofacial disease accounted for more than half the cases in earlier series, although it is believed to be less common at present.[423,427]

Thoracic Actinomycosis. The usual route of infection is believed to be aspiration of the organisms in mouth contents; underlying pulmonary disease such as atelectasis or other infection may be a predisposing factor. Occasionally there is direct extension from cervicofacial disease, from the esophagus, or from subdiaphragmatic disease.[428] Patients usually have the indolent onset of cough, sputum production, hemoptysis, and systemic symptoms of fever and weight loss. The roentgenographic picture is nonspecific: pneumonitis, more commonly involving the lower lobes, or an abscess. There may be pleural involvement with empyema. Diagnosis is quite difficult with this presentation; even the isolation of *A. israelii* from the sputum must be interpreted with caution, since it may be part of the normal flora. In a collection of 28 cases in which surgical procedures were performed on the thorax, the diagnosis of actinomycosis was made in only one prior to surgery.[429] The presence of chest-wall lesions or bone lesions with or without draining sinuses increases suspicion of this disease and provides a source of documentation. Thoracic actinomycosis has a greater predilection to disseminate than other forms. Lesions may involve skin, subcutaneous tissue, and muscle. These peripheral lesions may be the presenting sign.[430]

Abdominal Actinomycosis. The disease usually results from perforation of the gastrointestinal tract, either internally or following trauma. There may be hepatic or gallbladder involvement. An abdominal mass and pain with systemic symptoms may be present. As with the pulmonary disease, in the absence of an abdominal wall lesion with sinus tract formation, the diagnosis is rarely made prior to surgery. Genital actinomycosis has been associated with intrauterine contraceptive devices.[431]

Diagnosis

The presence of sulfur granules permits a tentative diagnosis; however, they may be seen in other infections. They are more easily seen if the pus is spread in a petri dish with a dark background. They appear grossly as yellowish-white 2- to 3-mm specks. The organism is *anaerobic* and therefore must be transported anaerobically and immediately cultured under anaerobic conditions. Inattention to this and the usual 4- to 8-day growth period may well contribute to the uncommon recognition of this disease. Human infections have almost invariably been associated with the growth of other microorganisms, particularly anaerobic organisms.[422–424]

With the use of an agar-gel double-diffusion test, antibodies were demonstrated in 21 of 24 (87.5%) of proven cases of disseminated actinomycosis, but were not found in localized (cervicofacial) or in normal controls. Cross-reactions were observed in patients with tuberculosis.

Management

Generally recommended therapy is penicillin in a dosage of 10 to 20 million units intravenously for 4 to 6 wk followed by oral penicillin in a dose of 2 to 5 million units for an additional 6 wk. Many authors, however, recommend that the oral medication be continued for a minimum of 6 mo, and some suggest that it should be continued for 12 to 18 mo, especially with thoracic or abdominal disease.[433]

In individuals who are allergic to penicillin, successful therapy has been achieved with lincomycin, erythromycin, tetracycline, chloramphenicol, streptomycin, clindamycin, and isoniazid.[434,435] There is one report of successful treatment of a perirectal abscess with hyperbaric oxygen when therapeutic antibiotics appeared to fail.[436] Surgical incision and drainage of abscesses and empyema spaces are required. There does not seem to be any role for pulmonary resection, although the diagnosis is commonly made at thoracotomy. If the organism is identified in tissue or culture at this time and the patient subsequently treated with penicillin, complications are unusual. Therapy has resulted in cure in 80 to 90% of patients when the disease is recognized in time to give adequate treatment.

Other actinomyces that have occasionally caused pleuropulmonary disease include *A. naeslundi* and *Bifidobacterium eriksonnii*.[437]

NOCARDIOSIS

Nocardiosis is a chronic suppurative disease caused by a *Nocardia asteroides* or *Nocardia brasiliensis*. The primary route of infection is respiratory; the organisms are distributed worldwide in soil. The disease was first described in 1888 by Nocard as glanders in cattle. Geppinger described the first patient with miliary lung disease and a brain abscess in 1890. Until 1957 it was considered a primary disease; however, since that time the majority of cases have been reported in association with underlying disease characterized by immunosuppression and the use of immunosuppressive drugs, in particular corticosteroids and with pulmonary alveolar proteinosis.[439–441]

In contrast to *A. israelii*, nocardia organisms are rarely identified in sputum in the absence of disease, occurring in .02% to .05% of two large series of sputum cultures.[441,443] Rarely, however, individuals have had positive cultures without evidence of either pulmonary or extrapulmonary disease due to nocardia. Neither person-to-person nor animal-to human transmission of the disease appears to occur. The disease is found in animals and particularly in cattle involving the udders. *N. asteroides* accounts for the great majority of pulmonary cases in the United States and Europe. *N. brasiliensis* is considered a more virulent organism and more likely to be a primary pathogen; it is isolated more commonly in Central and South America. Rare cases of primary infection through the gastrointestinal tract, at the site of ulceration, or in the appendix may occur. In addition percutaneous inoculation may occur in tropical areas, causing Madura foot.

Pathology

The nocardiosis lesion is characteristically a pyogenic process characterized by multiple abscesses with central necrosis and relatively little surrounding fibrosis. Sinus tract formation is less common than in actinomycosis. Granuloma formation or caseation is unusual. The organisms cannot be identified with hematoxylin and eosin stains but can be seen with modifications of the Gram stain such as the Brown-Brenn or MacCallum-Goodpasture. It may also be identified with the Gomori methenamine-silver stain, if the staining time is extended. In addition to the organism being gram-positive, it also stains with modifications of the Ziehl-Neelsen stain such as the Putt modification. It appears as delicate hyphae with branching usually at right angles. Typical sulfur granules characteristic of Actinomyces do not occur in lung lesions, but loosely formed structures may be seen.

The lung is involved in approximately 30% of reported cases; the central nervous system, usually a brain abscess, multiple or singular, in 5%; a combination of brain and lung in an additional 5%; the skin and subcutaneous tissue in 15%; and generalized dissemination in about 30%.[438–441]

Clinical Patterns of Nocardiosis

While subclinical pulmonary involvement has been recognized, the most common presentation is that of a chronic pneumonia with symptoms of cough, mucopurulent sputum with occasional blood streaking, and systemic symptoms of malaise, fever, and weight loss, not unlike that found in tuberculosis (double infections occur). In the presence of a cavity there may be massive hemoptysis. An acute pneumonic presentation with evidence of fulminant dissemination is seen particularly in the immunosuppressed host. The chest wall is not commonly involved. Since the presentation is so nonspecific it is often recognized only at autopsy.

Roentgenographic patterns are nonspecific, including segmental or nonsegmental pneumonic infiltrates, fibronodular and cavitary disease, pleural effusion or empyema, and solitary nodules. Mycetoma formation within a cavity due to nocardia has also been reported.

A brain abscess usually presents with constitutional symptoms and the neurologic findings of an enlarging mass lesion (*i.e.*, focal neurologic deficits, headache, nausea and vomiting, seizures and coma). Because the meninges are not commonly involved, identification of the organism in cerebrospinal fluid is rarely successful.

With systemic disease there may be cutaneous involvement or sinus-tract formation; in these lesions sulfur granules have been identified.

Diagnosis

Direct examination of sputum or purulent material reveals gram-positive delicate hyphae with branching at right angles. They are acid-fast with a modified Ziehl-Neelsen stain. When the organisms have broken up into coccoid or bacillary forms this acid-fast property may create confusion with acid-fast mycobacteria. Nocardia organisms are *aerobic* and grow readily on ordinary laboratory media without antibiotics, optimally at 37°C. Growth may be quite slow, taking 2 to 4 wk, although colonies may be identified earlier. The organisms will also grow on the usual mycobacterial media if the concentration and decontamination procedures have not been too stringent; they may be mistaken for mycobacteria other than *M. tuberculosis*. Skin tests and serologic studies of clinical usefulness are not available.

Management

Prior to the advent of specific chemotherapy, nocardiosis as a primary disease was stated to be fatal in 75% (probably a reflection of the autopsy series).[439] The most commonly used therapy since the mid-1940s has been sulfadiazine in a dose of 4 to 8 g per day in divided doses every 6 hr to obtain a serum level of 10 to 15 mg/dl. In more severe disease blood levels up to 20 mg/dl have been recommended. Triple sulfa combinations have been recommended to decrease renal toxicity. Blood levels rather than specific doses should be used to monitor therapy. Many authors have suggested the use of an additional drug such as ampicillin (2 g/day), streptomycin (2 g/day), and minocycline, tetracycline or chloramphenicol during the initial treatment.[439,440,444,445] Cycloserine is also effective and has been recommended as a second drug in presence of brain abscess.[446] Recently the combination of sulfamethoxazole (2.5 g/day) and trimethoprim (480 mg/day) appears to be the combination of choice in the presence of cerebral involvement.[447] Sulfa or trimethoprim-sulfa therapy should be continued for a minimum of 3 mo. With the use of sulfa drugs overall mortality approximates 50%. It is in excess of 80% with a brain abscess and less than 10% with pulmonary involvement alone. In a review of 147 cases up to 1967 the presence of one of the following correlated with an 85% mortality: (1) symptoms of less than 3 wk, (2) use of corticosteroids (or Cushing's disease) or antineoplastic agents, and (3) disseminated nocardiosis involving two or more contiguous organs.[448]

REFERENCES

1. DROLET GJ: Epidemiology of tuberculosis. In Goldberg B (ed): Clinical Tuberculosis. Philadelphia, F. A. Davis, 1936
2. LOWELL AM: Tuberculosis morbidity and mortality and its control. In Tuberculosis, Vital Health Statistics Monograph Series, Part I, p 1. American Public Health Association, Cambridge, Mass, Harvard University Press, 1969
3. US Department of Health, Education and Welfare: Tuberculosis Statistics: States and Cities, 1974. Public Health Service, Publication No. (CDC) 76–8249, July, 1975
4. US Department of Health, Education and Welfare: Tuberculosis Statistics: States and Cities, 1978. Publication No. (CDC) 80-8249, December, 1979
5. FALK A et al: Diagnostic Standards and Classification of Tuberculosis. New York, National Tuberculosis and Respiratory Disease Association, 1969
6. WEG JG et al: Diagnostic standards and classification of tuberculosis and other mycobacterial diseases, 14th ed. Am Rev Respir Dis 123:343, 1981
7. EDWARDS LB, PALMER CE: Tuberculosis infection. In Tuberculosis. Part II, Vital and Health Statistics Monograph Series, p 123. Cambridge, Mass, American Public Health Association, Harvard University Press, 1969
8. US Department of Health, Education and Welfare: Public Health Service: Tuberculosis Program Reports. II. Tuberculin Testing Data, 1967–1968 School Year, p 15. Atlanta, National

Communicable Disease Center, Tuberculosis Branch, Statistical Services Unit, 1968
9. US Department of Health, Education and Welfare: Tuberculosis Programs, 1973. Public Health Service, Publication No. (CDC) 75–8189, December, 1974
10. US Department of Health & Human Services: Tuberculosis in the United States, 1978. Public Health Service, Center for Disease Control, Publication No. (CDC) 80–8322, June, 1980
11. COMSTOCK GW: Frost revisited: The modern epidemiology of tuberculosis. Am J Epidemiol 101:363, 1975
12. US Department of Health, Education and Welfare: Public Health Service: Weekly report for year ending December 28, 1974. Morbidity and Mortality, 23(53), July 15, 1975
13. EDWARDS LB et al: An atlas of sensitivity to tuberculin, PPD-B and histoplasmin in the United States. Am Rev Respir Dis 99:1 (April, Part 2), 1969
14. RHOADES ER, ALEXANDER CP: Reactions to the tuberculin tine test in Air Force Recruits. Am Rev Respir Dis 98:837, 1968
15. US Department of Health, Education and Welfare: Illness Among Indians. Public Health Service, Publication No. (HSM) 72–507, July, 1971
16. TEMPEST P, POSANTI E: Community wide tuberculosis case finding program in the Navajo reservation. Am Rev Respir Dis 110:760, 1974
17. KECK CW et al: Tuberculosis in the Yungas area of Bolivia. Health Serv Res 88:499, 1973
18. HERSHFIELD ES: Tuberculosis in the world. Chest (December Suppl) 76:805, 1979
19. World Health Organization: Expert Committee on Tuberculosis, Ninth Report. Geneva, WHO Technical Report Series, 552, 1974
20. GRIGG ERN: The arcana of tuberculosis with a brief epidemiologic history of the disease in the U.S.A., Part III. Am Rev Tuberc 78:426, 1958
21. SBARBARO JA: Tuberculosis: The new challenge to the practicing clinician. Chest [Suppl] 68:436, 1975
22. ASHLEY MJ, ANDERSON TW, LERICK WH: The influence of immigration on tuberculosis in Ontario. Am Rev Respir Dis 110:137, 1974
23. ENARSON D et al: Tuberculosis in immigrants to Canada. A study of present-day patterns in relation to immigration trends and birthplace. Am Rev Respir Dis 119:11, 1979
24. RILEY RL: Airborne transmission. In Johnson JE (ed): Rational Therapy and Control of Tuberculosis. Gainesville, University of Florida Press, 1970
25. OLSON AM et al: Infectiousness of tuberculosis: A Report of the National Tuberculosis Association Ad Hoc Committee on Treatment of Tuberculosis Patients in General Hospitals. Am Rev Respir Dis 96:836, 1967
26. WELLS WF: Droplets and droplet nuclei: Study II. Am J Hygiene 20:611, 1934
27. PERKINS JE: Airborne infection and tuberculosis. Arch Environ Health 16:738, 1968
28. O'GRADY F, and RILEY RL: Experimental airborne tuberculosis. Adv Tuberc Res 12:150, 1963
29. HOUK VN et al: The Byrd study: An in-depth analysis of a micro-outbreak of tuberculosis in a closed environment. Arch Environ Health 16:4, 1968
30. HOUK VN et al: The epidemiology of tuberculosis in a closed environment. Arch Environ Health 16:26, 1968
31. RILEY RL: Airborne infection. Am J Med 57:466, 1974
32. SHAW JB, WYNN-WILLIAMS N: Infectivity of pulmonary tuberculosis in relation to sputum status. Am Rev Respir Dis 69:724, 1954
33. LOUDON RG, SPOHN SK: Cough frequency and infectivity in patients with pulmonary tuberculosis. Am Rev Respir Dis 99:109, 1969
34. Tuberculosis Chemotherapy Centre, Madras: A Review on Research Activities 1956–1966. New Delhi, Indian Council of Medical Research, 1967
35. GUNNELS JJ, BATES JH, SWINDOLL H: Infectiousness of culture-positive tuberculosis patients on chemotherapy. Am Rev Respir Dis 109:323, 1974
36. GUYTON HG, DECKER HM: Respiratory protection provided by five new contagion masks. Appl Microbiol 11:66, 1963
37. RICH AR: The Pathogenesis of Tuberculosis. Springfield, Charles C Thomas, 1944
38. CANETTI G: The Tubercle Bacillus in the Pulmonary Lesion of Man. New York, Springer-Verlag, 1955
39. DUBOS RJ: Biologic and epidemiologic aspects of tuberculosis. Am Rev Respir Dis 68:1, 1953
40. STEAD WW: The pathogenesis of pulmonary tuberculosis among older persons. Am Rev Respir Dis 91:811, 1965
41. STEAD WW: Pathogenesis of a first episode of chronic pulmonary tuberculosis in man: Recrudescence of residuals of the primary infection or exogenous reinfection? Am Rev Respir Dis 95:729, 1967
42. MEDLAR EM: The behavior of pulmonary tuberculous lesions: A pathological study. Am Rev Tuberc 71(2):1, 1955
43. AUERBACH O, GERE JB, PAWLOWSKI JM et al: The rate of healing of pulmonary tuberculosis as affected by chemotherapy. Am Rev Tuberc 76:988, 1957
44. AUERBACH O et al: Effect of degree of healing upon persistence of tubercle bacilli within pulmonary lesions. Am Rev Tuberc 72:386, 1955
45. AUERBACH O, SMALL MJ: The syndrome of persistent cavitation and noninfectious sputum during

chemotherapy and its relation to the open healing of cavities. Am Rev Tuberc 75:242, 1957

46. KOCH R: Die Aetiologie der Tuberculose. Klin Wochenschr 19:221, 1882 (English translation in Kelly EC (ed): Medical Classics, vol 2, no. 8, p 853. Baltimore, Williams & Wilkins, 1938)
47. SBARBARO JA et al: American Thoracic Society Statement: Preventive therapy of tuberculous infection. Am Rev Respir Dis 110:371, 1974
48. GROTH-PETERSON E, KNUDSEN J, WILBEK E: Epidemiologic basis of tuberculosis eradication in an advanced country. Bull WHO 21:5, 1959
49. COMSTOCK GW, PALMER CE: Long-term results of BCG vaccination in the southern United States. Am Rev Respir Dis 93:171, 1966
50. Medical Research Council, Tuberculosis Vaccines Clinical Trial Committee, Third Report: BCG and vole bacillus vaccines in the prevention of tuberculosis in adolescence and early adult life. Br Med J 1:973, 1963
51. KAPLAN M, ARMSTRONG D, ROSEN P: Tuberculosis complicating neoplastic disease: review of 201 cases. Cancer 33:850, 1974
52. GREEN RA: Clinical patterns of pulmonary tuberculosis. In Johnson JE (ed): Rational Therapy and Control of Tuberculosis, p 56. Gainesville, University of Florida Press, 1970
53. REICHMAN LB: Tuberculin skin testing—the state of the art. Chest (Suppl) 76:764, 1979
54. Committee on Diagnostic Skin Testing of the American Thoracic Society: Statement—What is PPDS? Am Rev Respir Dis 99:460, 1969
55. LANDI S et al: Disparity of potency between stabilized and nonstabilized dilute tuberculin solutions. Am Rev Respir Dis 104:385, 1971
56. LANDI S, HELD HR: Effect of light on tuberculin purified protein derivative solutions. Am Rev Respir Dis 111:52, 1975
57. MACLEAN RA: Tuberculin testing antigens and techniques. Chest [Suppl] 68:455, 1975
58. NASH DR, DOUGLASS JE: Anergy in active pulmonary tuberculosis—a comparison between positive and negative reactors and an evaluation of 5TU and 250TU skin test doses. Chest 77:32, 1980
59. HOLDEN M et al: Frequency of negative intermediate strength tuberculin sensitivity in patients with active tuberculosis. N Engl J Med 285:1506, 1971
60. KENT DC: Tuberculous lymphadenitis: Not a localized process. Am J Med Sci 254(6):866, 1967
61. SMITH DT: The diagnostic and prognostic value of the second strength dose of PPD (5.0 micrograms)—its use in detecting pseudo converters from blood transfusions and from the booster effects of previous tuberculin tests. Am Rev Respir Dis 101:317, 1970
62. MUNDT PW: Miliary tuberculosis in the chemotherapy era: With a clinical review in 69 American adults. Medicine 51:139, 1971
63. KENT D, SCHWARTZ R: Active pulmonary tuberculosis with negative tuberculin skin test reactions. Am Rev Respir Dis 95:411, 1967
64. PALMER CE, EDWARDS LB: Identify the tuberculosis infected: the dual-test technique. JAMA 205:167, 1968
65. HYDE L, HYDE CI: Skin testing with multiple PPD antigens in the differential diagnosis of mycobacterial diseases. Chest 66:108, 1974
66. COMSTOCK GW: False tuberculin test results. Chest [Suppl] 68:465, 1975
67. MCMURRAY DN, ECHEVERRI A: Cell mediated immunity in anergic patients with pulmonary tuberculosis. Am Rev Respir Dis 118:827, 1978
68. MCMURRAY DN: Mechanisms of anergy in tuberculosis. Chest 77:4, 1980
69. MOHR JA et al: The transfer of delayed hypersensitivity. JAMA 207(3):517, 1969
70. THOMPSON NJ et al: The booster phenomenon in serial tuberculin testing. Am Rev Respir Dis 119:587, 1979
71. US Department of Health, Education and Welfare: Guidelines for Prevention of TB Transmission in Hospitals. Atlanta, Public Health Service, Center for Disease Control, January, 1979 (revised)
72. PALMER PES: Pulmonary tuberculosis—Usual and unusual radiographic presentations. Semin Roentgenol 14:204, 1979
73. WEBER AL, BIRD KT, JANOWER ML: Primary tuberculosis in childhood with particular emphasis on changes affecting the tracheobronchial tree. Am J Roentgenol 103:123, 1968
74. STEAD WW, KERBY GR, SCHLEUTER DP et al: The clinical spectrum of primary tuberculosis in adults. Ann Intern Med 68:731, 1968
75. JACOBSON HG, SHAPIRO JH: Pulmonary tuberculosis. Radiol Clin North Am 1:411, 1963
76. KITTREDGE RD, FINBY N: Bilateral tuberculous mediastinal adenopathy in the adult. Am J Roentgenol 96:1022, 1966
77. DERHAM RJ: Postprimary intrathoracic tuberculosis in childhood: With special references to its sequelae. Texas State J Med 52:583–588, 1956
78. ADLER H: Phthisiogenetic studies by means of tomography in cases of localized pulmonary tuberculosis in adults. Acta Tuberc Scand [Suppl] 47:13, 1959
79. BURKE RM, WIER JA: Review of cases of nontuberculous disease originally diagnosed as pulmonary tuberculosis. Am Rev Tuberc 75:921, 1957
80. SIMPSON DG, KUSHER M, MCCLEMENT JH: Respiratory function in pulmonary tuberculosis. Am Rev Respir Dis 87:1, 1963
81. BATES DV, MACKLEM PT, CHRISTIE RV: Respiratory Function in Disease, 2nd ed, p 410. Philadelphia, WB Saunders, 1971
82. HOMAN W et al: Miliary tuberculosis presenting as acute respiratory failure: Treatment by mem-

brane oxygenator and ventricle pump. Chest 67:366, 1975

83. BRISCOE WA, SMITH JP, BERGOFSKY E et al: Castastrophic pulmonary failure. Am J Med 60:248, 1976
84. GOREN MB et al: Some observations on mycobacterial acid-fastness. Am Rev Respir Dis 118:151, 1978
85. STRUMPF IJ, TSANG AY, SCHORK MA et al: The reliability of gastric smears by auramine-rhodamine for the diagnosis of tuberculosis staining technique. Am Rev Respir Dis 113:(4):51, 1976
86. DANEK SJ, BOWER JS: Diagnosis of pulmonary tuberculosis by flexible fiberoptic bronchoscopy. Am Rev Respir Dis 119:677, 1979
87. WEG JG, BREWER LM: Percutaneous needle biopsy of the lung: A valuable diagnostic procedure in diffuse and localized disease. Am Rev Respir Dis 96:150, 1967
88. RAY JF et al: Open pulmonary biopsy: Nineteen year experience with 416 consecutive operations. Chest 69:43, 1976
89. KUBICA GP, DYE WE: Laboratory methods for clinical and public health mycobacteriology. Atlanta, US Department of Health, Education and Welfare, Public Health Service, 1967
90. VESTAL AL: Procedures for the isolation and identification of mycobacteria. Atlanta, Department of Health, Education and Welfare, US Public Health Service, 1969
91. BLAIR JE, LENNETTE EH, TRUANT JP (eds): Manual of Clinical Microbiology. Bethesda, American Society for Microbiology, 1970
92. Handbook of Tuberculosis Laboratory Methods: Veterans Administration—Armed Forces Cooperative Study on the Chemotherapy of Tuberculosis. Washington, DC, US Government Printing Office, 1962
93. HOBBY GL, JOHNSON PM, BOYTAR-PAPIRNYIK V: Primary drug resistance: A continuing study of drug resistance in tuberculosis in a veteran population within the United States. X. September 1970 to September 1973. Am Rev Respir Dis 110:95, 1974
94. WAYNE LG, DOUBEK JR: Diagnostic key to mycobacteria encountered in clinical laboratories. Appl Microbiol 16:925, 1968
95. KOPANOFF DE et al: A continuing survey of tuberculosis primary drug resistance in the United States: March 1975 to November 1977—a USPHS cooperative study. Am Rev Respir Dis 118:835, 1978
96. KUBICA GP: Differential identification of mycobacteria. VII. Key features for identification of clinically significant mycobacteria. Am Rev Respir Dis 107:9, 1973
97. RUNYON EH: Identification of Acid-Fast Pathogens Utilizing Colony Characteristics. 3rd ed. Salt Lake City, Veterans Administration Hospital and University of Utah, 1972
98. CASHMAN HH et al: Bacteriologic standards for the discharge of patients: A statement by the Committee on Bacteriologic Standards for the Discharge of Patients. Am Rev Respir Dis 102:470, 1970
99. RUNYON EH, WAYNE LG, KUBICA GP: Mycobacteriaceae. In Buchanan RE, Gibbons NE (eds): Bergy's Manual of Determinative Bacteriology. 8th ed. Baltimore, Williams & Wilkins, 1974
100. SNIDER DE: Extrapulmonary tuberculosis in Oklahoma, 1965 to 1973. Am Rev Respir Dis 111:641, 1975
101. LUNDIN AP et al: Tuberculosis in patients undergoing maintenance hemodialysis. Am J Med 67:597, 1979
102. JOHNSON JE: Generalized (miliary) tuberculosis. In Johnson JE (ed): Rational Therapy and Control of Tuberculosis. Gainesville, University of Florida Press, 1970
103. SAHN SA, NEFF TA: Miliary tuberculosis. Am J Med 56:495, 1974
104. BERGER HW, SARNORTIN TG: Miliary tuberculosis: Diagnostic methods with emphasis on the chest roentgenogram. Chest 58:686, 1970
105. SLAVIN RE, WALSH TJ, POLLACK AD: Late generalized tuberculosis. Medicine 59:352, 1980
106. BIEHL JP: Miliary tuberculosis: A review of sixty-eight adult patients admitted to a municipal general hospital. Am Rev Respir Dis 77:605, 1968
107. PETERSDORF RG, BEESON PB: Fever of unexplained origin: Report on 100 cases. Medicine 40:1, 1961
108. PROUDFOOT AT, AKHTAR AJ, DOUGLAS AC et al: Miliary tuberculosis in adults. Br Med J 2:273, 1969
109. LINELL F, OSTBERG G: Tuberculosis in an autopsy material. Scand J Respir Dis 47:200, 1966
110. GRIECO MH, CHMEL H: Acute disseminated tuberculosis as a diagnostic problem—a clinical study based on twenty-eight cases. Am Rev Respir Dis 109:554, 1974
111. CORR WP, KYLE RA, BOWIE EJ: Hematologic changes in tuberculosis. Am J Med Sci 248:709, 1964
112. TWOMEY JJ, LEAVELL BS: Leukemoid reactions to tuberculosis. Arch Intern Med 116:21, 1965
113. GOLDFINE IA, SCHACTER H, BARCLAY WR et al: Consumption coagulopathy in miliary tuberculosis. Ann Intern Med 71:755, 1969
114. CHUNG DK, HUBBARD WW: Hyponatremia in untreated active pulmonary tuberculosis. Am Rev Respir Dis 99:595, 1969
115. SHALHOUB RJ, ANTONIOUS LD: The mechanisms of hyponatremia in pulmonary tuberculosis. Ann Intern Med 70:943, 1969
116. VORHERR H et al: Antidiuretic principle in tuberculous lung tissue of a patient with pulmonary tuberculosis and hyponatremia. Ann Intern Med 72:383, 1970
117. SMITH HV, DANIEL P: Some clinical and pathologi-

cal aspects of tuberculosis of the central nervous system. Tubercle 28:64, 1947
118. O'TOOLE R, THORNTON GF, MUKHERJEE MK et al: Dexamethasone in tuberculous meningitis. Ann Intern Med 70:39, 1969
119. WEISS W, FLIPPEN HP: The prognosis of tuberculosis meningitis in the isoniazid era. Am J Med Sci 242:423, 1961
120. LEPPER MH, SPIES HW: The present status of the treatment of tuberculosis of the central nervous system. Ann NY Acad Sci 106:106, 1963
121. FITZSIMONS JM: Tuberculous meningitis: A follow-up study on 198 cases. Tubercle 44:87, 1963
122. FALK A: US Veterans Administration Armed Forces cooperative Study on the chemotherapy of tuberculosis. XIII. Tuberculous meningitis in adults, with special reference to survival, neurologic residuals, and work status. Am Rev Respir Dis 91:823, 1965
123. ROPER WH, WARING JJ: Primary serofibrinous pleural effusion in military personnel. Am Rev Tuberc 71:616, 1955
124. LOWELL JR: Pleural effusion: A study of the literature. J Okla State Med Assoc 52(8):510, 1959; 52(9):582, 1959
125. RAO NV et al: Biopsy of parietal pleura in 124 cases. Arch Intern Med 115:34, 1965
126. LEVINE H, METZGER W, LACERA D et al: Diagnosis of tuberculosis pleurisy by culture of pleural biopsy specimen. Arch Intern Med 126:269, 1970
127. MEDLAR EM: Cases of renal infection in pulmonary tuberculosis. Am J Pathol 2:401, 1926
128. BRANSCOMB BV, LESTER W, MACDONALD F et al: The present status of genitourinary tuberculosis: a statement of the committee on therapy. Am Rev Respir Dis 92:505, 1965
129. SIMON HB et al: Genitourinary tuberculosis. Am J Med 63:410, 1977
130. WECHSLER H, WESTGALL M, LATTIMER JK: Earliest signs and symptoms in 127 male patients with genitourinary tuberculosis. J Urol 83:80, 1960
131. ROYLANCE J, PENRY JB, DAVIES ER et al: The radiology of tuberculosis of the urinary tract. Clin Radiol 21:163, 1970
132. SUTHERLAND AM: Genital tuberculosis in women. Bull Sloan Hosp 13:127, 1967
133. KENNEY M, LOESCHEL AB, LOVELOCK FJ: Urine cultures in tuberculosis. Am Rev Respir Dis 82:564, 1960
134. BENTZ RR et al: The incidence of urine cultures positive for mycobacterium tuberculosis in a general tuberculosis patient population. Am Rev Respir Dis 111:647, 1975
135. MEDLAR EM, SASANO KT: Experimental renal tuberculosis with special reference to excretory bacilluria. Am Rev Tuberc 62:48, 1950
136. BURKE HE: The pathogenesis of certain forms of extrapulmonary tuberculosis. Am Rev Tuberc 62:48, 1950
137. DAVIDSON PT, HOROWITZ I: Skeletal tuberculosis—a review with patient presentations and discussion. Am J Med 48:77, 1970
138. TATELMAN M, DROUILLARD EJP: Tuberculosis of the ribs. Am J Roentgenol Radium Ther Nucl Med 70:923, 1953
139. FELDMAN F, HUERBACH R, JOHNSTON A: Tuberculous dactylitis in the adult. Am J Roentgenol Radium Ther Nucl Med 112:460, 1971
140. CHAPMAN M, MURRAY RO, STOKER DJ: Tuberculosis of the bones and joints. Semin Roentgenol 14:266, 1979
141. PAUL B: Tumour, tuberculosis and osteomyelitis of the spine—differential diagnostic aspects. Acta Orthop Scand 44:372, 1973
142. KEMP HBS, JACKSON JW, JEREMIAH JD et al: Pyogenic infections occurring primarily in intervertebral discs. J Bone Joint Surg 55B:698, 1973
143. MCTAMMANY JR, MOSER KM, HOUK VM: Disseminated bone tuberculosis—review of the literature and presentation of an unusual case. Am Rev Resp Dis 87:889, 1963
144. BERHEY S, GOLDSTEIN M, BISHKO F: Clinical and diagnostic features of tuberculous arthritis. Am J Med 53:36, 1972
145. SCHLESS JM, WIER JA: The current status and treatment of lymphatic tuberculosis—a review based on the experience with 120 cases. Am Rev Tuberc 76:811, 1957
146. CHAPMAN JS, GUY LR: Scrofula caused by atypical mycobacteria. Pediatrics 23:323, 1959
147. ROONEY JJ, CROCCO JA, LYONS HA: Tuberculous pericarditis. Ann Intern Med 72:73, 1970
148. KNOLL SM, SLOVIN SM: Tuberculosis in uremic pericarditis. Chest 66:205, 1974
149. SCHEPERS GWH: Tuberculous pericarditis. Am J Cardiol 9:248, 1962
150. HAGEMAN JH, D'ESOPO NC, GLENN WWL: Tuberculosis of the pericardium, a long term analysis of forty-four proved cases. N Engl J Med 270:327, 1964
151. SINGH MM, BHARGAVE AN, JAIN KP: Tuberculous peritonitis—an evaluation of pathogenetic mechanisms, diagnostic procedures, and therapeutic measures. N Engl J Med 281:1091, 1969
152. BORHARMANESH F, HEKMAT K, VAEZZADEH K et al: Tuberculous peritonitis—prospective study of 32 cases in Iran. Ann Intern Med 76:567, 1972
153. BROWNRIGG GM: Tuberculous peritonitis and salpingitis. N Engl J Med 282:1209, 1969
154. THIRUVENGADAM KV et al: Tuberculous peritonitis complicating portal cirrhosis. A study of 75 cases by peritoneal biopsy. J Indian Med Assoc 45:180, 1965
155. BURACK WR, HOLLISTER RM: Tuberculous peritonitis. A study of forty-seven cases encountered by a general medical unit in twenty-five years. Am J Med 28:510, 1960
156. UGHES HJ, CARR DT, GERACI JE: Tuberculous peri-

tonitis: A review of 34 cases with emphasis on diagnostic aspects. Dis Chest 38:42, 1960

157. GONELLA JS, HUDSON EK: Clinical patterns of tuberculosis peritonitis. Arch Intern Med 117:164, 1966
158. SOCHOCKY S: Tuberculous peritonitis—a review of 100 cases. Am Rev Respir Dis 95:398, 1967
158a. SHERMAN S, RAVIKRISHNAN KP, ROHWEDDER JJ, WEG JG: Tuberculosis enteritis and peritonitis: A review of 36 cases. Arch Intern Med 140:506, 1980
159. ROHWEDDER JJ: Upper respiratory tract tuberculosis—sixteen cases in a general hospital. Ann Intern Med 80:708, 1974
160. JOHNSTON RF, WILDRICK KH: State of the art review: The impact of chemotherapy on the care of patients with tuberculosis. Am Rev Respir Dis 109:636, 1974
161. GLASSROTH J et al: Medical progress. Tuberculosis in the 1980s. N Engl J Med 302:1441, 1980
162. BATES JH: Treatment of tuberculosis. Adv Intern Med 20:1, 1975
163. CANETTI J: Present aspects of bacterial resistance in tuberculosis. Am Rev Respir Dis 92:687, 1965
164. SENCER DJ et al: BCG vaccines for tuberculosis: Official ATS–CDC statement. Am Rev Respir Dis 112:478, 1975
165. NAGANNA K: Some of the BCG trials and certain aspects involved in them. Am Rev Respir Dis 109:497, 1974
166. OSEASOHN R: Current use of BCG. Am Rev Respir Dis 109:500, 1974
167. BCG: Bad news for India. Lancet 1:73, 1980
168. FEREBEE SH: Controlled chemoprophylaxis trials in tuberculosis. A general review. Adv Tuberc Res 17:28, 1969
169. ISEMAN MD: Containment of tuberculosis preventive therapy with Isoniazid, and contact investigation. Chest (Suppl) 76:801, 1979
170. COMSTOCK GW, WOOLPERT S, FEREBEE S et al: Isoniazid prophylaxis among Alaskan Eskimos: a progress report. Am Rev Respir Dis 110:195, 1974
171. HSU KHK: Isoniazid in the prevention and treatment of tuberculosis: A 20-year study of the effectiveness in children. JAMA 229:528, 1974
172. SNIDER DE JR: Editorial: The relationship between tuberculosis and silicosis. Am Rev Respir Dis 118:455, 1978
173. Editorial: Tuberculosis in patients having dialysis. Br Med J 1:349, 1980
173a. FISHER JR: Tuberculosis after gastrointestinal surgery. Ann Intern Med 87:792, 1977
174. SCHARER L, SMITH JP: Serum transaminases elevations and other hepatic abnormalities in patients receiving isoniazid. Ann Intern Med 71:1113, 1969
175. GARIBALDI RA, DRUSIN RE, FEREBEE SH et al: Isoniazid associated hepatitis. Am Rev Respir Dis 106:357, 1972
176. MADDREY WC, BOITNOTT JK: Isoniazid hepatitis. Ann Intern Med 79:1, 1973
177. MITCHELL JR et al: Isoniazid liver injury: Clinical spectrum, pathology, and probable pathogenesis. Ann Intern Med 84:181, 1976
178. COMSTOCK GW, EDWARDS PQ: The competing risks of tuberculosis and hepatitis for adult tuberculin reactors. Am Rev Respir Dis 111:573, 1975
179. WEG JG: Current concepts of tuberculosis control and treatment. J Occup Med 12:497, 1970
180. DOSTER B, MURRAY FJ, NEWMAN R et al: Ethambutol in the initial treatment of pulmonary tuberculosis. Am Rev Respir Dis 107:177, 1973
181. DUTT AK et al: Follow-up of patients with tuberculosis treated in a general hospital program—treatment largely as outpatients by community physicians. Chest 74:19, 1978
182. FOX W: The chemotherapy of pulmonary tuberculosis: A review. Chest (Suppl) 76:785, 1979
183. BYRD RB et al: Treatment of tuberculosis by the non-pulmonary physician. Ann Intern Med 86:799, 1977
184. STEINER M et al: Primary drug-resistant tuberculosis: Report of an outbreak. N Engl J Med 283:1353, 1970
185. FAIRSHTER RD, RANDAZZO GP, GARTIN J et al: Failure of isoniazid-resistant tuberculosis. Am Rev Respir Dis 112:37, 1975
186. BRENNAN RW, DEHAJIA M, KUTT H et al: Diphenylhydantoin intoxication attendant to slow inactivation of isoniazid. Neurology 18:183, 1968
187. GOOD AE, GREEN RA, ZARAFONETIS CJD: Rheumatic symptoms during tuberculosis therapy—a manifestation of isoniazid toxicity. Ann Intern Med 63:800, 1965
188. CAMERON WM: Isoniazid overdose. Can Med Assoc J 118:1413, 1978
189. GOLDMAN A, BRAMAN SS: Isoniazid: a review with emphasis on adverse effects. Chest 62:71, 1972
190. BOBROWITZ ID: Ethambutol in pregnancy. Chest 66:20, 1974
191. NEWMAN R, DOSTER BE, MURRAY JF et al: Rifampin in initial treatment of tuberculosis. Am Rev Respir Dis 109:216, 1974
192. ISEMAN MD et al: American Thoracic Society statement—guidelines for short course chemotherapy. Am Rev Respir Dis 121:611, 1980
193. AQUINAS SISTER M et al: Adverse reactions to daily and intermittent rifampicin regimens for pulmonary tuberculosis in Hong Kong. Br Med J 1:765, 1972
194. O'REILLY RA: Interaction of chronic daily warfarin therapy and rifampin. Ann Intern Med 83:506, 1975
195. BOLT HM, KAPPUS H, BOLT M: Rifampicin and oral contraceptives. Lancet 1:1280, 1974
196. LITWIN A, BROOKS SM, CLAES F: A pilot study concerning the early immunosuppressive effects of rifampin in man. Chest 65:548, 1974
197. MCLAUGHIN JS, HANKINS JR: Current aspects of

surgery for pulmonary tuberculosis. Ann Thorac Surg 17:513, 1974

198. CROCCO JA et al: Massive hemoptysis. Arch Intern Med 121:498, 1968
199. LATTIMER JK: Current concepts: Renal tuberculosis. N Engl J Med 273:208, 1965
200. Editorial: Tuberculosis of the spine. Br Med J 4(5945):613, 1974
201. Editorial: Genitourinary tuberculosis. Br Med J 1:183, 1971
202. BYRD RB, BOPP RK, GRACEY DR: The role of surgery in tuberculous lymphadenitis. Am Rev Respir Dis 103:816, 1971
203. SNIDER DE, LAYDE PM, JOHNSON MW et al: Treatment of tuberculosis during pregnancy. Am Rev Respir Dis 122:65, 1980
204. RALEIGH JW: The late results of prolonged multiple drug therapy for pulmonary tuberculosis. Am Rev Tuberc 76:540, 1957
205. LESTER W: Treatment of drug resistant tuberculosis. In Dowling HG (ed): Disease-a-month. Chicago, Year Book Medical Publishers, 1971
206. SIMPSON DG, HUBAYTAR RT: Hypersensitivity to drugs in the treatment of tuberculosis—rapid desensitization using cortisone acetate. Am Rev Respir Dis 86:738, 1962
207. Short course chemotherapy in pulmonary tuberculosis—a controlled trial by the British Thoracic Society and Tuberculosis Association. Lancet 1:119, 1975
208. MITCHISON DA: Basic mechanisms of chemotherapy. Chest (Suppl) 76:771, 1979
209. SBARBARO JA, HUDSON LD: High dose ethambutol; an oral alternate for intermittent chemotherapy. Am Rev Respir Dis 110:91, 1974

209a. WHITCOMB ME, ROCKLIN RE: Transfer factor in a patient with progressive primary tuberculosis. Ann Intern Med 79:161, 1973

210. WEG JG: Tuberculosis and the generation gap. Am J Nurs 71:495, 1971
211. RILEY RL, MOODIE AS: Infectivity of patients with pulmonary tuberculosis in inner city homes. Am Rev Respir Dis 110:810, 1974
212. American Thoracic Society's Ad Hoc Committee on the Treatment of Tuberculosis in General Hospitals: Guidelines for the general hospital in the admission and care of tuberculosis patients. Am Rev Respir Dis 99:631, 1969
213. US Department of Health, Education and Welfare: Guidelines for Prevention of TB Transmission in Hospitals. Atlanta, Public Health Service, 1974
214. CASHMAN HH et al: Bacteriologic standards for the discharge of patients. Am Rev Respir Dis 102:470, 1970
215. EDSALL J et al: Guidelines for work for patients with tuberculosis. Am Rev Respir Dis 108:160, 1973
216. BATES JH et al: Standards for tuberculosis treatment in the 1970's. Am Rev Respir Dis 102:992, 1970
217. MACGREGOR RR: A year's experience with tuberculosis in a private urban teaching hospital in the post sanatorium era. Am J Med 58:221, 1975
218. NAKIELNA EM, CRAGG R, GRZYBOWSKI S: Lifelong follow-up of inactive tuberculosis: Its value and limitations. Am Rev Respir Dis 112:765, 1975
219. SNIDER DE: Reactivation of tuberculosis in Oklahoma, 1970–1973. Chest 68:36, 1975
220. EDSALL J, COLLINS G: Routine follow-up of inactive tuberculosis, a practice to be abandoned. Am Rev Respir Dis 107:851, 1973
221. HOPEWELL PC et al: Discharge of tuberculosis patients from medical surveillance. Am Rev Respir Dis
222. RUNYON EH: Anonymous mycobacteria in pulmonary disease. Med Clin North Am 43:273, 1959
223. JENKINS DE et al: The clinical problem of infection with atypical acid-fast bacilli. Trans Am Clin Climatol 71:21, 1959
224. CURRY FJ: Atypical acid-fast mycobacteria. N Engl J Med 272:415, 1965
225. LESTER WL: Unclassified mycobacterial diseases. Annu Rev Med 17:351, 1966
226. CHAPMAN JS: The Atypical Mycobacteria and Human Mycobacteriosis. New York, Plenum Press, 1977
227. WOLINSKY E: State of the art—Nontuberculous mycobacteria and associated diseases. Am Rev Respir Dis 119:107, 1979
228. FALKINHAM III JD et al: Epidemiology of infection by nontuberculous mycobacteria—1. geographic distribution in the eastern United States. Am Rev Respir Dis 121:931, 1980
229. EDWARDS LB, PALMER CE: Isolation of 'atypical' mycobacteria from healthy persons. Am Rev Respir Dis 80:747, 1959
230. SCHAEFER WB, DAVIS CL: A bacteriologic and histopathologic study of skin granuloma due to Mycobacterium balnei. Am Rev Respir Dis 84:837, 1961
231. WOLINSKY F, GOMEZ F, ZIMPFER F: Sporotrichoid Mycobacterium marinum infection treated with rifampin ethambutol. Am Rev Respir Dis 105:964, 1972
232. KILBRIDGE TM, GONNELLA JS, BOLAN JT: Pancytopenia and death-disseminated anonymous mycobacterial infection. Arch Intern Med 120:38, 1970
233. BATES JH: A study of pulmonary disease associated with mycobacteria other than M. tuberculosis: Clinical characteristics. XX. A report of the Veterans Administration Armed Forces Cooperative Study on the Chemotherapy of Tuberculosis. Am Rev Respir Dis 96:1151, 1967
234. SCHAEFER WB, BIRN KJ, JENKINS PA et al: Infection with the Avian–Battey group of mycobacteria in England and Wales. Br Med J 2:412, 1969

235. BAILEY WC et al: Silico-mycobacterial disease in sandblasters. Am Rev Respir Dis 110:115, 1974
236. HARRIS GD, JOHANSON WG, NICHOLSON DP: Response to chemotherapy of pulmonary infection due to Mycobacterium kansasii. Am Rev Respir Dis 112:31, 1975
237. WOLINSKY E: The role of scotochromogenic mycobacteria in human disease. Ann NY Acad Sci 106:67, 1963
238. SALYER KE, VOLTELER TP, DORMAN GW: Surgical management of cervical adenitis due to atypical mycobacteria in children. JAMA 204:1037, 1968
239. CORPE RF, LIANG JL, SANCHEY ES: Early and late results in persons with atypical group III tuberculosis. Am Rev Respir Dis 111:915, 1975
240. ROSENZWEIG DY: Pulmonary mycobacterial infections due to *Mycobacterium intracellular-avium* complex. Clinical features and course in 100 consecutive cases. Chest 75:115, 1979
241. DUTT AK, STEAD WW: Long-term results of medical treatment in Mycobacterium intracellulare infection. Am J Med 67: 449, 1979
242. DARLING ST: Protozoon general infection producing pseudotubercles in lungs and focal necrosis in liver, spleen, and lymph nodes. JAMA 46:1283, 1906
243. DARLING ST: The morphology of the parasite (*Histoplasma capsulatum*) and the lesions of histoplasmosis, a fatal disease of tropical America. J Exp Med 11:515, 1909
244. DODD K, TOMPKINS EH: A case of histoplasmosis of Darling in an infant. Am J Trop Med 14:127, 1934
245. DEMOMBREUN WA: The cultivation and cultural characteristics of Darling's *Histoplasma capsulatum*. Am J Trop Med 14:93, 1934
246. LONG ER, STEARNS WH: Physical examination at induction: Standards with respect to tuberculosis and their application by review of 53,400 x-ray films of men in the army of the United States. Radiology 41:144, 1943
247. CHRISTIE A, PETERSON JC: Pulmonary calcification in negative reactors to tuberculin. Am J Public Health 35:1131, 1945
248. PARSON RJ, ZARAFONETIS CJD: Histoplasmosis in man: Report of 7 cases and review of 71 cases. Arch Intern Med 75:1, 1945
249. SCHWARZ J, BAUM GL: The history of histoplasmosis, 1906 to 1956. N Engl J Med 256:253, 1957
250. GOODWIN RA JR, DESPREZ RM: State of the art—histoplasmosis. Am Rev Respir Dis 117:929, 1978
251. TOSH FE et al: Primary cutaneous histoplasmosis: Report of a case. Arch Intern Med 114:118, 1964
252. SILLS M, SCHWARTZ A, WEG JG: Conjugal histoplasmosis. Ann Intern Med 79:221, 1973
253. LOSSLI CG et al: Pulmonary histoplasmosis in a farm family: a three-year follow-up. J Lab Clin Med 43:669, 1954
254. EDWARDS PQ, KLAER JH: Worldwide geographic distribution of histoplasmosis and histoplasmin sensitivity. Am J Trop Med Hyg 5:235, 1956
255. FURCOLOW ML: Epidemiology of histoplasmosis. In Sweany HC: Histoplasmosis, p 113. Springfield, Charles C Thomas, 1960
256. WILCOX KR JR, WAISBREN BA, MARTIN J: The Walworth, Wisconsin, epidemic of histoplasmosis. Ann Intern Med 49:388, 1958
257. LEHAN PH, FURCOLOW ML: Epidemic histoplasmosis. J Chron Dis 5:489, 1957
258. SAROSI GA et al: Histoplasmosis outbreaks, their patterns. In Ajellow L et al: Histoplasmosis, Proceedings of Second National Conference, pp 123–128. Springfield, Charles C Thomas, 1971
259. DRUTZ DJ: Urban coccidioidomycosis and histoplasmosis—Sacramento and Indianapolis. N Engl J Med 301:381, 1979
260. CAMPBELL CC: Histoplasmosis outbreaks: Recommendation for mandatory treatment of known microfoci of *H. Capsulatum* in soils. Chest 77:6, 1980
261. PROCKNOW JJ et al: Early pathogenesis of experimental histoplasmosis. Arch Pathol 69:413, 1960
262. SCHWARZ J: The primary lesion in histoplasmosis. In Sweaney HC: Histoplasmosis, p 292. Springfield, Charles C Thomas, 1960
263. SWEANY HJ: Histoplasmosis, p 268. Springfield, Charles C Thomas, 1960
264. PUCKETT TF: Pulmonary histoplasmosis: A study of 22 cases with identification of *H. capsulatum* in resected lesions. Am Rev Tuberc 67:453, 1953
265. STRAUB M, SCHWARZ J: The healed primary complex in histoplasmosis. Am J Clin Pathol 25:727, 1955
266. SCHWARZ J et al: The relation of splenic calcification to histoplasmosis. N Engl J Med 252:887, 1955
267. DODGE HJ, AJELLOW L, ENGELKE OK: The association of a bird-roosting site with infection of school children by *Histoplasma capsulatum*. Am J Public Health 55:1203, 1955
268. WHITEHOUSE WM, DAVEY WN, ENGELKE OK et al: Roentgen findings in histoplasmin-positive school children. J Michigan State Med Soc 58:1266, 1959
269. RUBIN R et al: The course and prognosis of histoplasmosis. Am J Med 27:279, 1959
270. RUBIN H, LEHAN PH, FURCOLOW ML: Severe nonfatal histoplasmosis. Report of a typical case with comments on therapy. N Engl J Med 257:599, 1957
271. FURCOLOW ML, BRASHER CA: Chronic progressive (cavitary) histoplasmosis as a problem in tuberculosis sanitoriums. Am Rev Tuberc Pulmonary Dis 73:609, 1956

272. CURRY FJ, WIER JA: Histoplasmosis. A review of one hundred consecutively hospitalized patients. Am Rev Tuberc Pulmonary Dis 77:749, 1957
273. BAUM GL, SCHWARZ J: Pulmonary histoplasmosis. N Engl J Med 258:677, 1958
274. GOODWIN RA et al: Disseminated histoplasmosis. Medicine 59:1, 1980
275. SILVERMAN FN et al: Histoplasmosis (review). Am J Med 19:410, 1955
276. HEYN RM, GIAMMONA ST: Disseminated histoplasmosis treated with amphotericin B. Am J Dis Child 98:253, 1959
277. REDDY P et al: Progressive disseminated histoplasmosis as seen in adults. Am J Med 48:629, 1970
278. SMITH JW, UTZ JP: Progressive disseminated histoplasmosis. A prospective study of 26 patients. Ann Intern Med 76:557, 1972
279. CONRAD FG, SASLAW S, ATWELL RJ: The protean manifestations of histoplasmosis as illustrated in twenty-three cases. Arch Intern Med 104:692, 1959
280. VANEK J, SCHWARZ J: The gamut of histoplasmosis. Am J Med 50:39, 1970
281. PICARDI JL et al: Pericarditis caused by *Histoplasma capsulum*. Am J Cardiol 37:82, 1976
282. DOZOIS RR et al: Sclerosing mediastinitis involving major bronchi. Mayo Clin Proc 43:557, 1968
283. SCHOWENGERDT CG, SUYEMOTO R, MAIN FB: Granulomatous and fibrous mediastinitis, a review and analysis of 180 case. J Thorac Cardiovasc Surg 57:365, 1969
284. GOODWIN RA, NICKELL JA, DESPREZ RM: Mediastinal fibrosis complicating healed primary histoplasmosis and tuberculosis. Medicine 51:227, 1972
285. KAUFMAN LR et al: Effect of a single histoplasmin skin test on serologic diagnosis of histoplasmosis. J Bacteriol 94:798, 1967
286. BUECHNER HA et al: The current status of serologic, immunologic and skin tests in the diagnosis of pulmonary mycoses. Chest 63:259, 1973
287. FURCOLOW JL: Tests of immunity in histoplasmosis. N Engl J Med 268:357, 1963
288. CAMPBELL, CC, BINKLEY GE: Serologic diagnoses with respect to histoplasmosis, coccidioidomycosis, and blastomycosis and the problem of cross reactions. J Lab Clin Med 42:896, 1953
289. HEINER DC: Diagnosis of histoplasmosis using precipitin reactions in agar gel. Pediatrics 22:616, 1958
290. PLOUFFE JF, FASS RJ: Histoplasma meningitis: Diagnostic value of cerebrospinal fluid serology. Ann Intern Med 92:189, 1980
291. SWEET GH et al: Antibodies in histoplasmosis detected by use of yeast and mycelial antigens in immunodiffusion and electroimmunodiffusion. Am Rev Respir Dis 120:441, 1979
292. COX R: Immunologic studies of patients with histoplasmosis. Am Rev Respir Dis 120:143, 1979
293. DAVIES SF et al: Trephine biopsy of the bone marrow in disseminated histoplasmosis. Am J Med 67:617, 1979
294. FURCOLOW MF et al: Course and prognosis of untreated histoplasmosis, a USPHS cooperative mycoses study. JAMA 177:292, 1961
295. FURCOLOW MF: Comparison of treated and untreated severe histoplasmosis, a CDC cooperative mycoses study. JAMA 183:823, 1963
296. GOODWIN RA JR et al: Early chronic pulmonary histoplasmosis. Am Rev Respir Dis 93:47, 1966
297. PARKER JD et al: Treatment of chronic pulmonary histoplasmosis, a national CDC cooperative mycoses study. N Engl J Med 283:225, 1970
298. DRUTZ DJ et al: Treatment of disseminated mycotic infections. Am J Med 45:405, 1968
299. UTZ JP et al: Amphotericin B toxicity (clinical staff conference of NIH) Ann Intern Med 61:334, 1964
300. MEDOFF G, KOBAYASHI GS: Strategies in the treatment of systemic fungal infections. N Engl J Med 302:145, 1980
301. SAROSI GA et al: Disseminated histoplasmosis: Results of long-term follow-up. A CDC cooperative mycoses study. Ann Intern Med 75:511, 1971
302. FIESE JM: Coccidioidomycosis. Springfield, Charles C Thomas, 1958
303. RIXFORD E, GILCHRIST TC: Two cases of protozoan (coccidioidal) infection of the skin and other organs. Johns Hopkins Med J 1:209, 1896
304. STEWART RH, MEYER KF: Isolation of *Coccidioides immitis* (Stiles) from soil. Proc Soc Exp Biol Med 29:937, 1932
305. DICKSON EC, GIFFORD MA: Coccidioides infection (coccidioidomycosis): The primary type of infection. Arch Intern Med 62:853, 1938
306. SMITH CE: Reminiscences of the flying chlamydospore and its allies. In Ajello L (ed): Coccidioidomycosis. Tucson, University of Arizona Press, 1967
307. AJELLO L (ed): Coccidioidomycosis. Current Clinical and Diagnostic Status. American College of Chest Physicians, Symposia Specialists. New York, Grune & Stratton, 1977
308. DRUTZ DJ, CATANZARO A: State of the Art—Coccidioidomycosis. Am Rev Respir Dis 117:559, 727, 1978
309. SMITH CE: Epidemiology of acute coccidioidomycosis with erythema nodosum. As J Public Health 30:600, 1940
310. SMITH CE, BEARD RR, SAITO MT: Pathogenesis of coccidioidomycosis with special reference to pulmonary cavitation. Ann Intern Med 29:623, 1948

311. ROTHMAN PE et al: Coccidioidomycosis—possible fomite transmission. Am J Dis Child 118:792, 1969
312. ECKMAN BH, SCHAEFER GL, HUPPERT M: Bedside interhuman transmission of coccidioidomycosis via growth on fomites. Am Rev Respir Dis 89:175, 1964
313. JOHNSON JE III et al: Laboratory-acquired coccidioidomycosis, a report of 210 cases. Ann Intern Med 60:941, 1964
314. PUCKETT TF: Hyphae of *Coccidioides immitis* in tissues of the human host. Am Rev Tuberculosis 70:320, 1954
315. FORBUS WD: Coccidioidomycosis: A study of 95 cases of the disseminated type with special reference to the pathogenesis of the disease. Milit Surg 9: 653, 1946
316. HUNTINGTON RW et al: Pathologic and clinical observations on 142 cases of fatal coccidioidomycosis with necropsy. In Ajellow L (ed): Coccidioidomycosis, p 143. Tucson, University of Arizona Press, 1967
317. SALKIN D: Clinical examples of reinfection in coccidioidomycosis. Am Rev Respir Dis 95:603, 1967
318. RICHTER HS: Coccidioidomycosis: A report of 300 new cases. GP Gen Practice 90:89, 1969
319. GREENDYKE WH: The varied roentgen manifestations of primary coccidioidomycosis. Am J Roentgenol 109:491, 1970
320. HYDE L: Coccidioidal pulmonary cavitation. Dis Chest [Suppl 1] 54:273, 1968
321. O'LEARY DJ, CURRY FJ: Coccidioidomycosis a review and presentation of 100 consecutive hospitalized patients. Am Rev Tuberc Pulmonary Dis 73:501, 1956
322. SIEVERS JL: Prognostic factors in disseminated coccidioidomycosis among southwestern American Indians. In Ajello L (ed): Current Clinical and Diagnostic Status, American College of Chest Physicians, Symposia Specialists. New York, Grune & Stratton, 1977
323. HARRIS RE: Coccidioidomycosis complicating pregnancy. Report of 3 cases and review of the literature. Obstet Gynecol 28:401, 1966
324. VAN BERGEN WS et al: Fetal maternal disseminated coccidioidomycosis in a nonendemic area. Am J Obstet Gynecol 124:661, 1976
325. DERESINSKI SC: Coccidioidomycosis in compromised hosts. Medicine 54:377, 1974
326. ROWLAND VS et al: Acute respiratory failure in miliary coccidioidomycosis. In Ajello L (ed): Current Clinical and Diagnostic Status. American College of Chest Physicians, Symposia Specialists. New York, Grune & Stratton, 1977
327. SMITHLINE NO et al: Disseminated coccidioidomycosis in renal transplant patients. In Ajello L (ed): Current Clinical and Diagnostic Status. American College of Chest Physicians, Symposia Specialists. New York, Grune & Stratton, 1977
328. LAND GA et al: The isolation of disseminated *Coccidioides immitis* by an improved blood culture technique. In Ajello L (ed): Current Clinical and Diagnostic Status, American College of Chest Physicians, Symposia Specialists. New York, Grune & Stratton, 1977
329. SMITH CE et al: Varieties of coccidioidal infection in relation to the epidemiology and control of the disease. Am J Public Health 36:1394, 1946
330. SMITH CE, SAITO MT, SIMMONS SH: Pattern of 39,500 serologic tests in coccidioidomycosis. JAMA 160:542, 1956
331. PAPPAGIANIS D, CRANE R: Survival in coccidioidal meningitis since the introduction of amphotericin B. In Ajello L (ed): Current Clinical and Diagnostic Status, American College of Chest Physicians, Symposia Specialists. New York, Grune & Stratton, 1977
332. CAUDILL RG, SMITH CE, REINARZ JA: Coccidioidal meningitis: A diagnostic challenge. Am J Med 49:360, 1970
333. SMITH CE et al: The use of coccidioidin. Am Rev Tuberculosis 57:330, 1948
334. WINN WA: A long-term study of 300 patients with cavitary abscess lesions of the lung of coccidioidal origin. Dis Chest [Suppl 1] 54:268, 1968
335. LEVINE HB et al: Derman sensitivity to *Coccidioides immitis:* A comparison of response elicited by spherulin and coccidioidin. Am Rev Respir Dis 107:379, 1973
336. WINN WA: Coccidioidal meningitis: A follow-up report. In Ajello L (ed): Coccidioidomycosis, p 55. Tucson, University of Arizona Press, 1967
337. EINSTEIN H: Some aspects of coccidioidomycosis therapy. In Ajello L (ed): Coccidioidomycosis, p 123. Tucson, University of Arizona Press, 1967
338. SAROSI GA et al: Chronic pulmonary coccidioidomycosis, a national CDC cooperative mycoses study. N Engl J Med 283:325, 1970
339. GRANT AR et al: Resectional surgery in pulmonary coccidioidomycosis: A review of 263 cases. In Ajello L (ed): Current Clinical and Diagnostic Status, American College of Chest Physicians, Symposia Specialists. New York, Grune & Stratton, 1977
340. DERESINSKI SC, STEVENS DA: Bone and joint coccidioidomycosis treated with miconazole. Am Rev Respir Dis 120:1101, 1979
341. GRAYBILL JR et al: Immunologic and clinical improvement of progressive coccidioidomycosis following the administration of transfer factor. Cell Immunol 8:120, 1973
342. CATANZARO A, SPITLER L, MOSER KM: Immunotherapy of coccidioidomycosis. J Clin Invest 54:690, 1974

343. PAPPAGIANIS D, LEVINE HB, SMITH CE: Further studies on vaccination of human volunteers with killed *Coccidioides immitis*. In Ajello L (ed): Coccidioidomycosis, p 201. Tucson, University of Arizona Press, 1967
344. GILCHRIST TC: A case of blastomycetic dermatitis in man. Johns Hopkins Hosp Rep 1:269, 1896
345. SCHWARZ J, BAUM GL: Blastomycosis. Am J Clin Pathol 21:999, 1951
346. MARTIN DS, SMITH DT: Blastomycosis: I. A review of the literature. Am Rev Tuberculosis 39:275, 1939
347. SMITH JG et al: An epidemic of North American blastomycosis. JAMA 158:641, 1955
348. BAUM GL, LERNER PI: Primary pulmonary blastomycosis: A laboratory acquired infection. Ann Intern Med 73:263, 1970
349. SAROSI GA et al: Clinical features of acute pulmonary blastomycosis. N Engl J Med 290:540, 1974
350. TOSH FE et al: A common source epidemic of North American blastomycosis. Am Rev Respir Dis 109:525, 1974
351. SAROSI GA, DAVIES SF: State of the art—blastomycosis. Am Rev Respir Dis 120:911, 1979
352. DENTON JF, DISALVO AF: Respiratory infection of laboratory animals with conidia of *Blastomyces dermatitidis*. Mycopathol Mycol Appl 36:129, 1968
353. CRAIG MW et al: Conjugal blastomycosis. Am Rev Respir Dis 102:86, 1970
354. SAROSI GA et al: Canine blastomycosis as a harbinger of human disease. Ann Intern Med 91:733, 1979
355. WILSON JW et al: Primary cutaneous North American blastomycosis. Arch Dermatol 71:39, 1955
356. FURCOLOW ML et al: Prevalence and incidence studies of human and canine blastomycosis. Am Rev Respir Dis 102:60, 1970
357. KEPRON MW et al: North American blastomycosis in central Canada. A review of 36 cases. Can Med Assoc J 106:243, 1972
358. VANEK J, SCHWARZ J, HAKIM S: North American blastomycosis: A study of ten cases. Am J Clin Pathol 54:384, 1970
359. WITORSCH P, UTZ JP: North American blastomycosis: A study of 40 patients. Medicine 47:169, 1968
360. CUSH R, LIGHT RW, GEORGE RB: Clinical and roentgenographic manifestations of acute and chronic blastomycosis. Chest 69:345, 1976
361. ABERNATHY RS: Clinical manifestations of pulmonary blastomycosis. Ann Intern Med 51:707, 1959
362. KAUFMAN L et al: Specific immunodiffusion tests for blastomycosis. Appl Microbiol 24:244, 1973
363. VARKEY B et al: Blastomycosis: Clinical and immunologic aspects. Chest 77:789, 1980
364. ABERNATHY RS, JANSEN GT: Therapy with amphotericin B in North American blastomycosis. Ann Intern Med 53:1196, 1960
365. BUSEY JF et al: Blastomycosis. I. A review of 198 collected cases in Veterans Administration hospitals. Am Rev Respir Dis 89:659, 1964
366. PARKER JD, DOTO IC, TOSH FE: A decade of experience with blastomycosis and its treatment with amphotericin B. A national CDC cooperative mycoses study. Am Rev Respir Dis 99:895, 1969
367. O'NEILL RP, PENMAN RWB: Clinical aspects of blastomycosis. Thorax 25:708, 1970
368. GONYEA EF: The spectrum of primary blastomycotic meningitis: a review of central nervous system blastomycosis. Ann Neurol 3:26, 1978
369. LOCKWOOD WR et al: The treatment of North American blastomycosis. Ten years' experience. Am Rev Respir Dis 100:314, 1969
370. ARNOW PM et al: Pulmonary aspergillosis during hospital renovation. Am Rev Respir Dis 118:49, 1978
371. PEPYS J: Pulmonary aspergillosis. In Monographs in Allergy, Vol 4, p 20. Basel, S. Karger, AC, 1969
372. TURNER-WARWICK M et al: Immunologic lung disease due to aspergillus. Chest 68:346, 1975
373. British Thoracic and Tuberculosis Association Report: Aspergilloma and residual tuberculosis cavities—The results of a resurvey. Tubercle 51:227, 1970
374. EDGE JRD et al: Pulmonary aspergillosis in an unselected hospital population. Chest 59:407, 1971
375. MEYER RD et al: Aspergillosis complicating neoplasms. Am J Med 54:6, 1973
376. TURNER-WARWICK M: Aspergillus fumigatus and lung disease. Postgrad Med J 55:642, 1979
377. GRIGOVIA D, DELACRATAZ J, BOMBULE J, Aspergillus sinusitis. Postgrad Med J 55:619, 1979
378. YOUNG RC et al: Aspergillosis, the spectrum of the disease in 98 patients. Medicine 49:147, 1970
379. PARKER JD et al: Pulmonary aspergillosis in sanitoriums in the south central United States. A national CDC cooperative mycoses study. Am Rev Respir Dis 101:551, 1970
380. FRUENDLICH I, ISRAEL IM: Pulmonary aspergillosis. Clin Radiol 24:248, 1973
381. MCCARTHY DS et al: The radiological appearances in allergic bronchopulmonary aspergillosis. Clin Radiol 21:366, 1970
382. MALO JL et al: Studies in chronic allergic bronchopulmonary aspergillosis: 2. Radiological findings. Thorax 32:262, 1977
383. SLAVIN RG et al: Allergic bronchopulmonary aspergillosis—A North American rarity. Am J Med 47:306, 1969
384. MALO JL et al: Studies in chronic allergic bronchopulmonary aspergillosis: 1. Clinical and physiologic findings. Thorax 32:254, 1977

385. ROSENBERG M et al: Clinical and immunologic criteria for the diagnosis of allergic bronchopulmonary aspergillosis. Ann Intern Med 86:405, 1977
386. GAGE AA et al: Aspergillus infection after cardiac surgery. Arch Surg 101:384, 1970
387. KILMAN JW et al: Surgery for pulmonary aspergillosis. J Thorac Cardiovasc Surg 57:642, 1969
388. VARKEY B, RAFF HD: Pulmonary aspergilloma a rational approach to treatment. Am J Med 61:626, 1976
389. RAMIREZ-RIVERA J: Pulmonary aspergilloma: Endobronchial treatment. N Engl J Med 271:1281, 1964
390. HARGIS JL et al: Intracavitary amphotericin B in the treatment of symptomatic pulmonary aspergillosis. Am J Med 68:389, 1980
391. PEPYS J et al: Inhibitory effects of disodium cromoglycate on allergen-inhalation tests. Lancet 2:134, 1968
392. AISNER J et al: Treatment of invasive aspergillosis: Relation of early diagnosis and treatment to response. Ann Intern Med 86:539, 1977
393. LEWIS JL, RABINOWICH S: The wide spectrum of cryptococcal infections. Am J Med 53:315, 1972
394. BAKER RD, HAUGEN RK: Tissue changes and tissue diagnosis in cryptococcosis—a study of 26 cases. Am J Clin Pathol 25:4, 1955
395. WARR W, BATES JH, STONE A: The spectrum of pulmonary cryptococcosis. Ann Intern Med 69:1109, 1968
396. TYNES B et al: Variant forms of pulmonary cryptococcosis. Ann Intern Med 69:1117, 1968
396a. KERKERING TM, DUMA RJ, SMITH S: The evolution of pulmonary cryptococcosis. Ann Intern Med 94:611, 1981
397. GOODMAN JL et al: Diagnosis of cryptococcal meningitis. N Engl Med 285:434, 1971
398. BATES JH: Pulmonary cryptococcosis: Special problems in diagnosis and treatment. In Utz JP, Gordon G (eds): Modern Treatment, Vol 7. Hagerstown, Harper & Row, 1970
399. BINDSCHADLER DD, and BENNETT JE: Serology of human cryptococcosis. Ann Intern Med 69:45, 1968
400. KAUFMAN L, BLUMER S: Value and interpretation of serological tests for the diagnosis of cryptococcosis. Appl Microbiol 16:1907, 1968
401. DIAMOND RD, BENNETT JE: Prognostic factors in cryptococcal meningitis. Ann Intern Med 00.176, 1974
402. VANDEVELDE AG, MAUCERI AA, JOHNSON JE, III: 5-fluoro-cytosine in the treatment of mycotic infections. Ann Intern Med 77:43, 1972
403. ROSE ND, VARKEY B: Deep mycotic infection in the hospitalized adult: A study of 123 patients. Medicine 54:499, 1975
404. WILLIAMS DM, KRICK JA, REMINGTON JS: Pulmonary infection in the compromised host. Am Rev Respir Dis 114:359, 1976
405. ROSE ND, SHETH NK: Pulmonary candidiasis. Arch Intern Med 138:964, 1978
406. MASUR H, ROSEN PP, ARMSTRONG D: Pulmonary disease caused by Candida species. Am J Med 63:914, 1977
407. KAPLAN W, GONZALEZ OCHOA A: Application of the fluorescent antibody technique to the rapid diagnosis of sporotrichosis. J Lab Clin Med 62:835, 1963
408. MOHR JA et al: Primary pulmonary sporotrichosis. Am Rev Respir Dis 106:260, 1972
409. RIDGEWAY NA et al: Primary pulmonary sporotrichosis: Report of two cases. Am J Med 32:153, 1962
410. BROOK CJ et al: Pulmonary and articular sporotrichosis. Am Rev Respir Dis 116:141, 1977
411. GONZALEZ OCHEA A: Contribuciones recientes al conaciemento de la esporotrichosis. Gac Med Mex 95:463, 1965
412. KARLIN JV, NIELSON HS: Serologic aspects of sporotrichosis. J Infect Dis 121:316, 1970
413. WILSON DE et al: Clinical features of extracutaneous sporotrichosis. Medicine 46:265, 1967
414. PARKER et al: Treatment of extracutaneous sporotrichosis. Arch Intern Med 125:858, 1970
415. ROHWEDDER JJ, ARCHER G: Pulmonary sporotrichosis: Treatment with miconazole. Am Rev Respir Dis 114:403, 1976
416. STRAATSMA BR, ZIMMERMAN LE, GASS JDM: Phycomycosis, a clinico pathologic study of fifty-one cases. Lab Invest 11:963, 1962
417. MEDOFF G, KOBOYOSHI GS: Pulmonary mucormycosis. N Engl J Med 286:86, 1972
418. MEYER RD, ROSEN P, ARMSTRONG D: Phycomycosis complicating leukemia and lymphoma. Ann Intern Med 77:871, 1972
419. MURRAY HW: Pulmonary mucormycosis with massive fatal hemoptysis. Chest 68:65, 1975
420. LEMLE A et al: Lung function studies in pulmonary South American blastomycosis. Correlation with clinical and roentgenographic findings. Am J Med 48:434, 1970
421. RESTREPO A et al: The gamut of paracoccidioidomycosis. Am J Med 61:33, 1976
422. COPE VZ: Actinomycosis. London, Oxford University Press, 1938
423. WEESE WC, SMITY IM: A study of 57 cases of actinomycosis over a 36-year period. Arch Intern Med 135:1562, 1975
424. KAY EB: Actinomyces in chronic bronchopulmonary infections. Am Rev Tuberculosis 57:322, 1948
425. ROBBOY SJ, VICKERY AL JR: Tinctorial and morphologic properties distinguishing actinomycosis and nocardiosis. N Engl J Med 282:593, 1970
426. BROWN JR: Human actinomycosis. A study of 181 subjects. Human Pathol 4:319, 1973
427. EVERTS EC: Cervicofacial actinomycosis. Arch Otolaryngol 92:468, 1970

428. BATES M, CRUICKSHANK G: Thoracic actinomycosis. Thorax 12:99, 1957
429. MCQUARRIE DG, HALL WH: Actinomycosis of the lung and chest wall. Surgery 64:905, 1968
430. VARKEY B et al: Thoracic actinomycosis dissemination to skin, subcutaneous tissue and muscle. Arch Intern Med 134:689, 1974
431. SCHIFFER MA et al: Actinomycosis infections associated with intrauterine contraceptive devices. Obstet Gynecol 45:67, 1975
432. GEORG LK, COLEMAN RM, BROWN JM: Evaluation of an agar gel precipitin test for the serodiagnosis of actinomycosis. J Immunol 100:1288, 1968
433. HARVEY JC, CANTRELL JR, FISCHER AM: Actinomycosis: Its recognition and treatment. Ann Intern Med 46:868, 1957
434. MOHR JA, RHOADES ER, MUCHMORE HG: Actinomycosis treated with lincomycin. JAMA 212:2260, 1970
435. FASS RJ, et al: Clindamycin in the treatment of serious anaerobic infections. Ann Intern Med 78:853, 1973
436. MANHEIM SD et al: Hyperbaric oxygen in the treatment of actinomycosis. JAMA 210:551, 1969
437. THOMAS AV, SODERMAN TH, BENTZ RR: *Bifidobacterium eriksonii* infection, report of a case. Am Rev Respir Dis 110:663, 1974
438. BALLENGER CN JR, GOLDRING D: Nocardiosis in childhood. J Pediatr 50:145, 1957
439. MURRAY JF et al: The changing spectrum of nocardiosis. Am Rev Respir Dis 83:315, 1961
440. KURUP PV, KANDHAWA HS, GUPTA NP: Nocardiosis: A review. Mycopathol Mycol Appl 40:193, 1970
441. FRAZIER AR, ROSENOW ED, III, ROBERTS GD: Nocardiosis. A review of 25 cases occurring in 24 months. Mayo Clin Proc 50:657, 1975
442. PALMER DL et al: Diagnostic and therapeutic considerations in *Nocardia asteroides* infection. Medicine 53:391, 1974
443. RAICH RA, CASEY F, HALL WH: Pulmonary and cutaneous nocardiosis: the significance of the laboratory isolation of nocardia. Am Rev Respir Dis 83:505, 1961
444. PEABODY JW, SEABURY JH: Actinomycosis and nocardiosis. Am J Med 28:99, 1960
445. BACH MC, MONACO AP, FINLAND M: Pulmonary nocardiosis therapy with minocycline and with erythromycin plus ampicillin. JAMA 224:1378, 1973
446. HOEPRICH PD, BRANDT D, PARKER RH: Nocardial brain abscess cured with cycloserine and sulfonamides. Am J Med Sci 57:671, 1974
447. MADERAZO E, QUINTILIANI R: Treatment of nocardial infection with trimethoprim and sulfamethoxazole. Am J Med 57:671, 1974
448. PRESANT CA, WIERNICK PH, SERPICK AA: Factors affecting survival in nocardiosis. Am Rev Respir Dis 108:1444, 1973

Chapter 10

Pulmonary Vascular Diseases

ISRAEL BELENKIE

PULMONARY EMBOLISM

THROMBOEMBOLISM

Incidence

Pulmonary thromboembolic disease is one of the major causes of in-hospital morbidity and mortality.[1] In various autopsy series of consecutive unselected cases, emboli were found in up to 64% of patients.[2–5] It was found to be the third most common cause of death at the Peter Bent Brigham Hospital, Boston, being the principal cause in 15% and a contributing factor in another 19% of 225 postmortem examinations. In one of the series,[4] 25% of the deaths from pulmonary embolism were considered to have been preventable, the others occurring in patients with terminal disease. It was also found to be the cause of death in 9 out of 19 autopsy cases of postoperative deaths following eye surgery.[6]

Pulmonary embolism is uncommon before adulthood and increases in incidence with age, so that at the age of 80, about 70% of autopsied patients have emboli.[4] Despite its frequency, the variety of presenting features are often easily confused with those of other diseases, so that the incidence of false-positive or false-negative diagnosis is extremely high, each about two-thirds in one autopsy study.[7] In another series, only 7.1% of patients with pulmonary embolism found at autopsy had the definitive diagnosis made prior to death.[8]

Since pulmonary thromboembolism often occurs as a sequela of thrombophlebitis, the factors predisposing to the latter condition are of interest. Using radioactively labeled fibrinogen, the frequency of thrombophlebitis in a variety of medical and surgical patients has been demonstrated to be very high (Table 10-1). Although only a small number of patient groups have been studied, a vast number of persons are at risk when the conditions that predispose to thrombophlebitis are considered (see list below).

TABLE 10-1. Frequency of Thrombophlebitis in High-Risk Patient Groups

Orthopaedic (fractured hip)	54%
Thoracotomy	51%
Urologic (prostatectomy)	25%
Surgical patients over the age of 40	28%
Gynecologic	18%
Acute myocardial infarction	39%
Obstetric	3%

Although pulmonary emboli are almost always due to thromboembolism, other materials occasionally found include tumor,[9] amniotic

Conditions Predisposing to Thrombophlebitis

- Postoperative states
- Trauma
- Congestive heart failure
- Cerebrovascular accidents
- Thrombocytosis
- Erythrocytosis
- Sickle cell anemia
- Systemic lupus erythematosus
- Oral contraceptives
- Pregnancy
- Prolonged bed rest
- Long periods of travel
- Underlying carcinoma
- Homocystinuria
- Antithrombin III deficiency

fluid, air, bone marrow and fat (see Chap. 11), a variety of foreign materials such as bullets, catheters, barium sulfate after barium enemas, talc, and oil after lymphangiography,[10,11] and other materials frequently injected by intravenous drug abusers (see below).

Thromboemboli most often originate in the deep veins of the legs or pelvis. Much less frequently, they come from more proximal locations, such as the arms or the right atrium.[12]

Pathogenesis and Pathology

Because of the dual circulation of the lung, pulmonary infarction is relatively uncommon, probably caused by about 10 to 15% of emboli. It had been thought to occur more often in patients with underlying cardiopulmonary disease and to be unusual in otherwise healthy persons, but this may be incorrect because the evidence was obtained primarily from pathologic studies which likely involved a disproportionately large number of patients with serious cardiac or pulmonary disorders. More recent clinical evidence suggests that emboli to more peripheral vessels are more likely to cause infarction and that larger ones that lodge in the central pulmonary arteries are less likely to do so, because the collateral blood flow from the bronchial circulation enters the pulmonary arterial circulation distal to the obstruction.[13] The patients without infarction often have more severe hemodynamic consequences, the embolic obstruction often being more central and extensive.

Pulmonary emboli are most frequently found in the lower lobes, because these regions receive the largest amounts of blood. They are almost always multiple. Infarcted areas are usually less than 5 cm in diameter and are roughly triangular in outline, with the base at the pleural surface. Hemorrhage into the alveolar tissue occurs in 24 to 48 hr, and the affected area becomes distinctly demarcated, hemorrhagic, and consolidated. There is some alveolar wall necrosis, so that the saccular partitions become shadowy or disappear. Within 2 weeks, repair begins, and new capillaries penetrate the affected side from the edge. Fibrosis advances rapidly, hemorrhages resorb, and the necrotic tissue is replaced by shrunken fibrotic scarring. In some cases, all evidence of the previous infarct disappears, whereas in others, pleural thickening and adhesions persist.

The use of radioactively labeled fibrinogen, and examination at autopsy,[14,15] have shown that the risk of pulmonary embolism and subsequent mortality are lowest when the veins of the calf alone are involved, and much higher when the more proximal leg veins and the iliac veins contain thrombus. Only about 50% of the patients with pulmonary embolism have premonitory clinical evidence of phlebitis. About 50% of the patients suffering from major embolism have had minor episodes preceding the more serious ones.

Venous thrombosis often begins with a white thrombus in the sinuses of the veins, in venous valves, in saccules, or at venous junctions. The initiating event appears to be an alteration in the endothelial wall of the vessel. Damaged cells release various substances, including thromboplastic materials, fatty acids, and adenosine diphosphate, that may initiate or accelerate coagulation or platelet aggregation. Exposed basement membrane may initiate platelet adhesion and activate the sequence of coagulation. Release of platelet components causes further aggregation and contributes to the coagulation process.

Just what causes the thrombus to dislodge is uncertain. Although there is little supportive evidence (mostly anecdotal), movement of the limb, straining at stool, or hyperventilation may play a role in causing a fresh, loosely anchored thrombus to break off. This unsettled question is important when considering that ambulation may be important in preventing further thrombi from forming.

The thrombus travels to the right side of the heart and is usually broken into smaller fragments by the churning action of the right ventricle. These fragments then travel to branches of the pulmonary artery, where they occlude vessels, either partially or completely. During systole, however, it is likely that the increased pressure forces some blood around the thrombus. Occasionally, at autopsy, one sees a single long thrombus extending from the right ventricle to the main pulmonary artery.

Little has been added to Virchow's original description, in 1846, of the predisposing factors in thrombophlebitis.[17] Vascular stasis, trauma, and hypercoagulability remain the three major considerations in most instances, although there are certainly many situations in which none of these is easily implicated. One or more of these factors is often considered important in some well-defined groups.

Many patient groups have been identified at risk for thromboembolic events.[18,19] Patients with acute myocardial infarction and all patients with congestive heart failure, regardless of cause, form a large group that is at significant risk. Long periods of bedrest, for whatever reason, predispose patients to thrombophlebitis and embolism by promoting stasis. Patients with acute paralytic disease appear to be at very high risk[20,21] (see also Chap. 6). Frequent pulmonary embolism in patients with respiratory failure is not well explained.[22,22a] The mechanism by which vascular stasis promotes thromboembolism is not well understood; several possibilities include the lack of dispersal and dilution of activated clotting factors, impaired neutralization of these factors by circulating inhibitors, their decreased clearance by the liver, or predisposition to clotting because of altered physical and chemical properties of blood that flows more slowly. Hypercoagulability is likely in neoplastic conditions,[18,19,23] particularly in carcinoma of the lung and pancreas. Hormonal changes, still incompletely explained, increase the risk in women taking oral contraceptives,[18,19] men receiving estrogens for prostatic carcinoma or after myocardial infarction,[24] and pregnant women.[25,26] Perhaps the best-explained group at risk are patients with familial antithrombin III deficiency. Antithrombin III is the main physiological inhibitor for thrombin and other clotting factors, and when it is deficient, patients are predisposed to more active clotting.[27] The interrelationships of stasis, measurable changes in levels of clotting factors, imbalance of inhibitors, and hormonal changes remain unclear in most clinical conditions at risk. Scientifically based therapeutic intervention will depend on further clarification.

Cardiorespiratory Responses to Acute Embolism

The response to acute pulmonary embolism varies considerably, depending on a number of factors.[28] Experimentally, if one entire pulmonary artery is occluded mechanically, there is little change in the pulmonary artery pressure and clinical state of the animal. If, however, an equivalent amount of vasculature is occluded by an embolus, the insult is not tolerated as well, and there may be marked hemodynamic and respiratory changes. Serotonin, histamine, prostaglandins, and possibly other pulmonary vasoconstrictors, such as bradykinin, are thought to originate from the platelets within the thrombus and to cause the increase in pulmonary artery pressure above that expected as a result of the mechanical blockage of the pulmonary vessels. This is supported by the finding that animals pretreated with heparin or sulfinpyrazone develop considerably less pulmonary hypertension following pulmonary embolism.[29] The mechanism of the protective effect of these and other drugs is not well understood and may involve an inhibition of platelet aggregation, or specific effects on the active substances. Other important factors include the number and size of the emboli and the previous state of the cardiovascular and respiratory systems. An embolus that might be well tolerated in a previously normal person could be the final insult in the patient with severe congestive heart failure.

In previously healthy persons, the magnitude of the cardiorespiratory effects correlates well with the extent of perfusion defects, as determined by lung scan. The cardiac index may be normal or slightly increased. A decrease is

TABLE 10-2. Hemodynamic Responses Following Pulmonary Embolism in Previously Healthy Patients

Cardiac output	N or ↑	↓ if >40–50% obstruction
Right atrial pressure	N or ↑	↑ suggests >30–35% obstruction
Pulmonary arterial pressure	N or ↑	↑ suggests >25% obstruction

N = normal.

usually associated with greater than 40 to 50% obstruction. The right atrial pressure may be elevated, particularly with obstruction greater than 30 to 35% and a mean pulmonary artery pressure greater than 30 mm Hg, but may be normal even in massive embolism. The pulmonary artery pressure is usually elevated if the defect exceeds 25%, but the mean pressure is almost always less than 40 mm Hg in this group of patients (Table 10-2). Modest elevations in pulmonary artery pressure in patients with 25% or less of the vasculature obstructed may be found, the level correlating somewhat with a fall in the arterial Po_2, suggesting that hypoxemia may contribute to the mechanism causing pulmonary hypertension in these patients.[30]

In patients with underlying cardiac or lung disease, the hemodynamic responses tend to be exaggerated. Greater degrees of pulmonary hypertension and a decrease in cardiac index are commonly seen in this group.

The most predictable effect of occlusion of a pulmonary vessel on gas exchange is the wasted ventilation of areas no longer perfused. This can be measured as an increase in physiologic dead space (Table 10-3).

The pulmonary airways are, however, also involved in the response to embolism. Experimental thromboembolism in animals is associated with increased resistance in the airways; reduction in lung volumes, including vital capacity and functional residual capacity; and reductions in static compliance. Furthermore, dynamic compliance is reduced with increasing breathing frequencies. Several studies have suggested that the reduction in airway size takes place predominantly at the level of alveolar ducts and very small bronchioles.[31] This effect on the airways has been ascribed to (a) the release of local vasoactive amines as a result of aggregation of platelets; (b) a reflex vagal effect; and (c) release of vasoactive substances circulating systemically. At present, the bulk of the evidence still favors the first of these hypotheses.[32]

TABLE 10-3. Pulmonary Function Following Pulmonary Embolism

Ventilatory effects	
Respiratory rate	↑
Vital capacity	N or ↓
Functional residual capacity	↓
Maximum expiratory flow rates	N or ↓
Lung compliance	↓
Frequency-dependent compliance	↓
Blood gas exchange	
Arterial Po_2	↓
Arterial Pco_2	↓
Alveolar-arterial O_2 gradient	↑
Alveolar-arterial CO_2 gradient	↑
Arterial *p*H	↑
Physiological dead space (wasted ventilation)	↑
Diffusing capacity	↓

N = normal.

The tachypnea so commonly associated with embolism is not entirely understood. Although hypoxemia may result in respiratory stimulation and an altered ventilatory pattern, it is likely that stimulation of irritant receptors in the bronchial walls also plays a role.

The impact of these ventilatory changes on the patient generally relates to abnormalities of gas exchange. Lung regions with low ventilation–perfusion ratios may result from a local decrease in ventilation or from increased perfusion as blood is directed away from obstructed vessels. In either situation, a high alveolar–arterial oxygen gradient results, with arterial hypoxemia.[33–36]

Several studies have suggested frank anatomical shunts due to the opening up of vessels in the pulmonary circulation during the course of pulmonary embolic disease. These have not generally been confirmed. A marked improvement in oxygenation and a reduction in the alveolo-arterial oxygen gradient occur during positive-pressure breathing and therapy with isoproterenol.[33] This suggests that dilation of the airways alone can result in reversal of the gas-exchange abnormalities.

Hypoxemia and perhaps stimulation of bronchial irritant receptors cause hyperventilation, with a reduced arterial Pco_2. This produces a respiratory alkalosis. Since substantial quantities of blood may bypass areas of effective ventilation, there may be a significant arterial-alveolar carbon dioxide gradient.[37,38] This was once suggested as a useful diagnostic aid; however, it is abnormal in other conditions with significant ventilation–perfusion inequalities. The diffusing capacity is characteristically decreased, owing to the loss of perfused vascular bed.

In chronic obstructive pulmonary vascular disease due to pulmonary embolism or primary pulmonary hypertension, an increase in the alveolar–arterial oxygen gradient has been shown to be caused by a combination of a relatively small ventilation–perfusion inequality plus a low mixed venous oxygen content resulting from low cardiac output. The dead space and diffusion capacity in those patients were shown to be normal.[34]

Common Symptoms in Acute Pulmonary Embolism

- Dyspnea
- Fatigability
- Chest pain
- Hemoptysis
- Fever
- Cough
- Syncope
- Symptoms of phlebitis
- Flu-like symptoms
- Headache
- Palpitations
- Anxiety

Clinical Manifestations

Patients with pulmonary embolism can present in many ways. Not infrequently, the disease is clinically silent (75% in one series).[16] It is sometimes surprising how much of the vasculature can be involved with few, if any, symptoms. If there are multiple recurrences of small emboli, chronic cor pulmonale might be the presenting feature, although this would be very unusual. At this end of the spectrum, the differentiation between recurrent pulmonary embolism and primary pulmonary hypertension might not be possible.

Patients without obvious underlying diseases frequently present with fairly characteristic findings: dyspnea, easy fatigability, pleuritic chest pain (usually not retrosternal, but it may be), hemoptysis, fever, cough, syncope, symptoms of phlebitis, and other nonspecific symptoms such as a flu-like illness, headache, vague chest pains, anxiety, and palpitations (see list above). A history of predisposing factors may be elicited (see Conditions Predisposing to Thrombophlebitis).

The diagnosis is frequently unsuspected in patients with underlying cardiovascular or respiratory disease. Although they may present with the characteristic symptoms outlined above, atypical features are often present. Increasing symptoms of congestive heart failure, fatigability, chest pain, unexplained fever, or tachycardia may be the only clues. Hemoptysis (occasionally massive) should suggest embolism. Pain that is indistinguishable from that of myocardial ischemia may occur. The mechanism of this is not well understood, and the previously postulated pulmonary–coronary artery reflex causing a decreased coronary arterial blood flow has been shown experimentally not to exist. Syncope is occasionally the major complaint (Fig. 10-1). Sometimes, the only symptom is that the patient is just not doing well. The diagnosis may not be suspected until the routine chest roentgenogram or electrocardiogram is done. Laboratory data obtained because of symptoms of phlebitis may reveal abnormalities that otherwise would have remained unsuspected.

Massive pulmonary embolism might cause symptoms similar to those described above, but certain ones are more prevalent.[39–41] Syncope and cardiorespiratory arrest are frequently the presenting features. Central chest pain and apprehension are also more common in this group. All too often, the diagnosis is made only at a routine autopsy following sudden death. In a group of 35 patients with massive pulmonary embolism (three of whom had previous cardiac disease, and none with previous pulmonary emboli),[39] central chest pain occurred in 12, pleurisy in 13, and hemoptysis in 4; 28 collapsed, and 10 experienced cardiac arrest (Table 10-4). In this group, it is of interest that several patients who had one half to two thirds of the vasculature occluded never complained of dyspnea; syncope was their only symptom. Twenty-four of these patients were postoperative, and 5 were

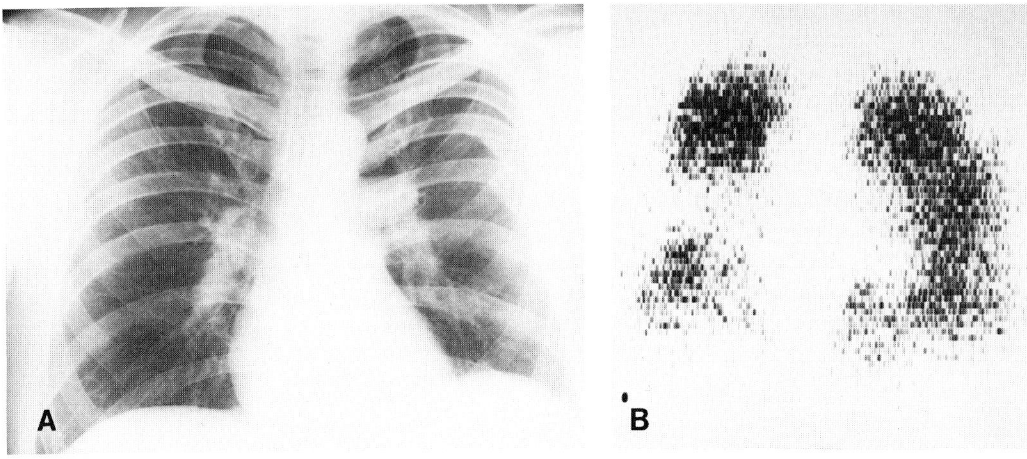

FIG. 10-1. **A.** Posteroanterior chest roentgenogram for a 34-year-old man who presented with shortness of breath, syncope, and fatigue. Note the prominent pulmonary arteries and the elevated left diaphragm. There are also old rib fractures. **B.** Rectilinear lung scan in the posterior projection demonstrates perfusion defects in both bases and the left mid-lung field.

TABLE 10-4. Common Symptoms in Massive Pulmonary Embolism

Collapse	80%
Dyspnea	72%
Central chest pain	34%
Pleurisy	37%
Cardiac arrest	28%
Hemoptysis	11%

(Sutton GC, Honey M, Gibson RV: Clinical diagnosis of acute massive pulmonary embolism. Lancet 1:271, 1969)

on oral contraceptives. In another series of 197 patients with massive embolism, syncope occurred in 20% and pleuritic chest pain in 64%, and none had a cardiac arrest.[41] The methods of patient selection and the presence of associated diseases may account for the variability of the symptoms in different series.

Physical Examination

The physical examination is frequently normal. However, if one searches carefully, subtle abnormalities may be found. Sinus tachycardia is common and, if otherwise unexplained, should lead one to suspect pulmonary embolism. Tachypnea is frequently, but not always, present, even in massive embolism; fever is fairly common and usually low grade, uncommon beyond six days, and rarely spiking.[42] The blood pressure and peripheral perfusion are usually well maintained, except in those most severely affected. Although the Po_2 is almost always decreased, cyanosis is often not clinically obvious. Signs of a pleural effusion or a pleural friction rub may be found. When pleuritic pain is present, splinting of the chest wall, with reduced ventilation of the affected side, is characteristic. A post-pulmonary infarction syndrome has been described, consisting of persistent fever, pleural effusion, and pericarditis.[43] Breath sounds are usually normal, although rhonchi are occasionally heard. Rales may be heard in some areas. Precordial palpation is frequently normal, but occasionally a right ventricular lift and the pulmonary artery pulsations are palpable. The second heart sound may be widely split, with a loud pulmonic component. A Grade II or III/VI systolic ejection murmur may be heard along the upper left sternal border. A continuous murmur, which suggests significant obstruction, is rarely heard. A right ventricular third or fourth heart sound might be audible. In patients with recurrent episodes, signs of pulmonary hypertension might be more obvious. Signs of phlebitis are present in less than 50% of cases and, even then, are frequently equivocal.

In massive pulmonary embolism, the patient might be in shock or have somewhat less dramatic evidence of poor peripheral perfusion.[39] Cyanosis is more common in this group and is occasionally position-related, suggesting mechanical obstruction of the tricuspid valve. Pulsus paradoxus is occasionally found and might erroneously suggest cardiac tamponade. Tachycardia is almost always present but might be absent even in severe cases. The jugular–venous pressure might be elevated, but in a surprising number of instances it is not (Fig. 10-2). Signs of right ventricular overload may be more prominent with audible right third and fourth heart sounds.

The pulmonic component of the second sound might be widely split and loud. Some patients, usually with underlying cardiac disease, might have increased left-sided failure, the pathophysiology of which is not well understood. The increased blood flow at higher pressures through a smaller number of patent pulmonary vessels may contribute to pulmonary edema. An increase in vascular permeability, perhaps due to local release of chemical mediators, might also play an important role.[43]

Physical Findings Following Acute Pulmonary Embolism

- Signs of hemodynamic disturbances
  - Sinus tachycardia
  - Tachypnea
  - Cyanosis
  - Hypotension
  - Diaphoresis
- Signs of pulmonary hypertension
  - Increased jugular-venous pressure
  - Right ventricular lift
  - Right ventricular gallop sounds
  - Palpable pulmonary artery
  - Loud P_2
  - Widely-split P_2
  - Pulmonary outflow tract murmur
- Signs of pulmonary infarction
  - Pleural effusion
  - Friction rub
  - Rales
- Others
  - Phlebitis
  - Fever
  - Pulsus paradoxus

Laboratory Findings

The most helpful laboratory tests commonly available are the blood gases, chest roentgenogram, lung scan, electrocardiogram, and, in selected cases, venography and pulmonary angiography. Biochemical tests, although frequently performed, are not usually as helpful. The frequently quoted triad of a raised bilirubin and lactate dehydrogenase with a normal serum glutamic-oxaloacetic transaminase (SGOT) is actually uncommonly found.[44] A rise in the lactic dehydrogenase (LDH) is usually seen in approximately 48 hr, and the level returns to normal in about 4 to 6 days. The lung is rich in LDH isoenzymes 2, 3, and 4, but LDH 5 may also increase. This is thought to be due to hepatic congestion. Occasionally, the creatine kinase is also elevated. The arterial oxygen tension is almost always decreased as a result of an increased alveolar-arterial oxygen gradient.[44] The partial pressure of carbon dioxide is often decreased, with a respiratory alkalosis. The small number of patients with pulmonary emboli who have a normal Po_2 generally are hyperventilating and still have an elevated alveolar-arterial gradient (see Chap. 5 for methods of calculating the A-a gradient). The leukocyte count is often mildly elevated.

Fibrin-split products are usually elevated, but unfortunately are not specific for pulmonary embolism. However, elevated levels provide supportive evidence of active thrombotic activity. A combination of an elevated ratio of fibrinogen/fibrin degradation products and an increased level of soluble fibrin complexes might help to separate patients with pulmonary embolism from normal and high-risk patients.[45] High initial values and subsequent increases of the former test, and later increases in the values in the latter test, might be useful in identifying patients at risk for further embolic episodes following acute embolism.[46]

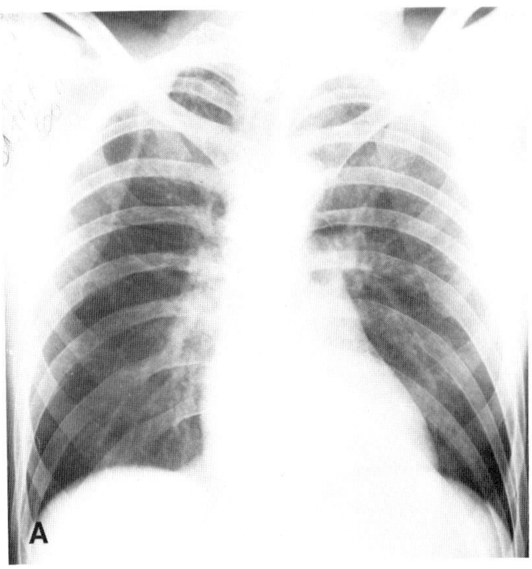

FIG. 10-2. A. Portable chest roentgenogram of a 35-year-old man who died after massive pulmonary embolism from cerebral complications. When first seen 1 hour after the episode, his jugular-venous pressure and systemic arterial pressure were normal, and his pulse rate was 76 beats per minute. The entire left lower lobe and smaller areas of the right lung were found to be infarcted at autopsy 2½ days following the acute episode. No emboli were found at that time. The chest roentgenogram shows minimal patchy infiltrates bilaterally and prominent central vessels on the left. **B.** Rectilinear lung scan in the posterior projection. There is very little perfusion to his entire left lung and to the right upper lobe of the right lung.

The chest roentgenogram might be entirely normal even if there is severe embolism. However, there frequently are subtle clues. The presence of an infiltrate or a pleural effusion is presumptive evidence of pulmonary infarction. The infiltrates are nonspecific; hump-shaped densities adjacent to the pleura (Hampton's hump), areas of consolidation with or without air bronchograms, platelike areas of atelectasis, a raised diaphragm (62% of cases), enlarged pulmonary arteries, a difference in the vascularity of the two sides (Westermark's sign), and, rarely, cavitation or pneumothorax may be seen. Cardiomegaly is uncommon and is due to right ventricular enlargement (Figs. 10-1 to 10-6, and 10-10). In septic pulmonary embolism, scattered areas of consolidation simulating bronchopneumonia are often seen, and they may extend rapidly or form wedge-shaped peripheral opacities. These are multiple in almost all cases. They might then excavate, producing thin-walled cavities resembling pneumatoceles (Fig. 10-12). The pleura might be involved, causing empyema, bronchopleural fistulas, and pneumothorax. Resolution might be complete, or pleural thickening or areas of fibrosis might remain.

Analysis of the pleural fluid can be helpful, but the findings vary greatly.[47] If the fluid is bloody in the absence of trauma or neoplasm, pulmonary embolism is suggested. However, it might be clear in about one third of patients with embolism. About 90% of bloody effusions are associated with infiltrates; if there is no blood, only 30% are associated with infiltrates. Approximately two thirds of the effusions have the characteristics of an exudate; therefore, the presence of a transudate does not rule out embolism. White blood cell counts vary widely and either neutrophils (more commonly) or lymphocytes might predominate.

Electrocardiographic changes, although generally nonspecific, occur in about 15 to 40% of cases[48] (see list, p. 486). Even massive embolism

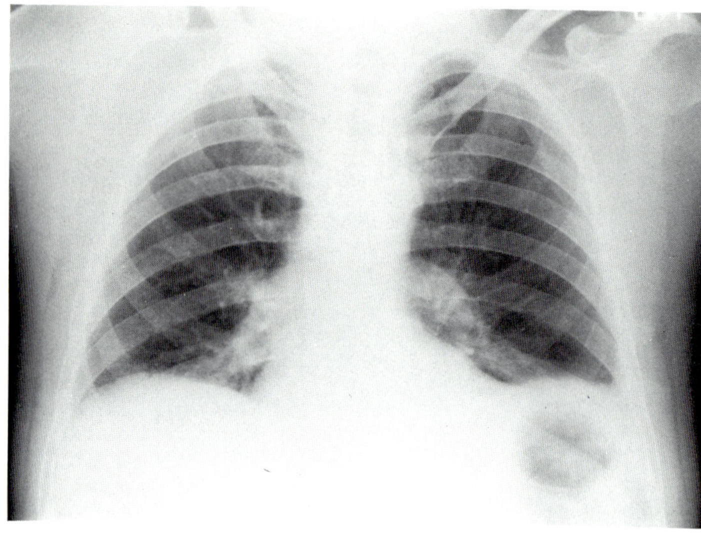

FIG. 10-3. Posteroanterior chest roentgenogram of a patient with acute pulmonary embolism. The pulmonary arteries are large, particularly the left one. The left hemidiaphragm is elevated, and there is a small left pleural effusion.

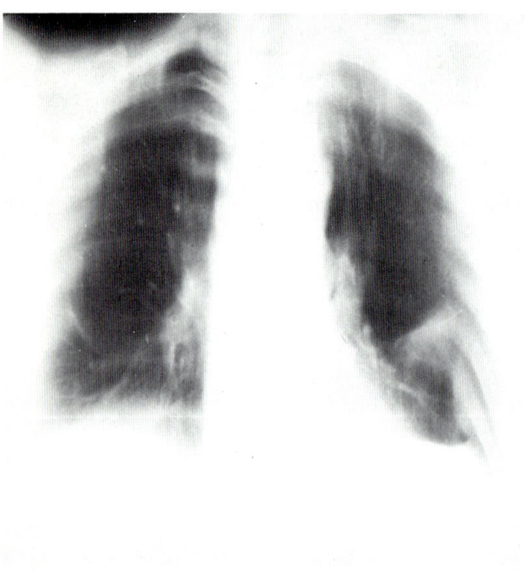

FIG. 10-4. Tomogram of a patient with acute pulmonary embolism. Note the opacities at the left lung base: the lower one may be pleural or parenchymal, and the upper one is a consolidated area.

may produce only nonspecific changes, or none at all. Signs of right ventricular strain suggest that 50% or more of the vasculature is obstructed. Complete right bundle branch block usually occurs only in massive embolism. Unexplained arrhythmias, especially atrial flutter, should alert one to the possibility of pulmonary embolism. In one series of 45 cases of atrial flutter, 25 were in patients with pulmonary embolism.[49]

Perfusion lung scans are currently available in most large centers and are extremely valuable in the diagnosis of pulmonary embolism (Figs. 10-1, 10-2, 10-5, 10-7 and 10-8). A variety of radioactively tagged macroaggregates can be injected intravenously and, in effect, act as microemboli to the lung. Decreased flow of blood to any portion of the lung results in decreased radioactivity over that same area. The distribution of radioactivity over the lung is usually displayed either on x-ray film by rectilinear scanners or on Polaroid film using a gamma or a scintillation camera. Scanning of radioactivity should be done in the anterior and posterior views, as well as the lateral and oblique projections. Occasionally, perfusion defects not evident on the first two projections are picked up in other views. There are no significant hazards associated with the procedure. The amount of radioactive exposure is minimal, and significant hemodynamic effects secondary to the relatively small number of microemboli that are injected have been reported only rarely. Repeated scans can be performed to follow patients (Fig. 10-7).

In order to interpret lung scans properly, one should obtain posteroanterior (PA) and lateral chest roentgenograms at the same time, and con-

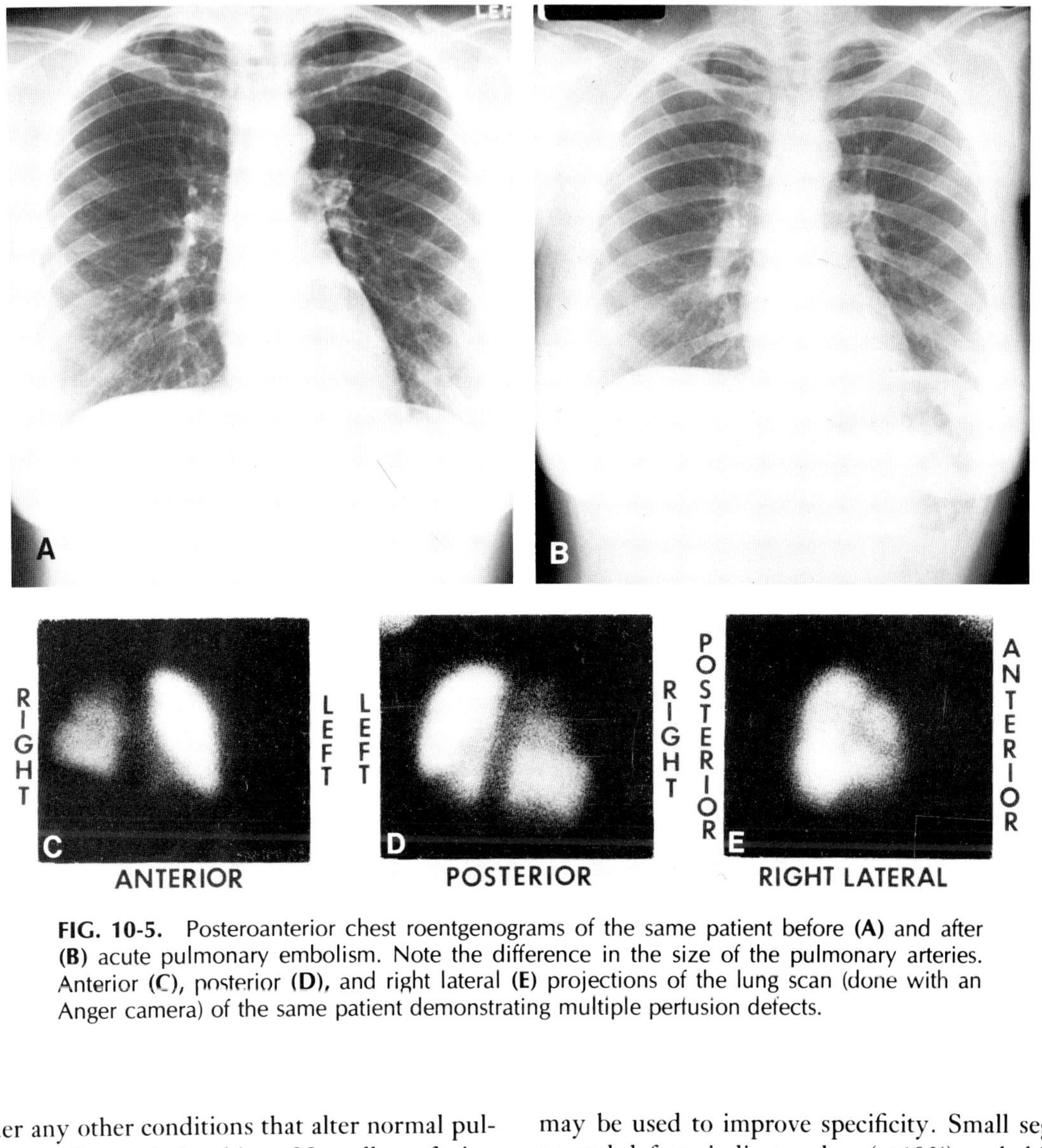

FIG. 10-5. Posteroanterior chest roentgenograms of the same patient before **(A)** and after **(B)** acute pulmonary embolism. Note the difference in the size of the pulmonary arteries. Anterior **(C)**, posterior **(D)**, and right lateral **(E)** projections of the lung scan (done with an Anger camera) of the same patient demonstrating multiple perfusion defects.

sider any other conditions that alter normal pulmonary flow relationships. Not all perfusion deficits are due to pulmonary embolism; they can result from any process that causes a decrease in blood flow to a portion of the lung, including bronchial asthma, chronic obstructive airway disease, emphysema, bullae (Fig. 10-8), pneumonia, atelectasis, pleural effusion, tumor, abscess, and a variety of other conditions. A normal lung scan virtually rules out the likelihood of demonstrating an embolus angiographically, although there is the occasional exception.[18,19]

In patients with normal chest roentgenograms, the pattern of perfusion abnormality may be used to improve specificity. Small segmental defects indicate a low (< 10%) probability. Single lobar or multiple segmental defects indicate an intermediate (25–50%) probability. Multiple segmental defects plus at least one lobar defect indicate a high (90%) probability.[50,50a,50b]

Simultaneous perfusion and ventilation scans may improve the diagnostic specificity of scanning in the presence of lung disease,[51] but experience with this technique suggests that it is of limited value.[22,52–54] In practice, both ventilation and perfusion are often similarly decreased in a diseased area of the lung, whether the primary disorder involves vessels or airways. Poor

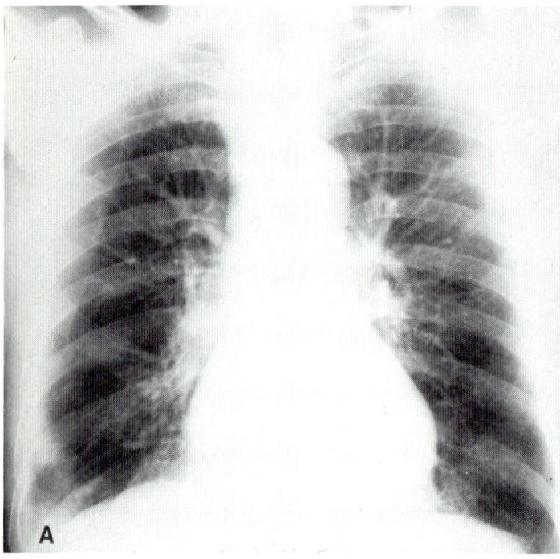

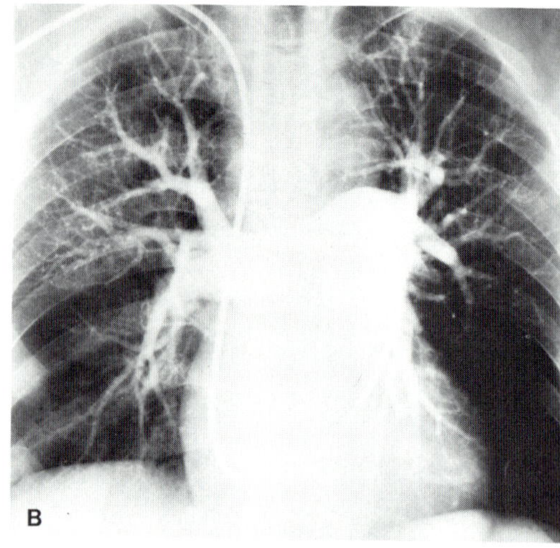

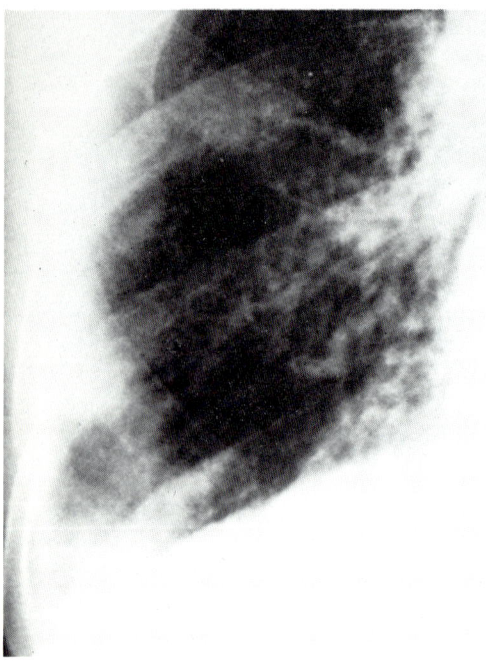

FIG. 10-6. A. Posteroanterior chest roentgenogram following acute pulmonary embolism. Note the peripheral hump-shaped densities in the right lower lung field (enlargement at left). **B.** Pulmonary angiogram done on the same patient. Note the scarcity of vessels to the right middle and lower lobes, but the lack of definitely distinguishable emboli on that side.

Electrocardiographic Changes in Acute Pulmonary Embolism

Normal or unchanged
Right axis deviation (S_1, Q_3, T_3 pattern)
Left axis deviation
Precordial transition shifted to the left
Increased R/S ratio in V_1
Right bundle branch block (complete or incomplete)
Nonspecific "ischemic" ST–T changes (especially downward T in 2, 3, AVF, V1-V5)
P-pulmonale
Pseudoinfarction (inferior and rarely anterior)
Atrial flutter, fibrillation, and ectopic beats
Ventricular arrhythmias
A–V dissociation
First degree heart block

Spodick DH: Electrocardiographic responses to pulmonary embolism: Mechanisms and sources of variability. Am J Cardiol, 30:695, 1972

perfusion in an area of normal ventilation, however, suggests that vascular disease is the cause.

When an infiltrate is present on chest roentgenogram, radioactive gallium (^{67}Ga) scanning may prove useful in differentiating embolism from pneumonitis as the cause.[52] Gallium tends to accumulate in areas of inflammation; in pulmonary embolism, the inflammatory component of the infiltrate is not large and therefore ^{67}Ga tends not to accumulate in the involved lung. A positive ^{67}GA scan strongly suggests that pneumonitis is the cause of the infiltrate; a negative scan may be found with other kinds of infiltrates so that angiography may be required for a definitive diagnosis. In septic pulmonary embolism, the ^{67}Ga scan may be positive.

Another recent development in lung scanning

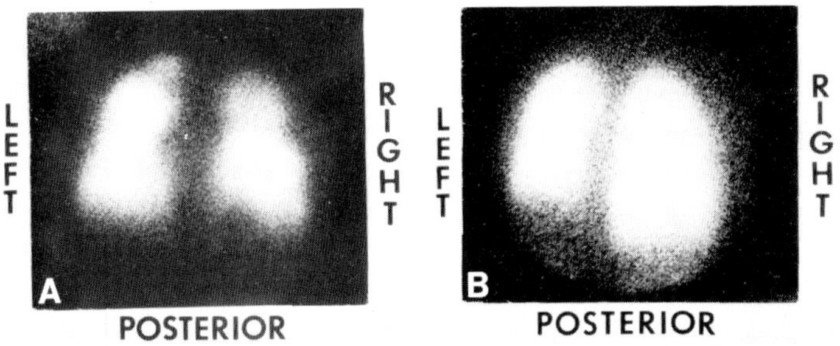

FIG. 10-7. Lung scans (done with an Anger camera) performed just after an episode of acute pulmonary embolism: **A** demonstrates several perfusion defects, and **B** shows nearly complete resolution 6 days later.

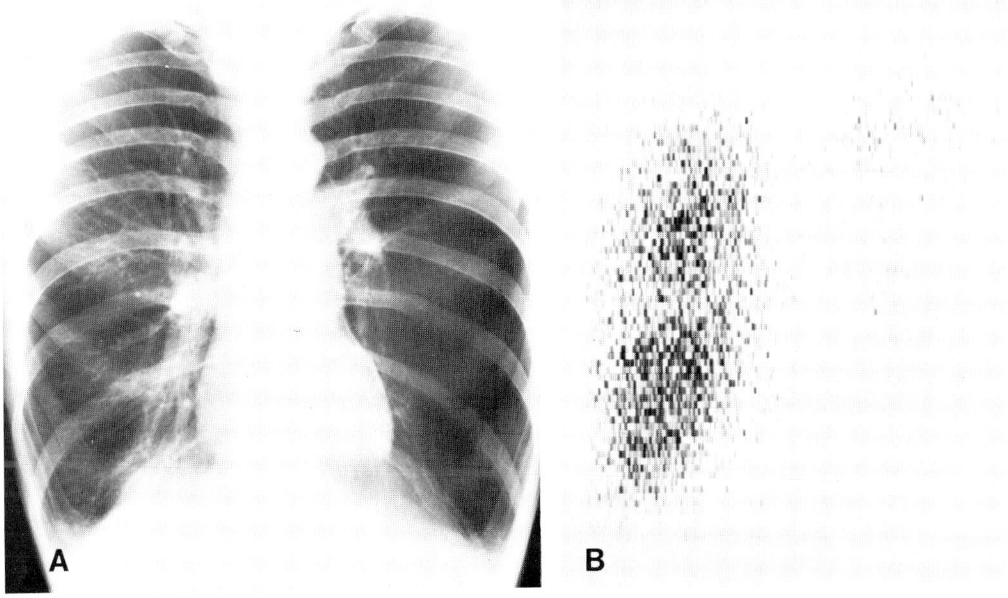

FIG. 10-8. A. Posteroanterior chest roentgenogram demonstrating hyperinflation, bronchial wall thickening with increased interstitial markings, and a very large bulla occupying the lower half of the left lung. **B.** Rectilinear lung scan in the anteroposterior projection demonstrates a gross lack of perfusion of the left lung due to bulla and not to pulmonary embolism.

involves the inhalation of radio-labeled carbon dioxide ($C^{15}O_2$). The $C^{15}O_2$ is inhaled, dissolved, and dissociated to HCO_3^- and $H_2{}^{15}O$ in the presence of carbonic anhydrase containing red blood cells.[55] If a pulmonary artery is obstructed, these products will not be perfused away, and "hot spots" will be demonstrated. The technique appears to be safe, relatively sensitive, but not as specific as angiography. Because of the short half-life of ${}^{15}O_2$, this scan can be performed only in institutions located near a cyclotron.

A fiberoptic angioscope is under active study for direct visualization of the pulmonary vessels, but its clinical role is not yet defined.[56]

Pulmonary angiography is the most definitive and reliable procedure short of seeing a thrombus at surgery or at autopsy.[57–59] It should be performed by experienced angiographers in a well-equipped laboratory. A catheter is introduced via a cutdown or percutaneously into a vein, and advanced to the main pulmonary artery, where a radiopaque fluid is injected rapidly. A single injection often suffices, but where there are questionable areas, selective angiograms, particularly with oblique views, can be

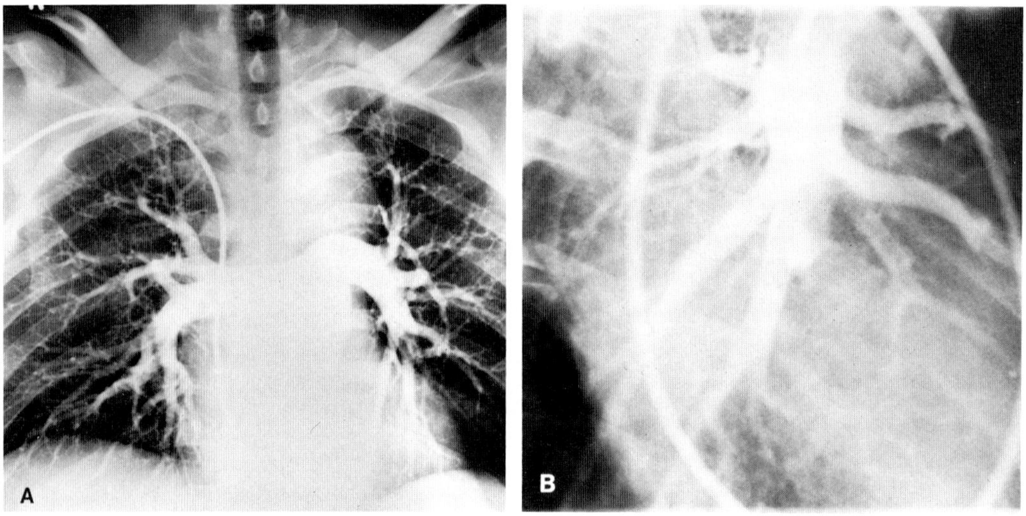

FIG. 10-9. A. Pulmonary angiogram demonstrating a suspicious area in the vessels leading to the lower portion of the left lung. **B.** A selective angiogram with a coned-down view in the left lateral projection demonstrates a filling defect caused by a clot blocking the vessels to the inferior segment of the lingula and the anteromedial segment of the left lower lobe. (Courtesy of Dr. R.F. Colapinto, Toronto General Hospital)

very helpful. (Fig. 10-9). As indicated above, it is rarely positive if the lung scan is normal. It should be considered when the diagnosis cannot be made with confidence using the lung scan, and it should always precede pulmonary embolectomy. This procedure should be done early where indicated, because of the potential rapid lysis of emboli (in as little as 4 hr in experimental emboli in rabbits). In one example, 2½ days following an episode of pulmonary embolism that caused infarction of the entire left lower lobe and smaller areas in other parts of the lungs, no emboli were found at autopsy (Fig. 10-2). The diagnosis is definitive if intraluminal filling defects or cutoff of arteries are seen (Figs. 10-10, 10-11). Areas of oligemia, asymmetry of flow, or pruning of vessels are suggestive but can occur in other conditions. The hazards of pulmonary angiography are surprisingly few; morbidity occurs in only a small percentage of patients, with only the very rare irreversible problem. Supraventricular and ventricular arrhythmias are not uncommon but are usually transient and easily managed. Right ventricular perforation by the catheter rarely occurs and might require surgical repair, although this is often not necessary. Reaction to the dye is not infrequent, but anaphylaxis is rare. It can even be done in very ill patients with relative safety. In selected instances, it might be desirable to obtain hemodynamic data at the same time. Bedside pulmonary angiography using a flow-directed (Swan-Ganz) catheter may be useful on occasion when the patient is too ill to be studied in a radiologic suite.[60] However, false negative examinations should be expected because film quality is usually less than optimal, and detailed studies normally cannot be done this way.

Ultrasound has been suggested to be a very useful and sensitive method for the diagnosis of pulmonary embolism. To date the application of this technique has not been widespread, but it may become more popular as more physicians learn to use it for other circulatory problems.[61]

In selected patients, venography can be performed to demonstrate the origin of the thrombus (for example, if contemplating inferior vena cava interruption). This is done by injecting radiopaque dye into a foot vein and occluding the superficial vein with a tourniquet, so that

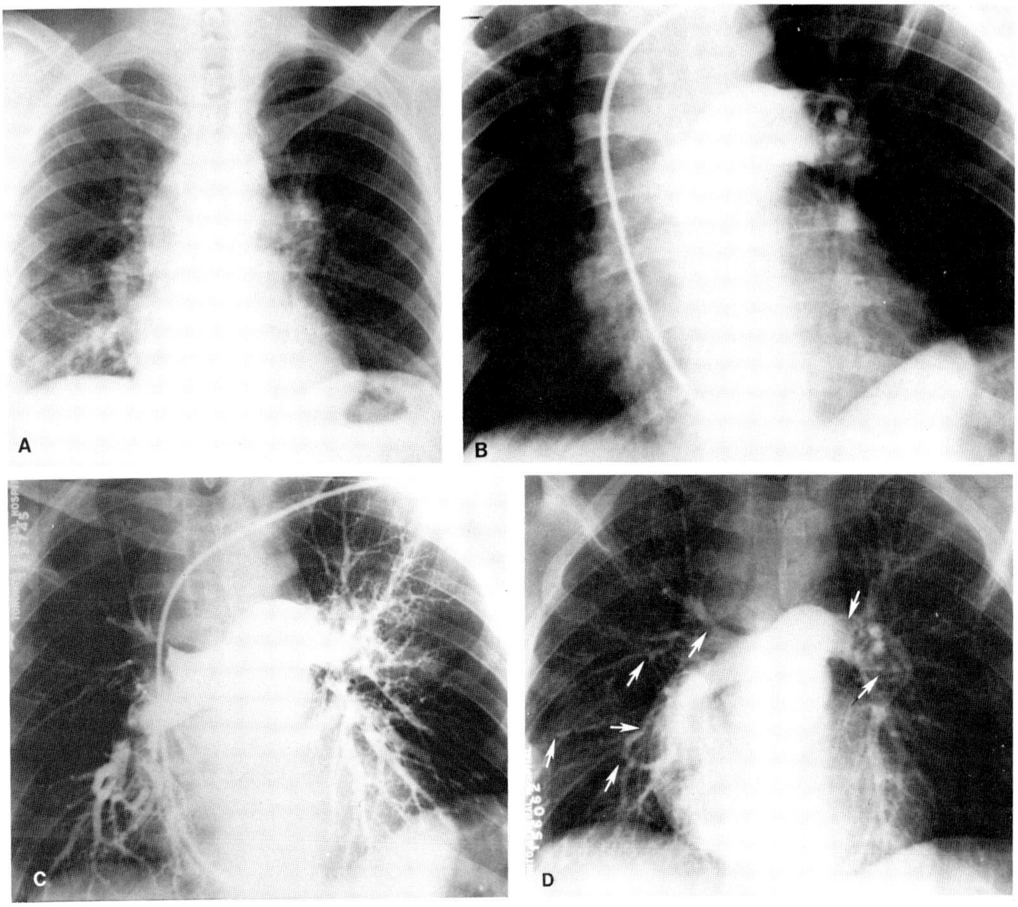

FIG. 10-10. **A.** Chest roentgenogram taken 5 days following acute massive pulmonary embolism. Note the large pulmonary arteries, particularly the left one; the decreased perfusion to the left lung field; and the infiltrate in the right middle lobe. **B.** Early roentgenogram of a pulmonary angiogram in the same patient, demonstrating a very large filling defect due to a clot in the left main pulmonary artery. **C.** A later roentgenogram, in the same sequence, demonstrating large emboli to the right upper, middle, and lower lobes. Small defects are present in both lung fields, and the difference in perfusion is readily appreciated. **D.** Repeat pulmonary angiogram done 10 days later. Notice that the large clots previously present in the left main pulmonary artery and in the larger branches of the right pulmonary artery have resolved almost completely. A number of smaller defects are seen more peripherally and probably represent fragments of the larger emboli (*arrows*). The lowest arrow points to an obstructed vessel that was previously patent. (Courtesy of Dr. R.F. Colapinto, Toronto General Hospital)

the dye flows through the deep system. Interpretation may be difficult and, not infrequently, the source is not demonstrated with this technique, presumably because the thrombus has already migrated proximally.

Detection of deep-vein thrombosis is facilitated by the use of ^{125}I labeled fibrinogen, which is incorporated into thrombus as it is formed. Leg scanning will be positive only if the thrombus is still forming. The procedure can be repeated frequently to detect formation or lysis of a thrombus.[62] The apparatus is portable so that bedside examination is simple. It is most accurate for distal deep-vein thrombosis and con-

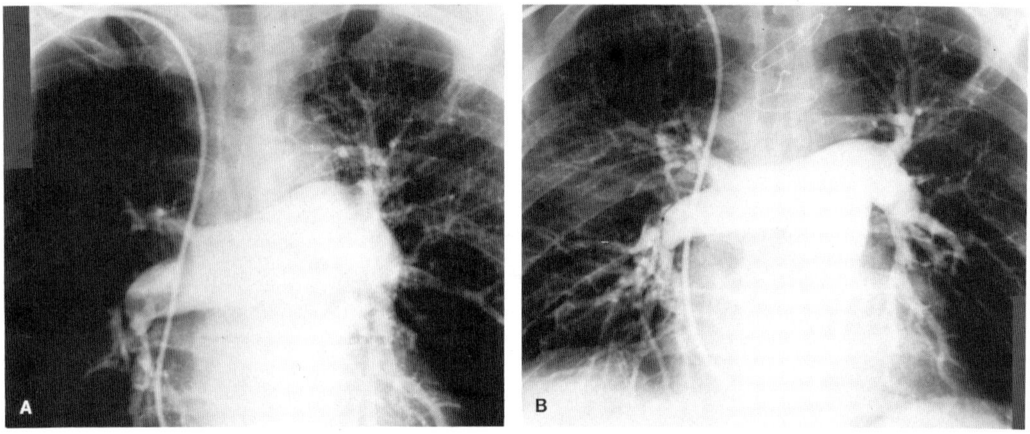

FIG. 10-11. A. Pulmonary angiogram demonstrating a very large clot in the right main pulmonary artery that extends into the major arteries to the three lobes. On the left side, there are clots in the vessels to the lingula. **B.** Following pulmonary embolectomy, this pulmonary angiogram demonstrates the much-improved perfusion, particularly to the right lung. (Courtesy of Dr. R.F. Colapinto, Toronto General Hospital)

siderably less so for proximal involvement.[63] This is a significant disadvantage, considering that most emboli originate in the more proximal veins. It is therefore a reasonable technique for screening patients at risk and should not be the sole method used to exclude the diagnosis of deep-vein thrombosis.

Impedance plethysmography, which detects deep venous disease, may identify hazardous proximal venous thrombi better than fibrinogen scans.[64–66] A combination of the two techniques may be accurate enough to reduce the need for venography.[67–69]

An ultrasonic method for the detection of venous obstruction, using the Doppler flowmeter, is also available.[62,70] Patency of the vessels is demonstrated by squeezing the leg distally, augmenting flow through the femoral vein.

Diagnosis

Conditions easily confused with pulmonary embolism include pneumonia, atelectasis, cardiac tamponade, pneumothorax, chest trauma, pleuritis of any etiology, pleurodynia, biliary tract disease, pericarditis, myocardial ischemia, sepsis, and a host of other diseases. Hyperventilation due to anxiety can occasionally be difficult to differentiate from pulmonary embolism without laboratory aids. Thromboembolic disease should be considered a possibility in any cardiorespiratory arrest, especially in hospitalized patients. It should be in the differential diagnosis in patients with unexplained fever or deterioration.

The high incidence of unsuspected pulmonary embolism continues to be a problem. Because pulmonary embolism is frequently inapparent and often occurs in patients with cardiovascular and respiratory disease that may mask its manifestations, one must remain alert to the possibility of this disease at all times. It is important to pursue the diagnosis aggressively as early as possible, preferably in the first 24 to 36 hr following pulmonary embolus, because it becomes increasingly difficult to establish a definitive diagnosis later.

The very low risk involved in laboratory tests should encourage physicians to investigate thoroughly those patients in whom pulmonary embolism is a serious consideration. However, the limitations of these tests, leading to false-positive diagnoses, must be understood.

Patients who were previously well and who present with characteristic symptoms, physical examination, blood gases, and lung scan, and with a normal chest roentgenogram usually do not require further investigation to establish a diagnosis. Those patients who have underlying cardiac or lung disease that might make interpretation of the lung scan difficult or impossible should be considered for pulmonary angiography if the diagnosis is in doubt. It should be remembered that if the alveolar–arterial oxygen gradient is normal and if the lung scan is normal, it is highly unlikely that an embolus will be demonstrated angiographically.

Course

It is possible that many persons who suffer transiently from pulmonary embolism are not seen by a physician and do well, with few, if any, recurrences. In previously healthy patients with proven embolic episodes, the ultimate prognosis is very good. If there is underlying cardiac, respiratory, or malignant disease the long-term outlook is not as good, partly owing to the limited survival rate of patients with the underlying disease, and the frequency of recurrent emboli.[71]

The majority of patients who die with massive pulmonary embolism do so in the first 30 to 60 min. Survival beyond this initial period means that they will usually do well with conservative treatment. The mortality rate in this group is about 15 to 20%.

Following a pulmonary embolus, the frequency of recurrences decreases exponentially with time and reaches a plateau at 4 months, with a slight further decrease in frequency by 3 years.[72] A history of this disease increases the risk two times. Anticoagulants reduce that risk to about 10% to 20%. Despite occasional recurrences, the long-term outlook is very good for patients with acute or subacute embolism. However, some patients initially present with chronic recurrent embolism and pulmonary hypertension, and frequently have recurrences (many of which are clinically silent), leading to chronic cor pulmonale, debility, and ultimately, death.[73,74] This course is, fortunately, uncommon.

Management

Deep venous thrombophlebitis of the lower limbs with no evidence of embolism should be treated initially in the hospital with bed rest and intravenous anticoagulants. Oral anticoagulants should be initiated and continued at least until all signs of phlebitis have disappeared, but the appropriate duration of therapy has not been documented. It is probable that 4 to 6 weeks is adequate. If signs persist for longer than several weeks, long-term anticoagulation might be advisable. Similar treatment of deep-vein thrombosis in the upper limbs is also necessary. Operative thrombectomy has been suggested,[12] but the benefits of this operation have not been established.

A recent trial has confirmed the efficacy of oral anticoagulants in preventing recurrent thrombosis or pulmonary embolism, and has suggested that low-dose heparin can be used after 14 days of full anti-coagulation when only the calf veins are involved.[75] Low-dose heparin (5,000 units every 12 hr) was also found to be as effective as warfarin when begun after four weeks of treatment with full doses of anticoagulants in patients with both deep-vein thrombosis and pulmonary embolism.[76] Confirmation of the benefits of low-dose heparin for the prevention of recurrences should be obtained before widespread application of this method of management.

When pulmonary embolism is being considered, arterial blood gases should be analyzed and an electrocardiogram (ECG) and chest roentgenogram done without delay. If the diagnosis is likely, the patient should be admitted immediately to the hospital and treatment commenced. Under normal circumstances, investigations can then be done while the patient is being treated as if the disease were present. A lung scan should be done, and pulmonary angiography, when indicated, should be performed within 24 hours if possible, because of the potential rapid dissolution of the emboli. Thus, the patient is treated for a potentially lethal disease immediately, instead of waiting for convincing evidence.

Patients presenting with pulmonary embolism without predisposing causes should be placed on heparin for 10 to 14 days and then kept on oral anticoagulants for 4 to 6 months, although low-dose heparin may prove to be a reasonable alternative after four weeks of full anticoagulation.[76] Supportive therapy such as oxygen could be life-saving, and analgesia should be used when indicated. Intravenous dexamethasone is occasionally useful when the usual narcotic analgesics are not effective.

The dosage of heparin varies in different patients and with the route of administration. The most common method is to give heparin intravenously, either by bolus injection or by continuous intravenous infusion, in doses that maintain either the Lee-White clotting time at about 2–2½ times normal or the activated partial thromboplastin time at 1½–2½ times the control.[77] In the case of bolus administration, it should be about 1½ times normal just before the next 4-hr dose. There is increasing evidence that anticoagulation with continuous infusion provides greater protection against recurrent emboli, with less risk of bleeding.[78] Subcutaneous heparin generally does not provide reliable anticoagulation, and should not be used for the acute episode.

Use of anticoagulants during pregnancy is associated with substantial increase in risk to the fetus as well as increased risk of excess bleeding at the time of delivery.[26] Rarely, patients with pulmonary infarction will develop massive hemothorax while on anticoagulants. The hemothorax requires drainage by tube thoracostomy, and temporary interruption of anticoagulant treatment.[79]

In patients with massive pulmonary embolism causing cardiorespiratory difficulty, heparin is given in much larger doses than that required to prevent thrombin-fibrinogen interaction. Experimental evidence suggests that the effect of heparin on platelet aggregation and release of serotonin might be beneficial. Ten thousand to 15,000 units per 4-hr period are given initially, with a reduction to the usual doses in 24 to 48 hours. If a patient is in shock, isoproterenol is usually considered the inotropic agent of choice because of its dilating effect on pulmonary vessels and bronchi. When contraindications to anticoagulation are present, the hazards of the disease must be balanced against the risks of treatment.

Treatment of pulmonary embolism with anticoagulants is usually very effective; recurrences are infrequent, compared with instances when anticoagulants are withheld because of contraindications.[80] Surgical removal of the emboli (pulmonary embolectomy), usually utilizing cardiopulmonary bypass, remains controversial, because there are no reliable criteria to predict which patients will improve without it.[81–83] Some authors suggest that embolectomy should be done in most cases of massive embolism, whereas others argue that few institutions are equipped to perform the operation early enough to save the majority of patients who die, that is, within 30 to 60 min. Because of the operative mortality (about 30 to 50%), it is suggested that the procedure might actually lower the survival. A seemingly rational approach is to do embolectomy on patients with persistent shock or where improvement in the hemodynamic status is not occurring. Another embolic episode in this latter group might be sufficient to cause death. However, there is still enough anecdotal experience to indicate that even this "middle-of-the-road" approach is not necessarily correct, since a number of these patients have survived with conservative treatment. Pulmonary angiography must be performed to ensure that the right diagnosis is made and that the size and location of the emboli are known prior to surgery. Transvenous embolectomy utilizing a catheter tip suction device has been evaluated and utilized extensively by Greenfield.[84,85] This exacting technique may hold particular promise if combined with angioscopic visualization of the embolus.

Persistent emboli in the main pulmonary arteries have been considered an indication for embolectomy if there is significant pulmonary hypertension, if there is significant respiratory disability, or if there is recurrent infection or hemoptysis.[86]

There is a significant mortality rate following surgical embolectomy, and not all patients improve.[87–90] Good results from the operation may depend on adequate bronchial artery collateral flow, which can be documented angiographically preoperatively.[88,89] Because medical treatment might be followed by a relatively benign course, it may be advantageous to attempt long-term anti-coagulation, and to operate only if the patient is seriously compromised or appears to be deteriorating.

Since the source of emboli is almost always

the inferior vena cava or an area distal to it, various methods of venous interruption to mechanically prevent travel of the emboli proximally have been evaluated, but the indications and methods unfortunately remain controversial. It is generally agreed that some form of interruption of inferior vena caval flow should be considered when there is recurrent embolization while the patient is being adequately anticoagulated, or when anticoagulation is contraindicated in a patient with pulmonary embolism. It is advocated by some in cases of massive pulmonary embolism, but there is evidence that the recurrence rate is low without venous interruption in these patients.[74] It should be noted that although the procedure may completely interrupt or partially occlude the inferior vena cava at the time of operation, large venous collaterals eventually form, so that thrombi of significant size can still embolize to the lungs.

There are a number of different methods of venous interruption.[91] Femoral vein ligation, commonly practiced in the past, is not considered to be effective, since there is still a 5 to 8% incidence of fatal recurrences. Inferior vena cava ligation caused a 20 to 50% mortality in patients who were already in congestive heart failure. The overall mortality in one series was 14%, with 6.3% recurrences and a fatality of 2.2% owing to recurrent pulmonary embolism. Inferior vena caval plication has been more commonly used recently and has approximately the same morbidity and mortality as ligation, but with a lower incidence of the postphlebitic sequelae that can be significant in some patients. Several umbrella-shaped filters are available; the Kim–Ray–Greenfield type have the highest patency rate and fewest recurrences.[50b,92] These devices can be introduced under local anesthetic, and, when placed by an experienced physician, the risks are acceptable. There is an obvious advantage to avoiding general anesthesia in critically ill patients, in whom the mortality rate, as mentioned above, is unacceptably high. The mortality rate of the procedure and the rate of recurrence of embolism must be considered in contemplating any of these procedures.

Trials designed to evaluate the thrombolytic drugs urokinase and streptokinase have provided a great deal of information about pulmonary embolism as well as the effects of those drugs.[93–95] Because of the relatively small numbers of patients involved, there was no demonstrable improvement in mortality for the patients treated with urokinase or streptokinase compared with the control patients who were treated with heparin. However, there were significant differences in most of the parameters measured. Accelerated resolution was demonstrated initially angiographically and by lung scans in the urokinase- and streptokinase-treated groups; however, both groups were similar by 7 days and continued to improve similarly to 12 months. The values for arterial oxygen saturation were not significantly different. Clinically, the dyspnea and the accentuation of the pulmonary component of the second sound improved faster in the urokinase-treated patients at 24 hours. Hemodynamic parameters, including mean right atrial, pulmonary artery, and right ventricular systolic and diastolic pressures improved faster when urokinase was administered. Streptokinase may be more effective than heparin in reducing the incidence of venous valvular insufficiency and its sequelae.[96,97]

Streptokinase and urokinase are equally effective. Both agents act by different mechanisms to convert the proenzyme plasminogen to plasmin, a proteolytic enzyme that digests and dissolves thrombus. Direct pulmonary artery infusions have no demonstrated advantage over infusions through peripheral veins. Since they dissolve clots indiscriminately, there are broad absolute and relative contraindications to their use (Table 10-5). The patient must be observed for serious bleeding (5–25% incidence) as well as other side-effects such as allergic reactions, most often with streptokinase. Fibrinolytic activity can be reversed if necessary by stopping the drug, by giving fresh frozen plasma or cryoprecipitate (usually effective in one hour), or by giving epsilon-aminocaproic acid, a plasmin inhibitor, for quicker results.

Although no statistical improvement in survival has been demonstrated, there appears to be sufficient evidence to warrant the use of fibrinolytic agents in acute massive embolism (obstruction of two or more lobar vessels) or where a lesser degree of vascular involvement has resulted in severe hemodynamic difficulty.[94,

TABLE 10-5. Contraindications to the Use of Fibrinolytic Agents

Risk of bleeding
- Recent surgery (7–10 days), biopsies, intra-arterial catheters
- Recent trauma (including external cardiac massage)
- Pregnancy (to 10 days post-partum)
- Severe hypertension
- Cavitating lung disease
- Active gastrointestinal ulcer
- Recent stroke
- Severe renal or hepatic disease
- Potential systemic emboli (bacterial endocarditis or mitral valve disease with atrial fibrillation)

Hypersensitivity to the enzyme

TABLE 10-6. Guidelines for Thrombolytic Agents

Patient selection
1. Consider contraindications (Table 10-5).
2. Select patients who require more benefit than provided by standard anticoagulation.
3. Ensure hemostatically competent state prior to treatment.

Monitoring of treatment
1. Ensured "lytic state"; thrombin time 2 to 5 times normal.
2. Careful observation for bleeding.

Drug administration
1. a) Urokinase: initial loading dose followed by 12-hr continuous infusion.
   b) Streptokinase: initial loading dose followed by 24 hr continuous infusion for pulmonary embolus; 12 hr for venous thrombosis.
2. Restart heparin one hour after completing infusion.

[95,98,99] Old thrombi are not as reliably dissolved by the drugs. More rapid resolution of the emboli and improvement in circulatory dynamics should provide a degree of protection from the effects of early recurrences and should play a beneficial role when the circulation is already compromised. It has been suggested that thrombolytic agents be used with patients in shock states before attempting a pulmonary embolectomy, because a significant number might improve, negating the need for the high-risk operation.[100] Reduction of the incidence of venous valvular insufficiency might reduce the frequency of post-phlebitis symptoms. The general guidelines for the use of these very costly drugs, urokinase and streptokinase, are listed in Table 10-6.

Prevention

Since there are well-defined groups of patients who are at increased risk of pulmonary embolism, special efforts must be made to prevent its occurrence. Some of the methods utilized to prevent stasis include early ambulation (particularly in postoperative, post-partum, and postmyocardial infarction patients), leg exercises, leg vibrators, electric calf muscle stimulation, and tensor bandages. It is likely that early ambulation is fairly effective, and it is routine when possible in most institutions. The other measures are only variably employed and have not been shown to be either very effective or practical.[101]

Attempts to modify blood coagulability with dextran, aspirin, or other antiplatelet drugs have their proponents, but the benefits and risks of these drugs must be better documented before they are widely used.[102] Earlier studies have clearly demonstrated the benefits of anticoagulants, but there is substantial resistance to fully anticoagulating large numbers of persons prophylactically, especially in the postoperative period because of the risk of bleeding.

The rationale for reduced anticoagulation using low-dose heparin has been tested widely in a variety of surgical and medical patients. Heparin-catalysed protease inhibition by antithrombin III takes place at drug levels that are lower than required to produce full anticoagulation.[103,104] Most clinical trials have demonstrated the efficacy of low-dose heparin in preventing deep-vein thrombosis in the lower limbs, but there are only a few well-controlled studies suggesting a significant decrease in pulmonary embolism in treated patients.[105–120] There is, however, some evidence to suggest that the clinical importance of this treatment might be minimal.[121–125] Significant bleeding complications are uncommon; there is also no need to follow the anticoagulant effects with laboratory tests.

Current recommendations are that 5000 units (USP) of heparin be administered subcutaneously 2 hr prior to surgery and at 12-hr intervals postoperatively until full ambulation or discharge in all patients over 40 years of age undergoing general thoracic or abdominal surgery.[102,123] They must not be on other anticoagulants or aspirin, and must have normal coagulation prior to surgery. Low-dose heparin is not recommended for eye or brain surgery, or when spinal anesthesia is used. It appears to be ineffective in hip surgery, above-knee amputations, repairs of femoral fractures, open prostatectomy, and trauma,[61,122–127] perhaps because of an increased stimulus to coagulation in patients with extensive tissue damage. Low-dose heparin combined with dihydroergotamine, a potent venoconstrictor that increases the velocity of blood flow, might be effective in patients undergoing total hip replacement.[128] Patients with acute myocardial infarction (particularly if there is heart failure), patients with severe respiratory failure,[22a] those with nonhemorrhagic strokes, those on estrogen therapy, and quadraplegics appear to be good candidates for low-dose heparin, although there is a paucity of clinical trials in these and other types of medical patients. It is important to recall that low-dose heparin is inadequate therapy for on-going thrombotic activity.

It is possible that the use of prophylactic anticoagulation will expand to include very large numbers of patients with predisposing risks. Since the disease may, in large part, be preventable, continuing clinical investigation along these lines is needed.

SEPTIC EMBOLISM

When septic pulmonary embolism occurs, there is usually a history of drug abuse, congenital heart disease, septic thrombophlebitis, or tricuspid valve endocarditis. The latter may both be found in intravenous drug abusers, in patients with indwelling catheters, or in those with cellulitis.[129–131] Other sources include septic phlebitis of the lower limbs or pelvis, jugular phlebitis owing to dental infection, ventricular atrial shunts, pacemaker wires, and arteriovenous shunts used for renal dialysis (see also Foreign Material Embolism below). These patients often present with severe sepsis and multiple pulmonary infiltrates that tend to cavitate.[130] (see Fig. 10-12.) Lung abscess, empyema (30%), and bronchopleural fistula are the most common severe complications. Hemoptysis is rare but was fatal in two of three patients in a series of over 60 patients with tricuspid valve endocarditis.[131] Because of the increased frequency of drug abuse and the use of chronic indwelling intravenous catheters, this disorder is becoming more common. It should be remembered that the nonmedical use of intravenous drugs is frequently denied by the drug abuser, so that evidence suggesting it should be carefully sought. When there is another obvious source for the septic emboli, right-sided bacterial endocarditis might co-exist and should be sought. Even when no murmur is heard, echocardiography might demonstrate a vegetation (Fig. 10-13).

Anticoagulants are not the major mode of therapy in septic embolization, especially when the source is endocarditis. Mycotic aneurysms predispose patients to hemorrhage from arterial vessels, which may be fatal.[131] If hemoptysis occurs, the source of the bleeding should be identified bronchoscopically, and the patient should be observed carefully, with matched blood available for transfusion. Intubation and suction equipment should be kept at the bedside. Urgent thoracotomy may be indicated in the event the hemoptysis becomes massive. Appropriate antibiotics and supportive therapy are the mainstays of treatment. Surgical treatment might be required if control of the infection is not achieved. Excision of the involved vein in an extremity, inferior vena cava interruption, or tricuspid valve surgery might be necessary.

FAT EMBOLISM

Fat embolism, an uncommon form of microembolic disease, occurs most often after trauma and is discussed in detail in Chapter 11. Bone marrow embolism occurs after trauma, and is seen pathologically after cardiopulmonary resuscitation.

AMNIOTIC FLUID EMBOLISM

Amniotic fluid embolism is a severe but rare complication of labor which causes 20 to 40% of maternal deaths.[132,133] The patients are usually older and multiparous. The onset is usually toward the end of the first stage of a difficult or

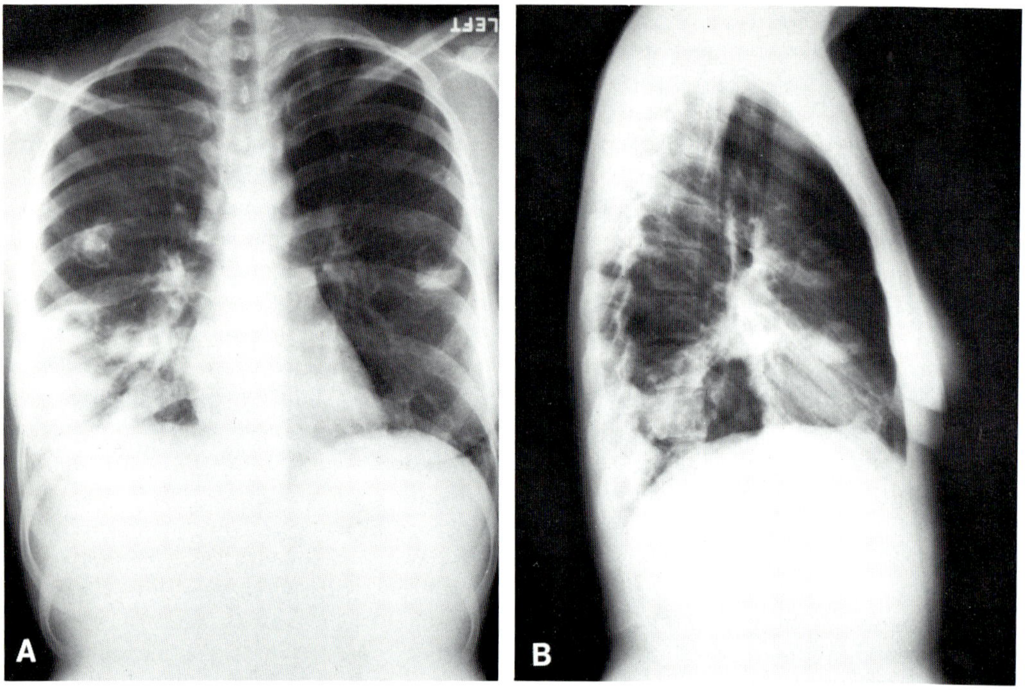

FIG. 10-12. Posteroanterior **(A)** and lateral **(B)** chest roentgenograms of a 22-year-old heroin addict. There are multiple cavities, mostly thin-walled, some with air-fluid levels, and an infiltrate in the right lower lobe.

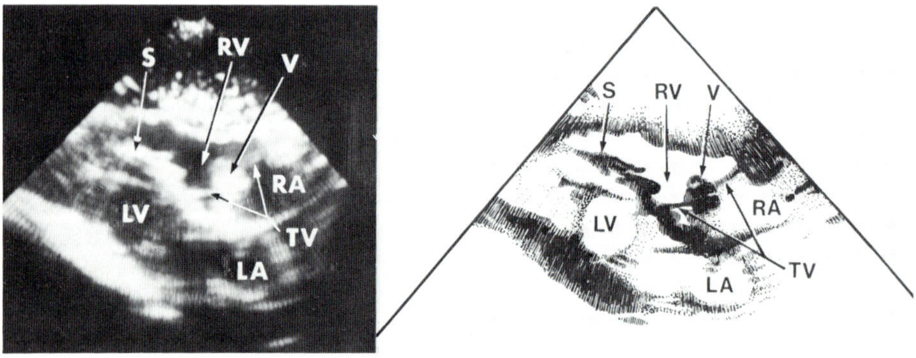

FIG. 10-13. This 29-year-old diabetic with a previous subclavian catheter had the clinical presentation of septic pulmonary emboli. Blood cultures grew *Staphylococcus aureus,* but there was no heart murmur. This two-dimensional echocardiogram (actual photo *left,* schematic positive tracing *right*) demonstrated tricuspid vegetations, diagnostic of endocarditis. RA and RV = right atrium and right ventricle; TV = tricuspid valve; LA and LV = left atrium and left ventricle; S = interventricular septum; V = vegetation posterior to tricuspid leaflet.

complicated labor. Rupture of the uterus is common. Amniotic fluid embolism has also been associated with saline- or glucose-induced abortions and, rarely, Cesarean sections. It is manifested by findings similar to those in acute thromboembolism, except that disseminated intravascular coagulation and occasionally severe bleeding may occur. Sometimes seizures lead erroneously to a diagnosis of eclampsia.

The diagnosis is usually based on the combination of the patient's hemodynamic deterioration, cyanosis, and disseminated intravascular coagulation in the absence of other causes. The chest roentgenogram may show bilateral pulmonary infiltration that is indistinguishable from other causes of pulmonary edema or only some of the subtle findings seen in pulmonary thromboembolism. Lung scans may demonstrate multiple small perfusion defects.[134] In general, the features are similar to those seen with fat embolism.

Amniotic fluid material is found in the lungs and most often consists of squamae and mucus, whereas hair and fat are found less often. Squamae and mucus are also often seen in other organs, including the heart, brain, and kidneys. Experimental amniotic fluid embolism produces pulmonary hypertension.

Management is directed at adequate oxygenation and the support of the circulation. In fully developed cases the mortality is high (86%). Serious long-term complications are uncommon in survivors. The optimal therapy for the intravascular coagulation remains controversial.[18]

AIR EMBOLISM

Air embolism occurs when air enters the venous system through an intravenous infusion, penetrating trauma, certain forms of surgical and gynecologic maneuvers, or rapid decompression. The atmospheric pressure must exceed the intravascular pressure at the site of entry; consequently, intrathoracic structures with subatmospheric pressure (*e.g.*, subclavian vein and central veins) are vulnerable and must always be connected to a fluid column during venipuncture. Barotrauma due to impact injuries, blast injuries, or positive-pressure breathing occasionally produces air embolism. The manifestations are similar to thromboembolism, except that a churning murmur may be heard over the precordium, and neurologic signs and symptoms may accompany cerebral air embolism. Death occurs owing to mechanical obstruction by the air in the right ventricle or in the pulmonary vessels. Five to 10 ml of air are generally safe, except in patients with congenital heart defects who are predisposed to paradoxical embolism. The lethal dose is about 5 to 55 ml/kg of air.[135–138]

The treatment of air embolism consists of turning the patient on the left side, so that the air will localize to the lateral wall of the right atrium. If the patient is positioned with the head and upper thorax lower down, the air can then be aspirated through a needle or catheter passed into the right heart. Where available, hyperbaric oxygen therapy is indicated and may dramatically reverse circulatory and neurologic manifestations.

TUMOR EMBOLISM

Mechanical obstruction of pulmonary vessels occurs with dislodgement of intravenous tumor fragments.[9,18] This phenomenon is suspected when a patient with a malignant tumor and clinical evidence of pulmonary thromboembolism fails to improve with anticoagulant treatment. It has been described most frequently with hypernephroma, hepatoma, pancreatic carcinoma, and atrial myxoma, and at autopsy, tumor can generally be seen invading the lumen of large veins.

Lymphangitic carcinomatosis probably also represents vascular tumor emboli. These are seeded diffusely to the extensive vascular bed, where they invade the interstitium and the lymphatics. Patients with this disease generally present with dyspnea, hypoxemia, and bilateral, finely nodular radiographic infiltrates[139] (see also Chap. 15).

FOREIGN MATERIAL EMBOLISM

Foreign material embolization is most commonly related to intravenous drug abuse.[140–147] Talc, hair, peanut butter, and mixing powders may produce lesions ranging from infarcts to diffuse granulomata with or without pulmonary hypertension.[18] Frequently the "mainliner" develops septic phlebitis or endocarditis with septic emboli. In patients in whom intravenous drug abuse has been controlled, there are frequently diffuse, finely nodular lung infiltrates, and a reduced diffusing capacity for carbon monoxide.

Lymphangiography occasionally results in pulmonary vascular embolism. Acute onset of dyspnea and cyanosis is associated with a reduced vital capacity and diffusing capacity. The alveolar–arterial oxygen gradient is increased. The chest film demonstrates diffuse, fine stippling. Treatment requires therapy for hypoxemic respiratory failure.[10,11]

Rarely, such substances as mercury have been injected intravenously and are apparent radiographically as tiny radio-opaque nodules distributed throughout the lungs.[148]

Iatrogenic embolism of polyethylene catheters, pacemaker wires, and disrupted ventricular atrial shunts is associated with a high risk of arrhythmias, infection, and thrombosis, and these devices generally require early removal.[149]

PULMONARY ARTERIAL HYPERTENSION

The pulmonary vascular bed is relatively silent clinically until late in the course of disease. Unlike the readily accessible systemic circulation, early detection, follow-up and treatment are not possible and have not been evaluated systematically. Consequently patients are rarely recognized as having significant pulmonary hypertension until marked physical signs, electrocardiographic changes, or frank right ventricular fail ure develops.

Factors affecting the pulmonary vascular resistance and pulmonary pressure are reviewed in Chapter 5. The major inter-relationships are summarized by the equation

$$\text{Pulmonary artery pressure} = \left\{ \begin{matrix} \text{Pulmonary} \\ \text{vascular} \\ \text{resistance} \end{matrix} \times \begin{matrix} \text{Pulmonary} \\ \text{blood} \\ \text{flow} \end{matrix} \right\} + \begin{matrix} \text{Pulmonary} \\ \text{venous} \\ \text{pressure} \end{matrix}$$

Pulmonary hypertension is mild when it occurs with increased blood flow during exercise, or in patients with left to right shunts but otherwise normal vascular beds. Only when the vascular bed is diseased, and pulmonary vascular resistance increased, does the increase in blood flow with exercise cause clinical problems. The vascular disease that may occur as a result of increased pulmonary blood flow is discussed under Secondary Pulmonary Hypertension. Pulmonary hypertension that occurs as a result of elevated pulmonary venous pressure begins as post-capillary pulmonary vascular disease with distinctive clinical features, and is dealt with separately.

PRIMARY PULMONARY HYPERTENSION

Primary pulmonary hypertension[150–154] is a rare disease of unknown etiology, manifested by various degrees of precapillary pulmonary hypertension. By definition, identifiable causes of pulmonary hypertension, such as diseases of the lung parenchyma, thromboembolism, intracardiac shunts, and left-sided heart disease (in particular mitral stenosis), have to be ruled out before the diagnosis is made.

Incidence

The disease can occur at any age, but the majority of cases occur in young adults, most of them females. However, in persons under the age of 16, the incidence is about equal in both sexes. Familial occurrences have been reported. An increased frequency of the disease was found in several European countries, apparently related to the use of aminorex fumarate, an anorexigenic drug.[153,155] About 1000 cases have been reported, but an active cardiac catheterization laboratory will make this diagnosis in 1% to 2% of cases.[153]

Pathology

The widespread changes in the pulmonary vascular bed include medial muscular hypertrophy, intimal proliferation and fibrosis, and thrombosis. The characteristic "plexiform lesion" is not pathognomonic. It consists of a highly cellular, intraluminal plexiform tuft, generally associated with distal dilatation. All varieties and stages of the lesions may be present in the same patient, and in the late stages may be associated with necrotizing arteritis. Since the disease generally presents clinically late in its course, the earliest histologic characteristics are not known. Clinically apparent pulmonary emboli are uncommon.

The etiology of primary pulmonary hypertension remains obscure. Any hypothesis must account for genetic predisposition, vasoconstrictive and vascular proliferative changes, and some autoimmune manifestations.

Clinical Manifestations

Patients with primary pulmonary hypertension usually present with the insidious onset of dyspnea on exertion, easy fatigability, and weakness. Syncope is frequent, particularly during effort. This is believed to be due to decreased cerebral perfusion caused by peripheral vasodilation in the face of a relatively fixed cardiac output. Chest pain, resembling that caused by coronary artery disease, might be due to the same mechanism that decreases coronary perfusion to the hypertrophied right ventricle. Raynaud's phenomenon is occasionally associated with primary pulmonary hypertension.

The physical findings are basically those of severe pulmonary hypertension, with the conspicuous absence of clues as to the cause. An increase in the height of the "A" wave of the jugular–venous pulse, and, later in the course, a large "V" wave (due to tricuspid regurgitation) might be seen. A right ventricular impulse is palpable. The pulmonary artery and the pulmonic component of the second sound are often palpable. There is usually a pulmonic ejection click and a systolic ejection murmur along the upper left sternal border. The pulmonic component of the second heart sound is usually very loud. Early in the course the second heart sound is narrowly split, but this widens as right ventricular failure develops.[154] The murmurs of tricuspid and pulmonic regurgitation, as well as a right ventricular gallop sound, might be heard. A pulsatile liver might be felt. Cyanosis, if present, is of the peripheral type, unless there is a right-to-left shunt through a patent foramen ovale.

The electrocardiogram usually shows right ventricular hypertrophy with a systolic overload pattern. The P waves might be large, suggesting right atrial hypertrophy. The chest roentgenogram shows large central pulmonary arteries, with tapering towards the periphery, and a large right ventricle.[156] Signs of left atrial hypertension or enlargement are absent. The lung scan demonstrates equal distribution of blood to upper and lower lung zones, in the upright position.

At cardiac catheterization, the important findings are pulmonary hypertension, with a normal pulmonary capillary wedge pressure and pulmonary angiogram. Mean pulmonary artery pressures are frequently in the 50 mm Hg to 80 mm Hg range, approaching systemic levels.[152] The pulmonary vascular resistance is characteristically high and relatively fixed; therefore, the pulmonary artery pressure rises precipitously with exercise.

Course

The course of primary pulmonary hypertension is usually a steady downhill progression to death within 3 or 4 years, although survival varies from several months up to 40 years. Signs of right ventricular failure or an increased frequency of syncopal episodes are usually ominous. The mortality rate during pregnancy may be as high as 50%. It should be noted that procedures ranging from cardiac catheterization to bone marrow aspirations have precipitated deaths. Angiography may be particularly hazardous because of the systemic vasodilating effects of the intravascular dye.[152,154]

Treatment

Until recently therapy was directed at the complications of the disease. There are now several reports of successful treatment with vasodilator drugs, including phentolamine,[157] diazoxide,[158] and hydralazine.[159] However, attempts to treat several patients with these drugs at our institution have not been successful. The true potential of this mode of treatment is still to be defined.[152,153] Anticoagulants are often administered without proof of their efficacy. Pregnancy should be avoided in advanced cases.

SECONDARY PULMONARY HYPERTENSION

Patients with increased pulmonary pressure tend to develop further increases in vascular resistance, regardless of the underlying cause. A wide range of diseases cause pulmonary hypertension, through loss of pulmonary vascular bed (emphysema, pneumonectomy), obliterative vascular disease, vasoconstriction, or increased resistance to venous outflow. Increased pulmonary vascular resistance with right ventricular hypertrophy or dilatation is broadly referred to as pulmonary heart disease or cor pulmonale.[160] Frequently, patients with this condition have distinctive clinical features that permit diagnosis of the underlying cause. Treatment programs may be more effective than those outlined for primary pulmonary hypertension.

Pulmonary Parenchymal Disease

Patients with chronic bronchitis and emphysema represent the most common cause of chronic cor pulmonale.[160,161] Cystic fibrosis and other forms of bronchiectasis frequently result in cor pulmonale in the late stages. Although anatomical loss of pulmonary parenchymal bed is of some importance, hypoxia and acidemia play a prominent vasoconstrictive role, particularly during episodes of respiratory decompensation. In one study of patients with stable obstructive lung disease due to pure emphysema, and in whom vascular destruction would be predicted, vasodilators and oxygen lowered pulmonary vascular resistance significantly, demonstrating a vasoconstrictive component.[162] Acute cor pulmonale has been well documented in bronchial asthma. Mean pulmonary artery pressures rarely increase above 50 mm Hg in the obstructive diseases (see detailed discussion, Chap. 14).

Diffuse parenchymal lung disease, particularly pulmonary fibrosis, is associated with pulmonary hypertension and right ventricular failure as a late manifestation of the disease (see Chap. 13). Recently, extensive vascular changes and increased pulmonary vascular resistance have been demonstrated in the adult respiratory distress syndrome (see Chap. 7).

Clinical examination is frequently misleading. Elevated venous pressure is reliable when present; however, clinical signs of pulmonary hypertension and right ventricular enlargement are commonly obscured by lung over-inflation in the obstructive diseases. The electrocardiogram may demonstrate right atrial enlargement (p pulmonale) and a vertical or right axis.

There is increasing evidence that hypoxemia and acidemia are worse during sleep, and this may be the time of greatest pulmonary hypertension (see Chap. 6).[163]

Pulmonary Vasculitis

The connective tissue diseases and autoimmune inflammatory diseases are frequently associated with pulmonary vascular disease. They represent a spectrum of clinical conditions better characterized by their clinical manifestations than by their pathogenesis.[164–166] The diffuse parenchymal lung involvement and the pathogenetic mechanisms are considered in detail in Chapter 13. Pulmonary hypertension with medial hypertrophy, and interstitial fibrosis of the vessels may develop. Although periarteritis nodosa, Wegener's granulomatosis, lymphomatoid granulomatosis and hypersensitivity vasculitis produce the most florid histologic inflammatory changes, sustained and severe pulmonary hypertension is more characteristic of scleroderma, mixed connective tissue disease, and their variants.[167–169] Lupus erythematosis is occasionally associated with severe pulmonary hypertension.

Treatment is directed at the underlying disease. If the pulmonary hypertension becomes the dominant clinical problem, treatment is the same as that for primary pulmonary hypertension. The role of immune suppression, plasmapheresis, or early institution of vasodilator therapy remains speculative.

Chest Wall Disease

Severe scoliosis, thoracoplasty, and restrictive pleuritis are frequently associated with pulmonary hypertension and right ventricular hypertrophy and failure.[170] The mechanisms postulated include "compression" of small vessels owing to small lung volumes; failure of pulmonary vessels to develop or grow when the deformity occurs in childhood; development of medial hypertrophy or intimal fibrotic proliferation secondary to long-standing hypoxemia and hypercapnia; and recurrent thromboembolism. Obesity, a special case of chest wall disease, causes pulmonary hypertension that is more marked in the supine position and during sleep (see also Chap. 6).

High Altitude Disease

The effects of hypoxia of altitude on the pulmonary circulation are discussed in detail in Chapter 1.

Congenital Left-to-Right Shunts

Congenital heart diseases that result in marked increase in pulmonary blood flow produce mild increases in pulmonary artery pressure. Unless the muscular vasculature of the fetal circulation persists, the pulmonary vessels become very distensible and tolerate the high flow rates. With increasing time, morphologic changes occur that are not entirely understood. Muscular hypertrophy and reduced branching might be important features.[154,171–173] Once the pulmonary vascular resistance is increased, the process tends to accelerate, and eventually pulmonary artery pressures may reach or exceed systemic levels.

Ventricular septal defects, patent ductus arteriosus, aortic pulmonary communications, atrial septal defects, and anomalous pulmonary venous drainage might all be associated with severe pulmonary vascular changes. The best treatment is early recognition of the increased pulmonary vascular resistance, because correction of the shunt at an early stage appears to arrest progression. The high pulmonary vascular resistance and the elevated right ventricular pressures account for reversed (right-to-left) shunts later in the clinical course.

Peripheral Pulmonic Stenosis

Congenital narrowing of the main, lobar, or peripheral pulmonary arteries is rarely seen. When the process is widespread or involves large vessels, pulmonary arterial hypertension occurs. Patients with this condition characteristically present because of unexplained murmurs that radiate along the direction of blood flow. They can be systolic or continuous, and can best be heard over the precordium or over the peripheral lung fields, depending on the site of the lesions.[154,171]

Even more rarely, mediastinal fibrosis might result in obstruction of the pulmonary arteries.[174]

Post-Capillary Pulmonary Vascular Disease

Cardiac Disease. In the early days of modern cardiology, it was recognized that the most common cause of right ventricular failure is left ventricular failure.[175] Today's physician can almost always elicit a history of recurrent pulmonary edema, and can demonstrate clinical or radiographic evidence of increased pulmonary venous pressure to assist in the correct diagnosis.[176]

Conditions with elevated left atrial or pulmonary venous pressure result in passive elevation of pulmonary capillary and pulmonary arterial pressure. This causes the "reactive" process of pulmonary vasoconstriction and muscular hypertrophy. Once initiated, the pulmonary vascular lesions, if untreated, progress to include widespread intimal proliferation, angiomatosis, plexiform lesions, acute angle branching, and ultimately fibrinoid necrosis. Although pulmonary venous stenosis, cor triatriatum and left ventricular failure can all cause the pulmonary vascular effects, the best descriptions center on the long course of patients with severe mitral stenosis.[152,175]

Pulmonary Veno-occlusive Disease. Pulmonary veno-occlusive disease is extremely rare, affecting patients mainly under the age of 16. There is no obvious predilection for either sex. The etiology of the disease is unknown. Thrombosis is likely an important factor, producing obstruction early in the course.[59,177] A viral infection might be the initiating event.

Small and medium-sized pulmonary veins are occluded or narrowed by variably loose or dense fibrous tissue. Major pulmonary veins are occasionally also affected. Recanalized veins and pulmonary infarction are often found. On occasion, only one lung is involved. The pulmonary arteries may show changes of pulmonary hypertension. Pulmonary congestion and right ventricular hypertrophy are usually found at autopsy.

Patients usually present with progressive effort dyspnea, and commonly show symptoms suggestive of pneumonia or pulmonary infarction. Cyanosis and syncope are unusual. The disease progresses relentlessly to death in one year, with few exceptions.

The chest roentgenogram provides the most important clues to the diagnosis. Pulmonary congestion is found without distended upper lobe veins, enlarged atrium, or enlarged ventricle. The pulmonary arteries are large centrally, tapering peripherally, and reflecting the severe pulmonary hypertension that is usually present. The lung scan is usually normal. The electrocardiogram shows right ventricular hypertrophy. Cardiac catheterization reveals severely elevated pulmonary artery pressures with normal or only slightly elevated capillary pressures because left atrial pressure is normal. This serves to exclude mitral stenosis, left atrial myxoma, cor triatriatum, and congenital obstruction of the pulmonary veins.

Treatment generally has been ineffective. Anticoagulants have been found to be temporarily beneficial. Azathioprine was beneficial in a patient who had autoimmune features associated with the disease.[178] A combination of antiocoagulants, aspirin, dipyridamole, and methylprednisolone was effective for two years up to the time it was reported.[179]

PULMONARY ARTERIOVENOUS MALFORMATIONS

Arteriovenous malformations, or fistulas, might occur only in the lung, but, in about 50% of the cases they are widespread throughout the body. They generally occur as part of the disorder known as *hereditary hemorrhagic telangiectasia* (Rendu–Osler–Weber disease)[180–183] The hereditary lesion is transmitted as a simple non-sex-linked dominant. In the lungs, they may be single or multiple, too small to see on plain chest films or large and easily recognized. One third of the lesions are multiple on plain chest films.

The malformations consist of shunts between pulmonary arteries and veins (occasionally bronchial arteries are involved) and are similar to hemangiomas. They are thin-walled vascular channels of different sizes lined with varying amounts of connective tissue. The degree of right-to-left shunting depends on the size and number of fistulas. This is a true anatomical right-to-left shunt; therefore, hypoxemia is not strikingly improved by increased concentrations of inhaled oxygen.

Pulmonary arteriovenous malformations are occasionally associated with pulmonary hypertension, with or without a known cause. This increases the pulmonary vascular resistance, increases the shunting, and lowers the arterial P_{O_2} further. Exercise may increase or reduce the shunt. Increased shunting is also present at total lung capacity (TLC) compared to functional residual capacity (FRC), presumably because of the higher pulmonary vascular resistance at TLC[184]; distension of the fistula so that it can accept a larger flow might also play a role. This should be considered when evaluating blood gases in patients with this disease.

Patients with pulmonary arteriovenous malformation commonly present in the third decade with a variety of manifestations, including an abnormal chest roentgenogram, cyanosis, dyspnea, clubbing, epistaxis, murmurs over the chest wall (which are louder with inspiration), cutaneous and mucosal hemangiomas (Fig. 10-14), hemoptysis, or central nervous system symptoms that might be secondary to polycythemia, thrombosis, abscess, cerebral malformations, or air embolism (Table 10-7). A family history, particularly of recurrent hemoptysis, epistaxis or gastrointestinal bleeding, might also be present.

Electrocardiographic abnormalities are unusual. Contrast echocardiography can be used to demonstrate right-to-left shunting, and perfusion lung scans can be used to locate the lesions.[185] The chest roentgenogram is usually abnormal, most often revealing well-defined opacities (Fig. 10-14). Rarely, multiple small

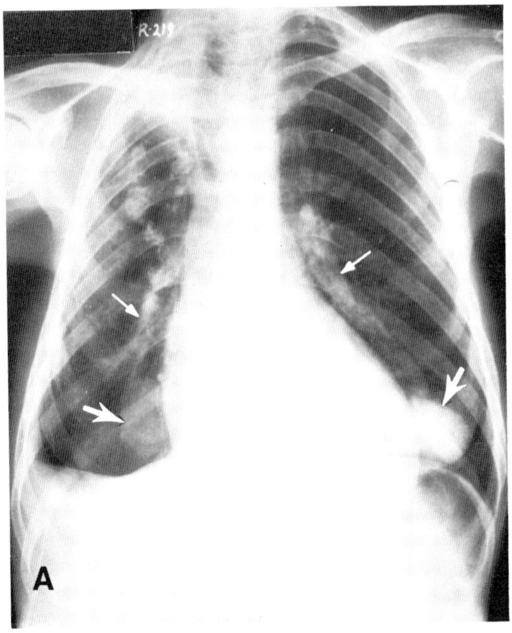

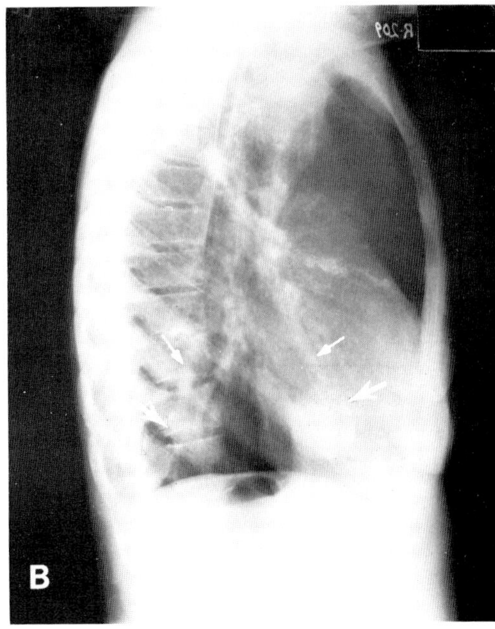

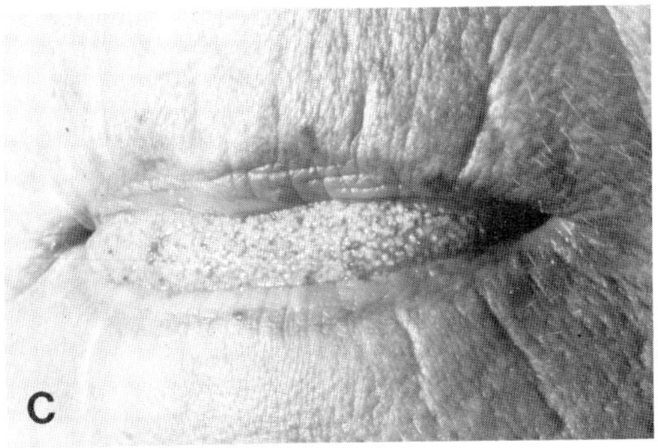

FIG. 10-14. Posteroanterior (**A**) and lateral (**B**) chest roentgenograms of a woman with hereditary hemorrhagic telangiectasia. There are two large malformations (*large arrows*), and the vessels (*small arrows*) leading to them are also visible. Note the old, calcified, granulomatous disease. **C.** Close-up of the same patient's face, showing multiple mucosal and cutaneous telangiectasia in the tongue and lips.

TABLE 10-7. Common Manifestations of Pulmonary Arteriovenous Malformations

Abnormality	Frequency
Dyspnea	60%
Cyanosis	70%
Epistaxis	50%
Respiratory tract bleeding	Common
Central nervous system symptoms	25%
Clubbing	75%
Cutaneous and mucosal hemangiomas	35%
Murmurs	50%
Abnormal chest roentgenogram	90%
Secondary polycythemia	55%

malformations are not visible but are apparent on pulmonary angiography. Fluoroscopic examination usually demonstrates that they are pulsatile and increase in size during Mueller's maneuver (forced inspiration against a closed glottis). They are usually easily identified angiographically. A pulmonary A–V malformation should be distinguished from a pulmonary varix, which is very rare and might be more benign (hemorrhage being the major complication). Pulmonary angiography will demonstrate the varix in the venous phase of the angiogram only, whereas an A–V malformation will be seen earlier in the arterial phase.

The course of the disease is variable. If cyanosis is absent or mild, there may be no progression at all. If cyanosis is severe, the outlook may be poor without surgery. Death is commonly due to rupture into a bronchus or pleural sac, a cerebral abscess, or gastrointestinal bleeding.

The indications for surgery are controversial. It would appear reasonable to observe small malformations, whereas the larger and enlarging ones probably ought to be removed, though frequent recurrence has been reported. If there are multiple bilateral lesions, they should be sufficiently localized so that conservative resection can be performed.[183] Pulmonary arteriovenous fistulas with systemic blood supply present a stronger case for surgical resection because of the risk of severe hemoptysis. If significant pulmonary hypertension is present, surgical resection might be contraindicated. Patients with large shunts and recurring hemoptysis have shown marked improvement after pulmonary arterial embolization therapy using occluding balloons or thrombogenic materials.[186,187]

REFERENCES

1. COON WW: Epidemiology of venous thromboembolism. Ann Surg 186:149, 1977
2. SMITH GT, DAMMIN GJ, DEXTER L: Postmortem arteriographic studies of the human lung in pulmonary embolization. JAMA 188:143, 1964
3. TEVIOTDALE BM, GWYNNE JF: Deep calf vein thrombosis and pulmonary embolism. A necropsy study. NZ Med J 66:530, 1967
4. MORRELL MT, DUNNILL MS: The postmortem incidence of pulmonary embolism in a hospital population. Br J Surg 55:347, 1968
5. FREIMAN DG, SUYEMOTO J, WESSLER S: Frequency of pulmonary thromboembolism in man. N Engl J Med 272:1278, 1965
6. KAPLAN MR, REBA RC: Pulmonary embolism as the leading cause of ophthalmic surgical mortalities. Am J Ophthalmol 73:159, 1972
7. MODAN B, SHARON E, JELIN N: Factors contributing to the incorrect diagnosis of pulmonary embolic disease. Chest 62:388, 1972
8. COON WW, COLLER FA: Clinicopathological correlation in thromboembolism. Surg Gynecol Ostet 109:259, 1959
9. WINTERBAUER RH, ELFENBEIN IB, BALL WC: Incidence and clinical significance of tumor embolization to the lungs. Am J Med 45:271, 1968
10. BRON KM, BAUM S, ABRAMS HL: Oil embolism in lymphangiography. Incidence, manifestations and mechanism. Radiology 80:194, 1963
11. FALLAT RJ, POWELL MR, YOUKER JE et al: Pulmonary deposition and clearance of I-131 labeled oil after lymphangiography in man. Correlation with lung function. Radiology 97:511, 1970
12. CAMPBELL CB et al: Axillary, subclavian, and brachiocephalic vein obstruction. Surgery 82:816, 1977
13. DALEN JE et al: Pulmonary embolism, pulmonary hemorrhage and pulmonary infarction. N Engl J Med 296:1431, 1977
14. KISTNER RL, BALL JJ, NOUDYKE RA et al: Incidence of pulmonary embolism in the course of thrombophlebitis of the lower extremities. Am J Surg 124:169, 1972
15. KAKKAR VV, FLANC C, HOWE CT: Natural history of post-operative deep vein thrombosis. Lancet 2:230, 1969
16. MORRELL MT: The relationship between leg–vein thrombosis and pulmonary emboli at autopsy. Br J Surg 60:306, 1973
17. VIRCHOW R: Weitere Untersuchungen uber die Verstopfung der Lungerarterie und ihre Folgen. Beitr Exp Pathol Physiol 2:21, 1846
18. MOSER KM: Pulmonary vascular obstruction due to embolism and thrombosis. In Pulmonary Vascular Disease Moser KM (ed): Chap. 5. New York, Marcel Dekker, 1979
19. MOSER KM: Pulmonary embolism. Am Rev Respir Dis 115:829, 1977
20. BRACH BB et al: Venous thrombosis in acute spinal cord paralysis. J Trauma 17:289, 1977
21. WARLOW C: Venous thromboembolism after stroke. Am Heart J 96:293, 1978
22. NEUHAUS A, BENTZ RR, WEG JG: Pulmonary embolism in respiratory failure. Chest 73:460, 1978

22a. PINGLETON SK, BONE RC, PINGLETON WW, RUTH WE: Prevention of pulmonary emboli in a respiratory intensive care unit. Chest 79:647, 1981

23. SACK GH, LEVIN J, BELL WR: Trousseau's syndrome and other manifestations of chronic disseminated coagulopathy in patients with neoplasms: Clinical, pathophysiologic and therapeutic features. Medicine 56:1, 1977
24. The Veterans Administration Co-operative Urological Research Group: Treatment and survival of patients with cancer of the prostate. Surg Gynecol Obstet 124:1011, 1967
25. HANDIN RI: Thromboembolic complications of pregnancy and oral contraceptives. Prog Cardiovasc Dis 16:395, 1974
26. HALL J, PAUL RM, WILSON KM: Maternal and fetal sequelae of antiocoagulation during pregnancy. Am J Med 68:122, 1980
27. HIRSH J: Hypercoagulability. Semin in Hematol 14:409, 1977
28. MACDONALD IG, HIRSH J, HALE AS et al: Major pulmonary embolism, a correlation of clinical findings, hemodynamics, pulmonary angiography

and pathologic physiology. Br Heart J 34:346, 1972
29. MLCZOCH J et al: Platelet-mediated pulmonary hypertension and hypoxia during pulmonary microembolism. Chest 74:648, 1978
30. ALPERT JS et al: Pulmonary hypertension secondary to minor pulmonary embolism. Chest 73:795, 1978
31. CLARKE SW, GRAF PD, NADEL JA: In vivo visualization of small airway constriction after pulmonary microembolism in cats and dogs. J Appl Physiol 29:646, 1970
32. HIROSE T, YASUTAKE T, TARABEIL A et al: Location of airway constriction following acute experimental pulmonary thromboembolism. J Appl Physiol 34:431, 1973
33. WILSON JE III et al: Hypoxemia in pulmonary embolism, a clinical study. J Clin Invest 50:481, 1971
34. DANTZKER DR, BOWER JS: Mechanisms of gas exchange abnormality in patients with chronic obliterative pulmonary vascular disease. J Clin Invest 64:1050, 1979
35. LEVY SE, SIMMONS DH: Mechanism of arterial hypoxemia following pulmonary thromboembolism in dogs. J Appl Physiol 39:41, 1975
36. DANTZKER DR et al: Gas exchange after pulmonary thromboembolization in dogs. Circ Res 42:92, 1978
37. ROBIN ED, JULIAN DC, TRAVIS DM et al: a physiological approach to the diagnosis of pulmonary embolism. N Engl Med 260:586, 1959
38. ROBIN ED et al: Alveolar gas exchange in clinical pulmonary embolism. N Engl J Med 262:283, 1960
39. SUTTON GC, HONEY M, GIBSON RV: Clinical diagnosis of acute massive pulmonary embolism. Lancet 1:271, 1969
40. WENGER ND, STEIN PD, WILLIS PW: Massive acute pulmonary embolism. The deceivingly non-specific manifestations. JAMA 220:843, 1972
41. BELL WR, SIMON TL, DEMETS DL: The clinical features of submassive and massive pulmonary emboli. Am J Med 62:355, 1977
42. MURRAY HW et al: Fever and pulmonary thromboembolism. Am J Med 67:232, 1979
43. SKLAROFF HJ: The post-pulmonary infarction syndrome. Am Heart J 98:772, 1979
43a. LEE BC, VAN DER ZEE H, MALIK AB: Site of pulmonary edema after unilateral microembolization. J Appl Physiol 47:556, 1979
44. SZUES MM et al: Diagnostic sensitivity of laboratory findings in acute pulmonary embolism. Ann Intern Med 74:161, 1971
45. BYNUM LJ, CROTTY CM, WILSON JE: Diagnostic value of tests of fibrin metabolism in patients predisposed to pulmonary embolism. Arch Intern Med 139:283, 1979
46. BYNUM LJ, PARKEY RW, WILSON JE: Tests of fibrin metabolism in recurrent venous thromboembolism. Arch Inter Med 137:1385, 1977
47. BYNUM LJ, WILSON JE III: Characteristics of pleural effusions associated with pulmonary embolism. Arch Intern Med 136:159, 1976
48. SPODICK DH: Electrocardiographic responses to pulmonary embolism: Mechanisms and sources of variability. Am J Cardiol 30:695, 1972
49. JOHNSON JD, FLOWERS NC, HORAN LG: Unexplained atrial flutter: A frequent herald of pulmonary embolism. Chest 60:29, 1971
50. MOSES DC, SILVER TM, BOOKSTEIN JJ: The complementary roles of chest radiography, lung scanning and selective pulmonary angiography in the diagnosis of pulmonary embolism. Circulation 49:179, 1974
50a. BIELLO DR et al: Ventilation–perfusion studies in suspected pulmonary embolism. Am J Roentgen 133:1033, 1979
50b. ROSENOW EC, OSMUNDSON PJ, BROWN ML: Pulmonary Embolism. Mayo Clin Proc 56:161, 1981
51. TAPLIN GW, CHOPRA SK: Lung perfusion–inhalation scintigraphy in obstructive airway disease and pulmonary embolism. Rad Clin North Am 16:491, 1978
52. NIDEN AH et al: ^{67}Ga lung scan, an aid in the differential diagnosis of pulmonary embolism and pneumonitis. JAMA 237:1206, 1977
53. ALDERSON PO, SECKER-WALKER RH, FORREST JV: Detection of obstructive pulmonary disease. Relative sensitivity of ventilation-perfusion studies and chest radiography. Nucl Med 112:643, 1974
54. SHARMA G, SASAHARA A: Diagnosis of pulmonary embolism in patients with chronic obstructive pulmonary disease. J Chronic Dis 28:253, 1975
55. NICHOLS AB et al: Scintigraphic detection of pulmonary emboli by serial positron imaging of inhaled ^{15}O-labelled carbon dioxide. N Engl J Med 299:279, 1978
56. MOSER KM, SHURE D, HARRELL JH et al: Angioscopic visualization of pulmonary emboli. Chest 72:2S:198, 1980
57. DALEN JE et al: Pulmonary angiography in acute pulmonary embolism: indications, techniques and results in 367 patients. Am Heart J 81:175, 1971
58. STEIN PD et al: The angiographic diagnosis of acute pulmonary embolism: evaluation of criteria. Am Heart J 73:730, 1967
59. MEISTER SG et al: Pulmonary cineangiography in acute pulmonary embolism. Am Heart J 84:33, 1972
60. LOOP JW, ARCHER G, NORTHROP CH: Bedside pulmonary arteriography. Radiology 114:469, 1975
61. SAGAR KB et al: Characterization of normal and abnormal pulmonary surface by reflected ultrasound. Chest 74:29, 1978

62. KAKKAR VV: Deep vein thrombosis detection and prevention. Circulation 51:8, 1975
63. SAUTTER RD et al: The limited utility of fibrinogen ^{125}I leg scanning. Arch Intern Med 139:148, 1979
64. NADEAU J, DEMERS R, SKINNER B et al: Impedance phlebography: accuracy of diagnosis in deep vein thrombosis. Can J Surg 18:219, 1975
65. HULL R et al: Impedance plethysmography using the occlusive cuff technique in the diagnosis of venous thrombosis. Circulation 53:696, 1976
66. HULL R et al: Impedance plethysmography: The relationship between venous filling and sensitivity and specificity for proximal vein thrombosis. Circulation 58:898, 1978
67. POLLOCK EW et al: Detection of anticoagulation therapy failures in patients with venous thrombosis. Am J Surg 134:214, 1977
68. DAY TK, FISH PJ, KAKKER VV: Detection of deep-vein thrombosis by Doppler angiography. Br Med J 1:618, 1976
69. HULL R et al: Combined use of leg scanning and impedance plethysmography in suspected venous thrombosis. N Engl J Med 296: 1497, 1977
70. JACQUES PF et al: Doppler ultrasonic screening prior to venography for deep venous thrombosis. Am J Roentgenol 129:451, 1977
71. PARASKOS JA et al: Late prognosis of acute pulmonary embolism. N Engl J Med 289:55, 1973
72. COON WW, PARK WW III: Recurrence of venous thromboembolism. Surgery 73:823, 1973
73. WILHELMSEN L, HAGMAN M, WERKO L: Recurrent pulmonary embolism: incidence, predisposing factors, and prognosis. Acta Med Scand 192:565, 1972
74. SUTTON GC, HALL RJC, KERR IH: Clinical course and late prognosis of treated subacute massive, acute minor, and chronic pulmonary thromboembolism. Br Heart J 39:1135, 1977
75. HULL R et al: Warfarin sodium versus low-dose heparin in the long-term treatment of venous thrombosis. N Engl J Med 301:855, 1979
76. BYNUM LJ, WILSON JE: Low-dose heparin therapy in the long-term management of venous thromboembolism. Am J Med 67:553, 1979
77. BASU D, GALLUS A, HIRSH J et al: A prospective study of the value of monitoring heparin treatment with the activated partial thromboplastin time. N Engl J Med 287:324, 1972
78. SALZMAN EW, DEYKIN D, SHAPIRO RM et al: Management of heparin therapy: Controlled prospective trial. N Engl J Med 292:1046, 1975
79. ROSTAND RA, FELDMAN RL, BLOCK ER: Massive hemothorax complicating heparin anticoagulation for pulmonary embolus. South Med J 70:1128, 1977
80. POLLAK EW, SPARKS FC, BARKER WF: Pulmonary embolism: An appraisal of therapy in 516 cases. Arch Surg 107:66, 1973
81. KRUNE WW: Operative therapy of venous thromboembolism. Mod Concepts Cardiovasc Dis 43:71, 1974
82. ALPERT JS et al: Treatment of massive pulmonary embolism: The role of pulmonary embolectomy. Am Heart J 89:413, 1975
83. BEALL AC, COLLINS JJ: What is the role of pulmonary embolectomy? Am Heart J 89:411, 1975
84. GREENFIELD LJ, REIF M, GUENTER CA: Hemodynamic and respiratory response to transvenous pulmonary embolectomy. J Thoracic Cardivasc Surg 62:890, 1971
85. GREENFIELD LJ et al: Transvenous pulmonary embolectomy for acute massive pulmonary embolism. Chest 71:213, 1977
86. SYMBAS PN, JACOBS WF, SCHLANT RC: Chronic pulmonary artery embolization or thrombosis. Am J Cardiol 28:342, 1971
87. TILKIAN AG, SCHROEDER JS, ROBIN ED: Chronic thromboembolic occlusion of main pulmonary artery or primary branches. Am J Med 60:563, 1976
88. CABROL C et al: Surgical correction of chronic post-embolic obstruction of the pulmonary arteries. J Thorac Cardiovasc Surg 76:620, 1978
89. SABISTON DC et al: Surgical management of chronic pulmonary embolism. Ann Surg 185:699, 1977
90. DAILY PO, JOHNSTON GG, SIMMONS CJ et al: Surgical management of chronic pulmonary embolism. J Thorac Cardiovasc Surg 79:523, 1980
91. GARDNER AMN: Inferior vena caval interruption in the prevention of fatal pulmonary embolism. Am Heart J 95:679, 1978
92. WINGERD M et al: Comparison of caval filters in the management of venous thromboembolism. Arch Surg 113:1264, 1978
93. The urokinase pulmonary embolism trial: A national co-operative study. Circulation [Suppl]47:47, 1973
94. The urokinase–pulmonary embolism trial. Phase 1 results. Urokinase–pulmonary embolism trial study group. JAMA 214:2163, 1970
95. Urokinase–streptokinase embolism trial. Phase 2 results. JAMA 229:1606, 1974
96. DUCKERT F et al: Treatment of deep-vein thrombosis with streptokinase. B Med J 1:479, 1975
97. KAKKER VV, SAGAR S, LEWIS M: Treatment of deep-vein thrombosis with intermittent streptokinase and plasminogen infusion. Lancet 2:674, 1975
98. BELL WR, MEEK AG: Guidelines for the use of thrombolytic agents. N Engl J Med 301:1266, 1979
99. MARDER VJ: The use of thrombolytic agents: Choice of patient, drug administration, laboratory monitoring. Ann Intern Med 90:802, 1979
100. MILLER GAH, HALL RJC, PANETH M: Pulmonary embolectomy, heparin, and streptokinase: Their

place in the treatment of acute massive pulmonary embolism. Am Heart J 93:568, 1977
101. SALZMAN EW: Physical methods for prevention of venous thromboembolism. Surgery 81:123, 1977
102. Prevention of venous thromboembolism in surgical patients by low-dose heparin. The American Heart Association Council on Thrombosis. Circulation 55:423A, 1977
103. FRATANTONI J, WESSLER S: Prophylactic therapy of deep-vein thrombosis and pulmonary embolism. DHEW Publication No. (NHIH)76-866, p 254, 1975
104. DOWNING MR: The interaction of proteases, antithrombin III, and heparin. J Lab Clin Med 95:777, 1980
105. SHARNOFF JB: Prevention of sudden cardiopulmonary arrest in the perioperative period with prophylactic heparin. Lancet 2:292, 1969
106. KAKKER VV et al: Low doses of heparin in prevention of deep-vein thrombosis. Lancet 2:669, 1971
107. KAKKER VV et al: Efficacy of low doses of heparin in prevention of deep-vein thrombosis after major surgery. Lancet 2:101, 1972
108. WARLOW C et al: A double-blind trial of low doses of subcutaneous heparin in the prevention of deep-vein thrombosis after myocardial infarction. Lancet 2:934, 1973
109. VAN VROONHOVEN TJMV, VAN ZIJL J, MULLER H: Low-dose subcutaneous heparin versus oral anticoagulants in the prevention of post-operative deep-venous thrombosis. Lancet 1:375, 1974
110. LAHNBORG G et al: Effect of low-dose heparin on incidence of postoperative pulmonary embolism detected by photoscanning. Lancet 1:329, 1974
111. SAGER S, MASSEY J, SANDERSON JM: Low-dose heparin prophylaxis against fatal pulmonary embolism. Br Med J 4:257, 1975
112. ROSENBERG IL, EVANS M, POLLOCK AV: Prophylaxis of postoperative leg vein thrombosis by low-dose subcutaneous heparin or preoperative calf muscle stimulation, a controlled clinical trial. Br Med J 1:649, 1975
113. MCCARTHY ST et al: Low-dose heparin as a prophylaxis against deep-vein thrombosis in patients undergoing total hip replacement. Lancet 2:800, 1977
114. SAGAR S et al: Efficacy of low-dose heparin in prevention of extensive deep-vein thrombosis in patients undergoing total hip replacement. Lancet 1:1151, 1976
115. GRUBER UF et al: Prevention of post-operative thromboembolism by Dextran, low doses of heparin, or xantinol nicotinate. Lancet 1:207, 1977
116. KILL J et al: Prophylaxis against post-operative pulmonary embolism and deep-vein thrombosis by low-dose heparin. Lancet 1:1115, 1978
117. NICOLAIDES AM et al: Small doses of subcutaneous sodium heparin in preventing deep vein thrombosis after major surgery. Lancet 2:890, 1972
118. GORDON-SMITH IC, LEQUESNE LP, GRUNDY DJ et al: Controlled trial of two regimens of subcutaneous heparin in prevention of postoperative deep-vein thrombosis. Lancet 1:1133, 1972
119. WILLIAMS HT: Prevention of postoperative deep vein thrombosis with perioperative subcutaneous heparin. Lancet 2:950, 1971
120. Prevention of fatal postoperative pulmonary embolism by low doses of heparin. An international multicenter trial. Lancet 2:45, 1975
121. BELL WR, ZUIDEMA GD: Low-dose heparin—concern and perspectives. Surgery 85:469, 1979
122. Failure of low-dose heparin to prevent significant thromboembolic complications in high risk surgical patients. Interim report of prospective trial. Groote Schuur Hospital Thromboembolus Study Group. Br Med J 1:1447, 1979
123. WESSLER S, GITAL SN: Low dose heparin: Is the risk worth the benefit? Am Heart J 98:1979
124. EYARTS CM, ALFIDI R: Thromboembolism after total hip reconstruction: Failure of low doses of heparin in prevention. JAMA 225:515, 1973
125. HAMPSON WGJ et al: Failure of low-dose heparin to prevent deep-vein thrombosis after hip replacement arthroplasty. Lancet 2:795, 1974
126. WILLIAMS JW et al: Failure of low-dose heparin to prevent pulmonary embolism after hip surgery or above the knee amputation. Ann Surg 188:468, 1978
127. BLAISDELL FW: Prevention of deep-vein thrombosis. Surgery 83:243, 1978
128. KAKKER VV et al: Prophylaxis for postoperative deep-vein thrombosis: Synergistic effect of heparin and dihydroergotamine. JAMA 241:39, 1979
129. MACMILLAN JC, MILSTEIN SH, SAMSON PC: Clinical spectrum of septic pulmonary embolism and infarction. J Thorac Cardiovasc Surg 75:670, 1978
130. JAFFE RB, KOSCHMANN EB: Septic pulmonary emboli. Radiology 96:527, 1970
131. WEBB DW, THADEPALLI H: Hemoptysis in patients with septic pulmonary infarcts from tricuspid endocarditis. Chest 76:99, 1979
132. LIBAN E, RAZ S: A clinicopathological study of fourteen cases of amniotic fluid embolism. Am J Clin Pathol 51:477, 1969
133. MORGAN M: Amniotic fluid embolism. Anesthesia 34:20, 1979
134. GREGORY MG, CLAYTON EM: Amniotic fluid embolism. J Obstet Gynaecol Br Commonwealth 43:236, 1973
135. BUTLER BD, HILLS BD: The lung as a filter for microbubbles. J Appl Physiol 47:537, 1979
136. GRACE DM: Air embolism with neurologic complications: A potential hazard of central venous catheters. Can J Surg 20:51, 1977

137. ALVARAN SE, TOUNG JK, GRAFF JE et al: Venous air embolism: comparative results of external cardiac massage, intracardiac aspiration, and left lateral decubitus position. Anesth Analg 57:166, 1978
138. ADORNATO DC et al: Pathophysiology of intravenous air embolism in dogs. Anesthesiology 49:120, 1978
139. THURLBECK WM: Neoplasia of the pulmonary vascular bed. In Moser KM (ed): Pulmonary Vascular Disease, Chapt 11. New York, Marcel Dekker, 1979
140. HOPKINS GB: Pulmonary angiothrombotic granulomatosis in drug offenders. JAMA 221:909, 1972
141. CAMARGO G, CULP C: Pulmonary function studies in ex-heroin users. Chest 67:331, 1975
142. ROBERTSON CH, JR, REYNOLDS RC, WILSON JE III: Pulmonary hypertension and foreign body granulomas in intravenous drug abusers. Am J Med 61:657, 1976
143. THOMASHOW D et al: Lung disease in reformed drug addicts: Diagnostic and physiologic correlations. Johns Hopkins Med J 141:1, 1977
144. JAFFE RB, KOSCHMANN EB: Intravenous drug abuse. Am J Radiol 109:107, 1970
145. SZWED JJ: Pulmonary angiothrombosis caused by "blue velvet" addiction. Ann Intern Med 73:771, 1970
146. PARE JAP et al: Pulmonary "mainline" granulomatosis: Talcosis of intravenous methadone abuse. Medicine 58:229, 1979
147. OVERLAND ES, NOLAN AJ, HOPEWELL PC: Alteration of pulmonary function in intravenous drug abusers. Am J Med 68:231, 1980
148. AMBRE JJ, WELCH MJ, SVARE CW: Intravenous elemental mercury injection. Ann Intern Med 87:451, 1977
149. FISHER R, FERREYRO R: Evaluation of current techniques for non-surgical removal of intravascular iatrogenic foreign bodies. Am J Roentgenol 130:541, 1978
150. VAGENVOORT CA: Vasoconstrictive primary pulmonary hypertension and pulmonary veno-occlusive disease. Cardiovasc Clin 42:98, 1972
151. EDWARDS WD, EDWARDS JE: Clinical primary pulmonary hypertension, three pathologic types. Circulation 56:884, 1977
152. VOELKEL N, REEVES JT: Primary pulmonary hypertension. In Moser KM (ed): Pulmonary Vascular Diseases, Chapt 10. New York, Marcel Dekker, 1979
153. FISHMAN AP, PIETRA GG: Primary pulmonary hypertension. Ann Rev Med 31:421, 1980
154. GREGORATOS G, KARLINER JS, MOSER KM: Mechanisms of disease and methods of assessment. In Moser KM (ed): Pulmonary Vascular Diseases, Chapt 4. New York, Marcel Dekker, 1979
155. GURTNER HP: Pulmonary hypertension produced by ingestion of substances. Bull Physiopathol Respir 5:435, 1969
156. KANEMOTO N et al: Chest roentgenograms in primary pulmonary hypertension. Chest 76:45, 1979
157. RUSKIN JN, HUTTER AM: Primary pulmonary hypertension treated with oral phentolamine. Ann Intern Med 90:772, 1979
158. KLINKE WP, GILBERT JAL: Diazoxide in primary pulmonary hypertension. N Engl J Med 302:91, 1980
159. RUBIN LJ, PETER RH: Oral hydralazine therapy for primary pulmonary hypertension. N Engl J Med 302:69, 1980
160. FISHMAN AP: Chronic cor pulmonale. Am Rev Respir Dis 114:775, 1976
161. HEATH D, SMITH P: Pulmonary vascular disease secondary to lung disease. In Moser KM (ed): Pulmonary Vascular Disease, Chap 6. New York, Marcel Dekker, 1979
162. STEIN PD, LEW JD, WELCH MH et al: Pathophysiology of the pulmonary circulation in emphysema associated with $alpha_1$ antitrypsin deficiency. Circulation 43:227, 1971
163. BOYSON PG et al: Nocturnal pulmonary hypertension in patients with chronic obstructive pulmonary disease. Chest 76:536, 1979
164. HUNNINGHAKE GW, FAWE AS: Pulmonary involvement in the collagen vascular diseases. Am Rev Respir Dis 119:471, 1979
165. FAUCI AS: Pulmonary vasculitis. In Kirkpatrick CH, Reynolds HY (eds): Immunologic and Infectious reactions in the Lung, Chapt 13. New York, Marcel Dekker, 1976.
166. FAUCI AS, HAYNES BF, KATA P: The spectrum of vasculitis. Ann Intern Med 89:660, 1978
167. YOUNG RH, MARK GJ: Pulmonary vascular changes in scleroderma. Am J Med 64:998, 1978
168. SALERNI R et al: Pulmonary hypertension in the CREST syndrome variant of progressive systemic sclerosis (scleroderma). Ann Intern Med 86:394, 1977
169. AGIA GA et al: Pulmonary involvement in mixed connective tissue disease. Am Rev Respir Dis 121S:105, 1980
170. BERGOFSKY EH: Respiratory failure in disorders of the thoracic cage. Am Rev Respir Dis 119:643, 1979
171. PERLOFF JK: Congenital heart disease and pulmonary hypertension. In Moser KM (ed): Pulmonary Vascular Diseases, Chapt 8. New York, Marcel Dekker, 1979
172. NIHILL MR, MCNAMARA DG: Magnification pulmonary wedge angiography in the evaluation of children with congenital heart disease and pulmonary hypertension. Circulation 58:1098, 1978
173. RABINOVITCH M: Lung biopsy in congenital heart diseases. Circulation 58:1107, 1978

174. ZORN SK et al: Pulmonary artery obstruction with fibrosing mediastinitis. Lung 155:91, 1978
175. THOMPSON WP, WHITE PD: Commonest cause of hypertrophy of the right ventricle—left ventricular strain and failure. Am Heart J 12:641, 1936
176. DEXTER L: Pulmonary vascular disease in acquired heart disease. In Moser KM (ed): Pulmonary Vascular Diseases, Chapt 7. New York, Marcel Dekker, 1979
177. VAGENVOORT CA: Pulmonary veno-occlusive disease, entity or syndrome? Chest 69:82, 1976
178. SANDERSON JE: A case of pulmonary veno-occlusive disease responding to treatment with azathioprine. Thorax 32:140, 1977
179. CHAWLA SK et al: Pulmonary veno-occlusive disease. Ann Thorac Surg 22:249, 1976
180. MURI J: Arterio-venous aneurysm of the lung. Dis Chest 24:69, 1953
181. LEROUX BT: Pulmonary arteriovenous fistulae. Q J Med 28:1, 1959
182. MARGER JH, GLANTZ G, BREST AN: Pulmonary arteriovenous fistulas. Am J Med 32:417, 1962
183. DINES DE, ARMS RA, BERNATZ RE et al: Pulmonary arteriovenous fistulas. Mayo Clin Proc 49:460, 1974
184. BRUYA TE et al: Longitudinal evaluation of a patient with arteriovenous fistulas: Use of FRC–TLC shunt technique. Chest 76:603, 1979
185. LEWIS AB, GATES GF, STANLEY P: Echocardiography and perfusion scintigraphy in the diagnosis of pulmonary arteriovenous fistula. Chest 73:675, 1978
186. TERRY PG et al: Balloon embolization for treatment of pulmonary arteriovenous fistulas. N Engl J Med 302:1189, 1980
187. TAYLOR BG, COCKERILL EM, MANFREDI F et al: Therapeutic embolization of the pulmonary artery in pulmonary arteriovenous fistula. Am J Med 64:360, 1978

Chapter 11

Chest Trauma

CLARENCE A. GUENTER

THORACIC INJURIES FROM PHYSICAL TRAUMA

IMPACT INJURIES

In previous generations, large numbers of physical injuries resulted from the Great Wars, and the surgeon with experience in the military arena became the most highly qualified to deal with major trauma in civilian life. As a consequence, the skillful management of severe head injuries, crush injuries to the chest, hemorrhagic shock, crush injuries of skeletal muscle, and most injuries involving blast or penetrating trauma was delivered most comfortably by the physician or surgeon with a background in the field of military conflict. Now, however, any physician practicing in an area with high-speed thoroughfares or large numbers of automobiles can be assured a substantial exposure to traumatic injuries. It is estimated that during the 1970s, trauma annually accounted for about 115,000 deaths and more than 11,200,000 disabling injuries in the United States. Approximately one half of the deaths were a result of automobile accidents.[1] In Canada, the figures are approximately proportional on a per-capita basis, with more than 6,000 deaths per year having been directly attributed to automobile accidents in the 1970s.[2,3] Since many more injured persons survive than die, the total number of patients who require care is very high. Furthermore, those persons who die frequently have prolonged periods of intensive, though eventually ineffective, care.

As with so many other ills of mankind, the medical profession is predominantly involved with provision of care for the suffering rather than with programs of prevention. Approximately 50% of automobile accidents appear to be alcohol-ingestion related and thus potentially avoidable, while a large number of the remaining 50% result from potentially avoidable human error or unnecessary travel.[4,5] Reduced speed limits and seat-belt legislation have resulted in reduction of mortality in certain regions. However, numerous new and exciting patterns of transportation are adding to the population at risk. In the northern, snow-covered portions of North America, the snowmobile takes its toll, with a substantially higher risk rate per mile than the automobile. Aggressive, adventure-seeking youths have accepted the hazards of motorcycles in spite of large numbers of deaths. The emphasis on physical fitness has resulted in joggers and cyclists using heavy traffic corridors, exposing themselves to impact injuries. It should be noted, however, that in groups of victims reported from large metropolitan centers, about 70% are injured as a result of motor vehicle accidents, and approximately 30% as a result of industrial accidents, falling from heights, and other types of impact injuries.[2,3,6–8] In most studies, 25% of deaths resulting from motor vehicle accidents are a result of thoracic trauma; however, the majority of these victims do not survive long enough to reach a hospital.

GENERAL ASSESSMENT OF PATIENTS WITH IMPACT INJURIES

Assessment of an impact injury is one of the most difficult tasks with which the physician is faced. Early diagnosis of the injury should be directed at identifying any immediately life-threatening problems. Table 11-1 lists factors that should preoccupy the physician in his systematic approach to the injured. In most in-

TABLE 11-1. Systematic Approach to Subjects of Impact Injury

Initial Evaluation (Immediate)	Early Secondary Evaluation (10–30 min later)	Subsequent Evaluation (30 min to 12 hr later)
1. Level of consciousness 2. Presence of cyanosis 3. Pulse rate, blood pressure 4. Respiratory rate, chest excursion and symmetry 5. Evidence of lacerations 6. Presence and location of pain 7. Deformity or inability to move limbs	1. Evidence of injuries that might be aggravated by movement 2. Examination for evidence of head injury 3. Evaluation of pulmonary air entry, chest-wall tenderness 4. Evaluation of cardiovascular status: venous pressure, rhythm disturbances, arterial pressure, friction rub, murmurs 5. Abdominal evaluation, urinalysis	1. Complete reevaluation, including history of previous health or disease 2. Repeat physical examination and careful search for new evidence of injuries 3. Repeat evaluation of cardiopulmonary status, with particular attention to late evidence of hypotension or respiratory failure

stances, the treatable injuries that may alter life expectancy relate to phenomena that are easily identified.

The physician faces a very urgent problem when the patient presents with unconsciousness, severe arrhythmias or hypotension, marked evidence of respiratory failure, or severe external bleeding, or is sufficiently obtunded to be unable to provide useful clinical information. Such a patient must be quickly evaluated, preferably by a team highly skilled in the urgent identification and management of injuries. All too frequently, when the injury suggests the obvious involvement of one organ system as an explanation for the major manifestations, the vigorous search for injuries involving other organ systems diminishes. However, recognition of a given cause for hypotension, for example, should not diminish the search for additional causes. Availability of nasotracheal suction and an oral or endotracheal airway, insertion of a large intravenous conduit for delivery of fluids, matching blood for possible transfusion, roentgenographic evaluation of the chest and other regions that may have been injured, and close monitoring of vital signs become mandatory. Cervical spine injuries should be assumed to be present until proven otherwise by clinical and/or roentgenographic examination.

The patient who is completely conscious, with no cyanosis, a near-normal pulse rate and blood pressure, a near-normal respiratory rate, symmetrical chest-wall excursion during respiration, no external evidence of major bleeding, and pain that is readily localized and evaluated will be more likely to survive for much more thorough evaluation and appropriate therapeutic intervention. Even the mildest evidence of significant injuries after high-impact trauma requires close observation and therapy in anticipation of additional problems.

If the initial examination reveals no evidence of major alterations in function or of discrete injury, a second examination should always be conducted soon after the initial cursory examination. Many patients suffering impact injury may, as a result of concussion, confusion, or anxiety, be less aware of pain and its location during the immediate postinjury period. Included in this secondary evaluation should be a careful search for injuries that may be aggravated if unrecognized. This includes a very cautious evaluation for evidence of injury to the cervical, thoracic, and lumbar spine, which might increase the possibility of neurologic damage during movement. At this point, the detailed search for evidence of head injury should include a history of concussion and a careful search for abrasion, superficial hematomas, periorbital or auditory canal and tympanic membrane hematomas, and cerebral spinal fluid drainage from the nose or ears. If any of the above are noted, skull roentgenograms and appropriate neurologic or neurosurgical consultation becomes mandatory. The evaluation of injury to the limbs and pelvis is less urgent, though important.

The more detailed evaluation of the thorax and lungs must include a directed search for evidence of injury. Cyanosis or marked tachypnea may be the earliest evidence of respiratory failure. The symmetry of the chest wall and evidence of soft tissue injury (hematoma and abrasion) should be noted during this early examination. Obvious asymmetry of respiratory movements generally indicates serious underlying disease. The position of the trachea and the apex beat of the heart help in identifying the position of the mediastinum. The conscious or even the semicomatose patient generally demonstrates pain on palpation of the chest-wall fractures. Palpation of the clavicles, the scapulae, the vertebral spines, the sternum, and each of the ribs, from anterior to posterior, generally elicits tenderness in the presence of fractures. In the absence of localized tenderness, evidence of rib fractures may be elicited by "springing the chest cage." This is accomplished in the anteroposterior diameter by placing the palm of the hand on the sternum and compressing toward the vertebral spine, with the patient lying flat in bed. The lateral diameter may be compressed by placing the palms of the hands, one on each side of the lateral chest cage, and pushing medially with each hand. Performing this maneuver in the midaxillary line over the lower ribs, the middle ribs, and the upper ribs frequently elicits pain not previously identified. Conversely, if this examination fails to reveal pain or tenderness in the conscious patient, the likelihood of significant fractures is markedly reduced. Obviously, the use of analgesics interferes with this evaluation. During the palpation, the distinctive, fine bubbly sensation of subcutaneous emphysema should be noted if present. *Subcutaneous emphysema* is air in the interstitial spaces and fascial planes, and, when present in large quantities, may result in severe swelling of the soft tissues. Percussion of the lung fields is particularly useful in the upright position and should permit identification of large accumulations of fluid or air in the pleural space. Auscultation of the lung fields permits more accurate definition of regional air entry and may identify the presence of airway obstruction or intrapulmonary fluid. This early examination is not complete without a chest roentgenogram, which may demonstrate the earliest evidence of disease, such as a pneumo- or hemothorax, aspiration pneumonia, pulmonary contusion, or widened mediastinum, and serves as a very important baseline for subsequent observation (Table 11-2). When at all possible, the chest roentgenogram should be obtained in the posteroanterior and lateral projections, with the patient as nearly upright as possible. Chest roentgenograms taken in the supine position, in the anteroposterior projection by portable equipment, frequently fail to demonstrate early evidence of pleural fluid, altered heart size, or retrocardiac disease. In most instances, an analysis of arterial blood gases is warranted to document problems with gas exchange and to serve as a baseline for subsequent complications.

Evaluation of the cardiovascular status is particularly critical. Hypovolemia may be recognized by increased pulse rate; decreased peripheral perfusion with cold, clammy, and perspiring skin; altered level of consciousness; or decreased urine output. A low venous pressure will be apparent under these circumstances. Injury to the heart may be evidenced by arrhythmia, electrocardiographic changes generally similar to those of ischemia, pericardial friction rub, or murmurs suggesting papillary muscle rupture or ventricular septal defect. Direct cardiac injury may result in increased central venous pressure, decreased cardiac filling, and hypotension. These findings most commonly result from pericardial tamponade, myocardial failure due to severe contusion, rupture of papillary muscle, or a traumatic ventricular septal defect. Evidence of mediastinal air is frequently first noted on auscultation of the heart.

Abdominal evaluation may be very difficult in these patients. Regardless of the degree of injury, bowel sounds are frequently present, with moderate generalized tenderness and some guarding related to the anxiety and pain resulting from other injuries. As a result, clinical assessment tends to be misleading, and roentgenographic evaluation is frequently of little help

TABLE 11-2. Clinical Features of Major Thoracic Injuries

Clinical Manifestations	Cause
Rib, sternal, clavicular fractures	Chest-wall trauma
Hemoptysis	Contusion of lung, laceration of trachea or bronchi
Hemothorax	Contusions or lacerations of parietal chest wall, visceral pleura, laceration of great vessels
Pneumothorax, pneumomediastinum, subcutaneous emphysema	Rupture of small airways, laceration of bronchi or trachea
Diffuse parenchymal pulmonary disease	See Table 11-5
Atelectasis	Obstruction by secretions, bronchial blood clots, lacerated bronchus
Consolidation	Contused lung, infection
Hypotension with low right atrial pressure	Blood loss: external or into body spaces
Hypotension with high right atrial pressure	Pericardial tamponade, myocardial contusion, heart-valve laceration, preexisting heart disease

during this early postinjury period. Even though the abdominal injury may not be apparent, a patient with hypovolemic hypotension without other obvious cause (or with other apparent cause but not responding to treatment of that cause) must be considered to have internal bleeding in the abdomen. The examination is not complete until a negative peritoneal lavage has been performed or until the abdomen has been explored.[9,10] A urinalysis must be obtained at this time to document urine output and identify hematuria, which demonstrates the presence of injury of the genitourinary tract.

Even with the most expert care of the initially apparent problems, a subsequent complete evaluation must be routinely conducted. When the life-sustaining and urgent matters have been dealt with, it becomes particularly important to know more about the patient's previous state of health and details regarding any previous disease, medications, or potential complications. Furthermore, because of the delayed evidence of some injuries, a new search for previously unrecognized problems and an analysis of the response to the initial therapeutic modalities are mandatory. Finally, with prolonged illness, metabolic and endocrine effects of the injury may become major considerations.[11]

Special problems must be considered in trauma to the pregnant woman. These have been reviewed in detail but will not be dealt with here.[10,11a]

The physician unwilling to commit this amount of time to the evaluation and management of the injured patient should not accept responsibility for his care. The multiplicity of injuries, their unpredictability, and the totally uncertain rate of development of overt clinical manifestations can only be dealt with by repetitive, completely comprehensive reevaluation.

CHEST-WALL INJURIES

Superficial Soft Tissue Injuries

Injuries involving the superficial soft tissues of the chest are generally important only if they are markers of more severe underlying injury. Abrasions, lacerations, and hematomas are of particular consequence when they suggest penetrating injury through the chest wall or associated blunt trauma to the underlying tissues. Where there is any question of deep penetrating injury, a thorough search for evidence of injury to underlying structures must be undertaken.

Rib Fractures

Table 11-3 is a classification of rib fractures that may be helpful in an approach to diagnosis and management.

Fracture of One Rib. *Clinical Manifestations.* Fracture of a single rib may occur in any location following minimal stress if the rib is dis-

TABLE 11-3. Classification of Rib Fractures

Injury	Major Manifestations, Related Injuries, and Common Complications
Fractures of One Rib	
Simple	Pain aggravated by deep breathing, coughing Localized tenderness Roentgenograms may or may not demonstrate fracture
Complicated	Pneumothorax, hemothorax Pulmonary infection or atelectasis
Multiple Rib Fractures	
With stable chest wall	Severe chest-wall pain Underlying lung contusion or contusion of opposite lung Decreased cough and accumulation of secretions Acute gastic dilatation Hemothorax, pneumomediastinum, and pneumothorax
With instability of chest wall	Generally involves fracture of each rib in two sites Panel of chest wall moves independent of thoracic cage (paradoxical respiration) Severely impaired cough and airway clearance Contusion of underlying lung Hemothorax and pneumothorax
Fractures of First Rib	Usually associated with fractures of clavicle and upper ribs May involve neurovascular structures of neck Intrathoracic injuries
Fractures of Lower Ribs (Seventh to twelfth)	Injuries to liver and spleen Acute gastric dilatation

eased. Thus, bone cysts and metastatic neoplasms involving ribs may result in fractures during very slight stresses that may have been completely unrecognized by the patient. Such fractures are referred to as pathologic fractures, indicating underlying rib pathology. An apparently normal rib may, however, be fractured with modest stress. The abrupt onset of chest pain after a severe bout of coughing or, occasionally, after a passionate embrace, suggests a fractured rib. Deep breathing, coughing, stooping, and lifting frequently elicit well-localized chest pain. This diagnosis is more likely when point tenderness can be elicited over the painful rib. Frequently, rib roentgenograms demonstrate the fracture; however, as indicated in Figure 11-1, this may be visible only when there is displacement of the ends of the fractures, or after 3 to 6 weeks when callus formation is established. Therefore, the diagnosis should be made on the basis of the history and clinical examination. The roentgenographic examination may confirm the diagnosis, but is particularly helpful in defining complications.

At one time, cough fractures of the rib were recognized most commonly in patients with pulmonary tuberculosis. In recent reports, the associated illness is less uniform. Large series of patients sustaining rib fractures without apparent underlying disease indicate that females under the age of 40 are most commonly affected (Table 11-4). The female predominance has not been explained; in fact, it is likely that many rib fractures go unreported, so that these figures may reflect physician visits rather than true occurrence of the problem. In this series, 30% of the patients had coughs without abnormal physical signs or roentgenographic abnormality suggesting underlying disease; 27% had chronic bronchitis; 13% had pneumonia; 10% had acute bronchitis; 8% had bronchiectasis; and 7% had other conditions, including pulmonary tuberculosis, bronchospasm, sarcoidosis, and pertussis. The final 5% included fractures caused by

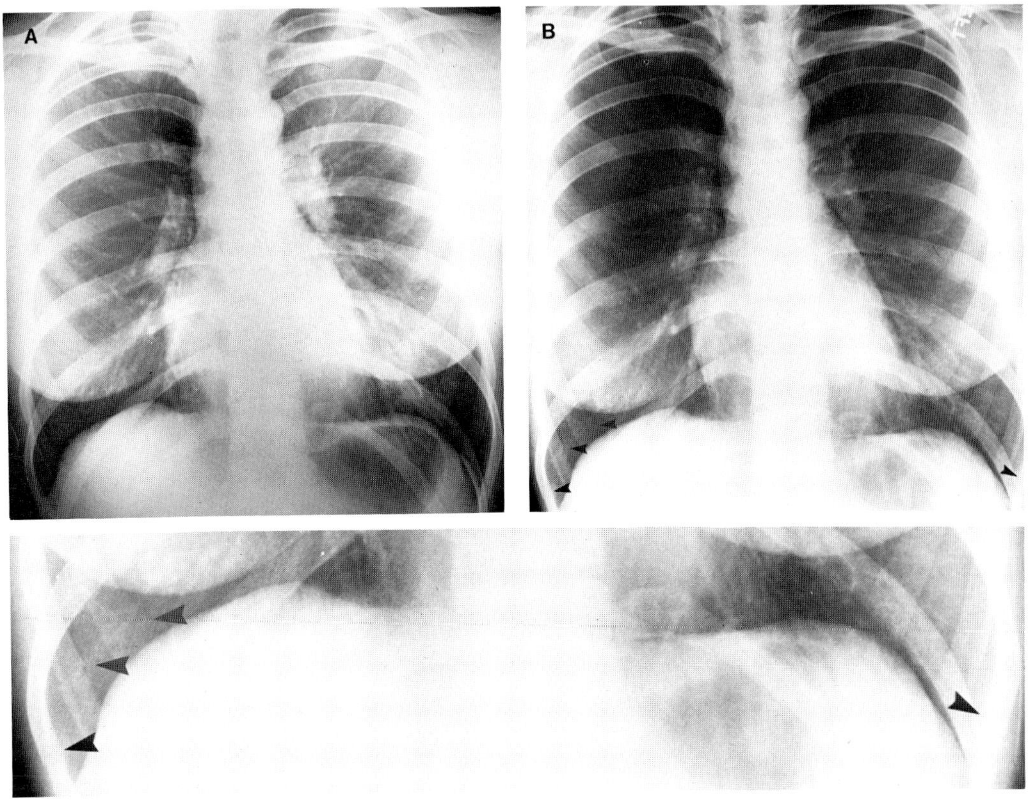

FIG. 11-1. Cough fractures of the ribs. **A.** This 29-year-old woman developed severe left-sided localized chest pain during a paroxysm of dry, hacking cough. In spite of well-demonstrated tenderness over the ninth rib in the mid-axillary line, no fracture was recognized on the initial chest roentgenogram. **B.** Within several days, the same patient developed similar severe chest pain on the right side during an episode of cough. This chest film, taken 5 weeks later, demonstrates the fracture of the ninth rib on the left, and the seventh, eighth, and ninth ribs on the right, as indicated by the arrows (*see enlargement*). Rib fractures are frequently best demonstrated roentgenographically when healing has begun. The physician should be prepared to make a clinical diagnosis of rib fractures when all the physical findings are present.

TABLE 11-4. Number of Persons with Cough Fractures Divided by Age and Sex

Age (years)	Men	Women	Total
0–19	0	1	1
20–29	0	10	10
30–39	2	16	18
40–49	9	9	18
50–59	11	4	15
60 +	6	3	9
Total	28	43	71

Wynn-Williams N, Young RD: "Cough" fracture of the ribs including one complicated by pneumothorax. Tubercle, 40:47, 1959

sneezing and by straightening up after stooping. Ten percent of patients had fractures on both sides at the same time, but in general, fractures were more common on the right than the left. Ninety-five percent of the fractures involved the fifth to tenth ribs. The seventh rib was affected most frequently, and the farther away a rib was from the seventh rib, the less likely it was to be fractured. The fracture generally occurs in the posterior axillary line. The first rib is most commonly fractured as a result of direct trauma that frequently results in fracture of the clavicle as well,[12] although stress fractures without gross trauma have been described.[13,14]

Fractures without significant trauma only occasionally result in pneumothorax or associated hemothorax. The patient with minor chest trauma and a single rib fracture generally has no related problems beyond those seen with the spontaneous fractures, although the incidence of hemo- and pneumothorax may be somewhat increased.

A syndrome of localized chest pain generally associated with subluxation of the lower costochondral junctions has been described, and frequently follows trauma. This slipping rib syndrome, occasionally called *traumatic intercostal neuritis*, is generally unilateral, involves the 8th to 10th ribs, and can be diagnosed by hooking the palpating fingers under the costal margin and springing the lower rib cage anteriorly. Surgical resection of the costochondral junction cures the pain.[3,15]

Management. The major concerns in the management of the rib fracture consist of alleviation of pain and prevention of secondary disease. Efforts to limit movement of the rib cage, and thus alleviate pain, may potentiate the development of retained secretions, inadequate clearance of the airways, and atelectasis or pneumonia (Fig. 11-2). Systemic analgesics may be used in doses that produce a minimum of respiratory depression, particularly in patients with underlying severe lung disease. Local analgesia may be provided by local anesthetic infiltrated at the site of the rib fracture or by an intercostal nerve block. The latter may be preferred, since the relief of pain tends to be more complete, and the procedure is quick and sure as described here. Utilizing a small-caliber needle (5 cm, 25-gauge is ideal) with a syringe containing the appropriate anesthetic solution, a small wheal is raised at the selected injection site. This is optimally in the region of the angle of the rib posteriorly and immediately adjacent to the paraspinal muscles. The needle is then advanced perpendicularly to the skin until the lower border of the rib is contacted. The needle is then withdrawn slightly, directed slightly inferiorly, and advanced about an eighth of an inch to enter the intercostal space. After withdrawing on the syringe to ensure that it is not in a vessel, the 5 ml of the anesthetic solution is injected. This generally provides relief of pain for several hours but frequently for much longer. Occasionally, two or three successive infiltrations permit sufficient relief of pain to require no further analgesia.

A paravertebral block is associated with substantially increased hazard as a result of involvement of the sympathetic chain and other nerves.

Chest strapping used to immobilize the ribs may be used, particularly in a patient with otherwise normal lungs. This should be performed by the placement of adhesive tapes, beginning well in front, covering and ending behind the site of the fracture, or by use of belts around the entire thorax. This is designed to immobilize the chest wall in that region, but is generally not very effective therapy.

Regardless of the treatment, pain and tenderness are generally much improved in 7 to 10 days; however, some pain on deep inspiration or cough may be experienced for 3 to 6 months. Healing is generally complete with stable ribs, free of pain, minimal displacement, and only roentgenographic evidence of the old fracture.

Multiple Rib Fractures with Stable Chest Wall. *Clinical Manifestations.* Chest trauma most commonly results in rib fractures in middle-aged or elderly persons, presumably because of decreased resilience of the bony and cartilaginous thorax. Children demonstrate rib fractures relatively infrequently. Thus, children frequently sustain major intrathoracic and intraabdominal injuries during the trauma without evidence of rib fractures.

Multiple rib fractures most commonly occur in the region of the seventh to tenth ribs.[3,12,16] In this location, particularly posteriorly, it is not uncommon to have laceration of the liver or spleen. Furthermore, acute gastric dilatation is common (Fig. 11-3). Multiple fractures are generally associated with severe localized chest-wall pain.

The major concern for patients with multiple rib fractures relates to impaired thoracic motion, injury to the underlying lung and pleura, and extrathoracic injuries (3).

The recognition of chest trauma may be dependent on the state of consciousness of the pa-

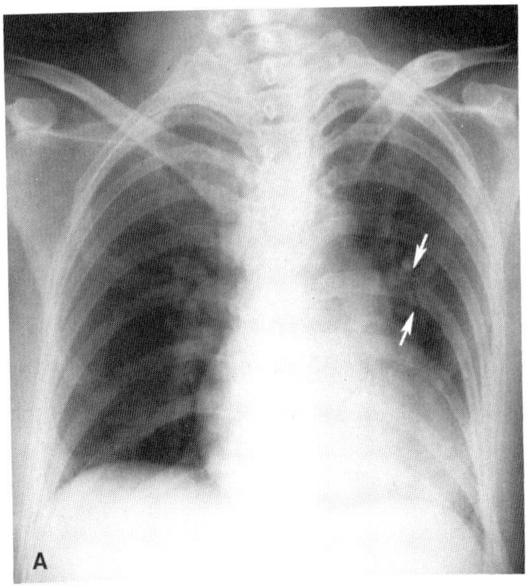

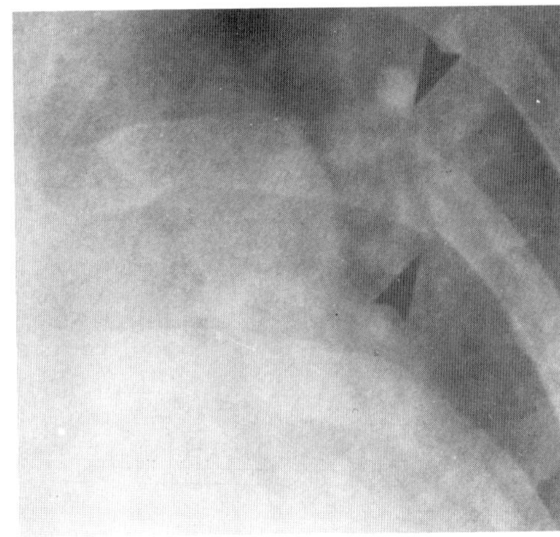

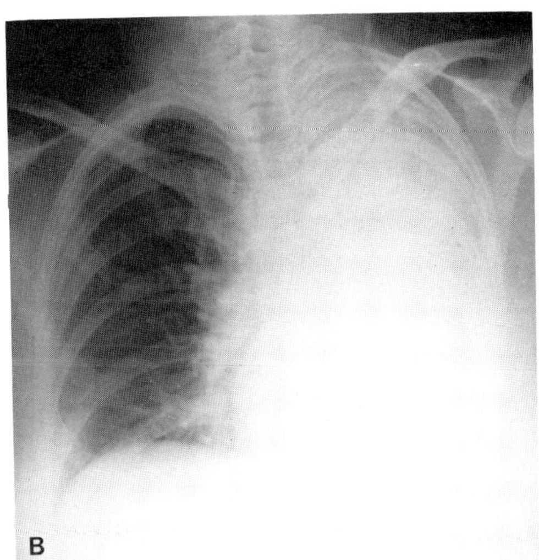

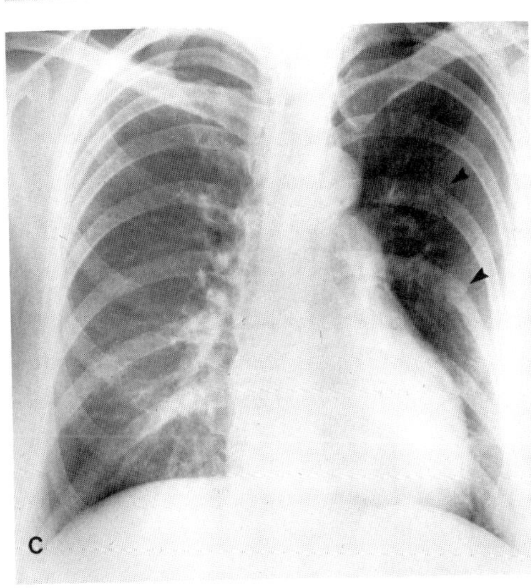

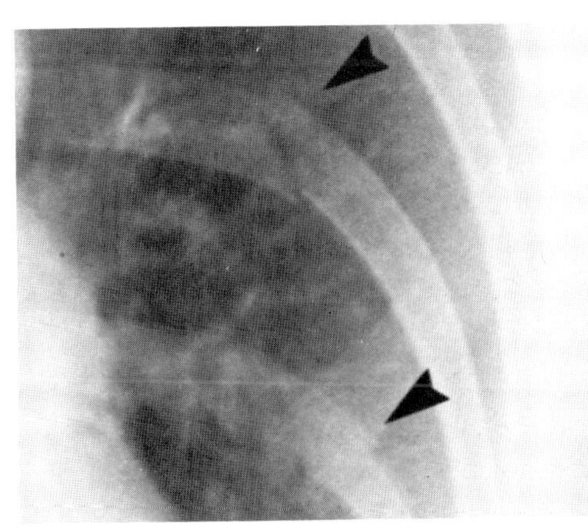

FIG. 11-2. Atelectasis as a result of rib fractures. **A.** This 32-year-old woman was admitted to the hospital after having been assaulted by her husband. In addition to widespread body abrasions and hematomas, she had an apparent clavicular fracture on the left and a left posterior rib fracture (*top arrows; see enlargement*). The initial chest film demonstrated probable atelectasis or consolidation of the left lower lobe. (Note the air bronchogram.) As a result of severe pain and systemic analgesia, she was immobile and lying flat in bed. **B.** Two days later, this film, demonstrating atelectasis of the entire left lung, suggested bronchial obstruction. She was bronchoscoped, and large amounts of tenacious purulent secretions were aspirated from the left main-stem bronchus and the left lower-lobe bronchus. A chest film taken within 3 hours of the bronchoscopy demonstrated approximately 90% reexpansion of the left lung. **C.** This film, taken 10 days later, reveals two fractured ribs (*bottom arrows*) with normal lung fields (*see enlargement*). This complication of infection and atelectasis can generally be avoided by vigorous tracheobronchial toilet, controlling the pain to permit adequate cough.

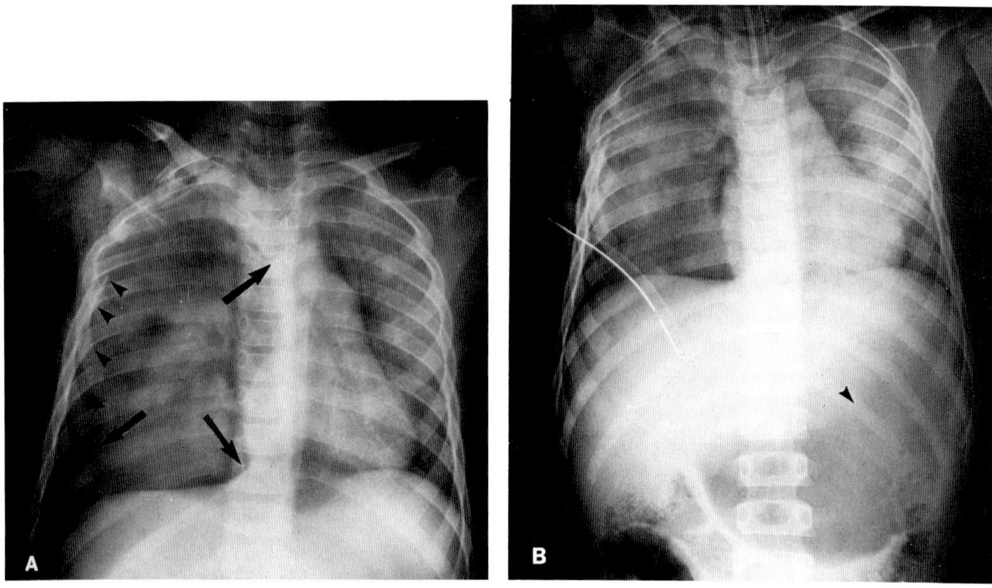

FIG. 11-3. Tension pneumothorax and acute gastric dilatation after severe blunt chest trauma. **A.** This 8-year-old lad was riding his bicycle across the freeway and was struck by an automobile. He was admitted to the hospital in severe respiratory distress, and the initial chest film demonstrated fracture of the right clavicle, multiple right rib fractures as indicated by the small arrows, and patchy density throughout both lung fields. In addition, a tension pneumothorax is apparent on the right, with shift of the mediastinum to the left. The margins of the pneumothorax are outlined by the large arrows. Note that the underlying contused lung has not completely collapsed, presumably as a result of the large fluid volume within the lung. Marked subcutaneous emphysema is apparent under the right shoulder joint, causing soft tissue swelling of the right lateral chest wall. **B.** Within 1 hour, a chest tube and an endotracheal tube are in position, but tremendous acute gastric dilatation is apparent in the region of the arrow. This complication could have been avoided by early insertion of a nasogastric tube.

tient at the time of injury. Thus, it is common for an alcoholic patient or one who has been transiently inebriated to present with chest pain without a history of trauma. When fully conscious, the major physical findings of chest-wall tenderness, localized pain, and soft tissue injury may be present. Roentgenograms of the chest (particularly oblique views taken with a high degree of penetration) delineate the bony structures in more detail. Occasionally, the documentation of the fracture will be complete only three to six weeks later, when healing has begun and callus formation around the site of the fracture is apparent roentgenographically. Frequently, in inveterate alcoholics, one can identify three to six old, healed, slightly misaligned fractures on the chest roentgenogram, although the patient is unaware of having sustained chest trauma. These "curb" fractures may have been sustained as a result of "curb," "lamp post," or "boot" impact.

With major impact injuries, it is not uncommon to have a line of fractures involving multiple ribs as evidence of the region of trauma. Complications are much more common with multiple than with single rib fractures, since the former generally reflect greater impact. Thus, 5% to 7% of such patients die as a result of cardiorespiratory complications, including pneumonia, atelectasis, and ventilatory failure.[3,12,16] There is evidence of pulmonary contusion in approximately 45%, pneumothorax in 12% to 25%, hemothorax in 4% to 12%, hemo- and pneumothorax in 9%, and evidence of myocardial contusion in 6%.

Fractures of the first two ribs frequently are

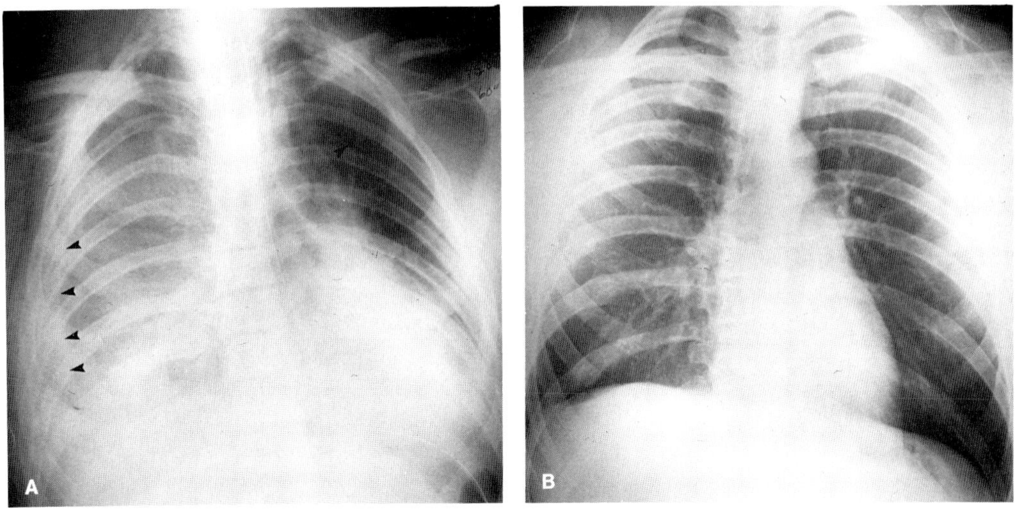

FIG. 11-4. Roentgenographic evidence of healing after major thoracic trauma. **A.** This 19-year-old motorcyclist was struck by an automobile. The initial chest films demonstrated the obvious left clavicular fracture, a large left pneumothorax as indicated by the arrow, a large right hemothorax as indicated by the arrows, and probable increased density of the lung parenchyma. Both pleural spaces were eventually drained with chest tubes, and he had a prolonged period of intenstive respiratory care. **B.** The follow-up film taken 1 year later demonstrates multiple healed rib fractures on the right, slight evidence of elevation of the right diaphragm, but otherwise entirely normal lung fields. This degree of recovery is characteristic, regardless of the severity of the initial apparent injuries.

associated with fractures of the clavicle, and may result in the thoracic outlet syndrome. This may be manifested by obstruction of the venous or arterial circulation or damage to the brachial plexus.[17] Whenever a first rib fracture is identified, multiple associated injuries should be sought.[14,18]

Management. As with single rib fractures, healing is almost always fairly quick and complete. Regardless of management, most rib fractures begin to be stable by 10 days to 3 weeks and are only tender on firm palpation by the end of 6 weeks. Healing appears to take place regardless of the degree of misalignment; presumably, the chest-wall tissues ensure adequate alignment in most instances. Even side-to-side displacement of fractured ends does not usually interfere with ultimate stability. Furthermore, it is uncommon for rib fractures to result in major degrees of deformity of the chest wall (Fig. 11-4).

The management of multiple rib fractures is similar to that outlined for fracture of a single rib, except that local analgesia tends to be less satisfactory, perhaps due to the increased mobility of the fractured bony thorax and the greater degree of surrounding tissue injury. The possibility of complications makes careful management of these patients urgent. Vigilant observation for the earliest evidence of respiratory failure is critical. Atelectasis, pneumonia, and retained secretions can generally be avoided by encouragement of deep breathing, support to the chest wall during spontaneous and requested coughing, nasotracheal suction if necessary, and treatment of underlying lung disease. In some patients, regular intermittent administration of systemic analgesics permits vigorous tracheal toilet and chest physiotherapy to be carried out more effectively.

Multiple Rib Fractures with Instability of the Chest Wall. *Clinical Manifestations.* The term *flail chest* is used to describe the condition in which a portion of the chest wall moves in a direction opposite to the rest of the thorax. During inspiration, when the thorax normally expands in all its diameters, the negative intrapleural pressure may cause indrawing of an unstable panel of the chest wall. Similarly, on exhalation, when the remainder of the thorax is decreasing in volume, the chest-wall panel tends to remain stable or appears to move in an outward direction if there is any degree of expiratory obstruction. This condition generally results from fractures of three or more ribs in at least two locations, so that the continuity of the bony thorax is interrupted. Most characteristically, this occurs as a result of bilateral rib fractures after a steering-wheel injury. Occasionally, the fractures involve ribs at one end and costochondral junctions at the other end of the unstable panel. Sternal fractures are particularly likely to result in increased mobility of a portion of the chest wall.

For many years, it was stated that instability of the chest wall affecting one hemithorax resulted in paradoxical ventilation. It was reasoned that the lung surrounded by the mobile panel would not fill during inhalation because of the mobility of the panel but would fill during exhalation when the positive pressure in the tracheobronchial tree and the normally functioning lung would force air into the side involved with the "flail chest." This phenomenon was referred to as *Pendelluft*,[19] a German term for pendulum-like action of the air. Although this concept is widely cited in standard textbooks, it does not follow physiologic principles. Regardless of what is happening to the chest-wall panel, the underlying lung remains inflated if there is a negative intrapleural pressure. The presence of flail chest may permit the intrapleural pressure to be less negative during inspiration, but this simply decreases the volume on inhalation of the affected portion of the lung and similarly decreases the amount that is left to be exhaled during expiration. Therefore, the unstable chest panel generally does not cause ventilation to be paradoxical, but simply reduced.

The major result of a flail panel is to diminish the effectiveness of ventilation. This has been clearly demonstrated in animals[19,20] and in humans.[21] Decreased thoracic motion resulting from pain and associated splinting of the chest wall also impairs ventilation. In addition, the unstable panel of the chest wall reduces the peak intrapleural pressure that can be generated during cough or maximum inflation of the lungs.

Studies in dogs have confirmed the clinical impression that a flail panel alone does not cause hypoxemia. The hypoxemia is related to underlying lung disease, generally contusion. Animals with a flail chest and contusion did not have greater hypoxemia than animals with contusion alone.[20]

Injury to the lung itself is very common when impact injuries are severe enough to cause a flail panel. These lung injuries include hemothorax, pneumothorax, and lung contusion. Clinical studies of lung function generally demonstrate reduced lung compliance, increased airway resistance, and hypoxemia probably resulting from regional low ventilation–perfusion ratios.[21,22]

Numerous centers have evaluated the incidence of the flail chest in patients suffering major blunt chest trauma.[2,3,8,22–24] A tabulation of approximately comparable patient groups will demonstrate that as many as 30% to 40% of patients admitted with major thoracic impact injuries can be expected to have this problem.

In general, the mortality rate among flail chest patients ranges from 20% to 50%. In a group of patients with flail chest who died acutely in the emergency room, the causes of death were multiple fractures, liver lacerations, or rupture of the spleen resulting in acute hypovolemia.[22] In the patients who died within two days of admission, craniocerebral trauma and acute hypovolemia related to intra-abdominal or retroperitoneal bleeding were the most common causes of death. Severe respiratory failure and pulmonary hemorrhage accounted for a small number of deaths. In patients who survived for two days with hospital care but ultimately died, acute bacterial bronchopneumonia, pulmonary edema, aspiration pneumonia, fat embolism, thromboembolism, tension pneumothorax, and intrapulmonary hemorrhage were pulmonary causes of death, whereas perforated duodenal ulcer, renal failure, complications of tracheostomy, and cerebral complications accounted for a small number of deaths.[12,22]

Equally interesting is an analysis of the course

of those who survived with flail chest trauma. The average stay in the hospital was 30 days. Associated injuries included multiple fractures (31%); blunt trauma to the abdomen, requiring laparotomy (29%); and associated craniocerebral injuries (18%). Thus, according to several studies,[6,8,19,22] it would appear that the major determinant of survival is the associated injury. In a recent report of 35 consecutive patients with flail chest, there was only one death, suggesting that mortality may have improved with modern management.[25]

Management. Managing patients with flail chest injury requires a great deal of skill and judgment. The patient with minimal movement of the chest wall panel and no underlying pleural or pulmonary disease tolerates the injury very well and, aside from mild degrees of hypoxemia, has local pain as his major problem. Such a patient requires careful observation, as with other rib fractures, in view of the fact that ventilatory embarrassment may result in atelectasis and infection.

Patients with more severe instability of the chest wall must be evaluated intensively. Unfortunately, due to the severity of injury and frequent alterations in sensorium (owing to head injury or analgesics), it is generally impossible to make a reliable measurement of ventilatory reserve (*e.g.*, the vital capacity). Hypoxia may be suspected clinically as a result of evidence of cerebral hypoxia or cyanosis, but it is best assessed by sequential determination of the arterial Po_2. In the most severe degrees of flail chest injury, the alveolar ventilation is substantially impaired, and the arterial Pco_2 rises. Hypoxemia may be managed by increased concentrations of inspired oxygen; however, when progressive respiratory failure is documented by decreasing arterial Po_2 or rising Pco_2, more dramatic intervention may be necessary.

In years gone by, mechanical aids were used to stabilize the chest wall.[26,27] Sandbags placed tightly along the bony thorax to decrease mobility or, in selected instances, insertion of screws into the appropriate portion of the bony thorax, permitted external traction to decrease mobility of the panel. This external immobilization was an effort to decrease the "paradoxical" movement of the chest. More recently, surgical reinforcement of the rib cage by metal plates or wires has been suggested for patients with severe anterior flail, which generally includes sternal fractures.[28,29] In most patients, internal splinting of the mobile chest-wall panel is very effectively provided by mechanical ventilation.[25,30,31]

The patient with chest-wall instability and severe respiratory failure is best managed by establishing a tracheal airway and by providing continuous controlled ventilation. For optimal care, the patient must not be permitted to make an inspiratory effort, since that creates a negative intrapleural pressure and retracts the mobile panel. When each breath is initiated by positive pressure from the respirator, the panel moves with the remainder of the chest wall, splinting the chest wall by inflation of the lung and thus permitting effective ventilation. Patients requiring this dramatic and sophisticated form of therapy occasionally require high levels of sedation and analgesia to eliminate their own respiratory drive, and occasionally are best controlled by the use of modest doses of muscle relaxants. Such complex respiratory care is discussed in detail in Chapter 7, and should be initiated only by those skilled in the management of respirator-dependent patients.

For several years, it was considered optimal to manage every patient with flail chest of notable size by use of an artificial ventilator. It now is apparent that, with good judgment, some patients may be spared this drastic form of therapy. In general, patients who are adequately oxygenated with supplemental oxygen in reasonable concentrations and who do not develop an increase in arterial Pco_2 do not require this form of ventilation, regardless of the size of the flail chest.[32,33] On the other hand, patients whose oxygenation deteriorates quickly after the injury, who are inadequately ventilated as indicated by their own sense of dyspnea and use of accessory muscles, or who have increasingly elevated arterial Pco_2 should have controlled ventilation established without delay. On general principles, anticipate that controlled ventilation, when instituted, will be necessary throughout the period of healing of rib fractures or until the mobile chest wall becomes fixed. Fortunately, when the effects of lung contusion, aspiration, pneumonia, and other acute injuries to pulmonary parenchyma are resolved during the first 7 to 10 days,[23] it is common to see a decrease in the pulmonary resistance and less severe degrees of paradoxical movement of the chest wall, thus permitting ventilation with lower intrapleural pressures. Since no evidence is available to indicate that ultimate healing of the chest wall, degree of deformity, or misalignment is substantially improved by prolonged controlled ventilation, the respirator may be discontinued at this stage. The clinical manifestations of respiratory failure, as commonly evaluated for other conditions, remain reliable criteria for instituting and discontinuing assisted ventilation.

Sternal Fractures

Clinical Manifestations. Fractures of the sternum are generally recognized by localized pain, soft tissue injury, and occasionally by displacement and mobility of the chest wall. Commonly, these symptoms are associated with the so-called steering-wheel injury and bilateral flail chest. The fracture of the sternum is rarely identified in the posteroanterior view of the chest roentgenogram; more commonly, the fracture can be localized in a good lateral roentgenogram of the chest. The fracture generally occurs in the body of the sternum or in the region just below the manubriosternal junction. It is uncommon for fractures to occur in the adult at the angle of Louis.[12]

Management. In general, the outcome is determined by the associated injuries. Respiratory failure is a common accompaniment if there is a marked degree of flail chest. In those persons with severe respiratory failure, the major therapeutic consideration is adequate ventilatory support. In general, the fracture heals in about the same time as rib fractures.[27]

PLEURAL SPACE DISEASE

Hemothorax

Clinical Manifestations. A marked unilateral decrease in movement of the chest wall during respiration should alert the examiner to the likelihood of pleural space disease. A large pneumothorax is more frequent than a large hemothorax, but the differentiation is generally not difficult clinically. Smaller amounts of fluid in the pleural space can be identified only by appropriate chest roentgenograms.

When clinical evidence of a pleural effusion is recognized by physical examination of the chest, by chest roentgenogram during the posttrauma period, or in patients with chest-wall injuries, the most likely diagnosis is a hemothorax. Various authors differ regarding the site of origin of blood in hemothorax. Bleeding may arise from contused visceral or parietal pleura, from avulsion and laceration at the site of pleural adhesions, or as a result of puncture and laceration of the lung by a protruding rib fracture.[34] It is likely that bleeding generally arises from venous vessels. This bleeding from low-pressure vessels is more likely to stop spontaneously than that from systemic arterial vessels. Penetrating chest wounds, discussed below, more frequently result in severe, continuing bleeding from systemic or pulmonary arterial vessels. Hemothorax with or without associated pneumothorax occurs in 25 % to 60% of patients with major chest trauma.[2,3,8,24]

The consequences of a hemothorax are debated. Although it has been clearly documented that pleural thickening, occasionally resulting in restriction of lung movement on the affected side, may follow the occurrence of a hemothorax, it has not been demonstrated that it is the presence of the blood in the pleural space that is responsible for this reaction (Fig. 11-5). Furthermore, aside from very large hemothoraces, it is not entirely clear that organization of the blood in the pleural space results in chronic thickening of the pleural tissue.[35] Animal experiments have demonstrated that the injection of blood into the pleural space results in minimal pleural reaction and reabsorption of the intact erythrocytes into the circulation.[35] When 30% of the animal's blood volume was injected into the pleural space, 61% was absorbed into the circulation in 90 hours. Furthermore, virtually the entire amount of blood was absorbed into the circulation in 5 to 6 days. These findings indicate that a normal pleura, presented with a large

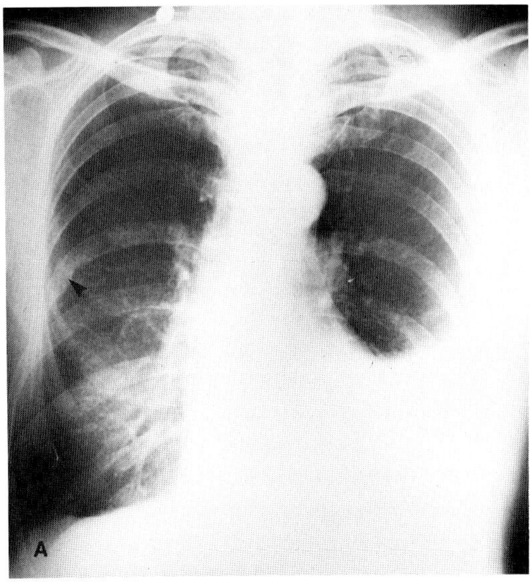

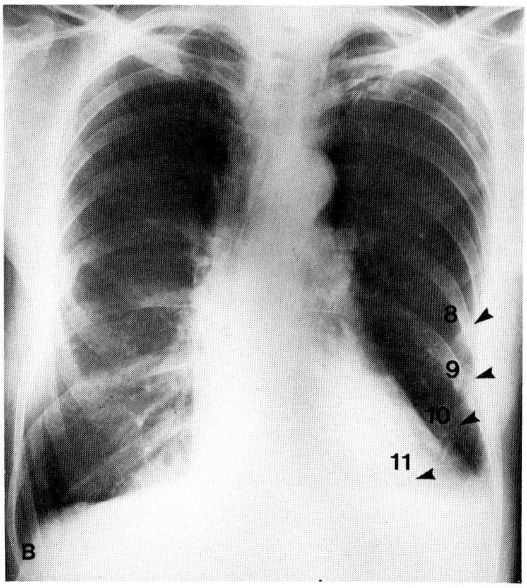

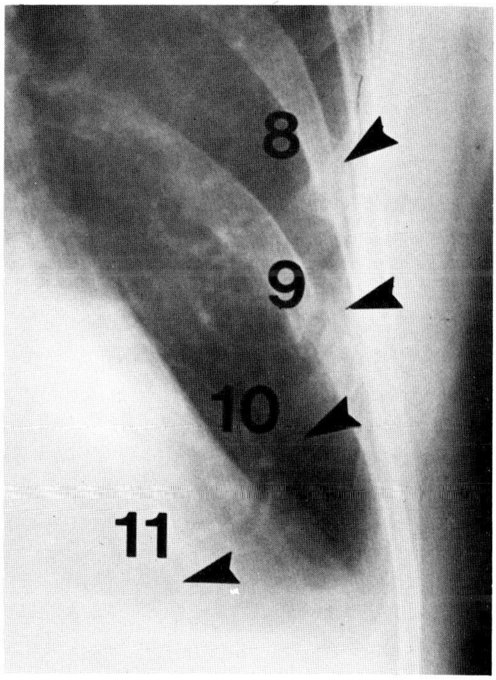

FIG. 11-5. Pleural thickening after hemothorax. This 65-year-old man presented with increasing dyspnea. He had all the clinical manifestations of chronic obstructive pulmonary disease. The chest film (**A**) demonstrates a large left pleural effusion. Thoracentesis was performed, aspirating more than 1,000 ml. of bloody fluid. Note the healed rib fracture on the right, indicated by the arrow. The postthoracentesis films demonstrated multiple rib fractures on the left. Careful review of his history indicated that he had sustained what he considered an inconsequential fall 6 weeks prior to the film. In spite of complete aspiration of the fluid, some organization of pleural fluid or pleural thickening had developed, and a film obtained 2 months later (**B**) reveals marked blunting of the left costophrenic angle, which was stable in the lateral decubitus position. This degree of pleural change is not uncommon when the hemothorax has not been initially evacuated. Note the callus formation around the healing rib fractures of the 8th, 9th, 10th, and 11th ribs (*see enlargement*).

amount of whole blood, is capable of complete reabsorption of the fluid and cells with no residual changes. It is not so certain, however, that a pleura that has been injured by trauma and whose drainage system may have been damaged as a result of an impact injury and associated inflammatory reaction will respond similarly. Extensive experience with penetrating wounds and blunt chest trauma suggests that a hemothorax in itself rarely causes long-term serious sequelae; however, empyema, residual hemothorax, and persistent atelectasis are complications in 5% to 10% of patients with hemothorax.[37–39]

Other uncommon causes of effusion in the post-traumatic patient include chylothorax as a result of trauma to the thoracic duct or other major lymphatic channels; empyema as a result of infection of the pleural space; and pleural effusions that may result from trauma to the pancreas and resultant acute pancreatitis (see Chap. 12).

Management. A minimal hemothorax with obliteration of the costophrenic angle (300–500 ml) is generally free of complications and will probably clear rapidly, leaving a normal chest roentgenogram, within 10 to 14 days. This primarily requires observation, because further accumulation and bleeding may occur. A moderate hemothorax, which fills about one third of the pleural space (500–1000 ml), occasionally with evidence of lung compression and loss of circulating blood volume, requires immediate drainage and replacement of intravascular volume. A large hemothorax, which fills half or more of the hemithorax, (more than 1000 ml) generally indicates that blood is coming from larger high-pressure vessels, such as the intercostal or internal mammary artery. This requires immediate drainage, and if the bleeding persists and continued infusion of blood is required, a thoracotomy to stop bleeding may become necessary. No fixed value can be stated for the amount of blood loss that warrants an early thoracotomy; however, the severity of continued bleeding, the general state of the patient, and the availability of highly skilled personnel to provide the surgical support should determine the indications.[34]

A large hemothorax should be evacuated to improve ventilation of underlying lung, to avoid any possibility of secondary pleural complications, and to prevent persistent atelectasis. The ideal method of evacuation has not been established. Repetitive thoracentesis, to provide as complete drainage as possible, and large-bore continuous tube drainage are both effective in preventing significant degrees of fibrothorax. Continuous tube drainage has the advantage of generally providing more complete drainage of the pleural space and allowing for careful monitoring of the degree of bleeding during the acute phase. Repetitive thoracentesis may be associated with a decreased incidence of infection, though this is not established. Concerns that pleural drainage may aggravate bleeding by creating a more negative pressure in the pleural space appear to be unwarranted.[12]

Several studies have suggested the use of fibrinolytic agents to decrease the degree of fibrin deposition and organization of blood in the pleural space. The results in those reports are no better than those reported in the absence of fibrinolytic agents with acceptable pleural drainage.[12]

The large experience with nondrained hemothorax as reported in the post-World War II literature suggested that fibrothorax was a late complication of untreated hemothorax. Although many of these patients had open wounds and infected hemothoraces, it is likely that some persons with an undrained hemothorax for a prolonged period of time develop severe pleural reaction and "organizing" hemothorax. Current experience indicates that empyema is no more common in patients treated by tube drainage than in those treated by thoracotomy.[38] Furthermore, surgical evacuation of residual hemothorax and early decortication are rarely indicated.[38–40]

Occasionally, in patients with an infected hemothorax, poor re-expansion of lung, and inadequate response to tube drainage, surgical evacuation of the pleural space and removal of early fibrothorax is necessary.[38,39]

Pneumothorax

Clinical Manifestations. Pneumothorax occurs after severe trauma to the thorax, in as high as 15% to 40% of patients.[2,3,8,24] The earliest manifestation may be the presence of subcutaneous emphysema, indicating that air has dissected through the fascial planes to the subcutaneous space. The most striking clinical manifestation of a large pneumothorax is that the affected hemithorax appears larger in volume than the unaffected side but moves less with respiratory movement. As discussed in Chapter 12, this is a result of an increased intrathoracic volume when air occupies the pleural space. Furthermore, hyperresonance to percussion and the classical auscultatory signs of decreased air entry are present on the affected side. Since the pneumothorax frequently arises as a result of laceration of the pleura or bronchi, the possibility of a valve-like mechanism developing, resulting in a tension pneumothorax, should constantly be borne in mind. Occasionally, the finding that raises suspicion regarding pneumothorax is the clinical detection of mediastinal emphysema. This may be recognized by the crunching or bubbling sound (frequently with distinct, high-pitched, almost metallic components), modified by respiration, but synchronous with the heartbeat. First described by Hamman in relation to spontaneous mediastinal emphysema,[41] it is likely that this sound is generated as a result of air being moved within the fascial planes of the mediastinum adjacent to the cardiac chambers. Although mediastinal emphysema may occur spontaneously,[42] it frequently accompanies trauma of the chest with or without gross evidence of pneumothorax. The mechanism of air entering the mediastinum is not established; however, most authors believe that it indicates trauma to alveoli or bronchi, with dissection of air along the vessels or bronchi to the mediastinal structures.

Occasionally, blunt chest trauma is associated with air embolism. Although this has been more frequently found in association with blast injuries and is difficult to establish in the individual patient, it is possible that high intrapulmonary pressures, resulting from an impact injury when the glottis is closed, result in dissection of air through traumatized vessel walls into systemic or pulmonary veins. Most commonly, air embolism is a result of penetrating lung injuries.[43]

Pneumoperitoneum may result from mediastinal air or pneumothorax, but is more likely to occur during artificial ventilation.[44] It is particularly important to distinguish this from a perforated hollow organ in the abdomen.

Management. The management of pneumothorax in association with trauma is generally the same as for pneumothorax that occurs spontaneously, as discussed in Chapter 12. Small pneumothoraces (less than 20%) may require no treatment. A large pneumothorax should be evacuated, permitting expansion of the underlying lung. A tension pneumothorax requires urgent intervention. Furthermore, the association of a pneumothorax with a hemothorax should generally be considered more ominous, and drained by continuous tube drainage until the rate at which the bleeding and air leak are occurring is established. In patients with a large pneumothorax who continue to have an air leak during continuous drainage, surgical closure of the lacerated lung may be required. Infrequently, the continued air leak is a result of a persistent penetration of lung by misaligned bony fragments of ribs.[23,24] These are usually clearly apparent by the character of the fractures seen on roentgenograms. A large persistent air leak should be evaluated for the possibility of a ruptured bronchus (discussed in detail below).

LUNG TRAUMA

Lung Laceration

Clinical Manifestations. Lung laceration may result in pneumothorax, hemothorax, pulmonary hematoma, traumatic pseudocyst, and massive hemoptysis.[3,45–49] Severe persistent pneumothorax and hemothorax are frequently associated with displaced rib fractures, but more frequently appear to result from sheering forces.[45]

Pulmonary hematomas are seen radiographically as localized densities. Post-traumatic pseudocysts or pneumatoceles occur most frequently in children or young adults. Although these patients may have associated hemoptysis or pneumothorax, the problem presents radiographically as single or multiple cavities, with or without fluid levels. The cavities generally have thick, irregular surrounding walls and may be multiloculated. They may be present immediately after trauma, or appear several days later. They are generally thought to result from laceration of lung parenchyma with surrounding hemorrhage or contusion, but occasionally represent loculated air in the oblique or horizontal fissures.[47–49]

Management. Lung lacerations require specific treatment only in the event of persistent bleeding or pneumothorax. The indications are summarized in the list below, and are discussed in relation to each condition.

Indications for Thoracotomy Following Blunt Chest Trauma

Emergency
- Sucking wounds of the chest
- Hemothorax with uncontrolled bleeding
- Severe persistent pneumothorax
- Bronchial laceration
- Ruptured diaphragm
- Cardiac or aortic tear
- Ruptured esophagus (rare)

Elective
- Residual large hemothorax or empyema

Pulmonary hematoma and pseudocyst should be recognized so as to avoid confusion with other causes of lung masses, or lung cavities. No specific treatment is required, and chest films clear in 2 to 6 weeks.

Lung Contusion

Clinical Manifestations. Respiratory failure can occur in the injured patient as a result of the mechanical effects of chest-wall and pleural injuries discussed to this point. Fractures and injuries involving the chest wall may result in muscle spasm or voluntary splinting of the chest, with decreased ventilatory effectiveness. Space-occupying material in the pleural cavity, including hemothorax and pneumothorax, may decrease aeration of the lungs. However, the hypoxemia that invariably occurs in these patients, the decrease in lung compliance, the increase in airway resistance, and the reduced diffusing capacity cannot be readily explained on the basis of the simple mechanical effects of chest-wall or pleural injury.[20,21,23] These additional functional derangements more likely result from parenchymal injury. Relatively minor degrees of parenchymal injury may be functionally more significant in the patient with an unstable chest wall or pleural-space disease.

Blunt chest trauma may result in lung contusion, with laceration of tissues, bleeding, hemoptysis, airways obstruction, and respiratory failure (Fig. 11-6).

Studies of closed-chest mechanical trauma to dog lungs[50] demonstrated roentgenographic findings within 24 to 48 hours, consisting of focal discoid atelectasis, peribronchial infiltration, and, in more advanced lesions, frank consolidation that did not follow lobar distribution patterns. These animals uniformly developed hypoxemia and hyperventilation when breathing spontaneously. Additional studies demonstrated decreased ventilation and perfusion of contused lobes.[47] Although hypoxemia improved, lung contusion was aggravated by continuous positive-pressure breathing. Studies on postmortem lungs demonstrated marked abnormalities of regional lung emptying, indicated by obstruction of airways, with poor deflation of some areas of lung. Surfactant levels were normal within the first 24 hours but had decreased by 48 hours. Pathologically, these lungs demonstrated fragmented alveolar walls, large amounts of interstitial and alveolar hemorrhage, and marked atelectasis alternating with areas of trapped air. Areas of lung with more extensive involvement showed marked intraalveolar, interstitial, and bronchial lumen edema.

In blast injuries, which occur most commonly in military combat, a very high energy release from an explosive source results in a pressure wave traveling radially through the atmosphere. It is postulated that when the pressure front travels from one medium to another of less density, such as when crossing the fluid-air interfaces of the delicate pulmonary alveoli, there occurs at the interface considerable local tension that results in fragmentation of tissues. Thus, edema and hemorrhage may occur. This is known as a *spalling effect*, and its relative importance, compared to simple pressure differentials that occur as a result of the pressure wave passing from the air to the liquid phase of the lung, is not certain. It is likely that marked pressure differentials occurring between the liquid and air phases in the lung may result in fragmentation of the tissues. Furthermore, pressure waves that strike the chest wall when the glottis is closed may result in significant tissue injury. Several studies have indicated that the presence of a

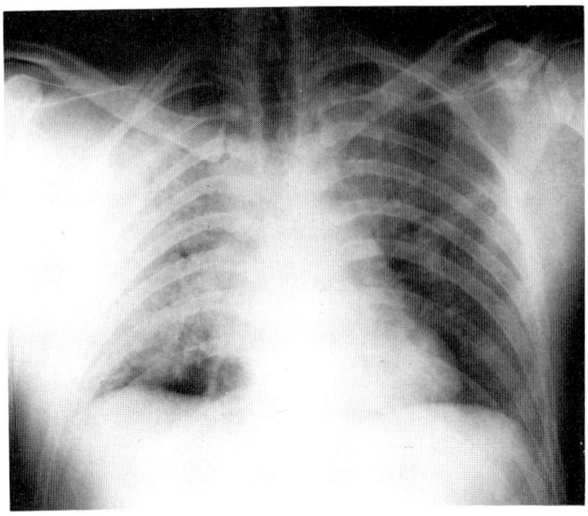

FIG. 11-6. Pulmonary contusion. This 33-year-old driver of a pickup truck struck an overpass abutment on a major highway. He sustained extensive cerebral, abdominal, and extremity injuries in addition to major thoracic trauma. This initial chest film demonstrates the asymmetrical pulmonary parenchymal densities commonly seen in pulmonary contusion. Aside from the early appearance of these densities, there are no categorically distinguishing features from other conditions that may have caused posttraumatic pulmonary infiltrates, as summarized in the section on contused lungs (Table 11-5).

pneumothorax actually protects the lungs from blast injury, perhaps owing to the compressibility of the pneumothorax, and it has been demonstrated that a tracheostomy (by-passing the glottis) may diminish damage to lung tissues in experimental studies.[51]

Table 11-5 illustrates the other factors that may be important in causing parenchymal abnormalities during the postinjury period[52–60] (Fig. 11-6).

Aspiration pneumonia is frequently a result of vomiting or regurgitation at the time of injury when the airway is not well controlled. This may subsequently be avoided by maintaining an empty stomach until the patient is well enough to cough in response to foreign material in the airway, or until a cuffed tracheal tube is in position. Aspiration results in abnormalities of lung function within minutes to hours.

Infection is generally not an early phenomenon, but tends to occur 3 to 7 days after the initial injury. The classical manifestations of pulmonary infection (including purulent sputum, fever, and leukocytosis) and the presence of infecting organisms, which may be demonstrated by microscopic examination and cultures of sputum, help to differentiate this process from other pulmonary lesions. There is no evidence that prophylactic antibiotics prevent secondary infections or improve the outcome of patients with contused lungs.[8]

Thromboembolism occurs in a significant number of patients who are immobilized for prolonged periods following injury. The incidence of this complication is totally unknown, and its significance in the respiratory outcome is not established. Only when the commonly recognized criteria are present can this diagnosis be entertained with confidence.

Fat embolism, notoriously difficult to establish except when the syndrome is florid, generally occurs within the first 18 to 72 hr after the injury. This is discussed below.

In persons developing progressive respiratory failure, with increased opacity of the lungs on chest roentgenogram, the possibility of pulmonary edema must always be entertained. Although the pulmonary edema may be on a classical hydrostatic hemodynamic basis, resulting from left ventricular failure or excessive fluid replacement,[58,59] there is substantial evidence accumulating that suggests the integrity of the pulmonary capillary may be altered, causing fluid to be lost from the lumen of the capillary in spite of normal hydrostatic pressures. This pulmonary edema may develop at any time in the course of the patient's disease, depending on the factors that are producing it. It is said that alterations in capillary permeability are more likely to occur in relation to contusion or immediately following a severe hypotensive period. Other studies have not confirmed hypotension as a potentiating feature of post-traumatic respiratory failure.[54] Microaggregates in transfused

TABLE 11-5. Factors Producing Stiff Lungs After Trauma

Pathological Process	Time of Onset of Respiratory Failure
Contusion	Within 24 hr of injury
Aspiration pneumonia	Immediate
Infection	3 days or more after injury
Thromboembolism	3 days or more after injury
Fat embolism	8 to 96 hr after injury
Pulmonary edema resulting from increased hydrostatic pressure	
Fluid overload	Anytime
Left ventricular failure	Anytime, depending on cardiovascular status
Central nervous system injury	Hours to days after injury
Decreased colloid/osmotic pressure: low serum albumin	Generally related to replacement of blood volume with crystalloids
Oxygen toxicity	5 or more days on high-inspired oxygen
Toxic factors from injury to other tissues	
Endotoxin	Unknown
Vasoactive peptides, kinins, prostaglandins	Unknown
Platelets, leukocytes, hemolysed erythrocytes	Unknown
Amniotic fluid	Unknown
Myoglobin	Unknown
Multiple transfusions	Unknown

blood may play a role in lung injury, a hypothesis that has resulted in increasing use and evaluation of blood filters.[59,60] Lungs with increased permeability are much more sensitive to changes in capillary hydrostatic pressure, and may develop severe edema with modest excess fluid.[57-62]

Injury to the central nervous system may be associated with pulmonary edema, which is not readily explained on the basis of other causes. Increased intracranial pressure is associated with pulmonary edema in animals,[63-67] which has been attributed to alpha-adrenergic constriction of pulmonary veins with increased hydrostatic pressure, and more recently to increased capillary permeability.[67] There are no convincing hemodynamic studies in humans to clarify the mechanism. Furthermore, the nature of central nervous system insult that may predispose humans to pulmonary edema has not been established.

We have observed one patient with severe respiratory failure owing to bilateral diaphragm paralysis following blunt chest trauma[68] and subsequent correspondence indicated this uncommon complication has been observed by others (see Chap. 6 for the effects of diaphragm paralysis).

In patients who have received very high concentrations of inspired oxygen for a prolonged period of time, oxygen toxicity is a serious consideration after the third to fourth day (see Chap. 7).

The patient developing post-traumatic pulmonary insufficiency may have one or more of the above factors contributing to lung damage; the specific factors are frequently impossible to delineate. Furthermore, the possibility of pulmonary parenchymal damage resulting from injurious agents released after nonpulmonary tissue damage has been considered. Endothelial damage has been attributed to a wide range of potentially injurious agents. Complement activation, platelet factors, vasoactive peptides, prostaglandins, histamine, fibrin deposition, and fibrinolysis have all been implicated in one scheme or other,[52-60] but none has been conclusively established as the dominant agent. Since intravascular leucocytes are sequestered in capillaries where they may degranulate and disintegrate, the release of leucocyte proteolytic enzymes or superoxide radicals may be important, but the evidence is incomplete.[55,69-73]

These uncertainties have given rise to terms such as *traumatic wet lung*, *shock lung*, *white lung syndrome*, and *acute respiratory distress syndrome*; that have no diagnostic significance. Each specific potential cause must be considered separately and treatment instituted appropriately.

Management. Management of the contused lung is similar to the management of other causes of the acute respiratory distress syndrome discussed in detail in Chapter 7. Survival rates depend on the nature of the underlying injury, the severity of associated injuries (particularly central nervous system injury) and complications such as renal failure and infection. Although many surgeons urge early institution of respirator management, this approach may aggravate lung contusion,[61] and there is no convincing data that suggests lung injury is reduced or survival improved by this treatment, when compared with treatment on the basis of respiratory failure.[52] Most patients who survive, recover normal or near normal function,[74] but occasionally progress to develop lung fibrosis.[75]

FAT EMBOLISM

Clinical Manifestations. Following the fracture of long bones, pelvis, or ribs, it is not uncommon for patients to develop a syndrome suggestive of diffuse small vessel disease. These patients may have evidence of central nervous system alterations including mild confusion, ranging through an entire spectrum of diffuse cerebral disease to coma and seizures. They usually exhibit respiratory distress characterized by tachypnea, dyspnea, and a marked decrease in arterial Po_2. Petechial hemorrhages occur in the skin, classically more prominently along the anterior axillary folds but also across the chest and in the flanks. Occasionally, petechiae are found in the subconjunctival area, the soft palate, and other areas of the skin.[76]

Characteristically, the patient is admitted to hospital because of other manifestations of trauma. Initially, he may be completely lucid, with no evidence of respiratory complications, but sometime in the ensuing 24 to 48 hr, the above manifestations become apparent. Several studies have demonstrated, however, that these features may appear anywhere from 1 to 96 hr after injury and occasionally appear only after manipulation of the long bones in order to improve alignment, days to weeks after the initial injury.

The incidence of fat embolism is not established. Estimates during World War I suggested that 10% of the battle-wounded suffered from fat embolism, whereas a study in World War II indicated that 65% of patients who died from battle wounds had evidence of fat embolism.[77] Prospective studies of patients with fractures of the extremities include one series in which 50 patients were evaluated. Seventy-four percent of these developed arterial hypoxemia, 46% had a low platelet count, and fat droplets were present in the urine in 76%. None of these, however, developed a fullblown syndrome as described above. Other studies of long bone fractures have indicated that 5% to 10% may develop the fat embolism syndrome.[78] A series of 5265 accident victims in Europe resulted in 855 deaths attributed to fat embolism.[77]

The patient with fat embolism who has transient cyanosis, tachypnea, and confusion, but rapidly improves when given oxygen, generally has no further difficulty.[79] The most severe problems are represented by those patients with severe hyperthermia, cerebral manifestations, tachycardia, pulmonary arterial hypertension, and pulmonary complications. These complications include diffuse bilateral pulmonary infiltrates roentgenographically consistent with diffuse interstitial pulmonary edema, a marked decrease in pulmonary compliance, life-threatening hypoxia, and clinical evidence of pulmonary hypertension.

There is no specific pathognomonic test to establish the diagnosis. Free fat may be found in the urine in approximately 50% of patients within 3 days after injury, but has no specificity. Increased lipase levels, thrombocytopenia, hypocalcemia, and hypoalbuminemia have been frequently documented but are nonspecific. Evidence of impaired gas exchange in the lungs, and microvascular disease are generally sufficient evidence for initiation of treatment in this problem.

The pathogenesis of the fat embolism syndrome continues to be a subject of controversy. Some believe that the origin of the emboli is mechanical, whereas others consider it to be chemical. The clinical observation that long bones are most frequently affected and the histologic observation of marrow emboli in the lungs support the notion that emboli are actually dislodged from the marrow of fractured bones. The observation that lipid may be found in the urine and may be microscopically demonstrable in the capillary beds of various tissues is similarly supportive. However, extensive experimental studies deny the hypothesis that all the embolic fat originates from traumatized depots. Furthermore, the mechanical theory does not provide a satisfactory explanation for fat embolism found in association with nontraumatic conditions such as burns, diabetic coma, pancreatitis, and intoxication.[80–83] Other explanations suggest that the stability of blood lipids is altered after trauma and that aggregation of platelets and chylomicrons occurs immediately after injury, with subsequent aggregation of erythrocytes and sludging of flow, or occlusion of capillary vessels with subsequent tissue hypoxia.[78] Perhaps neutral fat embolism occurs first followed by local lipolysis with release of free fatty acids, and endothelial injury.[84]

Detailed studies of patients with trauma indicate that levels of free fatty acids, catecholamines, and glucocorticoids are elevated, perhaps all reflecting the severity of the stress.[85]

The experimental canine oleic acid model, recently explored in detail,[86–88] demonstrates that fatty acids infused into the experimental animal result in increased pulmonary artery pressure, decreased lung compliance, decreased arterial Po_2, and evidence of intravascular consumption coagulopathy. Thus, fibrinogen, platelets, and other factors are depleted, resulting in appropriate abnormalities of clotting. This has led to the hypothesis that free fatty acids result in injury to the endothelium of systemic capillaries as well as of pulmonary capillaries, producing a "chemical edema." Perhaps the normal person who develops increased neutral fat in the circulating blood as part of the condition of fat embolism, mobilizes lipase and lipolytic processes with the production of free fatty acids and glycerol. These circulating fatty acids may then become the agents of injury at the local tissue level, particularly in the lungs. Such a sequence would explain the increase in lipase frequently found in patients with the fat embolism syndrome. Observations of lung microvasculature in living dogs through a thoracic window confirmed that emboli of free fatty acid globules were impacted within small vessels, in areas with obstruction. In areas where the fatty acid embolus passed slowly through the arteriole and only transiently occluded the vessel, there was soon evidence of interstitial edema and hemorrhage. This was interpreted as indicating a "toxic vasculitis."[84,89]

Management. The incidence of fat embolism is related to the frequency of major impact injuries; however, there is some evidence that careful efforts to decrease the mobility of the fractured sites may decrease the risk. The most important aspect of management, once the syndrome is established, is adequate oxygenation. This should be undertaken with the same systematic approach as for other causes of the acute respiratory distress syndrome in the adult, outlined in Chapter 7. Most patients treated vigorously in this manner survive. Those who survive generally have little evidence of residual lung injury after convalescence.[79,90]

Numerous other therapeutic modalities have been tried on various theoretical bases. Heparin was used as a lipolytic agent and to decrease intravascular coagulation; low-molecular-weight dextran may improve capillary perfusion by decreasing sludging. Ethyl alcohol, once advocated as a lipolytic agent, is no longer in vogue.[77]

Recent enthusiasm for the use of massive doses of corticosteroids in the management of severe fat embolism is based on the anti-inflammatory properties of these steroids, which may decrease local tissue injury and pulmonary edema. Doses ranging from 100 mg of cortisone to 30 mg/kg of methyl prednisolone sodium succinate have been recommended. In one study ,[91] the use of corticosteroids and vigorous respiratory care including artificial respirators where necessary resulted in 100% survival in a series of 31 cases; however, the most effective components of the therapeutic program were not defined. More recently, we reported 54 patients treated with oxygen, careful fluid balance, and other supportive care with a small number of patients receiving steroids. All patients survived.[79] We were impressed with the likelihood that associated injuries determine the prognosis if aggressive modern respiratory management is carried out. Prophylactic hypertonic glucose has been reported to reduce circulating fatty acids and prevent fat embolism, but this has not been confirmed.[92]

It is generally conceded that the most important aspect of the management of the fat embolism syndrome is adequate oxygenation and respiratory support, and that most patients spontaneously demonstrate marked improvement within 48 hr of the onset of the syndrome.[79,90,93] Since the diagnosis is never absolutely certain (or, at least, the pulmonary components of this problem cannot be distinguished with absolute certainty from other causes of respiratory insufficiency), the physician must constantly entertain a broad differential diagnosis when planning the management program.

INJURIES OF THE TRACHEOBRONCHIAL TREE

Clinical Manifestations. Trauma to the larynx, the cricoid cartilage, and the extrathoracic trachea should always be considered when blunt injury to the neck has occurred. These frequently present as obstruction of the upper airway, or later, as respiratory tract infection. The contents of the thorax are unusually well protected from direct injury by the thoracic cage; therefore, injuries to the intrathoracic trachea and major bronchi are infrequent.

After the age of 30, traumatic rupture of the bronchus rarely occurs without associated rib fractures. These fractures generally involve upper ribs and are generally on the same side as the ruptured bronchus. Prior to age 30, rib fractures are frequently not demonstrable. Approximately 20% of tracheobronchial ruptures affect the intrathoracic trachea, and 80% involve the bronchi.[94] Of these, the right main-stem bronchus is involved approximately twice as frequently as the left main-stem, and the most common site of laceration or amputation of the bronchus is at the first cartilaginous ring beyond the carina. Laceration or amputation of the bronchus should be considered in any traumatized patient with cervical subcutaneous emphysema, pneumothorax, or pneumomediastinum associated with hemoptysis or atelectasis. This should be of particular concern in patients with tension pneumothorax and large air leaks. The most specific diagnostic aid in early recognition is bronchoscopy.[95–100]

The precise mechanism by which the bronchus becomes lacerated or amputated has not been determined. Animal experiments support the suggestion that impact injuries with the glottis closed result in dramatic increases in intrathoracic pressure and may cause perforation of the bronchial wall. It seems unlikely that this would result in frank amputation of the bronchus; additional factors such as sudden deceleration of the intrathoracic tissues at the time of impact may be important.[95–97]

The air leak may seal before being recognized, and the diagnosis delayed until the patient develops distal pulmonary infection and atelectasis as a result of poor clearance of bronchial secretions and blood. Recurrent unilateral lung infection in a patient with a history of chest trauma should raise the suspicion of post-traumatic bronchostenosis.[98]

Management. The mortality rate in unrecognized amputation of the bronchus is high, but in patients who receive early surgical treatment (thoracotomy and primary repair with anastomosis of the severed bronchus), the prognosis is very good.[99,100]

CARDIOVASCULAR INJURIES

Injuries of the heart and great vessels are classified in the list on p. 534. These lesions may occur in the absence of other recognizable chest injuries or in the presence of such severe injuries to the rest of the body that the cardiac injuries are overlooked.

Injuries of the Heart

Clinical Manifestations. The most common lesions in fatal cardiac trauma are myocardial rupture, myocardial contusion, pericardial laceration, and pericardial hemorrhage (Table 11-6).[101]

The earliest suspicion of myocardial injury may result from acute evidence of righ heart failure, increasing heart size demonstrated roentgenographically, low cardiac output, development of a murmur, or evidence of left ventricular failure and pulmonary edema. When these findings are absent, however, electrocardiographic studies may be the only clues that myocardial contusion has occurred.[102] Nonspecific ST and T abnormalities are the most common accompaniment of contusion but may not reflect specific cardiac injury. Similarly, the use of enzymes indicating tissue necrosis is generally unsatisfactory because of widespread injury to other organs. Minor, clinically insignificant contusion of the right ventricle is the most frequent traumatic injury.

Occasionally, arrhythmias are the major manifestation of myocardial contusion. With more extensive myocardial contusion, the electrocardiographic changes characteristic of myocardial infarction may be present. This may be a particularly troublesome finding in the age group in which patients are prone to coronary artery disease, because the question will arise (for example, with the driver of a motor vehicle) whether the myocardial damage preceded or was a consequence of the impact; that is, might the myocardial event have been the cause of the accident?

Management. The importance of recognition of the heart injury is demonstrated by the beneficial effect of surgical treatment of many of these lesions.[103,104] More than 80% of persons with hemodynamic disturbances as a result of major cardiac injuries survive if the conditions are recognized early and treated appropriately. The physician who is not a thoracic surgeon needs to recognize the cardiac injury and initiate definitive diagnostic evaluation as soon as possible. Although definitive treatment will often have to await the thoracic or cardiovascular surgeon, pericardial fluid can be confirmed by cardiac ultrasound and tamponade as a result of bleeding, managed by pericardiocentesis.[105]

TABLE 11-6. Predominant Injury in Fatal Nonpenetrating Cardiac Trauma

Predominant Type of Injury	Incidence
Myocardial rupture, including septum	65%
Myocardial contusion or laceration	24%
Pericardial laceration	6%
Hemopericardium	5%
Valvular laceration, papillary muscle laceration or rupture, coronary artery laceration or rupture, coronary artery thrombosis	Less than 1% except when combined with other serious cardiac injury

Nonpenetrating Trauma of the Heart and Great Vessels

- Pericardial injury
  - Hemopericardium
  - Serofibrinous or suppurative pericarditis
  - Constrictive pericarditis (late)
  - Recurrent pericarditis with effusion
- Myocardial injury
  - Contusion
    - Anginal syndrome
    - Infarction
    - Aneurysm
    - Delayed rupture
    - Systemic thromboembolism
  - Laceration
  - Rupture, including septal rupture
- Coronary artery injury: laceration or thrombosis with or without myocardial infarction
- Valvular injury
  - Laceration, rupture, contusion
  - Papillary muscle or chordae tendineae tears
- Disturbances of rhythm or conduction
- Great vessel injury
  - Laceration, rupture
  - Aneurysm formation
  - Thrombotic occlusion

Injuries of the Great Vessels

Clinical Manifestations. Rupture of the thoracic aorta is the most frequent and serious injury to the great vessels. This most commonly occurs just below the take-off of the left subclavian artery; however, the next most common site is the root of the aorta just above the aortic sinuses. The most popular explanation for this site of injury suggests that, when the body decelerates suddenly, the inertia of the blood within the lumen of the aorta provides a strong impact at the site where the aorta traverses posteriorly behind the mediastinal reflections. Automobile and airplane accidents, and falling from a great height, are the most common causes.[3,6,7,14,106–113] As many as one of every six fatal traffic accident victims sustains aortic rupture. More than 80% are immediately fatal, but an additional 10% to 20% live long enough to benefit from surgical treatment.[106]

The earliest manifestation of a ruptured aorta may be severe hypovolemia, with circulatory shock. When this is not present, roentgenographic findings may raise suspicion. A widened superior mediastinum, displacement of the trachea, abnormal contour of the aortic knob and a bulging mass displacing the left upper lobe should be carefully sought. The presence of a widened superior mediastinum or the combination of a widened superior mediastinum with a pleural effusion should raise suspicion (Fig. 11-7). The effusion is hemorrhagic and generally is located in the left pleural space. In one series, 92% of patients with blunt injuries to the aortic arch or its branches had a widened mediastinum. Less than 50% had a difference in pulse pressure between upper and lower extremities.[109] The only definitive method of diagnosis is an ascending aortic angiogram.

Not infrequently, a false aneurysm is formed with a mediastinal hematoma. This generally results in some widening of the mediastinum, which might only be recognized incidentally on subsequent chest roentgenograms. Occasionally, the injury is first recognized when complications such as late rupture with hemorrhage, bacterial endocarditis, or peripheral embolism from this false aneurysm develop.

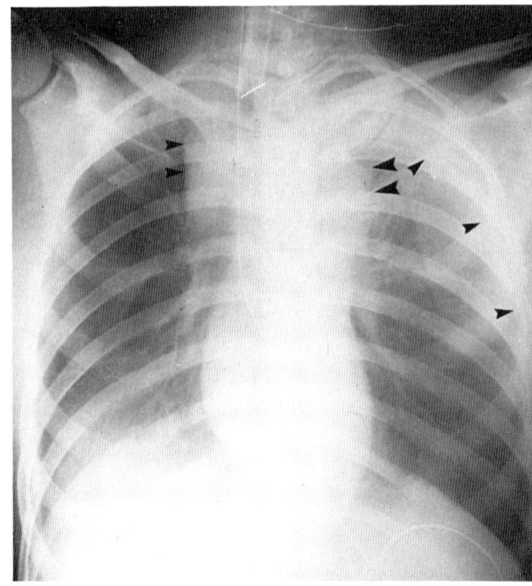

FIG. 11-7. Ruptured thoracic aorta. This 17-year-old girl was a passenger on a motorcycle that was struck by an automobile, and her body was thrown at least 50 feet from the site of impact. She presented slightly confused, complaining of discomfort in her extremities, and mildly hypotensive. The supine chest film demonstrates marked widening of the superior mediastinum, a significant pleural effusion, and a small heart frequently seen when the intravascular blood volume is reduced. She died before definitive surgical therapy could be undertaken for what at autopsy was confirmed to be rupture of the thoracic aorta just below the take-off of the subclavian vessels. The large arrows mark the site of the aortic tear. The small arrows mark the widened mediastinum on the right, and pleural fluid on the left.

Management. The serious suspicion of a ruptured aorta should lead to early definitive angiography and surgical correction.[3,106,110,112] This is true for the early phase commonly associated with evidence of acute blood loss, as well as for delayed recognition which may occur months to years after the trauma. The accuracy of ultrasound or the usefulness of computerized axial tomography for these lesions has not been established.

Although other injuries must be assessed and treated, first priority in investigation and management must generally go to the aortic injury.

INJURIES OF THE DIAPHRAGM

Clinical Manifestations. Traumatic rupture of the diaphragm is most commonly caused by stab wounds. However, it is becoming more common as a result of trauma to the abdomen and lower chest in high velocity accidents. Diaphragm tears result in a loss of the membrane function that divides the negative pressure pleural space from the positive pressure abdominal space, and abdominal contents move into the thorax to whatever extent the size of the tear will permit.[114–120]

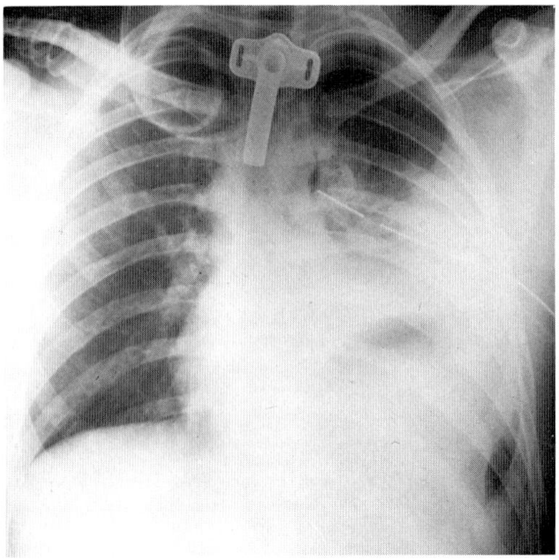

FIG. 11-8. Traumatic diaphragmatic hernia. A 56-year-old man was in severe respiratory distress 3 hours after a motor vehicle accident. The density in the left lower lung field was thought to represent hemothorax and atelectasis. A thoracostomy tube drained minimal blood. The left diaphragm is not well visualized on this film. Laparotomy confirmed that the gas-filled viscus, which is seen here above the level of the right diaphragm, was in the thorax, having passed through a ruptured diaphragm.

The patient, having suffered an impact injury, generally presents with dyspnea and epigastric or subcostal pain. Physical examination may demonstrate decreased air entry on the side of the diaphragmatic rupture. The mediastinum may be shifted away from the side of the herniation. The rupture of the leaflets of the diaphragm, associated with blunt trauma, is on the left side in 90% of the cases. The mechanism of this predilection has not been determined.[114,115] Some authors suggest that the liver prevents direct transmission of pressure on the right, and others have argued that right sided tears are more often overlooked.[116,117] A ruptured diaphragm is commonly associated with severe abdominal organ trauma, and this appears to be greater in right-sided diaphragm tears.

Although the chest roentgenogram would be expected to make the diagnosis, this frequently may not be definitive, because the differential diagnosis includes atelectasis with marked elevation of a diaphragm, phrenic nerve palsy, and other intrathoracic disease (Fig. 11-8). Only when bowel is clearly identifiable, located within the thoracic space, with clear evidence of mediastinal shift to the opposite side, can the diagnosis be made with certainty from the plain chest roentgenogram. On the other hand, contrast roentgenographic studies can be carried out for definitive diagnosis when the lesion is suspected. Diagnostic pneumoperitoneum will outline the diaphragm, and a resultant pneumothorax proves the diaphragmatic tear.[120] Occasionally, acute bowel obstruction may raise the suspicion of diaphragmatic rupture. Since diaphragmatic hernia generally is associated with multiple injuries, the lesion is frequently detected incidentally at laparotomy or overlooked at the time of the acute injury. Occasionally, the patient presents with bowel obstruction months to years later.[121]

Bilateral paralysis of the diaphragm, probably a result of mediastinal phrenic nerve injury, has been observed after blunt chest trauma, and resulted in severe respiratory failure.[68]

Management. Surgical repair of the diaphragmatic herniation is highly successful and should be undertaken as soon as the patient's condition stablizes or as an emergency procedure if necessary to maintain adequate respiratory exchange.

INJURIES OF THE ESOPHAGUS

Clinical Manifestations. Rupture of the esophagus occurs rarely with blunt chest trauma,[122,123] but is more frequent with penetrating thoracic wounds. Most frequently it results from instrumentation such as endoscopy, or dilatation of strictures. Spontaneous rupture has been associated with vomiting (Boerhaave's syndrome), maternal labor, vigorous exercise, and severe asthma.[123–125]

Perforation from blast injuries and penetrating wounds generally involves the more exposed cervical esophagus; spontaneous rupture generally occurs in the lower third.

Patients with rupture of the esophagus develop severe retrosternal chest pain and mediastinal emphysema. This may progress to include cervical and subcutaneous emphysema, pneumothorax, hydropneumothorax with or without empyema, and acute mediastinitis with a severe febrile illness. Patients with the fully developed syndrome have a high mortality (see also Chap. 12).

Management. Patients suspected of esophageal rupture should have appropriate drainage of the pleural space, endoscopy to establish the diagnosis, surgical correction of the tear, and, if appropriate, surgical drainage of the mediastinum. Antibiotic therapy including agents effective against oral anaerobic organisms should be initiated immediately. Surgical drainage of mediastinal abscesses may be required.

INJURIES OF THE ABDOMINAL ORGANS

Clinical Manifestations. Lacerations of the liver and spleen are common following impact injuries and are frequently present in patients with blunt trauma to the thorax. Patients with rib fractures over the lower thorax more frequently have lacerations of the liver or spleen on the affected side, but contra-coup effects may result in lacerations of the spleen with right-sided fractures or vice versa. Mesenteric lacerations may result in intra-abdominal bleeding. Rupture of the stomach or bowel, lacerations or contusions of the kidney, and contusion of the pancreas may all play a prominent role in determining the management of the patient.[2,3,14]

Intra-abdominal bleeding might not be associated with abdominal pain, tenderness, or ileus, but it can be readily diagnosed by peritoneal lavage.[9,10] This should be performed in any patient with extensive impact injuries and evidence of hypovolemia, even if other sites of blood loss have been identified. All too often, evidence of external blood loss or a significant hemothorax are accepted as sufficient explanation for hypovolemia, and the diagnosis of silent abdominal bleeding is overlooked until the patient deteriorates severely.

Many reports have emphasized the danger of delayed splenic rupture, but this, in most patients, reflects delayed diagnosis.[126] Late splenic rupture is a rare diagnosis if vigorous diagnostic approaches are pursued during the acute phase.

Management. Management of abdominal injuries with bleeding is generally surgical.

CHEST TRAUMA RESULTING FROM EXTERNAL CARDIAC MASSAGE

Clinical Manifestations. Since external cardiac massage was introduced in 1960 for the resuscitation of patients with acute pulselessness,[127] this procedure has gained wide acceptance and is used with variable skill. Rib fractures have been reported in 75% of patients being resuscitated in this manner. These fractures generally increase in number in proportion to the duration of the external massage. Although young persons tend to have few fractures, they increase markedly in the older age groups, in whom the thoracic cage is less resilient. Sternal fractures occur less frequently. In some intensive care units, multiple rib fractures sustained during external cardiac massage are the most common cause of "flail chest."[128]

Additional thoracic complications of external cardiac massage include pneumothorax, hemothorax, subcutaneous and mediastinal emphysema, and frank pulmonary lacerations.

Bone marrow pulmonary emboli are reported in up to 50% of cases of external massage subsequently subjected to autopsy.[129]

Several reports have indicated contusion of myocardium, rupture of myocardium, pericardial tamponade, laceration of liver and spleen, rupture of the stomach wall, and pneumoperitoneum incurred during the course of cardiopulmonary resuscitation.[130,131]

No convincing evidence is available to indicate that patients in the hands of a highly skilled resuscitator show fewer complications; however, it is clear that the least trauma compatible with the appropriate therapeutic response should be assured. Compression of the chest wall should be sufficient to provide adequate circulation as detected by pulses in the major vessels. A firm support for the chest cage posteriorly, with well-controlled systematic pressure applied to the lower portion of the sternum rather than to the entire anterior chest wall, minimizes injury to the thoracic cage.

The frequency of these injuries makes it mandatory that, following successful resuscitation, the patient be evaluated as if he had undergone an impact injury. Futhermore, during the course of resuscitation, signs of developing traumatic complications should be constantly considered and, if necessary, treated.

Management. The management of the complications of external cardiac massage must be dealt with in the same fashion as those for any other traumatic impact injury.

PENETRATING THORACIC INJURIES

Clinical Manifestations. Penetrating wounds are often inflicted deliberately by a variety of devices for stabbing, or by gunshot; stab wounds tend to cause less damage than gunshot wounds.[132–134] Patients with penetrating injuries must be observed closely and treated vigorously until the severity of the injury has declared itself.[135] Lacerations of intercostal and internal mammary arteries, lung laceration, or injury to the mediastinal great vessels may cause severe hemothorax. Cardiac laceration may result in pericardial tamponade. Lacerations of the lung or bronchus may cause severe pneumothorax, and occasionally air embolism.[136] Other injuries include laceration of the diaphragm, abdominal organs, esophagus, or injury to the spinal column.

High-velocity missiles commonly cause bleeding and contusion of surrounding lung, resulting in the acute respiratory distress syndrome.[137]

Management. Initial management should include tube drainage of the pleural space, hemodynamic support, radiographic investigation, and careful monitoring for blood loss and evidence of cardiac tamponade. The stable patient rarely requires immediate surgery, but may need late surgery for complications of hemothorax or infection. Indications for emergency thoracotomy include rapid blood loss, clinical evidence of pericardial tamponade, and diaphgram or esophageal injuries. In view of the high incidence of great vessel or cardiac injury with upper mediastinal entrance wounds, the location of the wound should be considered in determining whether or not surgery is necessary.[133–135]

Gunshot wounds frequently result in extensive lung injury and may require prolonged management of respiratory failure.

SHOCK IN PATIENTS WITH MULTIPLE TRAUMA

Clinical Manifestations. Shock that occurs within 12 hr following trauma is usually a result of hypovolemia. Cardiac tamponade, cardiac arrhythmias, massive fat embolism, air embolism and neurologic injury with vasomotor instability or diabetes insipidus are uncommon but must be considered. Internal bleeding is frequently at the site of major fractures, intra-abdominal or intrathoracic lacerations, or contusion. The patient who is slightly vasoconstricted on admission commonly develops frank hypotension after administration of analgesics. Postural changes in blood pressure may demonstrate hypovolemia when the resting blood pressure is normal. Heart rate may be within the normal range, perhaps a result of increased vagal tone associated with pain. Frequent measurements of blood pressure, pulse rate, and urine output are essential if precipitous drops in blood pressure owing to silent bleeding are to be detected early or avoided.[2,3,14,138] Metabolic acidosis generally occurs after significant hypotension.

Patients with shock develop a higher rate of sepsis, acute respiratory distress, and disseminated intravascular coagulation, and in spite of treatment have a higher mortality. Descriptions of the shock lung placed unnecessary emphasis on the role of the hemodynamic status. The acute respiratory distress syndrome is not specifically caused by or dependent on a period of shock.[54]

Management Hypovolemic shock represents a genuine medical emergency. Several large intravenous lines should be established and large volumes of fluid administered immediately. The

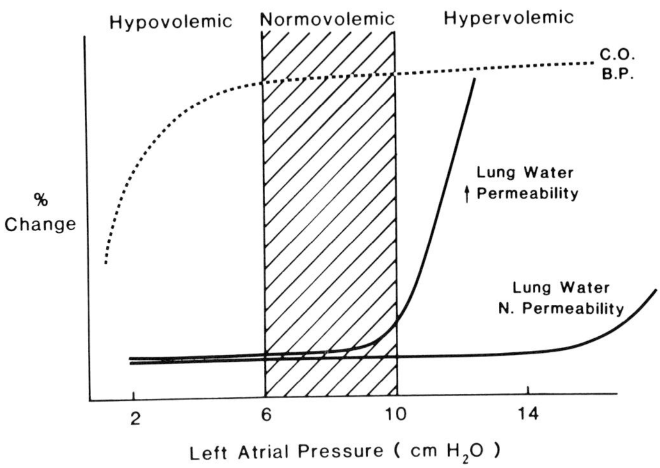

FIG. 11-9. This schematic drawing demonstrates the response of cardiac output and blood pressure to infused fluids when the left atrial pressure is raised in a hypovolemic patient (*interrupted line*). As the vascular volume is replaced, the cardiac output and blood pressure increase greatly until the patient is normovolemic. With further fluid administration, the cardiac output and blood pressure increase little, but significant hypervolemia is tolerated in the patient with normal lung vessels. Patients with lung injury and increased capillary permeability develop increased lung water and clinical pulmonary edema soon after the hemodynamic parameters have stabilized, occasionally within the normovolemic range.

feet should be elevated and the head lowered to a horizontal position to ensure maximum venous return and cerebral perfusion. While whole blood is being crossmatched, large volumes of crystalloid (normal saline or Ringer's lactate) should be administered. Experimental evidence indicates substantial losses of extravascular fluids in the hypovolemic patient. If the first liter of saline, administered over 15 to 30 min, raises the blood pressure and urine output, the total volume loss is modest and the search for the site of bleeding may be undertaken over the next few hours. If such rapid administration of fluid fails to produce a significant and sustained improvement, the site of bleeding must be identified and corrected immediately.

When large volumes of fluid replacement are required, about half to two thirds should be whole blood, the remainder crystalloid.[138] Massive fluid replacement should be performed, with fresh blood, if possible, to ensure adequate clotting factors and near normal oxygen affinity for hemoglobin. When large volumes are infused, or in patients with evidence of cardiac disease, fluid administration should be monitored by measurements of pulmonary venous pressure, using a flow-directed catheter (see Chap. 7). Use of filters may be helpful in avoiding lung injury from infused macroaggregates[59–60]; however, effective filters cause slow flow and result in hemolysis.

Administration of vasoactive drugs or corticosteroids has no clear scientific basis in early hypovolemic shock.[138] Bicarbonate administration may be necessary if metabolic acidosis is severe as indicated by a *p*H less than 7.20 or serum bicarbonate less than 15. Excess fluid replacement may precipitate pulmonary edema, even at relatively low left atrial pressure in patients with pulmonary capillary injury (Fig. 11-9).

PULMONARY EFFECTS OF SURGICAL PROCEDURES

Surgical procedures may be associated with pulmonary effects ranging from transient alterations in lung function to life-threatening complications. Many factors influence the risk to a given patient. Surgery involving the extremities is associated with a lower risk than surgery involving the upper abdomen, and neither of these has the severe adverse effects of resectional lung surgery (see list, p. 540). Obesity, respiratory tract infections, smoking, obstructive lung disease, and aging all increase the risk of pulmonary complications. Patients and procedures with increased risk should be identified, since appropriate management beginning in the preoperative period improves the outcome.

The respiratory consequences of surgery have been summarized here with special emphasis on predictable effects and avoidable risk factors, because surgery is not a naturally occurring illness.

Operative Sites That Result in Impaired Respiratory Function (Decreasing Order of Severity)

Bilateral thoracic
Unilateral thoracic
Intrapleural
Upper abdominal
Lower abdominal
Pelvic
Extremities and superficial

EFFECTS OF NONTHORACIC SURGERY

The changes in respiratory function after upper abdominal surgery have been well documented (Table 11-7).[139–144] A drop in vital capacity and functional residual capacity is common during the intraoperative period. Marked variability, averaging a 35% decrease from preoperative volumes, occurs by the first postoperative day. The closing volume may be normal or increased, but because the functional residual capacity is reduced, tidal breathing may actually occur at volumes below the closing volume, resulting in large areas of the lung being hypoventilated. This regional hypoventilation predictably results in hypoxemia and an elevation in the alveolar-arterial oxygen gradient. Studies performed during the intraoperative period demonstrate that when the functional residual capacity is maintained above the closing volume,[141,142] the increase in alveolar-arterial oxygen gradient does not occur.

TABLE 11-7. Effects of Upper Abdominal Surgery on Lung Function

Lung volumes	
Total lung capacity	↓
Functional residual capacity	↓
Inspiratory capacity	↓
Residual volume	↔ ↓
Closing volume	↔ ↑
Lung compliance	↓
Diffusing capacity	↔ ↓
Arterial blood gases	
*p*H	↑
P_{CO_2}	↓
P_{O_2}	↓
A-a gradient	↑

During this phase of reduced functional residual capacity, each anatomical focus of alveolar closure is small and the resulting lesions may not produce physical or roentgenographic abnormalities. The concept of microatelectasis is ascribed to Mead and Collier,[145] who observed that anesthetized dogs, whether breathing spontaneously or mechanically ventilated in a resting tidal volume range, had a progressive fall in pulmonary compliance. That is, the dogs' lungs became progressively stiffer, requiring higher inflation pressures to achieve the same tidal volume. These changes could be due to progressive atelectasis.

It was soon demonstrated[146] that normal unanesthetized humans develop a progressive fall in compliance when breathing at normal but monotonously regular tidal volumes and that this fall in compliance is reversed when the subjects are allowed to take larger tidal volumes. That is, the lung becomes less stiff following deep breaths. This study suggests that, without periodic hyperinflation, there is a closing of lung units even in normal persons when the lung is ventilated at low tidal volumes adequate to excrete carbon dioxide.

In a series of investigations, Bendixen and his co-workers at the Massachusetts General Hospital demonstrated the effects of microatelectasis on the oxygenation of surgical patients.[142–152] They related the changes in compliance caused by constant, small tidal volume ventilation to changes in arterial oxygenation. In patients undergoing surgery with general anesthesia and controlled ventilation, the anesthesiologists maintained normal CO_2 exchange and a constant low tidal volume. The average period of study was 76 min. There was an average fall of compliance of 15% and an average fall in oxygen tension of 22%. At the end of surgery, the patients were hyperinflated with three breaths: the first to 20 cm of water for 10 sec, the second to 30 cm of water for 15 sec, and the third to 40 cm of water for 15 sec. With hyperinflation, compliance returned to control values, and Pa_{O_2} increased progressively with successive hyperinflation until it also returned to control values.

This microatelectasis, described commonly in postoperative states,[153] is widely held to be the major cause of persistent hypoxemia. Several mechanisms whereby this occurs have been suggested: obstruction of peripheral airways attributed to hypocapnia, producing bronchoconstriction[154]; decreased production of surfactant as a result of inhalation of high oxygen concentrations or altered ventilating patterns[155]; inhalation of 100% oxygen with complete resorption of alveolar gases[156]; and all the usual factors resulting in postoperative lung infections or pulmonary edema.

The more severe effects of upper abdominal surgical procedures may be related to the intraoperative effects on tidal volume, postoperative pain inhibiting deep inspiration, or alterations in diaphragmatic function[156a] discussed below under Postoperative Respiratory Complications.

These predictable changes in respiratory function occur in persons whose lungs are normal preoperatively. The time course of improvement toward normal values is variable, but generally ranges from 4 to 8 days. Patients with pulmonary disease often have more severe adverse effects.[153]

EFFECTS OF THORACIC SURGERY AND LUNG RESECTION

Surgical resection of lung results in a predictable loss of lung function (see list at right). Consideration for resectional surgery requires analysis of the risk of the operative procedure, the loss of function that will result from resection of the specific portion of lung, and the function of the remaining lung tissue. Loss of lung function may be most apparent as ventilatory failure or as increased pulmonary vascular resistance with right ventricular failure. For example, a person with a normal left lung may tolerate removal of the entire right lung with only minimal increases in pulmonary artery pressure and strain on the heart. On the other hand, a person with abnormal function of his left lung may not survive removal of the entire right lung, or may develop severe pulmonary hypertension or cor pulmonale. If the portion of lung to be removed is nonfunctioning, then resection will not reduce pulmonary function further and will be tolerated as well as a nonresectional procedure.[157] In spite of numerous studies, no firm guidelines are available for criteria that prohibit resectional surgery. As with nonresectional surgery, the risk appears to increase approximately in proportion to the impairment of function.

Patients requiring resectional surgery, whose total pulmonary function is reduced prior to resection, should have evaluation of the function in the portion of lung to be removed. This can be estimated by studies of regional ventilation and perfusion. Analysis of regional ventilation, oxygen uptake, and carbon dioxide removal may be performed by bronchospirometry,[158] but is generally not necessary because less cumbersome techniques are now available.

Effects of Resectional Surgery on Pulmonary Function

- One lobe or less
  - Minimal measurable changes except with severe pulmonary disease
- Pneumonectomy
  - Decreased ventilatory function measured by:
    - Total lung capacity
    - Functional residual capacity
    - Residual volume
    - Vital capacity
    - Maximum expiratory flow rates
  - Decreased vascular bed measured by:
    - Diffusing capacity
  - Increased pulmonary vascular resistance, particularly apparent
    - During exercise
    - During hypoxemia
    - With increasing age

If a region of lung is obviously abnormal, owing to atelectasis or bullous emphysema as seen on the routine chest roentgenogram, it is probably nonfunctional. In such patients, studies of regional lung function are important to assess the remaining lung. Regional ventilation may be assessed in detail by radioisotope ventilation scans.[159–161] Simple numerical estimates of regional perfusion permit accurate prediction of loss of function after resection. If perfusion to the region is absent, it is nonfunctioning. Using a macroaggregate lung scan, the proportion of blood perfusing each lung may be established. If a diseased lung, to be resected, demonstrates 35% of the total perfusion, then the loss of ventilatory function after surgery will be proportional; the vital capacity, expiratory flow rates, maximum voluntary ventilation, functional residual capacity and total lung capacity will all be reduced by about 35%.[162,163] When the resection is predicted to cause loss of lung function to a level at which the postoperative, 1-sec vital capacity is less than 800 ml, the mortality has been reported as 15%, and is generally considered prohibitive.[163]

A simple laboratory procedure for assessment of unilateral lung function has been shown to correlate well with radioisotope studies. This test is based on the principle that when a person moves from the supine to the lateral lying position, the upper lung has an increase in FRC and the lower lung has no significant change. Therefore, measuring the volume change in FRC when comparing the two lateral positions to the supine position provides information on the function of the upright lung. This data, which can be obtained using a simple spirometer, may be useful in preoperative evaluation.[164,165]

A lobectomy is associated with a small decrease in total lung capacity, vital capacity, and flow rates, and is well tolerated even by patients with moderately severe obstructive lung disease.[166]

Pneumonectomy results in a reduced vascular bed with increased pulmonary vascular resistance, particularly during exercise. If a large portion of lung must be removed, some indication of the immediate pulmonary vascular response can be obtained by inserting a balloon catheter into the appropriate pulmonary artery, occluding that vessel, and analysing the pulmonary hemodynamic response in the remaining perfused lung.[168] Additional precision may be gained if assessment of regional lung function is carried out during exercise.[159,167–170] The acute test, however, does not necessarily indicate the postoperative course.

An overall assessment of respiratory function may be made by preoperative exercise evaluation. In one study, patients who were able to progress through a graded exercise program and complete the final stage, walking for 2 min at 3 mph at a 10% incline, suffered no morbidity or mortality from the pneumonectomy.[171]

Postoperative complications of major resectional surgery include the development of acute cor pulmonale, atrial arrhythmias,[172] and subsequently the development of chronic cor pulmonale.[173] Post-thoracotomy infections include bronchitis, pneumonia, empyema, and bronchopleural fistula.[173a]

Few studies have analyzed the long-term effects of pulmonary resection. Most pneumonectomies performed for malignant tumors are associated with short survival and characteristically are associated with widespread airways disease secondary to cigarette smoking. Similarly, the many patients who previously underwent pneumonectomies for tuberculosis probably had bilateral disease. In one study, a high incidence of cor pulmonale occurred 10 to 12 years following pneumonectomy.[174] Another small series of pneumonectomies for tuberculosis demonstrated the predicted decrease in vital capacity and total lung capacity early after resection, but marked increase in residual volume and reduction in expiratory flow rates occurred during a 20-year follow-up. The arterial oxygen saturation remained normal. The diffusing capacity, which was initially reduced in proportion to the loss of lung volume, returned to normal during the 20-year follow-up.[175]

Pneumonectomies performed in childhood during the period of lung growth may result in further growth of the remaining lung. Experimental animals with pneumonectomies performed early in life developed normal lung volumes and diffusing capacities, whereas animals that had a lung removed as adults developed the predicted loss of lung volume.[176]

EFFECTS OF GENERAL ANESTHESIA

Premedication

Patients undergoing general surgery are usually given preanesthetic medication to allay anxiety and atropine or other parasympathetic blocking agents to minimize respiratory secretions. Although such drugs cause several changes in pulmonary function, they do not lead to preoperative hypoxemia.[153,177–179] Similarly, preanesthetic doses of barbiturates do not alter PaO_2.[156,180] Both meperidine and morphine have been demonstrated to decrease PaO_2 significantly in doses that are used for preanesthesia.[152,180,181] Normal persons at rest take deep breaths on the average of ten times an hour, but following morphine, such deep breathing is suppressed.[150] It has been suggested that this hypoxemia is a result of uniformly small tidal volumes and the absence of deep breathing. These data suggest that preanesthetic regimens that include narcotics should be avoided in patients already known to be hypoxemic, or that oxygen should be given from the time of preanesthetic administration until induction of anesthesia. In addition, the respiratory depressant effects of narcotics may be harmful to patients with severe airways obstructive disease and hypercapnia.

Recent insights into mechanisms of hypoxemia during sleep are summarized in Chapter 6. Drug-induced sleep will require similar evaluation which should shed further light on narcotic-induced hypoxemia.

Intraoperative Period

The administration of general anesthetics is commonly associated with severe depression of respiratory control mechanisms. The skilled anesthetist supports ventilation as required, and controls ventilation when muscle relaxants are used. Because of concern for adequate oxygenation, arterial hypoxemia is less likely to occur during general anesthesia than at other times during the perioperative period. Although the mechanisms of microatelectasis described above lead to excessive intrapulmonary shunting during the course of anesthesia, satisfactory arterial oxygenation can be maintained by administering high concentrations of oxygen in the inspired gas. Because the anesthetized patient is given supplemental oxygen during the course of surgery with most anesthetic techniques, there is little likelihood of hypoxemia during surgery.

With the exception of the asthmatic patient, there is no apparent advantage to any particular anesthetic technique in patients with or without lung disease either during surgery or in the postoperative interval.[153,182–188] In the patient with asthma, it has been suggested that halothane or ketamine anesthesia may have some advantage, but there is insufficient evidence to support this position.[189,190]

The intraoperative period probably initiates the alterations in lung function so characteristic of the postoperative state. In spite of conflicting reports, it is probably accurate to conclude that general anesthesia is accompanied by an increased alveolar-arterial oxygen gradient, but the extent of the change is variable. Furthermore, the changes are minimal when tidal volumes exceed 8 ml/kg of patient weight, providing the benefits of hyperinflation.[181]

Postoperative Period

Hypoxemia while breathing room air is exceedingly frequent in the postoperative patient. Premedication with narcotics may lead to mild hypoxemia, and although the potential for intraoperative hypoxemia exists if the patient is not ventilated with high concentrations of inspired oxygen, it is during the postoperative period that the potential for serious hypoxemia is most marked. It is clear that serious hypoxemia can exist in persons without antecedent lung disease, but is more likely to occur in older patients, in those with pre-existing lung disease, in the obese, and in patients undergoing abdominal surgery. Immediately at the end of surgery, two factors may lead to arterial hypoxemia in addition to the microatelectasis and airway closure already discussed. These are posthyperventilation and diffusion hypoxemia.[181] If the anesthetic technique has employed hyperventilation, body stores of carbon dioxide are depleted. These stores of CO_2 are gradually refilled from endogenous CO_2 production. During this time, alveolar ventilation (and therefore, alveolar oxygen) is reduced. Many anesthetic techniques employ the use of nitrous oxide–oxygen mixtures for maintenance of sleep. When nitrous oxide–oxygen is abruptly replaced by air at the end of anesthesia, nitrogen replaces nitrous oxide in the blood. Because nitrous oxide is 31 times more soluble than nitrogen, there is a dilution of the alveolar gas with the excess volume of nitrous oxide as it escapes from the tissues to the lungs; hence, alveolar oxygen decreases. Both posthyperventilation and diffusion hypoxemia should be of relatively brief duration, and hypoxemia can be prevented by administration of high concentrations of inspired oxygen during the immediate postoperative interval.

Aspiration of gastric contents is a well-recognized and serious complication of general anesthesia.[191] Regurgitation of gastric juice into the pharynx was observed in 14% to 26% of patients undergoing general anesthesia.[192,193] The regurgitated material was observed in the tracheobronchial tree in 7% to 16% of patients. Aspiration is frequently silent at the time of surgery and is diagnosed only retrospectively. The clinical consequences depend on the volume and the *p*H of the material aspirated.[194] If a sufficient volume of juice with a *p*H of 2 or less is aspirated, predictable capillary injury results. The clinical presentation is that of noncardiogenic pulmonary edema, frequently referred to as the *adult respiratory distress syndrome.* Skillful anesthetic technique is generally effective in preventing this complication. Management is similar to that for other causes of the adult respiratory distress syndrome. In spite of controversy, some physicians believe intra- and postoperative aspiration is best avoided by use of a nasogastric suction tube, particularly following upper abdominal surgery.[195]

POSTOPERATIVE RESPIRATORY COMPLICATIONS

Following laparotomy in about 30% of patients, postoperative complications may be superimposed on the predictable alterations in lung function and may result in discrete pulmonary disease (see list, above).

Segmental or lobar collapse can be recognized clinically by the regional change in lung volume and by auscultatory findings. Often, it is best demonstrated roentgenographically during the early postoperative period. Such collapse is commonly ascribed to retained secretions resulting from impaired mucous transport.[196,197] However, bronchoscopy frequently fails to reveal a discrete occlusion by mucous plugs.

Postsurgical Pulmonary Complications

- Without pulmonary resection
  - Segmental or lobar atelectasis
  - Infection: tracheobronchitis, pneumonia
  - Bronchospasm
  - Pulmonary edema
  - Pulmonary embolism
  - Complications of endotracheal intubation
- With pulmonary resection (all of above plus)
  - Right heart failure
  - Atrial arrhythmias

The reported incidence of postoperative atelectasis varies widely, depending on the criteria for diagnosis and the region of surgery. Frequently it is impossible to distinguish between atelectasis and infection. In the current literature, fever, cough, dyspnea, and leukocytosis have been used to support both diagnoses. Table 11-8 illustrates the uniform incidence of postoperative atelectasis/infection over a 35-year period. Upper abdominal surgery has a much higher risk than lower abdominal surgery or nonabdominal procedures. Recent observations suggest that diaphragm dysfunction may play an important role in the loss of lung function and contribute to the lower lung zone atelectasis after upper abdominal surgery.[156a,201] Our clinical observations also demonstrate obstructed and central sleep apnea during the early postoperative period.

Infection of the tracheobronchial tree with development of increased sputum production may result in bronchospasm and obstruction of airways. This acute bronchitis commonly occurs without pulmonary parenchymal infiltrates.

Bacterial pneumonia, which complicates surgery, occurs with increased frequency in those with preceding cardiopulmonary disease. The organism involved is characteristically the organism present in the oropharynx at the time. In otherwise healthy persons, this is commonly the pneumococcus; however, with increased time in the hospital, the incidence of penicillin-resistant staphylococci and gram-negative enteric organisms increases.[201a]

Pulmonary edema occurs in the postoperative state with greater frequency than would be pre-

TABLE 11-8. Postoperative Pulmonary Complications

Year	Reference	Total	Nonabdominal	Site of Surgery Abdominal (Incidence, %)	Upper Abdominal
1933	198	8.9	1.2	14	27
1949	199	4.0	0.7	13	19
1968	200	6.2	0.6	10	21

dicted on the basis of fluid replacement therapy. The supine position, renal sodium and water retention, rapid intravenous fluid administration, and changes in pulmonary capillary permeability may all play a role. The characteristic decrease in serum albumin that follows surgical procedures and intravenous electrolyte administration may play some role through its effect on osmotic pressure in pulmonary capillaries.[202]

It has long been recognized that postoperative patients have a high incidence of venous thrombosis and pulmonary embolism.[203] Utilizing the ^{135}I-labeled fibrinogen technique, it has been demonstrated that up to 74% of postoperative patients have deep venous thrombosis.[204–207] Deep venous thrombosis is especially prevalent among men, older patients, patients with varicose veins, those with malignant neoplasms, and those with surgery for fractured hips. Prophylaxis is discussed in detail in Chapter 10.

Complications of endotracheal intubation are discussed in Chapter 7.

Systematic Approach to Respiratory Care in Surgical Patients

- Preoperatively
  - Identify risk factors (smoking, obesity, etc.)
  - Defer elective surgery to correct risk factors
  - Initiate airway care and physical therapy in high-risk groups
  - Determine optimal preoperative medication
  - Consider low-dose heparin
- Intraoperatively
  - Ensure adequate oxygenation and ventilation (endotracheal tube for all high-risk general anesthetics)
  - Keep tidal volumes in excess of 8 ml/kg
  - Carefully monitor supplemental oxygen
  - Continue oxygen, and ventilation into postoperative period, if necessary
- Postoperatively
  - Encourage frequent, deep, sustained inhalations
  - Supply supplemental oxygen if necessary
  - Encourage early mobilization (in bed and out)
  - Initiate vigorous airway care, coughing, postural drainage, and chest physiotherapy in patients with prior disease.

MANAGEMENT OF POSTOPERATIVE RESPIRATORY FAILURE

Patients undergoing major surgical procedures must be evaluated preoperatively, and management planned for the entire pre-, intra-, and postoperative periods as outlined in the list at right.

Identifying Risk Factórs

Prevention of postoperative pulmonary complications can best be carried out by careful identification of patients at increased risk (see list on p. 546.

A higher incidence of postoperative complications among men than among women is evidently related to the higher prevalence of smoking among men. In men and women with similar smoking histories, complications are as frequent among women as men.[200]

Some, but not all, series have found that obesity is associated with an increased incidence of postoperative complications.[208–212] Since extreme obesity causes small lung volumes and increased hypoxemia in the absence of surgical procedures, the data suggesting increased postoperative risk in obese patients seem reasonable.

By suppressing the normal sighing mechanism, narcotics tend to promote atelectasis and hypoxemia.[213] Bunker and associates found that men given more than four doses of narcotic fol-

Additional Risk Factors of Postoperative Pulmonary Complications

Sex (men at higher risk)
Smoking
Obesity
Recent upper respiratory tract infection
Excessive narcotics
Advancing age
Abnormal pulmonary function tests
Previous thromboembolic disease

lowing upper abdominal surgery were more likely to develop atelectasis than men given four or less doses.

Many investigators have found that aging affects postoperative complications. It has been suggested that this is due to the increased prevalence of obstructive airways disease in older patients, but older patients may well experience greater difficulties even in the absence of overt airways disease or smoking.

The increased incidence of postoperative pulmonary complications among smokers has been noted for many years. The importance of the amount of smoking is indicated by the data of Chalon and coworkers.[214] When patients were graded from nonsmokers (0) to very heavy smokers (4), it was found that there was a steady rise in the number of complications after operation as cigarette consumption increased. Thus, nonsmokers had a morbidity rate of 7.9%, whereas very heavy smokers had a rate of 43%. Unfortunately, the article does not contain sufficient data to determine the types of operations among the various groups. Smoking bore a strong correlation with postoperative complications, even though chronic bronchitis was not severe enough to cause a reduction in the forced expiratory volume in 1 sec (FEV_1).

Persons undergoing surgery in the presence of an upper respiratory infection, including only mild pharyngitis, are more likely to experience postoperative pulmonary complications.[215,216]

The most important single factor leading to postoperative pulmonary complications is the presence of chronic obstructive lung disease.[139,217–223] When the 1-sec vital capacity is less than 2 liters, and the maximum midexpiratory flow or maximum voluntary ventilation is less than 50% of predicted, the risk is said to be significantly increased. When the vital capacity is less than 1 liter, the 1 sec vital capacity less than 0.5 liter, or the maximum voluntary ventilation less than 50 liters, the morbidity and mortality are high.[224] Some studies indicate that complications are increased in patients with abnormal lung function, but not related to the degree of abnormality.[225] An elevated arterial P_{CO_2} and pulmonary hypertension indicate a significant increase in risk.[222,223]

Recent reviews[168,222,223] point out the degree of conflict regarding these data. Although prior cardiopulmonary disease increases the risk, this cannot be quantitated in relation to a single pulmonary function test, and vigorous, intensive, postoperative respiratory care frequently overcomes the statistical increase in risk otherwise present.

In emergency situations, adequate postoperative care should be sufficient to sustain the patient through almost any degree of abnormal function previously compatible with life. The presence of a "spring in the step and a glint in the eye" is generally a positive predictive factor.

Risk factors should preferably be dealt with before surgery. Patients should be encouraged to stop smoking 3 to 6 weeks prior to the procedure. Excessive weight should be lost by dieting, and elective surgery postponed until this has been accomplished. Any evidence of congestive heart failure should be treated well in advance to avoid sudden shifts in fluids and electrolytes during the postoperative period. Patients with bacterial bronchitis or bronchiectasis should receive a course of appropriate antibiotics and tracheal drainage. Asthmatics should be treated vigorously to obtain their best lung function before surgery; bronchodilation must be continued through the intraoperative and postoperative periods. Upper respiratory infections are an indication for postponement of elective surgery. In persons whose surgery is an emergency or who are considered acceptable risks, vigorous postoperative care may dramatically influence the postoperative complications.

Prophylactic systemic penicillin G or Ampicillin, for 6 hours before and 24 hours after lung resection, reduces the incidence of empyema and bronchopleural fistula.[173a,225a]

Postsurgical Care

If a patient is identified as having severe pulmonary impairment, surgery should be delayed, if possible, until expectorated secretions are at minimum. Preanesthetic regimens probably should not include narcotics. The type of anesthesia is not important.[185–187] An endotracheal tube should be used to provide control of the airway for mechanical ventilation in the postoperative period. Following surgery, the patient should be maintained on mechanical ventilation in the recovery room until he is fully awake and alert. At that time, an assessment should be made of the patient's ventilatory capacity. If it is thought to be adequate, the patient should be taken off the ventilator, given supplemental oxygen, and observed. If respiratory and heart rates remain low and if the patient is capable of attempting to cough, he should be observed for several minutes, and arterial blood gases should be obtained. If the clinical status and the blood gases are determined to be satisfactory, the patient may be extubated; if not, mechanical ventilation should be continued until such determinations are satisfactory. It is preferable to transfer either type of patient from the recovery room to an intensive care unit, where such parameters can be carefully monitored and good ventilatory therapy will be possible.

In all postoperative patients, efforts should be made to increase the functional residual capacity toward normal levels. Numerous maneuvers can be implemented. Expiratory maneuvers such as coughing (voluntary, encouraged, or catheter-stimulated) have been reported to be successful. The benefits probably result from the maximum inspiration that occurs prior to the cough rather than from the expiratory maneuver. Blowing into a balloon, glove, tube, or blow bottle has not been demonstrated to have any salutary effects in controlled studies.[155]

Carbon-dioxide-induced hyperventilation and intermittent positive pressure breathing (IPPB), as conventionally practiced in postoperative wards, had no beneficial effects in several controlled studies.[144,155] Because IPPB is generally carried out with pressure-cycled respirators, the restriction of the chest cage by pain may limit the excursion of the thorax. Perhaps a volume-cycled ventilator would be more effective, though this has not been adequately studied. Persons whose ventilation is severely limited, who have prior understanding of the use of positive-pressure ventilation, and who are in need of bronchodilator medications delivered by aerosol may benefit from this therapy.

The most effective means of preventing postoperative pulmonary complications include the upright position and frequent maximum voluntary inhalations.[144,155,226] Encouragement of maximum inhalation, with breath-holding at deep inhalation for as long as possible every hour or two through the first postoperative days, results in a 50% reduction of complications, including fever, atelectasis, and pneumonia. This mechanism for reversing the predictable abnormalities of pulmonary function has become a part of postoperative care in patients undergoing abdominal or thoracic surgery, although its scientific basis is not fully established.[229]

Postsurgical Care

1. Patients with increased risk of postoperative complications should be identified.
2. Patients in a low-risk category probably need only careful instruction concerning what to expect in the post-operative period, instructions in deep breathing pre- and postoperatively, and supplemental oxygen administration postoperatively until it can be demonstrated that such is no longer necessary.
3. Patients who are at high risk should be as free of respiratory secretions as possible before surgery. A reasonable regimen to achieve this includes cessation of smoking, inhaled bronchodilators, postural drainage, chest percussion following bronchodilators, and antibiotics if appropriate.
4. High-risk patients should be instructed in coughing while the site of operation is supported.
5. Deep-breathing procedures found to be most successful preoperatively should be continued postoperatively.
6. The patient should be as mobile as possible while in bed and should be forced into ambulation at the earliest possible date.
7. If severe respiratory failure occurs postoperatively, detailed management must be undertaken in the manner discussed in Chapter 7.

The type of anesthetic used has been studied extensively in relation to the incidence of postoperative pulmonary problems. As recently reviewed,[228,228a] the type of postoperative analgesia may be important to the mobility and convalescence of the patient in general, but this is not predictably associated with decreased pulmonary complications.

When one reviews the many approaches that have been used in the treatment of postoperative patients and the varying results reported, one must agree with Hamilton's evaluation[229]: "With a complication such as atelectasis which appears dependent on immobility, hypoventilation, and lack of cleansing of the lower respiratory tract, any therapy which increases attention to the patient as a whole may effect cures in atelectasis." A reasonable regimen is outlined in the list on page 547.

LUNG TRANSPLANTATION

Patients with many forms of end stage bilateral lung disease have been considered eligible for lung transplantation. Extensive animal work and experience with 38 human transplants have demonstrated that lung transplantation must still be considered experimental. One of the two longest survivors lived 10 months and the other lived 6 months. The average survival of a recipient was 18 to 21 days. It is clear that a single lung transplant can sustain a recipient; however, rejection, infection, imperfect bronchial anastomotic healing, and availability of suitable donor lungs for immediate transplantation remain the major problems.[230,231]

There has been recent interest in bilateral lung and heart transplantation, which has some technical advantages but also remains experimental.

REFERENCES

1. LUCAS CE, LEDGERWOOD A, WALT AJ: A scientific basis for medical student education in trauma. J Trauma 13:520, 1973
2. DOUGALL AM, et al: Chest trauma—Current morbidity and mortality. J Trauma 17:547, 1977
3. WILSON RF, MURRAY C, ANTONENKO DR: Nonpenetrating thoracic injuries. Surg Clin North Am 57:17, 1977
4. BAKO G, MACKENZIE WC, SMITH ESO: Case-control study of recidivist drivers involved in fatal highway accidents in Alberta in 1970-72. Can Med Assoc J 116:149, 1977
5. Impaired driving—Technical Report No 8. Health and Welfare Canada, 1978
6. PERRY JF, GALWAY CF: Chest injury due to blunt trauma. J Thorac Cardiovasc Surg 49:684, 1965
7. DRUMMOND DS, CRAIG RH, DOW E: Non-penetrating thoracic trauma: A statistical survey and analysis. Can J Surg 9:332, 1966
8. ASHBAUGH DG, et al: Chest trauma, analysis of 685 patients. Arch Surg 95:546, 1967
9. FISHER RP, et al: Diagnostic peritoneal lavage: Fourteen years and 2,586 patients later. Am J Surg 136:701, 1978
10. ROTHERBERGER DA, et al: Diagnostic peritoneal lavage for blunt trauma in pregnant women. Am J Obst Gynecol 129:479, 1977
11. HUME DM: Endocrine and metabolic responses to injury. In Schwartz SI, et al: Principles of Surgery. New York, (eds) McGraw-Hill, 1974

11a. BUCHSBAUM JN, (ed): Trauma in Pregnancy. Philadelphia, WB Saunders Co., 1979

12. NACLERIO EA: Chest Injuries. New York, Grune & Stratton, 1971
13. WYNN-WILLIAMS N, YOUNG RD: "Cough" fracture of the ribs including one complicated by pneumothorax. Tubercle 40:47, 1959
14. WILSON JM, THOMAS AN, GOODMAN PC et al: Severe chest trauma. Arch Surg 113:846, 1978
15. HEINZ GJ, ZAVALA DC: Slipping rib syndrome. JAMA 237:794, 1977
16. RAPPORT RL, ALLEN RB, CURRY GJ: The fractured rib—a significant injury. Arch Surg 71:7, 1955
17. MULDER DS, GREENWOOD FAH, BROOKS CE: Posttraumatic thoracic outlet syndrome. J Trauma 13:706, 1973
18. RICHARDSON JD, MCELVEIN RB, TRINKLE JK: First rib fracture: A hallmark of severe trauma. Ann Surg 181:251, 1975
19. MALONEY JV, SCHMUTZER KJ, RASCHKE E: Paradoxical respiration and "pendelluft." J Thorac Cardiovasc Surg 41:291, 1961
20. CRAVEN KD, OPPENHEIMER L, WOOD LDH: Effects of contusion and flail chest on pulmonary perfusion and oxygen exchange. J Appl Physiol 47:729, 1979
21. DUFF JH, et al: Flail chest: A clinical review and physiological study. J Trauma 8:63, 1968
22. RELIHAN M, LITWIN MS: Morbidity and mortality associated with flail chest injury: A review of 85 cases. J Trauma 13:663, 1973
23. GARZON AA, SELTZER B, KARLSON KE: Physiopathology of crushed chest injuries. Ann Surg 168:128, 1968

24. CONN JH, HARDY JD, FAIN WR et al: Thoracic trauma: Analysis of 1022 cases. J Trauma 3:22, 1963
25. CHRISTENSSON P, et al: Early and late results of controlled ventilation of flail chest. Chest 75:456, 1979
26. VIRSHUP M: The anteriorly crushed chest or "steering wheel injury." J Thorac Cardiovasc Surg 39:579, 1960
27. GIBSON LD, CARTER R, HINSHAW DB: Surgical significance of sternal fracture. Surg Gynecol Obstet 114:443, 1962
28. THOMAS AN, BLAISDELL FW, LEWIS FR et al: Operative stabilization for flail chest after blunt trauma. J Thorac Cardiovasc Surg 75:793, 1978
29. GUERNELLI N, et al: Technique for the management of anterior flail chest. Thorax 34:247, 1979
30. BLAIR E, MILLS E: Rationale of stabilization of the flail chest with intermittent positive pressure breathing. Am Surg 34:860, 1968
31. RANSDELL HT: Treatment of flail chest injuries with a piston respirator. J Trauma 5:412, 1965
32. TRINKLE JK, et al: Management of flail chest without mechanical ventilation. Ann Thorac Surg 19:355, 1975
33. SHACKFORD SR, et al: The management of flail chest: A comparison of ventilatory and nonventilatory treatment. Am J Surg 132:759, 1976
34. HANKINS JR: Extensive pulmonary laceration caused by blunt trauma. J Thorac Cardiovasc Surg 74:519, 1977
35. LANGSTON HT, TUTTLE WM: The pathology of chronic traumatic hemothorax. J Thorac Surg 16:99, 1946
36. WILSON JL, et al: The absorption of blood from the pleural space. Surgery 48:766, 1960
37. MALONEY JV: The conservative management of traumatic hemothorax. Am J Surg 93:533, 1957
38. WILSON JM, BOREN CH JR., PETERSON SR et al: Traumatic hemothorax: is decortication necessary? J Thoracic Cardiovasc Surg 77:489, 1979
39. Editorial: Traumatic hemothorax. Lancet ii:290, 1979
40. COLLINS MP, SCHUCK JM, WACHTEL TL et al: Early decortication after thoracic trauma. Arch Surg 113:440, 1978
41. HAMMAN L: Spontaneous mediastinal emphysema. Bull Johns Hopkins Hosp 64:1, 1939
42. BODEY GP: Medical mediastinal emphysema. Ann Intern Med 54:46, 1961
43. THOMAS AN: Air embolism following penetrating lung injuries. J Thorac Cardiovasc Surg 66:533, 1973
44. SUMMERS B: Pneumoperitoneum associated with artificial ventilation. Br Med J 1:1528, 1979
45. HANKINS JR, et al: Extensive pulmonary laceration caused by blunt trauma. J Thoracic Cardiovasc Surg 74:519, 1977
46. MOORE EE, MOORE JB, GALLOWAY AC et al: Postinjury thoracotomy in the emergency department: A critical review. Surgery 86:590, 1979
47. ELLIS R: Traumatic lung cysts. JAMA 236:1976, 1976
48. FAGAN CJ, SWISCHUK LE: Traumatic lung and paramediastinal pneumatoceles. Radiology 120:11, 1976
49. SANTOS GH, MAHENDRA T: Traumatic pulmonary pseudocysts. Ann Thorac Surg 27:359, 1978
50. NICHOLS RT, PEARCE HJ, GREENFIELD LJ: Effects of experimental pulmonary contusion on respiratory exchange and lung mechanics. Arch Surg 96:723, 1968
51. COPPEL DL: Blast injuries of the lung. Br J Surg 63:735, 1976
52. BLAISDELL FW, LEWIS FP JR: Respiratory distress syndrome of shock and trauma. In Major Problems in Clinical Surgery. Philadelphia, WB Saunders, 1977
53. MURRAY JF: Conference Report: Mechanisms of Acute Respiratory Failure. Am Rev Respir Dis 115:1071, 1977
54. CARRICO CJ, HOROVITZ JH: Postinjury acute pulmonary failure. Chapter 32. In Shires GT (ed): Care of the Trauma Patient, 2nd ed. New York, McGraw-Hill, 1979
55. JACOB HS, et al: Complement-induced granulocyte aggregation: An unsuspected mechanism of disease. N Engl J Med 302:789, 1980
56. COLLINS JA: The acute respiratory distress syndrome. Adv Surg 11:171, 1977
57. OVERLAND ES, SEVERINGHAUS JW: Non-cardiac pulmonary edema. Adv Intern Med 23:307, 1978
58. MUIR AL, et al: Cardiorespiratory effects of rapid saline infusion in normal man. J Appl Physiol 38:786, 1975
59. REUL GJ, BEALL AC, GREENBERG SD: Protection of the pulmonary microvasculature by fine screen blood filtration. Chest 66:4, 1974
60. DURTSCH MB, et al: Effect of micropore filter on pulmonary function after massive transfusion. Am J Surg 138:8, 1979
61. OPPENHEIMER L, et al: Pathophysiology of pulmonary contusion in dogs. J Appl Physiol 47:718, 1979
62. PREWITT RM, MCCARTHY J, WOOD LDH: Treatment of acute low pressure pulmonary edema in dogs. J Clin Invest 67:409, 1981
63. BEAN JW, BECKMAN DL: Centrogenic pulmonary pathology in mechanical head injury. J Appl Physiol 27:807, 1969
64. BRASHAER RE, PAMINTUAN RL: Increased pulmonary diffusing capacity and elevated cerebrospinal fluid pressure. J Appl Physiol 30:844, 1971
65. MOSS G: Shock, cerebral hypoxia, and pulmonary vascular control: The centrineurogenic eti-

ology of the respiratory distress syndrome. Bull NY Acad Med 49:689, 1973

66. MARON MD, DAWSON CA: Adrenal component to pulmonary hypertension induced by elevated cerebrospinal fluid pressure. J Appl Physiol 47:153, 1979

66a. FISHMAN AP, PIETRA GG: Stretched pores, blast injury, and neurohemodynamic pulmonary edema. Physiologist 23:53, 1980

67. BOWERS RE, et al: Increased pulmonary vascular permeability follows intracranial hypertension in sheep. Am Rev Respir Dis 119:637, 1979

68. SANDHAM JD, SHAW DT, GUENTER CA: Acute supine respiratory failure due to bilateral diaphragmatic paralysis. Chest 72:96, 1977

69. TSAO C, et al: Disseminated leukocyte injury during open heart surgery. Arch Pathol 95:357, 1973

70. FOUNTAIN SW, et al: Pulmonary leukostasis and its relationship to pulmonary dysfunction in sheep and rabbits. Circulation Research 46:175, 1980

71. HUMLER F, LEVIN NW: Leucopenia and hypoxemia. Arch Intern Med 139:1103, 1979

72. KUX M, et al: Pulmonary effects of E. coli endotoxin: Role of leukocytes and platelets. Ann Surg 175:26, 1972

73. PINGLETON WW, COALSON JJ, GUENTER CA: Significance of leukocytes in endotoxin shock. Exp Mol Pathol 22:183, 1975

74. LEWIS FR, BLAISDELL FW, SCHLOBOHM RM: Incidence and outcome of posttraumatic respiratory failure. Arch Surg 112:436, 1977

75. ZAPOL WM, MARK EJ: Post-traumatic pulmonary insufficiency. N Engl J Med 296:1279, 1977

76. PAZELL JA, PELTIER LF: Experience with sixty-three patients with fat embolism. Surg Gynecol Obstet 135:77, 1972

77. EVARTS CM: The fat embolism syndrome: A review. Surg Clin North Am 50:493, 1970

78. MCCARTHY B, MAMMEN E, LEBLANC LP et al: Subclinical fat embolism: A prospective study of 50 patients with extremity fractures. J Trauma 13:9, 1973

79. GUENTER CA, BRAUN T: Fat embolism: Changing prognosis. Chest 79:143, 1981

80. ROKKANEN P, LAHDERSUU M, KATAJA J et al: The syndrome of fat embolism: Analysis of 30 consecutive cases compared to trauma patients with similar injuries. J Trauma 10:299, 1970

81. HARDISTY RM, INGRAM GIC: Bleeding Disorders: Investigation and Management. Philadelphia, FA Davis, 1965

82. POLLAK R, MYERS RAM: Early diagnosis of the pet embolism syndrome. J Trauma 18:121, 1978

83. CURTIS AM, et al: The three syndromes of fat embolism: Pulmonary manifestations. Yale J Biol Med 52:149, 1979

84. JACOBOVITZ-DERKS D, DERKS CM: Pulmonary neutral fat embolism in dogs. Am J Pathol 95:29, 1979

85. BAKER PL, PAZELL JA, PELTIER LF: Free fatty acids, catecholamines, and arterial hypoxia in patients with fat embolism. J Trauma 11:1026, 1971

86. KING EG, WEILLY HS, GENTON E et al: Consumption coagulopathy in the canine oleic acid model of fat embolism. Surgery 69:533, 1971

87. KING EG, NAKANE PK, ASHBAUGH DG: The canine oleic acid model of fibrin localization in fat embolism. Surgery 69:782, 1971

88. PARKER FB, WAX SD, KUSAJIMA K et al: Hemodynamic and pathologic findings in experimental fat embolism. Arch Surg 108:70, 1974

89. KING EG, et al: Alterations in pulmonary microanatomy after fat embolism. Chest 59:524, 1971

90. GOSSLING HR, ELLISON LH, DEGRAFF AC: Fat embolism. The role of respiratory failure and its treatment. J Bone Joint Surg 56:1327, 1974

91. FISCHER JE, TURNER RH, HERNDON JH et al: Massive steroid therapy in severe fat embolism. Surg Gynecol Obstet 1:677, 1971

92. HORNE RH, HORNE JH: Fat embolization prophylaxis. Arch Intern Med 133:288, 1974

93. MURRAY D, RACZ G: Fat embolism syndrome (respiratory insufficiency syndrome). J Bone Joint Surg 56:1338, 1974

94. HOOD RM, SLOAN HE: Injuries of the trachea and major bronchi. J Thorac Cardiovasc Surg 38:458, 1959

95. BATTERSBY JS, KILMAN JW: Traumatic injuries of the tracheobronchial tree. Arch Surg 88:644, 1964

96. WILKINS EW, MARK EJ: Hypoxemia and pneumomodiastinum after a vehicular accident. N Engl J Med 304:1155, 1981

97. BURKE JF: Early diagnosis of traumatic rupture of the bronchus. JAMA 181:682, 1962

98. LOTZ PP, MARTEL W, ROHWEDDER JJ et al: Significance of pneumomediastinum in blunt trauma to the thorax. Am J Roentgenol 132:817, 1979

99. GUEST JL, ANDERSON JN: Major airway injury in closed chest trauma. Chest 72:63, 1977

100. GROVER FL, et al: Diagnosis and management of major tracheobronchial injuries. Ann Thorac Surg 28:384, 1979

101. HURST JW, LOGUE RB, SCHLANT RC et al: The Heart, Arteries, and Veins, 4th ed. New York, McGraw-Hill, 1978

102. PEARCE W, BLAIR E: Significance of the electrocardiogram in heart contusion due to blunt trauma. J Trauma 16:136, 1976

103. TRUEBLOOD HW, WUERFLEIN RD, ANGELL WW: Blunt trauma rupture of the heart. Ann Surg 177:66, 1973

104. MADOFF IM, DESFORGES G: Cardiac injuries due to nonpenetrating thoracic trauma. Ann Thorac Surg 14:504, 1972

105. STEIN L, SHUBIN H, WEIL MH: Recognition and management of pericardial tamponade. JAMA 225:503, 1973
106. KIRSH MM et al: The treatment of acute traumatic rupture of the aorta. Ann Surg 184:308, 1976
107. BROSS W: Injuries of the thoracic aorta. J Cardiovasc Surg 12:95, 1971
108. FISHBONE G, ROBBINS DI, OSBORN DJ et al: Trauma to the thoracic aorta and great vessels. Radiol Clin North Am 11:543, 1973
109. CASTAGNA J, NELSON RJ: Blunt injuries to branches of the aortic arch. J Thorac Cardiovasc Surg 69:521, 1975
110. BODILY K, PERRY JF JR, STRATE RG et al: The salvageability of patients with post-traumatic rupture of the descending thoracic aorta in a primary trauma center. J Trauma 17:754, 1977
111. BOLANOWSKI PJP, SARKERIA JS, NEVILLE WE: Traumatically widened mediastinum. N Y State J Med 78:2194, 1978
112. PLUME S, DE WEESE JA: Traumatic rupture of the thoracic aorta. Arch Surg 114:240, 1979
113. SANDOR F: Incidence and significance of traumatic mediastinal hematoma. Thorax 22:43, 1967
114. BEKASSY SM, DAVE KS, WOOLER GH et al: "Spontaneous" and traumatic rupture of the diaphragm: Long-term results. Ann Surg 177:320, 1973
115. WISE L, CONNORS J, HWAN YH et al: Traumatic injuries to the diaphragm. J Trauma 13:946, 1973 13:946, 1973
116. JARRETT F, BERNHARDT LC: Right-sided diaphragmatic injury. Arch Surg 113:737, 1978
117. MEADS GE, CARROLL SE, PITT DF: Traumatic rupture of the right hemidiaphragm. J Trauma 17:797, 1977
118. FATAAR S, RAD FF, SCHULMAN A: Diagnosis of diaphragmatic tears. Br J Radiol 52:375, 1979
119. ESTRERA AS, PLATT MR, MILLS LJ: Traumatic injuries of the diaphragm. Chest 75:306, 1979
120. CHRISTIANSEN LA, STAGE P, BRAHE EB et al: Rupture of the diaphragm. Thorax 29:559, 1974
121. GOURIN A, GARZON AA: Diagnostic problems in traumatic diaphragmatic hernia. J Trauma 14:20, 1974
122. BRIGGS JN, GERMANN TD: Traumatic perforations of the esophagus. Surg Clin North Am 48:1297, 1968
123. MARSTON EL, VALK HL: Spontaneous perforation of the esophagus: Review of the literature and report of a case. Ann Intern Med 51:590, 1959
124. CRADDOCK DR, LOGAN A, MAYELL M: Traumatic rupture of the esophagus and stomach. Thorax 23:657, 1968
125. ROGERS LF, PUIG AW, DOOLEY BN et al: Diagnostic considerations in mediastinal emphysema. Am J Roentgenol 115:495, 1972
126. BENJAMIN CI, ENGRAU LH, PERRY JF JR: Delayed rupture or delayed diagnosis of rupture of the spleen. Surg Gynecol Obstet 142:171, 1976
127. JUDE JR, KOUWENHOVEN WB, KNICKERBOCKER GG: Closed chest cardiac massage. JAMA 173:1064, 1960
128. HENRIKSEN H: Rib fractures following external cardiac massage. Acta Anaesthesiol Scand 11:57, 1967
129. GROSSMAN JI, RUBIN IL: Cardiopulmonary resuscitation. Am Heart J 78:569, 1969
130. POULSON H: Discussion on complications of cardiopulmonary resuscitation. Acta Anaesthesiol Scand [Suppl] 29:319, 1968
131. Complications of cardiac massage. Br Med J 5636:68, 1969
132. GRAY AR, HARRISON WH, COUVES CM et al: Penetrating injuries to the chest. Am J Surg 100:709, 1960
133. LOVE JW: Chest injuries. JAMA 232:385, 1975
134. SANDRASAGRA FA: Management of penetrating stab wounds of the chest. Thorax 33:474, 1978
135. SIEMENS R, et al: Indications for thoracotomy following penetrating thoracic injury. J Trauma 17:493, 1977
136. GRAHAM JM, BEALL AC, JR, MATTOX KI et al: Systemic air embolism following penetrating trauma to the lung. Chest 72:449, 1977
137. WANEBO H, VAN DYKE J: The high-velocity pulmonary injury. J Thorac Cardiovasc Surg 64:537, 1972
138. SHIRES GT: Principles and management of hemorrhagic shock. In Shires GT (ed): Care of the Trauma Patient, 2nd ed, Chapt 1. New York, McGraw-Hill Book, 1979
139. LATIMER RG, et al: Ventilatory patterns and pulmonary complications after upper abdominal surgery determined by preoperative and postoperative computerized spirometry and blood gas analysis. Am J Surg 122:622, 1971
140. PECORA DV: Predictability of effects of abdominal and thoracic surgery upon pulmonary function. Ann Surg 170:101, 1969
141. DON HF, WAHBA WM, CRAIG DB: Airway closure, gas trapping, and the functional residual capacity during anesthesia. Anesthesiology 36:533, 1972
142. WEENIG CS, PIETAK S, HICKEY RF et al: Relationship of preoperative closing volume to functional residual capacity and alveolar–arterial oxygen difference during anesthesia with controlled ventilation. Anesthesiology 41:3, 1974
143. VAN DE WATER JM, et al: Prevention of post-operative pulmonary complications. Surg Gynecol Obstet 135:229, 1972
144. MEYERS JR, LEMBECK L, O'KANE H et al: Changes in functional residual capacity of the lung after operation. Arch Surg 110:576, 1975
145. MEAD J, COLLIER C: Relation of volume history of

lungs to respiratory mechanics in anesthetized dogs. J Appl Physiol 14:669, 1959

146. FERRIS BG JR, POLLARD DS: Effect of deep and quiet breathing on pulmonary compliance in man. J Clin Invest 39:143, 1960

147. EGBERT LD, LAVER MB, BENDIXEN HH: Intermittent deep breaths and compliance during anesthesia in man. Anesthesiology 24:57, 1963

148. BENDIXEN HH, HEDLEY-WHYTE J, CHIR B et al: Impaired oxygenation in surgical patients during general anesthesia with controlled ventilation: A concept of atelectasis. N Engl J Med 269:991, 1963

149. HEDLEY-WHYTE J, LAVER MB, BENDIXEN HH: Effect of changes in tidal ventilation on physiologic shunting. Am J Physiol 206:891, 1964

150. BENDIXEN HH, SMITH GM, MEAD J: Patterns of ventilation in young adults. J Appl Physiol 19:195, 1964

151. BENDIXEN HH, BULLWINKEL B, HEDLEY-WHYTE J et al: Atelectasis and shunting during spontaneous ventilation in anesthetized patients. Anesthesiology 25:297, 1964

152. EGBERT LD, BENDIXEN HH: Effect of morphine on breathing pattern, a possible factor in atelectasis. JAMA 188:113, 1964

153. TSI GM: Preoperative evaluation of pulmonary function. Am Rev Respir Dis 119:293, 1979

154. TRIMBLE C, SMITH DE, ROSENTHAL MH et al: Pathophysiologic role of hypercarbia in post-traumatic pulmonary insufficiency. Am J Surg 122:633, 1971

155. BARTLETT RH, GAZZANIGA AB, GERAGHTY TR: Respiratory maneuvers to prevent post-operative pulmonary complications: A critical review. JAMA 224:1017, 1973

156. PONTOPPIDAN H, GEFFIN B, LOWENSTEIN E: Acute respiratory failure in the adult. N Engl J Med 287:690, 1972

156a. FORD GT, WHITELAW WA, CRUSE PJ et al: Diaphragm function after upper abdominal surgery. Amer Rev Resp Dis (Suppl) 123:2, 186, 1981

157. PIANETTO MB, HARRIS HA, SWEET HC: Changes in pulmonary function before and after pneumonectomy for pulmonary tuberculosis. Am Rev Respir Dis 95:189, 1967

158. NEUHAUS H, CHERNIACK NS: A bronchospirometric method estimating the effect of pneumonectomy on the maximum breathing capacity. J Thorac Cardiovasc Surg 55:111, 1968

159. WAGNER HN JR: The use of radioisotope techniques for the evaluation of patients with pulmonary disease. Am Rev Respir Dis 113:203, 1976

160. KRISTENSSON S, LINDELL SE, SWANBERG L: Prediction of pulmonary function loss due to pneumonectomy, using Xe^{133} radiospirometry. Chest 47:589, 1972

161. KRISTENSSON S, et al: Prediction of ventilatory function after lobectomy. Scand J Respir Dis 54:315, 1973

162. OLSEN GV, BLOCK AJ, TOBIAS IA: Prediction of postpneumonectomy pulmonary function using quantitative macroaggregate lung scanning. Chest 66:13, 1974

163. BOYSEN PG, BLOCK AJ, OLSEN GN et al: Prospective evaluation for pneumonectomy using the 99m technetium quantitative perfusion lung scan. Chest 72:422, 1977

164. MARION JM, et al: Unilateral lung function. Comparison of the lateral position test with radionuclide ventilation–perfusion studies. Chest 69:5, 1976

165. WALKUP RH, VOSSEL LF, GRIFFIN JP,: Prediction of post-operative pulmonary function with the lateral position. Chest 77:24, 1980

166. BEREND N, WOOLCOCK AJ, MARLIN GE: Effects of lobectomy on lung function. Thorax 35:145, 1980

167. LINDELL SC: Xe^{133} radiospirometry: Prediction of lung function after pulmonary resection. Scand J Clin Lab Invest 34:289, 1974

168. OLSEN GN, BLOCK AJ, SWENSON EW et al: Pulmonary function evaluation of the lung resection candidate: A prospective study. Am Rev Respir Dis 111:379, 1975

169. UGGLA LG: Indications for and results of thoracic surgery with regard to respiration and circulatory function tests. Acta Chir Scand 3:197, 1956

170. SODERHOLM B: The hemodynamics of the lesser circulation in pulmonary tuberculosis: Effect of exercise, temporary unilateral pulmonary artery occlusion and operation. Scand J Clin Lab Invest (Suppl) 9:1, 1957

171. REICHEL J: Assessment of operative risk of pneumonectomy. Chest 62:570, 1972

172. STOUGAARD J: Cardiac arrhythmias following pneumonectomy. Thorax 24:568, 1969

173. STANEK V, WIDIMSKY J, HURYCH J et al: Pressure flow and volume changes during exercise within pulmonary vascular bed in patients after pneumonectomy. Clin Sci 37:11, 1969

173a. COOPER DKC: The incidence of postoperative infection and the role of antibiotic prophylaxis in pulmonary surgery. Br J Dis Chest 75:154, 1981

174. QUINDON JJ, SCHAFFNER VD, HILTZ JE: Pneumonectomy for tuberculosis: Appraisal of results in 143 cases. Am Rev Respir Dis 97:193, 1968

175. GIMENO F, KRAAN JK, ORIE NGM et al: Pulmonary gas transfer 20 years after pneumonectomy for pulmonary tuberculosis. Thorax 32:80, 1977

176. WILCOX BR, MURRAY GF, FRIEDMAN M et al: The effects of early pneumonectomy on the remaining pulmonary parenchyma. Surgery 85:294, 1979

177. DON HF, ROBSON JG: The mechanics of the respiratory system during anesthesia: The effects of atropine and carbon dioxide. Anesthesiology 26:168, 1965

178. GARDINER AJS, PALMER KNV: Effect of premedication and general anesthesia on arterial blood gases. Br Med J 2:1433, 1964

179. MEDRADO V, STEPHEN CR: Effect of premedication with atropine sulphate on arterial blood gases and pH. Lancet 1:734, 1966

180. PIERCE JA, GAROFALO ML: Preoperative medication and its effect on blood gases. JAMA 194:99, 1965

181. MARSHALL BE, WYNCHE MQ JR: Hypoxemia during and after anesthesia. Anesthesiology 37:178, 1972

182. EGBERT LD, TAMERSOY K, DEAS TC: Pulmonary function during spinal anesthesia: The mechanism of cough depression. Anesthesiology 22:882, 1961

183. ASKROG V, SMITH TC, ECHENHOFF JE: Changes in pulmonary ventilation during spinal anesthesia. Surg Gynecol Obstet 119:563, 1964

184. BOUTROS AR: Effects of nitrous oxide, curare, ether and cyclopropane on post-operative respiratory adequacy. Anesthesiology 26:743, 1965

185. PASKING S, RODMAN T, SMITH TC: The effect of spinal anesthesia on the pulmonary function of patients with chronic obstructive pulmonary disease. Ann Surg 169:35, 1969

186. BOUTRSO AR, WEISEL M: Comparison of effects of three anesthetic techniques on patients with severe pulmonary obstructive disease. Can Anaesth Soc J 18:286, 1971

187. RAVIN MB: Comparison of spinal and general anesthesia for lower abdominal surgery in patients with chronic obstructive pulmonary disease. Anesthesiology 35:319, 1971

188. BRIDENBAUGH PO, BRIDENBAUGH LD, MOORE DC et al: The role of intercostal block and three general anesthetic agents as predisposing factors of post-operative pulmonary problems. Anesth Analg 51:638, 1972

189. GOLD MI: Anesthesia for the asthmatic patient. Anesth Analg 49:881, 1970

190. CORSSEN G, GUTIERREZ J, REVES JG et al: Ketamine in the anesthetic management of asthmatic patients. Anesth Analg 51:588, 1972

191. BANNISTER WK, SATTILARS AJ: Vomiting and aspiration during anesthesia. Anesthesiology 23:251, 1962

192. CULVER GH, MAKEL HP, BEECHER HK: Frequency of aspiration of gastric contents by the lungs during anesthesia and surgery. Ann Surg 133:289, 1951

193. BERSON W, ADRIANI J: "Silent" regurgitation and aspiration during anesthesia. Anesthesiology 15:644, 1954

194. JONES JG, BERRY M, HULANDS GH et al: The time course and degree of change in alveolar–capillary membrane permeability induced by aspiration of hydrochloric acid and hypotonic saline. Am Rev Respir Dis 118:1007, 1978

195. EDLUND G, GEDDA S, VAN DER LINDEN W: Intraperitoneal drains and nasogastric tubes in elective cholecystectomy. Am J Surg 137:775, 1979

196. GAMSU G, SINGER MM, VINCENT HH: Post-operative impairment of mucous transport in the lung. Am Rev Respir Dis 114:673, 1976

197. FORBES AR, GAMSU G: Lung mucociliary clearance after anesthesia with spontaneous and controlled ventilation. Am Rev Respir Dis 120:857, 1979

198. KING DS: Post-operative pulmonary complications. I. A statistical study based on two years' personal observation. Surg Gynecol Obstet 56:43, 1933

199. POOLER HE: Relief of post-operative pain and its influence on vital capacity. Br Med J 2:1200, 1949

200. WIGHTMAN JAK: A prospective survey of the incidence of post-operative pulmonary complications. Br J Surg 55:85, 1968

201. GUENTER CA, WHITELAW WA: The role of diaphragm function in disease. Arch Intern Med 139:806, 1979

201a. GARIBALDI RA et al: Risk factors for postoperative pneumonia. Am J Med 70:617, 1981

202. PETERS RM: Pulmonary physiologic studies of the perioperative period. Chest 76:576, 1979

203. BARKER NW, NYGAARD KK, WALTERS W et al: A statistical study of post-operative venous thrombosis and pulmonary embolism. I. Incidence of various types of operations. Proc Staff Meetings Mayo Clin 15:769, 1940

204. KAKKAR VV, et al: Low doses of heparin in prevention of deep-vein thrombosis. Lancet 2:669, 1971

205. WOOD EH, PRENTICE CRM, MCNICOL GP: Association of fibrinogen–fibrin-related antigen (FR-antigen) with post-operative deep-vein thrombosis and systemic complications. Lancet 1:166, 1972

206. BUTTERFIELD WJH [Chairman, Steering Committee on a Trial Sponsored by the Medical Research Council]: Effect of aspirin on post-operative venous thrombosis. Lancet 2:441, 1972

207. CLAGETT GP, SALZMAN EW: Prevention of venous thromboembolism in surgical patients. N Engl J Med 290:93, 1974

208. DRIPPS RD, DEMING MVN: Post-operative atelectasis and pneumonia: Diagnosis, etiology and management based upon 1,240 cases of upper abdominal surgery. Ann Surg 124:94, 1946

209. GOULD AB JR: Effect of obesity on respiratory complications following general anesthesia. Anesth Analg 41:448, 1962

210. ZOLLINGER RM, PASSI R: Observations on pre- and post-operative care. Am J Surg 122:716, 1966

211. CAHILL JM: Respiratory problems in surgical patients. Am J Surg 116:362, 1968

212. WISE L: Post-operative hypoxemia in obese patients. Ann Surg 180:877, 1974

213. BUNKER JP, et al: A comparison of either anesthesia with thiopental–nitrous oxide succinylcholine for upper abdominal surgery. Anesthesiology 20:745, 1959

214. CHALON J, TAYYAB MA, RAMANATHAN S: Cytology

of respiratory epithelium as a predictor of respiratory complications after operation. Chest 67:32, 1975

215. ROVENSTINE EA, TAYLOR IB: Post-operative respiratory complications: Occurrence following 7,874 anesthesias. Am J Med Sci 191:807, 1936
216. STEWARD DJ, STOAN IAJ: Recent upper respiratory infection and pulmonary artery clamping in the etiology of post-operative respiratory complications. Can Anaesth Soc J 16:57, 1969
217. MENEELY GR, FERGUSON JL: Pulmonary evaluation and risk in patient preparation for anesthesia and surgery. JAMA 175:1074, 1961
218. STEIN M, KOOTA GM, SIMON M et al: Pulmonary evaluation of surgical patients. JAMA 181:765, 1962
219. ROTHFELD EL, et al: Pulmonary function testing in geriatric surgical patients. Dis Chest 47:20, 1965
220. DIAMENT ML, PALMER KNV: Spirometry for preoperative assessment of airways resistance. Lancet 1:1251, 1967
221. SCHLENKER JD, HUBAY CA: The pathogenesis of post-operative atelectasis: A clinical study. Arch Surg 107:846, 1973
222. FEIGAL DW, BLAISDELL FW: The estimation of surgical risk. Med Clin North Am 63:1131, 1979
223. HARMAN E, LILLINGTON G: Pulmonary risk factors in surgery. Med Clin North Am 63:1289, 1979
224. GRACEY DR, DIVERTIE MB, DIDIEV EP: Preoperative pulmonary preparation of patients with chronic obstructive pulmonary disease. Chest 76:123, 1979
225. CAIN HD, STEVENS PM, ADANIGA R: Preoperative pulmonary function and complications after cardiovascular surgery. Chest 76:130, 1979
225a. Committee Report: Prophylaxis in Surgery. JAMA 237:1003, 1977
226. DOHI S, GOLD MI: Comparison of two methods of post-operative respiratory care. Chest 73, 592, 1978
227. BELMAN M, MITTMAN C: Incentive spirometry: The answer is blowing in the wind. Chest 79:254, 1981
228. PFLUG AE, MURPHY TM, BUTLER SH et al: The effects of post-operative peridural analgesia on pulmonary therapy and pulmonary complications. Anesthesiology 41:8, 1974
228a. WALTERING EA et al: Evaluation of bupivacaine nerve blocks in the modification of pain and pulmonary function changes after thoracotomy. Ann Thorac Surg 30:122, 1980
229. HAMILTON K: Atelectasis, pneumothorax, and aspiration as post-operative complications. Anesthesiology 22:708, 1961
230. VEITH FJ, KOERNER SK: The present status of lung transplantation. Arch Surg 109:734, 1979
231. VEITH FJ: Lung Transplantation. Surg Clin North Am 58:357, 1977

Chapter 12

Pleural Disease

ALAN K. PIERCE

The pleura consists of a thin layer of connective tissue covered by a single layer of mesothelial cells. It contains generous vascular and lymphatic networks, and the parietal pleural is supplied with nerve endings. The pleura covers the surface of the chest wall, the superior surface of the diaphragm and the mediastinum (parietal pleura), and the entire surface of both lungs (visceral pleura). The parietal pleura can be stripped from the chest wall with relative ease, but the visceral pleura is intimately connected to the lung parenchyma.

The visceral and parietal pleural surfaces are separated by a potential space that is filled with a layer of fluid a few angstroms thick. The two pleural spaces are completely enclosed and completely separated. Because of the inward elastic recoil of the lungs and the outward elastic recoil of the chest wall, the intrapleural pressure is subatmospheric. The intrapleural pressure becomes more subatmospheric (more negative) during inspiration and remains subatmospheric during passive expiration, but pleural pressure is supra-atmospheric (positive) during forceful expiratory maneuvers.

PLEURITIC PAIN

Patients with disorders of the pleura most commonly present to a physician because of pain, fever, dyspnea, or an incidentally discovered roentgenographic abnormality. Of the symptomatic presenting manifestations, only pleuritic pain is sufficiently specific to indicate the presence of pleural disease during the initial history. Without this symptom, the physician may not recognize pleural involvement until the physical or chest roentgenographic examination.

As with other symptoms, pleuritic pain is not described in the same way by every patient. Nevertheless, it tends to present in a relatively specific manner. Most commonly, pleuritic pain is abrupt in onset; at times, the patient can date the onset to a specific minute, whereas in other patients it begins over a period lasting from minutes to hours. It is usually severe enough to cause the patient to present to the physician within hours of onset. Pain in the chest that lasts for days before the patient seeks medical advice is not usually pleuritic. Pleuritic pain is almost always unilateral and tends to be in the lower and lateral part of the chest. Although the pain may be referred to the shoulder or the abdomen, it tends not to be central in location; that is, it is not usually paravertebral or substernal. It is usually well localized. The pain is made worse by deep breathing or coughing and may be accentuated by body movements that cause movement of the chest cage. The patient may receive partial relief by splinting the area of involvement.

Patients with pleuritic pain may demonstrate characteristic physical findings. Since deep breathing is painful, tidal volumes are small, and the respiratory rate is rapid. There is usually splinting of the affected side, causing a lesser excursion than the opposite hemithorax. If such unilateral decreased motion is not apparent on inspection, it may be determined by finding a lag to respiration on the affected side by palpation.

Other types of chest pain may be confused with pleuritic pain. Perhaps the most difficult differential is pain due to musculoskeletal disorders, since such pain may also be associated with respiratory motion. Musculoskeletal pain is not usually as severe as pleuritic pain and may be present for a protracted time before medical aid is sought. Certain patterns of musculoskeletal pain may reveal the correct diagnosis. One type is the pain caused by frequent, forceful coughing. This pain is frequently bilateral, an uncommon event for pleuritic pain. It is located at the inferior costochondral margins, where the abdominal muscles insert into the anterior rib cage. It is commonly made worse by motions that cause contraction of the abdominal muscles, such as rising from a lying to a sitting position. Also, it is frequently associated with tenderness to palpation along the affected muscles. A second type of common chest-wall pain is located along the costochondral junctions anteriorly. There is frequently tenderness to palpation of the affected area, although palpation of the intercostal spaces contiguous to the costochondral junction does not cause pain. This type of pain may be aggravated by movement of the shoulder girdle.

A second type of pain frequently confused with pleuritic pain is that caused by irritation of major bronchi, commonly associated with bronchitis. This type of pain is substernal, is dull or burning rather than sharp, may be of prolonged duration before the patient seeks medical advice, and is frequently associated with severe respiratory motions such as coughing but not with normal breathing.

Myocardial pain usually can be differentiated from pleuritic pain by its substernal location, its quality of a pressure sensation, and its lack of association with respiratory movements. However, pericardial pain may be associated with respiratory motion and may be impossible to differentiate from pleuritic pain. Its tendency to a substernal location and its relief by assuming a sitting and leaning-forward posture may suggest the correct diagnosis.

Mediastinal pain of other origins such as tumors may also have a respiratory component. These pains, however, tend to be less severe than pleuritic pain (with the exception of dissecting aortic aneurysm), tend to a midline location, and may radiate through to the back.

The exact pathogenesis of pleuritic pain is not known but it is caused by conditions that affect the parietal pleura. The visceral pleura does not contain pain fibers and may be manipulated without causing unpleasant sensations. The pain fibers of the parietal pleura are derived from the intercostal nerves.

Although most analgesic or narcotic drugs may make the patient less aware of pleuritic pain, they usually do not entirely relieve the pain or allow the patient to take deep breaths or to cough. An apparent exception to this is the anti-inflammatory drug, indomethacin. In one study, it was found that indomethacin, 100 to 200 mg given as a rectal suppository every 6 to 8 hr, was dramatic in relieving the pain and allowed the patients to cough effectively.[1] In our hospital, the use of indomethacin orally seems to confirm these findings in at least some patients. In other patients, however, the only way to relieve pleuritic pain sufficiently to allow normal respiratory excursions is to perform an intercostal nerve block.

The first step in performing an intercostal block is to determine the site of pain and hence to determine which intercostal nerves must be anesthetized. At least three nerves must usually be anesthetized in order to obtain complete relief of pain. The block is performed in an area of the chest wall between the midscapular and posterior axillary lines, where the ribs are relatively superficial, but before the intercostal nerves have arborized extensively. Although the anesthetic agent only lasts for a finite interval, usually 2 to 4 hr, many patients have permanent relief of pain from one intercostal block.

DIFFERENTIAL DIAGNOSIS OF PLEURITIC PAIN

When dealing with a patient with pleuritic pain, the differential diagnostic possibilities group into two large categories: those patients who do and those who do not have physical or roentgenographic abnormalities of the chest. The most common processes in these categories are indicated in the list on p. 558.

Physical and Roentgenographic Abnormalities Absent

Herpes zoster is an acute infectious disease thought to be caused by a reactivation of latent

Differential Diagnosis of Pleuritic Pain

- Physical and Roentgenographic Abnormalities Absent
  - Herpes zoster
  - Epidemic pleurodynia
  - Pulmonary emboli
  - Connective tissue disease
  - Subdiaphragmatic abscess
- Physical and Roentgenographic Abnormalities Present
  - Pneumothorax
  - Primarily parenchymal disease
    - Infectious
      - Acute aerobic bacterial pneumonia
      - Anaerobic bacterial pneumonia
    - Pulmonary embolus with infarction
    - Neoplasm
  - Primarily pleural effusion
    - Infectious
      - Tuberculosis
      - Septicemic aerobic bacterial empyema
      - Subdiaphragmatic abscess
    - Pulmonary emboli
    - Neoplasm

varicella virus in a partially immune person. It causes a unilateral, segmental inflammation of the posterior nerve-root ganglions, with a painful vesicular eruption of the skin along the distribution of the involved nerve. Over 75% of cases involve the area between the second thoracic and the second lumbar vertebrae. The disease is unusual in children and increases in frequency and in severity with age. Most patients give histories of previous attacks of varicella.

The incubation period varies from 1 to 3 weeks. During the preeruptive stage, which may last for 2 to 4 days, the patient may have fever and constitutional symptoms, with pain over the distribution of intercostal nerves that is, in essence, pleuritic pain. During this preeruptive stage, the cause of the pain is frequently not apparent. On some occasions, the patient has hyperesthesia over the area of involvement, which allows the physician to make a presumptive diagnosis. There are no other positive physical or roentgenographic findings.

Following the preeruptive phase, a dermatitis appears with papules and vesicles on an erythematous base. Once the eruption has occurred, almost always unilaterally, the diagnosis becomes apparent. Treatment of herpes of the chest wall is directed at pain relief with analgesic or narcotic drugs. Early administration of adrenal steroids may reduce the incidence and duration of postherpetic neuralgia.[2] However, steroids may be contraindicated in patients with underlying serious disease.

Epidemic Pleurodynia. Pleurodynia is an acute infectious disease most commonly caused by Coxsackie B virus infection but occasionally the syndrome may be caused by Coxsackie A, ECHO virus, and perhaps other viruses. It is characterized by fever and other systemic symptoms in association with pleuritic pain. It tends to be a disease of children and young adults, occurring predominantly in the summer and the fall. Pleurodynia most commonly occurs in epidemics; a third of all patients report that other persons living in their households also have the disease.[3]

After an incubation period of 2 days to 2 weeks, the patient frequently experiences mild prodromal symptoms such as malaise, sore throat, or myalgia, for a few days. There is then the abrupt onset of severe, unilateral pleuritic chest pain. Muscle tenderness is not usually a feature of pleurodynia. The disease may be accompanied by severe systemic symptoms, with fever as high as 105°F. Complications of viremia, including meningitis, arthralgias, jaundice, or orchitis, may occur. Respiratory symptoms other than pain are not common, except for a mild, nonproductive cough. Physical and roentgenographic examinations of the chest are negative, except that up to 25% of the patients have pleural friction rubs.

Routine laboratory examinations are not helpful in diagnosis. The leukocyte count may be low, normal, or mildly elevated. In cases with meningitis, the cerebral spinal fluid findings are those of an aseptic process (a moderate number of lymphocytes, elevated protein and normal glucose).

The illness usually lasts for 4 or 5 days, but many patients have much more protracted courses and relapses after a few symptom-free days are common. In such cases, recovery may take weeks.

Treatment is directed at relieving the patient's symptoms with analgesics, narcotics, or intercostal nerve block.

Pleurodynia may occur concurrently with Coxsackie B pericarditis. In such cases, the pain may be primarily pleural or pericardial, or both. The patient may also have a pericardial friction rub and physical and roentgenographic evidence of pericardial effusion. There may also be a small amount of pleural effusion.

Pulmonary emboli may cause pleuritic pain in the absence of parenchymal infiltrate or pleural effusion. Patients commonly have dyspnea in addition to the pleuritic pain and they may have such associated findings as cough and hemoptysis. The chest pain is usually unilateral.

The reader is referred to Chapter 10, for a more complete description of this syndrome.

Connective tissue disease, most commonly lupus erythematosus, may cause recurrent pleuritic pain in the absence of associated physical or roentgenographic abnormalities. On other occasions, the pleuritic pain may be associated with small pleural effusions or with nondescript, alveolar infiltrates. Any pain or effusion tends to subside spontaneously but either may recur. Effusions and pain tend to be ameliorated by adrenal cortical steroid drugs.

Subdiaphragmatic (subphrenic) abscess, most commonly on the right side, may also cause pleural pain without associated thoracic findings. Usually, however, a small pleural effusion is present, and this process will be discussed in a later section.

Physical and Roentgenographic Abnormalities Present

In arriving at a differential diagnosis in patients with pleuritic pain, it may be helpful to consider whether the disease is predominantly of the lung parenchyma or whether it is predominantly a pleural effusion. These diseases are considered more extensively in this and other chapters; this section is intended to indicate only a differential diagnostic approach to pleuritic pain. In addition, pleuritic pain is a common presenting symptom of spontaneous pneumothorax. This syndrome will be discussed subsequently.

Primarily Parenchymal Disease. Many patients with pleuritic pain have associated symptoms suggestive of infection, such as chills, fever and cough productive of purulent sputum. When, in addition, physical examination reveals signs of consolidation of the lung parenchyma and the chest roentgenogram demonstrates an extensive alveolar infiltrate with little or no pleural effusion, a diagnosis of acute bacterial pneumonia due to aerobic or anaerobic organisms is most likely. The likelihood of viruses, mycoplasma, or organisms that cause granulomatous disease causing such a presentation is not great, since such infections rarely cause pleuritic pain.

If there is also a significant amount of pleural effusion, it may be difficult to determine whether the process is primarily parenchymal or pleural. If it can be determined that the disease is primarily parenchymal with additional pleural effusion, the reasonable presumptive diagnosis is acute bacterial pneumonia complicated by a pleural effusion that may be an empyema. The differential diagnosis of bacterial organisms remains the same, except that the pneumococcus, the most common cause of bacterial pneumonia, is not likely to produce a pleural effusion that is evident at the time the patient presents to the physician.

When a patient presents with pleuritic pain and a process that is primarily parenchymal, it may be difficult to separate pulmonary infarction from an infectious process. Helpful findings include the roentgenographic characteristics that suggest pulmonary infarction (see Chap. 10, thromboembolism). Patients with lung infarctions usually do not have chills and fever as marked as those seen in patients with infectious processes. An additional helpful observation may be the absence of purulent sputum. In many patients, however, a definitive separation of infection from infarction can be made only with more specific studies such as a radioactive macroaggregated albumin lung scan or a pulmonary angiogram.

Patients with neoplasms involving the lung parenchyma without extensive pleural effusion may occasionally present with pleuritic pain. The correct diagnosis can usually be made on the basis of lack of signs of infection, historic features suggesting a neoplastic process, and the roentgenographic appearance of the lesion.

Primarily Pleural Effusion. In many patients presenting with pleuritic pain, the physical and roentgenographic findings are predominantly those of a pleural effusion. In such patients, it is common to have moderate degrees of parenchymal infiltrate, caused by atelectasis secondary to the effusion and the pleuritic pain. In some cases, the physician may not be able to determine whether the antecedent process is the pleural effusion or the parenchymal infiltrate, but most commonly a reasonable determination can be made.

If pleural effusion dominates the picture, the etiologic process is much less likely to be an acute aerobic or anerobic bacterial lung infection. Although one encounters an occasional empyema without marked parenchymal infiltrate which is arising from a partially treated bacterial process, or a subdiaphragmatic infection, such an event is not common. Instead, in the patient presenting with pleuritic pain with primarily a pleural effusion and signs of infection such as fever, the probability becomes much greater that one is dealing with a tuberculous pleural effusion.

Patients presenting with pleuritic pain and primarily a pleural effusion may have pulmonary embolization without lung infarction. As with other presentations of pulmonary embolization, the diagnosis may be most difficult. One must usually rely on techniques such as lung scan or pulmonary angiography.

Patients with neoplastic diseases, most commonly bronchogenic carcinoma, may present with pleuritic pain and primarily a pleural effusion. The differentiation of the neoplastic effusion from an infectious effusion will be considered subsequently.

PNEUMOTHORAX

A pneumothorax is an accumulation of gas in the pleural space. It may occur spontaneously or may be secondary to trauma, surgery, or therapy. Although the physiologic consequences may be similar, the clinical circumstances differ enough to consider these categories separately.

SPONTANEOUS PNEUMOTHORAX

CLINICAL MANIFESTATIONS

Primary spontaneous pneumothoraces occur most commonly in young, previously healthy adults. The greatest prevalence is among men 20 to 40 yr old.[4,5] In such patients, the air leaks from the lung into the pleural space because of the rupture of blebs on the visceral pleural surface, most commonly located near the apex of the lung. The cause of such apical blebs is not known but they are found frequently at thoracotomy in persons operated on for unrelated reasons.[6,7] The cause of rupture of the blebs is similarly unknown. It would be reasonable to believe that pressures placed on the lung by vigorous exercise might lead to lung rupture. Such is not the case, however, because most spontaneous pneumothoraces occur at rest, frequently during sleep.[8] Although it was believed at one time that spontaneous pneumothoraces were generally the result of pulmonary tuberculosis, this is not correct. Most patients have entirely normal chest roentgenograms after recovery from the pneumothorax.

Spontaneous pneumothoraces also may occur in the presence of some antecedent pulmonary disease (*secondary spontaneous pneumothorax*). The only community-based study in the United States assessing the incidence of spontaneous pneumothorax in a general population reported the following age-adjusted rates: primary spontaneous pneumothorax, 7.4/100,000/yr for males and 1.2/100,000/yr for females; secondary spontaneous pneumothorax, 6.3/100,000/yr for males and 2.0/100,000/yr for females.[9] Thus, spontaneous pneumothoraces were no more common among persons with pulmonary disease. Most secondary spontaneous pneumothoraces occurred in persons with chronic obstructive pulmonary disease. Catamenial pneumothoraces (recurrent pneumothoraces associated with menstruation) have been reported in a small number of women.[10,10a]

The most common presenting manifestation of a primary spontaneous pneumothorax is pleuritic pain that begins without prodromal symptoms in a previously healthy person. Many patients experience mild to moderate dyspnea, but this symptom is not usually severe in patients with otherwise normal lungs. There is usually no other associated symptom.

Physical examination typically reveals tachypnea with small tidal volumes. Since the pneumothorax allows the lung to recoil to a smaller volume, the lung's retractile force is less than normal. The more nearly atmospheric intrapleural pressure allows the chest wall on the affected side to assume a more inspiratory position than normally present at functional residual capacity. The resting position of the chest wall unopposed by the elastic recoil of the lungs is approximately 80% of total lung capacity. In a large pneumothorax, the physician may appreciate the asymmetry of the chest, the affected side appearing larger. In a small pneumothorax, such asymmetry may be appreciated as a lag in inspiration on the affected side which does not begin to move until the contralateral side reaches the same degree of inspiration. Percussion demonstrates a more hyperresonant note over the affected side, since the water-to-air ratio of thoracic contents has been decreased. The mediastinal structures are shifted away from the side of the pneumothorax toward the more subatmospheric intrapleural pressure of the unaffected side. On auscultation, one finds decreased breath sounds over the area of the pneumothorax, since the vibrations of the lung produced by respiration are not easily transmitted to the chest wall through the column of air. Similarly, fremitus is decreased over the pneumothorax.

Unless the pneumothorax is large, physical findings may be entirely normal or only suggestive of the correct diagnosis and a definitive diagnosis can be made only by roentgenograms of the chest. The visceral pleural edge must be visualized with lung markings medial but not lateral to the edge (Fig. 12-1). Although one would anticipate the collapsed lung to have increased water density because of the decrease in the amount of air in the lung, this is not strikingly apparent until the lung has lost considerable volume. The lack of increased water density is related to two factors. As ventilation decreases in the affected lung, blood flow to the lung also decreases, shifting to the contralateral side.[11] Thus, air and water densities remain relatively constant. In addition, the gas in the pneumothorax anterior and posterior to the lung further decreases the water-to-air ratio. On standard posteroanterior (PA) and lateral chest roentgenograms, the diagnosis may be subtle, and additional views may be necessary.

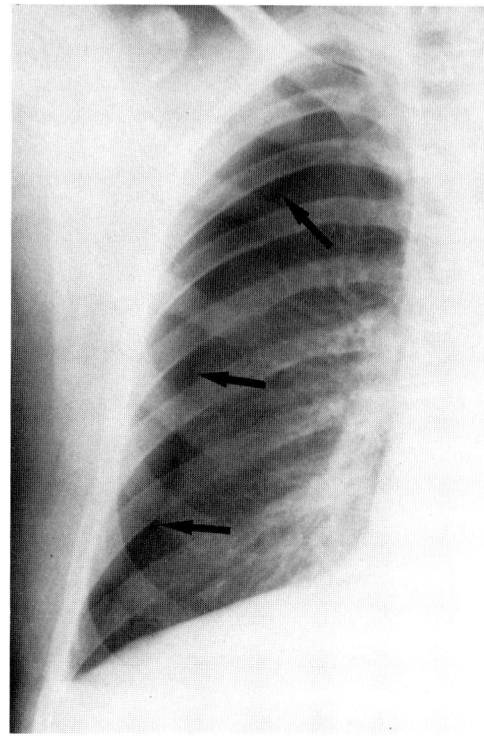

FIG. 12-1. Chest roentgenogram of the right hemithorax demonstrates the characteristics of a typical pneumothorax. The arrows indicate the visceral pleural edge, which generally parallels the chest wall. Parenchymal lung markings may be seen medial, but not lateral, to the visceral pleural edge. The roentgenographic density of the lung parenchyma adjacent to the pleural edge is not strikingly different from the density of the pneumothorax, owing to a decrease in blood flow to the affected lung and to the decrease in water-to-air ratio caused by the pneumothorax anterior and posterior to the lung.

If the visceral pleural edge cannot be outlined with certainty, a PA chest roentgenogram taken during a full expiration may be helpful (Fig. 12-2).

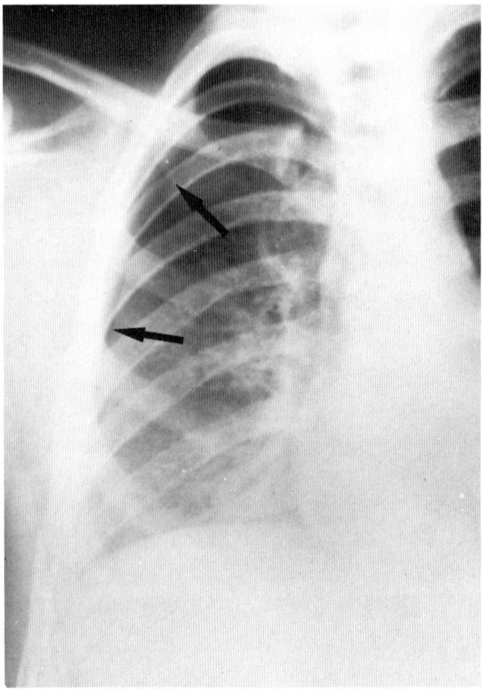

FIG. 12-2. Chest roentgenogram taken during expiration in a patient with a small pneumothorax. The roentgenogram taken during inspiration had not been diagnostic. During expiration, there was a sufficient increase in the water density of the lung parenchyma to allow the visceral pleural edge to become apparent (*arrows*).

During expiration, gas leaves the lung parenchyma but not the pleural space; the resulting increase in water density of the lung may help outline the pneumothorax, which now occupies a relatively greater fraction of the hemithorax. If an expiratory film is not definitive, a lateral decubitus film with the affected side up may be helpful. The pneumothorax should shift from the apex in the upright film to the lateral chest wall in the decubitus film, making the definition of the visceral pleural edge clearer, unimpeded by the bony structures near the apex.

Although most spontaneous pneumothoraces are not accompanied by pleural effusion, some patients develop small serous or bloody effusions. Since the effusion forms an air-fluid interface with the pneumothorax at approximately atmospheric pressure, the effusion forms a horizontal, straight edge on an upright chest roentgenogram (Fig. 12-3). Such a straight water density should lead the observer to search for a pneumothorax if such has not been previously apparent.

Immediately after a large pneumothorax, arterial hypoxemia occurs.[12] Over the next few hours, vasoconstriction in the affected lung causes the pulmonary arterial blood flow to be shifted to the contralateral lung, resulting in more appropriate ventilation-perfusion relationships. By 24 hr following pneumothorax, the arterial oxygen saturation returns to normal, although uniform airway closure may remain throughout the collapsed lung.[13] This mechanism may explain the clinical observation that a patient experiencing dyspnea following pneumothorax may no longer have this symptom the following day, even though the pneumothorax persists at approximately the same size.

The pleural leak allowing the pneumothorax usually seals by the time the patient presents to the physician, so that the pneumothorax usually is not progressive by the time the diagnosis has been established. Even without treatment, the gas ultimately is reabsorbed into the blood stream. This occurs because the amount of oxygen removed from arterial blood at the tissue level is greater than the amount of carbon dioxide diffused from the tissues into the blood. This results in the sum of the partial pressures of all of the gases in end capillary blood being lower than the sum of all the partial pressures of the gases in the pleural space. On the average, the pressure difference amounts to approximately 60 mmHg. This small pressure gradient allows for the reabsorption of the gas with time.

MANAGEMENT

There is some disagreement about the most appropriate therapy for patients with primary spontaneous pneumothorax.[14,15] Since most pneumothoraces are not progressive and since the gas is spontaneously reabsorbed, many physicians treat small pneumothoraces with only observation and repeated chest roentgenograms. Most physicians feel, however, that larger pneumothoraces should be removed in order to lessen morbidity. This can be performed by aspirating the gas from the pneumothorax into a syringe through a large bore needle placed into the pleural space through the second anterior intercostal space. Fearing further pleural laceration by the needle point as the lung reexpands, others aspirate through a plastic catheter placed into the pleural space through a metal needle that is withdrawn before aspiration begins. Realizing that up to a third of spontaneous pneumothoraces subsequently recur on the same side of the chest,[14] many physicians treat pneumothoraces with an indwelling thoracostomy tube, in the hope that the tube will incite sufficient inflammation of the visceral and parietal pleurae that symphysis will occur, thus preventing future pneumothorax. The thoracostomy tube is connected to a simple underwater seal system that acts as a oneway valve, allowing air out of the pleural space. The patient must raise the pressure in the pleural space to above atmospheric pressure in order for gas to escape from the pleural space. This is easily done by periodically coughing or performing forceful expirations. It is not necessary to attach the chest bottle seal to an aspiration pump. When gas ceases to flow from the pleural space for a period of a few hours, and if the lung is completely expanded, one can assume that the pleural leak has sealed and the thoracostomy tube may be removed.

Unilateral pulmonary edema has been reported to occur following rapid reexpansion of lungs which are chronically atelectatic because of large pneumothoraces.[16,16a] In an animal model, the requirements for producing pulmonary edema included a complete pneumothorax of 3 day's duration and rapid reexpansion by markedly negative intrapleural pressure.[17] Although the pathogenesis of edema formation is unknown, such reports suggest that markedly negative intrapleural pressures should be avoided when treating a pneumothorax. Initial evacuation of approximately half of the pneumothorax, allowing gradual re-expansion, should prevent this problem.

A patient who has had two spontaneous pneumothoraces on one side of the chest may continue to have many recurrences. Although authorities disagree on how many pneumothoraces should prompt therapy in addition to that already indicated, most agree that obliteration of the pleural space is indicated for repeated episodes of pneumothorax. This is probably best carried out by thoracotomy, with abrasion of the pleural surfaces or with parietal pleurectomy; these procedures lead to symphysis of the visceral and parietal pleurae as the patient recovers from thoractomy. Such a surgically produced fibrothorax does not usually significantly interfere with lung function permanently,[18] and the patient is relieved from the fear and morbidity of subsequent pneumothoraces.

A patient with a secondary spontaneous pneumothorax, usually associated with chronic obstructive lung disease, frequently has a more se-

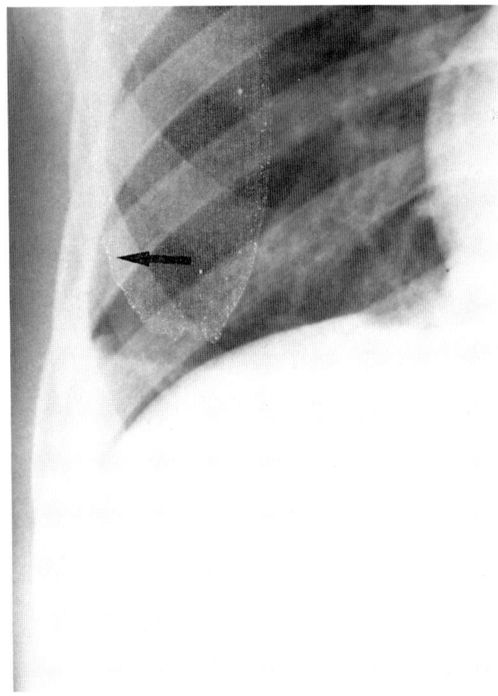

FIG. 12-3. In this chest roentgenogram taken in the upright position, the small pleural effusion in the right costophrenic sulcus has a horizontal upper edge, suggesting that the pressure in the pleural space is approaching atmospheric pressure. Such a straight water density should lead to a careful search for a visceral pleural edge, indicating a pneumothorax (*arrow*).

rious therapeutic problem. The air leaks from the visceral pleura are often diffuse and do not seal promptly.[19] Such a patient may need prolonged thoracostomy tube drainage and the underwater seal system must usually be attached to an aspiration pump in order to maintain lung expansion. If the air leak continues for approximately 2 weeks, this mode of therapy is not likely to be successful, and more aggressive measures are indicated. If the patient's pulmonary function is adequate, thoracotomy with excision of bullae and surgical pleurodesis is indicated.

Occasionally, the lung will completely expand, as seen on the chest roentgenogram, but air will continue to leak through the thoracostomy tube. After several days of maintaining complete expansion of the lung by continuous suction, a cautious trial of clamping the tube, and re-evaluating for evidence of recurrent pneumothorax, is warranted. If the pneumothorax does not recur in spite of a leak through the chest tube, pleural symphysis has occurred. The air is probably passing through a small tract from the lung to the chest tube, which will close spontaneously, and the chest tube can be safely removed.

Repetitive pneumothoraces or pneumothoraces which persist despite chest tube drainage may be treated successfully by chemical pleurodesis rather than surgery.[19a,b] This is discussed below under Pleural Effusions, Neoplasms. Our lack of experience with long-term sequelae and the lack of data regarding effects of the fibrothorax on pulmonary function suggest that this form of treatment should be reserved for patients whose underlying lung disease is too severe to allow surgery or that it should be performed in centers where the effects of the procedure will be carefully studied by long-term follow-up. It is encouraging to note, however, that the once popular talc pleurodesis did not predispose to the development of mesothelioma or bronchogenic carcinoma.[19c]

SECONDARY PNEUMOTHORAX

Pneumothorax may be caused by penetrating or nonpenetrating chest trauma. In nonpenetrating trauma, the pneumothorax is sometimes caused by fracture and dislocation of ribs with penetration of the visceral pleura. In such circumstances, there is usually an accompanying hemothorax. In most nonpenetrating traumas, however, a different mechanism must be evoked, since there is either no rib fracture or no displacement of fractured ribs. In these cases, the most likely explanation is the dissection of air from alveoli into interstitial spaces, with subsequent dissection into either the pleural space or the mediastinum. A patient may have pneumothorax, pneumomediastinum, or both. Because the air may dissect into the mediastinum without dissecting into the pleural space many patients with closed-chest trauma present with subcutaneous emphysema without evidence of pneumothorax. The air leak from the lung may remain patent for hours to days, with leakage of the air through the interstitial space to the mediastinum and subsequently to the subcutaneous tissues, resulting in progressive and marked subcutaneous emphysema without pneumothorax at any time.

Occasionally, particularly in patients on artificial ventilators, the pneumothorax is associated with a pneumoperitoneum, presumably caused by dissection of air through diaphragmatic orifices.[20] This may pose a dilemma when the diagnostic considerations include a perforated abdominal viscus.

In patients with chest trauma, pneumothorax may occur rarely from one of two additional complications, both of which are indications for immediate thoracic surgery. One of these is fracture of the trachea or a major bronchus, and the other is traumatic rupture of the esophagus. Bronchial tears most commonly occur in the presence of an anterior or lateral fracture of one or more of the first three ribs, evidently because the direction of force necessary to produce both of these events is similar.[21] The torn bronchus may dislocate completely, immediately resulting in a massive pneumothorax, or the bronchus may be held together by the peribronchial connective tissue for minutes to hours following the traumatic episode. On other occasions, the fractured bronchus remains intact without ever causing a pneumothorax. However, such bronchi tend to heal with excessive scarring, the encroachment on the bronchial lumen resulting in a partially obstructed bronchus that usually leads to infection in the distal lung. Bronchial tears should be searched for, most conveniently by means of fiberoptic bronchoscopy, when there is fracture of the first three ribs, hemoptysis associated with pneumothorax, or a large pneumothorax with continual leakage of air into the pleural space after treatment with a thoracostomy tube.

Rupture of the esophagus commonly leads to a pleural effusion in association with a pneumothorax and the effusion may contain gastric contents. Its diagnosis is best made by means of contrast roentgenographic studies.

Pneumonia caused by *Staphylococcus aureus* or by hospital-acquired gram-negative bacilli may lead to pneumothorax. In either case, the pneumothorax tends to occur through large air passages in the visceral pleura, caused by necrosis of lung tissue by the infecting organisms. Such bronchopleural fistulas frequently drain infected material into the pleural space, resulting in empyema as well as pneumothorax. These air leaks tend to close very slowly, resulting in the necessity for thoracostomy tubes for protracted intervals.

Pneumothorax is not a common complication of ventilator therapy, since inflation pressures and volumes are usually modest compared with those necessary for lung rupture. In the case of patients with the diffuse alveolar injury syndrome, most of whom have markedly decreased compliance, ventilatory therapy may be associated with pneumothorax. Such is evidently particularly true if the patient requires positive end expiratory pressure (PEEP) rather than only intermittent positive pressure breathing.[22,23] As in the case of nonpenetrating chest injury, air may leak into the mediastinum rather than into the pleural space, resulting in subcutaneous emphysema rather than pneumothorax.

Most patients with pneumothorax secondary to nonpenetrating chest trauma, infection, or to diffuse alveolar injury syndrome with ventilator therapy are extremely ill. Thus, physical findings are often difficult to interpret, and it is easy to miss a pneumothorax in this clinical setting. Unfortunately, chest roentgenograms are frequently taken with portable equipment with the patient in a recumbent position, resulting in poor-quality roentgenograms. On such roentgenograms, the air of a pneumothorax does not accumulate at the apex of the lung preferentially, since in these the circumstances this is not the highest part of the chest. Instead, the air may collect anteriorly and no visceral pleural edge will be demonstrated. In some patients, the air collects along the diaphragm, and films should be carefully scrutinized for a visceral pleural edge at the base of the lung or for exceptional clarity of the air-fluid interface of the diaphragm and the thoracic contents (Fig. 12-4). If

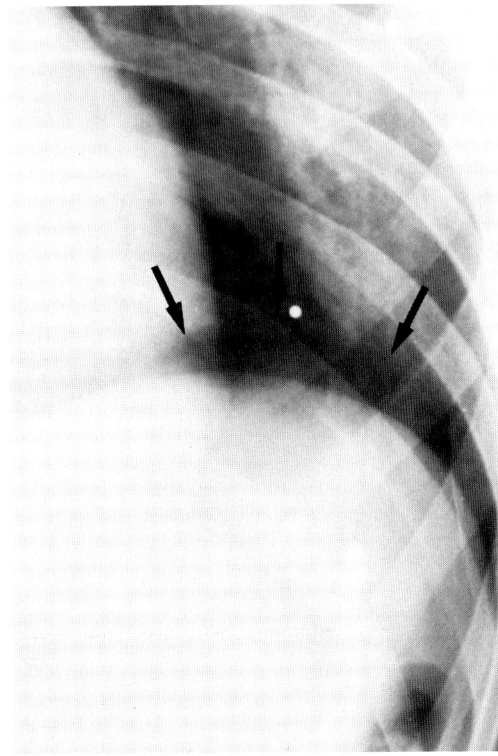

FIG. 12-4. This chest roentgenogram was taken in a recumbent position, because of the critical illness of the patient, caused by a shotgun wound injury. Several shotgun pellets appear in the roentgenogram as small, round, well-defined metallic densities. In the recumbent position, a pneumothorax may collect anteriorly and along the diaphragm. In this roentgenogram, a visceral pleural edge (*arrows*) may be seen, paralleling the diaphragm.

the usual film suggests the presence of a pneumothorax, most patients can be manipulated into a lateral decubitus position with the suspected side up, and a cross-bed horizontal beam used to confirm the diagnosis.

Virtually every patient with a secondary pneumothorax needs a thoracostomy tube since the visceral pleura does not seal promptly in such cases. In addition to a tube in the second anterior intercostal space to relieve the pneumothorax, many patients also need a posterior tube because of associated pleural fluid. Because the air leak into the pleural space is frequently large, simple underwater seal drainage may not be sufficient. In such cases, the port of the drainage bottle that is usually left open to atmospheric pressure is connected instead to a formal chest suction system. This arrangement allows gas to leave the pleural space continuously instead of only when pleural pressure is above atmospheric pressure. Reexpansion of the lung usually occurs.

In a patient with a secondary pneumothorax, the air leak may continue for a protracted interval. Tube drainage must continue until the air leak seals or until the visceral and parietal pleuras fuse around the bronchopleural fistula and the pneumothorax becomes localized.

TENSION PNEUMOTHORAX

A tension pneumothorax is gas in the pleural space at greater than atmospheric pressure during the entire respiratory cycle.[5] This is disastrous to cardiopulmonary function both because ventilation is severely compromised and because the positive pressure is transmitted to the mediastinum, resulting in decreased venous return of blood to the heart and the potential of low cardiac output shock. Therefore, tension pneumothorax most commonly presents as an acute medical emergency, with marked dyspnea, hypoxemia, and hypotension. Although spontaneous pneumothorax occasionally leads to a tension pneumothorax, this complication is more common in patients with pneumothoraces secondary to trauma or infection or during the course of ventilator therapy for the acute respiratory distress syndrome.

Physical findings in the chest are similar to those for simple pneumothorax except that the affected hemithorax may be more significantly larger than the nonaffected side and signs of mediastinal shift are likely to be more dramatic. Roentgenograms of the chest may not indicate that the pneumothorax is under positive pressure although mediastinal shift and depression of the diaphragm are likely to be more marked.

Rapid deterioration of the patient's clinical status may require that therapy be instituted, based on the physical findings, even though such findings may not be definitive. If no thoracostomy tube is immediately at hand, one places as large a bore needle as possible into the pleural space through the second anterior intercostal space. A rush of gas outward through the needle during the entire respiratory cycle indicates that a correct diagnosis has been made. Observing this phenomenon is made easier by attaching the needle to a syringe or connecting it by tubing to an underwater seal. The needle is left in place until a thoracostomy tube can be inserted, since a simple pneumothorax at atmospheric pressure is less detrimental to cardiopulmonary function than a tension pneumothorax. On the other hand, should air pass through the needle into the pleural space, the pneumothorax is not under tension, and the needle is immediately withdrawn. A thoracostomy tube is then inserted as soon as possible in the usual way. A third possibility consists of gas passing out through the needle during expiration, but air passing into the chest during inspiration. In this case, the patient has a simple pneumothorax. Forceful expiration, usually because of dyspnea, causes a positive intrapleural pressure only during this phase of respiration. In such patients, the needle is withdrawn, and one proceeds rapidly with a thoracostomy tube.

When the thoracostomy tube has been inserted and connected to an underwater seal bottle, an aspiration pump is connected to the bottle. The pressure in the bottle is maintained at subatmospheric levels, usually minus 40 cm H_2O, in order to hasten gas removal from the pleural space. In some patients, even this procedure does not allow full lung expansion, and a second thoracostomy tube must be inserted.

PLEURAL EFFUSIONS

The pleural cavity is normally moistened by a small amount of fluid that allows the visceral and parietal surfaces to move without friction during respiration. In healthy persons, the fluid film is only a few angstroms thick and cannot be seen on upright roentgenograms or detected on physical examination. However, a small amount of fluid may be seen along the dependent chest wall on lateral decubitus roentgenograms of some healthy persons.[24,25] When the fluid in the pleural space exceeds this small amount, a pleural effusion is said to exist.

In an effort to systematically approach the diagnosis of pleural effusions, it is common to divide them into the categories of transudates and exudates. In this regard, it is helpful to consider the mechanisms by which pleural fluid is formed and reabsorbed.[26,27]

DYNAMICS OF PLEURAL FLUID

The blood supply of the parietal pleura is from intercostal-artery capillaries that have a hydraulic pressure similar to that of other systemic capillaries, approximately 30 cm H_2O (Fig. 12-5). The pressure in the pleural space, against which the capillary wall is situated, is subatmospheric; at functional residual capacity, pleural pressure is approximately minus 5 cm H_2O, and it decreases further during inspiration. Thus, the net hydraulic pressure driving the fluid from within parietal pleural capillaries into the pleural space is approximately 35 cm H_2O. The blood supply of the visceral pleura is predominantly from pulmonary-artery capillaries that have a hydraulic pressure of approximately 11 cm H_2O. Since these capillaries also are affected by pleural-space pressure, the net hydraulic pressure across the visceral pleura is approximately 16 cm H_2O. This pressure also tends to drive fluid from within the capillary into the pleural space.

Capillaries are not freely permeable to the larger molecules in blood that create an osmotic pressure, tending to hold water within the capillaries. Albumin is the most important molecule in this regard. The colloid osmotic pressure of blood is approximately 34 cm H_2O and is the same in visceral and in parietal pleural capillaries. The capillary endothelium is not entirely impermeable to large molecules and a small amount of protein leaks into the pleural space. This pleural fluid protein exerts an osmotic pressure of approximately 8 cm H_2O. Thus, the balance of osmotic pressures from within capillaries to within the pleural space creates a gradient of approximately 26 cm H_2O, which would, if unbalanced by hydraulic pressures, cause water to move from within the pleural space into either the parietal or the visceral pleural capillaries.

The effects of hydraulic and osmotic pressures are to create a pressure of approximately 9 cm H_2O, causing water to flow from parietal capillaries into the pleural space, and of approximately 10 cm H_2O, causing the reabsorption of fluid from the pleural space into visceral pleural capillaries. Since the pressures are similar and fluctuate with respiration, the balance between filtration and reabsorption is determined by the relative resistances of the two capillary membranes. The visceral pleura is more vascular than the parietal pleura and its capillaries have a much larger surface area and hence are less resistant to fluid movement. Thus, the reabsorptive capacity of the visceral pleura exceeds the transudative capacity of the parietal pleura, resulting in a dynamic equilibrium. The turnover of water in the pleural space is 35 to 75% per hour,[28] a figure comparable to that of ascitic fluid, which turns over at 40% to 80% per hour.[29] Viewed in different terms, approximately 700 ml of pleural fluid are formed and absorbed in 24 hours in a 70-kg person, representing about 20% of the plasma volume per day. The turnover rate of small molecules such as sodium and chloride is essentially the same as that of water and their concentrations are equal in the pleural fluid and plasma.

As in other tissue spaces, lymphatics play an important role in the reabsorption of extravascular fluid. Both the visceral and parietal pleuras are rich in lymphatic vessels. However, the lymphatics of the visceral pleura do not regularly reabsorb fluid in experimental animals.[30] The majority of lymphatic reabsorption takes place in the lower mediastinal pleura and in the parietal pleura at the inferior margins of the thorax.

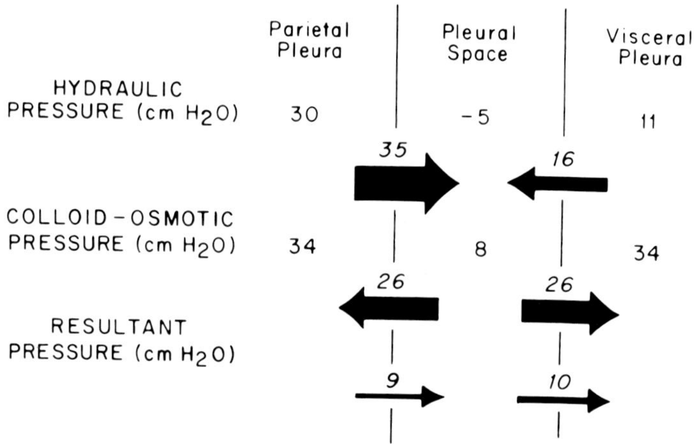

FIG. 12-5. Pleural fluid dynamics. This schematic representation is an approximation of the hydraulic and osmotic pressure gradients across parietal and visceral pleural capillaries adjoining the pleural space. The resultant of forces is such that fluid is driven into the pleural space from the parietal pleural capillaries and is reabsorbed from the pleural space into visceral pleural capillaries.

Lymphatic vessels also transport large-molecular-weight substances, such as protein, that have diffused from capillaries into the pleural fluid. Even cells, such as erythrocytes and leukocytes, may be reabsorbed intact through lymphatics.[31]

Lymphatic vessels of the parietal pleura drain to the parasternal lymph nodes anteriorly or to the paravertebral lymph nodes posteriorly. The lymph from the lower mediastinum drains primarily to the parasternal lymph nodes. Both of these lymphatic chains drain centrally through superior mediastinal nodes and empty ultimately through the bronchomediastinal lymph trunk into the right subclavian vein. A smaller fraction of the lymph flow drains into the left subclavian vein.

The pleural lymphatic channels transmit liquid from the pleural space, which has subatmospheric pressure, to the venous system, which, on the average, has an above-atmospheric pressure. Work must be performed to transport fluid against this pressure gradient. This energy is supplied by the respiratory movements of the chest. Hyperventilation causes an augmentation of lymph flow, whereas hypoventilation causes a reduction in lymph flow.[32] In the only measurements performed in humans, lymph flow from one hemithorax averaged 0.36 ml/kg of body weight per hour.[33] Lymph flow can probably increase during disease states by as much as 3 to 12 times the normal value. However, there is probably a maximum flow that cannot be exceeded.

The mechanisms of normal control of pleural fluid indicate two potential means of excessive fluid accumulation. First, there may be excessive hydraulic or insufficient osmotic pressure, either of which may cause excessive pleural fluid. Such effusions (filtrates of plasma across intact capillary walls) are generally termed *transudates*. Second, effusions may occur because of some breakdown in the normal formation-reabsorption pathway. Such effusions, which are generally termed *exudates*, might occur because of damage to pleural capillaries, allowing a leak of excessive protein-rich fluid into the pleural space. The altered osmotic pressure gradient causes more fluid to pour into the pleural space than might be accounted for by the original capillary leak. Alternately, a normal amount of protein leak into the pleural space may occur, but the lymphatics responsible for reabsorption of large molecules may be blocked by mediastinal disease. These mechanisms of exudate formation produce approximately the same type of fluid, but the difference in underlying mechanisms may be helpful in differential diagnosis.

EFFECTS ON RESPIRATION

Depending on the size of the pleural effusion, some portion of the lung may be compressed by the effusion and may not ventilate normally. Since this fraction of the lung may continue to have pulmonary arterial blood flow, there may be mismatching of ventilation and blood flow, with resultant hypoxemia. In some cases, there is virtual atelectasis of the lung involved. Blood flow to this nonventilating fraction of a lung constitutes a right-to-left "shunt," and the resultant hypoxemia may not be correctable even by a high concentration of inspired oxygen. Nevertheless, many patients with relatively large pleural effusions experience few symptoms. In some patients, dyspnea exceeds that which would be expected from the amount of lung displaced.

In some patients, the weight of a pleural effusion may cause descent of the dome of the diaphram. If the effusion is in the left hemithorax, diaphragmatic flattening may be recognized roentgenographically by the contour of the upper border of the stomach bubble on a film made in the upright position.[34] When the diaphragm is flattened, the initial vector of force is medial and may cause the lower thoracic cage to decrease in size during inspiration (see Chap. 2).

In a minority of patients, the weight of the pleural effusion may invert the diaphragm. This may be demonstrated roentgenographically by inversion of the stomach bubble (Fig. 12-6). On physical examination, the diaphragm may present as a mass in the left upper quadrant.[35] The inverted hemidiaphragm may be observed fluoroscopically to move upward, causing expiration on the affected side, while the normal hemidiaphragm is moving downward, causing inspiration on the normal side. During expiration, when the diaphragm relaxes, the normal hemidiaphragm moves upward, allowing gas to leave the normal lung, while the inverted hemidiaphragm moves downward, causing inspiration to occur on the side of the effusion. This series of events may allow gas to move from the affected lung into the normal lung during inspiration and allow the converse to occur during expiration. Such shifting of gas back and forth between the two lungs is catastrophic to ventilation. In patients with a flattened or inverted hemidiaphragm, removal of enough effusion to allow the diaphragm to resume a normal contour may markedly relieve dyspnea.

In patients studied before and after removal of 600 to 1800 ml of fluid by thoracentesis, there was a small increase in functional residual capacity and total lung capacity, but no immediate improvement in intrapulmonary shunt. These physiologic changes were considered inadequate to explain the improvement in symptoms.[34a]

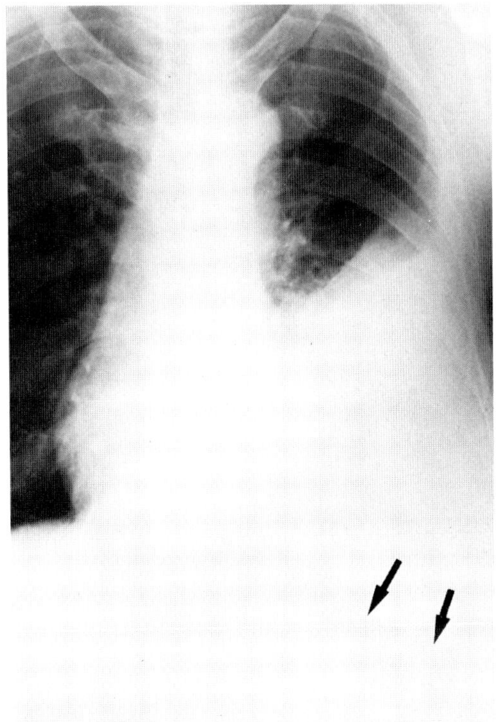

FIG. 12-6. In this chest roentgenogram taken in the upright position, the massive left pleural effusion has caused a downward sagging of the left hemidiaphragm, as indicated by a downward convexity of the upper margin of the stomach bubble (*arrows*).

DIAGNOSTIC PROCEDURES

PHYSICAL EXAMINATION

On observation, the patient with a large pleural effusion may have tachypnea due to dyspnea. There may be mild outward bulging of the intercostal spaces and a lag on inspiration on the affected side. If the effusion has flattened or inverted the diaphragm, the affected side may not have the normal outward movement of the chest wall during inspiration or the rib cage may move inward with inspiration.

Palpation confirms the movements of the

chest wall suggested by observation. Fremitus is decreased in the area of the chest occupied by the pleural effusion. If the effusion has caused significant atelectasis of the lung under it, the increased transmission of vibration caused by atelectasis may balance the decreased transmission caused by the effusion and fremitus may approach normal. If the atelectasis extends along the upper border of the effusion, there may be an area of decreased fremitus inferiorly with increased fremitus superiorly.

Percussion reveals dullness to flatness of the area of the effusion. The level of dullness may not fluctuate with inspiration and expiration, as would be expected from normal diaphragmatic excursions.

Auscultation reveals decreased transmission of breath sounds in the area of the effusion. If there is significant atelectasis under the effusion, breath sounds may be bronchovesicular. As in all other forms of the physical examination, comparison with the opposite hemithorax may be necessary in order to allow the examiner to appreciate subtle changes. The upper border of the effusion may have sufficient underlying atelectasis to cause bronchial breath sounds.

ROENTGENOGRAPHIC EXAMINATION

On an upright PA or lateral chest roentgenogram, the normal diaphragm meets the lateral chest wall at a sharp angle. The most common appearance of a pleural effusion is the accumulation of water which has a concave superior air-fluid interface with the lung and which obscures this angle (Fig. 12-7). When the effusion is small, this sign is best appreciated on the lateral film. In many instances, a small effusion cannot be clearly differentiated from a fibrous tissue scar caused by previous inflammatory disease or trauma.

In the case of larger effusions, the water density may occupy a much larger fraction of the hemithorax, but it tends to maintain the upward concave air-fluid interface unless the entire hemithorax is filled with fluid. The differentiation of fluid from infiltrative diseases of the lungs, most commonly pneumonia or atelectasis, may be difficult. Fluid tends to cause a very homogenous water density whereas infiltrative lung diseases most commonly have some mixture of air with the water density (air bronchograms or air alveolograms).

Many effusions are trapped in a subpulmonic location between the inferior margin of the lung and the superior surface of the diaphragm and do not demonstrate the usual appearance. The diagnosis of such a subpulmonic effusion can only be suggested by an upright posteroanterior chest roentgenogram. In such a view, the normal diaphragm is typically arched so that its major convexity is approximately in the middle of the hemithorax. As fluid collects between the base of the lung and the diaphragm, the major convexity frequently is shifted laterally (Fig. 12-8). In addition, if the effusion is in the left hemithorax, there may be excessive water density separating the top of the stomach bubble from the top of the apparent diaphragm.

Although the PA view may be only suggestive of a subpulmonic effusion, the lateral roentgenogram may be diagnostic. The normal diaphragm is a continuously arching structure with no straight air-fluid interface between the diaphragm and the lung (Fig. 12-9). It is also possible to follow each diaphragm to its costophrenic sulcus, where it forms an acute angle. In the presence of a subpulmonic effusion, the anterior margin of the diaphragm may form a straight, horizontal air-fluid interface with the lung. This causes the anterior and middle portions of the diaphragm to meet at an angle instead of an arch. In some cases, fluid also runs superiorly into the long fissure that meets the diaphragm at this angle. This angulation of the diaphragm, indicating a subpulmonic effusion, is sometimes referred to as the "Rock of Gibraltar" sign. In many cases, the subpulmonic effusion may have the typical, upward concavity of the water density at the posterior margin of the diaphragm.

It may be difficult to position acutely ill patients for standard roentgenographic procedures and anteroposterior (AP) recumbent films are frequently all that are obtained. In the recumbent position, a pleural effusion may lie along the posterior chest wall and may cause only a diffuse "ground glass" appearance. Since there is no characteristic air-fluid interface, the effusion may be misinterpreted as a parenchymal lung infiltrate. An effusion should be suggested,

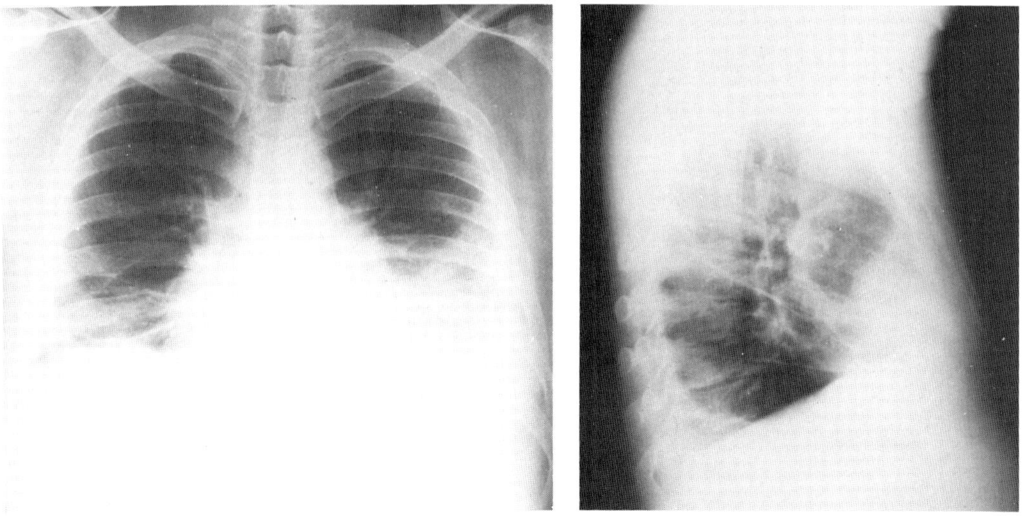

FIG. 12-7. Posteroanterior (*left*) and lateral (*right*) chest roentgenograms taken in the upright position of a patient with a relatively typical left pleural effusion. The water density in the left costophrenic sulcus has a concave superior air-fluid interface, which may be seen on both the PA and lateral projections.

however, by the homogeneity of the water density, with no air alveolograms apparent.

Whenever a diagnosis of a pleural effusion is not clear, a lateral decubitus roentgenogram should be obtained. Most pleural effusions run freely in the pleural space and hence settle to the most dependent part of the chest. On the lateral decubitus film, therefore, the water density may be seen along the lateral margin of the dependent hemithorax (Fig. 12-10). Even relatively small effusions may be detected with this technique. When such a film is ordered, the technician should be informed that the major area of interest is the dependent hemithorax, in order that this area not be obscured by the roentgenographic technique.

ULTRASONIC EXAMINATION

The diagnosis of small amounts of pleural fluid, the differentiation of free fluid from pleural fibrosis, and the localization of fluid within a loculated pleural effusion may be facilitated by ultrasonic techniques.[36–40] If the amount of fluid obtained at subsequent thoracentesis is 50 ml or less, ultrasound may be used to detect the fluid in approximately 85% of the patients with a false-

FIG. 12-8. Posteroanterior chest roentgenogram taken in the upright position of a patient with bilateral subpulmonic effusions. On the right, the major upward convexity of the apparent diaphragm has been shifted toward the lateral chest wall. On the left, the upper margin of the apparent diaphragm has been separated by several centimeters from the top of the stomach bubble.

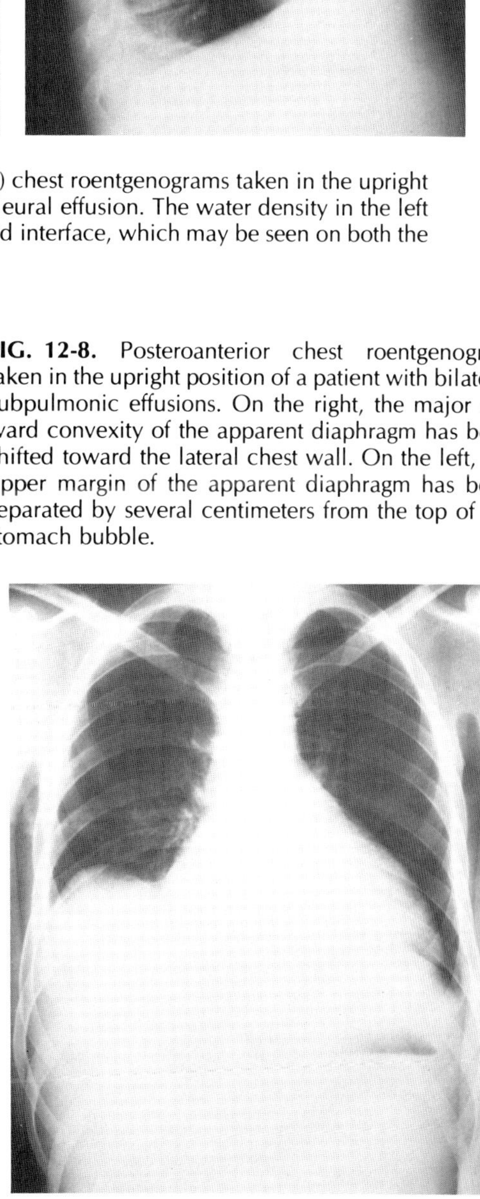

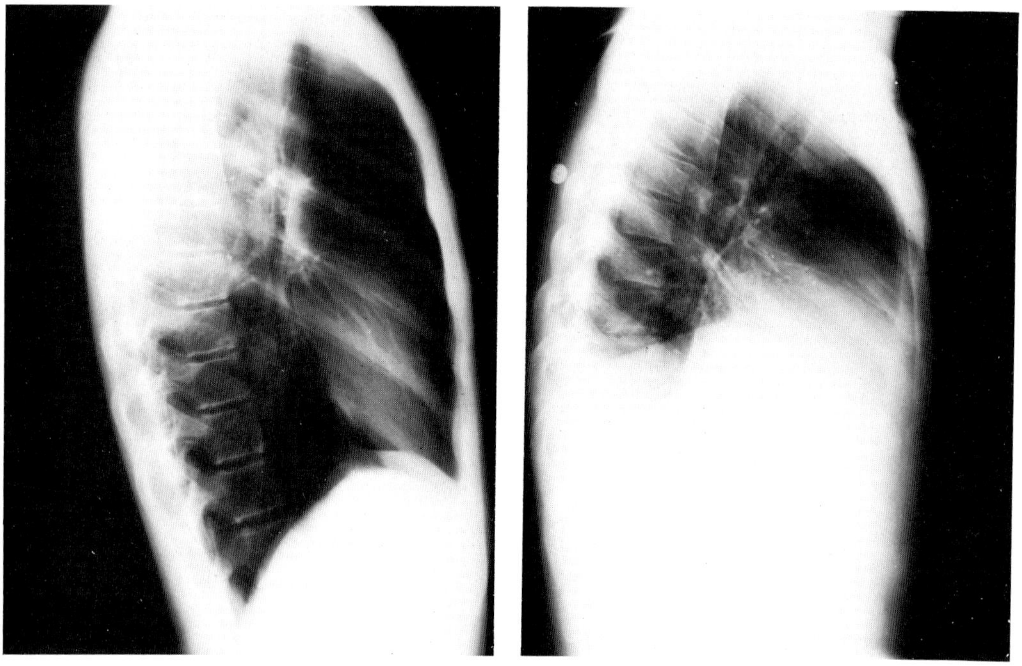

FIG. 12-9. Lateral chest roentgenograms of two separate patients. The one on the left demonstrates the normal, continuously arching contours of the diaphragms. The patient on the right has a subpulmonic effusion, as indicated by the straight anterior margin of the right diaphragm, the relatively straight middle portion of the diaphragm meeting the anterior portion at an angle instead of an arch, and the upward concavity of the water density against the posterior chest wall.

FIG. 12-10. Right lateral decubitus roentgenogram of the patient in Figure 12-8. The subpulmonic effusion has layered against the lateral chest wall, making it easily apparent.

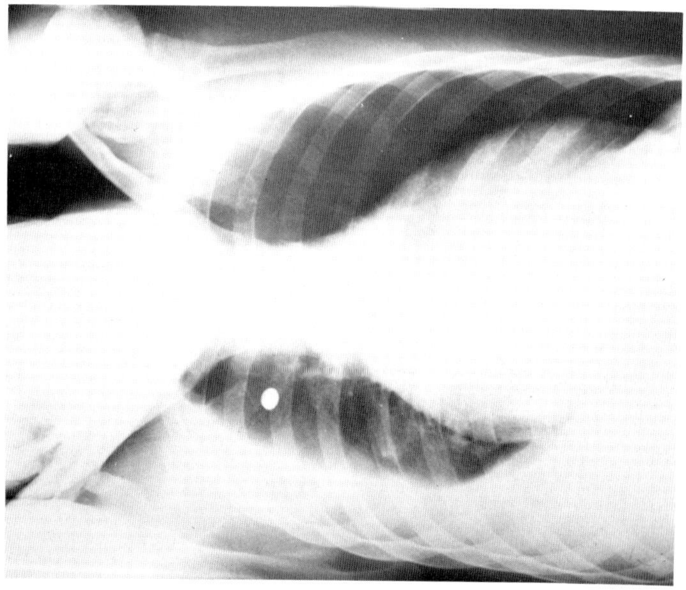

negative rate of 5%.[38] Radiologic techniques detect such small amounts of fluid in about 60% of instances with 15% false-negative studies. The ultrasonic technique is almost always positive when the amount of fluid exceeds 100 ml, while the amount of fluid must exceed 500 ml for radiographic techniques to achieve such accuracy.

Ultrasound may also be useful for determining where to perform a thoracentesis in a patient with a loculated effusion. The ultrasonographer can indicate the best location on the chest wall to attempt thoracentesis and can indicate the depth at which the fluid can be expected. In some instances, pockets of fluid containing no more than 10 ml have been aspirated using this technique.[40]

THORACENTESIS

Whenever the etiology of a pleural effusion is not clear or when an effusion is causing dyspnea, a thoracentesis should be performed. The procedure usually is performed with the patient seated and the effusion is at the base of the thorax. When the effusion is small, however, the physician may be unsure of its level relative to the diaphragm; thoracentesis then may be carried out with the patient in a lateral decubitus position with the dependent thorax exposed between two beds or by an aperture in an examination table. The physician then approaches the patient from below. With either position, the physician estimates the point at which to insert the thoracentesis needle by means of dullness to percussion on physical examination.

A surgical aseptic technique is used, and includes preparing the skin with suitable antiseptics, draping the area with sterile towels, and using sterile gloves while handling all equipment. Local anesthesia is provided by injection of a suitable agent such as lidocaine, first intradermally and then subcutaneously and into the intercostal muscles. For instillation of the anesthetic, a small-gauge needle (*e.g.*, 21 gauge) is used, and the anesthetic agent is injected all the way down to the pleural space. The needle is inserted in the intercostal space immediately over the superior margin of the rib below in order to avoid the intercostal vessels and nerve that run in the inferior sulcus of each rib. During injection of anesthesia, aspiration is attempted each time the needle is moved, in order to insure that the anesthetic agent is not injected into a blood vessel.

Once anesthesia has been accomplished, a large-bore needle (*e.g.*, 16 gauge) is used for the thoracentesis. It is convenient to place a sterile three-way stopcock between the needle and a syringe, so that fluid aspirated into the syringe may be emptied repeatedly into appropriate containers without having to remove the syringe from the needle. The needle is advanced into the pleural space along the same path as the previously injected anesthetic agent. The needle is advanced, taking care to keep it perpendicular to the chest wall. Continuous aspiration is performed while the needle is being advanced; usually, one can determine when the pleural space is entered both by a sudden lessening of the force necessary to advance the needle and by the aspiration of fluid into the syringe.

If the procedure has been traumatic, the first fluid obtained may be slightly bloody but it clears as more is withdrawn. If the fluid is bloody because of the underlying disease process, it continues to be bloody during the entire procedure. Part of the fluid should be transferred from the syringe into tubes containing an anticoagulant solution so that appropriate chemistries and cell counts may be performed. Part of the fluid should be saved in sterile containers for subsequent Gram stain and culture. If fluid is to be used for cytologic examination, as large a volume as possible should be sent for this procedure. In most instances, one can continue to aspirate fluid as long as it flows freely. With extremely large effusions, rapid removal of fluid may be associated with pain, hypotension, and rarely, pulmonary edema. It is generally safer to remove only about half a hemithorax of fluid in one sitting.

PLEURAL BIOPSY

The procedure for needle biopsy of the pleura should be mastered by all physicians who care for patients with pleural effusions. Hook-type biopsy needles that allow both thoracentesis and pleural biopsy with the same instrument have been devised by Abrams and by Cope, and the needles are usually referred to by these men's names.[41,42] The Abrams' needle also may be referred to by the name of the hospital in which it was first introduced, Harefield. The operative procedures used with these needles are clearly described by Abrams[41] and Cope.[42] The larger series reporting pleural biopsy indicate that adequate specimens are obtained about 85% of the time.[43–63] Among over 1400 reported biopsies in which information is available, there have been only 57 complications, an incidence of 4%, and in only 3 cases was the complication serious enough to require treatment. In only 1 reported case was the biopsy thought to contribute to the patient's death and that patient was moribund from carcinoma before the biopsy was performed. Thus, the procedure carries no more risk than a thoracentesis without biopsy.

Of 526 reported biopsies in patients who were ultimately proven to have tuberculosis, 341 (65%) were diagnostic of the underlying condition. Similarly, of 461 biopsies reported in patients proven to have carcinoma, 270 (59%) were diagnostic.

CONSTITUENTS OF PLEURAL FLUID

Separation of Transudates and Exudates

The differentiation of transudates due to hydraulic or osmotic abnormalities and exudates due to capillary damage or lymphatic blockage is of considerable diagnostic importance in any patient with a pleural effusion. Measurement of several properties of pleural fluid has been advocated; unfortunately, no one test has proven infallible. The first advocated procedure was the measurement of the specific gravity of the effusion fluid. Hydrometers and refractometers in clinical use are usually calibrated for urine, however, and are not entirely satisfactory for determinations in pleural fluid.[64]

The most widely used test is the measurement of the pleural-fluid protein concentration. The original report indicated that 85% of patients with congestive heart failure had fluid protein levels of less than 3g/dl, and that 90% of fluids due to cancer and tuberculosis had levels of more than 3g/dl.[65] It was also indicated that transudates and exudates of other causes could be differentiated by their protein content. Unfortunately, subsequent studies have indicated that the overlap of values above and below 3 g/dl may be greater than originally indicated.[66,67] In patients with congestive heart failure, the pleural-fluid protein may be elevated during periods of diuresis, when fluid is mobilized more rapidly than protein from the pleural space. Moreover, the longer the duration of the pleural effusion due to heart failure, the higher the pleural-fluid protein tends to be. Indeed, one study found that of 27 patients with long-standing congestive heart failure, 21 had pleural-fluid protein levels of greater than 3 g/dl.[68] Similarly, effusions due to malignancy have been found to have pleural-fluid protein levels as low as 1.2 g/dl and have been found to be below 3 g/dl up to 20% of the time. Since pleural fluid proteins are derived from serum proteins, variations in the latter may effect the pleural concentration. It has been found that a ratio of pleural fluid to serum protein of more or less than 0.5 is a better index of exudates or transudates than the absolute pleural protein concentration.[69] Thus, pleural protein levels, although useful, cannot be considered an absolute indicator of the mechanism causing the pleural effusion.

Another method for differentiating between transudates and exudates is the pleural-fluid lactic dehydrogenase (LDH) activity. In 1957, it was noted that pleural-fluid water turns over rapidly, but pleural globulin tends to reach equilibrium with that of the plasma at a considerably slower rate (2 or more days).[70] Lactic dehydrogenase activity is a constituent of plasma globulin, and presumably it is a globulin constituent of the effusion protein. This suggests that the LDH of an effusion does not come into equilibrium with the serum LDH when lactic dehydrogenase is being added directly to the effusion. It was originally felt that since malignant cells contribute LDH to the medium that bathes them, they would cause the LDH of malignant effusions to be consistently greater than that of the serum of the same patient. However, any type of fluid that contains cellular debris of benign or malignant origin may have a high LDH activity, and the ratio of effusion to serum LDH may be high.[71] Thus, although not helpful to specifically diagnose malignancy, measurement of the LDH of pleural fluid and serum simultaneously may be the best differentiator between transudates and exudates since the latter tend to have much more cellular debris. One group of investigators has found that none of their patients with a transudative pleural effusion had LDH activity of greater than 550 units in the pleural fluid, whereas patients with exudative pleural effusions regularly did.[67] In a separate investigation, it was found that a pleural-fluid LDH concentration of greater than 220 units or a pleural fluid to serum LDH ratio of greater than 0.6 indicated an exudative cause for the effusion.[69] The combination of elevated protein and LDH concentrations offers the greatest evidence of an exudative cause of an effusion at present.

Pleural fluid acidosis is associated with exudates, as described below.

Biochemical Abnormalities

Other noncellular substances have been assayed for their value in diagnosis. One of these is the *pleural-fluid glucose*. The glucose concentration in the pleural space follows the plasma glucose concentration and averages two-thirds to three-quarters of that value.[72] The pleural-fluid glucose concentration is usually low in infections of the pleural space (empyema), but this diagnosis is made on the basis of organisms in the fluid. The only condition in which the pleural-fluid glucose concentration is frequently of diagnostic value is rheumatoid arthritis; effusions frequently have a strikingly low glucose concentration.[73] On some occasions, no glucose may be detected at all and commonly it is less than 10 to 20 mg/dl. The cause of the low glucose concentration in rheumatoid effusions has not been completely ellucidated, but it has been demonstrated to be a transport rather than a utilization defect.[74] In the absence of an infection of the pleural space, an exceedingly low glucose concentration in the pleural fluid is almost always diagnostic of an effusion associated with rheumatoid arthritis. However, in a few cases, exceedingly low glucose concentrations in pleural effusions may be due to other causes, especially cancer.[75]

The *pleural-fluid amylase* concentration is a useful diagnostic test in cases of pleural effusion associated with diseases of the pancreas. The amylase concentration is usually elevated to 500 to 2000 units/ml when the effusion is due to such diseases, and may reach exceedingly high levels (*e.g.*, 50,000 units/ml).[76] The pleural-fluid amylase concentration may be significantly higher and frequently remains elevated for considerably longer than the serum amylase concentration. The pleural-fluid amylase may also be elevated in patients with perforation of the esophagus (see Intra-abdominal Disease: Pancreatitis, below).

It has been reported that the amounts of whole hemolytic *complement* and its components C3 and C4 in pleural fluid from patients whose effusion is due to systemic lupus erythematosus or rheumatoid arthritis are smaller than those in other effusions.[77] The reduced levels of complement components are thought to be due to complement conversion in the pleural fluid by immune complexes.[78] Whole hemolytic complement is usually undetectable (less than 5 CH_{50} units/ml) in such effusions. The concentration of C3 and C4 in pleural effusions caused by lupus or rheumatoid arthritis may overlap with concentrations found in effusions from other causes. The low whole-hemolytic-complement concentration occurs in the pleural space despite normal concentrations in serum of the same patient.

The *abnormal serum proteins* in some patients with connective tissue diseases may also be found in pleural effusions due to these diseases. Rheumatoid factor, antinuclear antibody, and lupus erythematosus cells have been found in pleural effusions. The positive rate of these abnormal tests in pleural effusions due to these diseases has not been carefully documented.

The tensions of *respiratory gases* (Po_2 and Pco_2) of pleural fluid have been found to be too variable to be of diagnostic use.[79] *Pleural fluid acidosis*, with a *p*H level of less than 7.3, may be found in empyema, hemothorax, esophageal rupture, fluids due to rheumatoid and tuberculous pleurisy, and carcinomatous effusion. Results of a series of experiments[80–83] have indicated that glucose metabolism by cells in the pleura or in the fluid generates lactic acid and carbon dioxide. The *p*H level of the fluid is determined by such acid production and by the character of the pleural lining which may prevent efflux of hydrogen ions and carbon dioxide. Results of attempts to relate these findings to coagulation and loculation of pleural fluid[84] are not definitive. Transudates usually have pleural fluid *p*H greater than 7.3.

Pleural Fluid Cytology

Approximately 5000 to 6000 erythrocytes/mm^3 are needed in order to impart a red tint to a pleural effusion and to lead to a description of the fluid as being bloody.[85] A bloody effusion is most commonly caused by malignancy, but is also relatively common in congestive heart failure, pulmonary infection, pulmonary infarction, and trauma.[86] Tuberculosis, however is not a frequent cause. When the count is more than 100,000/mm^3, the cause is most likely trauma, pulmonary embolus, or neoplasia.

The total leukocyte count may add to circumstantial diagnostic evidence, but it is not specific. Generally, exudates have leukocyte counts of over 500/mm^3, and frequently of over 1000. Empyema usually causes a much higher count, frequently exceeding 10,000/mm.^{3} Transudates tend to have fewer leukocytes, but there is no absolute level differentiating the two types of fluid. In most tuberculous effusions, more than 60% of the leukocytes are lymphocytes, and lymphomas causing effusion are almost always associated with lymphocytosis.[87,88] Acute infectious diseases are usually associated with a polymorphonuclear leukocytosis, with less than 50% lymphocytes. However, in the acute phase of tuberculous pleurisy, the majority of cells may be polymorphonuclear, with a shift towards lymphocytes as the effusion becomes more chronic. Other infectious processes also may shift from polys to lymphocytes when the effusion has been present for a protracted interval.

Eosinophilia in pleural effusions is of no diagnostic value. Several recent reports have emphasized that effusions with high eosinophil counts generally have characteristics of exudates and may be associated with sheets of pleural histiocytes and eosinophils in biopsy, and in the absence of identifiable associated disease, these patients generally have a good prognosis.[89,89a]

A variety of additional components of pleural fluid have been assayed in an attempt to improve diagnostic accuracy. These include chromosome examination,[90] "living cytology,"[91] carcinoembryonic antigen[92–94] for the diagnosis of malignancy, lysozyme[95] for the diagnosis of tuberculosis, and the distribution of T and B lymphocytes.[96,97] Further study is needed in order to determine the value of these tests in clinical practice.

Thus, of the various constituents of effusions that have been analyzed, the protein and LDH concentrations are the most helpful, although not infallible, means of separating exudates and transudates. The concentrations of glucose, amylase, and whole hemolytic complement may be helpful in specific conditions. Abnormal proteins associated with connective tissue diseases may be found in the pleural effusions caused by such diseases. Pleural fluid acidosis may suggest empyema, and that the fluid will loculate. Finally, the cellular constituents of the effusion may give suggestive evidence as to etiology.

PLEUROSCOPY

Direct visualization of the pleural space (pleuroscopy) may be performed with a fiberoptic instrument such as that used for bronchoscopy[98–101] or arthroscopy.[102,103] Using appropriate local anesthesia and sterile technique, the fiberscope is introduced percutaneously into the pleural space in much the same manner as a thoracostomy tube is inserted. The pleural effusion is removed and a controlled pneumothorax is induced through the aspiration channel so that the instrument may be freely moved over a substantial portion of the pleural surfaces. Loculated effusions may prevent adequate visualization. Areas which appear to be abnormal may be biopsied by introducing forceps through the aspiration channel.

This technique is most useful for diagnosing lesions with a definite histologic appearance although the absence of any visualized pleural abnormality may be useful information in the care of some patients. Thus, neoplasms causing pleural effusions have been reported as the most frequent finding at pleuroscopy, although infectious lesions such as tuberculosis may also be identified. An insufficient number of procedures has been reported to be sure of the rate of false-negative results.

SPECIFIC ETIOLOGIES OF PLEURAL EFFUSIONS

Hydraulic Osmotic Causes (Transudates)

Cardiovascular Causes. As indicated in the section on dynamics of pleural fluid the fluid normally present in the pleural space is a filtrate of plasma, primarily from parietal pleural capillaries; the fluid is reabsorbed from the pleural space through the visceral pleural capillaries and pleural lymphatics which return the fluid to the circulation through central veins. Left ventricular failure alters the steady state by increasing pressure in visceral pleural capillaries, tending to diminish reabsorptive forces. Right ventricular failure augments transudation by increasing pressure in the parietal pleural capillaries and diminishes reabsorption by increasing central venous pressure. These events may lead to an excessive accumulation of fluid. Although it has been demonstrated in experimental animals that elevation of the systemic venous pressure causes significantly more pleural fluid accumulation than does similar pressure elevation in pulmonary veins,[104] pleural effusions are not a manifestation of cor pulmonale with only right ventricular failure. Both ventricles usually are compromised in patients with pleural effusion associated with congestive heart failure.

Pleural effusions caused by congestive heart failure usually are associated with other manifestations of heart failure, if the patient is examined before therapy is initiated. In most instances, cardiomegaly is evident on physical and roentgenographic examination. The absence of cardiomegaly should be taken as strong evidence against heart failure as the cause.[105] In addition, most patients demonstrate pulmonary parenchymal changes such as inspiratory rales, on physical examination and alveolar infiltrates on chest roentgenograms. There may also be findings of right ventricular failure, such as an elevated central venous pressure, hepatomegaly, and pedal edema. Following appropriate treatment, other findings of heart failure may be minimal although the effusion remains. On some occasions, the effusion remains only in a very localized area of the pleura such as the oblique fissure, and the roentgenographic appearance may simulate a lung mass. Such "phantom tumors" regress with additional compensation of the heart failure.

Effusions from congestive heart failure are frequently bilateral and such a finding in the presence of a large heart strongly suggests this cause; most effusions due to exudative causes are unilateral. If an effusion due to heart failure is unilateral, it is most frequently in the right hemithorax. The cause for this right-sided preference is not known.

Pleural effusions sometimes occur in patients with markedly elevated systemic venous pressure and without clinical evidence of elevated pulmonary venous pressure. In cases of constrictive pericarditis, where systemic and pulmonary venous pressures are elevated approximately equally, evidence of right heart failure generally dominates the clinical findings. Pleural effusions are uncommon in cases of superior vena caval obstruction where very high systemic venous and elevated lymphatic pressures may be of pathogenetic importance. The characteristics of such effusions are similar to those caused by congestive heart failure.

The chemical and cytologic constituents of a pleural effusion from heart failure are most commonly those suggestive of a transudate. However, a significant number have a pleural fluid protein level of greater than 3 g/dl, especially if the effusion is long-standing or if recent therapy has included a brisk diuresis.[68] Heart failure effusions may also be blood-tinged[86]; the mechanism of this finding is not known.

Treatment of pleural effusions caused by heart failure is directed at the primary derangement. No specific therapy for the effusion is necessary unless the patient is dyspneic. In such a patient, removing a relatively small amount of effusion may produce dramatic relief of symptoms. This is usually accomplished by needle thoracentesis; tube thoracostomy is rarely necessary.

Overexpanded Fluid Volume. Patients with markedly overexpanded body water due to excess fluid administration, most frequently from marked hypoalbuminemia, may develop pleural effusions. These pleural effusions may be unilateral or bilateral. Most commonly, the heart is enlarged in these syndromes, but such may not

Specific Etiologies of Pleural Effusions

Hydraulic-Osmotic (Transudates)
Cardiovascular
- Congestive heart failure
- Constrictive pericarditis
- Superior vena caval obstruction

Overexpanded fluid volume
- Hypoalbuminemia
- Salt-retaining syndromes

Intra-abdominal disease
- Cirrhosis with ascites
- Peritoneal dialysis

Exudates
Tuberculosis
Neoplasm
- Bronchogenic carcinoma
- Metastatic carcinoma
- Lymphoma
- Mesothelioma
- Intra-abdominal tumors
- Chest-wall neoplasms

Pulmonary embolus
Connective tissue diseases
- Lupus erythematosus
- Rheumatoid arthritis

Intra-abdominal diseases
- Subdiaphragmatic abscess
- Pancreatitis
- Abdominal surgery
- Hepatitis

Miscellaneous
- Familial Mediterranean fever
- Lymphedema
- Post myocardial infarction syndrome

Myxedema
Idiopathic

Infections
Bacterial empyema
Tuberculosis
Fungi
Parasites
Viruses and mycoplasma

Trauma
Hemothorax
Chylothorax
Esophageal rupture

be the case if the fluid overload has taken place rapidly, so that the pericardium prevents myocardial expansion. With or without cardiomegaly, this syndrome does not represent true heart failure, since the force of myocardial contraction is appropriate for the end diastolic ventricular pressure.[106] The effusion may occur with or without symptoms of pulmonary vascular congestion being evident on physical or roentgenograph examination.

In this syndrome, pleural effusions occur later than edema elsewhere in the body. The low-pressure vessels in the visceral pleura cause the pleural space to have an advantage for fluid reabsorption over the dependent parts of the body, so that patients virtually always have massive systemic edema before accumulating pleural fluid.

Intra-abdominal Disease. Hydrothorax occurs in 5 to 10% of patients with cirrhosis of the liver,[107] almost always in patients with ascites. However, hydrothorax may occasionally occur in cirrhotic patients without demonstrable ascites on physical examination.[108] The pleural fluid is most commonly unilateral on the right side, but it may occur on the left side alone or bilaterally. The pleural effusion may sometimes be massive and recurrent even though the amount of ascitic fluid is minimal. The type of cirrhosis leading to ascites is evidently not important for determining whether a pleural effusion will occur.

In patients with ascites, the constituents of the pleural effusion mimic those of the ascitic fluid, although the protein concentration and other elements may not be identical. It has been demonstrated by radioactively labeled albumin techniques that although fluid may pass from the peritoneal space into the pleural space, pleural fluid does not pass into the peritoneal space.[107] It is not clear whether the fluid traverses the diaphragm through lymphatic channels or through minor holes in the diaphragm.

The management of patients with hepatic hydrothorax is directed at treating the primary disease. If the pleural effusion interferes with ventilation, thoracentesis may be necessary. However, if a large amount of ascites remains, the pleural fluid tends to reaccumulate rapidly. Cautious paracentesis may result in more sustained improvement. When the pleural effusion is refractory to all such therapy and results in continued or recurrent respiratory distress, it has been suggested that a chemically induced pleurodesis may relieve the patient's symptoms by preventing subsequent pleural fluid accumulation.[109]

Patients undergoing peritoneal dialysis may develop small pleural effusions that may be unilateral, on either side, or bilateral. The pleural fluid tends to have a similar composition as the dialysate, and regresses rapidly when dialysis is terminated.

Exudates

Postprimary Tuberculous Effusion. Tuberculosis causes two types of pleural effusions. One type, tuberculous empyema, is an infection of the pleural space that occurs in the course of overt pulmonary tuberculosis. This syndrome will be considered in the section on infections (below). The other type, and by far the more common, presents as a pleural effusion in the absence of roentgenographically demonstrable pulmonary parenchymal disease. Such an effusion is most likely caused by the incidental spillage of tubercle bacilli into the pleural space from subclinical pulmonary parenchymal lesions adjacent to the visceral pleura. Alternately, the bacilli may reach the pleural surface during the silent bacteremia that occurs in the primary phase of tuberculosis. The effusion is most likely to occur within months of the primary, subclinical infection.

The postprimary tuberculous effusion is a manifestation of delayed hypersensitivity.[110] Marked effusions may be produced in experimental animals by injecting viable or nonviable tubercle bacilli into the pleural space after the animal has been immunized with tuberculoprotein. Viable tubercle bacilli in the pleural space of nonimmunized animals cause granulomas but little effusion. Since the effusion is a manifestation of delayed hypersensitivity, the tuberculin skin test is almost invariably positive. Most patients with tuberculous effusions are reactive to intermediate-strength purified protein derivative (PPD; 5 TU), but some are reactive only to second-strength PPD (250 TU).[111] Since an effusion is caused by bacilli that are fortuitously deposited in an immunized pleural space, bilateral effusions due to tuberculosis are rare. Occasionally, an effusion occurs on one side and is followed by one on the opposite side at a later date. When a patient subsequently develops clinical pulmonary tuberculosis, the parenchymal lesion may not develop on the same side as the effusion.

The clinical manifestations of postprimary tuberculous pleural effusions vary greatly.[112] Some patients are asymptomatic and the effusion is diagnosed only because of an incidental roentgenogram. More commonly, however, systemic symptoms of fever, lethargy, and weight loss have been present for several days or weeks. Still other patients present with an acute febrile illness accompanied by pleuritic pain and generalized symptoms of toxicity. In none of the presentations is cough likely to be a prominent symptom, and sputum production is unlikely. The occurrence of dyspnea depends on the volume of effusion present. The physical examination usually reveals nothing other than the finding of an effusion. Roentgenograms of the chest similarly indicate an effusion without significant parenchymal disease, except that the effusion may cause some lung compression or discoid atelectasis. Routine laboratory examinations are normal. If sputum can be obtained, acid-fast organisms usually are not demonstrable on smear, and tubercle bacilli usually are not cultured.

Fluid analyzed after thoracentesis usually is typical of an exudate, although in some samples the protein level is less than 3 g/dl. The effusion usually contains few erythocytes and a moderate number of leukocytes (1000 to 2000/mm^3). The leukocytes usually are predominantly lymphocytes, frequently in excess of 95% of the cells.[87] Direct smear of the effusion fluid rarely reveals acid-fast organisms. Series of cases vary in the number of effusions from which tubercle bacilli are cultured but rarely exceed 25%. Pleural biopsy is much more likely to be diagnostic; granulomas have been found in up to 65% of patients with tuberculosis.[62] The diagnostic accuracy of biopsy may be increased by culturing part of the specimen for Mycobacterium tuberculosis.[63] It should be stressed that although a positive biopsy is diagnostic, a negative biopsy does not exclude the possibility of tuberculosis. Indeed, any patient with an undiagnosed pleural effusion and a positive tuberculin skin test should be treated as if the effusion has been caused by tuberculosis.

The course of tuberculosis pleural effusions varies but most tend to resolve spontaneously in weeks or months. If the fluid is removed by thoracentesis, the condition does not usually recur; if it does recur, it usually is not of the same magnitude as the original effusion. With or without thoracentesis, the effusion may resolve completely with no residual pulmonary impairment or there may be mild scarring remaining in the pleural space. Such pleural fibrosis usually is not a cause of significant pulmonary restriction.[113] Thoracostomy tube drainage is rarely indicated.

Although the effusion tends to resolve spontaneously without residua, it is mandatory to treat these patients with antituberculosis chemotherapy. In a series of patients with undiagnosed pleural effusions who were tuberculin-positive, up to 65% developed overt apical granulomatous pulmonary tuberculosis following the episode of effusion.[111] Of the cases of pulmonary tuberculosis, 80% occur within 5 yr of the pleural effusion. Appropriate antituberculous chemotherapy for active disease, as outlined in Chapter 9, virtually prevents the subsequent development of clinical pulmonary tuberculosis.

Neoplasms commonly cause pleural effusions, especially in older persons. In five large series,[85,86,114–116] malignancy accounted for 40% of all pleural effusions. It is apparent that neoplasms must be considered in any patient with an undiagnosed effusion.

Bronchogenic carcinoma is the most common malignancy that leads to a unilateral pleural effusion.[117] Bilateral pleural effusions are not common in patients with bronchogenic carcinoma, and when such occur, roentgenograms typically manifest a mediastinal mass.[105] This malignancy most commonly causes pleural effusion by direct involvement of the pleura. Thus, patients with bronchogenic carcinoma and pleural effusions are generally regarded as inoperable, especially if malignant cells are recovered from the fluid.[118,118a] However, some patients do not have direct pleural involvement and in these cases the effusion is probably secondary to obstructive pneumonia or to obstruction of lymphatic drainage of the pleural space.

Most commonly, patients with a pleural effusion due to bronchogenic carcinoma do not have symptoms directly referable to the effusion, and their presentation is dependent on the primary process (see Chap. 15, on bronchogenic carcinoma). The symptom most referable to the pleural effusion is dyspnea, caused by the volume of the fluid and its effect on the mechanics of the diaphragm. Occasionally, a malignant pleural effusion causes pleuritic pain. The physical examination reveals the presence of the effusion; other physical findings depend on the location and the extent of the primary neoplasm. Roentgenographically, there is frequently an abnormality of the lung parenchyma in addition to the effusion. There may be a peripheral lung mass, an obstructive pneumonia, or a hilar mass (which may be the primary carcinoma or due to metastatic disease to the hilar lymph node). Routine laboratory and sputum cytologic examinations are described elsewhere.

Fluid obtained at thoracentesis may be yellow and clear or may be grossly bloody.[86] In the majority of cases, the fluid has the findings suggestive of an exudate.[58] The number of erythrocytes present varies from a few to greater than 100,000/mm^3. The number of leukocytes tends to be in the 2500/mm^3 range, and there is a tendency for these cells to be lymphocytes. The pleural fluid glucose is usually normal, but occasionally it may be extremely low.[75,119] A definitive diagnosis may be obtained by cytologic examination of the pleural fluid in a large fraction of patients.[118a,120] The number of definitive diagnoses probably depends not only on the extent of pleural involvement by tumor but also on the adequacy of the specimen presented to the cytologist and on the experience of the cytologist. Pleural biopsy may also reveal a definitive diagnosis in approximately 60% of cases.

The course of a pleural effusion due to bronchogenic carinoma is usually discouraging for the patient and the physician, for there is a marked tendency for the fluid to progress; when the fluid is removed by thoracentesis, there is a tendency for it to recur promptly. This tendency toward rapid reaccumulation of fluid is not common for other causes of exudative effusions, and such a course suggests malignancy in a patient without a definitive diagnosis. Since it is not possible to cure the cancer in a patient with a malignant effusion, the least aggressive approach that will alleviate the patient's symptoms is used. If the effusion reaccumulates slowly after the initial thoracentesis, it may be possible to manage the patient with occasional thoracenteses. If reaccumulation is rapid, however, obliteration of the pleural space, (pleurodesis) is attempted through instillation of irritating substances or chemotherapeutic agents or operative pleurectomy or closed thoracostomy tube drainage to allow the pleural space to be obliterated by cancer cells.[121–125]

A chemical approach to pleurodesis with a sound experimental rationale[126,127] and demonstrated clinical effectiveness[128,129] is the instillation of tetracycline. This approach has the highest success rate and the lowest morbidity of any method currently in use.

The technique of tetracycline instillation is important for its success.[124,125,129] A tube thoracostomy should be inserted so as to drain all pleural fluid as confirmed by chest roentgenogram. Since the pleural reaction causes severe pain, premedication with narcotic analgesics is desirable. This is followed by injecting 500 mg of tetracycline in 50 ml of saline into the pleural space and flushing the tube with 20–30 ml of saline. The tube should be clamped for 30 min to 1 hr in order to permit the patient to rotate through a range of body positions and thus ensure fluid dispersal. The chest tube is then connected to suction drainage for 24 hr and until all fluid has been drained, as demonstrated by chest roentgenograms. Any reaccumulation of loculated fluid may require an additional chest tube. When all fluid has been drained for 24 hr, the chest tube is removed. With this method, approximately 90% of patients will achieve pleurodesis.

Metastatic carcinoma may also produce pleural effusions, and all types of carcinoma added together have equaled bronchogenic carcinoma in frequency in some series.[85,86] If a malignant pleural effusion is bilateral, the cause is much more likely to be metastatic carcinoma than bronchogenic carcinoma.[105] By far the most common metastatic malignancy to produce pleural effusion is carcinoma of the breast followed by carcinoma of the ovary, kidney, stomach, pancreas, and other sites in the gastrointestinal and urinary tracts.

Effusions caused by metastic malignancy evidently may be caused by two separate mechanisms. One of these is direct involvement of the pleura by metastic foci; such foci almost invariably involve the visceral pleura, although the parietal pleura may be involved as well.[130] The second mechanism of fluid production is obstruction of mediastinal lymph nodes, causing poor reabsorption of fluid from the pleural space. Such obstruction may occur without obvious roentgenographic changes, at least at the time the patient first presents to the physician.

Parenchymal metastases usually do not cause significant symptoms. If the pleural effusion associated with the metastasis is large, the patient may present with dyspnea as a primary complaint. Pleuritic chest pain is not common. The physical examination reveals the finding of the effusion and other findings depend on the site of the primary carcinoma and its metastases. Chest roentgenograms most commonly reveal diffuse pulmonary densities in addition to the pleural effusion, which may be unilateral or bilateral. Chest roentgenograms may also reveal mediastinal masses.

Fluid obtained by thoracentesis may be yellow or grossly bloody. Chemical findings are usually those of an exudate. Erythrocytes vary in number from a few to in excess of 100,000/mm^3. The leukocyte count is not likely to be more than 2,500/mm^3, and typically these are lymphocytes.[87] Cytologic preparations may reveal malignant cells if the mode of fluid formation is direct involvement of the pleura; if the effusion is caused by mediastinal lymphatic obstruction, no malignant cells are likely to be found. Pleural biopsy may yield the correct diagnosis, but generally adds little to the results of cytologic examination.[118a,120]

As with patients with pleural effusions from bronchogenic carcinoma, patients with metastatic carcinoma are likely to have progressive effusions that recur after thoracentesis. Treatment is similar to that for bronchogenic carcinoma, insofar as the effusions are concerned. Overall patient management depends on the primary site of the carcinoma and its mode of therapy. When treatment of the primary tumor is successful and the tumor regresses the pleural effusion is commonly less troublesome.

Lymphomas and leukemia frequently cause pleural effusions that may be unilateral or bilateral. As a group, lymphomas are the third most common causes of malignant pleural effusions, after bronchogenic carcinoma and carcinoma of the breast.[86,124] If the effusion is bilateral, lymphoma is a more likely cause than bronchogenic carcinoma.

The mechanism by which lymphomas produce pleural effusions is not clear.[131–133] It seems most reasonable to believe that the mechanism may be either a direct involvement of the visceral pleura or may be the result of lymphatic obstruction, with failure of fluid removal from the pleural space.

Pleural effusions do not typically occur early in the course of a lymphoma and the diagnosis usually has already been established when the effusions are first detected.[131] If associated with enlarged mediastinal lymph nodes, there may be no symptoms, cough, or retrosternal ache. If associated with pulmonary parenchymal disease, the patient commonly has cough and dyspnea. Pleuritic pain is rare. Effusions frequently are small and may not be detected on physical examination. Large effusions usually are associated with parenchymal disease, and the findings of both fluid and increased transmission of breath sounds. Other physical findings depend on the extent of other organ involvement. Roentgenograms of the chest most commonly reveal hilar or mediastinal lymph node involvement, and in addition, there may be pulmonary parenchymal changes. Parenchymal changes include irregular lung masses, linear and reticulonodular lung infiltrates, isolated multiple alveolar infiltrates, segmental or lobar consolidation with air bronchograms, or subpleural masslike densities. The combination of pleural, parenchymal, and lymph node involvement suggests the correct diagnosis.

Thoracentesis may reveal a serous or serosanguinous fluid. The fluid may have the characteristics of either a transudate or an exudate. Erythrocytes may be few or numerous, and leukocytes tend to be of the same order of magnitude as in other malignant processes. The differential count of the leukocytes almost always reveals in excess of 90% lymphocytes.[87] Occasionally, the effusion is a chylous fluid.[134]

In the absence of parenchymal disease, pleural effusions tend to be small and without serious clinical significance. The effusions may clear after irradiation therapy of the mediastinal nodes. Large effusions associated with parenchymal disease are a bad prognostic sign.[131] Thoracentesis, with removal of as much of the fluid as possible, may relieve the patient while therapy is being directed at the underlying neoplasm.

Mesotheliomas are rare tumors that arise from either the visceral or parietal pleura. There are two types of mesotheliomas.[135] The solitary, benign mesothelioma is a localized growth in the pleural space that does not usually produce a pleural effusion and that usually may be cured by surgical removal. The diffuse, malignant mesothelioma spreads widely in the pleural space and usually is associated with an extensive pleural effusion; direct invasion of thoracic structures prevents surgical cure. The histologic picture of these tumors has led to considerable controversy in the medical literature and may lead to difficulty in patient management. One group of tumors has the histologic appearance of connective tissue origin. In some, the appearance is histologically benign, and these tumors may be reported as fibromas. In others, the histologic picture is that of a malignant tumor, and the term *fibrosarcoma* is more likely to be used. Other tumors have a histologic appearance characterized by tubes lined by cells; these tumors resemble carcinomatous glands; that is, the tumor appears to be an adenocarcinoma. In many tumors, there is a mixture of fibrous and tubular elements. A variety of special staining and histochemical techniques may be used to differentiate mesotheliomas from adenocarcinomas,[136] but none is entirely specific. Electron microscopy also may be helpful. There is a tendency for the localized tumors to have the histologic appearance of a fibroma or fibrosarcoma and for the diffuse tumors to appear glandular or mixed. In any case, however, the histologic appearance cannot be used to predict the clinical behavior of the tumor. Localized tumors that do not recur after surgical removal, and aggressively invading diffuse tumors, may have the same histologic picture.

Local benign or diffuse malignant mesotheliomas may occur at any age and in either sex, although there is a higher prevalence among older men. An increased incidence of malignant pleural and peritoneal mesotheliomas among persons with a heavy exposure to asbestos was first reported in 1960.[137] This association has been substantiated in several geographic areas,[138,139] and has been further substantiated by the finding of asbestos bodies in the lungs of some patients and by the experimental observation that intrapleural injection of asbestos in experimental animals induces pleural mesotheliomas.[140] The average period between excessive exposure to asbestos and the development of tumors is prolonged, perhaps 20 to 40 yr. The patient has not necessarily been continuously exposed to asbestos during this interval. The exposure does not require that the patient has actually worked with asbestos, for many patients have only lived in the vicinity of asbestos mines or mills.[141]

Many patients with localized tumors are asymptomatic, even when the tumors are quite large; others with local disease may experience cough, chest pain, or weight loss. Only a few patients with localized mesothelioma develop pleural effusions. Most patients with diffuse tumors are symptomatic; chest pain and dyspnea are the most frequent symptoms. The chest pain is due to invasion of chest wall muscles and is usually described as dull; it is rarely pleuritic.[135] Less frequent symptoms are fever, weight loss, weakness, hemoptysis, and digital clubbing. Migratory polyarthralgias, pulmonary osteoarthropathy, and hypoglycemia have all been reported in some series. Most patients with diffuse mesotheliomas have a significant volume of pleural effusion.

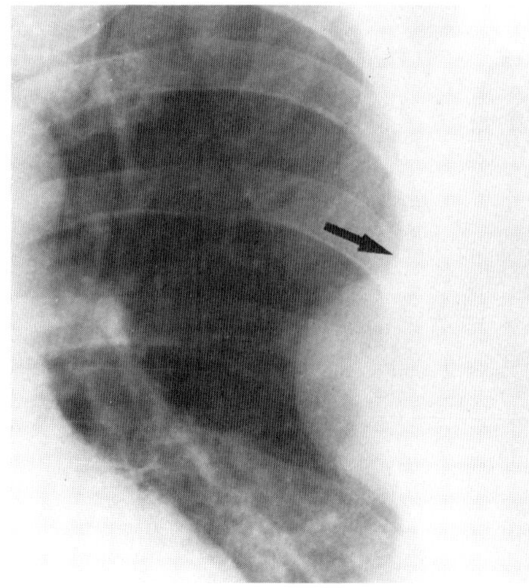

FIG. 12-11. Roentgenogram of a patient with multiple myeloma of the chest wall. The tumor indents the lung by pushing the visceral pleura ahead of it, causing the water density to form an obtuse angle with the chest wall (*arrow*), the extrapleural sign.

Roentgenographically, the local benign mesothelioma appears as a homogenous mass of water density situated peripherally in the lung fields contiguous to the pleura or in the interlobar fissure. Lesions arising in the fissure may simulate a solitary lung nodule or an encapsulated effusion. Lesions arising from pleural surfaces against the chest wall usually indent the lung in such a way that the water density forms an obtuse angle with the chest wall when viewed in profile, known as the *extra-pleural sign* (Fig. 12-11). This roentgenographic sign of an obtuse angle may help in distinguishing lesions arising in the pleural space from those arising in the lung parenchyma, which tend to meet the chest wall at an acute angle (Fig. 12-12). Diffuse mesotheliomas may be hidden by the accompanying pleural effusion, although pleural densities in a non-gravity-dependent location overlying the pleural effusion may suggest the correct diagnosis. Furthermore, even a large effusion associated with a mesothelioma tends not to displace the mediastinum to the contralateral thorax, as commonly occurs in large pleural effusions of

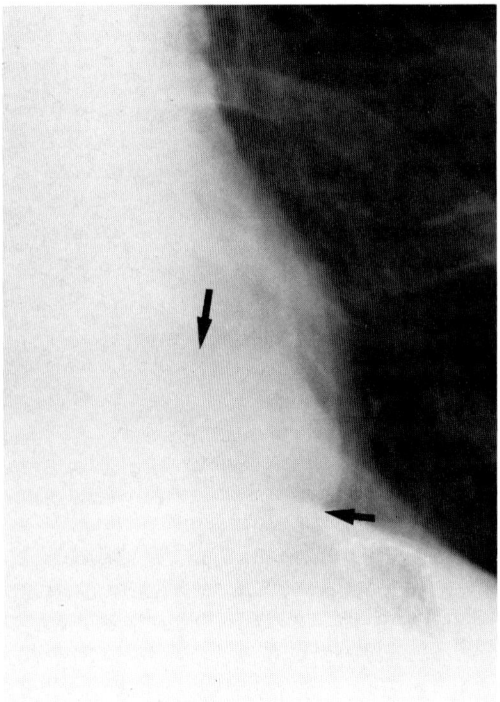

FIG. 12-12. Roentgenogram demonstrating a bronchogenic carcinoma in the left lower lobe posterior to the heart. A tumor arising from the lung parenchyma tends to meet the chest wall at an acute angle (*arrows*).

other causes.[142] Such a roentgenographic finding does not necessarily differentiate mesothelioma from bronchogenic carcinoma with a pleural effusion, however, since the latter may cause the same finding when it is associated with obstructive atelectasis.

Thoracentesis may reveal either serous or serosanguinous fluid, which may have from few to many erythrocytes. The effusion tends to have the characteristics of an exudate and malignant cells may be observed. Pleural biopsy by a needle technique may yield the correct diagnosis. However, the variable histologic picture may lead to the diagnosis of metastatic adenocarcinoma. The correct diagnosis of mesothelioma may require a thoracotomy in order to obtain sufficient tissue from several sites. However, the issue in some cases is resolved only at the time of autopsy.

Treatment for local lesions is thoracotomy with surgical excision. Such therapy is usually curative, even though the histologic appearance of the tumor is malignant. Conversely, the prognosis for patients with diffuse, malignant mesothelioma is poor, with the usual survival from 4 to 12 months after diagnosis or 8 to 14 months after onset of symptoms.[135,143,144] Women have somewhat longer survival times and the symptom of chest pain is more ominous than dyspnea.[143] Although no treatment regimen is satisfactory at present, surgical resection of as much of the disease as possible followed by high-dose radiotherapy and a chemotherapeutic regimen containing doxorubicin apparently offers the best opportunity for prolonged survival and occasional cure.[143,145,146]

Intraabdominal Tumors. Pelvic neoplasms in women may be associated with ascites and pleural effusions (Meig's syndrome).[147,148] The syndrome has been reported most frequently with fibromas, thecomas, granulosa cell tumors, and Brenner tumors, but it has also been reported with cystadenomas, adenocarcinomas, and fibromyomas of the uterus. These women usually present with a history of abdominal pain, progressive enlargement of the abdomen, and dyspnea. Physical findings reveal a pleural effusion, ascites, and a pelvic mass. Roentgenograms of the chest indicate only the pleural effusion, which varies from a small to a massive amount of fluid. The effusion is most commonly unilateral on the right side, but it may be left-sided or bilateral.

The effusion is usually serous and demonstrates the typical findings of an exudate. The pleural fluid evidently arises from transdiaphragmatic movement of the abdominal fluid; the constituents of the fluid in the two spaces are similar, and carbon particles injected into the peritoneal space subsequently may be recovered from the pleural space.[149] Cytology of the pleural effusion does not reveal malignant cells, nor is a pleural biopsy rewarding.

After removal by thoracentesis, the pleural effusion may recur rapidly, even if there is only a moderate amount of ascites. Both the ascites and the pleural effusion promptly disappear, however, following removal of the pelvic neoplasm.

Such a salutary course is to be expected even if the neoplasm is malignant.

Other intraabdominal neoplasms have been associated with pleural effusions in the absence of direct chest involvement.[149,150] These, also, are associated with ascites. In the case of retroperitoneal lymphomas, the effusions have been due to chylothorax (discussed subsequently). Irradiation of the abdomen without direct therapy to the thorax may result in regression of the pleural effusion.[150]

Chest-Wall Neoplasms. Occasionally, malignant tumors of the chest wall cause a pleural effusion. The tumors may arise from ribs or from the tissue of the intercostal space. On physical and roentgenographic examination, the chest wall may be expanded, and lytic lesions of bone may be apparent. Occasionally, the effusion may be caused by multiple myeloma invading one or more ribs[151] and the involved ribs may be expanded, a finding highly suggestive of myeloma. Although malignant plasmacytes may sometimes be found in the pleural fluid,[152,153] this finding is inconstant, and diagnosis depends on adequate biopsy of the primary lesion in most cases.

Pulmonary embolism may be accompanied by a pleural effusion. Various series estimate that the incidence of effusion accompanying embolism is 17% to 56% of the cases.[154–160] These data must be interpreted with caution, however, since the incidence of effusion depends on the criteria by which embolism was diagnosed. The highest incidence reported was from a series with very stringent diagnostic criteria, which may have led to underdiagnosis of pulmonary embolism in the patient population studied.[160] It is clear, however, that pleural effusions are relatively common manifestations of pulmonary embolism.

The pathogenesis of effusion accompanying embolism is not known. It is clear, however, that effusion may occur with or without lung infarction, as manifested by a roentgenographic infiltrate. That is, the effusion may be the only roentgenographic abnormality.

The pleural effusion is most commonly unilateral in either hemithorax, but bilaterality is not rare. Effusions resulting from embolism usually are not large, and they usually do not lead to symptoms directly. Symptomatology is dependent on the primary process. The effusion usually is not progressive and following removal by thoracentesis, it usually does not recur unless there is a subsequent episode of embolization. Physical findings are those of a small unilateral or bilateral effusion without other abnormalities on the chest exam. Roentgenographically, the effusion may or may not be associated with a pulmonary parenchymal infiltrate, which may or may not have the characteristics of a "Hampton's hump."[161] The diagnosis of thromboembolism is based on pulmonary angiography or radioactive scan (see section on thromboembolism, Chap. 10).

There is no typical effusion in pulmonary embolism, since the pleural fluid findings are remarkably variable.[160] There is a tendency for the fluid to be an exudate, but a significant minority are transudates when no concomitant cause for transudation exists. Erythrocyte counts vary from nil to more than 200,000/mm^3. There is a strong correlation between bloody effusions and the appearance of parenchymal infiltrates, suggesting that pulmonary infarction may in part determine whether the effusion accompanying an embolus is bloody.[160] Leukocyte counts likewise vary from nil to 25,000/mm^3. There is a tendency for the leukocytes to be polymorphonuclear but in a significant fraction of the patients, lymphocytes may exceed 70% of the total leukocyte count. The constituents of the pleural effusion may relate, in part, to the chronicity of the effusion; there is no direct correlation between treatment with anticoagulant drugs or lack thereof.

Occasionally, the effusion may be large enough to cause dyspnea, and thoracentesis for removal of the fluid may be indicated. More commonly, however, no specific therapy need be directed at the effusion.

Connective Tissue Disease. *Lupus Erythematosus (LE).* Pleural changes occur in the course of systemic lupus erythematosus in a significant fraction of patients with this disease. Such has been reported in as high as 74% of cases.[162] These changes may be a pleuritis manifested primarily by transient episodes of pleuritic pain with no roentgenographic abnormalities, or there may be pleural effusion with or without pleuritic chest pain. Effusions have been reported in up to 55% of patients with lupus erythematosus at some time during their course.[163] Such pleural disease may be the first manifestation of lupus erythematosus, but more commonly, pleural changes occur after other signs or symptoms have become manifested.[164]

Although pleural effusions from lupus erythematosus tend to be small, they may sometimes dominate the clinical picture. Effusions may be unilateral or bilateral, or they may transiently occur in one hemithorax and then the other. The effusion may be the only abnormality on chest roentgenograms, but frequently the cardiac silhouette is enlarged in a nonspecific way.[162] There may also be nonspecific alveolar infiltrates of the lung parenchyma, which tend to be basilar. The effusions tend to clear over a brief interval, even in the absence of specific therapy, and usually there are no roentgenographic residua.

The pleural effusions due to lupus erythematosus are usually exudates, although they may be transudates, especially in the presence of complications such as renal or cardiac failure. The cellular constituents are not distinctive, and the fluid is rarely bloody. It has been reported that the whole hemolytic complement and its components C3 and C4 are present in lesser amounts (less than 5 CH_{50} units per ml) in these patients, that there is complement conversion in the pleural fluid, and that an immune complex vasculitis may be observed in the pleural blood vessels.[77,165,166] The LE cell phenomenon may be observed in some pleural effusions.

Specific therapy usually is not necessary, since effusions are characteristically small and transient. In the case of large effusions, adrenal cortical steroids are beneficial. It usually is not necessary to perform a thoracentesis unless the diagnosis is in doubt.

Rheumatoid Arthritis. Pleural effusions occur in from 2% to 5% of patients with rheumatoid arthritis.[73,167–171] The effusions may accompany rheumatoid disease of the lung parenchyema, either nodular infiltrates or fibrosis (see Chap. 13 on connective tissue diseases), but usually they occur independent of other thoracic changes. Most commonly, the effusion is unilateral, although bilateral effusions are reported.

Despite the fact that rheumatoid arthritis is more common in women, rheumatoid pleural effusion is much more common in men. Characteristically, it occurs in middle age. The patient has most commonly had arthritis for several years, and the diagnosis of rheumatoid arthritis has usually been established. Subcutaneous rheumatoid nodules are present in a large fraction of the patients. Occasionally, the pleural effusion antedates any other symptoms of rheumatoid disease, or the onset of arthritis and effusion are simultaneous.

The pleural fluid has been described as turbid and greenish yellow in many patients,[73] but it may be a clear yellow. The fluid has the constituents of an exudate. Erythrocytes are not likely to be numerous, and any leukocytes are predominantly lymphocytes. A unique feature of rheumatoid pleural effusion is the exceedingly low glucose concentration,[73,74] which is frequently less than 20 mg/dl and may be undetectable. Such low values are almost diagnostic of rheumatoid pleural effusion, but an occasional malignant effusion has been reported with similarly low glucose values.[75] Rheumatoid factor may also be found in the pleural fluid, but this finding is not specific, since rheumatoid factor or rheumatoid-factor-like activity has been demonstrated in the effusion fluid from patients with bacterial pneumonia, carcinoma, and tuberculosis.[172]

A unique cytologic picture has been observed in pleural fluids from patients with rheumatoid arthritis.[173] The characteristic cytologic elements of a background of orange or red granular material, large elongated cells, and giant round or oval multinucleated cells are thought to be derived from the breakdown products of palisades of histiocytes, which are a part of the inflammatory reaction in rheumatoid pleuritis. Pleural biopsy may reveal an appearance similar to that of a rheumatoid nodule that has been opened out, exposing the fibrinoid zone to the serous cavity.[174] This appearance is diagnostic of rheumatoid pleural effusion.

Rheumatoid effusions tend to persist for months or years. They apparently are not affected by steroid therapy. Since they most commonly do not lead to significant symptoms, aggressive therapy by repeated thoracentesis or thoracostomy tube drainage usually is not indicated.

Intra-abdominal Disease. *Subdiaphragmatic (subphrenic) abscess* produces symptoms that are as likely to be referable to the thorax as to the abdomen.[175] The disease is more common in men and is most prevalent in middle age. Approximately two-thirds of such abscesses are on the right side, approximately 25% are left-sided, and a small percentage are bilateral. Subdiaphragmatic abscess develops as a complication of abdominal disease in almost all cases. Gastrointestinal perforations and surgery on the upper gastrointestinal tract are the most common causal factors; liver and biliary tract diseases or operations are second most common. Trauma and appendiceal disease make up the majority of the remainder, although any intra-abdominal surgery may be associated with this complication.

Thoracic symptoms and signs occur in a very high percentage of these patients.[175-178] Pain may be typically pleuritic or may be pleuritic in nature but referred to the shoulder (diaphragmatic pleurisy). There may be symptoms of an acute pneumonia, dyspnea due to altered diaphragmatic function, or expectoration of purulent material from a bronchial-abscess fistula. Other patients have symptoms predominantly of abdominal origin, including flank pain, tenderness, or a mass in the region of the abscess. Less specific symptoms of anorexia, nausea, vomiting, and weight loss are common. Fever is present in approximately 85% of cases. It is not uncommon for such symptoms to be longstanding before the patient seeks medical aid.

Roentgenographic findings suggestive of subdiaphragmatic abscess are generally present, and diagnostic findings occur in approximately a third of cases.[179] There is almost always an elevation of the hemidiaphragm on the affected side, and fluoroscopy reveals the diaphragm to have a limited range of motion. In approximately half of the cases, the diaphragm does not move at all. These diaphragmatic changes are associated with a pleural effusion in approximately 80% of patients and basilar pneumonia or atelectasis in approximately 70%. The effusion tends not to be large. A diagnostic sign present in approximately a third of patients is an air-fluid level below the diaphragm (Fig. 12-13). Various roentgenographic maneuvers may be necessary to insure that the air lies outside of the gastrointestinal tract. Of less importance is the roentgenographic finding of displacement of intra-abdominal viscera, which is most commonly observed when the abscess is on the left side. Radionucleotide scanning of the liver and spleen and sonographic examination of the abdomen are usually helpful when a subdiaphragmatic abscess is suspected.

Thoracentesis most commonly reveals a clear serous fluid with the characteristics of an exudate. Although the fluid may have a relatively high leukocyte count, it is usually sterile. In some instances, there may be a frank empyema, with organisms similar to those in the abscess cavity. In such instances, there has been a perforation of the diaphragm by the abscess. There is often a mixture of organisms found on culture of the abscess and empyema fluid. The most common offending organisms are staphylococcus, streptococcus, *E. coli*, other gram-negative bacilli, and anaerobic organisms.

In most cases, no direct therapy is necessary for the pulmonary manifestations of subdiaphragmatic abscess. Treatment is directed at surgical drainage of the abscess and broad-spectrum antimicrobial agents. Most commonly, drainage of pleural fluid is not necessary, since the fluid is sterile. If the pleural space is infected, drainage of both abscess and pleural pus by surgical means may be necessary. Even with adequate antimicrobial drugs and surgical drainage, the mortality of diaphragmatic abscess remains high. If the correct diagnosis is made and surgical drainage carried out, the mortality rate is approximately 25%.[176,176a] If drainage is not performed, the mortality rate approaches 100%.

Pancreatitis. Pleuropulmonary complications have been detected roentgenographically in from 15 to 55% of patients with acute pancreatitis or with pancreatic pseudo-cyst.[180] Abnormalities have included elevated hemidiaphragm, basilar atelectasis, pleural effusion, and pleural reaction. Pleural effusions have been reported in between 3 and 17% of cases. Pleural effusions are much more commonly on the left than on the right, and a significant fraction are bilateral.[76] Although such findings are not specific for pancreatic disease, they are certainly suggestive in the presence of an appropriate clinical setting, including epigastric pain radiating through to the back, nausea and vomiting, fever, and the presence of a predisposing cause such as alcoholism.

Pleural effusions due to pancreatitis tend to occur early in the course of the disease. The effusion usually is not large. Most commonly, it is a serous yellow fluid, but it may be blood-tinged in up to a third of cases. The findings are those of an exudate. A nearly diagnostic feature is the presence of a high concentration of amylase, which is usually raised out of proportion to the serum amylase. The high concentration of amylase in the pleural fluid may remain for a protracted interval, even though the serum amylase has returned to normal. This finding is not observed in all patients whose effusion is caused by pancreatitis. Likewise, it is not absolutely diagnostic of pancreatitis, since it has been reported in effusions due to neoplasms or infection.[75] A high amylase concentration of salivary origin has also been reported in pleural fluid associated with esophageal rupture.[181]

Pleural effusions from pancreatitis do not require specific therapy. They tend to regress as the primary disease improves.

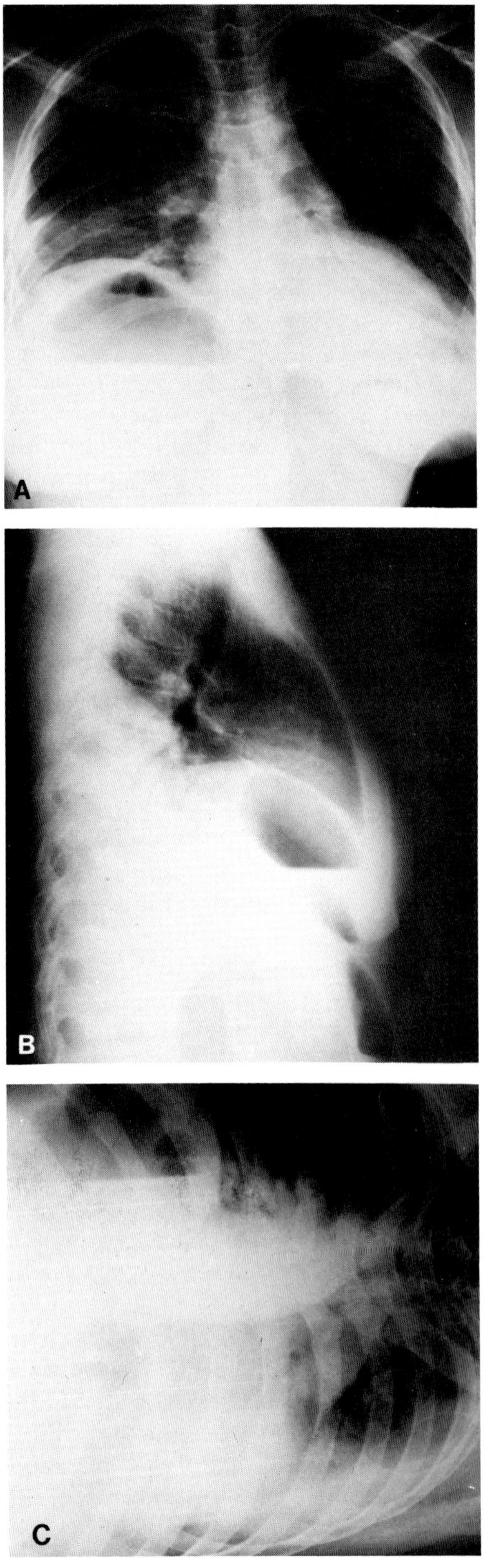

FIG. 12-13. A. Anteroposterior chest roentgenogram of a patient with a peritonitis and bilateral subdiaphragmatic abscesses. The right hemidiaphragm is markedly elevated, and there is a pleural effusion and parenchymal infiltrate in the right lower lobe. Note the large air pocket, with an air-fluid level below the diaphragm. **B.** Lateral chest roentgenogram demonstrating the upward bowing concavity of fluid posteriorly in the thorax, and several collections of air under the diaphragm, with a large air space demonstrating the horizontal air-fluid level. **C.** The left lateral decubitus chest film demonstrates the mobility of the fluid in the right subdiaphragmatic space and confirms that it is not in a normal gastrointestinal structure. Incidentally, the left-sided pleural effusion is seen much more clearly in this lateral decubitus view.

Abdominal Surgery. Approximately 50% of patients who undergo abdominal surgery have small pleural effusions demonstrable by lateral decubitus radiographs during the first few postoperative days.[182] In some patients, the thickness of fluid may exceed 10 mm. Fluid is more likely to be present following upper-abdominal surgery, when free fluid is present in the abdomen, on the side on which the surgery was performed, and when postoperative atelectasis occurs. The fluid has the characteristics of an exudate. The occurrence of fluid in this setting requires no diagnostic procedures in an uncomplicated patient and resolves spontaneously over the course of a few days.

Hepatitis. Pleural effusions have been reported in a few patients with hepatitis[183,184]; hepatitis B antigen, hepatitis B surface antigen, and viral particles have been demonstrated in the pleural fluid.[185] Insufficient data are available to determine the frequency of this event. However, the infectivity for medical personnel is highly probable; relief of dyspnea is likely the only indication for intervention.

Miscellaneous. *Familial Mediterranean fever* (familial paroxysmal polyserositis) is an uncommon disease, occurring most frequently in patients of Sephardic Jewish, Armenian, or Arabic ancestry.[186,187] The exact etiology is unknown, but it is inherited as an autosomal recessive trait in approximately 50% of reported patients. It is characterized by recurrent attacks of fever and polyserositis, with the average age of onset between 5 and 15 yr.

Attacks occur with an exceedingly varying frequency, but most commonly every 2 to 4 weeks. There may be spontaneous remission lasting for months or years, and patients tend to get better with age. A single attack usually lasts for 24 to 48 hr but may be protracted for up to 10 days. It may begin with a chill, and there is always fever. More than 95% of the patients have abdominal pain that usually begins in one area and progresses to involve most of the abdomen. The pain may be referred to the shoulders in a typical diaphragmatic radiation. The abdomen usually is tender and frequently mimics the findings in an acute surgical emergency. The pain may be accompanied by nausea and vomiting. Approximately 75% of the patients have pleuritic pain, either alone or associated with abdominal pain. During the course of the pleuritic pain, there may be small, transient pleural effusions that may be unilateral or bilateral. The fluid tends to have the properties of an exudate, with no identifying characteristics. Many patients have arthritis, and approximately 25% develop erythematous skin lesions on their legs during attacks. Some develop colloid-body-like dots in the optic fundi, and some have splenomegaly or hepatomegaly. Most patients have mild leukocytosis and an elevated sedimentation rate during attacks.

Approximately 25% of patients in the Middle East develop amyloidosis involving arterioles, venules, glomeruli, and the spleen, without cardiac or hepatic involvement. In North America, amyloidosis is rare. Those patients who develop amyloidosis frequently develop nephrotic syndrome, which may be a cause of death. In the absence of amyloidosis, the prognosis for longevity is good.

The pleural effusions and pleuritic pain may lead to difficulty in differential diagnosis, but the family history of similar illness and the recurrent nature of the symptoms should suggest familial Mediterranean fever. In addition, the pleural effusions are very transient, which is not common in most other etiologies of effusions.

Lymphedema. Patients with recurrent pleural effusions associated with lymphedema have been reported.[188–192] These patients have chronic lymphedema of the legs, hands, and face, which tends to appear during adult life. Several patients have been reported to have yellow discoloration of their fingernails.[189,190] The pleural effusions associated with this syndrome have been chronic, recurrent, and bilateral. The effusions have the properties of an exudate, and pleural biopsy has been unrewarding. One patient has been reported with extremely low glucose concentrations in the pleural fluid.[191] The only available data suggest that the effusions are due to abnormalities of pleural and mediastinal lymphatics, leading to poor absorption of fluid and protein from the pleural space.

Post Myocardial Infarction Syndrome. Dressler originally described a clinical syndrome which occurs in approximately 3% of patients following myocardial infarction.[193] The syndrome typically begins within weeks of the infarction and is characterized by recurrent episodes of fever, pericardial or pleural pain, and pericarditis; it may recur over several years. Up to 85% of patients have pleural effusions which are usually small and in the left hemithorax. The effusions typically have the characteristics of an exudate. At times, the pleural effusions occur without pericarditis.[194] The syndrome is thought to be caused by immunologic mechanisms, but the pathogenesis is poorly understood.

Each episode of pericarditis is self-limiting. Symptoms frequently may be controlled with aspirin or indomethacin. Adrenocortical steroids are administered when symptoms are severe.

Myxedema. Pleural effusion in the absence of pericardial effusion and of recognizable causes of fluid retention may occur in the course of myxedema.[195] There are no particular identifying characteristics of the fluid. The effusions tend to be small and not to lead to disability.

Idiopathic Effusions. Despite reasonable diagnostic efforts, the cause of pleural effusion is not determined in up to 25% of patients.[85,86,114–116a] A definitive diagnosis may not be reached even if an exploratory thoracotomy is performed.[196,197,197a] Since the causes of such effusions are likely to be diverse, the clinical presentations of patients with idiopathic pleural effusions are varied. The effusion may be discovered incidentally at the time of a routine physical examination or chest roentgenogram. In those patients with symptoms, the clinical picture tends to be similar to that of patients with tuberculous effusions.[197] The duration of the effusion may be transient or protracted. The pleural fluid is likely to be an exudate, without other identifying characteristics.

In those patients studied by open thoracotomy, the pleura was found to consist of a smooth, glistening, and opalescent fibrous peel.[197] Microscopically, the pleura was fibrotic and edematous. There was generally mesothelial cell enlargement and hyperchromasia. There were foci of lymphocytes and occasional plasma cells. The underlying lung parenchyma was most commonly normal. In one study, 60% of patients had no recurrence, but of the remainder, malignancy, connective tissue diseases, and other causes eventually became evident.[197a]

Patients who have a pleural effusion that cannot be diagnosed by the procedures outlined in this chapter and who have positive tuberculin skin tests should be treated with antituberculosis chemotherapy, as outlined in the section on tuberculosis effusions (see Chap. 9)

Infections

Parapneumonic Effusions and Bacterial Empyema. By strict definition, the term *empyema* refers to a collection of pus in the pleural space, but since the appearance of some fluids associated with infection is serous, a broader definition of infection of the pleural space is probably more desirable. Recently, the term *parapneumonic effusion* has been suggested.[75,198–201] A parapneumonic effusion is defined as a pleural effusion in association with an acute febrile illness in which pulmonary infiltrates and purulent sputum are present. This definition includes pleural effusions secondary to pneumonia whether the effusion is serous or frankly purulent. The purpose of this nomenclature is to emphasize that pleural effusions in association with pneumonia do not necessarily indicate that the pleural space is infected and hence do not connote an illness more serious than the primary pneumonia. Thus, all empyemas in association with pneumonia are parapneumonic effusions, but not all parapneumonic effusions are empyemas. An uncomplicated parapneumonic effusion which will regress with antimicrobial therapy without the need for aggressive drainage procedures is suggested by clear or turbid, freely moving fluid which may be easily aspirated, absence of bacteria on Gram stain of the fluid, a pleural fluid *p*H level of greater than 7.3, and a pleural fluid glucose level of greater than 60 mg/dl.[198–201] Conversely, findings which suggest that the parapneumonic effusion is an empyema and will require aggressive drainage procedures for cure are indicated in the following list (p. 591).

In adults, pleural infection is secondary to

Features Suggesting Empyema

1. Loculated fluid or air-fluid levels in pleural space
2. Grossly purulent fluid or foul smell
3. Bacteria demonstrable by gram stain
4. Pleural fluid *p*H less than 7.3
5. Pleural fluid glucose less than 60 mg/dl
6. Fluid rapidly reaccumulates after thoracentesis

pulmonary parenchymal infection in approximately 55 to 65% of cases,[202,203] whereas in children, empyema is an extension of underlying pulmonary infection in 75% of cases.[204] Approximately 15 to 25% of pleural infections are secondary to surgery, and other causes include posttraumatic esophageal lesions, spontaneous pneumothorax, postthoracentesis, subdiaphragmatic abscess, and unknown cause. It is customary to divide empyema into acute and chronic cases, although the differentiation on a purely chronologic basis is not entirely satisfactory. In acute cases, the pleura is lined by infected fibrin, and the material may be drained without resorting to extensive surgical procedures. In chronic empyema, the pleural space contains fibrous tissue which can be removed only by thoracotomy. In an individual case, such a differentiation may be made only by the response to initial management by aspiration.[205]

Aerobic bacteria most commonly implicated as the etiology of empyema in adults include staphylococci in 17 to 45% of cases; gram-negative bacilli, most commonly klebsiella or psuedomonas, 13 to 56%; streptococci, 4 to 26%; and pneumococci, 4 to 15%.[202,203,206–208] Other aerobic bacteria are less common. It has been suggested, however, that inadequate methods for detecting anaerobic bacteria in many hospitals have led to underdiagnosis of these organisms as a cause of empyema, and that this accounts for the high incidence of "sterile empyema" reported from several laboratories.[209,210] When meticulous techniques have been used to preserve anaerobes during transfer to the laboratory and culture, these organisms have been recovered in up to 75% of cases studied, and they have been the exclusive isolates in 35% of cases.[209] Variability in bacterial etiology among different series may also result from the selection of cases. *Staphylococcus aureus* is the most prevalent pathogen in young children with empyema, and anaerobic organisms are not likely in pediatric patients.[208] In cases of empyema occurring after thoracic surgery, gram-negative bacilli, especially pseudomonas, are the most frequent offenders.

In patients with empyema due to underlying pulmonary parenchymal infection, the onset of symptoms frequently is insidious, and the disease is present for days to weeks before the patient seeks medical attention.[208,210,211] The most common presenting complaint is chest pain. The patients have almost always been febrile, and many complain of dyspnea. Significant weight loss has occurred in 25 to 50% of patients. Many patients also complain of cough, chills, hemoptysis, night sweats, and chest tenderness. Physical examination usually reveals a relatively high fever, 102 to 103°F, and confirms the presence of a pleural effusion. Chest roentgenograms typically reveal both a parenchymal infiltrate and a pleural effusion. Routine laboratory examination indicates a leukocytosis in most patients with counts commonly over 20,000/mm^3. Anemia is common.

Thoracentesis usually reveals thick, purulent fluid. However, it is not uncommon for the fluid to be thin and serous, and it may be blood-tinged. In some patients, the fluid is serous initially and becomes more purulent with time; in others, the fluid is loculated, and some spaces yield serous and other purulent fluid.[210] Leukocyte counts are most commonly above 5,000 mm^3 and may range over 30,000 cells/mm^3; an average leukocyte count is approximately 15,000 mm^3. Most commonly, in excess of 80% of the cells are neutrophils. Pleural-fluid protein is usually in excess of 3 g/dl. Pleural-fluid glucose is usually low, less than 20 mg/dl, and the *p*H less than 7.3. The causative organism usually can be seen on Gram stain of the fluid; bacterial morphology may be better demonstrated by a methylene blue stain. Anaerobic bacteria are suggested if more than one type of bacterial morphology is observed.

Successful therapy depends on appropriate antimicrobials and adequate drainage of the pleural space. The initial choice of antimicrobial is dependent on the results of Gram stain of the empyema fluid. If the organisms present the unambiguous appearance of streptococci or pneumococci, penicillin is indicated. A penicillinase-resistant synthetic penicillin (*e.g.*, methicillin) is indicated for organisms appearing to be staphylococci. Gentamicin is a reasonable choice for all gram-negative bacilli, and high-dose penicillin is the initial drug of choice for apparent anaerobic infections. If there is any doubt about the likely bacterial etiology, combined antimicrobial therapy is reasonable in severely ill patients. The combination of high-dose penicillin and gentamicin is reasonable initial therapy in such instances. In all cases, antimicrobial therapy is adjusted when specific cultural and sensitivity data become available. Reliable data on bacterial etiology include culture of the empyema fluid or blood. Pathogens cultured from sputum may not indicate the correct cause of the empyema.[211] Antimicrobials are continued until the patient is clinically well and until chest roentgenograms indicate complete resolution or a minimal stable residue. Patients with empyema usually require protracted antimicrobial therapy; 3 weeks is apparently the minimum duration,[211] and 6 to 12 weeks is not unusual.[210] A part of this therapy may be as an outpatient, but hospitalization is usually prolonged.

Adequate drainage of the empyema fluid is mandatory for a successful outcome. Adequate drainage occasionally may be achieved by repeated thoracentesis, if the fluid is thin and easily drained. However, this procedure is not often successful, especially if the empyema fluid is purulent. More commonly, attempts at repeated thoracentesis drainage only lead to delayed adequate drainage, with increased patient morbidity and mortality.[212] In almost all cases, more aggressive drainage procedures should be instituted immediately upon making the diagnosis of empyema. Closed thoracostomy tube drainage is the procedure of choice for most patients. Care should be taken to ensure that the tube is at the most dependent part of the empyema, and more than one tube may be necessary for loculated empyemas. Occasionally, tube placement under fluoroscopy or with the aid of ultrasound may be necessary to localize fluid. Adequate drainage is indicated by defervescence and general clinical improvement. If such does not occur within four days, more extensive drainage is indicated.[211] In some patients, reinsertion of a closed thoracostomy tube into a loculated area may yield adequate drainage. More commonly, however, limited thoracotomy, with rib resection and manual lysis of fibrinous adhesions, is necessary. A few patients respond to neither, and more radical thoracotomy with decortication of the pleural space is necessary. If drainage has not been successful, secondary decortication probably should be performed without delay in order to minimize prolonged disability. A few patients who have not received adequate drainage reasonably early in their course require a serious and disabling operation—thoracoplasty. For physicians unfamiliar with these procedures the concise review by Samson is recommended.[213]

Despite antimicrobials, the mortality rate of patients with empyema continues to be approximately 20%. The prognosis is worse in older patients, in those with severe underlying conditions, in patients not demonstrating a febrile response or leukocytosis at the time of admission, and in those with a prolonged delay in adequate drainage of the empyema fluid.

Tuberculous Empyema. In addition to the hypersensitivity pleural effusions that some patients experience during the postprimary phase of tuberculosis, *Mycobacterium tuberculosis* occasionally produces an infection of the pleural space. Tuberculous empyema is associated with a very high bacterial count in the pleural fluid. The fluid has the properties of an exudate and a high leukocyte count, characteristically predominantly lymphocytes.

Tuberculous empyema is invariably associated with active pulmonary tuberculosis, most characteristically far-advanced pulmonary disease with bronchopleural fistulas. Patients with this complication of pulmonary tuberculosis are rare because of the success of antituberculosis chemotherapy in preventing progressive lung destruction. The principles of management include adequate chemotherapy and drainage or obliteration of the pleural space. These principles are discussed in Chapter 9, in the section on pulmonary tuberculosis.

Fungi. Most fungi that cause pulmonary disease are not often associated with pleural effusions. Diseases due to *Histoplasma capsulatum*,[214] *Blastomyces dermititidis*,[215] and *Cryptococcus neoformans*[216] rarely cause pleural effusions. *Coccidioides immitis*[217] and aspergillosis[218] only occasionally cause empyema in the course of pulmonary parenchymal disease. However, infections with *Actinomyces israelii* and *Nocardia asteroides* regularly cause empyema in the course of pulmonary suppuration.[219,220] There is invariably a pulmonary parenchymal infiltrate in addition to the pleural effusion. Most commonly, the infiltrate is of a relatively homogeneous density with nonsegmental distribution; abscess formation is common. In some patients, the parenchymal infection has an appearance similar to that associated with pulmonary tuberculosis, and in others, the infiltrate appears roentgenographically like a mass lesion.

Empyema caused by actinomycosis has a tendency to burrow through the chest wall, producing subcutaneous abscesses and chronic draining sinuses in the skin (empyema necessitatis). In the pus draining from such pleural-cutaneous fistulas, there is a tendency for actinomyces to form dense clusters that are grossly visible as yellowish brown particles (sulphur granules).

The diagnosis and management of patients with fungal infections are discussed in Chapter 9, in the section on chronic infections. The management of patients with empyema does not differ from the prolonged administration of appropriate antimicrobials necessary in patients with pulmonary infections without empyema. Drainage of the fluid, as for bacterial empyema, is indicated, especially in patients with nocardiosis. It has been suggested that drainage is not as critical in patients with actinomycosis and that results of prolonged antimicrobial therapy are satisfactory.[220]

Parasites. Amebiasis is the only parasitic disease occurring in residents of North America that is likely to cause a pleural effusion. The intrathoracic disease caused by *Entamoeba histolytica* is almost always secondary to amebic abscess of the liver, which occurs in from 3 to 9% of all patients with amebiasis. Approximately 75% of patients with an amebic liver abscess demonstrate abnormalities on routine chest roentgenograms.[221,222,222a] Most commonly, the abnormality is an elevated right hemidiaphragm. Less frequently, there are infiltrates in the lower lobe of the right lung or a right pleural effusion. Similar findings on the left are much less common.

Patients with an amebic pleural effusion may present with symptoms suggestive of either an acute inflammatory process or a chronic disease. In various series, the duration of symptoms have ranged from 1 day to 3 yr; 75% of the patients have an acute course, with symptoms lasting less than 3 weeks.[221] Most patients are febrile, and approximately a third have had chills. Weight loss is common, and most patients have had diarrhea that was frequently bloody. Pain in the right upper abdominal quadrant is described by most patients. Ten to 15% of patients have pleuritic pain, and a similar percentage have symptoms of respiratory tract infection, with cough and sputum. Physical examination reveals the signs of a right-sided pleural effusion and frequently signs of consolidation of lung parenchyma over the effusion. The liver is characteristically enlarged and tender. Jaundice is relatively uncommon, and it is generally mild when present.

Laboratory examination in patients with an amebic pleural effusion does not differ from that described for patients with pulmonary parenchymal amebiasis in Chapter 8. The pleural effusion fluid may be serofibrinous, with the characteristics of an exudate; amebic trophozoites may or may not be demonstrated in the fluid. In some patients, there is a fistula between the hepatic abscess and the pleural space; in these cases, thoracentesis yields fluid with a chocolate appearance. This fluid contains blood, digested liver tissue, and small solid particles of liver parenchyma. Such fluid is likely to show trophozoites. Some amebic liver abscesses become secondarily infected with aerobic or anaerobic bacteria, and the pleural effusion in these patients has the characteristics of a bacterial empyema.

Drug therapy with metronidazole (Flagyl)[223] is indicated. The effusion is drained by simple needle thoracentesis as often as necessary to keep the pleural space dry, if there is no secondary bacterial infection. If bacterial empyema coexists, the principles of management outlined in the section on bacterial empyemas are followed.

Mortality is generally listed at 10 to 20%. However, if the correct diagnosis is made promptly and if appropriate antiamebic therapy is instituted, the mortality rate is significantly less.[221]

Pleural effusions may also occur in patients infected with *Paragonimus westermani* or *Echinococcus granulosis*.

Viruses and Mycoplasma. Pneumonias caused by viruses or *Mycoplasma pneumoniae* are not often associated with significant amounts of pleural effusion.[224–226] However, there may be small collections of pleural fluid in association with these pneumonias.[227] The fluid is characteristically so small in amount that lateral decubitus views are necessary to demonstrate it convincingly. The fluid collections are transient, lasting 5 days or less. In the few effusions due to virus or mycoplasma that have been analyzed after thoracentesis, the fluid was found to be serous, with a protein level of more then 3 g/dl and a leukocyte count of 100 to 6,000/mm^3.[227] It should be emphasized, however, that a significant amount of pleural fluid in association with pneumonia is evidence against a viral or mycoplasmal etiology.

It has been reported that patients with sickle-cell or sickle-cell hemoglobin C disease may have a much more severe pneumonia associated with mycoplasma than normal persons.[228,229] Severe pleuritic chest pain and rapidly developing massive effusion may occur in such patients. The cause of these unusual manifestations of mycoplasmal pneumonia is not known (see also Chap. 8).

Trauma

Hemothorax. Pleural effusions associated with malignancy and pulmonary emboli are frequently blood-tinged; however, the term *hemothorax* is reserved for frank bleeding into the pleural space. Hemothorax most frequently results from trauma, although it occasionally occurs during a spontaneous pneumothorax and in rare cases from a hematologic disorder.[230] Hemothorax or hemopneumothorax may occur with either penetrating or blunt chest trauma.[231]

Patients with chest trauma frequently have additional nonthoracic injuries, and total patient care may include several procedures in addition to care of the hemothorax. Patients with small amounts of hemothorax occasionally may be managed by simple thoracentesis, with removal of all blood and repeated observation. However, almost all patients, especially those with concurrent pneumothorax, are managed by thoracostomy tubes in order to promote as complete drainage of blood and air as possible.[232,233] It is important to use large tubes in order to assure adequate drainage. Hemothorax per se is not an indication for immediate thoracotomy. If the patient continues to hemorrhage briskly, if the blood cannot be totally removed from the pleural space, if a very large air leak into the pleural space exists, or if it is not possible to alleviate shock, immediate thoracotomy may be indicated. Immediate operation is indicated in only a small fraction of patients with either penetrating or closed chest trauma.

Some fraction of patients with traumatic hemothorax, probably less than 5%, may not resolve the hemothorax in the usual way.[232] These are most commonly patients in whom adequate early drainage has not been carried out. The blood may coagulate in the pleural space and lead to a loculated fibrothorax. It is not clear what factors other than delayed drainage promote formation of fibrothorax in some patients; experimental hemothorax has not produced this lesion despite a variety of additional manipulations.[234–236] It is usually possible to predict during the first few days that a patient's hemothorax is unlikely to resolve with thoracostomy tube drainage. If the chest radiograph demonstrates a large amount of residual blood and the patient continues febrile and clinically toxic, early thoracotomy is probably indicated.[232]

A left-sided hemothorax occasionally may indicate rupture of the aorta, a lesion almost universally fatal if immediate thoracotomy is not undertaken. This lesion should be suspected if chest roentgenograms indicate a widened superior mediastinum, sternal fracture, anterior fracture of the first three ribs, or posteriorly displaced clavicular fractures, or in patients with pulse deficits involving branches of the aortic arch or with massive hemothorax with continued bleeding.[237,238] Such patients should have aortography in order to confirm the suspected aortic rupture (see also Chap. 11 on chest trauma).

Chylothorax is a pleural effusion due to leakage of thoracic duct lymph, or chyle, into a pleural space. Approximately 50% of the cases are due to some type of traumatic damage to the thoracic duct. Such trauma may be penetrating chest trauma, closed chest injury, or trauma induced by a variety of thoracic surgical procedures.[239] However, a high fraction of cases of chylothorax is due to tumor. Lymphomas are most commonly implicated, but mediastinal metastasis of carcinoma, especially bronchogenic carcinoma, is also frequent.[240] Tumors causing chylothorax are almost always malignant. Other causes of chylothorax include congenital malformations of the thoracic duct, tuberculous nodes, mediastinal fibrosis, thrombosis of great veins, and a variety of miscellaneous lesions.[239]

The thoracic duct originates in the cisterna chyli located on the body of the second lumbar vertebra. It passes through the esophageal hiatus of the diaphragm and extends extrapleurally in the posterior mediastinum along the anterior surface of the vertebral column, between the azygos vein and the descending aorta in the right side of the mediastinum. At the level of the fifth or sixth thoracic vertebra, it veers to the left into the superior mediastinum, ascending behind the aortic arch. In the neck, it empties into the venous system near the angle of the internal jugular and subclavian veins. There is considerable anatomic variability and there are a number of collateral circulations.[241] The general course of the thoracic duct, however, is thought to explain why trauma to the duct low in the thorax results in a right-sided chylothorax, whereas higher trauma results in a left-sided chylothorax. Occasionally, effusions are bilateral.

The symptoms of chylothorax are those of the underlying disorder, in addition to dyspnea if the effusion is large enough to compromise respiratory function. Following rupture of the duct, chyle accumulates in the posterior mediastinum until it finally ruptures the mediastinal pleura. The appearance of a chylothorax may be delayed for some time after trauma; the latent interval is usually from 2 to 10 days, but in some patients it may be weeks or even months.[241] Physical and roentgenographic findings are no different than for other forms of pleural effusion. The roentgenographic appearance of the mediastinum frequently is normal, even in cases due to malignancy. Laboratory abnormalities depend on the underlying condition.

The diagnosis of chylothorax usually is made during thoracentesis, when the aspirated fluid is observed to have a milky white appearance. Traumatic chylothorax may be blood-tinged initially, leading to a delay in diagnosis, but on subsequent thoracentesis, the characteristic milky appearance usually is evident. The fluid is alkaline and odorless, and the milky appearance clears when the emulsification is shaken with ether.[242] When the fluid is allowed to stand, a creamy top layer forms. Fat globules may be observed microscopically when the fluid is stained with Sudan III dye. The fluid usually is an exudate, although the total protein concentration is less than 3 g/dl in some cases. Cellular constituents are usually lymphocytes, which range from 400 to 7,000/mm^3. A few erythrocytes are usually present. The total fat content ranges from 0.4 to 6.0 g/dl, with total cholesterol 65 to 220 mg/dl and cholesterol esters 25 to 185 mg/dl.

Chylothorax of any cause usually recurs promptly after initial drainage. Traumatic lymph fistulas may close spontaneously, but this is quite unpredictable. Conservative management with repeated aspiration of fluid or thoracostomy tube drainage is attempted initially. However, the massive loss of fat and protein leads to rapid weight loss, and such therapy cannot be protracted. During this interval, the flow of chyle is reduced to a minimum by discontinuing oral feedings and maintaining the patient on intravenous fluids. Authorities vary on how long to persist in conservative therapy, but a period of a week is a reasonable maximum trial, unless there is clear evidence that the volume of drainage is becoming progressively less.[241] If it is determined that the patient is not likely to respond to conservative therapy, a thoracotomy on the side of the chylothorax is performed, and the thoracic duct is ligated at the site of rupture.[242a] Lymphangiograms may be helpful in locating the site of rupture; some surgeons advocate preoperative oral administration of fat stained with a lipophilic dye. If the site of duct rupture cannot be localized, the thoracic duct is ligated near the diaphragm. In patients with chylothorax due to malignancy, conservative management is rarely successful. Radiation therapy results in adequate control of chylothorax in over 50% of patients with lymphoma or metastatic carcinoma.[240] In the remainder of cases, thoracic surgery is indicated.

Pseudo-chylothorax. Some patients with pleural effusions may be incorrectly classified as having a chylothorax on the basis of a cloudy, chylous-appearing fluid with a high fat content, who instead have the syndrome of cholesterol pleural effusion. This condition occurs in patients with long-standing pleural effusions; the average duration of effusion is 5 yr, with a few cases developing within 1 yr of the onset of effusion.[243] The majority of cholesterol pleural effusions are thought to be due to tuberculosis or rheumatoid lung disease.[244] Many patients are asymptomatic; others have symptoms attributable to the underlying disease process or to impairment of pulmonary function due to the effusion. The effusion is usually unilateral, although a few instances of bilateral effusion have been reported. The pleura is invariably thickened from the longstanding disease process, and it may be calcified. There are no distinctive physical or roentgenographic features, and laboratory examination depends on the underlying process.

The pleural fluid typically is thick and yellow. It exhibits a sheen like that of a metallic paint. It is an exudate, with varying numbers of degenerating leukocytes and erythrocytes. Microscopically, cholesterol crystals with a rhomboid configuration may be seen. Cholesterol concentrations varying from 140 to 4500 mg/dl have been reported, and 40 to 50% is esterified. The cholesterol level decreases with repeated aspiration of the pleural fluid. Biopsy of the pleura reveals a thickened, fibrotic membrane, with cholesterol crystals observed in clefts.

The origin of the cholesterol in such effusions is not known. It most probably originates from degenerating leukocytes in longstanding effusions, with a liberation of cholesterol that diffuses poorly from the pleural space, owing to the thickened pleural membrane.[243] The patient's prognosis depends on the underlying cause of the cholesterol effusion, and specific therapy for the effusion frequently is not indicated. A few patients may have improved pulmonary function after thoracotomy and pleural decortication, which may result in cessation of fluid formation.

Esophageal Rupture. A left-sided pleural effusion or hydropneumothorax may occasionally result from traumatic perforation of the esophagus. Perforation due to blunt trauma or penetrating wounds is rare; rupture is usually due to forceful vomiting (Boerhaave syndrome) or perforation at the time of an endoscopic procedure.[245] The signs and symptoms caused by this acute catastrophe may be tabulated from three surgical series of 71 patients with spontaneous esophageal perforation.[246–248] In almost all cases, there is an acute onset of chest or abdominal pain. Chest pain is commonly substernal or in the left side of the chest, and abdominal pain is epigastric. Radiation of the pain is common, involving the areas already mentioned and the shoulder or the back. Most patients experience vomiting, but any sudden change in intrabdominal pressure can initiate the series of events that terminates with esophageal rupture. Abdominal trauma, uncontrolled seizures, the act of parturition, defecation, and lifting heavy objects have all been reported to result in esophageal rupture. Serious dyspnea is reported by approximately two-thirds of the patients. Fever is experienced by only 60% of the patients initially, frequently being delayed by up to 12 hr. Approximately half the patients developed subcutaneous emphysema in the neck. This physical finding is clearly the most specific for this condition. If a combination of these signs or symptoms suggests the diagnosis, a radiograph of the chest should be obtained in the shortest possible interval. Only about 5% of patients will have a normal chest roentgenogram. Lower lobe infiltrates, especially retrocardiac discoid atelectasis on the left, is very common. Almost all patients will have some combination of fluid and extraparenchymal air in the chest. About 80% of patients have a pleural effusion or pneumothorax or both. About 15% have only pneumomediastinum or subcutaneous emphysema or both. About 75% of those with hydro- or pneumothorax have this finding on the left, and the remainder are equally divided between unilateral right sided and bilateral findings. The diagnosis can be confirmed in almost all cases by an esophagogram which is usually carried out with Lipiodol.

The pleural fluid may reveal recently ingested food. It is likely to be bloody and frequently contains a high leukocyte count with a predominance of polymorphonuclear leukocytes. A pleural-fluid *p*H, performed at the bedside with standard reagent paper, demonstrating a *p*H less than 6 is highly suggestive of esophageal rupture, with contamination of the pleural space by gastric juice; a higher *p*H, however, may be observed.[249] The fluid also may demonstrate a high concentration of amylase, which has been demonstrated to be of salivary origin.[250]

Therapy for patients with esophageal rupture includes early thoracotomy with repair of the perforation; antimicrobial therapy; and complete drainage of the pleural space. Delayed therapy is associated with a high mortality rate, with 25% of patients dying within 12 hr and 65% within 24 hr,[251] but if the condition is recognized early, therapy is usually successful.

FIBROTHORAX

Fibrothorax is a fusion of the pleural surfaces by layers of fibrin, hyalin, and connective tissue composed of collagen, but not elastic, fibers. Calcification may develop. Fibrothorax may result from healing of a previous hemothorax, tuberculous effusion, or empyema; however, in at least 50% of the cases, no specific cause can be demonstrated at the time of thoracotomy.[252]

The most common complaint is dyspnea on exertion. Typically, dyspnea has been slowly

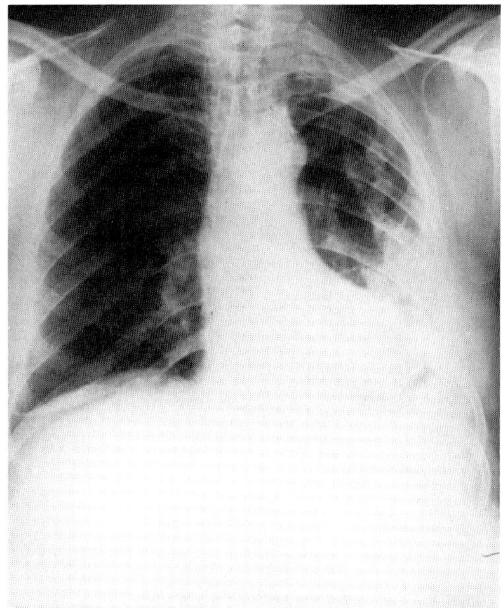

FIG. 12-14. Chest roentgenogram of a patient with a left fibrothorax. The water density along the lateral chest wall is in an antigravity distribution, and mottled calcification is present within the water density of the thickened pleura.

progressive over a protracted interval before it is severe enough for the patient to seek medical advice. Associated symptoms depend on the presence or absence of pulmonary parenchymal disease in addition to fibrothorax. Symptoms of right ventricular failure occur in extreme cases. The physical examination reveals a unilateral fixation of the chest, with absent or diminished respiratory excursions. There is dullness to percussion, diminished or absent breath sounds, and decreased fremitus. Roentgenographically, there is a markedly thickened water density surrounding the lung in an antigravity distribution (Fig. 12-14). Mottled calcification may be present within the water density of the pleural peel. If the pulmonary parenchyma can be distinguished under the thickened pleura, it may or may not be normal, depending on the cause of the fibrothorax. Laboratory examination is normal. Usually, it is not possible to obtain free fluid by thoracentesis.

Fibrothorax causes a restriction in lung volumes without functional changes of airways obstruction. It has been emphasized that pleural lesions are more detrimental to lung function than are unilateral parenchymal lesions.[253] The function of the lung is frequently overestimated by the roentgenographic appearance, because the fibrothorax appears on the film as only a rim of pleural thickening. Ventilation is depressed on the side of the fibrothorax, but the oxygen uptake of the affected side is depressed out of proportion to reduced ventilation.[254] In the absence of hypoxemia, this relationship is indicative of decreased perfusion with respect to ventilation on the affected side. It is not clear why perfusion is so depressed in the absence of pulmonary parenchymal disease. In addition, some patients with fibrothorax have marked pulmonary hypertension that cannot be explained by the anatomical or physiological alterations that have been measured.[255] Such pulmonary hypertension may lead to cor pulmonale, if long-standing.

The management of symptomatic patients with fibrothorax is by thoracotomy and pleural decortication. The degree of improvement following decortication is related to the extent of parenchymal lung disease that exists under the pleural peel.[256] The cause of fibrothorax is evidently not important. The duration of fibrothorax before decortication is likewise not critical, and good results have been reported in a patient who had a fibrothorax for 20 years before decortication.[257]

REFERENCES

1. SACKS PV, KANAREK D: Treatment of acute pleuritic pain. Am Rev Respir Dis 108:666, 1973
2. EAGLSTEIN WH, KATZ R, BROWN JA: The effects of early corticosteroid therapy on the skin eruption and pain of herpes zoster. JAMA 211:1681, 1970
3. FINN JJ JR, WELLER TH, MORGAN HR: Epidemic pleurodynia: Clinical and etiologic studies based on one hundred fourteen cases. Arch Intern Med 83:305, 1949
4. HYDE L: Benign spontaneous pneumothorax. Ann Intern Med 56:746, 1962
5. KILLEN DA, GOBBEL WG: Spontaneous Pneumothorax. Boston, Little, Brown & Co, 1968
6. GRIMES DF, FARBER SM: Air cysts of the lung. Surg Gynecol Obstet 113:720, 1961
7. LICHTER I, GWYNNE JF: Spontaneous pneumothorax in young subjects. Thorax 26:409, 1971
8. BROOKS JW: Open thoracotomy in the management of spontaneous pneumothorax. Ann Surg 177:798, 1973
9. MELTON LJ III, HEPPER NGG, OFFORD KP: Incidence of spontaneous pneumothorax in Olmsted County, Minnesota: 1950 to 1974. Am Rev Respir Dis 120:1379, 1979
10. LILLINGTON GA, MITCHELL SP, WOOD GA: Catamenial pneumothorax. JAMA 219:1328, 1972

10a. LAWS HL, FOX LS, YOUNGER BJ: Bilateral catamenial pneumothorax. Arch Surg 112:627, 1977

11. DORNHORST AC, PIERCE GW: Pulmonary collapse and consolidation: The role of collapse in the production of lung field shadows and the significance of segments in inflammatory lung disease. J Faculty Radiol 5: 276, 1954
12. NORRIS RM, JONES JG, BISHOP JM: Respiratory gas exchange in patients with spontaneous pneumothorax. Thorax 23:427, 1968
13. ANTHONISEN NR: Regional lung function in spontaneous pneumothorax. Am Rev Respir Dis 115:873, 1977
14. RUCKLEY CV, MCCORMACK RJM: The management of spontaneous pneumothorax. Thorax 21:139, 1966
15. STRADLING P, POOLE G: Conservative management of spontaneous pneumothorax. Thorax 21:145, 1966
16. SAUTTER RD et al: Fatal pulmonary edema and pneumonitis after re-expansion of chronic pneumothorax. Chest 60:399, 1971

16a. PEATFIELD RC, EDWARDS PR, JOHNSON N: Two unexpected deaths from pneumothorax. Lancet 1:356, 1979

17. MILLER WC: Experimental pulmonary edema following re-expansion of pneumothorax. Am Rev Respir Dis 108:664, 1973
18. ANDERSEN I, POULSEN T: Surgical treatment of spontaneous pneumothorax. Acta Chir Scand 118:105, 1959
19. LICHTER I: Long-term follow-up of planned treatment of spontaneous pneumothorax. Thorax 29:32, 1974

19a. GOLDSZER RC et al: Intrapleural tetracycline for spontaneous pneumothorax. JAMA 241:724, 1979

19b. LARIEU AJ et al: Intrapleural instillation of quinacaine for treatment of recurrent spontaneous pneumothorax. Ann Thorac Surg 28:146, 1979

19c. CHARLES J: A study of the long term effects of talc pleurodesis. Br J Dis Chest 72:251, 1978

20. GLAUSER FL, BARTLETT RH: Pneumoperitoneum in association with pneumothorax. Chest 66:536, 1974
21. REYNOLDS J, CHRISTENSEN EE: Early radiologic signs of bronchial rupture. Tex Med 64:50, 1968
22. KUMAR A et al: Continuous positive pressure ventilation in acute respiratory failure: Effects on hemodynamics and lung function. N Engl J Med 283:1430, 1970

23. LATORRE FJ et al: Incidence of pneumothorax and pneumomediastinum in patients with aspiration pneumonia requiring ventilatory support. Chest 72:141, 1977
24. MULLER R, LOFSTEDT S: The reaction of the pleura in primary tuberculosis of the lungs. Acta Med Scand 122:105, 1945
25. HESSEN I: Roentgen examination of pleural fluid: A study of the localization of free effusions, the potentialities of diagnosing minimal quantities of fluid and its existence under physiological conditions. Acta Radiol [Diag] [Suppl] 86:1, 1951
26. AGOSTONI E, TALLIETTI A, SETNIKAR I: Absorption force of the capillaries of the visceral pleura in determination of the intrapleural pressure. Am J Physiol 191:277, 1957
27. BLACK LF: The pleural space and pleural fluid. Mayo Clin Proc 47:493, 1972
28. BURGEN ASV, STEWART PB: A method for measuring the turnover of fluid in the pleural and other serous cavities. J Lab Clin Med 52:118, 1958
29. PRENTICE TC, SIRI W, JOINER EE: Quantitative studies of ascitic fluid circulation with tritium-labelled water. Am J Med 13:668, 1952
30. BURKE HE: The lymphatics which drain the potential space between the visceral and the parietal pleura. Am Rev Tuberculosis 79:52, 1959
31. WILSON JL et al: The absorption of blood from the pleural space. Surgery 48:766, 1960
32. STEWART PB, BURGEN ASV: The turnover of fluid in the dog's pleural cavity. J Lab Clin Med 52:212, 1958
33. STEWART PB: The rate of formation and lymphatic removal of fluid in pleural effusions. J Clin Invest 42:258, 1963
34. MULVEY RB: The effect of pleural fluid on the diaphragm. Radiology 84:1080, 1965
34a. BROWN NE, ZAMEL N, ABERMAN A: Changes in pulmonary mechanics and gas exchange following thoracentesis. Chest 74:540, 1978
35. SWINGLE JD, LOGAN R, JUHL JH: Inversion of the left hemidiaphragm. JAMA 208:863, 1969
36. DOUST BD, BAUM JK, MAKLAD NF et al: Ultrasonic evaluation of pleural opacities. Radiology 114:135, 1975
37. SANDWEISS DA, HANSON JC, GOSINK BB et al: Ultrasound in diagnosis, localization, and treatment of loculated pleural empyema. Ann Intern Med 82:50, 1975
38. GRYMINSKI J, KRAKOWKA P, LYPACEWICZ G: The diagnosis of pleural effusion by ultrasonic and radiologic techniques. Chest 70:33, 1976
39. RAVIN CE: Thoracocentesis of loculated pleural effusions using grey scale ultrasonic guidance. Chest 71:666, 1977
40. ADAMS FV, GALATI V: M-mode ultrasonic localization of pleural effusion. JAMA 239:1761, 1978
41. ABRAMS LD: A pleural-biopsy punch. Lancet 1:30, 1958
42. COPE C: New pleural biopsy needle. JAMA 167:1107, 1958
43. DEFRANCIS N, KLOSK E, ALBANO E: Needle biopsy of the parietal pleura. N Engl J Med 52:948, 1955
44. HELLER P, KELLOW WF, CHOMET B: Needle biopsy of the parietal pleura. N Engl J Med 255:684, 1956
45. DONOHOE RF, KATZ S, MATTHEWS M: Pleural biopsy as an aid in the etiologic diagnosis of pleural effusion: Review of the literature and report of 132 biopsies. Ann Intern Med 48:344, 1958
46. WEISS W: Needle biopsy of the parietal pleura in tuberculosis. Am Rev Tuberculosis 78:17, 1958
47. SAMUELS ML, OLD JW, HOWE CD: Needle biopsy of pleura. Cancer 2:980, 1958
48. MISRA SS, SHARMA UC: Pleural biopsy with the Vim–Silverman needle. Tubercle 40:54, 1958
49. MESTITZ P, PURVES MJ, POLLARD AC: Pleural biopsy in the diagnosis of pleural effusion. Lancet 2:1349, 1958
50. LEGGAT PO: Needle biopsy of the parietal pleura in malignant disease. Br Med J 2:478, 1959
51. RICHERT JH, WIER JA, SALYER JM et al: The reliability of tissue diagnosis of pleurisy: A preliminary report. Ann Intern Med 52:320, 1960
52. SHAW RK, HALLETT WY: Biopsy of the parietal pleura. Am J Med Sci 241:593, 1961
53. NIDEN AH, BURROWS B, KASIK JE et al: Percutaneous pleural biopsy with a curetting needle. Am Rev Respir Dis 84:37, 1961
54. CARPENTER RL, LOWELL JR: Pleural biopsy and thoracentesis by a new instrument. Dis Chest 40:182, 1961
55. HAMPSON F, KARLISH AJ: Needle biopsy of the pleura in the diagnosis of pleural effusion. Q J Med 30:249, 1961
56. REESE D JR, MCCLEAN RL, RAAEN TD: Acid fast bacilli in pleural biopsy specimens. Arch Intern Med 108:160, 1961
57. THIRUVENGADAM KV, ANGULI VC, MADANAGOPALAN N et al: Etiologic diagnosis of pleural effusion by punch biopsy of the parietal pleura. Dis Chest 42:529, 1962
58. SISON BS, WEISS W: Needle biopsy of the parietal pleura in patients with pleural effusion. Br Med J 2:298, 1962
59. HANSON G, PHILLIPS T: Pleural biopsy in diagnosis of thoracic disease. Br Med J 2:300, 1962
60. LEVINE H, CUGELL DW: Blunt-end needle biopsy of pleura and rib. Arch Intern Med 109:516, 1962
61. SCHOOLS GS: Needle biopsy of parietal pleura. Tex State J Med 59:1056, 1963
62. RAO NV et al: Needle biopsy of parietal pleura in 124 cases. Arch Intern Med 115:34, 1965
63. SCHARER L, MCCLEMENT JH: Isolation of tubercle

bacilli from needle biopsy specimens of parietal pleura. Am Rev Respir Dis 97:466, 1968

64. LIGHT RW: Falsely high refractometric readings for the specific gravity of pleural fluid. Chest 76:300, 1979
65. CARR DT, POWER MH: Clinical value of measurements of concentration of protein in pleural fluid. N Engl J Med 259:926, 1958
66. FELDSTEIN AM, SAMACHSON J, SPENCER H: Levels of calcium phosphorous, alkaline phosphatase, and protein in effusion fluid and serum in man. Am J Med 35:530, 1963
67. CHANDRASEKHAR AJ, PALATAO A, DUBIN A et al: Pleural fluid lactic acid dehydrogenase activity and protein content. Arch Intern Med 123:48, 1969
68. PILLAY VKG: Total proteins in serous fluids in cardiac failure. S Afr Med J 39:142, 1965
69. LIGHT RW, MACGREGOR MI, LUCHSINGER PC et al: Pleural effusions: The diagnostic separation of transudates and exudates. Ann Intern Med 77:507, 1972
70. WROBLEWSKI F: The clinical significance of alterations in lactic dehydrogenase activity of body fluids. Am J Med Sci 234:301, 1957
71. HORROCKS JE, KING J, WAIND APB et al: Lactic dehydrogenase activity in the diagnosis of malignant effusions. J Clin Pathol 15:57, 1962
72. RUSSAKOFF AH, LEMAISTRE CA, DEWLETT HJ: An evaluation of pleural fluid glucose determination. Am Rev Respir Dis 85:220, 1962
73. CARR DT, MAYNE JG: Pleurisy with effusion in rheumatoid arthritis, with reference to the low concentration of glucose in pleural fluid. Am Rev Respir Dis 85:345, 1962
74. CARR DT, MCGUCKIN WF: Pleural fluid glucose. Am Rev Respir Dis 97:302, 1968
75. LIGHT RW, BALL WC JR: Glucose and amylase in pleural effusions. JAMA 225:257, 1973
76. HAMMARSTEN JF, HONSKA WL JR, LIMES BJ: Pleural fluid anylase in pancreatitis and other diseases. Am Rev Tuberculosis 79:606, 1959
77. HUNDER GG, MCDUFFIE FC, HEPPERN NG: Pleural fluid complement in systemic lupus erythematosus. Ann Intern Med 76:357, 1972
78. HUNDER GG et al: Pleural fluid complement, complement conversion, and immune complexes in immunologic and nonimmunologic diseases. J Lab Clin Med 90:971, 1977
79. FUNAHASHI A, SARKAR TK, KORY RC: Measurements of respiratory gases and pH of pleural fluid. Am Rev Respir Dis 108:1266, 1973
80. POTTS DE et al: The acidosis of low-glucose pleural effusions. Am Rev Respir Dis 117:665, 1978
81. SAHN SA, POTTS DE: Turpentine pleurisy in rabbits: A model of pleural fluid acidosis and low pleural fluid glucose. Am Rev Respir Dis 118:893, 1978
82. SAHN SA, TARYLE DA, GOOD JT JR: Experimental empyema: Time course and pathogenesis of pleural fluid acidosis and low pleural fluid glucose. Am Rev Respir Dis 120:355, 1979

82a. GOOD JT JR et al: The diagnostic value of pleural fluid pH. Chest 78:55, 1980

83. TARYLE DA, GOOD JT JR, SAHN SA: Acid generation by pleural fluid: Possible role in the determination of pleural fluid pH. J Lab Clin Med 93:1041, 1979
84. GOOD JT JR, TARYLE DA, HYERS TM et al: Clotting and fibrinolytic activity of pleural fluid in a model of pleural adhesions. Am Rev Respir Dis 118:903, 1978
85. TINNEY WS, OLSEN AM: The significance of fluid in the pleural space: a study of 274 cases. Proc Staff Meetings Mayo Clin 20:81, 1945
86. LEUALLEN EC, CARR DT: Pleural effusion, a statistical study of 436 patients. N Engl J Med 252:79, 1955
87. YAM LT: Diagnostic significance of lymphocytes in pleural effusions. Ann Intern Med 66:972, 1967
88. LIGHT RW, ENOZAN YS, BALL WC: Cells in pleural fluid. Arch Intern Med 132:854, 1973
89. VERESS JR, KOSS LG, SCHREIBER K: Eosinophilic pleural effusions. Acta Cytologica 23:40, 1979

89a. ASKIN FB, MCCANN BG, KUHN C: Reactive eosinophilic pleuritis. Arch Pathol Lab Med 101:187, 1977

90. DEWALD G, DINES DW, WEILAND LH et al: Usefulness of chromosome examination in the diagnosis of malignant pleural effusions. N Engl J Med 295:1494, 1976
91. MONIF GRG, STEWART BN, BLOCK AJ: Living cytology. Chest 69:626, 1976
92. BOOTH SN et al: Cancer-associated proteins in effusion fluids. J Clin Pathol 30:537, 1977
93. NYSTROM JS et al: Carcinoembryonic antigen titers on effusion fluid. Arch Intern Med 137:875, 1977
94. RITTGERS RA et al: Carcinoembryonic antigen levels in benign and malignant pleural effusions. Ann Intern Med 88:631, 1978
95. KLOCKARS M et al: Pleural fluid lysozyme in human disease. Arch Intern Med 139:73, 1979
96. PETTERSSON T et al: T and B lymphocytes in pleural effusions. Chest 73:49, 1978
97. MOISAN T et al: Distribution of lymphocyte subpopulations in patients with exudative pleural effusions. Am Rev Respir Dis 117:507, 1978
98. SENNO A et al: Thoracoscopy with the fiberoptic bronchoscope. J Thorac Cardiovasc Surg 67:606, 1974
99. DECAMP PT, MOSELEY PW, SCOTT ML et al: Diagnostic thoracoscopy. Ann Thorac Surg 16:79, 1973
100. KERBY GR, PIERCE G, RUTH WE: Clinical experience with pleuroscopy utilizing the bronchofiber-

scope. Ann Otol Rhinol Laryngol 84:602, 1975

101. GWIN E et al: Pleuroscopy and pleural biopsy with the flexible fiberoptic bronchoscope. Chest 67:527, 1975
102. ASH SR, MANFREDI F: Directed biopsy using a small endoscope. N Engl J Med 201:1398, 1974
103. BOUSHY SF, NORTH LB, HELGASON AH: Thoracoscopy: Technique and results in eighteen patients with pleural effusion. Chest 74:386, 1978
104. MELLINS RB, LEVINE OR, FISHMAN AP: Effect of systemic and pulmonary venous hypertension on pleural and pericardial fluid accumulation. J Appl Physiol 29:564, 1970
105. RABIN CB, BLACKMAN NS: Bilateral pleural effusion, its significance in association with a heart of normal size. J Mount Sinai Hosp 24:45, 1975
106. SCHLANT RC: Heart failure: Altered physiology of the cardiovascular system in heart failure. In Hurst JW, Logue RB (eds): The Heart, 4th ed. New York, McGraw-Hill, 1978
107. JOHNSTON RF, LOO RV: Hepatic hydrothorax. Ann Intern Med 61:385, 1964
108. CASTLEMAN B (ed): Correlation records of the Massachusetts General Hospital weekly clinicopathological exercises. N Engl J Med 268:320, 1963
109. FALCHUK KR, JACOBY I, COLUCCI WS et al: Tetracycline-induced pleural symphysis for recurrent hydrothorax complicating cirrhosis. Gastroenterology, 72:319, 1977
110. ALLEN JC, APICELLA MA: Experimental pleural effusion as a manifestation of delayed hypersensitivity to tuberculosis PPD. J Immunol 101:481, 1968
111. ROPER WH, WARING JJ: Primary serofibrinous effusion in military personnel. Am Rev Tuberculosis 71:616, 1955
112. LEVINE H, SCANTO PB, CUGELL DW: Tuberculous pleurisy. Arch Intern Med 122:329, 1968
113. FILLER J: Comparison of pulmonary function following tuberculous pleural effusion treated with or without adrenal corticosteroids. Am J Dis Child 102:735, 1961
114. ENGELHARDT HT, WILSON JL: Some observations on the etiological significance of fluid in the pleural spaces. South Med J 40:1023, 1947
115. SAHN SH, LEICHTLING M, BASS HE: The significance of pleural effusion in patients past the age of 50. N Engl J Med 246:927, 1952
116. MYERSON RM: Pleural effusion: A statistical analysis of 100 cases in which thoracentesis was performed. Del Med J 28:87, 1956
116a. HIRSCH A et al: Pleural effusion: Laboratory tests in 300 cases. Thorax 34:113, 1979
117. CHERNOW B, SAHN SA: Carcinomatous involvement of the pleura. Am J Med 63:695, 1977
118. BRINKMAN GL: The significance of pleural effusion complicating otherwise operable bronchogenic carcinoma. Dis Chest 36:152, 1959
118a. DECKER DA et al: The significance of a cytologically negative pleural effusion in bronchogenic carcinoma. Chest 74:640, 1978
119. CARR DT, SOULE EH, ELLIS FH JR: Management of pleural effusions. Med Clin North Am 48:961, 1964
120. FRIST B, KAHAN AV, KOSS LG: Comparison of the diagnostic values of biopsies of the pleura and cytologic evaluation of pleural fluids. Am J Clin Pathol 72:48, 1979
121. ADLER RH, SAYEK I: Treatment of malignant pleural effusion: A method using tube thoracostomy and talc. Ann Thorac Surg 22:8, 1976
122. GREENWALD DW, PHILLIPS C, BENNETT JM: Management of malignant pleural effusion. J Surg Oncol 10:361, 1978
123. FRIEDMAN MA, SLATER D: Malignant pleural effusions. Cancer Treat Rev 5:49, 1978
124. LEFF A, HOPEWELL PC, COSTELLO J: Pleural effusion from malignancy. Ann Intern Med 88:532, 1978
125. AUSTIN EH, FLYE MW: The treatment of recurrent malignant pleural effusion. Ann Thorac Surg 28:190, 1979
126. SAHN SA, POTTS DE: The effect of tetracycline on rabbit pleura. Am Rev Respir Dis 117:493, 1978
127. SAHN SA, GOOD JR JR, POTTS DE: The pH of sclerosing agents. Chest 76:198, 1979
128. RUBINSON R, BOLOOKI H: Intrapleural tetracycline for control of malignant pleural effusion. South Med J 65:847, 1972
129. WALLACH HW: Intrapleural tetracycline for malignant pleural effusions. Chest 68:510, 1975
130. MEYER PC: Metastatic carcinoma of the pleura. Thorax 21:437, 1966
131. FISHER AMH, KENDALL B, VAN LEUVEN BD: Hodgkin's disease: A radiological survey. Clin Radiol 13:115, 1962
132. STOLBERG HO et al: Hodgkin's disease of the lung. Am J Roentgenol Radium Ther Nucl Med 92:96, 1964
133. WEICK JK et al: Pleural effusion in lymphoma. Cancer 31:848, 1973
134. LOWE DK, FLETCHER WS, HOROWITZ JJ et al: Management of chylothorax secondary to lymphoma. Surg Gynecol Obstet 135:35, 1972
135. LEGHA SS, MUGGIA FM: Pleural mesothelioma: Clinical features and therapeutic implications. Ann Intern Med 87:613, 1977
136. WAXLER B, EISENSTEIN R, BATTIFORA H: Electrophoresis of tissue glycosaminoglycans as an aid in the diagnosis of mesotheliomas. Cancer 44:221, 1979
137. WAGNER JC, SLEGGS CA, MARCHAND P: Diffuse pleural mesothelioma and asbestos exposure in N W Cape Province. Br J Ind Med 17:260, 1960
138. SELIKOFF IJ: Cancer risk of asbestos exposure. In Hiatt HH, Watson JD, Winston JA (eds): Ori-

gins of Human Cancer. Cold Spring Harbor, Cold Springs Laboratories 1977, pp 1765–1784

139. BECKLAKE MR: Asbestos-related diseases of the lungs and other organs: Their epidemiology and implications for clinical practice. Am Rev Respir Dis 114:187, 1976

140. WAGNER JC, SKIDMORE JW: Asbestos dust deposition and retention in rats. Ann NY Acad Sci 132:77, 1965

141. WAGNER JC: Epidemiology of diffuse mesothelial tumors: Evidence of an association from studies in South Africa and United Kingdom. Ann NY Acad Sci 132:575, 1965

142. HUTCHINSON WB, FRIEDENBERG MJ: Intrathoracic mesothelioma. Radiology 80:937, 1963

143. ANTMAN KH et al: Multimodality therapy for malignant mesothelioma based on a study of natural history. Am J Med 68:356, 1980

144. AISNER J, WIERNIK PH: Malignant mesothelioma: current status and future prospects. Chest 74:438, 1978

145. WANEBO HJ et al: Pleural mesothelioma. Cancer 38:2481, 1978

146. ANTMAN KH: Malignant mesothelioma. N Engl J Med 303:200, 1980

147. MEIGS JV, CASS JW: Fibroma of the ovary with ascites and hydrothorax: With a report of seven cases. Am J Obstet Gynecol 33:249, 1937

148. MEIGS JV, ARMSTRONG SH, HAMILTON HH: A further contribution to the syndrome of fibroma of the ovary with fluid in the abdomen and chest, Meig's syndrome. Am J Obstet Gynecol 46:19, 1943

149. ROTHSTEIN E: Benign pleural effusion and ascites associated with adenocarcinoma of the body of the pancreas. Dis Chest 15:603, 1949

150. SWENSSON NL, KUROHARA SS, GEORGE FW III: Complete regression, following abdominal irradiation alone, of chylothorax complicating lymphosarcoma with ascites. Radiology 87:635, 1966

151. KINTZER JS JR, ROSENOW EC III, KYLE RA: Thoracic and pulmonary abnormalities in multiple myeloma. Arch Intern Med 138:727, 1978

152. SCULLIN DC JR, COHEN HJ: Myelomatous pleural effusion: clinical course and immunologic characterization of the pleural fluid cells. Am J Hematol 6:267, 1979

153. HUGHES JC, VOTAW ML: Pleural effusion in multiple myeloma. Cancer 44:1150, 1979

154. SMITH GT, DAMMIN GJ, DEXTER L: Postmortem arteriographic studies of the human lung in pulmonary embolization. JAMA 188:143, 1964

155. HILDNER FJ, ORMOND RS: Accuracy of the clinical diagnosis of pulmonary embolism. JAMA 202:567, 1967

156. GRINER PF: Bloody pleural fluid following pulmonary infarction. JAMA 202:947, 1967

157. MCINTYRE KM, SASAHARA AA, SHARMA GVRK: Pulmonary thromboembolism: Current concepts. Adv Intern Med 18:199, 1972

158. TALBOT S, WORTHINGTON BS, ROEBUCK EJ: Radiographic signs of pulmonary embolism and pulmonary infarction. Thorax 28:198, 1973

159. MOSES DC, SILVER TM, BOOKSTEIN JJ: The complementary roles of chest radiography, lung scanning, and selective pulmonary angiography in the diagnosis of pulmonary embolism. Circulation 49:179, 1974

160. BYNUM LJ, WILSON JE III: Characteristics of pleural effusions associated with pulmonary embolism. Arch Intern Med 136:159, 1976

161. HAMPTON AO, CASTLEMAN B: Correlation of postmortem chest teleroentgenograms with autopsy findings, with special reference to pulmonary embolism and infarction. Am J Roentgenol Radium Ther Nucl Med 43:305, 1940

162. GOULD DM, DAVES ML: A review of roentgen findings in systemic lupus erythematosus (SLE). Am J Med Sci 235:596, 1958

163. DUBOIS EL: The effect of the LE cell test on the clinical picture of systemic lupus erythematosus. Ann Intern Med 38:1265, 1953

164. WINSLOW WA, PLOSS LN, LOITMAN B: Pleuritis in systemic lupus erythematosus: Its importance as an early manifestation in diagnosis. Ann Intern Med 49:70, 1958

165. HUNDER GG et al: Pleural fluid complement, complement conversion, and immune complexes in immunologic and nonimmunologic diseases. J Lab Clin Med 90:971, 1977

166. SCHOCKET AL, LAIN D, KOHLER PE et al: Immune complex vasculitis as a cause of ascites and pleural effusions in systemic lupus erythematosus. J Rheumatol 5:33, 1978

167. EMERSON PA: Pleural effusion complicating rheumatoid arthritis. Br Med J 1:428, 1956

168. HORLER AR, THOMPSON M: The pleural and pulmonary complications of rheumatoid arthritis. Ann Intern Med 51:1179, 1959

169. LEE PR, SOX HC, NORTH FS et al: Pleurisy with effusion in rheumatoid arthritis. Arch Intern Med 104:634, 1959

170. WARD R: Pleural effusion and rheumatoid disease. Lancet 2:1336, 1961

171. BERGER HW, SECKLER SG: Pleural and pericardial effusions in rheumatoid disease. Ann Intern Med 64:1291, 1966

172. LEVINE H et al: Rheumatoid factor in non-rheumatoid pleural effusions. Ann Intern Med 69:487, 1968

173. NOSANCHUK JS, NAYLOR B: A unique cytologic picture in pleural fluid from patients with rheumatoid arthritis. Am J Clin Pathol 50:300, 1968

174. CHAMPION GD, ROBERTSON MR, ROBINSON RG: Rheumatoid pleurisy and pericarditis. Ann Rheumatol 27:521, 1968

175. CARTER R, BREWER LA: Subphrenic abscess: A

thoracoabdominal clinical complex. Am J Surg 108:165, 1964
176. ALTEMEIER WA, SCHOWENGERDT CG, WHITELEY DH: Abscesses of the liver: Surgical considerations. Arch Surg 101:258, 1970
176a. BONFILS-ROBERTS EA, BARONE JE, NEALON TF JR: Treatment of sub-phrenic abscess. Surg Clin North Am 55:1361, 1975
177. PITT HA, ZUIDEMA GD: Factors influencing mortality in the treatment of pyogenic hepatic abscess. Surg Gynecol Obstet 140:228, 1975
178. DECASSE JJ, POULIN TL, FOX PS et al: Subphrenic abscess. Surg Gynecol Obstet 138:841, 1974
179. MILLER WT, TALMAN EA: Subphrenic abscess. Am J Roentgenol Radium Ther Nucl Med 101:961, 1967
180. KAYE MD: Pleuropulmonary complications of pancreatitis. Thorax 23:297, 1968
181. SHERR HP et al: Origin of pleural fluid amylase in esophageal rupture. Ann Intern Med 76:985, 1972
182. LIGHT RW, GEORGE RB: Incidence and significance of pleural effusion after abdominal surgery. Chest 69:621, 1976
183. GROSS PA, GERDING DN: Pleural effusion associated with viral hepatitis. Gastroenterology 60:898, 1971
184. COCCHI P, SILENZI M: Pleural effusion in HB Ag-positive hepatitis. J Pediatr 89:329, 1976
185. TABOR E et al: Hepatitis B surface antigen and e antigen in pleural effusion: A case report. Gastroenterology 73:1157, 1977
186. EHRENFELD EN, ELIAKIM M, RACHMILEWITZ M: Recurrent polyserositis (familial Mediterranean fever; periodic disease). Am J Med 31:107, 1961
187. SOHAR E, GAFNI J, PRAS Met al: Familial Mediterranean fever. Am J Med 43:227, 1967
188. HURIVITZ PA, PINALS DJ: Pleural effusion in chronic hereditary lymphedema (Nonne, Milroy, Meige's disease). Report of two cases. Radiology 82:246, 1964
189. EMERSON PA. Yellow nails, lymphedema and pleural effusions. Thorax 21:247, 1964
190. HILLER E, ROSENOW EC, OLSEN AM: Pulmonary manifestations of the yellow nail syndrome. Chest 61:452, 1972
191. ANGELILLO VA, O'DONOHUE WJ JR: Yellow nail syndrome with reduced glucose level in pleural fluid. Chest 75:83, 1979
192. RUNYON BA, FORKER EL, SOPKO JA: Pleural-fluid kinetics in a patient with primary lymphedema, pleural effusions, and yellow nails. Am Rev Respir Dis 119:821, 1979
193. DRESSLER W: The post-myocardial infarction syndrome. Arch Intern Med 103:28, 1959
194. DOMBY WR, WHITCOMB ME: Pleural effusion as a manifestation of Dressler's syndrome in the distant post-infarction period. Am Heart J 96:243, 1978
195. SCHNEIERSON SJ, KATZ M: Solitary pleural effusion due to myxedema. JAMA 168:1003, 1958
196. SCHLESS JM, HARRISON HN, WIER JA: The role of thoracotomy in the differential diagnosis of pleural effusion. US Armed Forces Med J 10:1055, 1959
197. ARRINGTON CW, HAWKINS JA, RICHERT JH et al: Management of undiagnosed pleural effusions in positive tuberculin reactors. Am Rev Respir Dis 93:587, 1966
197a. RYAN CJ et al: The outcome of patients with pleural effusion of indeterminate cause at thoracotomy. Mayo Clin Proc 56:145, 1981
198. LIGHT RW, MACGREGOR MI, BALL WC JR et al: Diagnostic significance of pleural fluid pH and Pco_2. Chest 64:591, 1973
199. POTTS DE, LEVIN DC, SAHN SA: Pleural Fluid pH in parapneumonic effusions. Chest 70:328, 1976
200. LIGHT RW: Management of parapneumonic effusions. Chest 70:325, 1976
201. POTTS DE, TARYLE DA, SAHN SA: The glucose–pH relationship in parapneumonic effusions. Arch Intern Med 138:1378, 1978
202. SNIDER GL, SALEK SS: Empyema of the thorax in adults: Review of 105 cases. Dis Chest 54:410, 1968
203. WEESE WC, SHINDLER ER, SMITH IM et al: Empyema of the thorax then and now. Arch Intern Med 131:516, 1973
204. BECHAMPS GL, LYNN HB, WENZL JE: Empyema in children: Review of Mayo clinic experience. Mayo Clin Proc 45:43, 1970
205. YEH TJ, HALL DP, ELLISON RG: Empyema thoracis: A review of 110 cases. Am Rev Respir Dis 88:785, 1963
206. COHN LH, BLAISDELL EW: Surgical treatment of non-tuberculous empyema. Arch Surg 100:376, 1970
207. SIMMONS EM et al: Review of nontuberculous empyema at the University of Missouri Medical Center from 1957 to 1971. J Thorac Cardiovasc Surg 64:578, 1972
208. SULLIVAN KM, O'TOOLE RD, FISHER PH et al: Anaerobic empyema thoracis. Arch Intern Med 131:521, 1973
209. BARTLETT JG, GORBACK SL, THADEPALLI H et al: The bacteriology of empyema. Lancet 1:338, 1974
210. BARTLETT JB, FINEGOLD SM: Anaerobic infections of the lung and pleural space. Am Rev Respir Dis 110:56, 1974
211. VIANNA NJ: Nontuberculous bacterial empyema in patients with and without underlying disease. JAMA 215, 1971
212. BRYANT CR et al: Management of thoracic empyema. J Thorac Cardiovasc Surg 55:850, 1968
213. SAMSON PC: Empyema thoracis. Ann Thorac Surg 11:210, 1971
214. GOODWIN RC JR, DES PREZ RM: State of the art:

Histoplasmosis. Am Rev Respir Dis 117:929, 1978
215. WITORSCH P, UTZ JP: North American blastomycosis: A study of 40 patients. Medicine 47:169, 1968
216. HAMMERMAN KJ et al: Pulmonary cryptococcosis: Clinical forms and treatment. Am Rev Respir Dis 108:1116, 1973
217. DRUTZ DJ, CATANZARO A: State of the art: Coccidioidomycosis, Part I and II. Am Rev Respir Dis 117:559, 727, 1978
218. ATKINSON GW, ISRAEL HL: 5-fluorocytosine treatment of meningeal and pulmonary aspergillosis. Am J Med 55:496, 1973
219. PEABODY JW JR, SEABURY JH: Actinomycosis and nocardiosis, a review of basic differences in therapy. Am J Med 28:99, 1960
220. SEABURY JH: Actinomycosis and nocardiosis. In Buechner HA (ed): Management of Fungus Diseases of the Lungs. Springfield, Charles C Thomas, 1971
221. BARBOUR GL, JUNIPER K JR: A clinical comparison of amebic and pyogenic abscess of the liver in sixty-six patients. Am J Med 53:323, 1972
222. HERRERA-LLERANDI R: Thoracic repercussions of amebiasis. J Thorac Cardiovasc Surg 52:361, 1966
222a. IBARRA-PEREZ C: Thoracic complications of amebic abscess of the liver. Chest 79:672, 1981
223. ANTANI J, SRINIVAS HV: Clinical evaluation of metronidazole in hepatic amebiasis. Am J Trop Med Hyg 19:762, 1970
224. GEORGE RB et al: Roentgenographic appearance of viral and mycoplasmal pneumonias. Am Rev Respir Dis 96:1144, 1967
225. BRYANT RE, RHOADES ER: Clinical features of adenoviral pneumonia in Air Force recruits. Am Rev Respir Dis 96:717, 1967
226. HEBERT DH: The roentgen features of Eaton agent pneumonia. Am J Roentgenol 98:300, 1966
227. FINE NL, SMITH LR, SHEDDY PF: Frequency of pleural effusions in mycoplasma and viral pneumonias. N Engl J Med 283:790, 1970
228. SHULMAN ST, BARTLETT J, CLYDE WA JR et al: The unusual severity of mycoplasmal pneumonia in children with sickle-cell disease. N Engl J Med 287:164, 1972
229. SOLANKI DL, BERDOFF RL: Severe mycoplasma pneumonia with pleural effusions in a patient with sickle cell-hemoglobin C (SC) disease. Am J Med 66:707, 1979
230. FROMKE VL, SCHMIDT WR: Hemothorax in idiopathic thrombocytopenic purpura (ITP). J Thorac Cardiovas Surg 63:962, 1972
231. REYNOLDS J, DAVIS JT: Injuries of the chest wall, pleura, pericardium, lungs, bronchi and esophagus. Radiol Clin North Am 4:383, 1966
232. MILFELD DJ, MATTOX KL, BEALL AC JR: Early evacuation of clotted hemothorax. Am J Surg 136:686, 1978
233. GRIFFITH GL et al: Acute traumatic hemothorax. Ann Thorac Surg 26:204, 1978
234. WILSON JL et al: The absorption of blood from the pleural space. Surgery 48:766, 1960
235. SHERMAN RT, PATE JW: The role of intrapleural blood in fibrothorax. Am Surg 31:1, 1965
236. CONDON RE: Spontaneous resolution of experimental clotted hemothorax. Surg Gynecol Obstet 126:505, 1968
237. STONEY RJ, ROE BB, REDINGTON JV: Rupture of thoracic aorta due to closed-chest trauma. Arch Surg 89:840, 1964
238. DE MEULES JE, GRAMER G, PERRY JF JR: Rupture of aorta and greater vessels due to blunt thoracic trauma. J Thorac Cardiovasc Surg 61:438, 1971
239. BREWER LA III: Surgical management of lesions of the thoracic duct. Am J Surg 90:210, 1955
240. ROY PH, CARR DT, PAYNE WS: The problem of chylothorax. Mayo Clin Proc 42:457, 1967
241. ROSS JK: A review of the surgery of the thoracic duct. Thorax 16:12, 1961
242. BOWER GC: Chylothorax, observations in 20 cases. Dis Chest 46:464, 1964
242a. STRAUSSER JL, FLYE MW: Management of nontraumatic chylothorax. Ann Thorac Surg 31:520, 1981
243. COE JE, AIKAWA JK: Cholesterol pleural effusion. Arch Intern Med 108:763, 1961
244. FERGUSON GC: Cholesterol pleural effusion in rheumatoid lung disease. Thorax 21:577, 1966
245. BRIGGS JN, GERMANN TD: Traumatic perforations of the esophagus. Surg Clin North Am 48:1297, 1968
246. ABBOTT OA et al: Atraumatic so-called "spontaneous" rupture of the esophagus. J Thorac Cardiovasc Surg 59:67, 1970
247. ROSOFF L SR, WHITE EJ: Perforation of the esophagus. Am J Surg 128:207, 1974
248. TRIGGIANI E, BELSEY R: Oesophageal trauma: Incidence, diagnosis, management. Thorax 32:241, 1977
249. DYE RA, LAFORET EF: Esophageal rupture: Diagnosis by pleural fluid pH. Chest 66:454, 1974
250. SHERR HP et al: Origin of pleural fluid amylase in esophageal rupture. Ann Intern Med 76:985, 1972
251. DERBES VJ, MITCHELL RE JR: Rupture of the esophagus. Surgery 39:688, 1956
252. FERGUSON TB, BURFORD TH: The role of surgery in the management of unilateral pleural effusion. Ann Intern Med 50:981, 1959
253. AUTIO V: The reduction of respiratory function by parenchymal and pleural lesions. A bronchospirometric study of patients with unilateral involvement. Acta Tuberc Scand 37:112, 1959
254. GAENSLER EA, WATSON TR JR, PATTON WE: Bron-

chospirometry. VI. Results of 1089 examinations. J Lab Clin Med 41:436, 1953

255. ROBIN ED, et al: Pulmonary hypertension and unilateral pleural constriction with speculation on pulmonary vasoconstrictive substance. Arch Intern Med 118:391, 1966

256. PATTON WE, WATSON TR JR, GAENSLER EA: Pulmonary function before and at intervals after surgical decortication of the lung. Surg Gynecol Obstet 95:477, 1952

257. PETTY TL, FILLEY GF, MITCHELL RS: Objective functional improvement by decortication after twenty years of artificial pneumothorax for pulmonary tuberculosis: Report of a case and review of the literature. Am Rev Respir Dis 84:572, 1961

Chapter 13

Chronic Noninfectious Parenchymal Diseases

JOHN G. WEG

GENERAL APPROACH AND CLASSIFICATION

A very large number of specific diseases present with the common and often signal finding of a diffuse abnormality on the chest roentgenogram. The pattern is usually that of bilateral disease involving all lobes but not necessarily to an equal extent; less commonly, diseases that are usually diffuse may involve only a localized area of lung; and, occasionally, interstitial disease may be present clinically, physiologically, and pathologically with a normal chest roentgenogram (up to 10% in a large but selected series[1]).

The roentgenographic patterns have been classified as (1) alveolar or acinar (rounded densities usually with fluffy, ill-defined margins that may be confluent with other densities); (2) interstitial or reticular (more linear, fairly discrete abnormalities); and (3) mixed (an acinar and interstitial pattern, which is most common). These patterns have been considered an aid in diagnosis.[2,3] We believe an attempt to ascribe specific patterns to individual diseases is unwarranted for the following reasons: (a) histologic evaluation documents that with few exceptions there is both an intra-alveolar and interstitial component; (b) at various "stages," any given disease may have a predominance of one or the other pattern roentgenographically and histologically; (c) most patterns are roentgenographically "mixed"; (d) roentgenographic classification into a pattern is quite subjective; and (e) reliance on such pattern reading may lead to a false sense of security as to the diagnosis. More distinctive is the pattern of honeycombing—the presence of multiple small nodular lesions and cystic spaces of varying sizes which correlates well with end-stage fibrosis. However, it too is nonspecific. Diffuse disease may also appear as multiple nodular lesions of varying size that may on occasion cavitate. A characteristic finding is that of small lungs with an elevated diaphragm (the superior border of the tenth posterior rib intersects the diaphragm on postero-anterior chest roentgenograms in normal persons).[4] Roentgenographic reduction in lung size reflects the physiologic pattern of restrictive disease and is also a very rough guide to progression or remission.

In addition to parenchymal abnormalities, other findings may lend strong support to a specific diagnosis. Thus symmetrical bilateral hilar adenopathy and right paratracheal adenopathy are characteristic of sarcoidosis but are also seen on occasion with mycotic disease, mycobacterial infections, and malignancy. Pleural effusion is more suggestive of a systemic disease such as a collagen disease or a superimposed infection or malignancy. An osteolytic bone lesion suggests mycotic disease or eosinophilic granuloma. Pneumothorax may complicate many of the diffuse diseases.

The clinical presentations of patients with most diffuse lung diseases are remarkably similar. A goodly portion may have no respiratory symptoms and their diseases are recognized because of abnormal chest roentgenograms. The respiratory symptoms are dyspnea, which may be progressive, and cough, which is usually nonproductive or productive of small amounts of mucoid sputum. The cough is commonly paroxysmal, and this may be associated intermittently with blood streaking in the sputum. Nonspecific constitutional symptoms of fatigue, malaise, weight loss, arthralgia, and fever (usually low-grade) are common. The most frequent physical finding is tachypnea. Examination of the chest is remarkable for the paucity or absence of abnormal findings in the majority of patients. There may be fine, discontinuous, crackling sounds, heard especially at the bases (i.e., fine, moist rales); these have been termed interstitial rales or "Velcro" rales because they are associated with diffuse interstitial fibrosis (DIF) and can be simulated by opening a Velcro fastener (or by rubbing strands of hair next to the ear). These rales are not specific for DIF; they may be heard in other conditions, and they are not always present even with DIF. Clubbing is present in the majority of patients with DIF, but again occurs with other diffuse diseases. If the disease is quite severe, there may be cyanosis and the physical findings of cor pulmonale. The presence of lymphadenopathy, hepatosplenomegaly, arthritis, or skin lesions suggests a systemic disease.

It is helpful when evaluating the patient with diffuse lung disease on the chest roentgenogram to ask the following questions: (1) Is this primary pulmonary disease? (i.e., no evidence of potentially related disease in another organ); (2) Is this a pulmonary manifestation of failure of another organ? (e.g., left heart failure, mitral stenosis, uremia); and (3) Is this a pulmonary manifestation of a systemic disease? (e.g., collagen disease, sarcoidosis, Wegener's granulomatosis). This should ensure recognition of extrapulmonary disease and serve as a reminder of the common pulmonary manifestations of systemic diseases.

General laboratory studies are usually unrewarding in contributing to the diagnosis of primary diffuse lung disease. However, they may suggest disease in another organ or systemic disease.

The pulmonary physiologic abnormalities are those of restriction (see also Chap. 4). The total lung capacity is reduced; the vital capacity and the other subunits of lung volume are reduced, usually in proportion to the decrease of total lung capacity. Air flow in large airways is usually quite well preserved: the ratio of the forced expired volume at 1 sec to the forced vital capacity is usually normal. Airways resistance is usually normal. However, small airways obstruction is common. This is manifested as decreased flow rates near residual volume on a maximum expiratory flow–volume curve or as frequency dependence of compliance. The lung compliance is reduced; the lung is stiff.[5–10]

Gas exchange is abnormal and may be measured as a decreased diffusing capacity for carbon monoxide. This interference with gas transfer was initially attributed to a thickened alveolar–capillary membrane, and commonly referred to as the "alveolar capillary block syndrome." It is, however, primarily a reflection of the mismatch of ventilation and perfusion in the lung and the actual loss of alveolar capillary membrane. A diffusion limitation may occur with exercise.[6] The diffusing capacity is a useful single-figure estimate of effective alveolar-capillary membrane interface; it is the most sensitive, noninvasive study for monitoring changes in the disease process or response to therapy. The alveolar-arterial oxygen gradient ($P(A\text{-}a)O_2$) is usually increased, and with more severe disease there is hypoxemia. Classically, hypoxemia increases with exercise, but occasionally, arterial oxygen tension may improve with exercise, a reflection of improved ventilation/perfusion relationships. The $P(A\text{-}a)O_2$ during exercise appears to correlate best with the degree of pathologic change and response to therapy.[5] The arterial carbon dioxide tension is usually decreased. Hypercarbia is usually only present with severe irreversible preterminal disease, but on occasion it is seen with cor pulmonale and may be reversible with aggressive therapy including oxygenation and diuresis.

Although the ventilatory and gas exchange abnormalities usually progress in tandem, one or the other may predominate; thus, it is preferable to obtain information about both initially and follow both serially. Although changes on the chest roentgenogram generally correlate in a rough fashion with physiologic abnormalities, they are inadequate for estimating the degree or even the presence of such abnormalities. The roentgenogram may be strikingly abnormal with little physiologic impairment or vice versa; it may show remarkable resolution with corticosteroid therapy without physiologic improvement.

A single comprehensive, logical, and rigorous classification of diffuse pulmonary disease has not yet been developed. The most useful criteria

Etiological Classification of Diffuse Diseases of the Lung*

Infections
Pyogenic bacteria
Mycobacteria
Fungi
Viruses
Parasites
Pneumocystis carinii

Specific Organ Failure
Cardiac (pulmonary edema, mitral stenosis)
Renal

Thromboembolic
Multiple pulmonary emboli
Fat emboli
Amniotic fluid emboli
Tumor emboli
Foreign body emboli
Air emboli

Neoplasms
Alveolar (bronchiolar) cell carcinoma
Metastatic (lymphangitic or hematogenous)
Lymphoma, leukemia

Endogenous
Shock
Disseminated intravascular coagulation
Sepsis

Drug Reactions
Oral or injected
Inhaled
Poisons

Radiation Injury

Inhalation Diseases
Inorganic dusts (classic pneumoconioses)
Organic dusts (allergic alveolitis)
Fumes and gases (including oxygen)
Aspiration

Uncertain Origin
Diffuse interstitial fibrosis (DIF)
  Idiopathic pulmonary fibrosis (IPF)
Sarcoidosis
Collagen vascular diseases
Granulomatous angiitis spectrum
Lymphocytic infiltrative disorders
Pulmonary hemorrhage and nephritis
Eosinophilic pneumonia
Miscellaneous

* Each of these diseases may result in an end-stage nonspecific diffuse interstitial fibrosis of varying degree, with the possible exception of neoplasms.

seem to be etiology, when known, and histopathologic features in the absence of a known specific cause. Such a classification is given at left.[3,8] The pulmonary diseases resulting from infection, heart and renal disease, thromboembolic phenomena, and neoplasms, and those of an "endogenous" nature are covered elsewhere (a reflection of the difficulties of classification). Even within this classification, overlap is inevitable. Should Goodpasture's syndrome or Wegener's granulomatosis be considered with renal disease? Where should drug reactions that produce a granulomatous angiitis be listed? A second classification relates to the histopathologic features (see outline, p. 611).

The diagnosis of specific diffuse lung diseases begins with a search for known etiologic agents. Careful questioning is mandatory concerning (1) exposure to inhaled inorganic or organic dusts, fumes, and gases; (2) exposure to infectious agents (contacts with tuberculosis, infective soil, chicken coops, etc., for histoplasmosis, or travel through an endemic area of coccidioidomycosis, etc.); (3) drug usage; and (4) other diseases. The physical examination may confirm the presence of disease in another organ, or systemic disease. Sputum should be evaluated for bacterial, mycobacterial, and fungal organisms. Skin tests for tuberculosis, coccidioidomycosis aspergillosis, and certain inhaled organic dusts may be helpful. Serologic studies for mycotic infections should be obtained (see Chap. 9, Chronic Respiratory Tract Infections), and serologic studies reflecting an immunologic response to organic dusts may confirm the clinical history. However, individuals with exposure to organic dusts may have reactive skin tests or serology without evidence of disease; immunologic reactions *per se* do not establish a diagnosis. If systemic or hematogenous infection is suspected, blood cultures and bone marrow biopsy and culture are warranted. Nonspecific skin lesions should be studied histologically, including special stains for fungi and mycobacteria, and cultured for these organisms.

If a thorough systematic evaluation for known etiologies is not rewarding, tissue is usually required in order to make a diagnosis and recom-

Histopathologic Classification of Diffuse Diseases of the Lung

Diffuse Interstitial Fibrosis (Fibrosing Alveolitis)
Usual interstitial pneumonitis (UIP)
Desquamative interstitial pneumonitis (DIP)
Lymphoid interstitial pneumonitis (LIP) (Pseudolymphoma)
Other patterns
  Bronchiolitis obliterans
  Giant cell interstitial pneumonitis
  Lymphoplasmacytic pneumonitis

Granulomatous Parenchymal Disease
Sarcoidosis
Eosinophilic granuloma

Granulomatous Angiitis
Bronchocentric (*allergic alveolitis*)
Angiocentric (Wegener's granulomatosis)

Angiitis (Periarteritis Nodosa)

Alveolar Filling Diseases
Alveolar proteinosis
Alveolar microlithiasis

Miscellaneous
Goodpasture's disease (antibasement membrane-induced glomerulonephritis and pulmonary hemorrhage)
Idiopathic hemosiderosis
Eosinophilic pneumonia

mend appropriate therapy. In a setting suggestive of sarcoidosis, Wegener's granulomatosis, or Goodpasture's disease, biopsy of lymph nodes, mucocutaneous lesions, or kidney, respectively, may be diagnostic. Lung tissue should be obtained directly if there is no evidence of other organ involvement. Studies to date indicate a diagnostic yield of 75% to 94% with both closed percutaneous cutting or drill needle biopsy and open lung biopsy. Closed biopsy techniques have the advantage of minor morbidity (pneumothorax, bleeding) and rare mortality; their disadvantage is the relatively small piece of tissue obtained, which may not be representative of the process and which limits diagnostic studies such as chemical analysis and X-ray diffraction studies. The larger specimen obtained at open biopsy is of particular value in identifying the extent of inflammation and fibrosis, which characteristically varies in small areas. It is generally necessary in order to identify vasculitis. However, it carries with it the morbidity of a thoracotomy and a slightly higher mortality rate. Using the transbronchoscopic biopsy technique, the amount of tissue obtained is smaller than with a needle biopsy and more subject to crush artifact. While the yield appears to be good in sarcoidosis, other granulomatous diseases, tumor, and infection, its yield in other diffuse diseases is variable. Because the procedure is simple and has a low morbidity rate, it should be used first unless there are contraindications. Multiple samples should be obtained during the procedure. The decision to proceed to open biopsy must integrate all clinical and laboratory evidence with the confidence of pathologic interpretations. In addition, there should be a reasonable conviction that the information obtained will enhance decision-making in the care of the patient.[11–16]

A special diagnostic problem is posed by the individual with a known systemic disease that may have pulmonary manifestations (e.g., systemic lupus erythematosus) but also predisposes to superimposed infections either of itself or because of the use of immunosuppressive agents. Such patients commonly require not only the usually thorough evaluation for infectious etiologies, but also prompt invasive diagnostic studies (see also Respiratory Infection in the Compromised Host, Chap. 8).

DIFFUSE INTERSTITIAL FIBROSIS

Clinical Features

Diffuse interstitial fibrosis (DIF) represents a common histologic end-stage response of the lung to a whole variety of insults.[17] The term *idiopathic pulmonary fibrosis* (IPF) is frequently applied when the etiology is unknown.[8,18] The outline above classifies the known causes and unknown processes that may produce this entity; it is reasonable to expect continued additions to this list. The findings are nonspecific and analogous to end stage renal or hepatic disease. Hamman and Rich initially described a rapidly fatal illness leading to death in approximately 6 months; this acute interstitial fibrosis is commonly called the Hamman-Rich syndrome. More patients today are seen with a chronic process that remains stable, may resolve, or is slowly progressive over many years.[9,19–23]

The clinical presentation is that of dyspnea and a usually nonproductive cough; this may be paroxysmal and associated with blood streaking. The presence of "interstitial" rales is common. Clubbing has been found in up to 70% of individuals at the time of initial evaluation. A familial predisposition may be present.[9,21,24]

The physiologic pattern is that of restriction with decreased lung volumes, decreased compliance, normal flow rates corrected for volume, abnormalities in gas transfer as determined by a decreased diffusing capacity, a widened alveolar to arterial oxygen gradient, and hypoxemia. [5–10]

Pathogenesis

In a syndrome defined by nonspecific histopathology with numerous known etiologies that account for less than half of the cases, a uniform concept of pathogenesis may ultimately prove to be unsatisfactory. However, a series of recent investigations support the hypothesis that a chronic ongoing alveolitis results in IPF or DIF.[8,25] It is believed that local production of specific cellular chemotactic factors recruit inflammatory and immune effector cells into the alveolar interstitium. This deranges lung connective tissue and damages parenchymal cells. Disruption of the epithelial and endothelial basement membranes—the scaffolding of the lung—results in irreversible DIF. The reason for the persistence of this alveolitis is unknown; it contrasts with the prompt resolution of the intense inflammatory reaction that accompanies the usual pneumonias such as pneumococcal pneumonia, mycoplasmal pneumonia, and so forth.

Bronchoalveolar lavage (BAL) has added a new dimension to the evaluation of lung disease over the last decade.[8,18,25–29] A flexible fiberoptic bronchoscope is wedged into a small bronchus and about 100 cc of sterile saline in divided doses is instilled; somewhat less than half is recovered by suction. The cells, proteins, and lipids collected are representative of conditions in the lung parenchyma, except in patients with inflammatory airways disease. Table 13-1 provides representative values in normal nonsmoking individuals and the changes reported in some disease states.[8,25–29] Although there is considerable variation in reports, there is general agreement.

In IPF there is an absolute increase in inflammatory and immune effector cells—alveolar macrophages, lymphocytes, and neutrophils. There is an increase in the proportion of lymphocytes and neutrophiles *vs.* alveolar macrophages. The proportion of T lymphocytes and activated T lymphocytes appears to be normal but the proportion of immunoglobulin-secreting lymphocytes is increased. The alveolar macrophages appear to be stimulated by immune complexes. This results in the local release of chemotactic factors for neutrophils. IgG-antigen immune complexes can stimulate macrophages and have been found in serum, lung, and BAL fluid from IPF patients.[30] The immune complexes may be produced locally by the B lymphocytes. Macrophage chemotactic factors also "activate" neutrophils to release preformed neutral proteases such as elastin, cathepsin G, and collagenase; collagenase is found in the lower respiratory tract of 70% of patients with IPF. The neutrophils also release oxidising radicals such as super oxide anion, H_2O_2, and the hydroxyl free radical; these can damage cell membranes. More than 95% of patients with IPF have circulating lymphocytes that release a lymphokine, migration inhibition factor, when exposed to Type I collagen.[31]

An acute hemorrhagic neutrophil-rich intra-alveolar and interstitial exudate that fades over 96 hours can be induced by the intrabronchial injection of heterologous antibody (rabbit IgG) and the intravenous injection of radiolabeled antigen (bovine serum albumin) in the rat.[25,32] Antigen–antibody alveolar and interstitial deposits are demonstrable by immunofluorescence. The reaction does not occur in the absence of C3 complement or polymorphonuclear leukocytes. It can be blocked by human chemotactic factor inhibitor.[29,33] Rabbits developing a hyperactive

TABLE 13-1. Bronchoalveolar Lavage (BAL)—Some Representative Findings in Normal Nonsmokers, in Smokers, and in Disease States[8,18,25–29]

	Normal	Smokers	DIF†	Hypersensitivity Pneumonitis	Sarcoidosis
Total Cells	2.53 × 109	↑	↑		
Macrophages*	93 ± 3	↑	↑		
Lymphocytes*	7 ± 1			↑	↑
T Lymphocytes‡	73 ± 4			↑	↑
Activated‡	6 ± 2				
B Lymphocytes‡	8 ± 3				
Neutrophils*	<1%	↑ (?)	↑		
Eosinophils*	<1%			↑	
Basophils*	<1%				
Total Protein	1–10 mg				
IgG§	0.1–0.6		↑	↑	↑
IgM‖	0			**	
Collagenase			**		

* As % total cells.
† Diffuse interstitial fibrosis including some with asbestosis, collagen vascular disease and histiocytosis-X.
‡ As % lymphocytes.
§ As mg/mg albumin.
‖ Rarely found in normals.
** = present.

antibody response to daily injections of bovine serum albumin, administered in sufficient doses to maintain a relative antigen–antibody equivalence, will develop histologic features of IPF, with associated deposits of antigen, host globulin, and complement in alveolar capillary walls and the interstitium.[34]

The intratracheal instillation of C5a complement into the hamster lung produces an acute diffuse confluent intralveolar neutrophilic inflammatory reaction, while intravenous infusion of C5a produces mainly vascular changes. Neutral proteases from neutrophils and perhaps alveolar macrophage not only damage structural elements, but also can cleave C3 and C5 complement, activating the complement pathway and thereby amplifying the inflammatory reaction. The presence of immunoglobulins and complement in irregular granular deposits along alveolar capillary walls, of circulating immune complexes, and of activated complement in BAL fluid in patients with IPF support a role for immune complex injury in at least some cases of IPF.[25]

Light-microscope evaluation of lung in IPF supports the hypothesis that increased amounts of collagen are present. The normal lung contains predominantly Types I and III collagen in a 2:1 ratio. Type I is fibrillar and also found in skin, bone, tendon, blood vessels, and lung. Type III is probably reticular and is also found in skin, blood vessels, intestine, and lung but not in bone and tendon. Earlier studies found no increase in lung collagen concentration from patients with IPF, but they did find an increase in the ratio of Type I to Type III. The higher ratio of Type I to Type III collagen is characteristic of less compliant tissues. In addition, no increase in collagen synthesis could be detected in open biopsy specimens from IPF.[18,35] More recently, however, increased collagen content has been documented in human lungs with IPF following severe respiratory failure and in animal models of bleomycin-induced fibrosis.[17,36] Increased collagen synthesis was demonstrated in the animal models. This fibrosis in animal models can be suppressed by indomethacin, antilymphocytic globulin, urokinase, certain proline analogues, and penicillamine.[17]

The recent extensive advances in our understanding of the pathogenesis of at least some forms of DIF clearly implicate a variety of immunologic mechanisms; some similar mechanisms have been identified in asbestosis, silicosis, coal workers' pneumoconiosis, collagen vascular diseases, and Goodpasture's syndrome. However, the trigger or triggers that result in an ongoing chronic phlogistic response have not been identified. (The history of antecedent viral illness in about one third of patients is tantalizing.) Experimental methods for suppression of fibrosis may lead to more effective therapy.

Pathology

Post mortem examination of end-stage lungs with DIF reveals a nodular pleural surface, which is similar in appearance to the surface of the liver in portal cirrhosis. The lungs are small, heavy, and stiff. On cut surfaces, the nodules correspond to dilated bronchioles and alveolar ducts which form microcysts between retracted areas of fibrosis.

The microscopic changes may be categorized in the following way:

1. *Acute (early) microscopic changes*, characterized by a increased number of mononuclear cells in alveolar spaces (lymphocytes, free alveolar macrophages, and Type II alveolar lining cells), and by an increased number of neutrophils; there is interstitial edema, fibrinous exudate, and fibroblast proliferation involving alveolar spaces and septa.
2. *Subacute (intermediate) microscopic changes*, characterized by interstitial infiltrates of lymphocytes, large mononuclear cells and neutrophils, obliteration of alveolar spaces, metaplastic cuboidal epithelium, hyperplastic columnar epithelium, and capillary obliteration.
3. *Chronic (late) microscopic changes*, characterized by marked parenchymal distortion, microcyst formation, interstitial smooth muscle hyperplasia, elastic fiber fragmentation, and hyperplastic columnar-alveolar epithelium with some atypia;[37] There is peribronchiolar fibrosis, perhaps explaining small airways obstruction; thickening of the muscular media of the pulmonary arteries and cholesterol clefts correlate with pulmonary hypertension.[18]

The implied chronology of these categories must be used with caution; for example, late changes may be seen acutely, and the same lung may demonstrate all stages simultaneously. Severe pulmonary fibrosis following acute respiratory failure (adult respiratory distress syndrome) may be seen in two weeks or less.[38]

Although the term DIF (or IPF) is well established in the United States, fibrosing alveolitis is the preferred term in Great Britain.[9,39] A variety of other expressions have also been used: cirrhosis cystica pulmonum, acute diffuse interstitial fibrosis, honeycomb lung, bronchiolar emphysema, familial fibrocystic displasia, peribronchiolar and interstitial muscular hyperplasia associated with bronchiolar dililation, and idiopathic bronchiolectasis.

Other Patterns

Liebow and colleagues have described potentially distinct categories of DIF that may be of some clinical usefulness.[40] *Desquamative interstitial pneumonitis (DIP)* is characterized primarily by an intra-alveolar collection of mononuclear cells (alveolar type II cells and macrophages), relatively intact alveolar walls without destruction or fibrinous exudates, and a fairly uniform pattern throughout. This pattern has correlated with a distinctly more benign course and a better response to corticosteroids in a prospective study. (However, if the patients with the usual interstitial fibrosis [UIP] or DIF are combined with those with DIP, overall outcome appears to match other series of DIF.)[4] Since a pattern of DIP very commonly coexists with UIP (or DIF), it is considered to more likely represent an "earlier" and perhaps more reversible stage of DIF. In Great Britain, desquamative fibrosing alveolitis and mural fibrosing alveolitis are preferred terms for DIP and UIP (or DIF), respectively.

Lymphoid interstitial pneumonia was also described by Liebow. In patients with this rare condition, the clinical, physiologic, and radiographic features are similar to DIF, but the histology consists of diffuse infiltration by lymphocytes without destruction of bronchi, lung vessels, or granuloma formation. The histology and clinical course should permit these patients to be distinguished from those with allergic alveolitis, pseudolymphoma, pulmonary lymphoma, and lymphomatoid granulomatosis. Patients have been described with subsequent development of extrapulmonary lymphoma, and with amyloid, myasthenia gravis Sjögren's syndrome, and a variety of dysgammaglobulinemias.[41–43]

Other patterns of histologic interest include DIF associated with *bronchiolitis obliterans* and a pattern of *giant cell interstitial pneumonia* with lymphocytic infiltrates and bizarre giant cells in the alveoli. Clinical correlations with these uncommon patterns have not been made.

Greenberg and coworkers have described a histologic pattern of *lymphoplasmacytic pneumonia with dysproteinemia*, characterized by both lymphocytic and plasma cell infiltration associated with hypergammaglobulinemia. The clinical course appears to be slowly progressive, and it is believed to represent a chronic inflammatory response to an unknown stimulant.[44]

Eosinophilic pneumonia is described below.

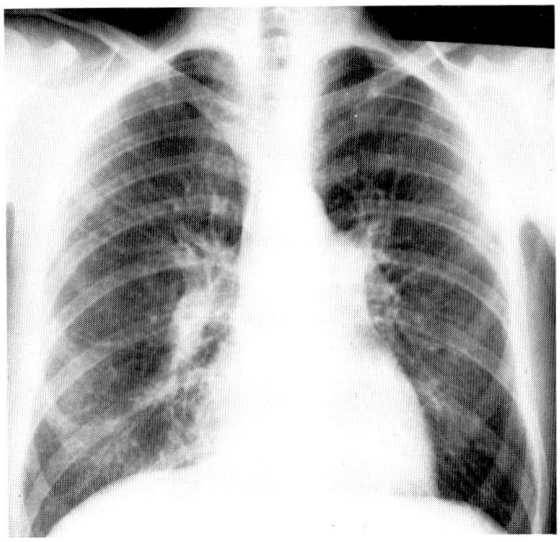

FIG. 13-1. Chest roentgenogram showing a diffuse bilateral reticular pattern. This 23-year-old man had rapidly progressive dyspnea and developed cor pulmonale over 3 months. Biopsy documented acute interstitial fibrosis with a prominent mononuclear cell infiltrate, without desquamation.

Diagnosis

Since this is the end-stage response to a whole host of insults, both known and unknown, including the evolution of the granulomatous angiitides to be discussed subsequently, a "diagnosis" of DIF is morphologic and nonspecific. However, some would call it a disease on the basis of its macrophage, lymphocyte, and neutrophil responses as determined by BAL, and on the basis of the evolving evidence of an immunologically mediated alveolitis.[8] Clinically, the diagnosis of DIF or IPF is useful in excluding other specific entities and providing a basis for recommending therapy. In general, lung biopsy is necessary to make this diagnosis, although some would rely on the clinical and roentgenographic picture.[45] In the presence of diffuse, quite stable radiographic abnormality documented roentgenographically for a year or more, biopsy for diagnosis is not recommended (see Management). In our studies of approximately 100 such patients, the histology was uniformly that of DIF (Figs 13-1, 13-2, and 13-3).

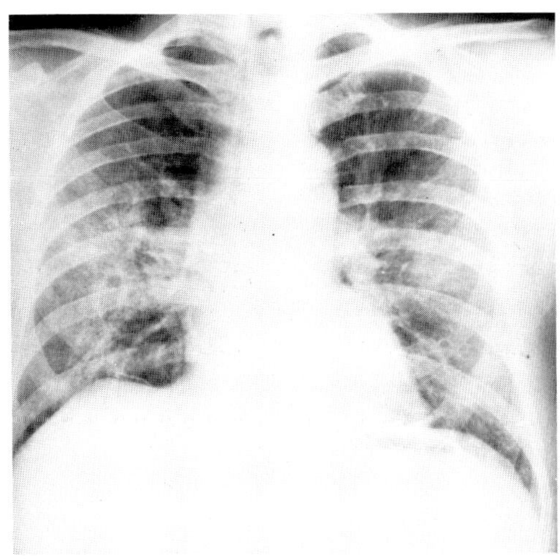

FIG. 13-2. Chest roentgenogram of a patient with diffuse interstitial fibrosis. There is soft, somewhat nodular infiltrate involving both lung fields, which is more evident in the midlung zones.

Somewhere between 10% and 20% of patients with DIF will have low titers of rheumatoid factor in their serum, and up to 40% will have antinuclear antibodies. Whether this indicates a *forme fruste* of rheumatoid disease or a nonspecific immunologic response is unclear.[19] Cryoimmunoglobulins have also been found in 40% of DIF patients. There is considerable

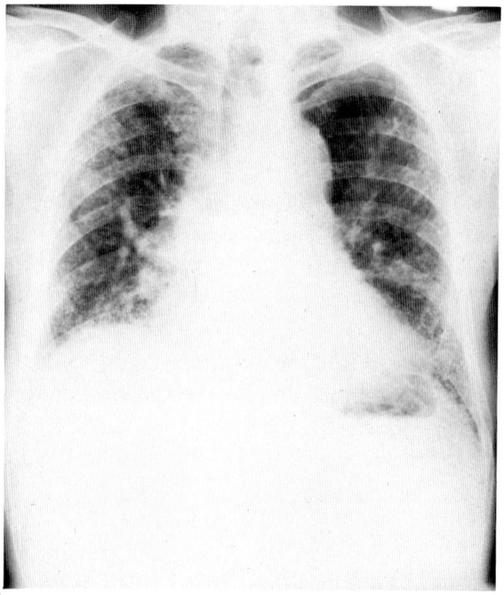

FIG. 13-3. Chest roentgenogram demonstrating bilateral reticular nodular shadows with multiple cystic areas (honeycombing). The diaphragms are elevated. The patient (shown in Fig. 13-2 at age 65) is seen here 18 years later. He gradually developed moderate exertional dyspnea, but continued calisthenics for 2 hours each day. Pulmonary function studies documented moderate restriction (forced vital capacity was 67% of predicted; single-breath diffusing capacity was 31% of predicted; resting PaO_2 was 91 mm Hg, and with 2 mph treadmill exercise, PaO_2 was 67 mm Hg).

variation in the incidence of serologic abnormalities in different series. The sedimentation rate is almost always elevated.

Management

No definitive guidelines for DIF therapy are available. Cases are reported with spontaneous remission. Those DIF cases having acute or early histologic patterns, with the presence of increased intra-alveolar cellularity and little damage to the alveolar walls, appear to have a better response to steroids and a better prognosis.[4] Some have suggested that corticosteroids may prevent the development of severe fibrosis, but this is not established.[19,20,39,46,47]

More recently, efforts have been directed at using BAL and ^{67}gallium lung scintigraphy to identify the presence of active alveolitis (rather than fibrosis), to follow the course of active inflammation, and to monitor the response to therapy.[7,8,18,26–29,48] It is generally agreed that the chest roentgenogram and pulmonary function studies correlate poorly, if at all, with the degree of alveolitis or the amount of fibrosis.

Alveolitis in which the proportion of neutrophils in lavage fluid is greater than 10% of the cells has been called "high-intensity alveolitis."[8] It has been proposed that patients with more than 10% neutrophils should be treated with corticosteroids, and that a neutrophil count that decreases indicates a good response to therapy and a better prognosis. In contrast, others have found a better response to corticosteroids in those patients with greater than 11% lymphocytes, irrespective of associated increases in neutrophils or eosinophils; they did not find a decrease in neutrophils with corticosteroids. These studies have not provided adequate physiologic documentation to correlate with criteria for treatment. They did caution that general changes in lavage counts should not necessarily be equated with a clinical response.[27,28] It seems reasonable to follow lavage information if available, along with clinical, radiographic, and most importantly, physiologic parameters. At present, clinical improvement substantiated in the pulmonary physiology laboratory is the criterion for a salutary response to corticosteroid therapy, and the reverse is an indication of disease progression. Although BAL findings do correlate reasonably well with different clinical diagnoses such as IPF, hypersensitivity pneumonitis, and so forth, they are not sufficiently specific to substitute for lung tissue biopsy in making a diagnosis.

Scintigraphy with ^{67}gallium citrate offers a noninvasive means of serially monitoring lung inflammation in IPF and sarcoidosis. Uptake also occurs in many other diffuse lung diseases, infections, and tumors. A Ga index that provides a semiquantitative index of alveolitis has been developed. A score of greater than 50 is considered abnormal and is found in 70% of patients with IPF. It correlates with BAL findings, but also suffers from the same lack of data that would provide physiologic correlation with disease. Its place in routine patient management is yet to be defined.

On the basis of available information, it seems reasonable to reserve a trial of corticosteroids for patients who have significant respiratory symptoms that interfere with reasonable levels of activity, or for those who demonstrate clinical and physiologic progression of disease. Prednisone in an initial dose of 60 mg daily, or its equivalent, is recommended. The response should be documented clinically and physiologically for 30–60 days. If a response is documented, the dose is slowly reduced, with careful physiologic monitoring, to 15 to 30 mg of prednisone daily or on alternate days, using a single morning dose. The appropriate duration of therapy is not known. If improvement is maintained for 6 to 12 months, a further slow taper with the intent of discontinuing corticosteroids may be considered. We recommend careful physiologic monitoring (lung volumes, diffusing capacity, and $P[A\text{-}a/O_2]$ at rest and exercise) at regular intervals during this period. If there is physiologic deterioration, the corticosteroid dose should be approximately doubled. There are anecdotal reports of relapse when corticosteroids are discontinued, with failure to respond to their reintroduction. An alternate approach is 1 mg/kg of prednisone daily for 6 weeks with a taper of 2.5 mg/week to 0.25 mg/kg day; the decision to increase, decrease, or discontinue corticosteroids is governed by changes in ^{67}Ga scanning and BAL.[8]

Scattered reports have suggested therapeutic benefit from immunosuppressive agents as well as concern for their side-effects.[8] Recently, 12 of 20 patients in a prospective study had physiologically documented improvement with azathioprine. Prednisone was initiated two weeks after open biopsy and azathioprine (3 mg/kg) was added at 3 months. All patients had progressive disease. The response was better if the illness was of one year's duration or less and when there was less fibrosis. Response did not correlate with the amount of alveolitis. Eight of the patients had a selective beneficial effect from azathioprine. While both drugs caused side-effects, they were reversible with discontinuation of the drugs.[49] A trial of azathioprine appears reasonable if steroids do not halt progressive illness.

Patients benefit symptomatically from supplemental oxygen when the PaO_2 is less than approximately 60 mm Hg (saturation of <90%) either at rest or exercise. The use of oxygen may also forestall the development of cor pulmonale.

A trial of bronchodilators (*e.g.*, aminophylline or beta-sympathetic agents) should be considered, since obstruction of small airways is common. Because the paroxysmal cough associated with DIF is often a major debilitating sympton, a trial of potent antitussives in effective doses is also recommended.

End-stage pulmonary fibrosis is associated with severe disability, cor pulmonale, and predilection to infection.[21] Treatment for these complications is similar to treatment of chronic respiratory failure outlined in Chapter 14. Lung cancer may be more common in patients with pulmonary fibrosis particularly if they are cigarette smokers.[23] Several patients with severe disease have developed severe associated obstructive lung disease.[50]

SARCOIDOSIS

Sarcoidosis is a systemic disease with protean manifestations of unknown etiology characterized by noncaseating granuloma involving multiple organs with varying frequency, although almost invariably the lung (see Table 13-2). While noncaseating granulomas are the hallmark of this disease, they are not pathognomonic. The clinical course may be brief, self-limited, and even asymptomatic (a chance roentgenographic finding), characterized by exacerbations and spontaneous remissions; there may be progressive disability in perhaps 10% of patients. Although specific therapy is not available, corticosteroids may be salutary for specific manifestations. In spite of the many challenging, unresolved problems of sarcoidosis, the competent clinician usually is able to recognize sarcoidosis, confirm the diagnosis with appropriate studies, and define those manifestations that require treatment. There will, however, be a goodly number of "borderline cases about

TABLE 13-2. Tissues Involved in Patients with Sarcoidosis

Organ	Percent Affected
Lung	95–100
Lymph nodes	75–80
Spleen	75
Liver	50
Skin	30
Eyes	15
Joints	10
Nervous system	5
Myocardium	>5

which the wise will accept the need to reserve judgement, and the disputatious will argue."[51] An exhaustive bibliography and several extensive reviews are available.[52–56]

Definition

The following descriptive definition provides a generally accepted and utilitarian foundation for sarcoidosis: "Sarcoidosis is a systemic granulomatous disease of undetermined etiology and pathogenesis. Mediastinal and peripheral lymph nodes, lungs, liver, spleen, skin, eyes, phalangeal bones, and parotid glands are most often involved, but other organs or tissues may be affected. The Kveim reaction is frequently positive and tuberculin-type hypersensitivities are frequently depressed. Other important laboratory findings are hypercalciuria and increased serum globulins. The characteristic histologic appearance of epithelioid tubercles with little or no necrosis is not pathognomonic, and tuberculosis, fungal infection, beryllium disease, and local sarcoid reactions must be excluded. The diagnosis should be regarded as established for clinical purposes in patients who have consistent clinical features, together with biopsy evidence of epithelioid tubercles or a positive Kveim test.[56] The primacy of noncaseating granuloma involving multiple organs and the importance of withholding judgments concerning potential etiologies have recently been re-emphasized.[51]

Incidence

Sarcoidosis has been recognized the world over, but more commonly in the United States, England, and Scandinavia. The annual incidence of new cases is approximately 05.0 per 100,000 in Great Britain and Denmark, the only areas with such data. It occurs most commonly between the ages of 20 and 35, is more frequent in women, and is 12 to 15 times more common in blacks, in whom it causes more disability than tuberculosis in the United States today.[57] Prevalence rates of 30 to 64 per 100,000 have been reported.

Pathology

The characteristic lesion is that of many similar, noncaseating granulomas involving multiple organs, composed predominantly of epithelioid cells with centrally placed giant cells surrounded by lymphocytes, macrophages, monocytes, and fibroblasts. In developing granuloma, these differentiated cells are more common than epithelioid cells. Crystalline or conchoidal (Schaumann) bodies are frequently seen. Occasionally there may be some central granular necrosis. Definite caseative necrosis strongly indicates a specific infectious granulomatous disease, generally mycobacterial or fungal. While a small number of cases of necrotizing granuloma with a nodular chest roentgenographic pattern have been attributed to sarcoidosis, specific infectious agents can generally be detected.[58] Over a varying period of time, the granulomas progress to nonspecific residual fibrotic lesions or may resolve with little or no residual scar. While it would appear that most lesions reach a fibrotic stage in about a year, continued "active" granulomas may be seen 20 or 30 years after the onset of illness. These active lesions are associated with accumulation of lymphocytes, macrophages, and monocytes seen predominantly in the interstitium of the lung.[51,59,60]

It must be emphasized that noncaseating granulomas are nonspecific. They may be found in mycobacterial and fungal disease (although rarely without caseating lesions in other areas of the specimen); as a response to trauma or foreign bodies; in lymphoma; and in the regional nodes draining malignant, mycobacterial, or fungal infections. However, the documentation of multiple organ involvement with noncaseating granulomas that do not reveal organisms with special stains and cultures for mycobacteria and fungi provides a solid basis for diagnosis. Although rare, berylliosis may simulate sarcoidosis not only histologically but also clinically; its recognition requires an exposure history. Areas in lung biopsy specimens of extrinsic allergic alveolitis may also have noncaseating granulomas, but the history and absence of other organ involvement should prevent confusion.

Clinical Manifestations

It is estimated that approximately 50% of patients with sarcoidosis will have some symptoms at the time of diagnosis. The percentage with symptoms varies greatly, from low figures in series in which screening chest roentgenograms were employed, such as in military populations or earlier tuberculosis surveys, to very high figures in series from inner city hospitals or referral centers. The signal finding is frequently the abnormal chest roentgenogram; when such patients are evaluated, a history of mild nonspecific respiratory and constitutional symptoms is often elicited. The individual with an abnormal roentgenogram, however, may be truly asymptomatic.

The most common respiratory symptoms of sarcoidosis are dyspnea and cough; the cough is usually nonproductive, but sputum is occasionally blood-streaked, especially when associated with paroxysmal coughing or extensive fibrosis. There may be substernal or central chest aching discomfort. With progressive disease, evidence of cor pulmonale and respiratory failure may develop. Nonspecific constitutional symptoms of fatigue, malaise, weight loss, and arthralgias are common. While fever may occur in sarcoidosis[61] (even up to 39° C), its presence warrants a careful search for superimposed infections or consideration of an alternative diagnosis in the patient undergoing initial evaluation. Some individuals may present acutely with arthralgias and erythema nodosum, which is associated with bilateral hilar adenopathy on the chest roentgenogram.

The physical examination may be normal. There may be an increased respiratory rate, rales (often interstitial and basilar), and rarely, wheezing which may indicate bronchial involvement. Generalized palpable lymphadenopathy is present in approximately 75% to 80% of patients. A palpable liver (in 50%) and spleen (in 75%) have been noted. There may be tenderness and swelling, particularly of the large joints and distal interphalangeal joints. A variety of nonspecific skin lesions may be found in about one-third of patients; these include macules, papules, or plaques with scaling or atrophic scarring; they may appear in previous scars, and are commonly seen about the face, ears, and neck. Anterior uveitis or chorioretinitis have been reported in up to 25% of patients; slit lamp examination may be required for its detection. Myocardial involvement is usually suspected because of arrhythmias or conduction defects[63]; however, one third of the patients show defects on thallium scans, and have impaired ventricular function[64] and small pericardial effusions.[65] These findings may result from the extensive myocardial lesions reported at autopsy.[66] The nervous system is involved in approximately 5% of patients. Central nervous system involvement has protean manifestations usually related to a basal granulomatous meningitis; the facial and optic nerves are the most commonly involved cranial nerves. Peripheral nerve involvement usually occurs late.[67–69] Nonspecific, usually self-limited electroencephalographic changes have been observed in about one-third of patients with intrathoracic sarcoidosis without clinical evidence of central nervous system involvement.[70] Diabetes insipidus and other evidence of hypothalamic–pituitary dysfunction may develop.[70a] Mucosal involvement of the ear, nose, throat, and bronchial tree is reported in one-half or more of patients who have been thoroughly evaluated for such lesions. The uveal tract, parotid glands, and cranial nerves may be involved and associated with fever (i.e., uveoparotid fever of Heerfordt), but this is uncommon. The relative incidence of specific organ involvement is quite variable in reported series. Data are undoubtedly biased by the presenting complaints of the patient and the special interest of the authors. These figures, however, do substantiate the multiple organ involvement characteristic of sarcoidosis.

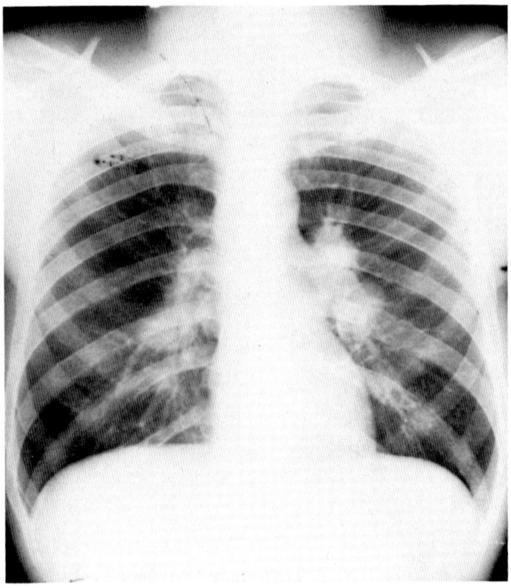

FIG. 13-4. Chest roentgenogram of a 25-year-old asymptomatic patient with sarcoidosis. Bilateral hilar adenopathy is apparent, but the parenchyma is normal ("potato nodes").

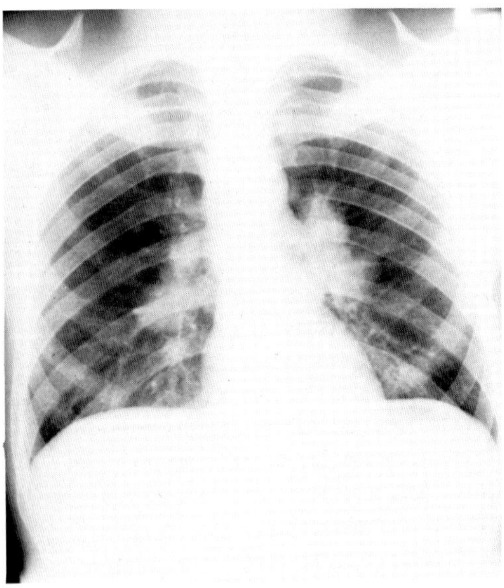

FIG. 13-5. Chest roentgenogram of a patient with sarcoidosis, bilateral hilar adenopathy, and bilateral nodular infiltrates in the lower lobes. This 30-year-old had a nonproductive cough, vague malaise, and a weight loss for 3 months.

Roentgenographic Manifestations

The classic roentgenographic pattern is that of symmetrical bilateral hilar and right paratracheal node adenopathy without evidence of pulmonary parenchymal involvement (Fig. 13-4). This pattern, however, is not pathognomonic; it may be seen in tuberculosis, mycotic infections, and less commonly, with lymphoma (where anterior mediastinal lymphadenopathy is also usually present) and metastatic carcinoma. Asymmetric or subcarinal lymphadenopathy is more commonly seen with specific granulomatous infections, lymphoma, or malignancy, although it occurs rarely in sarcoidosis. A second pattern is that of bilateral hilar adenopathy associated with diffuse symmetric pulmonary involvement (Figs 13-5, and 13-6). The parenchymal lesions display an almost infinite variety of reticular and nodular patterns; the nodules vary from very small to 1 cm or more, which may suggest metastatic disease. Unilateral or localized pulmonary involvement is rare and warrants very careful evaluation for other etiologies. In particular, a biopsy of a lymph node draining such a lesion that has noncaseating granulomas most commonly accounts for the "false diagnosis" based on a histologic appearance. A third pattern is that of diffuse pulmonary involvement without lymphadenopathy (Fig. 13-7). In addition to the previously described variations, more linear, "hard" patterns compatible with fibrosis may be seen. There may be honeycombing or volume loss, especially of the upper lobes, simulating tuberculosis. Cystic lesions may be found, and may be complicated by the development of an aspergilloma.[53,71–73]

Some authors have viewed these patterns as stages: Stage I, bilateral hilar adenopathy; Stage II, hilar adenopathy and pulmonary infiltrates; and Stage III, parenchymal involvement alone.[74] They have then described a natural history of the disease, indicating that Stage I is followed by Stages II and III. While this may generally correlate with chronologic progression, our data and that of others do not support so rigid a classification (Fig. 13-8). Patients are seen with just parenchymal involvement with documented new disease, and the histologic variations from granuloma to fibrosis do not correlate with the roentgenographic patterns. Thus, the use of a term such as Class or Group to refer to these patterns is preferable.[51,59]

Physiologic Changes

The most common abnormalities of pulmonary function in sarcoidosis demonstrate the restrictive pattern, including a decreased vital capacity, total lung capacity, and other subunits of volume, and reduced static compliance. Large airways obstruction is seldom found in early and uncomplicated sarcoidosis;[75] however, small airways obstruction is common. Excessive reactivity to methacholine challenge has also been demonstrated.[76] Some patients with Stage I disease develop obstruction that is not responsive to bronchodilators, probably as a result of bronchial mucosal lesions.[77] With severe chronic disease and extensive lung fibrosis, retraction of lung with compensatory areas of emphysema develop. These patients also demonstrate marked airways obstruction that is not responsive to bronchodilators. When inspiratory and expiratory flow rates are reduced, particularly in the presence of audible stridor or persistent localized wheezing, bronchostenosis should be considered.

The diffusing capacity for carbon monoxide is characteristically reduced in sarcoidosis. There may be a widened alveolar–arterial oxygen gradient or hypoxemia, and an increased dead space–tidal volume ratio, predominantly on the basis of abnormal ventilation–perfusion relationships; with extensive disease, there may be loss of alveolar capillary membrane. The arterial oxygen tension usually falls with exercise but may improve, reflecting an improvement in ventilation–perfusion ratios. The diffusing capacity, a noninvasive procedure, and the alveolar–arterial oxygen gradient at rest and with exercise are the most sensitive studies in following the disease process or its response to therapy.[59,78,79]

Diagnosis

The diagnosis of sarcoidosis generally requires a characteristic clinical and roentgenographic picture, the presence of noncaseating granulomas in a biopsy of one or more organs, and the exclusion of other disease processes. Even when these criteria are met, it is prudent to reserve final judgment until longitudinal follow-up excludes the presence of other diseases, particularly specific granulomatous infections. Thus one must use extreme caution in attributing to sarcoidosis (1) asymmetric hilar or paratracheal, subcarinal, or anterior mediastinal adenopathy; (2) asymmetric or localized parenchymal disease; (3) fever, draining sinuses or mucosal ulcerations; or (4) any other unusual manifestations.[51,59,79,80]

A thorough evaluation for specific granulomatous infection is mandatory. It should include a tuberculin and coccidioidin skin test (a significant reaction indicates infection, remote or current, and does not exclude the diagnosis of sarcoidosis), fungal serologies, sputum cultures for mycobacteria and fungi, and most importantly, careful histologic study with special stains and cultures of granulomatous tissue for mycobacteria and fungi. Direct biopsy of localized pulmonary disease or asymmetric hilar or mediastinal nodes is advisable (see also Chap. 9).

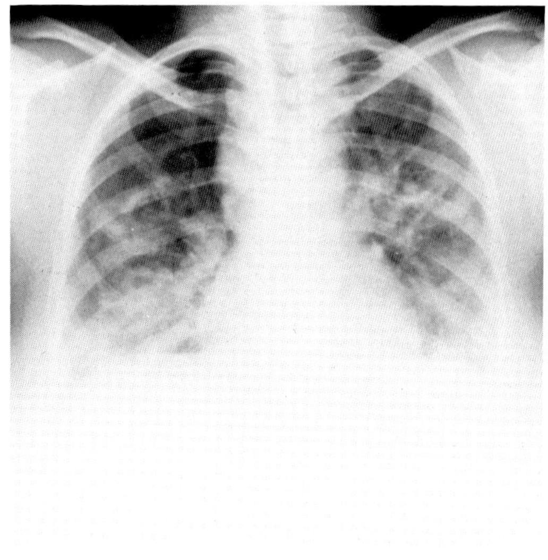

FIG. 13-6. Chest roentgenogram of a 28-year-old black woman with sarcoidosis, bilateral hilar adenopathy, paratracheal adenopathy, extensive diffuse confluent infiltrates (predominantly in the lower two-thirds of the lung), and small lung volumes. The patient had an inexorable downhill course, developing cor pulmonale and respiratory failure that did not respond to corticosteroid therapy. She died 15 months after the onset of symptoms.

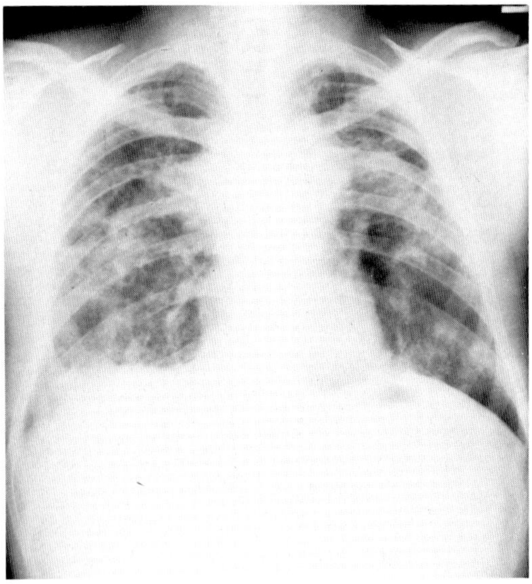

FIG. 13-7. Chest roentgenogram of a 45-year-old dyspneic man with sarcoidosis. There is predominantly a reticular or linear pattern with some nodules. The hilar shadows are markedly elevated and some adenopathy persists. Scalene lymph node and lung biopsies confirmed the diagnosis. Extensive studies over several years did not identify a specific infectious etiology.

FIG. 13-8. Chest roentgenogram of a 22-year-old patient with sarcoidosis. Multiple bilateral nodules without discrete margins, hilar adenopathy, and paratracheal adenopathy returned to normal over 2 years. This is a somewhat unusual roentgenographic presentation.

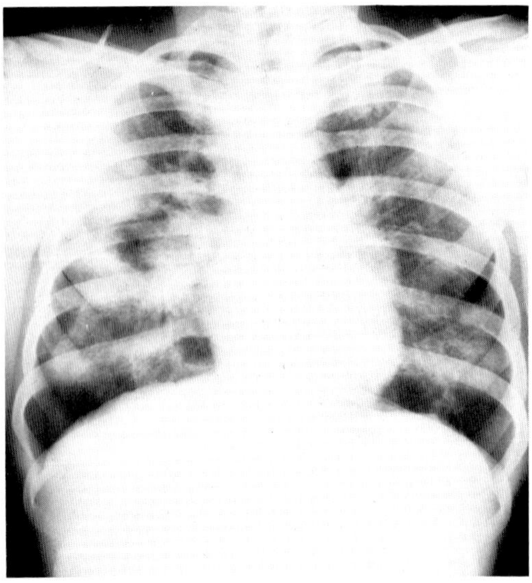

The diagnostic yield of noncaseating granulomas from various tissue sites varies with the duration of disease; the yield is considerably greater in disease of 1 to 2 years duration, although granulomas may be present many years later. Choice of biopsy sites should be governed by both the yield and the potential for morbidity of the procedure. In disease of recent origin (e.g., less than 2 years or with evidence of activity), scalene node biopsy, even without palpable nodes or mediastinoscopy, has a yield of 80 to 90%; percutaneous or needle lung biopsy yields approach 100%; the transbronchial biopsy yield is variable, 57% to 90%; salivary gland, 58%[81]; skin 30% (7%–60%); bronchus, 30% to 60%; and conjunctiva with follicles, 25%.[16,51,53,55,59] Clearly, a skin biopsy is least meddlesome, but may pose a problem with foreign body reactions. Although liver biopsy may yield noncaseating granuloma in about 70% of patients, diagnosed as sarcoidosis, we do not recommend it because so many diseases (in particular, the granulomatous infections) may cause nonspecific granuloma in liver. Tissue confirmation from one organ with evidence of disease in another is generally satisfactory.

The Kveim test may be a satisfactory alternative form of tissue diagnosis. A suspension of sarcoidal spleen is injected intradermally. The development of typical noncaseating granuloma in a biopsy of the site some 4 to 8 weeks after injection, whether or not a papule occurs, is positive. With the use of specified, carefully certified antigens such as that of Siltzbach, positive reactions occur in about 89% of patients with disease of less than 2 years duration, and less frequently in disease that has been present for longer periods and is inactive. False positives are rare (2%–4%). The specificity (selectivity) and sensitivity of reliable antigens have been repeatedly well documented.[82–84] However, the use of antigens subsequently shown to lack specificity has produced false-positive reactions in a high proportion of individuals with lymphadenopathy, and perhaps in those with other diseases.[51,85,86] The major problem with the Kveim test is the lack of a ready source of a certified or validated antigen for general use. Unless this is available, the test is of only academic interest. A second disadvantage is the 4- to 8-week delay required for the reaction to develop; this may be obviated if *in vitro* tests using the Kveim antigen with a patient's serum or cells are perfected.[87]

A variety of other laboratory abnormalities may be found in sarcoidosis. They are nonspecific and thus do not contribute to the diagnosis. They include anemia, leukopenia, hyperglobulinemia, hypercalcemia, hypercalciuria, bone lesions, positive serologic studies for rheumatoid factor, and abnormal liver function studies.

It has been suggested that tissue confirmation is not necessary when bilateral hilar adenopathy is found in the asymptomatic individual with a normal physical examination and normal screening laboratory studies, or when associated with erythema nodosum, fever and arthritis.[88] The latter presentation occurs with some fungal infections or occasionally with tuberculosis. While such a presentation permits a reasonable working diagnosis when other diseases have been excluded by thorough noninvasive studies, we believe it is preferable to obtain tissue.

Etiology

The etiology of sarcoidosis is not known. Significant elevations of serum antibody to virulent atypical mycobacteria have been reported in 80% of patients with sarcoidosis, as opposed to approximately 30% of other patients and controls.[80] Mycobacterial phages have been found in stools of all patients with histologically proven sarcoidosis. These phages produced morphologic and growth alterations in *M. tuberculosis in vitro* so that they no longer resembled tubercle bacilli; the altered tubercle bacilli produced noncaseating granuloma in guinea pigs. Although the phages were present in the stool of sarcoid patients, phage-neutralizing antibody could not be demonstrated in their serum although it is present in high concentrations in the serum of tuberculous patients. Strains of atypical mycobacteria have been cultured from sarcoid biopsies in medium containing phage antisera.[90,91] An apparent, unusual lack of skin test reactivity to antigens of atypical mycobacteria has been noted. These and other studies tend to support a potential etiologic role for mycobacterium, perhaps modified in a host with an altered immunologic response.[51,92] However, they have not been confirmed by others. Other serologic studies have shown reactivity to herpes-like viruses. There is some evidence of a genetic predisposition and a relationship to specific HL-A histocompatibility antigens.[51,87]

In searching for a specific transmissible agent, Mycobacteria, Mycoplasma, Nocardia, Cryptococcus, Blastomyces, Propionibacterium, and Yersinia organisms have been isolated by individual workers (and apparently not found by others).[51,93] Controlled experiments in mice indicate the presence of a transmissible agent in human sarcoid tissue that produces a delayed systemic noncaseating granulomatous reaction and a positive Kveim reaction. This agent can be repeatedly transferred and is approximately the size of a virus; acid-fast organisms were seen in mice but not in the original sarcoid homogenate.[94] Electron microscopic studies of lung biopsies from sarcoid patients have demonstrated inclusion bodies that might represent mutants of mycobacteria[95]; however, they may represent cell-derived organelles.[96] Despite this provocative evidence, the etiology remains unknown.

Immunology

Patients with sarcoidosis have a generalized hyporeactivity to skin tests, which produce a delayed, cellular, or Type IV reaction. This reactivity tends to vary inversely with disease activity. When patients are studied longitudinally with serial skin tests, their reactivity to common antigens approaches that of the general population.[92] Because tuberculin reactions are generally uncommon in people in developed nations, the evaluation of hypersensitivity by skin tests may require a battery of antigens such as tuberculin (intermediate and second-strength), trichophytin, *Candida albicans*, mumps, and streptokinase-streptodornase. Occasionally, induction of hypersensitivity may be necessary by sensitization with dinitrochlorobenzene. It appears that superinfection with tuberculosis in patients with sarcoidosis will result in a significant tuberculin reaction. *In vitro* studies support the hypothesis of a depression of cellular or delayed hyperreactivity, as follows: (1) a poor response of cultured blood lymphocytes to phytohemagglutinin and other mitogens, and (2) depressed blood T-cell numbers and activity (and increased blood B-cell activity).[97,98] Recent studies of BAL fluid have documented an increase of lung lymphocytes in patients with sarcoidosis to 33% ± 6% (*vs.* a normal level of less than 10%) and, with clinical "activity," to 55% ± 8%. Others have found less striking elevations.[99] (High lymphocyte counts have also been seen in hypersensitivity pneumonitis, tuberculosis, and lung lymphoma.) The total number of cells was also increased. The percentage of T-lymphocytes was 90% ± 4% (*vs.* a normal level of 65% – 80%), and no patient with other evidence of lung disease had less than 80%. It is believed that monocytes and macrophages are recruited from the bloodstream under the influence of a monocyte chemotactic factor elaborated by activated large T-lymphocytes. These cells also produce a leukocyte inhibitory factor, and the elevated serum lysozyme in sarcoid patients also inhibits neutrophil migration. Tissue neutrophils are not a feature in sarcoid alveolitis. Blood monocytes of sarcoid patients have increased numbers of IgG-Fc and C3 receptors; contain more lysozyme, B galactosidase, and angiotensin-converting enzyme; and show increased spreading. These factors are considered to be evidence of mononuclear phagocytic activation.[60,87] Sarcoid tissue suspensions (Kveim antigen) have produced (1) lymphocyte transformation, (2) leukocyte migration inhibition, and (3) release of migration inhibition factor.[87]

In contrast, there is an increase in circulating immunoglobulins IgG, IgA, IgM, and IgE in sarcoid patients as compared with controls, but some decrease in IgD. There are increased circulating antibodies to Epstein-Barr, herpes simplex, rubella, rubeola, and parainfluenza viruses. There is also increased serum complement activity, increased lysozyme levels, increased antibody response to mismatched blood, occasional false-positive Wassermann reactions, and increased serum angiotensin-converting enzyme (ACE). The possible role of these immunologic alterations in the pathogenesis of sarcoidosis remains unclear.[87]

Prognosis and Therapy

The great majority of patients with sarcoidosis require no therapy. In particular, up to 90% of patients with the acute bilateral hilar adenopathy syndrome spontaneously resolve. Overall, approximately 30% to 40% have complete clinical roentgenographic and physiologic resolution of the disease in a period of months to 1 to 2 years; another 30% to 40% are left with some residual symptoms, roentgenographic changes, or physiologic abnormality, usually involving the lungs, eyes, or skin; some 10% to 20% are left with severe impairment and disability, usually involving the lungs or the eyes; and sarcoid is the cause of death in about 10%. These figures are necessarily fairly gross approximations because reported data are skewed by their sources.[51,53–56,84,100–102]

Recent efforts have been directed at identifying the patient with active lung disease who presumably is at the greatest risk of developing further pulmonary physiologic impairment (*e.g.*, high-intensity alveolitis) and clinical deterioration. A high-intensity alveolitis has been defined as a level of T lymphocytes in bronchoalveolar lavage fluid of greater than 28% of the cells. The percentage of lymphocytes and the percentage of T lymphocytes correlate well with abnormal ^{67}Ga lung scans. Presumably these should return to normal if therapy results in improvement. However, as with IPF, documentation of clinical and physiologic improvement correlating with remission of the alveolitis has not been convincing. In fact, the lack of correlation among these parameters, even without treatment, is not surprising since pulmonary physiologic impairment can be expected from alveolitis, fibrosis, and granulomas.[60,103]

Angiotensin-converting enzyme (ACE) is elevated in sarcoid lymph nodes and mononuclear cells but not in lung tissue. Elevated serum ACE levels have been reported in Gaucher's disease, leprosy, asbestosis, berylliosis, primary biliary cirrhosis, Hodgkin's disease, silicosis, coccidioidomycosis, and tuberculosis in varying percentages in different centers; thus, the test is not diagnostically useful.[104,105] ACE was elevated in about half the sarcoidosis patients, with varying correlation with other evidence of disease activity. Serum ACE levels frequently decrease when corticosteroid therapy is given. There has been no correlation with BAL and ^{67}GA scans.[104]

Pulmonary Treatment. Controlled prospective studies do not support the efficacy of corticosteroids in preventing the development of fibrosis, or in altering physiologic changes or the ultimate course of the disease.[51,106] Although there is evidence of symptomatic and radiographic improvement with their use, documentation of physiologic improvement in controlled studies is not available.[109–110] In individuals with significant symptoms and physiologic abnormalities, especially with evidence of progression, corticosteroids are almost invariably recommended. When corticosteroid therapy is instituted, a regime similar to that described above for diffuse interstitial fibrosis is appropriate. The use of immunosuppressive and other agents has not been well studied.[8]

Extrapulmonary Treatment. Ocular sarcoidosis generally responds to the topical instillation of steroids. Systemic low-dose steroids will control hypercalcemia. While skin lesions frequently respond to topical steroids, low-dose systemic steroids may be necessary with troublesome or disfiguring lesions. Although controlled data are again not available, corticosteroids (along with antiarrhythmia agents[110]) are recommended for myocardial and central nervous system manifestations.[68,70]

Hydroxychloroquine may also be effective against skin lesions but has the potential of ocular toxicity. Immunosuppressive drugs have not been adequately studied.[51]

WEGENER'S GRANULOMATOSIS

Clinical Manifestations

Wegener's granulomatosis is a systemic disease of unknown etiology characterized by necrotizing granulomatous vasculitis of the upper and lower respiratory tract, focal and segmental glomerulonephritis, and widespread disseminated vasculitis involving small arteries and veins.[111,112] Prior to effective therapy, it ran a rapidly fatal course with an 82% mortality in 1 year, a 90% mortality in 2 years, and a mean survival of 5 months; the usual cause of death was renal failure.[113] A "limited" form of the disease which spares the kidney has had a more favorable course even without therapy.[114,115]

Wegener's granulomatosis fits approximately midway in the spectrum of granulomatosis and the necrotizing angiitides.[116–118] It must be differentiated from (1) polyarteritis nodosa, which usually involves the larger medium-sized arteries, less commonly involves the lungs, and does not cause necrotizing granuloma; (2) hypersensitivity angiitis, which is usually associated with a drug reaction, involves small arterioles with similar-appearing lesions, and does not produce granuloma; (3) the vasculitis of the collagen diseases, which may usually be differentiated clinically, tend to have more evidence of angiitis, and usually do not involve the upper and lower respiratory tract and kidney; (4) Goodpasture's syndrome, the pulmonary-renal syndrome with pulmonary hemorrhage and glomerulonephritis, which does not produce granuloma and can be identified by the presence of linear antiglomerular basement membrane deposits; (5) allergic granulomatosis, which usually occurs in an atopic individual having dense lung infiltration with eosinophils and often with peripheral eosinophilia, and is associated clinically with wheezing; (6) the specific infectious granulomatous diseases*, in which there may be granuloma and angiitis together in respiratory tract tissue, and which may involve the upper respiratory tract and, uncommonly, the kidney; (7) the nonspecific, noncaseating granulomatous diseases such as sarcoidosis and berylliosis, in which vasculitis is extremely rare; and (8) neoplastic disease, which may simulate the clinical presentation of Wegener's granulomatosis but which is definitive histologically.

* Identification of the organism is required for recognition, although the clinical pattern is usually different and, with infectious granuloma, vasculitis is generally limited to the area of granulomatous disease.

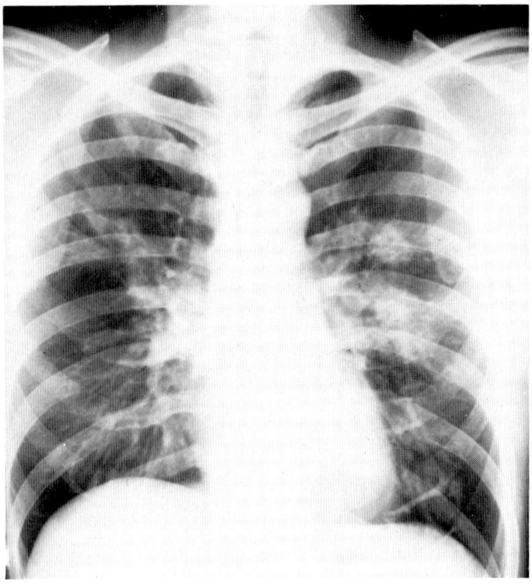

FIG. 13-9. Chest roentgenogram of a patient with Wegener's granulomatosis. Note the bilateral nodular densities and cavitation in the uppermost density on each side. Prior to therapy with cyclophosphamide, new nodular lesions appeared and some old ones cleared. This 45-year-old had sinus and renal involvement. The response to therapy was satisfactory.

The disease most commonly affects individuals in the fourth and fifth decades of life, but the age distribution is from infancy to the eighth decade. The usual presenting complaint is referable to the upper respiratory tract: persistent, often purulent rhinorrhea, nasal ulcerations with crusting, sinus drainage, pain, and bleeding. These symptoms are usually associated initially with respiratory tract symptoms including cough, purulent sputum production, hemoptysis, and pleuritic chest pain. There are usually constitutional symptoms of fever, which may be secondary to superimposed infection, and anorexia. Evidence of systemic vasculitis is commonly manifested by arthralgia or arthritis, skin lesions, otitis media, eye involvement, or neurologic abnormalities. Renal involvement is manifested by abnormal urinary sediment with or without functional impairment initially. There may be ulcerative lesions in the oral pharynx or larynx, and evidence of destruction of nasal cartilage with a "saddle nose." Eye involvement includes corneal and scleral ulcerations, keratitis, uveitis, proptosis, and pseudotumor of the orbit. Skin lesions include papules, vesicles, subcutaneous nodules, and ulcerations. The upper and lower respiratory tracts are almost always involved. Bronchostenosis with obstruction and recurring infection is common. The joints, skin, eye, nervous system, and middle ear are involved in 40% to 50% of patients. The heart is less often involved, as with myocarditis, pericarditis, or coronary vasculitis. Neurologic disease may result from direct extension of upper respiratory tract lesions, from the development of granulomas in the meninges or brain, and from vasculitis, which is most common and may manifest as polyneuritis or mononeuritis multiplex.[112]

The chest roentgenographic pattern characteristic of Wegener's granulomatosis is the presence of multiple, usually bilateral nodules of varying size that may change or disappear fairly rapidly; they frequently cavitate and may have thick, shaggy walls or thin ones; the nodules usually have discrete borders (Fig. 13-9). Endobronchial disease and pleural involvement have been reported.[120] Sinus films may show mucosal changes, air fluid levels (usually secondary to *Staphylococcus aureus* infection), or bony destruction.

The diagnosis requires the documentation of granulomatous disease and angiitis. This may be confirmed in tissue from the upper or lower respiratory tract, the skin, or the kidney. The kidney is less likely to have granuloma.

Management

While it appears that the "limited" form of the disease (without renal involvement) may be relatively indolent and not require therapy, the course of disease with renal involvement is characteristically rapidly progressive, resulting in a uremic death. Corticosteroids may ameliorate severe constitutional symptoms and local evidence of inflammation or vasculitis in the skin, eyes, joints, or pericardium; however, they do not alter the outcome. With renal involvement, the treatment of choice is a cytotoxic agent. The most experience has been obtained with cyclophosphamide, which has produced favorable results in up to 90% of patients, as manifested by reversal of upper and lower respiratory tract involvement, systemic evidence of vasculitis, and most importantly, control or even resolution of the renal lesion. The dosage regimen recommended is 1 to 2 mg per kg of body weight, orally, for about 2 weeks. The dosage in the responding patient is adjusted to maintain the white count above 3000/mm. If there is no response, the dose should be increased by 25 mg every two weeks until there is either a clinical response or drug toxicity. With fulminant disease involving the cerebrum, lung, peripheral nerves, or kidney, cyclophosphamide is recommended at a dose of 4 mg/kg of body weight per day, orally or intravenously, for 3 days; it should then be reduced to 1 mg to 2 mg/kg of body weight per day over 3 days. Thereafter, the program for nonfulminant disease should be followed. Corticosteroids (the equivalent of 60 mg/day of prednisone in divided doses) are also given until a response is seen. A rapid conversion to a single morning dose and then alternate day therapy for several weeks is recommended. It is recommended that therapy be continued for 1 year after complete resolution of disease activity, or longer if disease persists or resolves slowly. Less dramatic responses have also been obtained with alkylating agents, purine metabolites, and folic acid antagonists. The advisability of obtaining renal tissue to assess kidney involvement if renal function and urinalysis are persistently normal is still unresolved. In such circumstances, renal biopsies have occasionally been abnormal. The use of a cytotoxic agent to prevent progression in the absence of manifest renal disease has not been documented, although the concept is attractive.[119,121–124]

LYMPHOMATOID GRANULOMATOSIS

Clinical Manifestations

Lymphatoid granulomatosis almost always involves the lung, producing angiocentric and angiodestructive lesions with lymphoreticular proliferation and granuloma formation. The granuloma are less frequent and the vasculitis lacks the leukocytoclastic or fibrinoid necrotic features which are characteristic of Wegener's vasculitis. The clinical presentation is that of cough, often productive, fever, and dyspnea. The roentgenographic presentation is that of nonspecific, usually lower-lobe infiltrates that commonly assume a nodular configuration and frequently cavitate. Skin lesions (macular or nodular) and renal involvement are present in about one-half the patients. The central nervous system is involved in about 25%, and this may dominate the clinical picture; peripheral neuritis occurs in about 15%. The clinical presentation is quite similar to that of Wegener's granulomatosis. The following manifestations contrast with those of Wegener's granulomatosis: (1) rare involvement of upper airways and sinus tracts; (2) nodular renal parenchymal infiltration; (3) leukopenia; (4) a normal sedimentation rate; and (5) anergy. Histologically, the lesions simulate malignant lymphoma and some cases have progressed to lymphoma, involving many organs. Some physicians have identified those patients with a more benign course and good response to chlorambucil as having "benign lymphocytic angiitis and granulomatosis."[123,124]

Management

Lymphomatoid granulomatosis does not seem to respond as well to therapy as does Wegener's granulomatosis, particularly when neurologic involvement is present and large numbers of atypical lymphoreticular cells are seen in lung biopsies. However, early initiation of corticosteroids and cyclophosphamide, as in Wegener's, is recommended.[117,118,123–126]

EOSINOPHILIC GRANULOMA

Clinical Manifestations

Eosinophilic granuloma of the lung is characterized by an interstitial granuloma composed of moderately large, pale histiocytes and eosinophiles, and an arteriolitis with eosinophiles. This histocytic process with eosinophiles then involves bronchioles, alveolar ducts, and alveolar septa, causing their destruction; the proliferative endarteritis leads to necrosis. End-stage diffuse interstitial fibrosis with cyst formation is

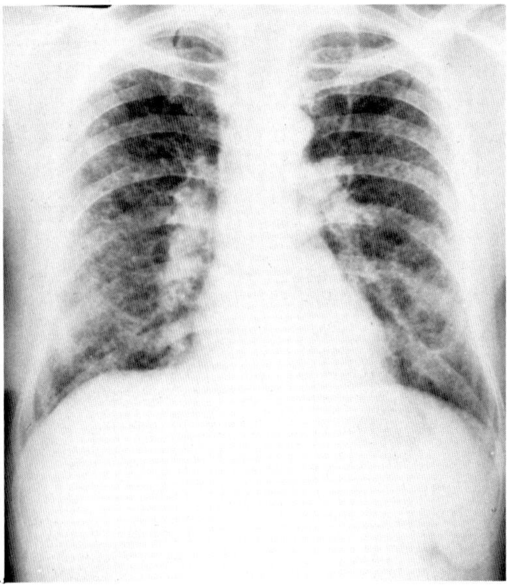

FIG. 13-10. Chest roentgenogram of a patient with eosinophilic granuloma. Note the bilateral nodular pattern with multiple cystic spaces (honeycombing). This man was 37 years old at the time of diagnosis. He had a modest nonproductive cough and no limitation with normal activities. He has remained clinically, roentgenographically, and physiologically stable for 20 years.

a prototype of honeycomb lung.[127] Intracytoplasmic rodlike structures of unknown significance have been identified with the electron microscope.[128] On the basis of similar histologic characteristics, Lichtenstein classified eosinophilic granuloma, a relatively benign disease involving bone, lung, and occasionally other sites, in a spectrum with the progressively more severe Hand–Schüller–Christian disease and the rapidly fatal Letterer-Siwe disease seen in infants; he designated all of these as histiocytosis-X.[129] Subsequently, others have had difficulty in fitting patients into this classification,[130] or consider it unwarranted.[131] The etiology is unknown; it has been considered a hypersensitivity reaction, a response to an infectious agent (not identified), or even a form of malignancy.[127–131] With current information, it seems most reasonable to consider this disease to be a specific entity which involves (1) bone or lung alone; (2) lung and bone; or (3) lung, bone, and hypothalamus, usually with diabetes insipidus (about 20%), and rarely panhypopituitarism. Occasional, involvement of other organs is seen, including the oropharynx, vulva, thyroid, prostate, and gastrointestinal tract.[131,132]

The radiographic pattern is that of fairly discrete, small nodular densities that have a tendency for greater involvement of the upper lobes (Fig. 13-10). A pattern of nodular and reticular densities may be seen. A very coarse reticular pattern representing multiple cystic lesions of varying sizes—a honeycomb appearance—is characteristic but not pathognomonic. Lung volumes are usually maintained. Mediastinal and hilar adenopathy has been reported in one series.[133] Pneumothorax is a complication in approximately 25%, of cases, again a characteristic finding,[134] but one that occurs with other diffuse diseases as well. The bone lesions are osteolytic.

Approximately 25% of patients are identified because of an abnormal roentgenogram. The disease most commonly affects males in the third and fourth decades. The usual symptoms are a nonproductive cough, chest pain that may reflect a pneumothorax or lesions in ribs, and dyspnea; nonspecific constitutional symptoms of fatigue, malaise, weight loss, or, less commonly, fever may be present. The course of the disease is quite variable, but spontaneous resolution or relatively mild symptomatic disease appears to be most common. Progressive pulmonary disease resulting in cor pulmonale and respiratory failure does occur.[128,132,135]

The characteristic physiologic pattern is that of a decreased diffusing capacity associated with hypoxemia; there is a tendency toward maintenance of fairly normal lung volumes and static compliance, which may reflect the combined processes of fibrosis and cyst formation. On occasion, obstructive airways disease may be a prominent feature.[105,136]

Management

Specific therapy for eosinophilic granuloma has not been defined. In an uncommon disease characterized by remissions and exacerbations and in which so-called end-stage fibrosis may be present early, or active histologic lesions (histiocytes and eosinophils rather than fibrosis) may be identified late, evaluation of responses to therapy is difficult. Since spontaneous remissions and nonprogressive disease are most common, it is appropriate to limit therapeutic trials to those who have significant symptoms and evidence of progression.[136] Corticosteroids have on occasion been helpful, and there may be a role for antimetabolites.[128,131,137]

CONNECTIVE TISSUE DISEASES

Classification of the connective tissue, or collagen vascular, disease is not entirely satisfactory and continues to change. This section deals with the vasculitis end of the spectrum[138]; the more granulomatous histologic patterns have already been reviewed.

RHEUMATOID DISEASE

The pulmonary involvement in patients with rheumatoid arthritis may affect airways, pleura, or lung parenchyma. The major clinical concern is the differentiation of these manifestations of a systemic disease from that of a superimposed process, particularly infection. The pleuropulmonary manifestations may precede the onset of arthritis or appear years later; males are more frequently affected than females.

Airways Involvement

Patients with hoarseness and occasionally dysphagia may have cricoarytenoid arthritis. Deformation of the larynx can be seen by means of direct laryngoscopy or at the time of fiber optic bronchoscopy.

Obstruction to expiratory air flow may be more common in patients with rheumatoid arthritis, particularly in cigarette smokers, and has been implicated as a cause of somewhat higher rates of lung infection.[139,140]

Pleural Involvement

The most common pulmonary finding in rheumatoid disease is nonspecific pleural scarring, which may correlate with a history of previous pleuritic chest pain. Pleural effusion has been reported in about 5% of retrospective studies of patients with definite or classic rheumatoid arthritis.[141,142] The patient is commonly asymptomatic but may have pleuritic pain and dyspnea. The pleural fluid is an exudate with a high protein level, a low *p*H, and a very low sugar level (i.e., less than 25 mg.%).[143,144] The cells are usually lymphocytes, but a polymorphonuclear response may occur.[145] "Rheumatoid arthritis" cells may be seen in microscopic examination of the fluid.[146] There is a unique picture with the Papanicolaou technique: a background of orange or red granular material, large, elongated cells, and giant, round or oval multinucleated cells.[147] Pleural biopsy usually discloses a nonspecific inflammation, but rheumatoid nodules are occasionally found.[148] The major concern is to search for specific infectious processes including tuberculosis, especially when immunosuppressive drugs have been used; infectious empyemas occurred in 50% of one series of rheumatoid pleural effusions.[149] Pneumothorax may also occur (see also Chap. 12).

Parenchymal Involvement

The most common form of parenchymal involvement is that of a diffuse nonspecific interstitial fibrosis, both roentgenographically and pathologically. Although Ellman proposed the term *rheumatoid disease* in 1947[150] to recognize its systemic nature, and Rubin in 1957 commented on the potential role of collagen disease (including rheumatoid disease) in the development of diffuse interstitial fibrosis,[20] this relationship has been a subject of controversy.[151]

In a prospective study of 41 consecutive patients with definite or classic rheumatoid disease who were seen for arthritis, we found a 41% incidence of abnormalities in diffusion studies, usually associated with a decreased vital capacity, decreased total lung capacity, and arterial hypoxemia; only half had roentgenographic abnormalities (6% parenchymal). Although 6 of the 17 patients with physiologic changes admitted to dyspnea on specific questioning, none volunteered such information. Each of the eight lung biopsies performed had nonspecific interstitial fibrosis; over 2 years there were slight decreases in diffusing capacity without new respiratory symptoms. Thus it would appear that physiologic diffuse disease is common, although often of uncertain clinical significance.[152–154]

Less commonly, diffuse interstitial fibrosis may be progressive, with dyspnea, cough, roentgenographic changes of volume loss or honeycombing, and hypoxemia with cor pulmonale and respiratory failure.[155]

Parenchymal involvement may also take the form of nodules,[156] and these may cavitate ("necrobiotic nodules").[157] Similar nodules may appear in association with the pneumoconioses as described by Caplan (see Pneumoconioses). Pulmonary arteritis and hypertension rarely may be the dominant manifestation of rheumatoid lung disease.[138]

The major clinical problem is to exclude superimposed infection: bacterial, mycobacterial, and opportunistic organisms. With the nodular form there is concern about tumor. Despite thorough evaluation, a definitive diagnosis is commonly obtained only by lung biopsy.

SYSTEMIC LUPUS ERYTHEMATOSUS (SLE)

Pleuropulmonary involvement in SLE occurs in 50% to 90% of various series.[138,158–160] The signal symptom of this systemic collagen vascular disease with polyserositis is often pleuritic pain. The identification of the etiology of pleuropulmonary disease in known SLE is most difficult because the disease itself may be responsible for changes in the lung and pleura resulting from pericardial disease, heart failure, uremia, or the nephrotic syndrome. Fever is common, superimposed infections at some point in time are almost invariable, and the predisposition to such infections is enhanced by use of immunosuppressive drugs.

Pleural Involvement

As a manifestation of polyserositis, pleural effusions have been reported in 40% to 60% of patients with SLE. They are more commonly bilateral. The fluid is an exudate with elevated protein, but the glucose is normal.[138,161]

Pulmonary Involvement

The most common roentgenographic abnormality is that of patchy nonspecific densities that may represent either acute infections or the underlying disease process (Fig. 13-11). Basilar linear or platelike atelectasis is also frequent and may be transient.[159] The roentgenographic pattern of diffuse interstitial fibrosis is uncommon, being estimated at less than 3%; it may progress to honeycombing and volume loss.[162] Pleural effusions and pulmonary infiltrates are seen in about half the cases of drug-induced SLE.[138,163]

Symptoms of dyspnea on exertion, cough, and mucoid sputum production are very common; they were present in more than half of a group of patients undergoing physiologic studies, over 60% of whom had a history of pneumonia or pleurisy.[163]

Physiologic surveys of SLE confirm the presence of restrictive disease as manifested by a decreased diffusing capacity in about 80% of patients, decreased lung volume in 65%, and reduced arterial oxygen saturation (below 95%) in about 55%.[160,163,164] Diaphragmatic dysfunction attributed to a diffuse myopathy of the diaphragm has been described. These patients have supine dyspnea, which is a characteristic feature of diaphragmatic paralysis.[165] Thus, physiologic evidence of disease is common.

The respective roles of repeated, localized, usually infectious parenchymal insults, pulmonary embolism, secondary changes due to uremia and heart failure, the contribution from pleural involvement, and diffuse parenchymal disease per se (although not roentgenographically common) have not been defined. The pathologic pattern is usually that of nonspecific diffuse interstitial fibrosis, commonly with evidence of superinfection or other changes associated with a terminal event.[166–170]

Acute lupus pneumonitis has been reported in those patients with exacerbation of their disease process. These patients have high antinuclear antibody titers, reduced levels of circulatory complement, and tissue binding of immunoglobulins or complement, suggesting an acute, immune mediated lung injury.[167,168] Occasionally, patients develop extensive nodular lymphocytic infiltrates that may be confused with lymphoma of the lung; these have been described as pseudolymphoma.[169]

PROGRESSIVE SYSTEMIC SCLEROSIS (SCLERODERMA)

Clinical and roentgenographic pulmonary involvement usually occurs after there is evidence of well-established systemic disease. The most common complaint is dyspnea in about two-thirds of patients; cough and sputum production may be present; cor pulmonale and respiratory failure occur, but death is usually related to renal or cardiac involvement. Basilar rales are heard in about 50% of patients.

The roentgenographic pattern is that of nonspecific diffuse interstitial fibrosis that tends to involve the lower lung fields predominantly. Pleural changes may be present. Pathologically, the picture is that of diffuse interstitial fibrosis that may be severe, with honeycombing; there is also prominent involvement of the pulmonary vasculature.[173]

The physiologic profile is that of restriction with decreased lung volumes, diffusing capacity, static compliance, and arterial oxygen tension. These findings usually antedate the onset of symptoms or roentgenographic abnormality.[174] We have commonly noted an unexplained increase in residual volume, either absolute or relative, as determined with body plethysmography. While a potential contribution from the thickening of skin over the chest wall has been considered, normal chest wall compliance has been reported.[175] Elevated pulmonary artery pressures and increased pulmonary vascular resistance are common. A group of patients who develop rapidly progressive respiratory failure with severe pulmonary hypertension has been identified.[176] Pulmonary hypertension without pulmonary fibrosis has been reported in the CREST syndrome (calcinosis, Raynaud's phenomenon, esophageal dysfunction, sclerodactyly, and telangiectasia), a supposedly benign form of scleroderma.[177]

Esophageal motility abnormalities are commonly associated with pulmonary aspiration. A roentgenographic pattern of lower lobe diffuse interstitial fibrosis and a widened esophagus with an air fluid level is strongly supportive of the diagnosis of scleroderma.

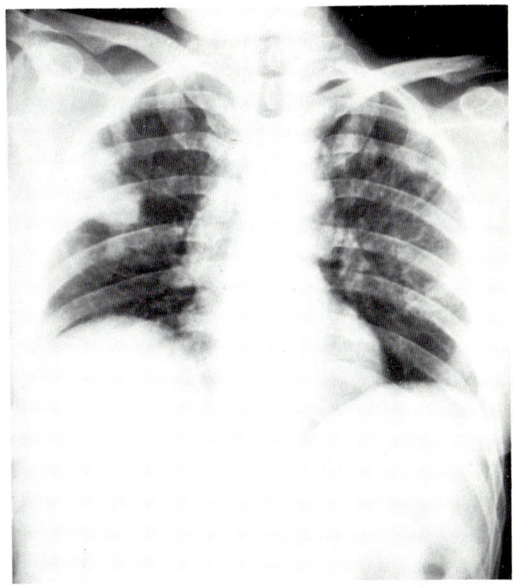

FIG. 13-11. Chest roentgenogram of a patient with systemic lupus erythematosus (SLE). There are bilateral nodular shadows throughout both lung fields and an infiltrate in the anterior segment of the right upper lobe. The costophrenic angles are blunted bilaterally. This 47-year-old woman with known SLE had been treated for recurrent systemic sepsis and was receiving corticosteroids. Brushings from the right upper lobe at fiberoptic bronchoscopy identified acid-fast mycobacteria.

Although an increased incidence of alveolar (bronchiolar) carcinoma in persons with scleroderma has been suggested,[175,178] others have not confirmed these findings.[171–173]

Specific therapy for this disease is not available. Corticosteroids do not appear to be of value for either the systemic or pulmonary manifestations.

POLYMYOSITIS/DERMATOMYOSITIS

Polymyositis is a diffuse inflammatory disorder of striated muscle that causes symmetric proximal extremity, neck, and pharyngeal weakness.

It is called dermatomyositis if the skin is involved. It is often associated with malignancy. The lung may be involved owing to aspiration or through quite uncommon nonspecific interstitial fibrosis. The latter has been reported to respond to corticosteroid therapy; immunosuppressive agents have also been used.[138,179,180]

SJÖGREN'S (SICCA) SYNDROME

Sjögren's, or sicca, syndrome overlaps with rheumatoid arthritis, systemic lupus erythematosus, and the other collagen diseases. It is characterized by exocrine gland dysfunction producing dryness. Glandular involvement can lead to keratoconjunctivitis sicca. Oral dryness and parotid gland swelling are common; severe dental caries occur. Involvement of the upper and lower respiratory tract glands results in persistant hoarseness, a nonproductive cough, recurrent upper respiratory tract infections, airways obstruction, and pneumonia. Lymphoid interstitial infiltrates in the lung and nonspecific diffuse interstitial fibrosis are occasional features.[138,181,182] Malignant lymphoma develops more commonly in patients with this syndrome.

POLYARTERITIS NODOSA

An uncommon systemic vasculitis, polyarteritis nodosa infrequently involves the lung.[138,183] It is characterized by a vasculitis of the medium-sized arteries and surrounding tissues (periarteritis). The roentgenographic pattern most commonly reported is that of patchy infiltrates that may be transient; nodules may occur and rarely cavitate; there may be cardiac enlargement or venous engorgement and rarely evidence of pulmonary infarction.[184] Intractable wheezing suggests the diagnosis, especially with evidence of systemic involvement. Hypertension, renal failure, abdominal pains, skin lesions, peripheral neuritis, unexplained fever, peripheral blood eosinophilia, and generalized weakness are among the common systemic manifestations.[138,185,186] Diagnosis usually requires histologic documentation from an involved extrapulmonary site. Circulating immune complexes, cryoglobulins, hepatitis B_s antigens, and reduced levels of complement all point to immunologic mechanisms for this poorly understood disease. The mortality rate is high, with approximately 50% of patients surviving at 5 years.[186]

Treatment with high-dose corticosteroids may provide symptomatic improvement. High-dose steroids and cytotoxic drugs (cyclophosphamide) combined have been reported to induce remissions of the disease. Treatment must be carefully monitored and generally prolonged.[187]

OTHER COLLAGEN VASCULAR DISORDERS

Some patients have features characteristic of several of the collagen disorders for which the terms "mixed connective tissue disease" and "overlap syndrome" have been used. The pulmonary involvement is similar to that seen in the connective tissue disorders described above.[188]

Ankylosing spondylitis may cause a restrictive pattern owing to spinal involvement. In addition, upper lobe fibrosis and bulla or cavities are seen in some patients. These spaces may become superinfected with mycobacteria and aspergilli or other fungi (188a; see also Chap. 6).

In Behçet's disease, bilateral pulmonary infiltrates with or without pleurisy and hemoptysis may occur in conjunction with disease exacerbation. Superior vena cava thrombosis has been reported in up to one-fourth of patients.[138]

Relapsing polychondritis commonly involves the upper respiratory tract and trachea. Tracheal stenosis may occur along with hoarseness and saddle-nose deformities. Pneumonia is frequent.[138]

ANGIOIMMUNOBLASTIC LYMPHADENOPATHY (AIL)

Angioimmunoblastic lymphadenopathy (AIL) affects older individuals with the mean age in the late sixties. The patients note acute onset of rapidly enlarging lymph nodes which may be tender and associated with malaise, fever, and weight loss. These patients appear acutely ill.

Often a generalized pruritic maculopapular or morbilliform rash precedes the acute onset by several months. Hepatosplenomegaly is usually present, along with anemia, a positive Coombs' test, and hypergammaglobulinemia. The features suggest a mixture of neoplastic and immunologic disorders. The chest roentgenogram reveals mediastinal and hilar lymphadenopathy. Although initially considered uncommon, diffuse parenchymal infiltrates with cough, dyspnea, and symptomatic pleural effusions are being reported more frequently.[189–191] The characteristic pathologic findings are best seen in the lymph nodes, athough they are present in other organs including the lung. Lymph nodes show capsular, pericapsular, and trabecular areas of infiltration with lymphocytes, plasma cells, and immunoblasts. There is marked small blood vessel proliferation that alters nodal architecture. Eosinophils, histiocytes, and giant cells are commonly found.

Initially, AIL was considered to be a benign deficiency of T-cell regulatory function resulting in a proliferative and auto-aggressive B-cell response; however, it progressed to malignancy in a third of one series. A similarity to the collagen vascular diseases is also evident.

Patients may have a rapidly progressive fatal course lasting less than 20 months or a relatively indolent course lasting 2 to 5 years. Corticosteroids and cytotoxic drugs have been recommended for patients with aggressive disease.[189–191]

PULMONARY HEMORRHAGE AND NEPHRITIS

In 1919, Goodpasture recognized the association of pulmonary hemorrhage and nephritis in a young man following influenza; in 1964, Benoit and coworkers reviewed 52 cases of what appeared to be a specific nosologic entity.[192] It occurred 5 times more commonly in males in their early twenties. The initial complaint was that of one or more episodes of hemoptysis followed by a latent period of 1 to 9 months, at which time progressive acute glomerulonephritis led either to uremia and death over a period of about 6 months, or to pulmonary hemorrhage where the average survival was less than 3 months. Subsequently, the linear deposition of IgG and beta-1-C globulin has been reported almost invariably on the glomerular basement membrane, and often on the alveolar capillary basement membrane, with antibasement membrane antibody (ABMA) in the serum[193–196] (see Table 13-3 for an overview of the immune mechanisms involved in lung disease). This immunologic marker has led to a reasonable classification of the various presentations of pulmonary hemorrhage (lung purpura) with or without nephritis: (1) Goodpasture's syndrome, in which there is pulmonary hemorrhage and glomerulonephritis with linear deposition, usually of IgG and beta-1-C globulin along the glomerular and alveolar basement membrane*; and (2) idiopathic pulmonary hemorrhage, in which there is pulmonary hemorrhage without vasculitis or granuloma, a histologically normal kidney without antibasement membrane antibody, and no ABMA in the serum.[197]

TABLE 13-3. Immunopathologic Mechanisms in Lung Disease

Type of Reaction	Major clinical Manifestation
I. IgE-dependent, release of chemical mediators	Bronchial asthma
II. Cytotoxic, tissue-specific antibody, with injury to basement membranes	Pulmonary hemorrhage and nephritis
III. Immune complex disease, local tissue reaction	Bronchial asthma, allergic alveolitis
IV. Cell-mediated, delayed hypersensitivity	Graft rejection, granulomatous tissue changes

GOODPASTURE'S SYNDROME

The following are the criteria to establish a diagnosis of Goodpasture's syndrome: (1) pulmonary hemorrhage (diffuse bilateral infiltrates, hemoptysis); (2) anemia; (3) glomerulonephritis, and (4) antiglomerular basement antibody (AGBMA).

* Goodpasture's syndrome is also termed antibasement membrane antibody-induced glomerulonephritis and pulmonary hemorrhage.

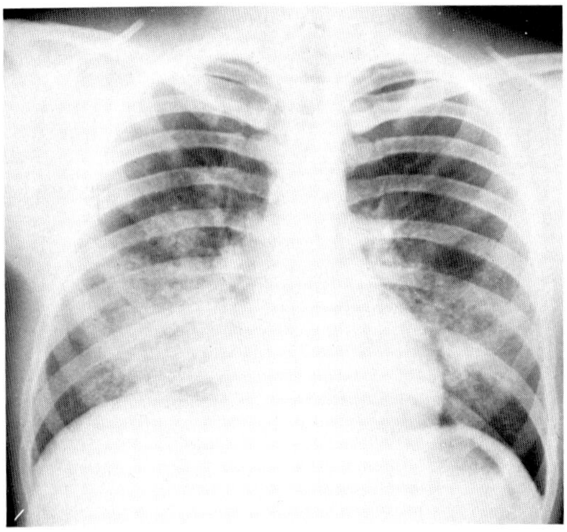

FIG. 13-12. Chest roentgenogram of a patient with pulmonary hemorrhage and nephritis. The bilateral fluffy infiltrate was predominantly perihilar. This 19-year-old man had an initial episode of slight hemoptysis 2 months earlier. At this time he had moderate hemoptysis and dyspnea; he was anemic and uremic.

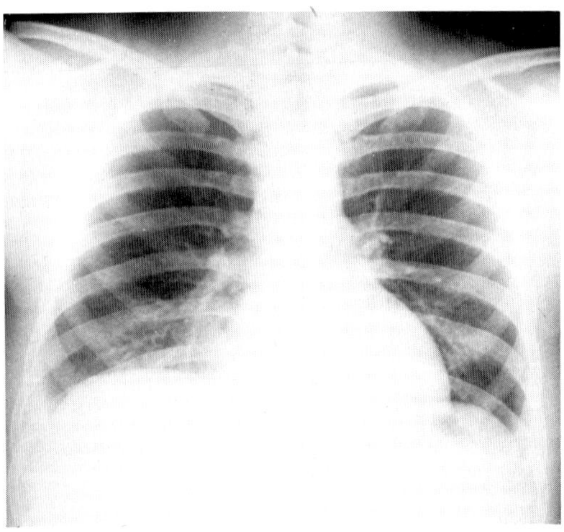

FIG. 13-13. Chest roentgenogram of the patient shown in Figure 13-12, taken 11 days later. There has been clearing of the infiltrates with control of the bleeding. There is residual reticular and nodular disease in both lower lobes. Despite continued prednisone and the addition of azathioprine, the patient died 1 month later.

While initially seen more frequently in young males, the mean age in reported series has risen from 21 to 30 years; patients have been identified in their late seventies, and the male predominance has been reduced to 2:1. In collected series, on first admission to the hospital, more than 90% of persons with Goodpasture's syndrome have hemoptysis, 75% have dyspnea; about 50% have fatigue, weakness and cough; and about 25% have a history of prior upper respiratory tract infection, nausea, vomiting, chills, or fever. Pallor and rales are common; hypertension, abnormal fundi, and liver and spleen enlargement are sometimes noted. Anemia is almost always present, averaging about 8 g/dl; azotemia is found in about 75%, and an abnormal urine (proteinuria, microscopic hematuria, granular casts, and occasionally, gross blood) in about 90%. The sputum contains hemosiderin-laden macrophages.

The chest roentgenogram is abnormal in about 90% of cases.[198] The early roentgenographic findings include patchy, acinar infiltrates that extend from the hilum and involve predominantly the lower and middle lobes; there may also be air bronchograms. This is the pattern of bleeding into the alveoli. Over 3 to 4 days, the pattern becomes more reticular and may clear entirely over 2 weeks (Figs. 13-12 and 13-13). With recurrent hemorrhage, diffuse, more linear shadows develop and resolution of acute hemorrhage is incomplete.

The immunopathologic hallmark of the disease can be identified in renal tissue by the linear deposition of IgG on the basement membrane; rarely, IgA has been found. Because of background immunufluorescence, this may be more difficult to demonstrate in the lung. Deposition of complement is seen in about 75% of cases, and antitubular basement membrane antibody in about 50%. The antibody should be eluted with acid citrate to avoid false-positive readings which may be found in the presence of diabetes, autolysis, a transplanted kidney, or systemic lupus erythematosis. Some laboratories report that the pattern is so distinctive that elution is not necessary. Alternatively, circulating antibody can be identified with radioimmune assay (94%) or indirect immunofluorescence (89%).

Nonlinear deposition of IgG has been reported with pulmonary hemorrhage and nephritis, and in patients who start with AGBMA-mediated nephritis and develop immune-complex nephritis (or vice versa). It has been estimated that 3% to 16% of all cases of glomerulonephritis are AGBMA-mediated; about half of these have a clinical picture compatible with Goodpasture's syndrome. The immunopathologic findings with the appropriate clinical picture usually distinguish this syndrome from systemic lupus erythematosus, microscopic polyarteritis, cryglobulinemia, Schönlein-Henoch purpura, uremic pneumonitis, immune complex glomerulonephritis, and idiopathic pulmonary hemorrhage.[197–204]

The lung lesion is characterized histologically by intra-alveolar hemorrhage with many hemosiderin-laden macrophages; with recurrent hemorrhage, diffuse interstitial fibrosis develops. The kidney lesion is that of acute glomerulonephritis. Cases are reported in which the urinalysis is normal and the renal biopsy documents focal glomerulonephritis, or in which a normal biopsy histologically had ABMA deposition.[205] There is a report of the identification of viral-like particles in renal epithelial cells.[206]

Management

There are no controlled studies to evaluate the treatment of Goodpasture's syndrome. The use of corticosteroids to control pulmonary hemorrhage has increased the median survival from 3.3 to 5.3 months. With the use of steroids and occasionally dialysis or renal transplantation, a mean survival of 12.7 months was calculated. Twelve of sixteen patients survived for 1 week to 5 years with the use of bilateral nephrectomy, transplantation, and dialysis. For the last several years, greater survival rates have been reported with the use of corticosteroids, cytotoxic agents, and plasmapheresis.[198,207–210] Therapy should be started *before* severe renal disease occurs (*i.e.*, creatinine levels of 2–5 mg%). Plasmapheresis reduces circulating AGBMA (although AGBMA is pathogenetically important, serum levels do not correlate with disease activity; cessation of pulmonary hemorrhage with clamping of the renal vessels at nephrectomy suggests other mediators). Usually, about 5000 cc of plasma is exchanged for 4000 cc of 5% serum albumin or plasma protein fraction and 500 ml of fresh frozen plasma over 3 hours; about 11 exchanges have been used in each series. The most commonly used cytotoxic agent is cyclophosphamide, 2 mg/kg/day initially (some believe intermittent intravenous dosing is more effective). The cytotoxic agent is continued for about 1 year (or 3–4 months beyond the disappearance of AGBMA from serum with clinically quiescent disease). Prednisone, 1 mg/kg/day, is given concomitantly with the cytotoxic agent. The dose of prednisone can be reduced after pulmonary hemorrhage ceases. For massive pulmonary hemorrhage, the equivalent of 3–3.5 gm of prednisone per day in divided doses has been recommended. Because spontaneous remissions have been reported, some physicians withhold therapy in mild disease until progression occurs.[207–210] Following the diffusing capacity may help differentiate hemorrhage from other causes of lung infiltrations. In the presence of diffuse pulmonary bleeding, the diffusing capacity increases about 50% from the usually low baseline level seen in renal failure.[210a]

IDIOPATHIC PULMONARY HEMOSIDEROSIS

As described prior to immunofluorescent studies, idiopathic pulmonary hemosiderosis occurred most commonly in children under 10 years of age and usually had a relatively slow onset characterized by recurrent hemoptysis and an indolent course, with a considerably better prognosis than Goodpasture's syndrome. However, the disease has also been reported in adults, and glomerulonephritis has been reported in some patients. It appears inevitable that there has been some crossover with Goodpasture's syndrome in reporting this disease, owing to the variable course of Goodpasture's syndrome, the absence of abnormal urinalysis even with nephritis, and the presence of normal kidney histology with ABMA. Further studies using immunofluorescent techniques may better define what appears to be separate entity in young children.[211]

Several recent reports of pulmonary hemorrhage in patients with occupational exposure to resins containing trimellitic anhydride suggest that inhaled substances may be a factor. No circulating immune complexes or antibasement membrane antibodies were identified in these patients.[212]

Corticosteroid and immunosuppressive drugs have been used in the management of this syndrome.

PULMONARY INFILTRATES WITH EOSINOPHILIA

EOSINOPHILIC PNEUMONIA

Chronic eosinophilic pneumonia is characterized by alveolar filling with eosinophiles, large mononuclear cells, and infiltration of the interstitium with these cells.[213] The characteristic roentgenographic pattern has been described as a "photographic negative" of pulmonary edema: dense pneumonic peripheral infiltrates that spare the perihilar areas. Localized infiltrates may also occur.[214,215] In individuals without asthma, the clinical presentation is that of a productive cough, weight loss, and dyspnea; there may be fever. The chest roentgenogram is more apt to show patchy localized disease, usually peripheral in location.

More commonly, the presentation is that of asthma for the first time, high fever, night sweats, weight loss, mucoid sputum production, and severe dyspnea. Physiologically there is restriction with decreased volumes, decreased diffusing capacity, and hypoxemia. The diagnosis is made histologically. The response to corticosteroid therapy has been good.[215]

HYPEREOSINOPHILIC SYNDROME

Eosinophilic pneumonia appears to be distinct from the rare hypereosinophilic syndrome, characterized by multiple organ involvement that includes the nervous system, heart, liver, kidneys, and skin. Although hypersensitivity to drugs has been suggested, the etiology is uncertain. The peripheral leucocyte count may range as high as 50,000 with 70% eosinophils. The prognosis for patients with this condition is poor, with a 75%, 3 year mortality. Corticosteroids and hydroxyurea have been used with some success in treatment programs.[216–219]

LOEFFLER'S SYNDROME

Transient idiopathic nonsegmental pulmonary infiltrates associated with cough and a peripheral blood eosinophilia were first described by Loeffler—hence, the designation *Loeffler's syndrome.* The condition is also described as benign pulmonary infiltrates with eosinophilia (PIE syndrome).[220] Light and electron microscopic study of one case demonstrated an interstitial eosinophilic pneumonia without tissue necrosis or vasculitis; the alveolar capillary membranes were intact and there were no immune deposits.[221] With increasing diagnostic skills, specific etiologies for this presentation or for more chronic forms of PIE have limited the use of this term.

TROPICAL EOSINOPHILIA

Tropical eosinophilia is the term applied to pulmonary infiltrations believed to be caused by microfilaria. Other parasites may also cause pulmonary infiltrates with eosinophilia—for example, ascaris, strongyloides, ancylostoma, and *Toxocara canis* (see Chap. 8).

Eosinophilia and pulmonary infiltration with various syndromes of the granulomatous angiitides and bronchopulmonary aspergillosis are described in Chapter 9. Numerous drugs which may result in infiltrates and eosinophilia are discussed below under Drug-Induced Lung Disease. The PIE syndrome may be classified as simple pulmonary eosinophilia (Loeffler's), pulmonary eosinophilia with asthma, tropical pulmonary eosinophilia, and pulmonary eosinophilia with periarteritis nodosa.[222]

PULMONARY ALVEOLAR PROTEINOSIS

Clinical Manifestations

Pulmonary alveolar proteinosis is a rare disorder of unknown etiology characterized by a diffuse bilateral pulmonary infiltrate, usually of the so-called acinar pattern in a butterfly distribution (Fig. 13-14), and the intra-alveolar deposition of an amorphous lipoprotein material. In the initial description of 27 patients by Rosen and coworkers, the pathologic pattern was noted to be so distinctive that it was considered a new disease,[223] although this has been questioned.[224] Since the lung alone is involved, it has been postulated that the disorder represents a response to an inhaled substance, but such a substance has not been identified. It has been postulated that this response may represent an excess production of surfactant that may be altered in nature. In association with an alveolar capillary membrane injury, plasma with its fibrogen may inactivate surfactant; these changes in surfactant may interfere with the normal alveolar clearing mechanisms including the alveolar macrophage. It is believed the macrophage abnormalities, which include a defect in bacterial phagocytosis, are secondary.[225–229]

Pulmonary alveolar proteinosis is more common in males and appears most frequently in the fourth decade. Commonly, the individual is asymptomatic and the lesion is a roentgenographic discovery. Symptoms of a usually quite mild, nonproductive cough associated with fatigue, malaise, weight loss, and occasionally fever may be found. Characteristically, the roentgenographic pattern is far more impressive than the symptoms. Physical examination is usually normal; specifically, altered breath sounds or rales are unusual. Clubbing has been reported.

Pulmonary function studies demonstrate a restrictive defect with severe hypoxemia resulting from a large physiologic shunt. Serum lactic dehydrogenase levels are generally elevated.[230]

Although sputum is usually absent and quite difficult to induce, the use of a series of special stains lends strong support to the diagnosis. The alveolar material is periodic acid–Schiff positive, Alcian-green and mucicarmine negative, pale blue or green with faint pink floccular regions with colloidal iron, and green with orange particles with Masson stain. In most patients, a lung biopsy is necessary to make the diagnosis. The alveoli are filled with a granular, flocculent material with acicular spaces; it stains pink with hematoxylin and eosin. This material is periodic acid–Schiff positive, and it can be seen in swollen alveolar macrophages. The interstitial space is usually normal, although varying amounts of interstitial fibrosis may be present with severe disease. This intra-alveolar pattern is quite similar to that of *Pneumocystis carinii* infection, which is identified by staining the organisms with a silver methenamine stain.

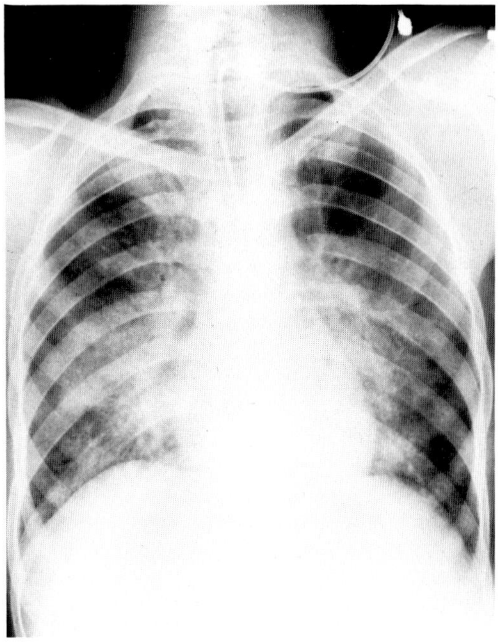

FIG. 13-14. Chest roentgenogram of a patient with pulmonary alveolar proteinosis. There are bilateral fluffy, confluent, predominantly perihilar densities that simulate pulmonary edema. A catheter for attempted segmental lavage is seen entering the left mainstem bronchus. (This form of lavage was unsuccessful; intubation with lavage of a *full* lung is preferable.) This 22-year-old had a nonproductive cough and dyspnea with heavy exercise. The lesions cleared over several years without therapy.

Pneumocystis carinii pneumonia generally occurs in the immune-compromised host, and is associated with dyspnea, nonproductive cough, and fever in the majority of patients. This diagnosis should be made as early as possible in order to institute therapy (see discussion of parasitic infections, Chap. 8).

Approximately one-third of reported patients with alveolar proteinosis have cleared spontaneously; another third have remained quite stable, usually with few or no symptoms; and about one-third died in earlier series.[231] Death not uncommonly has been related to superinfection, particularly with *Nocardia*.

Management

The only effective treatment of pulmonary alveolar proteinosis is pulmonary lavage. The technique has been refined and its physiologic consequences during the procedure reported. It appears to be quite effective in reversing the clinical and physiologic manifestations of the disease for variable periods of time. It is recommended only for those patients with progressive symptomatic disease.[230,232–234] A recent case report indicated successful treatment by aerosolized trypsin.[235]

PULMONARY ALVEOLAR MICROLITHIASIS

Pulmonary alveolar microlithiasis is characterized by the intra-alveolar deposition of microliths of calcium and phosphorus. It has a characteristic roentgenographic picture of a myriad of small nodules (3 mm or less) with the density of calcium; they may be so profuse that the lung appears diffusely white, especially over the lower lobes.

There is a strong familial occurrence, particularly in siblings. Patients may be asymptomatic, or they may present with a stable chronic cough with or without mild dyspnea, or slowly progressive dyspnea with fibrosis leading to cor pulmonale. The physiologic pattern is restrictive.[236–239]

Metastatic calcifications of the lungs may occur in a variety of diseases associated with prolonged hypercalcemia. These rarely result in clinically or radiographically significant changes, but postmortem examination may reveal extensive calcium deposits around blood vessels and in alveolar septae. Patients with renal failure undergoing chronic hemodialysis frequently demonstrate these deposits in the lungs.[240–243]

INHALATION LUNG DISEASES

The lung may respond adversely to a variety of inhaled materials such as infectious agents, inorganic and organic dusts, noxious fumes and gases, and physical insults (extreme cold and heat).[244–247] A careful and detailed occupational history is the essential first step in identifying inhalation lung disease. Specific questions should be asked about the following: (1) the material in tools used as well as the material that is being processed on the job; (2) the actual work performed rather than the name of the firm or job title; (3) other occupational activities occurring in the same work place as well as in adjacent "factories," and even the work of household contacts (especially in the case of asbestos and sensitizing agents); (4) remote and brief exposures (*e.g.*, at a summer job while in school); and (5) recreational activities (*e.g.*, hobbies).

A recent symposium addressed the problems of separating impairment (physiologic abnormality) from disability (inability to perform certain tasks). It emphasized the problems of attributing a specific disease to a given exposure and the role of the physician in decision making, and it provided guidelines for appropriate resolution of these vexing problems.[248]

PNEUMOCONIOSES

Pneumoconioses are diagnosable diseases of the lung produced by the inhalation of dust (dust being understood to be particulate matter in the solid phase, excluding living organisms). Many classic texts limit the term to inorganic dust exposure, which will be discussed first. The response of the lung to the inhalation of inorganic dusts will vary with (1) the chemical nature of the dust (nonreactive dusts such as coal, tin, iron, barium, and cement may be contrasted with fibrogenic dusts such as silica and the silicates); (2) the solubility of the dust; (3) concentration and length of exposure to the dust (as the number of particles increases, lung clearance mechanisms become less effective); and (4) the size of the dust particles. The deposition of particles in the lung is a function of sedimentation, inertial impaction, and diffusion. Particles in the 0.5μ to 5μ range are most likely to produce damage. A great majority of particles that are larger are cleared by the lung defense mechanisms, the nasopharyngeal airway, and the mucociliary escalator. Smaller particles that reach the alveoli may be engulfed by alveolar macrophages, and some particles will be removed through the lymphatics. Filamentous particles in the range of 30μ to 60μ, such as asbestos and talc, also reach the alveoli because such long, narrow fibers have a low settling velocity. Particles greater than 10μ in diameter do not reach the peripheral parts of the lung; particles in the 1μ to 3μ range are most likely to be deposited in the peripheral lung units, while smaller particles may be exhaled without settling (see discussion of lung clearance mechanisms, Chap. 8).

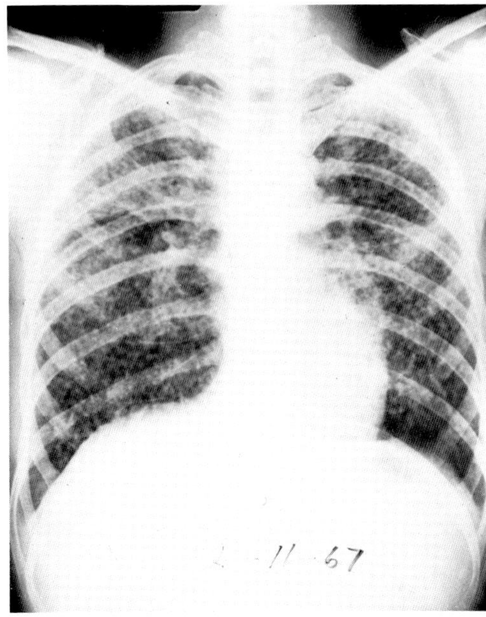

FIG. 13-15. Chest roentgenogram of a patient with silicosis. Note the bilateral hard discrete nodular shadows. In both upper lobes, beginning progressive massive fibrosis is evident. This 27-year-old had worked approximately 70 hours per week for less than 9 months as a sand-blaster. He was severely dyspneic and had cor pulmonale. This acute presentation of silicosis is unusual.

Silicosis

Silicosis is caused by the inhalation of free silicon dioxide particles. This dust is fibrogenic, producing nodular lesions diffusely throughout the lungs, and may involve the hilar nodes. These nodules are whorled, laminated masses of hyalinized material with silica particles that may be seen by using polarizing microscopy. With time and continued exposure, the nodules enlarge and coalesce, forming dense masses typically in the upper portions of the lung (progressive massive fibrosis, or PMF).[249]

The major symptom of silicosis is shortness of breath; this is commonly associated with cough and sputum production, probably related to cigarette smoking. Usually there is exposure of some 20 years to silica before the onset of symptoms. The roentgenographic manifestations of silicosis have been categorized in a detailed grading system progressing from simple to complicated, depending on the size of the nodules and evidence of mass formation.[250] The presence of small diffuse nodules involving usually the upper lobes is termed a simple pneumoconiosis. The hilar nodes may be enlarged and have a ring of peripheral calcification ("eggshell calcification"). Such roentgenographic changes are usually not associated with either clinical symptoms or physiologic changes. The term *complicated pneumoconiosis* is used when lesions 1 cm or greater appear; such lesions may continue to enlarge and may be associated with volume loss, particularly involving the upper lobes (Fig. 13-15). The presence of cavitation strongly suggests superimposed mycobacterial infection. This is commonly associated with progressive dyspnea, cough and sputum production, hemoptysis, and chest pain. At this stage, superinfection with mycobacteria including *M. tuberculosis*, *M. kansasii*, or *M. intracellulare* occurs frequently (Fig. 13-16). As the disease progresses, cor pulmonale

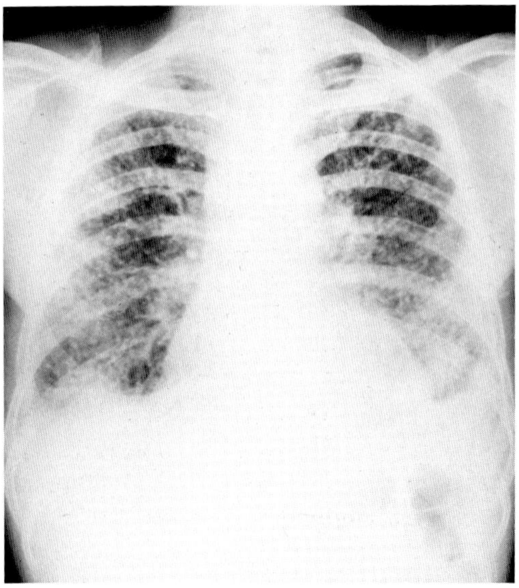

FIG. 13-16. Chest roentgenogram of a patient with silicotuberculosis. There are bilateral discrete nodular densities; just above both diaphragms are areas of confluence; there is a left pleural effusion. This 47-year-old man had worked in a foundry for more than 20 years. He sought medical attention for dyspnea and fever. *M. tuberculosis* was cultured from sputum and pleural fluid; organisms were identified in caseating granuloma in a pleural biopsy.

and respiratory failure may develop. Respiratory failure may be precipitated by a pneumothorax. The disease may be complicated by the development of connective tissue disorders such as systemic lupus erythematosus, rheumatoid arthritis, or scleroderma.

A similar pattern is seen in accelerated silicosis in which the onset of disease occurs within 4 to 5 years of initial dust exposure. Superimposed mycobacterial infection appears to be more common in this group. Acute silicosis may occur with exceptionally heavy exposure; symptoms and roentgenographic changes appear within a period of 1 to 4 years of initial exposure (and rarely, with massive exposure, in days).

The diagnosis of silicosis can usually be made on the basis of the history of exposure and the roentgenographic picture. The following is a list of principal industrial exposures to free silica: (1) mining of gold, tin, copper, sandstone, and mica; (2) quarrying and tunneling; (3) stone cutting or finishing; (4) use and manufacture of abrasives, including sand paper and scouring powders containing flint and quartz, and abrasive blasting; (5) glass manufacture; (6) foundry work including the use of sand molds, particularly their blasting, hammering, and chiseling; (7) manufacture of pottery, porcelain, and lining bricks; (8) boiler scaling; (9) manufacture of vitreous enamel; and (10) the use of free silica in a variety of other combinations such as asbestos cement, tile or roofing, silica brick, kiln linings, or the heating of amorphous silica such as diatomaceous earth to near the temperature of crystallization. If the history of silica exposure is not recognized, the diffuse roentgenographic pattern may be attributed to such conditions as sarcoidosis, diffuse interstitial fibrosis, and lymphangitic carcinoma. The large masslike lesions of PMF may simulate a primary lung carcinoma.

In patients with simple silicosis, ventilatory function is usually normal. The roentgenographic pattern of complicated silicosis correlates with physiologic evidence of restriction; there may be obstruction or both patterns of ventilatory impairment. At this stage, the diffusing capacity is decreased and there may be hypoxemia, increased by exercise; lung compliance is also decreased.

There is no specific therapy for silicosis. Since superinfection with mycobacteria is such a serious and common occurrence, careful evaluation for such infection is mandatory. A tuberculin skin test should be given and sputum should be cultured for mycobacteria. If the skin test reaction is significant, many recommended initiation of antituberculous therapy while awaiting results of cultures. In areas where superinfection with *M. kansassii* is most common, the use of isoniazid and rifampin is preferable. If repeated cultures for mycobacteria are negative, then preventative therapy with INH for 1 year should be given. With the presence of extensive silicosis or progressive massive fibrosis, some recommended continuation of antituberculous therapy for periods beyond 3 years, especially if there is residual cavitation or roentgenographic progression.[249] There appears to be an increased incidence of the collagen vascular diseases in patients with chronic accelerated silicosis. Patients with silicosis have been reported with positive antinuclear and antilung antibodies, rheumatoid factor, and increased serum and secretory IgA.

The incidence of silicosis in developed countries is decreasing owing to strict enforcement of preventive measures such as the use of masks, wetting techniques, improved ventilation, and blasting hoods. Since masks and hoods are cumbersome and uncomfortable, ongoing monitoring is usually necessary to assure their use, especially where heavy physical activity is required. It has recently been reported that, when threshold limits are regularly exceeded, the prevalence of silicosis in exposed workers can be as high as 37%.[251]

Asbestosis

Asbestosis is a pulmonary disease characterized by fibrosis caused by exposure to asbestos. Asbestos is a fibrous, flexible, crystalline silicate of magnesium, sometimes in combinations with calcium, chromium, or sodium. In addition to the production of pulmonary fibrosis, asbestos exposure is associated with an increased incidence of bronchogenic carcinoma, mesothelioma, and gastrointestinal tract neoplasms.[248,252]

Asbestosis is characterized by a diffuse basilar bilateral pulmonary fibrosis; with increasing exposure, the fibrosis extends up from the bases but usually spares the apices. With the progression of the pulmonary fibrosis, there may be honeycomb formation. Fibrous pleural thickening and pleural plaque formation are common; the plaques may calcify. They are commonly located on the parietal pleura and in particular on its diaphragmatic surface. Asbestos bodies may be found in the lesions. These bodies are 20μ to 50μ long and 2 μ to 10μ wide; with hematoxylin and eosin stain, a golden brown iron protein complex surrounds the asbestos fiber; one end is usually bulbous and the other narrow. Since other fibers may be engulfed by a similar iron protein complex, it is more appropriate to call the surrounded asbestos fiber a *ferruginous body*. The presence of ferruginous bodies in sputum correlates well with asbestosis pulmonary fibrosis. However, using a variety of pathologic techniques, ferruginous bodies may be found in from 40% to 100% of postmortem lung specimens from the general population. Using an alkali digestion technique, all specimens in a cross section of rural and urban Michigan residents had such bodies. Thus, their presence in tissue does not necessarily correlate with disease.[253]

Recognition of asbestosis requires the identification of exposure. Occupations with the potential for such exposure include asbestos mining and manufacturing, plumbers, electricians, demolition workers, shipyard workers (particularly those working in the holds and around engine rooms), and pipe insulators. Materials that may expose workers to asbestos include roofing shingles, cement, vinyl asbestos tile, fireproof paint, fireproof clothing and sheets, brake linings, acid-resistant filters, valve packing, lagging material used around steam pipes and electrical wiring, ship bulkhead coating, ropes, theater curtains, air filtration systems, paint filters, asbestos boards, and laboratory hoods. The risk is in the manufacture, cutting, or demolition of these materials rather than exposure to finished products.

The characteristic presenting complaint is the insidious onset of progressive dyspnea on exertion, often associated with a dry cough; in a cigarette smoker, the cough may be productive. There may be mild to moderate chest pain, on occasion pleuritic. Clubbing is common. There are usually interstitial basilar rales bilaterally, or areas of decreased breath sounds in relation to pleural fibrosis. Hemoptysis is unusual and suggests a complicating neoplasm. Anorexia, weight loss, cor pulmonale, and respiratory failure occur with progressive disease. The chest roentgenogram initially shows a fine diffuse homogeneous or "ground-glass" infiltrate involving the lower lobes. There may be pleural fibrosis or pleural plaques that may calcify (Fig. 13-17). The heart borders have an irregular "shaggy" appearance and, with extensive disease, may be difficult to identify. The presence of a pleural effusion warrants strong consideration of a superimposed malignancy; pleural effusions have been reported in asbestosis without malignancy.

The usual physiologic pattern is that of restrictive disease with decreased lung volumes, decreased gas transfer, widening of the alveolar-

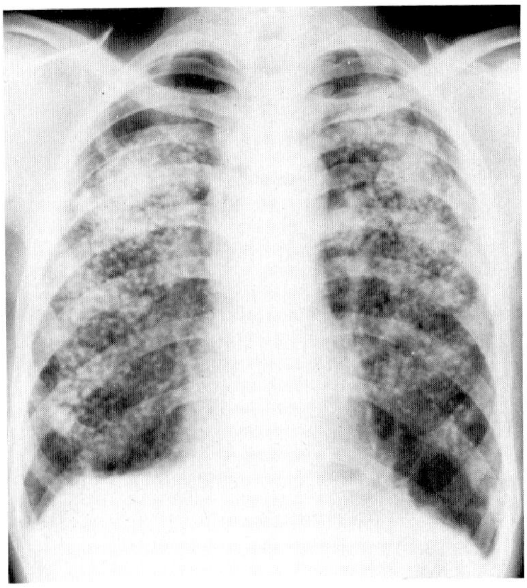

FIG. 13-17. Chest roentgenogram demonstrating the changes resulting from asbestosis. The multiple hard nodular densities throughout both lung fields and the large confluent densities in both upper lobes (progressive massive fibrosis) are parenchymal lesions. The left heart border is "shaggy." There are several pleural plaques along the lateral lung margins and bilateral pneumothoraces. This 57-year-old man had worked with pipe insulation for 20 years. He had cor pulmonale and was hospitalized with respiratory failure precipitated by the pneumothoraces.

to-arterial oxygen gradient, hypoxemia, and decreased static lung compliance. Usually the clinical, roentgenographic, and physiologic manifestations parallel each other, but on occasion the physiologic abnormality may be present without significant roentgenographic findings.

Significant asbestos exposure produces a definite increase in incidence of lung carcinoma. In various studies this has ranged from 7 to 10 times in excess of predicted. In one study almost all such patients were cigarette smokers, and the increased incidence of carcinoma, with what appears to be cocarcinogens, was approximately 100-fold. However, the incidence is definitely increased in nonsmokers and appears to be greater with exposure to crocidolite as opposed to chrysotile asbestos.[252,254] The incidence of carcinoma of the stomach, colon, and rectum is increased. There is also an increased incidence of mesothelioma of both the pleura and peritoneum.[255,256] There appears to be an inverse relationship between the extent of asbestos exposure and the development of carcinoma such that with severe asbestos exposure, fibrosis intervenes with progression leading to cor pulmonale and death prior to the development of carcinoma. With a lesser exposure, bronchogenic carcinoma is more likely to be the cause of death, ranging from 17% to in excess of 50% of deaths in patients with asbestosis[257]; with perhaps even smaller exposures, there appears to be a greater incidence of mesothelioma. In fact, persons who have lived in the vicinity of asbestos plants or mines or who have handled the clothes of asbestos workers have developed mesothelioma.[257,258] Asbestosis does not appear to predispose to mycobacterial disease.

An exposure of 7 to 20 years usually precedes the onset of symptoms of asbestosis. However, with heavy exposure such as spraying, the disease may become evident in as little as 3 years.

Talcosis

Pneumoconiosis related to exposure to talc, a hydrated magnesium silicate, produces a fibrotic and granulomatous reaction. In infants and small children the accidental inhalation of large amounts of "talcum powder" may lead to an acute diffuse, often fatal pneumonia;[259] recently talc has been removed from many such products for infants and children. Drug addicts may develop the disease by injecting solutions of drug tablets which have talc as a filler.[260] Occupational exposure may occur in the mining or milling of talc and in rubber and cable manufacturing. Talc is also used to insulate steam pipes, in the manufacture of electric switchboards, and as a filler in drug tablets, paper, paint, and soaps.[261] The clinical presentation with occupational exposure is that of insidious dyspnea with cough and sputum production; there may be clubbing. The roentgenographic pattern is that of nonspecific diffuse interstitial disease, more prominent in the middle lung zones. There may be pleural plaques with calcification that may involve the pericardium. Progressive massive fibrosis may develop.[261]

Other Silicates Causing Pneumoconioses

Exposure to other silicates has on occasion caused similar patterns of pneumoconioses. These include kaolin (China clay), mica, sillimanite, sericite, Fuller's earth, amorphous silica, feldspar, and pumice. The potential role for fiberglass or glass wool in producing lung disease has been suggested.

Respiratory Disease in Coal Workers

A variety of terms have been used to describe respiratory disease in coal miners and other coal workers, including anthracosis, anthrosilicosis, coal worker's pneumoconiosis, miner's lung, and "black lung." The general use of the term "black lung" to encompass any pulmonary disease in a coal worker, while quite popular, creates additional confusion in a complex area that is the subject of considerable controversy.[248,262,263] Respiratory disease in coal workers can be subdivided as follows: (1) coal worker's pneumoconiosis (CWP), referring to the clinical, roentgenographic, and pathologic pattern of coal dust deposition in the lung; (2) silicosis, which is a function of the amount of silica in or around the coal or exposure to free silica in a variety of mining operations; and (3) industrial bronchitis, characterized by cough and sputum production with or without evidence of airways obstruction.[262] The contribution of chronic bronchitis and emphysema due to cigarette smoking must be assessed in evaluating the clinical and physiologic evidence for either disease or disability, both in an individual and in the many studies related to respiratory disease in miners.

Coal worker's pneumoconiosis (CWP) is characterized by the roentgenographic evidence of carbon deposition in the lung. Miners who work at the coal face using a cutting machine or "continuous miner" have the greatest dust exposure, followed by roof bolters and those involved in transportation of coal from the mine face to the surface. There is a general correlation between years underground, roentgenographic evidence of dust deposition, and the amount of dust found in lung specimens. A recent estimate of the prevalence of CWP in miners in the United States is approximately 10%, of which 0.4% develop complicated CWP or progressive massive fibrosis (PME). This is an appreciable decrease from previous reports of a 30% prevalence. While this reduction may in part represent improved mining practices, it also reflects the increased number of workers who have been classified as disabled from CWP.

Simple CWP is characterized by pinpoint or finely reticular nodulation throughout the lung fields. With greater dust inhalation over a period of time, the size of these lesions may increase. Histologically the primary lesion of coal worker's pneumoconiosis (CWP) is the coal macule. This develops around first- or second-order respiratory bronchioles with their associated alveoli and consists of coal dust, macrophages, fibroblasts, and some reticulin, but without collagen formation. There may be focal emphysema around such lesions.

Complicated CWP or progressive massive fibrosis is defined on the basis of the roentgenographic abnormality with nodules of 1 cm or greater. These are present in usually one or the other upper lobe and tend to appear first at the periphery and migrate toward the hilum with enlargement. The nodules are composed of dense acellular collagenous tissue containing black pigmentation. The mechanism of formation of progressive massive fibrosis is unclear. In earlier studies, when tuberculosis was more common, histologic or bacteriologic evidence of mycobacterial disease was found in 40% of PMF lesions at autopsy.[264] Others have suggested an antibody reaction with support obtained from an increased incidence of rheumatoid factor or antinuclear antibody. Still others have related the development of PMF to the total amount of dust or to other infections.

The roentgenographic deposition of carbon in the nodular pattern of a simple pneumoconiosis does not appear to correlate with respiratory symptoms or physiologic impairment that indicates disability. In carefully controlled studies, especially those in nonsmoking miners, there is evidence of a slight increase in total lung capacity, a modest decrease in forced vital capacity, forced expired volume at 1 sec, forced expired flow near residual volume and frequency dependence of compliance, a modest increase in alveolar–arterial oxygen gradient and dead space/tidal volume ratio, and a decrease in diffusing capacity. A study of underground miners in Utah with a mean age of 56 years and a mean of 29 years in coal mining found a prevalence of chronic bronchitis in 57% and CWP in 25%; only one worker had PMF. Significant impairment of pulmonary function was found in smokers. Chronic bronchitis or CWP was not associated with physiologic impairment.[265] Assessment for disability benefits remains complex and controversial.[266]

Individuals with complicated CWP or PMF do develop symptoms of progressive dyspnea, cough, and sputum production. They may expectorate large amounts of black fluid (melanoptysis). The disease progresses to cor pulmonale and respiratory failure. Such individuals have evidence of both severe restrictive and obstructive lung disease.

Caplan's syndrome, seen in coal workers, is characterized by the development of nodules from 0.5 to 5 cm in diameter, which may appear rapidly and disappear only to recur over a period of time, and which on occasion cavitate. These usually occur with the onset of rheumatoid arthritis, although they have been known to antedate or follow the disease by considerable periods of time. Many such patients have rheumatoid antinuclear factors in their serum.[267] The role of coal dust in development of these nodules is uncertain, and the syndrome is not uniformly accepted.

Silicosis in Coal Miners. Coal miners working with anthracite (hard coal) are likely to have notable exposure to silica in the surrounding rock formation. Roof bolters and motormen or brakemen who sand the rails may also have an increased exposure. The incidence of silicosis is generally quite low in US miners.

Industrial Bronchitis. There is good evidence that exposure to increasing amounts of coal dust correlates with cough and sputum production and a slight decrease in FEV_1. Years underground also correlate with a decrease in peak flow and flow at high lung volumes, indicating changes in large airways that do not correlate with radiographic evidence of CWP.[265]

Berylliosis

Berylliosis may present as an acute diffuse pulmonary disease with evidence of systemic involvement. It is due to the inhalation of metallic beryllium or its soluble salts. Exposure may occur in the extraction, mining, smelting, or fabrication of beryllium or its alloys. Beryllium is used in certain plastics and ceramics, in the aerospace and atomic energy industries, and in the manufacture of x-ray tubes. Owing to its high toxicity, beryllium is no longer used in fluorescent light bulbs.

With heavy exposure, the presentation is that of an acute chemical pneumonitis beginning shortly after exposure. The patient has cough, often paroxysmal, with blood streaking and a diffuse bilateral infiltrate on chest roentgenogram. A history of exposure is necessary for diagnosis.

Chronic berylliosis presents with a latency period of 1 to 20 years after exposure. The clinical, roentgenographic, physiologic, and pathologic findings simulate those of sarcoidosis very closely. Berylliosis, however, does not involve the eyes, salivary glands, or bone, and the Kveim reaction is negative. Chemical identification of beryllium in tissue or urine supports the diagnosis. Corticosteroid therapy may be of benefit.[268]

Other Pneumoconioses

Tungsten carbide may produce a severe interstitial fibrosis or intermittent episodes of cough and wheezing.[269,270] Cadmium may produce an acute chemical pneumonitis or a chronic illness involving the lung and kidneys[271] with development of emphysema. Aluminum oxide or its fumes may produce an interstitial fibrosis.

Benign pneumoconioses may result from the inhalation of barium, tin (stannosis), carbon, and iron (siderosis), calcium-containing materials, antimony, and titanium.[244–246,248]

IRRITANT GASES

The following highly irritant gases may cause an acute chemical pneumonitis: chlorine, ammonia, sulfur dioxide, ozone, nitrogen dioxide, phosgene, and smoke (see also Chap. 1). Most exposures occur in an industrial setting. Chlorine is used in the chemical and plastic industries and to disinfect water. Ammonia is used in commercial refrigeration. Sulfur dioxide exposure may occur in paper manufacture and smelting of sulfide ores. Ozone may be generated in welding and is used in the manufacture of bleaches and peroxides. Nitrogen dioxide may be liberated after exposure of nitric acid to air and may be released from fresh silage as a reddish brown gas (silo filler's disease).[272] Phosgene is used in the production of analine dyes. Hydrogen sulfide may cause acute, fatal pulmonary edema.[272a]

All of these gases are highly irritant and usually result in the immediate onset of tracheobronchitis or bronchiolitis manifested by cough, usually paroxysmal, dyspnea, chest pain, and signs of ocular and oropharyngeal mucous membrane irritation. Symptoms may be rapidly progressive. However, not uncommonly they partially or completely resolve for periods of 24 to 48 hours only to rapidly recur with even greater intensity. There may be rhonchi or wheezing. Forced expiration usually provokes a paroxysmal cough. There may be basilar rales. The roentgenogram initially may be normal but with progression a diffuse bilateral infiltrate like that seen in pulmonary edema occurs (Fig. 13-18). Physiologically there may be evidence of airways obstruction, but the major problem is that of hypoxemia. With severe disease the findings are those of the acute respiratory distress or wet lung syndrome.

Since there may be a period of temporary improvement, close observation for a period of 24 to 48 hours is prudent.

Therapy consists of adequate oxygenation and bronchodilators. We recommend the use of corticosteroids with 60 to 100 mg of Prednisone per day, usually for several days or until there is reversal of physiologic and roentgenographic abnormalities. The role of corticosteroids, however, has not been established in controlled studies.

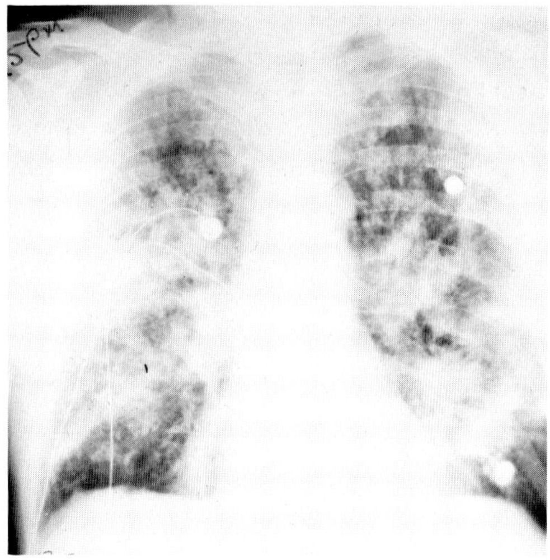

FIG. 13-18. Chest roentgenogram of a patient with silo-filler's disease (exposure to nitrogen). There are confluent, diffuse, bilateral soft fluffy infiltrates involving all lung fields; ECG monitoring leads are evident. This 68-year-old man attempted to descend through his silo a day after it was filled. After inhaling brownish fumes that irritated his eyes, nose, and throat, he almost immediately developed a paroxysmal cough followed by shortness of breath. He was hospitalized in florid respiratory failure 4 hours later and was treated with mechanical ventilation, oxygen, corticosteroids, and constant positive pressure. After an initial improvement and extubation, he developed progressive bronchiolitis obliterans and emphysema, confirmed at autopsy several months later.

Late sequellae of irritant gas exposure may include bronchiectasis or bronchiolitis obliterans with diffuse emphysematous changes. These entities are discussed in Chapter 14.

ORGANIC "DUST" EXPOSURE

Over the last four decades there has been increasing recognition of several different pulmonary responses to the inhalation of an ever-increasing number of organic compounds, usually as dusts.[273–275] These exposures have most commonly been related to occupation, such as "farmer's lung" (described clinically by Ramazinni in 1713), but also to avocations such as bird breeding and, more recently, to the ubiquitous thermophilic actinomycetes disseminated through air conditioners.[276] It is now recognized that an endless variety of naturally occurring and synthetic substances may cause lung disease.

Byssinosis

Byssinosis occurs with exposure to cotton, flax, and soft hemp. A similar disease occurs with exposure to sisal. In US cotton mills, carders and spinners have the most exposure to dirty or raw cotton; cotton pickers, however, are not affected. Workers with byssinosis complain of chest tightness, wheezing, and cough within a few hours on the first work day after several days of absence ("Monday morning asthma"). The disease has been classified as follows: Grades ½ to 1 (Monday symptoms only), Grade 2 (symptoms on other workdays), and Grade 3 (continuous dyspnea and chronic cough). A second pattern of illness is bronchitis with cough and sputum production on a chronic basis independent of cigarette smoking. Smoking increases the grade of the classic variable byssinosis and also adds to the clinical and physiologic evidence of bronchitis.

The chest roentgenogram is usually normal but may show hyperinflation. Airways obstruction may be documented by a decreased FEV_1 or a decrease in various flow rates. Some workers have functional abnormalities without symptoms. Airways obstruction is initially reversible, but with continued exposure becomes fixed. Older workers have greater airways obstruction and greater disability when matched for age and smoking history.[277] Postmortem studies have not shown a greater amount of emphysema.[278]

It is believed that an agent in the cotton dust is responsible for immune release of mediators with resultant bronchoconstriction. Gram-negative bacteria and endotoxin have been implicated.[279] Inhalation challenge with dust will produce symptoms and decreased flow rates within 20 to 30 min, even in a person not previously exposed. Steam cleaning of the cotton, dust control, and pretreatment with disodium cromoglycate reduce the amount of bronchospasm.[246,277–281,282]

Industrial Asthma

Exposure to a variety of organic substances may produce clinical asthma with wheezing, dyspnea, chest tightness, and cough (see also Chap. 14). A prototype is seen in laundry workers exposed to the proteolytic enzymes of *B. subtilis*. They usually develop symptoms several hours after leaving the plant. However, symptoms or physiologic changes may occur shortly after exposure as expected in an IgE-mediated reaction, or may only be noted by the patient many hours after exposure ("midnight" asthma for the day worker); this late reaction may recur for several nights. Airways obstruction may be persistant, along with hyperreactivity to a variety of nonspecific irritants.

The chest roentgenogram is normal or may show hyperinflation. Physiologically, there is airways obstruction and air trapping. This group of diseases appears to share both a Type I or immediate reaction and a Type III, Arthus, or delayed reaction. Both an immediate and a delayed response can be provoked in a sensitized individual with an inhalation challenge.[283,284] A diagnosis of industrial asthma rests on the history of exposure that produces symptoms, with relief on removal from exposure. However, as noted, this may not be easy to ascertain. The most reliable confirmation is obtained with an inhalational challenge to the specific antigen (if known) or to a simulated occupational exposure. Such exposures must be carefully supervised to avoid unnecessary risk.

The key to management is removal from exposure. This sometimes creates such financial havoc that a person will refuse (at least initially) to avoid exposure.

Similar diseases have occurred with the inhalation of toluene diisocyanate used in the manufacture of polyurethane,[285,286] with exposure to the wheat weevil (*Sitophilus granarius*) in grain or dust, and with exposure to platinum salts, piperazine dihydrochloride, and aminoethanolamine. They have also occurred in animal handlers, apiarists (bee handlers), bakers (with inhalation of flour and dust), chemical and plastic workers (with inhalation of formalin, chloramine, trypsin chromium, piperazine, and polyvinyl chloride), coffee workers and roasters, oyster culture workers, electricians (with exposure to aluminum soldering flux, and aminoethanolamine), grain storage workers, metal workers (with exposure to vanadium and nickle sulfate), printers (with inhalation of fragacanth gum arabic), and welders (with inhalation of acetylene). They have occurred with exposure to medications (penicillin, sulfathiazole, salvarsan, psyllium, pyrethrum, iris, and disinfectants) and dyes (phenylene diamine and diazonium salts). They have occurred with castor bean poisoning, and in photo studios with inhalation of potassium chloroplatinate. They have occurred in parents of children with cystic fibrosis as a result of exposure to pancreatic extracts, and with exposure to vinyl chloride and polyvinyl chloride. These latter two appear to be responsible for a roentgenographic and histologic pattern of diffuse fibrosis, or a granulomatous reaction, in addition to the role of vinyl chloride as a carcinogen.[287–289] Farmers and grain workers are exposed to a wide variety of organisms, organic dusts, and chemicals. Asthma, hypersensitivity pneumonitis, acute toxic laryngotracheobronchitis, and noncardiac pulmonary edema may result from inhalation of the appropriate substances.[289a]

Extrinsic Allergic Alveolitis

The term extrinsic allergic alveolitis is used to describe a syndrome resulting from exposure to a variety of organic materials including dusts, organic compounds, and several fungi contained in dusts. (See Table 13-4 for a list of currently recognized exposures and their known antigenic association.)

The prototype of this syndrome is *farmer's lung*, which occurs with exposure to moldy hay containing thermophilic actinomycetes such as *Microspora faeni* or *Thermoactinomyces vulgaris*.[290] These same thermophilic fungi grow in many warm, damp places including air conditioners, home humidifiers, hot air furnaces, and flues of fireplaces.

Early studies emphasized Type I and Type III immunologic reactions underlying the lung response. The pathogenesis seems more complex, however with elements of all four major immune mechanisms in different patients with different features of the illness.[284,291,292]

Three clinical presentations are recognized. They vary with the amount of antigen to which the individual is exposed and with the chronicity of exposure. Some 4 to 8 hr after heavy expo-

TABLE 13-4. Known Causes of Allergic Alveolitis

Disease	Source	Antigen	Reference
Farmer's lung	Moldy hay	*Microsporum faeni, Thermoactinomyces vulgaris*	290
Mushroom worker's lung	Mushroom compost		293
Bagassosis	Moldy bagasse (sugar cane)	*Thermoactinomyces vulgaris*	294
Maple bark disease	Maple bark	*Cryptostroma corticale*	295
Sequoiosis	Redwood sawdust	Graphium, *Aureobasidium pullulans*	296
Wood pulp worker's disease	Wood pulp, sawdust	*Alternaria*	297
Malt worker's disease	Moldy barley	*Aspergillus clavatus*	298
Mill worker's disease (wheat weevil disease)	Wheat flour	*Aspergillus fumigatus, Sitophilus granarius*	299
Cheese washer's lung	Moldy cheese	*Penicillium casei*	300
"Doghouse disease"	Moldy straw	*Aspergillus versicolor*	301
Suberosis	Cork dust	Cork dust	302
Coffee worker's lung	Coffee bean	Coffee bean dust	303
Bird fancier's lung (Pigeon breeder's lung)	Pigeon, parrot, and other bird droppings	Bird sera, protein, and droppings	304, 305
Pituitary snufftaker's lung	Pituitary snuff	Pituitary snuff	306

sure, the individual develops fever up to 40°C, extreme malaise, myalgia, arthralgia, chest tightness, dyspnea, and usually a dry cough. He will be tachypneic, and there may be rales over the lower lobes. Wheezing is absent or slight. Improvement usually occurs over 12 to 24 hr. If the exposure is less intense, there may be dyspnea, a dry cough, and fatigue without other systemic symptoms. If an individual has repeated exposures over extended periods of time (each usually quite light), the pattern is that of progressive dyspnea with chronic cough and sputum production. The chest roentgenogram with acute exposure usually shows bilateral, increased bronchovascular markings, occasionally Kerly's B lines, and small nodular densities involving the lower lobes. With light exposures the chest film may be normal. With chronic exposures a more dense fibrotic and linear pattern with or without nodulation develops; in some with chronic exposure there is only evidence of hyperinflation compatible with emphysema.

With an acute heavy exposure there will be a reduction in vital capacity and total lung capacity and little or no airways obstruction. Diffusing capacity and static compliance are reduced. There is usually hypoxemia, which may be severe. These abnormalities tend to improve gradually over 3 to 4 weeks. With less intense exposures, similar but milder abnormalities occur.[307] With chronic exposure the initial pattern, that of restriction, may become fixed or may progress.[308] Some patients, however, develop a pattern of airways obstruction with decreased flow rates, increased airways resistance, hyperinflation, a decreased diffusing capacity, and a loss of elastic recoil; this is a pattern indistinguishable from that of emphysema.[305]

The pathologic response to acute intense exposure is mixed. There is evidence of an acute vasculitis involving alveolar capillaries with fibrin thrombi and an influx of neutrophiles and eosinophiles compatible with an Arthus or Type III reaction. In addition, there is an influx of many macrophages, foreign-body giant cells, and neutrophiles. Subsequently granuloma formation, either noncaseating or with central necrosis, occurs, compatible with a Type IV or delayed hypersensitivity reaction. This process may continue with the development of diffuse interstitial fibrosis with honeycombing, with or without residual granuloma. Intense bronchiolitis obliterans may develop; this may represent the histologic corollary to the physiologic findings of emphysema in some patients.

For many of these clinical syndromes, antigens are now available that will produce a significant skin test response in 4 to 8 hr. Most individuals will have precipitating antibodies in their serum. However, individuals without any evidence of disease may have skin test reactivity and precipitating antibodies to several of the known antigens. Thus, the skin tests are not helpful diagnostically because of their nonspecificity.

The most important therapy is removal from further exposure once the disease is recognized. Some individuals, however, cannot or will not take this step. They may diminish their exposure by using high efficiency masks that exclude most particles of 2μ or less; this, however, is a compromise. Treatment with corticosteroids in a dose equivalent to 60 mg a day of prednisone appears to decrease systemic toxicity and hasten the resolution of pulmonary disease. The drug is usually continued for 2 or more weeks or until there is resolution of clinical, roentgenographic, and physiologic abnormalities. In addition, adequate oxygenation should be maintained and bronchodilators may be of benefit. The role of corticosteroids in treating the effects of chronic disease has not been defined. In the presence of severe symptomatic disease with physiologic impairment, a trial of steroids with careful clinical and physiologic monitoring may be warranted.[308]

RADIATION INJURY

The use of radiation therapy for malignancies of the chest and chest wall may result in radiation injury to the lung. If the dose of radiation is less than 2000 rads, lung injury is rare. Doses in excess of 6000 rads over 6 weeks almost uniformly produce disease. Extension of the period of treatment lessens the likelihood of lung damage. In the most commonly used intermediate range, radiation damage is variable.[309,319]

Acute radiation pneumonitis presents with a paroxysmal, hacking, often quite severe nonproductive cough and dyspnea. Heartburn and dysphagia are common. These symptoms usually begin some 6 to 14 weeks after completion of therapy; they may begin even up to 6 months later. However, some patients clearly have the onset of symptoms shortly after completing therapy and occasionally during therapy. Some patients develop insidious cough and dyspnea after an extended latent period of 6 or more months without a history of an acute episode. Roentgenographic changes may precede symptoms. There is usually a fairly homogeneous density that may have strikingly linear rectangular borders matching the radiation ports (Fig. 13-19). The lesion may be patchy or may extend beyond the area of radiation. Volume loss associated with dense fibrosis may occur. Radiation damage produces a restrictive pattern with decreased lung volumes, diffusing capacity, and arterial oxygen tension.[311] Localized radiation causes volume loss in the affected lobes and hypertrophy of adjacent nonradiated lobes.[312]

The acute tissue reaction of "radiation pneumonitis" is that of alveolar capillary endothelial damage and edema formation; there may be hyaline membranes. This is a nonspecific acute injury pattern. The process may resolve or progress to severe diffuse interstitial fibrosis obliterating airways and small vessels; this, too, is a nonspecific pattern.

Other than the judicious use of radiation therapy and supportive measures such as potent antitussives and oxygen when appropriate, there is no specific therapy. Corticosteroids improve lung compliance by increased surfactant production in experimental animals.[313] Their use in the presence of an underlying malignancy, the immunosuppressive effect of radiation, and the possible concurrent use of antimetabolites may potentiate the risks for opportunistic infection. However, in the presence of progressive and severe radiation lung disease, a trial of steroids is recommended.[312,313]

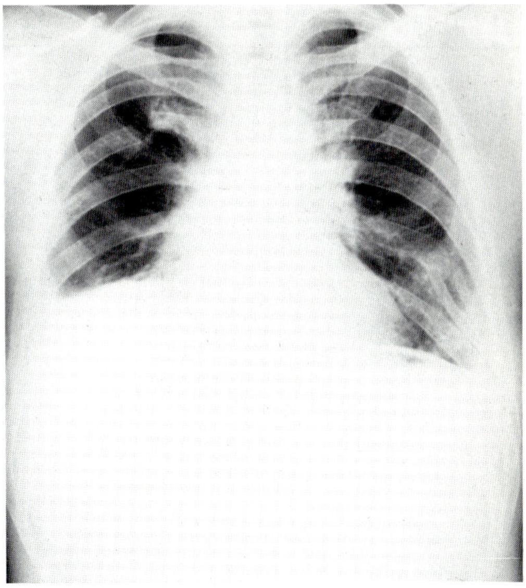

FIG. 13-19. Chest roentgenogram demonstrating radiation pneumonitis. There is a rectangular infiltrate affecting both lung fields, centered on the mediastinum at the level of the carina. The left hemidiaphragm is elevated from previous surgery. The eighth rib on the left is deformed due to previous empyema drainage. This 43-year-old man had a primary lymphoma of the right lower lobe resected, followed by radiation therapy to the mediastinum. While receiving radiation he had a paroxysmal cough and esophagitis. The mediastinum and surrounding lung parenchyma were normal until 7 weeks after radiation when this pattern developed.

DRUG-INDUCED DISEASE

Numerous drugs may be responsible for a wide range of pulmonary abnormalities as listed in Table 13-5. The pulmonary effects include lung parenchymal, airways, and vascular lesions; pleural disease; lymphadenopathy and hilar lipomatosis; and respiratory muscle paralysis. The effects may be apparent within days after initiating drug treatment, or after many years.[314–316] Specific mechanisms are poorly defined for most drugs but include direct cellular toxicity, hypersensitivity and other immune mechanisms, vascular injury, and neuromuscular blockade.

TABLE 13-5. Drug-Induced Pulmonary Diseases

Disease	Agents	
Diffuse interstitial fibrosis	Bleomycin Busulfan Carmustine Chlorambucil Cyclophosphamide Gold salts Hexamethonium	Mecamylamine Melphalan Methotrexate Methysurgide Mitomycin Nitrofurantoin Paraquat
Pulmonary edema	Ethchlorvynol Heroin Hydrochlorothiazide Hypaque Leukoagglutinins (blood transfusions) Methadone	Nitrofurantoin Oxyphenylbutazone Penicillamine Phenylbutazone Propoxyphene Salicylates (See also Chap. 7)
Systemic lupus erythematosus (SLE)	Aminosalicylic acid Diphenylhydantoin Hydralazine	Isoniazid Methyldopa Procainamide
Pulmonary infiltrates with eosinophilia	Carbamazepine Chloropropamide Imipramine Mephenesin carbamate	Para-aminosalicylate Penicillin Sulfa drugs Tetracycline
Angiitis and angiitic granulomatosis	Hydralazine Penicillin Phenylbutazone	Promazines Sulfa drugs Thiouracil
Metastatic calcifications	Excess calcium Vitamin D (high doses)	
Pleural effusions	Drug-induced SLE Methysurgide Nitrofurantoin (See also Chap. 12)	
Hilar adenopathy, or mediastinal widening	Diphenylhydantoin Steroids	
Bronchoconstriction	(See Chap. 14)	
Muscle paralysis	(See Chap. 6)	
Pulmonary hypertension	(See Chap. 10)	

This section will emphasize those drugs that cause diffuse lung disease; other lung reactions have been dealt with in the appropriate chapters as listed in Table 13-5.

Patients with drug-induced, nonspecific infiltrates commonly present with slowly progressive dyspnea and nonproductive cough. Roentgenographic changes may precede symptoms, and pose the difficult problem of defining their etiology. Because patients on drug treatment generally have underlying (frequently malignant) disease, the possibilities of disease progression, superimposed infection, or drug reaction must be assessed. The clinical presentation as well as the radiographic, pulmonary function and histologic abnormalities are all nonspecific. The diagnosis is frequently based on "guilt by association" and only established by the improvement seen with discontinuation of the medication. The diagnosis of drug-induced lung disease can rarely be made unequivocally.

Busulfan may cause a pattern of DIF with an insidious onset even as late as 3 to 10 years after starting treatment. Large atypical hyperchromatic cells suggesting malignancy may be found on cytological examination of sputum. Cyclophosphamide produces a similar pattern; atypical cells can also be seen after radiation therapy, although far less frequently. Pulmonary toxicity is the most significant side-effect of therapy with bleomycin; there is a pattern of DIF. The estimated incidence of 10% and mortality of 1% in earlier studies was reduced when a dose of 400 to 450 units or less was established. Patients with prior radiation and those over 70 years of age are predisposed to pulmonary toxicity from bleomycin. There is no known effective treatment other than limiting dosage and stopping the drug with onset of disease. Patients can be followed by measuring forced vital capacity and diffusing capacity (which is more sensitive).[317]

Methotrexate pulmonary toxicity is characterized by dyspnea, nonproductive cough, fever, eosinophilia, hypoxemia, a diffuse bilateral infiltrate, and a restrictive defect. Histologically there is DIF and granuloma. Corticosteroids may be of value in treatment. A mortality of 11% with the acute disease has been reported.[318]

Carmustine (BCNU) may also cause diffuse interstitial fibrosis that is more likely to occur with increased dose, increased number of cycles, a history of lung disease, and increasing age. Symptomatic lung disease has been reported in 1 to 20%.[319,320] Nitrofuratoin may cause an acute reaction, with fever, chills, cyanosis, and dyspnea (almost simulating pulmonary edema), with onset in a few hours to 10 days. There are diffuse bilateral infiltrates with or without effusions, and eosinophilia. It also causes a chronic DIF pattern with onset at 6 or more months. The histology is that of DIF (or occasionally DIP). Discontinuation of the drug usually results in resolution.[321,321a]

Diffuse interstitial fibrosis has also been caused by cromolyn, and perhaps by inhaled beclomethasone, hexamethonium, mecamylamine, pentolinium, methysergide (which more commonly causes retroperitoneal and mediastinal fibrosis, and may also cause pleural effusion), gold salts, paraquat, and tocainamide.[314,315,322,323] This list continues to grow.

The following drugs may produce acute pulmonary edema with very rapid onset after ingestion (or injection): heroin, nitrofurantoin (acute), methadone, propoxyphene, leukoagglutinins (blood transfusions), hydrochlorothiazide, phenylbutazone, oxyphenylbutazone, penicillamine, and salicylates.

The following drugs have been associated with a syndrome of systemic lupus erythematosus: isoniazid, diphenylhydantoin, hydralazine, methyldopa, and procainamide (quite commonly). The following drugs have been associated with an allergic angiitis or angiitic granulomatosis: sulfa drugs, penicillin, thiouracil, hydralazine, phenylbutazone, quinidine, promazine, and hydantoins. The syndrome of pulmonary infiltrates with eosinophilia has been associated with sulfa drugs, para-aminosalicylate, penicillin, chlorpropamide, mephenesin carbamate, imipramine, carbamazepine, and tetracycline.[322,324] Metastatic calcification of the lung has been related to high doses of vitamin D, calcium, and inorganic phosphorus, and to milk-alkali syndrome.[314,315]

OXYGEN TOXICITY

Excess oxygen may cause impaired clearance mechanisms, microvascular injury, and potentiate lung fibrosis in patients with the adult respiratory distress syndrome. Oxygen toxicity is reviewed in Chapter 7.

MISCELLANEOUS DISEASES

A variety of poorly understood and uncommon conditions that are associated with chronic parenchymal pulmonary disease have been reported.

Amyloidosis, whether primary or secondary, commonly involves the chest. Patients with this rare condition may be asymptomatic, or they may complain of cough, dyspnea, or hemoptysis; respiratory failure has been reported. On chest roentgenogram there may be the following: (1) single or multiple, discrete or ill-defined nodules of variable size, which may calcify; nodules may be bilateral; (2) parenchymal involvement that may be localized or diffuse; (3) endotracheal or endobronchial disease producing obstruction; (4) mediastinal or hilar adenopathy; (5) cardiomegaly. The lesions may be fairly stable or slowly progressive, but the life expectancy is highly variable. Diagnosis requires appropriate staining of tissues with Congo red and a search for green birefringence with polarized light. It often simulates primary or metastatic malignancy.[325–329]

Tuberous Sclerosis is characterized by mental retardation, epileptic seizures, and adenoma sebaceum (dermalangiofibroma). Hamartomatous proliferative lesions occur in many organs; there are sclerotic bone changes, renal involvement, and intracranial calcifications. It is inherited as an autosomal dominant trait. The lungs are diffusely involved, with fibrosis and cystic changes that cause honeycombing. Pneumothorax is common. Airways obstruction is common; in one case, there was loss of elastic recoil and increased static compliance compatible with emphysema.[330,331]

Lymphangioleiomyomatosis is characterized by smooth muscle proliferation in the pulmonary, retroperitoneal, and mediastinal lymphatics. It usually affects women of childbearing age. Dyspnea, repeated pneumothoraces, hemoptysis, and chylothorax occur. The chest roentgenogram has the pattern of DIF with honeycombing, but with increased lung volumes. There is airways obstruction, hyperinflation, air trapping, and a reduced diffusing capacity compatible with emphysema, despite the fibrosis. Corticosteroid and immunosuppressive therapy have not been helpful.[332,333]

Storage Disease. *The Hermansky–Pudlack syndrome* is a ceroid storage disorder inherited as an autosomal recessive trait. It is characterized by oculocutaneous albinism and hemorrhage resulting from a qualitative platelet defect. The symptoms, the chest roentgenogram, and the results of pulmonary function studies are those of diffuse interstitial fibrosis. Histologically, there are macrophages filled with ceroidlike material and extensive fibrosis. Inflammatory bowel disease also occurs.[334] *Gaucher's disease*[335] and *Fabry's disease*[336] are rare hereditary storage diseases with occasional diffuse pulmonary involvement.

Hematologic Malignancies. Leukemia and lymphoma may cause diffuse or nodular infiltrates owing to tumor. Generally, other manifestations characteristic of the disease will dominate the clinical picture. Patients undergoing chemotherapy may present with extensive infiltrates resulting from drug-induced lung fibrosis, diffuse hemorrhage, or infection.[337–340] These clinical presentations are discussed in Chapter 8, Infections of the Compromised Host, and Chapter 15, Neoplastic Disease.

Neurofibromatosis (Recklinghausen's disease) is frequently associated with thoracic manifestations including kyphoscoliosis, superficial skin lesions, and neurofibromas on intercostal nerves and in the posterior mediastinum. Furthermore, diffuse interstitial fibrosis has been reported.[341,342]

REFERENCES

1. EPLER GR et al: Normal chest roentgenograms in chronic diffuse infiltrative lung disease. N Engl J Med 298:934, 1978
2. FELSON B: Chest Roentgenology, p 299. Philadelphia, WB Saunders, 1973
3. FRASER RG, PARE JAP: Diagnosis of Diseases of the Chest, Vol I, 2nd ed, p 341. Philadelphia, WB Saunders, 1977
4. CARRINGTON CB, et al: Natural history and treated course of usual and desquamative interstitial pneumonia. N Engl J Med 293:801, 1978
5. FULMER JD et al: Small airways in idiopathic pulmonary fibrosis. Comparision of morphologic and physiologic observations. J Clin Invest 60:595, 1977
6. WAGNER PD et al: Distribution of ventilation–perfusion ratios in patients with interstitial lung disease. Chest [Suppl] 69:257, 1976

7. FULMER JD et al: Morphologic–physiologic correlates of the severity of fibrosis in idiopathic pulmonary fibrosis. J Clin Invest 63:665, 1979
8. CRYSTAL RG et al: Interstitial lung disease: Current concepts of pathogenesis staging and therapy. Am J Med 70:542, 1981
9. SCADDING JG: Diffuse pulmonary alveolar fibrosis. Thorax 29:271, 1974
10. GIBSON GJ, PRIDE NB: Pulmonary mechanics in fibrosing alveolitis. Am Rev Respir Dis 116:637, 1977
11. KRUMHOLZ RH, MANFREDI F, WEG JG, ROSENBAUM D: Needle biopsy of the lung: Report of its use in 112 patients and review of the literature. Ann Intern Med 65:29, 1966
12. WEG JG, BREWER LM: Percutaneous needle biopsy of the lung: A valuable diagnostic procedure in diffuse and localized disease. Am Rev Respir Dis 96:150, 1967
13. STEEL SJ et al: Trephine biopsy for diffuse lung lesions. Br Med J 2:30, 1967
14. GAENSLER EA, MOISTER MVB, HAMM J: Open-lung biopsy in diffuse pulmonary disease. N Engl J Med 270:1319, 1964
15. LEVINE DC, WICKS AB, ELLIS JH JR: Transbronchial lung biopsy via the fiberoptic bronchoscope. Am Rev Respir Dis 110:4, 1974
16. WALL CP et al: Comparison of transbronchial and open biopsies in chronic infiltrative lung diseases. Am Rev Respir Dis 123:280, 1981
17. KARLINSKY JB, GOLDSTEIN RH: Editorial: Fibrotic lung disease: A perspective. J Lab Clin Med 96:939, 1980
18. CRYSTAL RG et al: Idiopathic pulmonary fibrosis: Clinical, histologic, radiographic, physiologic, scintigraphic, cytologic and biochemical aspects. Ann Int Med 85:769, 1976
19 TURNER-WARWICK M: A perspective view on widespread pulmonary fibrosis. Br Med J 2:371, 1974
20. RUBIN E, LUBLINER R. The Hamman–Rich syndrome: Review of the literature and analysis of cases. Medicine 36:397, 1957
21. TURNER-WARWICK M, BURROWS B, JOHNSON A: Cryptogenic fibrosing alveolitis: Clinical features and their influence on survival. Thorax 35:171, 1980
22. EDITORIAL: Prognosis of cryptogenic fibrosing alveolitis. Br Med J 2:849, 1978
23. TURNER-WARWICK M, LEBOWITZ M, BURROWS B et al: Cryptogenic fibrosing alveolitis and lung cancer. Thorax 35:496, 1980
24. JAWAHERI S, LEDEVER DH, PELLA JA et al: Idiopathic pulmonary fibrosis in monozygotic twins. Chest 78:591, 1980
25. JOHNSON KJ, CHAPMAN WE, WARD PA: Immunopathology of the lung: A review. Am J Pathol 95:795, 1979
26. HUNNINGHAKE GW et al: Inflammatory and immune processes in the human lung in health and disease: Evaluation of bronchoalveolar lavage. Am J Pathol 97:149, 1979
27. GEE JBL, FICK RB JR: Editorial: Bronchoalveolar lavage. Thorax 35:1, 1980
28. HASLAM PL et al: Bronchoalveolar lavage fluid cell counts in cryptogenic fibrosing alveolitis and their relation to therapy. Thorax 35:328, 1980
29. DAVIS GL et al: Quantitation of inflammatory activity in interstitial pneumonitis by bronchofiberscopic pulmonary lavage. Chest [Suppl] 69:265, 1976
30. DREISEN RB et al: Circulating immune complexes in the idiopathic interstitial pneumonias. N Engl J Med 298:353, 1978
31. KRAVIS TC et al: Pathogenic mechanisms in pulmonary fibrosis. Collagen-induced migration inhibition factor production and cytotoxicity mediated by lymphocytes. J Clin Invest 58:1223, 1976
32. JOHNSON KJ, WARD PA: Acute immunologic pulmonary alveolitis. J Clin Invest 54:349, 1974
33. JOHNSON KJ, ANDERSON TP, WARD PA: Suppression of immune complex induced inflammation by the chemotactic factor inactivator. J Clin Invest 59:951, 1977
34. BRENTJENS JR et al: Experimental immune complex disease of the lung: The pathogenesis of a laboratory model resembling certain human interstitial lung diseases. J Exp Med 140:105, 1974
35. FULMER JD et al: Collagen concentration and roles of synthesis in idiopathic pulmonary fibrosis. Am Rev Resp Dis 122:289, 1980
36. MADRI JA, FURTHMAYR H: Collagen polymorphism in the lung. Human Path 11:353, 1980
37. FRAIRE AE et al: Diffuse interstitial fibrosis of the lung. Am J Clin Pathol 59:636, 1973
38. ZAPOL WM et al: Pulmonary fibrosis in severe acute respiratory failure. Am Rev Resp Dis 119:547, 1979
39. SCADDING JG, HINSON KFW: Diffuse fibrosing alveolitis (diffuse interstitial fibrosis of the lungs): Correlation of histology at biopsy with prognosis. Thorax 22:291, 1967
40. LIEBOW AA, STEER A, BILLINGSLEY JG: Desquamative interstitial pneumonia. Am J Med 39:369, 1965
41. GREENBERG SD et al: Pulmonary lymphoma vs. pseudolymphoma: A perplexing problem. South Med J 65:775, 1972
42. STRIMLAN CV, ROSENOW EC III, WEILAND LH et al: Lymphocytic interstitial pneumonitis. Ann Int Med 88:616, 1978
43. O'BRODOVICH HM, MOSER MM, LU L: Familial lymphoid interstitial pneumonia: A long-term follow-up. Pediatrics 65:523, 1980
44. GREENBERG SD et al: Lymphoplasmacytic pneumonia with accompanying dysproteinemia. Arch Pathol 96:73, 1973

45. SCADDING JG: Lung biopsy in the diagnosis of diffuse lung disease. Br Med J 2:557, 1970
46. STACK BHR, CHOO-KANG YFF, HEARD BE: The prognosis of cryptogenic fibrosing alveolitis. Thorax 27:535, 1972
47. BENSON MK, HUGHES DTD: Serial pulmonary function tests in fibrosing alveolitis. Br J Dis Chest 66:33, 1972
48. LINE BR et al: Gallium-67 citrate scanning in the staging of idiopathic pulmonary fibrosis: Correlation with physiologic and morphologic features and bronchoalveolar lavage. Am Rev Respir Dis 118:355, 1978
49. WINTERBAUER RH et al: Diffuse interstitial pneumonitis: Clinicopathologic correlations in 20 patients treated with prednisone/azathiaprine. Am J Med 65:661, 1978
50. MCCARTHY DS, OSTROW DN, HERSCHFIELD ES: Chronic obstructive pulmonary disease following idiopathic pulmonary fibrosis. Chest 77:473, 1980
51. MITCHELL DN, SCADDING JG: State of the art—sarcoidosis. Am Rev Respir Dis 110:774, 1974
52. MANDEL W et al: Bibliography on Sarcoidosis, 1878–1963. Washington DC, US Public Health Service, Publication No. 1213, 1964
53. SCADDING JG: Sarcoidosis. London, Eyre and Spottiswoode, 1967
54. CUMMINGS MM, HAMMARSTEN JF: Sarcoidosis. Ann Rev Med 13:19, 1962
55. MAYOCK RL et al: Manifestations of sarcoidosis. Am J Med 33:67, 1963
56. Proceedings of the international conference on sarcoidosis. Am Rev Respir Dis (Suppl) 2:1–183, 1967
57. ISRAEL HL et al: Granulomatous lung diseases. In Respiratory Diseases. National Heart and Lung Institute, Task Force on Research on Respiratory Diseases. Washington DC, US Department of Health, Education and Welfare, Publication No. (NIH) 73–432:101, 1972
58. CHURG A et al: Necrotizing sarcoid granulomatosis. Chest 76:406, 1979
59. YOUNG RL et al: Pulmonary sarcoidosis. I. Pathophysiologic correlations. Am Rev Respir Dis 97:997, 1968
60. CRYSTAL RG et al: Pulmonary sarcoidosis: A disease characterized and perpetuated by activated lung T-lymphocytes. Ann Int Med 94:73, 1981
61. NOLAN JP, KLATSKIN G: The fever of sarcoidosis. Ann Intern Med 61:455, 1964
62. JAMES DG, NEVILLE E, CARSTANS LS: Bone and joint sarcoidosis. Semin Arthritis Rheum 6:53, 1976
63. GOZO EG: The heart in sarcoidosis. Chest 60:379, 1971
64. KINNEY EL, JACKSON GL, REEVES WC et al: Thallium-scan myocardial defects and echocardiographic abnormalities in patients with sarcoidosis without clinical cardiac dysfunction. Am J Med 68:497, 1980
65. KINNEY E, MURTHY R, ASCUNCE G et al: Pericardial effusions in sarcoidosis. Am Rev Respir Dis 76:476, 1979
66. ROBERTS WC, MCALLISTER HAJ, FERRANS VJ: Sarcoidosis of the heart: A clinicopathologic study of 35 necropsy patients (Group I) and review of 78 previously described necropsy patients (Group II). Am J Med 63:86, 1977
67. SILVERSTEIN A, FEUER NM, SILTZBACH LE: Neurologic sarcoidosis. Arch Neurol 12:1, 1965
68. DOUGLAS A: Sarcoidosis of the central nervous system. In Proceedings of the Sixty International Conference on Sarcoidosis, p 340. Baltimore, University Park Press, 1974
69. DELANEY P: Neurologic manifestations in sarcoidosis: Review of the literature with a report of 23 cases. Ann Int Med 87:336, 1977
70. NIITU Y: Electroencephalography in patients with intrathoracic sarcoidosis. In Proceedings of the Sixth International Conference on Sarcoidosis, p 344. Baltimore, University Park Press, 1974
70a. STUART CA et al: Disordered control of thirst in hypothalamic–pituitary sarcoidosis. N Engl J Med 303:1078, 1980
71. ELLIS K, RENTHAL G: Pulmonary sarcoidosis: Roentgenographic observations on course of disease. Am J Roentgenol Radium Ther Nucl Med 88: 107, 1962
72. BACSA S, MANDI L: Abdominal lymphography in thoracic sarcoidosis. Scand J Respir Dis 47:244, 1967
73. ISRAEL HC, OSTROW H: Sarcoidosis and aspergilloma. Am J Med 47:243, 1969
74. BOUSHY ST et al: The course of pulmonary function in sarcoidosis. Ann Intern Med 62:939, 1965
75. RIZZATO G et al: Impaired airway function and pulmonary hemodynamics in sarcoidosis. In Williams WJ, Davies BH (eds): Proceedings of the Eighth International Conference on Sarcoidosis and other Granulomatous Diseases, p 349. Cardiff, Wales, UK, Alpha Omega Publishing, 1980
76. BECHTEL J et al: Airways hyper-reactivity in sarcoidosis. Am Rev Respir Dis (Suppl) 121:110, 1980
77. DINES DE, STUBBS SE,MCDOUGALL JG: Obstructive disease of the airways associated with stage I sarcoidosis. Mayo Clin Proc 53:788, 1978
78. YOUNG RC et al: Sarcoidosis: Relationship between changes in lung structure and lung function. Am Rev Respir Dis 95:224, 1967
79. KENT DC et al: The definitive evaluation of sarcoidosis. Am Rev Respir Dis 101:721, 1970

80. ISRAEL HL: The diagnosis of sarcoidosis. Ann Intern Med 68:1323, 1968
81. NESSAN VJ, JACOWAY JR: Biopsy of minor salivary glands in the diagnosis of sarcoidosis. N Engl J Med 301:922, 1979
82. SILTZBACH LE: The Kveim test in sarcoidosis. JAMA 178:476, 1961
83. KENNEY M, STONE DJ: Objective evaluation of the Kveim test in a "double blind" study. Am Rev Respir Dis 87:504, 1963
84. SILTZBACH LE et al: The course and prognosis of sarcoidosis around the world. Am J Med 57:847, 1974
85. ISRAEL HL, GOLDSTEIN RA: Relation of Kveim antigen reaction to lymphoadenopathy. N Engl J Med 284:345, 1971
86. IWAI K et al: Kveim reaction disagreement in results and tentative criteria. In Proceedings of the Sixth International Conference on Sarcoidosis, pp 57–107. Baltimore, University Park Press, 1974
87. JAMES DG, NEVILLE E, WALKER A: Immunology of sarcoidosis. Am J Med 59:388, 1975
88. WINTERBAUER RH, BELIC N, MOORES KD: A clinical interpretation of bilateral hilar adenopathy. Ann Intern Med 78:65, 1973
89. CHAPMAN JS, SPEIGHT M: Further studies of mycobacterial antibodies in the sera of sarcoidosis patients. Acta Med Scand 176:61, 1964
90. MANKIEWICZ E, VAN WALBECK M: Mycobacteriophages: Their role in tuberculosis and sarcoidosis. Arch Environ Health 5:122, 1962
91. MANKIEWICZ E: The relationship of sarcoidosis to anonymous bacteria. Acta Med Scand 176:68, 1964
92. LORDON RE et al: Sarcoidosis. II. A clinical evaluation of the alteration in delayed hypersensitivity. Am Rev Respir Dis 97:1009, 1968
93. HO Y et al: The production of granulomas in animals and men by a propionibacterium suspension and yersina. Williams WJ, Davies BH (eds): Proceedings of the Eighth International Conference on Sarcoidosis and Other Granulomatous Diseases, p 142. Cardiff, Wales, UK, Alpha Omega Publishing, 1980
94. MITCHELL DN, REES RJW: Further observations on the nature of physical characteristics of transmissible agents from human sarcoid and Crohn's disease tissues. Williams WJ, Davies BH (eds): Proceedings of the Eighth International Conference on Sarcoidosis and Other Granulomatous Diseases, p 121. Cardiff, Wales, UK, Alpha Omega Publishing, 1980
95. GREENBERG SD et al: The ultrastructure of the pulmonary granuloma in "sarcoidosis". Am Rev Respir Dis 102:648, 1970
96. LEAKE ES, MYRVIK QN: Osmophilic structures in granulomatous macrophages and the problem of intracellular mycobacteria. Ann Rev Respir Dis 104:132, 1971
97. GOODWIN JS, DEHORATIUS R, ISRAEL H et al: Suppressor cell function in sarcoidosis. Ann Intern Med 90:169, 1979
98. DANIELE RP, DAUBER JH, ROSSMAN MD: Immunologic abnormalities in sarcoidosis. Ann Intern Med 92:406, 1980
99. DAUBER JH, ROSSMAN MD, DANIELE RP: Bronchoalveolar cell populations in acute sarcoidosis. J Lab Clin Med 94:862, 1979
100. HOYLE E: Prognosis of pulmonary sarcoidosis. Lancet 2:611, 1961
101. RUDBERG-ROOS I: The course and prognosis of sarcoidosis as observed in 296 cases. Acta Tuberc Pneumol Scand [Suppl 51] 41:5, 1962
102. RAISNER D: Course and prognosis of sarcoidosis. Am Rev Respir Dis 96:361, 1967
103. LINE BR et al: Gallium-67 scanning to stage the alveolitis of sarcoidosis: Correlation with clinical studies, pulmonary function studies, and bronchoalveolar lavage. Am Rev Respir Dis 123:440, 1981
104. STUDDY P et al: Serum angiotensin-converting enzyme (SACE): Experience in ten centres. Williams WJ, Davies BH (eds): Proceedings of the Eighth International Conference on Sarcoidosis and Other Granulomatous Diseases, p 241. Cardiff, Wales, UK, Alpha Omega Publishing, 1980
105. SHARMA OP: Diagnosis of sarcoidosis. Arch Intern Med 138:689, 1978
106. YOUNG RL et al: Pulmonary sarcoidosis: A prospective evaluation of glucocorticoid therapy. Ann Intern Med 73:207, 1970
107. STONE DJ, SCHWARTZ A: A long-term study of sarcoid and its modification by steroid therapy. Am J Med 41:528, 1966
108. SHARMA OP, COLP C, WILLIAMS MH: Course of pulmonary sarcoidosis with and without corticosteroid therapy as determined by pulmonary function studies. Am J Med 49:541, 1966
109. EMIRGIL G, SOBOL BJ, WILLIAMS MH: Long-term study of pulmonary sarcoidosis: The effect of steroid therapy as evaluated by pulmonary function studies. J Chronic Dis 22:69, 1969
110. SELROOS O et al: XI Therapy. Proceedings of the Sixth International Conference on Sarcoidosis, pp 525–550. Baltimore, University Park Press, 1974
111. FAHEY JL et al: Wegener's granulomatosis. Am J Med 17:168, 1954
112. FAUCI AS, WOLFF SM: Wegener's granulomatosis: Studies in eighteen patients and a review of the literature. Medicine 52:535, 1973
113. WALTON EW: Giant-cell granuloma of the respiratory tract (Wegener's granulomatosis). Br Med J 2:265, 1958

114. CARRINGTON CB, LIEBOW AA: Limited forms of angiitis and granulomatosis of Wegener's type. Am J Med 41:497, 1966
115. CASSAN SM, COLES DT, HARRISON EG: The concept of limited forms of Wegener's granulomatosis. Am J Med 49:366, 1970
116. ALARCON-SEGOVIA P, BROWN HL: Classification and etiologic aspects of necrotizing angiitides: An analytical approach to a confused subject with a critical review of the evidence for hypersensitivity in polyarteritis nodosa. Mayo Clin Proc 39:207, 1964
117. LIEBOW AA: The J Burns Amberson Lecture: Pulmonary angiitis and granulomatosis. Am Rev Respir Dis 108:1, 1973
118. KATZENSTEIN AL, LIEBOW AA, FRIEDMAN PJ: Bronchocentric granulomatosis, mucoid impaction, and hypersensitivity reactions to fungi. Am Rev Respir Dis 111:497, 1975
119. WOLFF SM et al: Wegener's granulomatosis (NIH Conference). Ann Intern Med 81:513, 1974
120. MAGUIRE R et al: Unusual radiographic features of Wegener's granulomatosis. Am J Roentgenol 130:233, 1978
121. REZA MJ et al: Wegener's granulomatosis: Long-term follow-up of patients treated with cyclophosphamide. Arthritis Rheum 18:501, 1975
122. ISRAEL HL, PATCHEFSKY AS: Treatment of Wegener's granulomatosis of lung. Am J Med 58:671, 1975
123. FAUCI AS, HAYNES BF, KATZ P: The spectrum of vasculitis: Clinical immunologic and therapeutic considerations. Ann Intern Med (Suppl) 89:660, 1978
124. ISRAEL HL, PATCHEFSKY AS, SALDANA MJ: Wegener's granulomatosis, lymphomatoid granulomatosis and benign lymphocytic angiitis and granulomatosis of lung: Recognition and treatment. Ann Intern Med 87:691, 1977
125. KATZENSTEIN A, CARRINGTON CB, LIEBOW AA: Lymphomatoid granulomatosis: A clinicopathologic study of 152 cases. Cancer 43:630, 1979
126. LIEBOW AA, CARRINGTON CRB, FRIEDMAN PJ: Lymphatoid granulomatosis. Hum Pathol 3:457, 1972
127. AULD D: Pathology of eosinophilic granuloma. Arch Pathol 63:113, 1957
128. SMITH M et al: "Primary" pulmonary histiocytosis X. Chest 65:176, 1974
129. LICHTENSTEIN L: Histiocytosis X: Integration of eosinophilic granuloma of bone, "Letterer-Siwe disease" and "Schüller-Christian disease" as related manifestations of a single entity. Arch Pathol 56:84, 1953
130. ENRIQUEZ P et al: Histiocytosis X: A clinical study. Mayo Clin Proc 42:88, 1967
131. LIEBERMAN PH et al: A reappraisal of eosinophilic granuloma of bone, Hand-Schüller-Christian syndrome and Letterer-Siwe syndrome. Medicine 48:375, 1959
132. LEWIS JG: Eosinophilic granuloma and its variants with special reference to lung involvement. A report of 12 patients. Quart J Med 33:337, 1964
133. WEBER WN, MARGOLIN FR, NIELSEN SL: Pulmonary histiocytosis X: A review of 18 patients with reports of 6 cases. Am J Roentgenol Radium Ther Nucl Med 107:280, 1969
134. TAKAHASKI M, MARTEL W, OBERMAN HA: The variable roentgenographic appearance of idiopathic histiocytosis. Clin Radiol 17:48, 1953
135. BASSET F, CORRIN B, SPENCER H et al: Pulmonary histiocytosis X. Am Rev Respir Dis 118:811, 1978
136. STANFORD W et al: Eosinophilic granuloma of the lung. Ann Thorac Surg 11:299, 1971
137. HOFFMAN L, COHN JE, GAENSLER E: Respiratory abnormalities in eosinophilic granuloma of the lung: Long-term study of five cases. N Engl J Med 267:577, 1962
138. HUNNINGHAKE GW, FAUCI AS: State of the art: Pulmonary involvement in the collagen vascular diseases. Am Rev Respir Dis 119:471, 1979
139. Editorial: Respiratory complications of rheumatoid disease. Br Med J 1:1437, 1978
140. Editorial: Airways in rheumatoid disease. Lancet 1:192, 1978
141. WALKER WC, WRIGHT V: Rheumatoid pleuritis. Ann Rheum Dis 26:467, 1967
142. MARTEL W et al: Pulmonary and pleural lesions in rheumatoid disease. Radiology 90:641, 1968
143. CARR DT, MAYNE JG: Pleurisy with effusion in rheumatoid arthritis, with reference to the low concentration of glucose in pleural fluid. Am Rev Respir Dis 85:345, 1962
144. SAHN SS, KAPLAN RL, MAULTIZ RM et al: Rheumatoid pleurisy. Arch Intern Med 140:1237, 1980
145. CAMPBELL GD, FERRINGTON E: Rheumatoid pleuritis with effusion. Dis Chest 53:521, 1968
146. BERGER HW, SECKLER SG: Pleural and pericardial effusions in rheumatoid disease. Ann Intern Med 64:1291, 1966
147. NOSANCHICK JS, NAYLOR B: A unique cytologic picture in pleural fluid from patients with rheumatoid arthritis. Am J Clin Pathol 50:330, 1968
148. GRUENWALD P: Visceral lesions in a case of rheumatoid arthritis. Arch Pathol 46:59, 1948
149. JONES FL, BLODGETT RC: Empyema in rheumatoid pleuropulmonary disease. Ann Intern Med 74:665, 1971
150. ELLMAN P: The etiology of chronic rheumatism. Proc R Soc Med 40:332, 1947
151. Editorial: Rheumatoid lung and rheumatoid piles. Br Med J 1:186, 1967
152. FRANK ST et al: Pulmonary dysfunction in rheumatoid disease. Chest 63:27, 1973
153. LAITENEN O, NISSILA M, SALORINNES et al: Pulmo-

nary involvement in patients with rheumatoid arthritis. Scand J Respir Dis 56:297, 1975

154. CERVANTES-PEREZ P, TORO-PEREZ AH, RODRIGUEZ-JURADO P: Pulmonary involvement in rheumatoid arthritis. JAMA 243:1715, 1980
155. PATTERSON CD, HARVILLE WE, PIERCE JA: Rheumatoid lung disease. Ann Intern Med 62:685, 1965
156. RUBIN EH, GORDON M, THELMO WL: Nodular pleuropulmonary rheumatoid disease. Am J Med 42:567, 1967
157. PORTNER MM, GRACIE WA JR: Rheumatoid lung disease with cavitary nodules, pneumothorax, and eosinophilia. N Engl J Med 275:697, 1966
158. HARVEY A MCG et al: Systemic lupus erythematosus: Review of the literature and clinical analysis of 138 cases. Medicine 33:291, 1954
159. BULGRIN JG, DUBOIS EL, JACOBSON G: Chest roentgenographic changes in systemic lupus erythematosus. Radiology 74:42, 1960
160. HUANG CT, HENNIGAR GR, LYONS HL: Pulmonary dysfunction in systemic lupus erythematosus. N Engl J Med 272:288, 1965
161. BLACK LF: The pleural space and pleural fluid. Mayo Clin Proc 47:493, 1972
162. EISENBERG H et al: Diffuse interstitial lung disease in systemic lupus erythematosus. Ann Intern Med 79:37, 1973
163. HUANG CT, LYONS HA: Comparison of pulmonary function in patients with systemic lupus erythematosus, scleroderma, and rheumatoid arthritis. Am Rev Respir Dis 93:865, 1966
164. GOLD WM, JENNINGS DB: Pulmonary function in patients with lupus erythematosus. Am Rev Respir Dis 93:556, 1966
165. GIBSON GJ, EDMONDS JP, HUGHES GRU: Diaphragm function and lung involvement in systemic lupus erythematosus. Am J Med 63:926, 1977
166. GLADMAN DD, UROWITZ MB: Venous syndromes and pulmonary embolism in systemic lupus erythematosus. Ann Rheum Dis 39:340, 1980
167. PERTSCHUK LP, MOCCIZ LF, ROSEN Y et al: Acute pulmonary complications in systemic lupus erythematosus. Am J Clin Pathol 68:553, 1977
168. MATTHAY RA, SCHWARTZ MI, PETTY TL et al: Pulmonary manifestations of systemic lupus erythematosus. Medicine 54:397, 1974
169. YUM MN, ZIEGLER JR, WALKER PD et al: Pseudolymphoma of the lung in a patient with systemic lupus erythematosus. Am J Med 66:172, 1977
170. PURNELL DC, BAGENSTOSE AH, OLSEN AM: Pulmonary lesions in disseminated lupus erythematosus. Ann Intern Med 42:619, 1955
171. PIPER WW, HELWIG EB: Progressive systemic sclerosis. Visceral manifestations as generalized scleroderma. Arch Dermatol 72:535, 1955
172. D'ANGELO WA et al: Pathologic observations in systemic sclerosis (scleroderma): A study of 58 autopsy cases and 58 matched controls. Am J Med 46:428, 1969
173. WEAVER AL, DIVERTIE MB, TITUS JL: Pulmonary scleroderma. Dis Chest 54:490, 1968
174. WILSON RJ, RODNAN GP, ROBINE ED: An early pulmonary physiologic abnormality in progressive systemic sclerosis (diffuse scleroderma). Am J Med 36:361, 1964
175. SACHNER MH et al: The pathophysiology of scleroderma involving the heart and respiratory system. Ann Intern Med 60:611, 1964
176. YOUNG RH, MARK GJ: Pulmonary vascular changes in scleroderma. Am J Med 64:999, 1978
177. SALERNI R et al: Pulmonary hypertension in the CREST syndrome variant of progressive systemic sclerosis (scleroderma). Ann Int Med 86:394, 1977
178. CAPLAN H: Honeycomb lungs and malignant pulmonary adenomatosis in scleroderma. Thorax 14:89, 1959
179. SCHWARZ MIet al: Interstitial lung disease in polymyositis and dermatomyositis: Analysis of six cases and a review of the literature. Medicine 55:89, 1955
180. PLOWMAN PN, STABLEFORTH DE: Dermatomyositis with fibrosing alveolitis: Response to therapy with cyclophosphamide. Proc R Soc Med 70:738, 1977
181. MOUTSOPOULOS HM et al: Sjögren's syndrome (Sicca syndrome): Current issues. Ann Int Med 92(1):212, 1980
182. NEWBELL HH, BRAHIM SA: Chronic obstructive airway disease in patients with Sjögren syndrome. Am Rev Respir Dis 115:295, 1977
183. ARKIN A: Clinical and pathological study of periarteritis nodosa: Report of five cases, one histologically healed. Am J Pathol 6: 401, 1930
184. GARLAND LH, SISSON MA: Roentgen findings in the "collagen" diseases. Am J Roentgenol Radium Ther Nucl Med 71:581, 1954
185. ROSE GA, SPENCER H: Polyarteritis nodosa. Q J Med 26:43, 1957
186. COHEN RD, CONN DL, ILSTRUP DM: Clinical features, prognosis and response to treatment in polyarteritis. Mayo Clin Proc 55:146, 1980
187. FAUCI AS, KATA P, HAYNES BF et al: Cyclophosphamide therapy of severe necrotising vasculitis. N Engl J Med 301:235, 1979
188. AGIS GA, ZEDDY UC, MALTBY J et al: Pulmonary involvement in mixed connective tissue disease. Am Rev Respir Dis 121(2):105, 1980
188a. KENTALA Æ, REPO UK, LEHTIPUU A-L et al: HLA-antigens and pulmonary upper lobe fibrocystic changes with and without ankylosing spondylitis. Scand J Respir Dis 59:8, 1978
189. FRIZZERA A, MORAN EM, RAPPOPORT H: Angioimmunoblastic lymphadenopathy diagnosis and clinical course. Am J Med 59:803, 1975

189a. MYERS TJ, COLE SR, TASTUSZAK WT: Angioimmunoblastic lymphadenopathy: Pleuropulmonary disease. Cancer 40:266, 1978

190. NATHWANI BN et al: Malignant lymphoma arising in angioimmunoblastic lymphadenopathy. Cancer 41:578, 1978

191. WEISENBERGER D, ARMITAGE J, DICK F: Immunoblastic lymphadenopathy with pulmonary infiltrates, hypocomplementemia and vasculitis. Am J Med 63:849, 1977

192. BENOIT FL et al: Goodpasture's syndrome: A clinicopathologic entity. Am J Med 37:424, 1964

193. LERNER RA et al: The role of antiglomerular basement membrane antibody in the pathogenesis of human glomerulonephritis. J Exper Med 126:989, 1967

194. MCPHAUL JJ et al: The presence of antiglomerular basement membrane antibodies in peripheral blood. J Immunol 103:1168, 1969

195. WILSON CB, DIXON FJ: Antiglomerular basement membrane antibody induced glomerulonephritis. Kidney Int 3:74, 1973

196. MCCOMBS RP: Diseases due to immunologic reactions in the lungs. N Engl J Med 286:1186, 1972

197. THOMAS HT III, IRWIN RS: Classification of diffuse intrapulmonary hemorrhage. Chest 68:483, 1975

198. TEAGUE CA et al: Goodpasture's syndrome: Analysis of 29 cases. Kidney Int 12:492, 1978

199. WILSON CB, DIXON FJ: Diagnosis of immunopathologic renal disease. Kidney Int 5:389, 1974

200. KOFFLER D et al: Immunologic studies concerning the pulmonary lesions in Goodpasture's syndrome. Am J Pathol 54:293, 1969

201. AGODOA LCY et al: The appearance of non-linear deposits of immunoglobulins in Goodpasture's syndrome. Am J Med 61:407, 1976

202. PASTERNACK A: Evidence of both anti-GBM and immune complex mediated pathogenesis in the initial phase of Goodpasture's syndrome. Clin Nephrol 9:77, 1978

203. REES AJ et al: Enhanced allergic tissue injury in Goodpasture's syndrome by intercurrent infection. Br Med J 2:723, 1977

204. BEIRNE GJ et al: Immunohistology of the lung in Goodpasture's syndrome. Ann Intern Med 69:1207, 1978

205. MATHEW TH et al: Goodpasture's syndrome: Normal renal diagnostic findings. Ann Intern Med 82:215, 1975

206. DUNCAN DA et al. Pulmonary hemorrhage and glomerulonephritis: A report of six cases and study of the renal lesion by the fluorescent antibody technique and electron microscopy. Ann Intern Med 62:920, 1965

207. PROSKEY AJ et al: Goodpasture's syndrome. A report of five cases and review of the literature. Am J Med 48:162, 1970

208. LOCKWOOD CM et al: Immuno-suppression and plasma-exchange in the treatment of Goodpasture's syndrome. Lancet 1:711, 1976

209. MUNK ZM, SKAMENE E: Goodpasture's syndrome: Effects of plasmapheresis. Clin Exp Immunol 36:244, 1979

210. ERIKSON SB et al: Use of combined plasmapheresis and immunosuppression in the treatment of Goodpasture's syndrome. Mayo Clin Proc 54:714, 1979

210a. GREENING AP, HUGHES JMB: Serial estimations of carbon monoxide diffusing capacity in intrapulmonary hemorrhage. Clin Sci 60:507, 1981

211. SOERGEL KH, SOMMERS SC: Idiopathic pulmonary hemosiderosis and related syndromes. Am J Med 32:499, 1962

212. HERBERT FA, ORFORD R: Pulmonary hemorrhage and edema due to inhalation of resin containing trimellitic anhydride. Chest 76:546, 1979

213. LIEBOW AA, CARRINGTON CB: The eosinophilic pneumonias. Medicine 48:251, 1969

214. CARRINGTON CB et al: Chronic eosinophilic pneumonia. N Engl J Med 280:787, 1969

215. PEARSON DJ, ROSENOW EC III: Chronic eosinophilic pneumonia. Mayo Clin Proc 53:73, 1978

216. ROGERS RM et al: Eosinophilic pneumonia physiologic response to steroid therapy and observations on light and electron microscopy. Chest 68:665, 1975

217. CHUSID MJ et al: The hypereosinophilic syndrome: Analysis of fourteen cases with a review of the literature. Medicine 54:1, 1975

218. PARILLO JE, FAUCI AS, WOLFF SM: Therapy of the hypereosinophilic syndrome. Am Intern Med 89:167, 1978

219. BRUSH RK, GELLER M, BUSSE WW et al: Response to corticosteroids in the hypereosinophilic syndrome. Arch Intern Med 138:1244, 1978

220. BEDROSSIAN CWM, GREENBERG SD, WILLIAMS LJ: Ultrastructure of the lung in Loeffler's pneumonia. Am J Med 58:438, 1975

221. REEDER WH, GOODRICH BE: Pulmonary infiltration with eosinophilia (PIE syndrome). Ann Intern Med 36:1217, 1952

222. CROFTAN JW et al: Pulmonary eosinophilia. Thorax 7:1, 1952

223. ROSEN SH, CASTLEMAN B, LIEBOW AA: Pulmonary alveolar proteinosis. N Engl J Med 258:1123, 1958

224. LARSON RK, GORDINIER R: Pulmonary alveolar proteinosis. Ann Intern Med 62:292, 1965

225. FRANK ST, MALONEY TR, WEG JG. Pulmonary alveolar proteinosis: Report on two cases and comments on its pathogenesis. South Med J 62:867, 1969

226. KUHN C et al: Pulmonary alveolar proteinosis: A study using enzyme histochemistry, electron microscopy, and surface tension measurements. Lab Invest 15:492, 1966

227. TAYLOR FB, ABRAMS ME: Effect of surface-active

lipoprotein on clotting and fibrinolysis and of fibrinogen on surface-active lipoprotein. Am J Med 40:347, 1966

228. HARRIS JO: Pulmonary alveolar proteinosis: Abnormal *in vitro* function of alveolar macrophages. Chest 76:156, 1979
229. GOLDE DW: Editorial: Alveolar proteinosis and the overfed macrophage. Chest 76:119, 1979
230. MARTIN RJ, ROGERS RM, MYERS NM: Pulmonary alveolar proteinosis. Am Rev Respir Dis 117:1059, 1978
231. BALA RM, SNIDAL DP: Pulmonary alveolar proteinosis. Dis Chest 49:643, 1966
232. RAMIREZ-RIVERA J, KIEFFER RF, BALL WC: Bronchopulmonary lavage in man. Ann Intern Med 63:819, 1965
233. ROGERS RM et al: Hemodynamic response of the pulmonary circulation to bronchopulmonary lavage in man. N Engl J Med 286:1230, 1972
234. ROGERS RM, BRAUNSTEIN MS, SHUMAN JF: Role of bronchopulmonary lavage in the treatment of respiratory failure: A review. Chest [Suppl] 62:95S, 1972
235. JAY SJ: Pulmonary alveolar proteinosis: Successful treatment with aerosolized trypsin. Am J Med 66:348, 1979
236. SOSMAN MC et al: The familial occurrence of pulmonary alveolar microlithiasis. Am J Roentgenol Radium Ther Nucl Med 77:947, 1957
237. CAFFERY PR, ALTMAN RS: Pulmonary alveolar microlithiasis occurring in premature twins. J Pediatr 66:758, 1965
238. O'NEILL RP, COHN JE, PELLERGRINO ED: Pulmonary alveolar microlithiasis. Ann Intern Med 67:957, 1967
239. OKA M et al: Pulmonary alveolar microlithiasis: Reports of three cases. Am Rev Respir Dis 93:612, 1966
240. JUSTRABO E, GENIN R, RIFLE G: Pulmonary metastatic calcification with respiratory insufficiency in patients on hemodialysis. Thorax 34:384, 1979
241. HEATH D, ROBERTSON AJ: Pulmonary calcinosis. Thorax 36:606, 1977
242. COHEN AM, MAXON HR, GOLDSMITH RC et al: Metastatic pulmonary calcification in primary hyperparathyroidism. Arch Intern Med 137:520, 1977
243. CONGER JD, HAMMOND WS, ALFREY AC et al: Pulmonary calcification in chronic dialysis patients. Am Intern Med 83:330, 1975
244. MORGAN WKC, SEATON A: Occupational Lung Diseases. Philadelphia, WB Saunders, 1975
245. PARKES WR: Occupational Lung Disorders. Edinburgh, Butterworth, 1974
246. BOUHUYS A, PETERS JM: Control of environmental lung disease. N Engl J Med 283:573, 1970
247. LEE DHK: Environmental Factors in Respiratory Disease. New York, Academic Press, 1972
248. MORGAN WKC: International conference on occupational lung diseases. Chest [Suppl] 2:352, 1980
249. ZISKIND M, JONES RW, WEILL H: State of the art: Silicosis. Am Rev Respir Dis 113:643, 1975
250. JACOBSON G, GILSON JC: Present status of the UICC/Cincinnati classification of radiographic appearances of the pneumoconioses. Ann NY Acad Sci 200:552, 1972
251. SILICOSIS—ILLINOIS. Morbidity and Mortality Weekly Report 29:206, 1980
252. BECKLAKE MR: State of the art: Asbestos-related diseases of the lung and other organs: Their epidemiology and implications for clinical practice. Am Rev Respir Dis 114:187, 1976
253. DICKE TE, NAYLOR B: Prevalence of "asbestos" bodies in human lungs at necropsy. Dis Chest 56:122, 1969
254. SELIKOFF IJ, HAMMOND EC, CHURG J: Asbestos exposure, smoking, and neoplasia. JAMA 204:106, 1968
255. SELIKOFF IJ, CHURG J, HAMMOND EC: Relation between exposure to asbestos and mesothelioma. N Engl J Med 272:560, 1965
256. BUCHANAN WD: Asbestosis and primary intrathoracic neoplasms. Ann NY Acad Sci 132:507, 1965
257. BOROW M et al: Mesothelioma following exposure to asbestos: A review of 72 cases. Chest 64:641, 1973
258. WAGNER JC, SLEGS CA, MARCHAND P: Diffuse pleural mesothelioma and asbestos exposure in the North-West Cape Province. Br J Ind Med 17:260, 1960
259. GOULD SR, BARNARDO DE: Respiratory distress after talc inhalation. Br J Dis Chest 66:230, 1970
260. HOPKINS GB, TAYLOR DG: Pulmonary talc granulomatosis: A complication of drug abuse. Am Rev Respir Dis 101:101, 1970
261. GAMBLE JF, TELLNER W, DIMEO MJ: An epidemiologic study of a group of talc workers. Am Rev Respir Dis 119:741, 1979
262. MORGAN WKC, LAPP NL: State of the art: Respiratory disease in coal miners. Am Rev Respir Dis 113:531, 1976
263. ZAHORSKI WW: Coal Workers' Pneumoconiosis: A Critical Review. Hanover, NH, University Press of New England, 1974
264. JAMES WRL: The relationship of tuberculosis to the development of massive pneumokoniosis in coal workers. Br J Tuberc 48:89, 1954
265. ROM WN et al: Respiratory disease in Utah coal miners. Am Rev Respir Dis 123:372, 1981
266. MORGAN WKC, LAPP NL, SEATON D: Respiratory disability in coal miners. JAMA 243:2401, 1980
267. CAPLAN A, PAYNE RB, WITHEY JL: A broader concept of Caplan's syndrome related to rheumatoid factors. Thorax 17:205, 1962
268. STOECKLE JD, HARDY HL, WEBER AL: Chronic beryllium disease: Long-term follow-up of 60 cases

and a selective review of the literature. Am J Med 46:545, 1969
269. COATES EO JR, WATSON JHL: Diffuse interstitial lung disease in tungsten carbide workers. Ann Intern Med 75:709, 1971
270. COATES EO JR et al: Hypersensitivity bronchitis in tungsten carbide workers. Chest 64:390, 1973
271. BETON DC et al: Acute cadmium fume poisoning: Five cases with one death from renal necrosis. Br J Ind Med 23:292, 1966
272. GRAYSON RR: Silage gas poisoning: Nitrogen dioxide pneumonia, a new disease in agricultural workers. Ann Intern Med 45:393, 1956
272a. OSBERN LN, CRAPO RO: Dung lung: A report of toxic exposure to liquid manure. Ann Intern Med 95:312, 1981
273. PEPYS J: Hypersensitivity diseases of the lung due to fungi and organic dusts. In Monographs in Allergy, Vol 4. Basel S. Karger, 1969
274. SCHLEUTER DP: Response of the lung to inhaled antigens. Am J Med 57:476, 1976
275. KALTREIDER HB: State of the art: expression of immune mechanisms in the lung. Am Rev Respir Dis 113:347, 1976
276. BANAZAK EJ, THIEDE WH, FINK JN: Hypersensitivity pneumonitis due to contamination of an air conditioner. N Engl J Med 283:271, 1970
277. BECK CJ et al: The relation of lung function to subsequent employment status and mortality in cotton textile workers. Chest [Suppl] 79:26, 1981
278. PRATT PC: Comparative prevalence and severity of emphysema and bronchitis at autopsy in cotton mill workers *vs.* controls. Chest [Suppl] 79:49S, 1981
279. RYLANDER R: Bacterial toxins and etiology of byssinosis. Chest [Suppl] 79:34S, 1981
280. OLENCHOCK SA et al: Cotton dust and complement *in vivo.* Chest [Suppl] 79:53S, 1981
281. SCHACTER EW et al: The effect of mediator modifying drugs in cotton bract-induced bronchospasm. Chest [Suppl] 79:73S, 1981
282. MERCHANT J, KILBURN KH et al: Byssinosis and chronic bronchitis among cotton textile workers. Ann Intern Med 76:423, 1972
283. WEILL H, WADDELL LC, ZISKIND M: A study of workers exposed to detergent enzymes. JAMA 217:425, 1971
284. PEPYS J: Clinical and therapeutic significance of patterns of allergic reactions of the lungs to extrinsic agents. Am Rev Respir Dis 116:573, 1977
285. PETERS JM et al: Acute respiratory effects in workers exposed to low levels of toluene diisocyanate (TDI). Arch Environ Health 16:642, 1968
286. BUTCHER BT et al: Longitudinal study of workers employed in the manufacture of toluene diisocyanate. Am Rev Respir Dis 116:411, 1977
287. LILLIS R: Vinylchloride and polyvinylchloride exposure and occupational disease. Chest 78:826, 1980
288. CORDASCO EM et al: Pulmonary manifestations of vinyl- and polyvinylchloride (interstitial lung disease). Chest 78:830, 1980
289. KARR RM et al: Occupational asthma. J Allergy Clin Immunol 61:54, 1978
289a. COCKCROFT D, DOSMAN J: Respiratory health risks in farmers. Ann Intern Med 95:380, 1981
290. EMANUEL DA et al: Farmer's lung. Clinical, pathologic and immunologic study of 24 patients. Am J Med 37:392, 1964
291. ROBERTS RC, MOORE VL: Immunopathogenesis of hypersensitivity pneumonitis. Am Rev Respir Dis 116:1075, 1977
292. OLENCHOCK SA: Animal models of hypersensitivity pneumonitis: A review. Ann Allergy 38:119, 1977
293. GRINGHURST LS, BRYNE RN, GERSHON-COHEN J: Respiratory disease of mushroom workers: Farmer's lung. JAMA 171:15, 1959
294. WEILL H et al: Bagassosis: A study of pulmonary function in 20 cases. Ann Intern Med 64:737, 1966
295. EMANUEL DA, WENZEL TJ, LAWTON BR: Pneumonitis due to cryptostroma corticale (maple bark disease). N Engl J Med 274:1413, 1966
296. COHEN HI et al: A granulomatous pneumonitis associated with redwood sawdust inhalation. Am J Med 43:785, 1967
297. SCHLUETER DP, FINK JN, HENSLEY GT: Wood-pulp workers disease: A hypersensitivity pneumonitis caused by alternaria. Ann Intern Med 77:907, 1972
298. RIDDLE HFV et al: Allergic alveolitis in a malt worker. Thorax 23:271, 1968
299. LUNN JA, HUGHES DTD: Pulmonary hypersensitivity to the grain weevil. Br J Ind Med 24:158, 1967
300. SCHLUETER DP: Cheese worker's disease: A new occupational hazard? Ann Intern Med 78:606, 1973
301. RHUDY J, BURNELL RG, MORGAN WKC: Yet another cause of allergic alveolitis. Scand J Respir Dis 52:177, 1971
302. AVILA R, VILLAR TG: Suberosis: Respiratory disease in cork workers. Lancet 1:620, 1968
303. VAN TOORN DW: Coffee worker's lung. Thorax 25:399, 1970
304. FINK FJ et al: Pigeon breeders' disease: A clinical study of a hypersensitivity pneumonitis. Ann Intern Med 68:1205, 1968
305. SCHLUETER DP, FINK JN, SOSMAN AJ: Pulmonary function in pigeon breeders' disease. Ann Intern Med 70:457, 1969
306. HARPER LO et al: Allergic alveolitis due to pituitary snuff. Ann Intern Med 73:581, 1970

307. ARNOW PM, FINK SN, SCHLUETER DP et al: Early detection of hypersensitivity pneumonitis in office workers. Am J Med 64: 236, 1978

308. BROWN SR, DEPICO GA, ISIATIS A et al: Farmer's lung disease: Long-term clinical and physiologic outcome. Am Rev Respir Dis 119:185, 1979

309. JENNINGS FL, ARDEN A: Development of radiation pneumonitis: Times and dose factors. Arch Pathol 74:351, 1969

310. GROSS NJ: Pulmonary effects of radiation therapy. Ann Intern Med 86:81, 1977

311. SMITH JC: Radiation pneumonitis, a review. Am Rev Respir Dis 87:647, 1963

312. COLLINS JF, JOHANSON WG, MCCULLOUGH B: Effects of compensatory lung growth in irradiation-induced regional pulmonary fibrosis in the baboon. Am Rev Respir Dis 117:1079, 1978

313. GROSS NJ: Radiation pneumonitis in mice. J Clin Invest 66:504, 1980

314. ROSENOW EC III: The spectrum of drug-induced pulmonary disease. Ann Intern Med 77:977, 1972

315. LIPPMANN M: Pulmonary reactions to drugs. Med Clin NA 61:1353, 1977

316. FORD GT, GILLETTE D: Drug-induced lung disease. In Thurlbeck WM, Abell MR (eds): In the Lung: Structure, Function and Disease. International Academy of Pathology. Baltimore, Williams and Wilkins Co, 1978

317. BENNETT JM, REICH SD: Diagnosis and treatment: Drugs five years later: Bleomycin. Ann Intern Med 90:945, 1979

318. SASTMAN HD et al: Methotrexate-induced pneumonitis. Medicine 55:371, 1975

319. WEISS EB, MUGGIA FM: Cytotoxic drug-induced pulmonary disease. Update 1980. Am J Med 68:259, 1980

320. ARANIN PA et al: Prediction of BCNU pulmonary toxicity in patients with malignant gliomas. N Engl J Med 303:1831, 1980

321. SOVIJARVI S et al: Nitrofurantoin-induced acute, subacute and chronic pulmonary reactions: A report of 66 cases. Scand J Respir Dis 58:41, 1977

321a. HOLMBERG L, BOMAN G, BÖTTINGOULE et al: Adverse reactions to nitrofurantoin. Am J Med 69:733, 1980

322. PERLOW GM et al: Tocamide-associated interstitial pneumonitis. Ann Intern Med 94:489, 1981

323. MCCORMIC J, COLE S, LAHIRRI B et al: Pneumonitis caused by gold salt therapy. Am Rev Respir Dis 122:145, 1980

324. IIO D et al: Pulmonary infiltrates with eosinophilia associated with tetracycline. Chest 76:33, 1979

325. RUSINOW A, CELL BR, COHEN AS et al: Localized amyloidosis of the lower respiratory tract. Am Rev Respir Dis 118:603, 1978

326. KANADA DJ, SHARMA OP: Long-term survival with diffuse interstitial pulmonary amyloidosis. Am J Med 67:879, 1979

327. HIMMELFARB E, WELLS S, RABINOWITZ JG: The radiologic spectrum of cardiopulmonary amyloidosis. Chest 72:327, 1977

328. CELLI BR et al: Patterns of pulmonary involvement in systemic amyloidosis. Chest 74:543, 1978

329. DESAI R et al: Pulmonary amyloidoma and hilar adenopathy: Rare manifestations of primary amyloidosis. Chest 76:170, 1979

330. DAWSON J: Pulmonary tuberous sclerosis and its relationship to other forms of disease. Q J Med 90:1, 1966

331. LIE JT, MULLER RD, WILLIAMS DE: Cystic disease of the lungs in tuberous sclerosis: Clinicopathologic correlation including body plethysmographic lung function tests. Mayo Clin Proc 55:547, 1980

332. CORRIN B, LIEBOW AA, FRIEDMAN PJ: Pulmonary lymphangiomyomatosis: A review. Am J Pathol 79:348, 1975

333. CARRINGTON CB et al: Lymphangioleiomyomatosis: Physiologic–pathologic–radiologic correlations. Am Rev Respir Dis 116:972, 1977

334. GARAY SM et al: Hermansky–Pudlack syndrome: Pulmonary manifestations of a ceroid storage disorder. Am J Med 66:737, 1979

335. SCHNEIDER EL, EPSTEIN CJ, KABACK MJ et al: Severe pulmonary involvement in adult Gaucher's disease. Am J Med 63:475, 1977

336. ROSENBERG DM et al: Chronic air flow obstruction in Fabry's disease. Am J Med 68:898, 1980

337. MANOHARAN A, PITUEY WR, SCHONELL ME et al: Intrathoracic manifestations in non-Hodgkins lymphoma. Thorax 34:29, 1979

338. MACDONALD JB: Lung involvement in Hodgkin's disease. Thorax 32:664, 1977

339. TENHOLDEN MF, HOOPER RG: Pulmonary hemorrhage in the immune-compromised host: An elusive reality. Am Rev Respir Dis 121(2S): 198, 1980

340. JENKINS PF, WARD MJ, DAVIES P et al: Non-Hodgkins lymphoma, chronic lymphatic leukemia and the lung. Br J Dis Chest 75:22, 1981

341. WEBB RW, GOODMAN PC: Fibrosing alveolitis in patients with neurofibromatosis. Radiology 122:289, 1977

342. MASSARO D, KATZ S: Fibrosing alveolitis: Its occurrence, roentgenographic and pathologic features in von Recklinghausen's neurofibromatosis. Am Rev Respir Dis 93:934, 1966

Chapter 14

Obstructive Diseases

MARTIN H. WELCH

CHRONIC BRONCHITIS AND DIFFUSE OBSTRUCTIVE EMPHYSEMA (COPD)

MAGNITUDE OF THE PROBLEM

During the past 25 years, the medical and public health significance of chronic obstructive pulmonary disease (COPD) has grown to assume major proportions. Prior to 1950, the disorders included under this classification were relatively uncommon. Since then, morbidity, disability, and death due to chronic bronchitis and emphysema have become increasingly common. The beginning of this trend was preceded by a substantial increase in consumption of cigarettes,[1] and a large amount of data suggests a cause-and-effect relationship between these events. Less well documented is an association between these diseases and other sources of pollution of the atmosphere, including the gasoline engine and a host of industrial processes.

Most readily accessible data documenting the increased importance of chronic obstructive lung disease in the United States include mortality rates from these disorders. The rise in deaths during the past decades is illustrated in Figure 14-1, along with the rise in cigarette consumption, which is widely believed to be causally related.

Death rates fail to describe in full the adverse effects of these diseases, since death is usually preceded by a prolonged period of suffering and disability.[2] In addition, prolonged and repeated hospitalizations for respiratory failure are often economically and emotionally devastating for families of patients, as well as costly to the community in the drain on medical care resources. Prevalence rates and disability rates therefore provide a more useful measure of the problem of chronic lung disease. The National Health Survey, from information collected by administration of questionnaires to a sample of 42,000 households representative of the population of the United States, estimates the 1970 prevalence of emphysema to have been 9.8 per 1000, and of bronchitis, 29.5 per 1000. Limitation of activity from these conditions was reported in 5% of persons with bronchitis, and 37.3% of those with emphysema.[3] In some segments of the population, the proportion of patients affected by these diseases is substantially larger.[4] A prospective study of a small sample of patients admitted to a midwestern VA hospital found the prevalence of obstructive lung disease, as defined by abnormal spirometry, to be 38%.[5]

Some measure of the disability caused by COPD can be obtained from the 1972 Social Security Administration Survey of Disabled and Nondisabled Adults.[6] Among 15.6 million disabled persons from 20 to 64 years of age identified in this survey, 1.1 million identified chronic bronchitis or emphysema as the cause of their disability. Musculoskeletal and cardiovascular diseases were more frequent causes of disability.

EPIDEMIOLOGY AND ETIOLOGIC CONSIDERATIONS

Cigarette Smoking

A great deal of the epidemiologic data available concerning COPD provides apparent associations with factors such as sex, occupation, and racial or ethnic origin, which on closer examination are found to influence smoking habits. Much of this information was reviewed and summarized in a series of documents issued between 1964 and 1979 by the US Department of

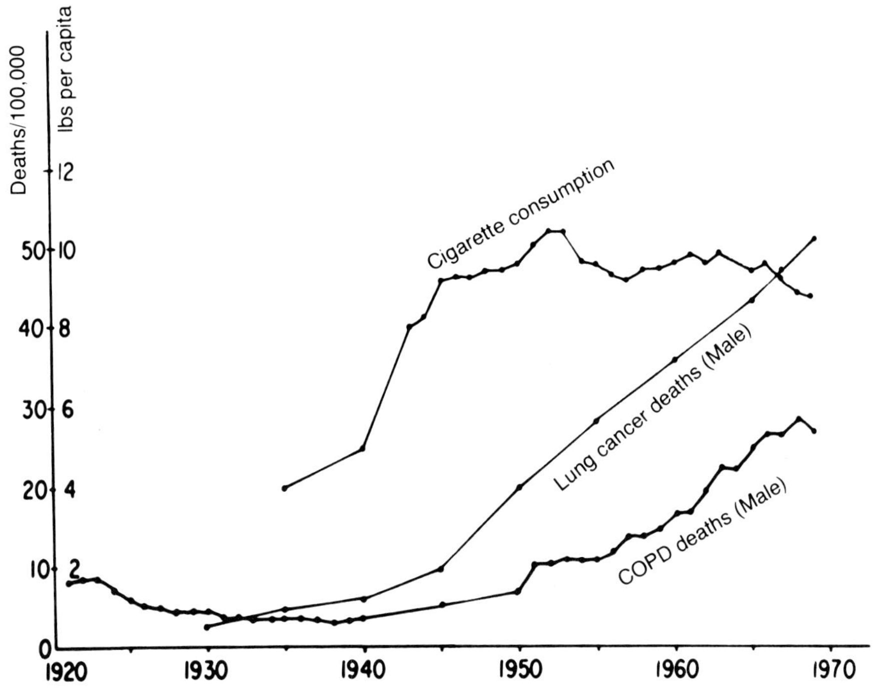

FIG. 14-1. Rise in cigarette consumption and deaths due to lung cancer and COPD. (Ayres, SM: Cigarette smoking and lung diseases: an update. Basics of RD 3(5), American Thoracic Society, 1975)

Health, Education and Welfare, Public Health Service, and available from the US Government Printing Office.[2,4,7–15] During this period, the total number of articles available for review in the world literature on smoking and health increased from 6,000 to 30,000. The first of these publications concluded: "A relationship exists between pulmonary emphysema and cigarette smoking, but it has not been established that the relationship is causal." Subsequent evidence includes documentation of so consistent an association between the disease and cigarette smoking within so many population subgroups that realistic doubt about cause and effect seems hardly possible. The 1974 document states: "Epidemiologic, autopsy, and experimental data presented in previous editions of this report indicate that cigarette smoking is the primary cause of chronic bronchitis and emphysema." The 1979 review strongly reaffirms this view.[2,14]

Evidence reviewed demonstrates a strong association between prevalence of COPD and resulting mortality in both men and women. These effects are more prominent in men, perhaps only because of longer exposure to cigarette smoking. Mortality from bronchitis in smokers was from 3.6 to 21.2 times that of nonsmokers, and from emphysema, 6.9 to 25.3 times greater.

Among both male and female cigarette smokers, there was a higher incidence of symptoms and pulmonary function impairment characteristic of COPD than among nonsmokers, and improvement in these parameters occurred with cessation of smoking. Pipe and cigar smokers were at greater risk than nonsmokers, but less than cigarette smokers. Certain trends in the overall death rate among smokers offer an encouraging note to preventive medicine. Former smokers have a declining mortality as the years pass, and after 15 years have no greater mortality than lifelong nonsmokers. Subsequent data confirm the benefits of smoking cessation in

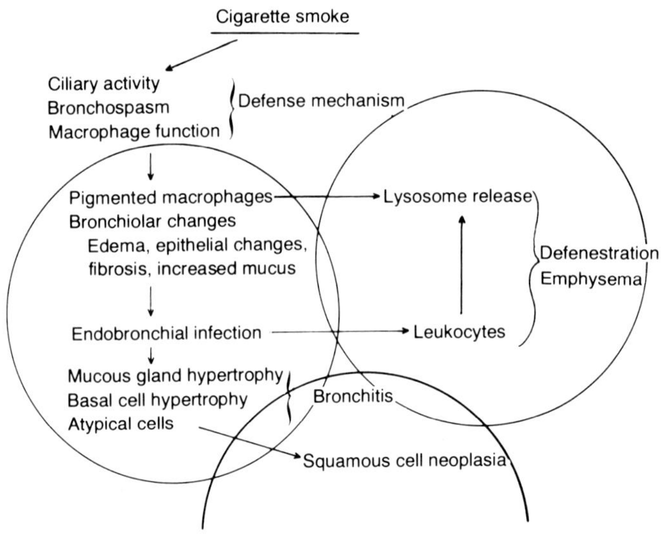

FIG. 14-2. Postulated mechanisms of production of chronic bronchitis and emphysema. (Ayres, SM: Cigarette smoking and lung diseases: an update. Basics of RD 3(5), American Thoracic Society, 1975)

terms of improved survival.[15a] Overall mortality rates are less for exposure to cigarettes with lower tar and nicotine content (see also Chapter 1 for specific components of cigarette smoke).

A summary of mechanisms by which smoking may produce chronic obstructive lung disease, based on currently available data, has been prepared by Ayres (Fig. 14-2).[1] He has suggested that smoke produces impaired ciliary activity and macrophage function, with early production of obstructive changes due to infection, inflammation, edema, increased mucus, and fibrosis in small bronchioles; similar changes in larger airways, resulting in productive cough; and finally, emphysema due to lysosomal enzymes released from macrophages and leukocytes which are increased in number due to inflammatory changes in the tracheobronchial tree. Subsequent studies suggest that cigarette smoke also impairs the antiprotease defense mechanism.[15b]

Environmental Pollution

The role of environmental pollution in the production of chronic lung disease is not so clearly defined as that of cigarette smoking,[16] although much attention has been devoted to it.[16a] The data concerning air pollution are more difficult to collect and to interpret (see also Chapter 1, Air Pollution). Modern industrial populations are mobile, and the components of "polluted" air numerous and variable. In an individual patient, a retrospective analysis of cumulative exposure to environmental pollutants is usually close to impossible, while an accurate estimate of smoking exposure is readily obtained. The potentially damaging components of the atmosphere of urban areas include nitrogen and sulfur oxides, and a host of particulate materials which can be quantitated; but concentrations of these materials vary greatly with climatic changes, and within geographical areas. A report of emphysema mortality (1963) exemplifies data which suggest that air pollution is less important than smoking as a cause of this disease.[17] Only 4 smoking-related deaths in 5 years occurred in a primarily nonsmoking population of 64,256 Seventh Day Adventists in California. Twenty-two deaths would have been expected at concurrent mortality rates for the state. The population studied presumably varied only in smoking habits, not in environmental exposure from the general California population. Of special interest is the fact that a history of smoking was obtained from families of three of the four deceased emphysema patients, and these were among the minority of members of this religious group who smoked heavily.

There have been studies, however, that suggest air pollution is not to be ignored as a cause of chronic respiratory disorders. The frequency of symptoms of chronic bronchitis has been shown to be twice as high in London men as in similarly employed inhabitants of rural England.[18] Similarly, an ingenious study of Boston policemen has shown a relation between chronic respiratory symptoms and traffic exposure.[19,20] Evidence that long-term grain workers develop airway symptoms and abnormal airway function suggests chronic changes result from organic particles.[202]

Whatever the role of air pollution in the cause of COPD, its contribution to exacerbations of the disease is clear. Symptoms have been shown to increase, and the death rate to rise, with abrupt increases in air pollution levels.[21–31] In one study, a post-exercise decrease in ventilatory function in normal children was shown to be related to pollutants.[32]

Hereditary Factors

In 1963, McKusick, in a review of genetic factors in respiratory disease, commented: "It is noteworthy that so little has been done by way of studying genetic factors in emphysema."[33] Since the time of that statement, a great amount of effort has been expended in investigation of hereditary factors in chronic lung disease, and some progress has been made.[34]

Most notable has been the discovery by Laurell and Eriksson, in Sweden, of the association of obstructive lung disease with a hereditary deficiency of alpha$_1$ globulin.[35,36] This discovery was made in the course of a survey of serum protein electrophoretic patterns, during which five subjects were found with near absence of alpha$_1$ globulin. Three had chronic obstructive lung disease.

The specific component of alpha$_1$ globulin which proved to be deficient in these subjects is a glycoprotein substance referred to as α_1 antitrypsin. This substance is responsible for much of the antiprotease activity of human serum. In early studies, 90% of the antitryptic activity of serum was shown to be localized in the alpha$_1$ globulin zone.[37,38]

Further studies by Eriksson led him to the conclusion that deficiency of α_1 antitrypsin is inherited, with a tendency toward development of lung disease in early adulthood.[39]

Since 1965, repeated confirmation and refinement of Eriksson's observations has appeared in the American and European literature. Reviews of this literature are available.[40–42,44] Alpha$_1$ antitrypsin has been found to be a polymorphic protein with more than 30 phenotypes which can be distinguished by specialized electrophoretic techniques.[43,43a,43b] Inheritance is hypothesized as being controlled by a single autosomal locus with multiple codominant alleles. The various proteinase inhibitor (Pi) alleles and phenotypes which result are represented by letters. Pi^M occurs most frequently, and phenotype MM has normal electrophoretic mobility. Pi^Z results in deficient amounts of protein with abnormal mobility. Homozygotes with phenotype ZZ have less than 10% of normal antitrypsin concentration, and have a 70–80% likelihood of development of obstructive lung disease, most characteristically panacinar emphysema. Heterozygotes MZ have antitrypsin concentrations in the range of 60% of normal. Some evidence suggests that these individuals have an increased susceptibility to the development of abnormalities of mechanical properties of lung, or even to clinical disease. The degree of this susceptibility, and its clinical and public health significance remains a subject of debate.[45–68]

Homozygotes (ZZ) are uncommon in all populations studied (4 in 6995 Swedes studied), and the predisposition to disease in them has little public health significance. Other phenotypes, including MZ, make up 5% or more of some populations. If these persons are predisposed to obstructive lung disease, the public health significance is substantial, particularly if cigarette smoking, or environmental or occupational exposure proves to accelerate development of clinical disease.

Identification of new varieties of genetically determined types of alpha$_1$ globulin continues as wider population studies with more sophisticated analytical techniques are reported.[41] At present, there is considerable evidence that severe deficiency and lung disease may be associated with phenotypes Z, SZ, Z null and null. The relationship of intermediate antiprotease levels to disease in persons with phenotypes MZ, M null, S and FZ remains controversial.[41,68a]

The observation that subtypes of the commonest group (*e.g.*, M_2) may be associated with reduced antiprotease levels and increased risk of industrial bronchitis may lead to further reassessment of previous studies which did not evaluate M protein subtypes.[68b,68c] Furthermore, the observation that phenotype B_{Sask}, which has normal antiprotease levels, may be associated with familial emphysema raises basic questions regarding the role of this protein in protection against disease.[68d]

Although all forms of chronic obstructive lung disease have been reported in association with homozygous (ZZ) antitrypsin deficiency,[39] a distinctive clinical presentation has been observed especially often: onset of the symptom of dyspnea on exertion, with little or no productive cough, is seen in the third or fourth decade of life, with slow progression to severe respiratory insufficiency; the chest is hyperinflated, with diminished breath sounds and low diaphragms; weight loss is frequent, and onset of severe blood gas derangement with erythrocytosis and cor pulmonale is delayed until late in the course of the disease.[69] The clinical picture, then, is one characteristic of primary emphysema. Pulmonary function abnormalities are those of relatively pure pulmonary emphysema,[69] and the chest roentgenograph reveals involvement of the lung bases bilaterally and symmetrically with the emphysematous process.[70,71] Pulmonary vessels are pruned and sparse in the lung bases, with relatively normal arborization in the upper lung zones. Radioisotope studies of lung ventilation and perfusion show bilateral lower zone decrease in these functions,[72] and angiograms confirm vascular abnormalities, most marked in the lower zones.[73]

Diagnosis of homozygous deficiency is often relatively simple, since alpha$_1$ globulin is so severely reduced as to appear nearly absent on a routine serum protein electrophoresis. Quantitative assessment should be carried out by radial immunodiffusion,[74] or assay of trypsin inhibitory capacity of serum (TIC) for confirmation.[39] These latter techniques are not adequate for certain identification of heterozygous (MZ) deficiency, since there is overlap of values with those for normal subjects and certain unusual Pi types. Phenotyping can be done with special electrophoretic techniques.[43a,43b,75,76]

Decreased levels of serum α_1 antitrypsin have been reported in infants with respiratory distress syndrome, apparently not on a hereditary basis.[77] Hereditary antitrypsin deficiency has been reported in association with cirrhosis in infants,[78,79] and in some adults with liver disease.[80–82a] Hepatoma and glomerulonephritis are reported to occur with increased frequency in patients with α_1 antitrypsin deficiency.[41] The reason for the variation in clinical abnormalities in association with the serological defect remains an enigma.

It has been hypothesized that α_1 antitrypsin (better referred to as α_1 antiprotease) is essential in protection of the lung against the destructive action of naturally occurring proteases.[83] The substance has been shown to inhibit several proteolytic enzymes other than trypsin; possible sources of such proteases include bacteria, leukocytes, macrophages, and serum. According to the theory, persons with normal serum trypsin inhibitory ability may be protected against these endogenous insults, while the lungs of deficient subjects undergo gradual dissolution. In normal and heterozygous deficient subjects, an increase in α_1 antitrypsin occurs in response to inflammation, and with administration of estrogen.[84–86] This ability to increase antitrypsin levels in response to stress may in itself be a protective mechanism. Homozygous (ZZ) deficient subjects lack this ability,[85–95] in addition to having low baseline values of serum antitrypsin. The preponderence of current evidence suggests that elastase from alveolar macrophages and/or leucocytes is the proteolytic enzyme most important in the production of emphysema.[88–92] Both cell sources may be important, but the production of emphysema by leukocytes in experimental animals,[92] and the demonstration of great individual variability of human leukocyte elastase content[88] would account for several clinical features. The ability of human serum to inhibit elastase may be its major property in protecting against emphysema. (See also Pathogenesis of Emphysema, to follow.)

Damage to the liver may have a somewhat different etiology, since deficient subjects have been shown to have abnormal collections of antitrypsin within hepatocytes.[81] It is possible that the defect in these subjects may be an inability to release, rather than to produce antitrypsin, and that the presence of abnormal collections of this material within the liver cells which produce it may somehow cause liver disease. No practical treatment is yet available either to disperse these abnormal collections of antitrypsin or to raise serum levels substantially for prolonged periods of time. If such treatment becomes available, its usefulness in preventing manifestations of disease will remain to be demonstrated, since the possible mechanisms of disease production described above are unproven. Although no practical treatment is available, several exciting advances have occurred. Patients with the ZZ phenotype and severe liver disease who survived liver transplantation developed normal levels of circulating α_1 antitrypsin.[93] This heroic treatment will clearly have limited clinical application. A potent anabolic drug, danazol, has been shown to cause modest but significant elevations of circulating α_1 antitrypsin, but the therapeutic role is entirely unclear.[94] Perhaps of most immediate interest is the demonstration that oral administration of a synthetic elastase inhibitor prevented elastase induced emphysema in experimental mice.[95] These studies point to the direction of future preventive treatment.

Hereditary factors other than antitrypsin deficiency influence the occurrence of chronic obstructive lung disease. Inheritance of fibrocystic disease is well known as a cause of bronchiectasis, as is deficiency of serum immunoglobulins. An increase in the occurrence of asthma in relatives of asthmatics is recognized,[87,96] and relatives of patients with other forms of COPD have an increased risk of developing these disorders apart from inheritance of antitrypsin deficiency.[49,97–100] Mechanisms of inheritance and of production of disease in these latter conditions are uncertain.

Infection

The possible role of infection in the natural history of chronic obstructive pulmonary disease presents a problem of great practical importance because of the implications it has for therapeutic intervention.[101]

Widespread current clinical practice involves administration of antibiotic drugs for treatment and even "prevention" of exacerbations of sputum purulence in patients with chronic bronchitis. This practice is based upon prevailing opinion that infection, though not of great importance as a cause of chronic bronchitis, does contribute substantially to morbidity from exacerbations. Evidence for an association of *Streptococcus pneumoniae* and *Hemophilus influenzae* with exacerbations is the basis for selection of antibiotic agents by many physicians. Demonstration of a decrease in duration, though not in number, of exacerbations in patients receiving continuous antibiotic therapy has been interpreted as evidence that viral infections cause many exacerbations which are then prolonged by superimposed bacterial infections.[102] A recent study provides additional support for the role of interaction between viruses and bacteria in chronic bronchitis.[103]

The possible role of infection in early life as a predisposing cause of chronic bronchitis and emphysema has received relatively little objective evaluation until recently. Tager and Speizer[101] have reviewed early studies suggesting an increased history of childhood, or early adult, respiratory illness in adult bronchitics as compared with normal controls.[104,105] More recent studies suggest an important role of viral infections in childhood.[106–109] Bronchiolitis, caused predominantly by respiratory syncytial virus, may be an especially frequent precursor of chronic respiratory disease.[110]

The association of *H. influenzae* and the pneumococcus with episodes of sputum purulence in patients with established chronic bronchitis was noted by May in 1953,[111] and subsequently by others. The interpretation of this finding is complicated by lack of evidence of antibody response to these organisms in many subjects in whom the organisms are cultured, and presence of the organisms in the upper respiratory tracts of many normal subjects and lower respiratory tracts of bronchitics not in exacerbation. Evidence for the role of viral and mycoplasmal agents in chronic bronchitis is even more poorly defined, as Tager and Speizer point out (see also Chap. 8).

The role of exacerbations of bronchitis in hastening progression of chronic obstructive lung disease is a matter of considerable importance which readily lends itself to investigation. Currently available data suggest that the pulmonary function decline in patients with COPD follows a somewhat predictable course which is not greatly influenced by periodic exacerbations of symptoms. These data, cited in the following discussion of natural history of COPD, fail to support a currently popular theory of the pathogenesis of emphysema, which postulates that proteolytic enzymes from bacteria, leukocytes, or macrophages associated with infection attack alveolar walls, resulting in their dissolution.

NATURAL HISTORY OF COPD

During the past 10 years, some knowledge of the natural history of chronic bronchitis and emphysema has begun to evolve. This knowledge is of obvious interest to the individual physician and his patient, but of still more importance to the investigator concerned with the cause and prevention of these diseases in large populations. Longitudinal studies, both of symptomatic subjects with established disease and of asymptomatic subjects thought to be at high risk or with abnormal pulmonary function tests, need to be considered.

Most of the available studies have not separated chronic bronchitis clearly from emphysema, and the relation of these disorders to airways obstruction is unclear, especially early in the course of the disease. Therefore, the natural histories of this group of diseases will be considered together.

The prognosis of patients with chronic respiratory insufficiency suffering an acute episode of respiratory failure is of particular importance to the clinician treating a patient with such an episode. Maximum treatment in such a case is often prolonged and costly in terms of the drain on medical care resources. Financial cost to the patient and his family is often overwhelming, and the discomfort and emotional impact may be devastating as well. The study of Asmundsson and Kilburn[112] published in 1969 permits some estimate of the benefits that may be expected from such costly effort.

These investigators analyzed 239 episodes of acute respiratory failure occurring in 146 patients with chronic respiratory failure. Patients survived 68% of the episodes: 55% survived 6 months, 20% survived 30 months, and the same percentage were alive at 48 months. Factors predicting a poor prognosis included old age, low body weight, edema and anemia, and severely abnormal spirometry or arterial oxygen or carbon dioxide tension.

Similarly, prognosis in a group of outpatients with chronic obstructive lung disease, studied by Burrows and Earle,[113] was related to severity of spirometric abnormality, and was adversely affected by resting tachycardia, chronic hypercapnia and severely abnormal diffusing capacity. In the absence of these latter factors, there was an 80% five-year survival if the FEV_1 exceeded 1.2 liters; a 60% survival when the FEV_1 was about 1 liter; and a 40% survival at FEV_1 less than 0.75 liter. In subjects who survived, a rather steady, predictable decline in ventilatory function occurred, with a loss of 56 ml per year in FEV_1.[114] A later study by Burrows and associates[115] added the observation that the measurement of FEV_1 after bronchodilator administration improved prediction of survival. Another recent study noted that a good response to bronchodilator was predictive of a better prognosis.[116]

Studies of subjects with much milder abnormalities of ventilatory function than Burrows' patients have demonstrated a similar slow, steady deterioration, which is nevertheless significantly different from the normal decline with age.[117–121] It is interesting that this excessive rate of decline appears to be related to cigarette smoking, but not clearly to chronic bronchitis, an observation which has been interpreted as evidence that it may be due to emphysema. The slowness and relative evenness of decline supports the validity of attempts to detect obstructive airways disease early, and hopefully institute measures to prevent its progression; but the need for extremely sensitive tests for early detec-

Natural History of Chronic Obstructive Pulmonary Disease (COPD)

Age 15 to 25	Age 25 to 35	Age 35 to 45	Age 45 to 55	Age 55 to 65
Smoking Asymptomatic	↓ Exercise tolerance Subtle function abnormalities ↑ A-a gradient (supine) ↑ closing volume ↑ slope of phase III Frequency dependence of compliance Abnormal helium vs. oxygen expiratory flow	Productive cough ↓ $FEF_{25-75\%}$ ↓ $FEV_{1.0}$	Dyspnea on exertion Loss of time from work Frequent chest colds Hypoxemia Abnormal spirometry	Cor pulmonale Respiratory failure Severe disability Death

tion has been questioned. Burrows[122] has pointed out that the FEV_1, which has been criticized as insensitive, should be detectably abnormal before the age of 30 in any subject who is likely to die of obstructive disease by age 70. In a similar vein, Bates[123] has suggested that seldom is the MMFR, a simple spirometric measurement, normal at age 40, or probably even at age 30, in a subject who will be severely disabled from obstructive lung disease at age 50. Fletcher[120,121] has added the observation that cessation of smoking converts the rapid pulmonary function decline of the COPD patient to a normal rate of decline. He has predicted, on the basis of data from an 8 year study by the British Medical Research Council, that the smoker at risk of COPD can be detected in early middle age by an abnormal FEV_1, or an abnormal rate of decline of FEV_1. Such a person, by ceasing smoking, might avert premature death, according to Fletcher's calculations.

If these observations are correct, as is likely, then widespread application of more difficult and more sensitive tests for obstructive airways disease may have little practical importance.

PATHOGENESIS OF CHRONIC BRONCHITIS AND EMPHYSEMA

The mechanisms by which the pathologic and pathophysiologic abnormalities of bronchitis and emphysema take place are incompletely understood. The variation in clinical presentation in this group of disorders suggests that alternate pathways may lead to ventilatory insufficiency and eventual respiratory failure from COPD.

CHRONIC BRONCHITIS

The mucus hypersecretion of chronic bronchitis can readily be superficially explained in terms of response of the secretory glands of the mucosal epithelium to a host of irritants. Details of the mechanisms by which this process is initiated have not been well explored, and the roles of particulate and gaseous environmental pollutants, the components of tobacco smoke, and of bacterial and viral infections are incompletely understood. Once the composition of tracheobronchial secretions has been altered, and ciliated mucosa has been disrupted, the lung defenses are altered in such a way that increased susceptibility to subsequent injury is easily envisioned. Productive cough is an easily explained sequel. Edema, viscid secretions, and even increased collapsibility of large airways could explain to some extent the decrease in maximum expiratory flow rates which occur.

Much of the early research relating volume of mucus-secreting glands to productive cough in bronchitis has been carried out on pathologic sections from large airways. However, more recent investigation suggests that airways less than 2 mm in diameter are an important site of obstruction to airflow in COPD.[124] Moreover, there is no clear quantitative correlation between episodes of productive cough and ventilatory impairment, or progression of ventilatory impairment in COPD.[123] A recent morphologic study of the lungs of smokers without clinically manifest COPD, who died of other causes, provides an insight into the early lesions associated with cigarette smoking.[125] The respiratory bronchioles of these subjects had undergone inflammatory changes which could be expected to produce the subtle physiologic abnormalities which other investigators have found in smokers.[126,127] The changes, if progressive, would explain the severe air flow obstruction seen in advanced COPD. That such progression does occur is suggested by the work of Matsuba and Thurlbeck, who found narrowing and mucus plugging of small airways associated with bronchitis and emphysema.[128]

These observations permit formulation of a hypothesis by which productive cough and small airways obstruction might be explained by related but not identical mechanisms. The effects of infection and inhaled irritants upon the trachea and large bronchi may be mucus gland hypertrophy and hypersecretion, with resultant productive cough. These same insults acting upon the smaller airways may primarily produce air flow obstruction. This theory would explain the imperfect correlation between the manifestations of large and small airway injury. The predominant manifestations might depend upon the level to which injurious agents penetrate the tracheobronchial tree, as well as the nature of the injury produced.

Theories of Pathogenesis of Emphysema

Partial airways obstruction with air trapping
Primary alteration of chest wall
Compensatory overdistention
Structural change in alveolar walls
Vascular loss
Proteolysis

EMPHYSEMA

Theories of the pathogenesis of emphysema over the past 150 years have considered a number of mechanical and biochemical possibilities. Laennec in 1819 proposed a theory of partial airway obstruction which has been repeatedly reexamined. The concept that air trapping, occurring distal to partial obstruction because of freer ingress than egress of air, is attractive in its simplicity. Lesions partially obstructing small bronchioles, proximal to areas of emphysema, have been interpreted as supporting this hypothesis.[129] The degree to which this mechanism is operative is still uncertain, but the occurrence of severe bronchial asthma without complicating emphysema, at least as defined as dilatation and destruction of walls of alveoli, mitigates against the theory.

The *protease-antiprotease* theory which currently appears most promising and widely applicable owes its popularity to the discovery by Eriksson of the pulmonary disease associated with α_1 antitrypsin deficiency.[39] This theory envisions emphysema as the result of an unfavorable balance between naturally occurring proteolytic enzymes and defense mechanisms, which include serum antiproteases such as alpha$_1$ antitrypsin.[83,130] Sources of such proteolytic enzymes that might induce dissolution of alveolar walls include bacteria, leukocytes, and macrophages. Inflammation within the tracheobronchial tree might result in release of protease from these sources at the level of the respiratory bronchioles and result in emphysema with a centriacinar distribution, such as is believed to occur secondary to chronic bronchitis. Panacinar emphysema, distributed more evenly within anatomic units of the lung, might result from a blood borne source of proteolytic insult, such as the trapping of leukocytes that is known to occur in the pulmonary capillaries under some circumstances. Support for this concept has resulted from the experimental production of emphysema by proteases instilled into the tracheobronchial tree[131,132] and following induction of leukocyte trapping within pulmonary capillaries.[92,133]

An excellent recent review of experimental emphysema includes a discussion of the protease-antiprotease concept of pathogenesis.[134] Much of the recent research suggests that leukocyte elastase is the naturally occurring protease important in production of emphysema, and that α_1 antitrypsin exerts its protective effect by its antielastase activity. Individual variation in leukocyte elastase and chemotactic activity may also be important. It has been suggested that the time is appropriate to develop methods for preparing an antitrypsin fraction of serum in sufficient quantity for administration to deficient subjects.[89] If the progress of emphysema in such patients could be slowed, administration to other emphysema patients without antitrypsin deficiency might follow.

CLINICAL PRESENTATION OF THE PATIENT WITH "MIXED" COPD

The typical patient with chronic obstructive lung disease presents with a mixed form of chronic bronchitis and emphysema, with a prominent element of wheezing similar to that seen in asthma, and often complicated by manifestations of right sided heart failure. As a result, even the most discriminating clinician is led into the habit of lumping these patients into a single diagnostic category and treating them all in a similar fashion. This habit results in overmedication of those with severe emphysema and little reversible disease and in inadequate therapy for those with predominant chronic bronchitis.

The classic mixed COPD patient with whom most readers will be familiar is a man in the fifth or sixth decade of life who presents with disabling shortness of breath on exertion, chronic productive cough, and a more or less predominant history of episodic wheezing. True bronchial asthma is often clinically easily distinguished from mixed COPD by its episodic nature, with complete remissions and with exacerbations in clear response to extrinsic allergens. Intrinsic asthma is sometimes perennial and unrelenting, however, and occasional bronchiectatics have dramatic bronchospasm that defies clear diagnostic definition. In these latter patients, the label *asthmatic bronchitis* is attractive since it carries useful therapeutic implications.

The patient with mixed COPD is usually a heavy smoker. He most often presents to his physician only when the symptoms of dyspnea become severe enough to limit activities which are critical to his daily life and necessary to his self-esteem. He may deny the presence of a chronic cough which is obvious to observers. Episodes of shortness of breath may occur at night in association with the recumbent posture, and simulate the symptoms of pulmonary edema, but on close questioning these episodes are usually initiated by productive cough, as thick secretions accumulate in the tracheobronchial tree during sleep. Acute episodes of bronchial or pulmonary infection may or may not be predominant in his history. Loss of body weight may be masked by the presence of edema.

Physical examination in the patient with advanced disease may reveal cyanosis, though this sign is notoriously unreliable as an indicator of arterial hypoxemia. Breathing is labored at rest or with exercise, and involves use of the accessory muscles of respiration. Intercostal and supraclavicular retraction is noted on inspiration, and expiration is prolonged and carried out through pursed lips. The overinflated chest moves poorly, and the lower ribs may retract paradoxically inward on inspiration. The thorax may be hyperresonant, and wheezing may be audible with or without a stethoscope. The diaphragms are low and fixed. Tobacco stained fingers and edema of the ankles are common indices.

At this advanced stage of the course of COPD, cure is not possible. There is even lack of convincing proof that treatment can reverse or slow the progress of the disease, or prolong life to an extent which would satisfy statisticians. It is clear to clinicians working with this disease, however, that in many cases, therapy can relieve symptoms, improve exercise tolerance, and reverse life-threatening complications. It is also clear that evaluation of the relative degrees of emphysema and bronchitis, along with a physiologic assessment of other factors in the individual patient, can guide therapy in a useful way. Maximum therapeutic benefit with minimum side-effects of therapy is the goal, and treatment must be individualized.

The approach to the patient with COPD, then, should be characterized by a careful attempt to establish a diagnosis which is as specific as possible. The diagnosis should include classification of the disease as chronic bronchitis, emphysema, or mixed COPD. It should include special attention to those features of the disease which are potentially reversible with treatment.

During the historical interview (Table 14-1), attention should be paid to the intensity and time and mode of onset of the central symptoms of dyspnea and chronic productive cough. Pulmonary emphysema in its purest form is characterized by the slow progressive onset of shortness of breath on exertion, uncomplicated in the early stages by cough, or by an effect of body position, or by episodes of worsening or remission. Productive cough, when it appears late in the course of disease, may be viewed as the result of secondary factors. Chronic bronchitis as a primary disease is characterized by productive cough. This may be present as an isolated symptom for many years before dyspnea results.

Episodes of wheezing associated with shortness of breath should be analyzed carefully. Such episodes in COPD patients usually represent bronchospasm which is potentially reversible with treatment. Wheezing may also indicate obstruction of airways by edema or excess secretions, or even fixed obstruction of major airways by tumors or other processes. When a striking episodic nature suggests bronchospasm, it may be part of the primary symptom complex in bronchial asthma, or a secondary event of obscure pathogenesis in bronchitis or emphysema. In the absence of wheezing or episodic dyspnea, with a subjective or objective response to bronchodilator drugs, these agents are probably not indicated. In a patient with stable and relatively pure emphysema, they may merely produce toxic side-effects without benefit.

Prognosis in COPD is most closely related to the degree of severity of ventilatory impairment in a given stable patient at a given time. Certain physical findings which are not closely related to severity of ventilatory impairment may help in establishing prognosis and guiding therapy, however (Table 14-2). Weight loss tends to be experienced by patients with emphysema rather than bronchitis and emaciation indicates a poor prognosis. Resting tachycardia has ominous significance in a stable patient. A rib cage fixed in the inflated position, and low, flat, fixed diaphragms tend to support a diagnosis of emphysema. Decreased or absent breath sounds in areas of aerated lung, especially symmetrically at the posterior lung bases, suggest pulmonary emphysema. The finding of prominent expiratory rhonchi is more suggestive of bronchitis, especially with bronchospasm.

Cor pulmonale, that is, right ventricular failure and pulmonary hypertension, may be evident on physical examination (Table 14-3). Cor

TABLE 14-1. Differential Diagnosis of COPD: Clinical History

Diagnostic indications	Chronic bronchitis	Emphysema	Asthma
Productive cough	Predominant symptom—early	May be absent, or develop late in course of disease	Common, nocturnal
Shortness of breath	May be absent early, severe in advanced stage of disease	Predominant symptom, early in course of disease, insidious onset, exertional	Episodic, may be brought on by exertion
Wheezing	Variable	Usually absent or minimal	Predominant symptom
Tendency to exacerbations and remissions	Strong tendency in some patients		Usual
History of allergy			Often present
Smoking history	Usual	Usual	

TABLE 14-2. Differential Diagnosis of COPD: Physical Examination

Physical signs	Chronic bronchitis	Emphysema	Asthma
Barrel chest	Sometimes present	Often dramatic	Usually absent
Slowed expiratory flow rates	Present	Present	Present
Rales	Usually absent	"Dry" crackling rales sometimes occur	Usually absent
Rhonchi	Often prominent	Often absent or minimal	Dramatic "musical" rhonchi
Decreased breath sounds	Only in severe attacks	Characteristic	Only in severe attacks
Signs of cor pulmonale	Often present in moderately advanced disease	May be present in far advanced disease	Usually absent
Cyanosis	Often dramatic	Often absent, even in presence of low arterial P_{O_2}	May be present in acute attack
Weight loss		May be severe in advanced disease	

TABLE 14-3. Differential Diagnosis of COPD: Complications

Complications	Chronic bronchitis	Emphysema	Asthma
Chronic hypercarbia	Frequent	Only in far advanced disease	Only in very severe attacks, signifies need for hospitalization and intensive care
Secondary erythrocytosis	Frequent	Only in far advanced disease	Seldom
Cor pulmonale	Frequent	Only in far advanced disease	Seldom

pulmonale occurs generally in rather severe obstructive lung disease, and is thus associated with a poorer prognosis. However, in pure chronic bronchitis, it may occur relatively early in the course of disease, due to pulmonary vasospasm, and in an untreated patient represents a potentially reversible complication. In pure pulmonary emphysema, cor pulmonale occurs in the most advanced cases, and is often the result of irreversible destruction of the pulmonary vascular bed. Therefore, in these patients especially, it indicates a poor outlook and responds poorly to treatment (see also Chap. 10, Pulmonary Hypertension).

The chest roentgenogram may be used with reasonable accuracy to establish the presence of emphysema, at least in advanced cases (Table 14-4).

Pulmonary function testing is extremely helpful in establishing the severity of obstructive lung disease and in following its course, and contributes greatly to understanding the disturbed physiology (Table 14-5). However, as carried out in the usual clinical laboratory, it

TABLE 14-4. Differential Diagnosis of COPD: Radiologic and Laboratory Findings

Chest radiograph	Chronic bronchitis	Emphysema	Asthma
Hyperinflation	May be present	May be present	May be present
Increased peribronchial & bronchiolar markings	May be present		
Patchy hyperlucency & fibrosis		May be present	
Vascular attenuation		Diagnostic if present	
Flat diaphragms		Diagnostic if present	
Functional Evaluation	**Chronic bronchitis**	**Emphysema**	**Asthma**
Expiratory flow rates	Decreased	Decreased	Decreased
Vital capacity	Decreased	Decreased	Decreased
Improvement in VC and flow rates with bronchodilator	Moderate	Minimal	Marked
Residual volume	Increased	Increased	Increased
Total lung capacity	Normal	Increased	Normal
Diffusing capacity	Normal	Decreased	Normal or increased
Arterial Po_2	Chronically decreased at rest, better with exercise	Chronically decreased at rest, worse with exercise	Decreased with acute attacks
Arterial Pco_2	Chronically increased in moderately severe disease	Chronically increased in late stages of disease	Increased in severe, acute attacks
Lung compliance (static)	Normal	Increased	Normal

TABLE 14-5. Differential Diagnosis of COPD: Therapeutic Implications

Therapeutic alternatives	Chronic bronchitis	Emphysema	Asthma
Antibiotics	Very useful	Limited usefulness	Useful in exacerbations
Bronchodilators (oral, IV, aerosol)	Very useful	Limited usefulness	Very useful
Humidification-nebulization	Useful	Limited usefulness	Useful
Postural drainage, percussion	Useful	Limited usefulness	Useful
Influenza prophylaxis	Useful	Useful	Useful
Specific treatment of cor pulmonale	Very useful	Limited value	Seldom needed
Avoidance of smoking, environmental pollution	Essential	Essential	Essential
Chronic oxygen supplementation	Most useful in cor pulmonale and secondary erythrocytosis	Useful	Seldom needed

may contribute surprisingly little to the distinction between chronic bronchitis, emphysema, and asthma in an acute exacerbation. The usual ventilatory studies show similar findings in all forms of obstructive disease: decreased vital capacity, decreased maximal expiratory flow rates, increased functional residual capacity, and residual volume. The patient with asthma may show a dramatic improvement in response to bronchodilators, while the bronchitic shows a more modest response and the emphysema patient improves not at all.

Arterial blood gas studies are of relatively little specific diagnostic help. Bronchitics may develop hypoxemia and hypercarbia with a milder spirometric defect than patients with emphysema.

In large groups of subjects, a decreased diffusing capacity has been found to correlate especially well with the extent of pulmonary emphysema. Destruction of the capillary bed in this disorder impairs diffusion predictably.

Other physiologic tests not generally available in the smaller clinical pulmonary laboratory are helpful in distinguishing the chronic obstructive lung diseases. Airways resistance measured by the plethysmographic technique is increased in bronchitis and bronchial asthma; and lung compliance is increased in pulmonary emphysema.

It should be apparent then that a very discriminating analysis of the patient with COPD can be made by a conscientious clinician with the tools readily available to him. This analysis can be of great help in assuring the patient optimal benefit from therapy without requiring him to pay the price of useless overmedication (Table 14-5).

CHRONIC BRONCHITIS

Chronic bronchitis is a disorder defined by general agreement in North America and Great Britain, by its most common clinical manifestation, chronic productive cough, present on most days for at least three months of the year, and for at least two successive years.[135–137] This definition presumes exclusion of the many other identifiable causes of productive cough which is, of course, a nonspecific symptom. By this simple definition the disease would seem to be innocuous enough, and indeed in its simplest form the manifestations are benign and easily ignored by the patient. Some persons may be troubled only by productive cough, uncomplicated by respiratory insufficiency for many years. In others, however, the disorder follows an aggressive course leading to respiratory failure and death.

So complex is the relationship between bronchitis and emphysema that prior to about 1960, use of the two terms was not uniform even among the clinical investigators most knowledgeable about COPD. In Great Britain, most patients with COPD tended to be diagnosed as bronchitics, while in the United States, the diagnosis of emphysema was more often made. This led to a comparison of clinical forms of the diseases in the two countries, which required a critical analysis of clinical manifestations.[138–140] The studies of Burrows and Fletcher led to the conviction that clinical forms of COPD really did not differ in the two countries but that diagnostic criteria did. It is now generally agreed that although bronchitis has been given a clinical definition, it has clearly definable morphologic correlates, and although emphysema is best defined by its pathologic picture, it can be recognized with reasonable accuracy by its clinical manifestations.

Clinical Presentation

Out of these and other studies of obstructive lung disease, two distinct, classic presentations of patients with advanced COPD have emerged. These two distinctive types occur less often than do the mixed forms, but seem to define two ends of a broad spectrum of disease ranging between pure emphysema and pure chronic bronchitis. In 1955, Dornhorst[141] presented one of the early attempts to separate distinctive clinical syndromes out of the heterogeneous population of patients with respiratory insufficiency. He is credited with having coined the terms *blue bloater* and *pink puffer* for patients with bronchitic and emphysemic presentations, respectively. Burrows[138–140,142,143] referred to *Type B* (bronchitic) and *Type A* (emphysemic) and Filley[144–147] to *BB* and *pp*. These various observers are in substantial agreement in their descriptive analyses.

The chronic bronchitic as blue bloater is much more than simply a fellow with chronic productive cough. He demonstrates the fully developed syndrome of advanced chronic bronchitis with its complications. Chronic productive cough is a prominent feature, however, characteristically present for many years prior to the onset of other clinical manifestations. Viral and bacterial infections of the tracheobronchial tree are frequent, with impaired lung clearance due to an excess of viscid secretions obstructing air passages and hindering mucociliary defenses. The infections are generally considered a result rather than a cause of chronic bronchitis. These tracheobronchial infections often lead to bronchopneumonia, especially if left untreated. Shortness of breath on exertion and finally even at rest may be less disabling and distressing in the chronic bronchitic than in a patient with comparable ventilatory defect due to emphysema. Seemingly, the bronchitic, with his less intense dyspnea, tends to permit respiratory gas exchange to be compromised, resulting in hypoxemia and carbon dioxide retention to a greater degree than in the emphysematous patient. The increased arterial P_{CO_2} can be explained on the basis of a characteristically rapid, shallow pattern of breathing.[148] Lethargy and somnolence may reflect breathing disorders during sleep (see Chap. 6). The hypoxemia is clinically manifested by cyanosis, more in the blue bloater than the pink puffer as the terms imply.

Other features of the bronchitic can be traced, at least in part, to this early failure to maintain normal arterial oxygen and carbon dioxide tensions. Cor pulmonale with its attendant peripheral edema is largely due to blood gas derangement in these patients. Hypoxemia and respiratory acidosis, both separately and in concert, cause pulmonary vasospasm with elevated pulmonary vascular resistance, placing an increased work load on the right ventricle, which eventually fails, and peripheral venous distention, edema, and hepatomegaly result. Arterial hypoxemia alone provides an adequate explanation for the erythrocytosis which occurs in the classic advanced bronchitic. Nocturnal hypoxemia may aggravate pulmonary hypertension and polycythemia.[149] In those who continue to smoke, carboxyhemoglobin accounts for part of the polycythemia. Bronchitics tend to maintain normal body weight well into the course of their disease, and not infrequently, are obese. The reasons for this tendency are entirely obscure.

Physical examination of the bronchitic with advanced airways obstruction reveals, in addition to the features described above, several other features of interest. Breathing may be labored, even at rest, with contraction of the accessory muscles of respiration (sternocleidomastoid). The chest may be overinflated and move poorly, but these features are less striking than in the patient with emphysema. The diaphragms tend to maintain relatively normal position and excursion. The expiratory phase of respiration is prolonged, even at rest, in severely diseased subjects; and in less ill patients a maximal forced expiration from full inspiration will be more prolonged than the 3 to 4 seconds required in a normal person. Normal vesicular breath sounds may be decreased, but inspiratory and expiratory rales and rhonchi replace them, so that auscultation reveals a noisy chest rather than the quiet one of emphysema. If pulmonary artery pressure is increased, the pulmonary component of the second heart sound may be increased, though the splitting of the second sound will be normal or decreased. An audible fourth heart sound may accompany pulmonary hypertension and a third heart sound may signify right ventricular failure.

Roentgenographic Findings

The chest roentgenogram in general is not helpful in identifying bronchitis *per se*. It does remain a basic part of the evaluation of the patient with bronchitis, however, primarily for its role in the diagnosis of other disorders which cause chronic cough and shortness of breath. Neoplastic and inflammatory pulmonary diseases and left ventricular failure with pulmonary edema, produce characteristic roentgenographic abnormalities which must be excluded. Pulmonary emphysema coexists with chronic bronchitis so frequently that evidence for this disorder should be sought in each case.

Chest roentgenograms have been reported to

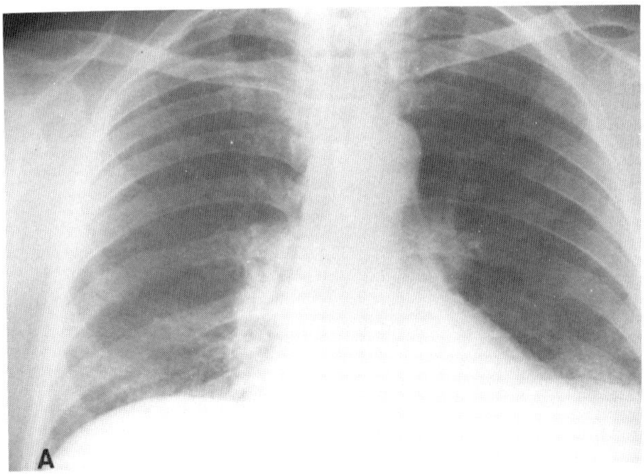

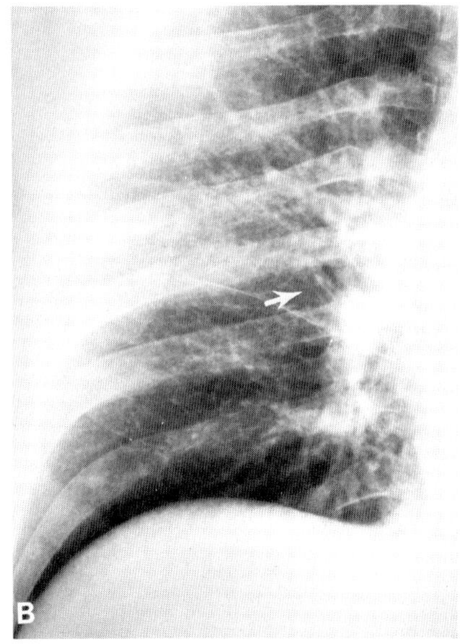

FIG. 14-3. Chest roentgenogram of patient with chronic bronchitis. **A.** Conventional posteroanterior view; **B.** enlargement for detail. Arrow indicates thickened bronchial walls, or "tram tracks."

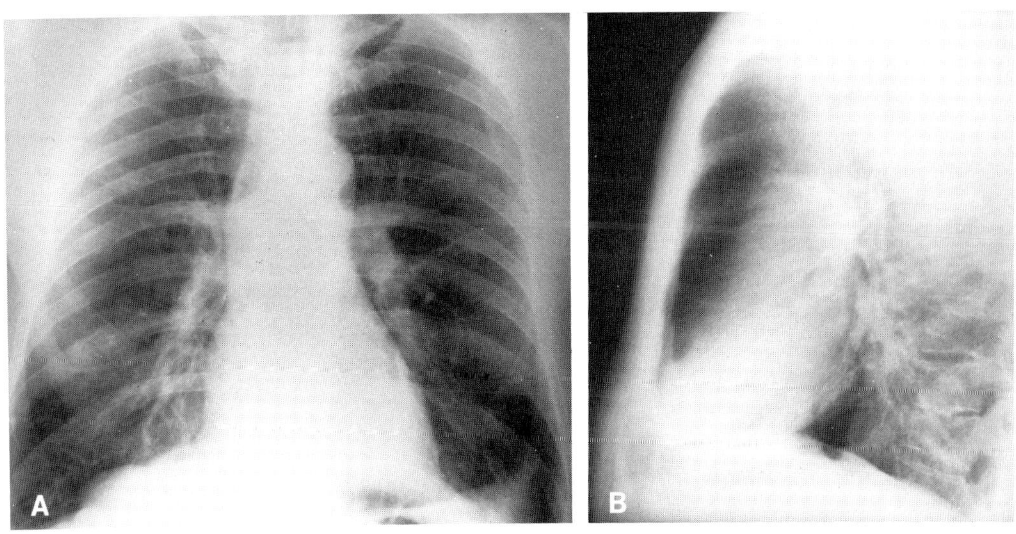

FIG. 14-4. Chest roentgenogram of patient with chronic bronchitis and emphysema. Note patchy increase in interstitial and peribronchial markings, commonly referred to as "dirty chest." Flattened diaphragms suggest presence of emphysema. **A.** Posteroanterior view; **B.** lateral view.

be abnormal in 60 to 80% of patients with clinical manifestations of chronic bronchitis.[150–152] The frequency with which abnormalities are due to the bronchitis itself is a matter of disagreement. Roentgenographic abnormalities which are considered by some authorities to be due to bronchitis include overinflation, parallel lines (*tramtracks*) which may represent thickened bronchial walls (Fig. 14-3), and increase in peripheral lung markings, known as *dirty chest* (Fig. 14-4). None of these findings has been shown by pathologic studies to be specific for chronic bronchitis. Bates and associates[150] found them to occur frequently in association with the clinical disorder, however. These investigators observed overinflation in 64.5%, visible bronchial walls in 43.5%, and increased peripheral markings in 17.9% of their subjects. Simon[151] and Simon and Galbraith[152] have not been impressed with the usefulness of these findings, and did not observe roentgenographic appearances which they could regard as characteristic of chronic bronchitis in a review of over 800 patients with chronic bronchitis.

FIG. 14-5. Electrocardiogram of patient with severe chronic bronchitis and emphysema, showing changes characteristic of cor pulmonale. Note tall, peaked P waves of right atrial enlargement. ST depression and T wave inversion in V_1-V_4 suggest right ventricular strain.

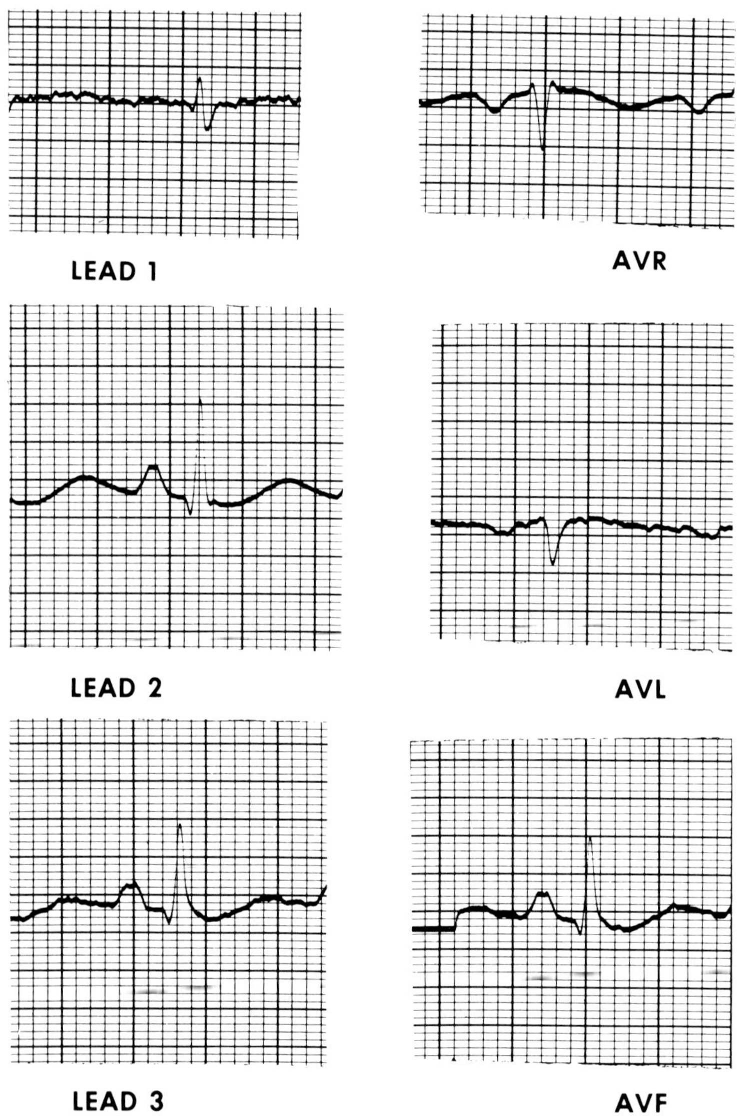

Fraser and co-workers[153] have combined the roentgenographic findings of increased peripheral bronchovascular markings, overinflation, and evidence of pulmonary arterial hypertension as a pattern highly predictive of morphologic emphysema, especially of the centrilobular sort. They have referred to this pattern as that of *increased marking emphysema*, but it seems likely that chronic bronchitis has a role in the production of the radiographic abnormalities.

Bronchographic findings characteristic of chronic bronchitis include pitting of the undersurfaces of the main and segmental bronchi due to dilation of mucous glands, a "broken bough"

FIG. 14-5. *(Continued)*

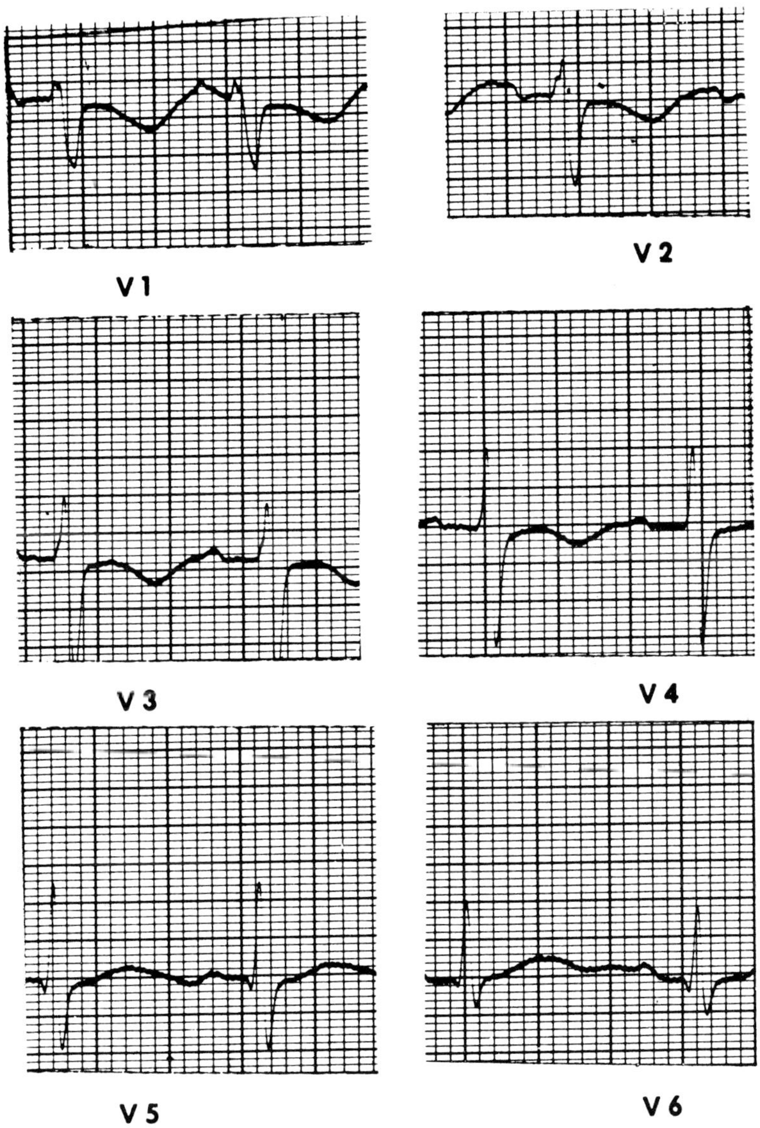

appearance resulting from occlusion of fifth to eighth generation bronchi, and pooling of radio-opaque medium in dilated bronchioles.[151,152] In usual clinical practice, performance of bronchography is not indicated to verify a diagnosis of bronchitis, though under certain circumstances it may be useful in excluding bronchiectasis or neoplasm in bronchitic patients.

Electrocardiogram

Electrocardiographic (ECG) abnormalities are frequent in chronic obstructive lung disease,[154–167] and in general relate more to the severity than the type of disease[157] (Fig. 14-5). One study has indicated correlation between ECG abnormalities and total pulmonary vascular resistance,[156] which would be expected to reflect severe airway obstruction as well as blood gas derangements. Tall, symmetrical, peaked P waves and rightward shift of the P-wave axis, and evidence of right ventricular hypertrophy are common in patients with severe obstructive disease. The electrocardiographic diagnosis of right ventricular hypertrophy is imperfect, however. The criteria proposed by various investigators have been recently reviewed,[158] and in the absence of conduction defects, four findings have been suggested as most helpful: S_1Q_3 pattern; right axis deviation $\geqq 110°$; S_1-S_2-S_3 pattern; and R to S ratio in $V_6 \leqq 1.0$. Combining these four findings provided criteria which reduced false-negative rates when autopsy correlation was examined. One of the best combinations of criteria, S_1Q_3 pattern and R to S ratio in $V_6 \leqq 1$, had a false-positive rate of 20% and a false-negative rate of 33%, however.

Arrythmias, both atrial and ventricular, are common in chronic obstructive lung disease severe enough to produce pulmonary hypertension and arterial blood gas derangement.[159–164] In COPD patients with acute respiratory failure, atrial arrhythmias appear to be especially common,[160,163] occurring in as many as 80 to 90% of such patients monitored for prolonged periods. When ventricular arrhythmias occur in this setting (about 24% of such patients),[163] they appear to be associated with severe hypoxemia and a poor prognosis.

Stable patients with COPD studied with ambulatory electrocardiographic monitoring also have a high frequency of arrhythmias (80 to 90%),[161,162] but in this setting, multifocal premature contractions predominate. The cause and clinical significance of these abnormal rhythms is not yet clear. Mechanical effects on heart muscle, hypoxemia, and drug side-effects have been proposed as causative, and it would seem that sudden death might be a result. One group of investigators has provided suggestive evidence that nocturnal hypoxemia may provoke ventricular rhythms and that oxygen administration may ameliorate them.[165,166]

When it occurs, multifocal atrial tachycardia should be identified as such, because it is most commonly confused with atrial fibrillation, and does not respond to known antiarrhythmic drugs. It consists of many ectopic atrial beats, commonly so frequent that only an occasional sinus beat can be seen. The only treatment available is correction of the underlying respiratory failure. Improvement in the arrhythmia is poorly correlated with improved blood gases.[167]

Other Laboratory Findings

The hemoglobin and hematocrit may be elevated in patients with secondary erythrocytosis, but correlation of these peripheral blood findings with total red blood cell mass is not perfect, since intravascular volume is variable. Plasma volume may increase in right heart failure, while diuretic use may decrease it.

Laboratory examination of sputum contributes in a limited way to the evaluation and management of these patients. The clinical history of a change in sputum volume, consistency, or color may be of great importance in defining an exacerbation of bronchitis related to viral or bacterial infection. Gross or microscopic examination of sputum for pus is useful. Examination of a Gram stain for organisms may contribute useful information if a predominance of gram-positive or gram-negative organisms is seen; and cultures may likewise be helpful in guiding therapy if predominance of a pathogen is found. More often, a mixture of organisms is identified, and the role of any one of them in producing symptoms remains doubtful. Pneumococcus and *Hemophilus influenzae* have been said to be the bacteria most often associated with exacerbations, but this is not necessarily so in patients receiving antibiotics frequently, in whom the tracheobronchial tree tends to become colonized with an assortment of gram-negative bacilli. These organisms often seem to have no role in exacerbating symptoms of bronchitis. When pneumonia occurs, identification of a specific bacterial cause assumes much greater importance than suggested above for exacerbations of bronchitis. Bacteremia is not uncommon in pneumonia, however, and blood cultures may be of great value in this circumstance (see Chap. 8, Acute Respiratory Tract Infections).

Pulmonary Function Evaluation

Early in the course of chronic bronchitis, there may be little or no functional impairment. A heavy cigarette smoker with chronic productive cough may warrant the diagnosis of chronic bronchitis, but exhibit normal values for routine tests of ventilatory function. Such subjects may, however, exhibit abnormalities in one or all of a group of tests currently believed to be exquisitely sensitive to patchy obstructive disease in the small peripheral airways[127] (see Chap. 4, Laboratory Screening for Subclinical Disease). It has been theorized that the *small airways disease* inferred by the demonstration of one of these abnormalities represents the earliest demonstrable form of the chronic obstructive lung disease caused by chronic bronchitis. It has not been shown that all (or indeed any) of such subjects progress to full-blown COPD. Likewise, it has not been shown that any or all COPD patients began the course of their disease with this group of abnormalities and otherwise functionally normal lungs. The theory is very attractive, however, and its elucidation will have high priority for future investigators.[168]

Progression of disease of small peripheral airways, or involvement of larger airways, may ultimately result in elevation of total resistance of the pulmonary airways with the symptoms of shortness of breath related to increase in work of breathing. Simple spirometry will reveal slowing of expiratory flow rates at this point. Since shortness of breath is a symptom likely to lead a patient to be examined by a physician, airways disease of this level of severity has been better studied. The functional abnormalities of clinically manifest obstructive lung disease are well characterized. The course of disease from this point until death is reasonably well understood.

Our knowledge of the physiologic abnormalities of chronic bronchitis is chiefly derived, however, from studies of patients in whom the absence of co-existent emphysema has not been proven morphologically. These studies for the most part correlate physiologic parameters with one another and with clinical observations in order to assess the role of bronchitis, as opposed to emphysema, in producing them.[142–147,169–171]

The small body of data on functional abnormalities of patients with bronchitis and absence of significant emphysema at autopsy has been reviewed by Thurlbeck and co-workers.[153]

The best-known functional abnormalities of chronic bronchitis with airways obstruction are those shown by measurements which reflect a decrease in maximum expiratory flow rates. These abnormalities include a decrease in timed forced-expiratory volumes, and a proportionate decrease in maximum voluntary ventilation. The flow-volume curve during a maximal forced expiratory effort shows concavity upward and instantaneous flow rates read from such a curve are decreased, as is peak flow obtained from a curve or from a Wright peak-flow meter. These abnormalities are probably due to disease in small peripheral airways in most patients with chronic bronchitis, though some observers believe that collapse of major airways during forced expiration is more important. At this stage, airways resistance as measured with a plethysmograph is elevated. These parameters of air flow obstruction are not specific for chronic bronchitis, of course. Maximal expiratory flow rates are decreased in asthma and emphysema, and airways resistance is elevated in asthma. These abnormalities are partially reversible in response to bronchodilators in bronchitis, entirely reversible in some patients with asthma, and entirely irreversible when due to emphysema alone.

Pure chronic bronchitis, uncomplicated by pulmonary emphysema, appears to cause an elevated residual volume with a reduced vital capacity and no change in total lung capacity. Functional residual capacity may be elevated or relatively normal in the face of increased residual volume, resulting in reduced expiratory reserve volume. This pattern may be helpful, though not definitive, in separating bronchitis from emphysema, in which total lung capacity tends to be increased.

Diffusing capacity tends to remain normal in chronic bronchitis, as in asthma, since the pulmonary capillary bed is not decreased. Emphysema results in destruction of pulmonary capillaries at the alveolar level, and thus a decrease in diffusing capacity. This distinction may be blurred by extreme degrees of ventilation-perfusion mismatching which may reduce the diffusing capacity, and by other sources of variation in this test, which is rather poorly reproducible in this group of subjects.

Chronic bronchitics tend to have rather extreme ventilation-perfusion imbalance with physiologic shunting related to maldistribution of ventilation, and to relatively well-preserved pulmonary blood flow. These patients tend not to increase tidal volume or total minute ventilation enough to compensate for ventilation-perfusion mismatching. Arterial hypoxemia and hypercarbia are therefore common.[148] Exercise of moderate degree with increased tidal volume may improve ventilation-perfusion relationships and arterial blood gas levels will tend to return toward normal. If the exercise is intensified to the extent that metabolic needs exceed the patient's ability to ventilate, hypercarbia will result, and hypoxemia may worsen. Inefficiency of ventilation is usual in these patients, at rest or with exercise, and will be measured as elevated physiologic dead space (another measure of ventilation-perfusion inequality), or as an increased ventilatory equivalent of oxygen consumption. Maximum oxygen consumption will be reduced, as will maximum exercise levels.

Static compliance of the lungs in chronic bronchitis is normal or reduced, providing an especially useful means of distinguishing bronchitis from emphysema, since in the latter disorder it is increased. Dynamic compliance is reduced, especially at rapid breathing frequencies.

Pathology

It has been pointed out elsewhere that the definition of chronic bronchitis is clinical, not pathologic. Pathologic findings which correlate with the clinical definition of chronic productive cough have been well described and recent reviews of these findings are available.[153,172] The relation between the pathologic changes which have been so carefully described and quantitated and the obstructive physiology of advanced chronic bronchitis, is reviewed in Chapter 3.

The secretions of the tracheobronchial tree are produced by goblet cells in the epithelial lining, and by tubular branching bronchial mucous glands which lie beneath the epithelium and discharge their secretory products through ducts opening onto the epithelial surface. Goblet cells are distributed in a patchy fashion throughout the tracheobronchial tree, chiefly in the larger central airways. They are present in smaller numbers in the bronchioles.[173] The bronchial glands are more evenly distributed throughout the tracheobronchial tree, and normally have a total volume some 40 times that of goblet cells.[174] For these reasons, the interest of pathologists has centered upon the bronchial glands in chronic bronchitis. Their volume suggests an important role in a clinical state associated with an increased sputum volume, and their more even distribution simplifies sampling for purposes of quantitation. The glands are increased in thickness in chronic bronchitis, and goblet cells appear to be present in increased number.

Reid has described a method of quantitating the increase in mucous glands which has gained wide acceptance for its simplicity and reproducibility.[174] The Reid index is simply the ratio of bronchial gland thickness to total thickness of the bronchial wall from epithelial basement membrane to the inner surface of the perichondrium. Measurements are usually made on main and lobar bronchi, since the cartilaginous rings are more readily sampled in these areas. The index was found by Reid to be increased (above 0.36) in most bronchitics, and to be below 0.36 in most normal subjects; and even to correlate to some degree with the volume of sputum produced. Other investigators have shown a bell shaped distribution curve of the Reid index, with somewhat higher values in normal subjects (mean, 0.44) and in bronchitics (mean, 0.52).[175]

These changes, along with an increase in the volume of tracheobronchial secretions and changes in their composition and physical properties, appear adequate to explain the chronic productive cough of chronic bronchitis.[172,176] They do not so readily explain the frequency dependence of dynamic compliance seen in advanced disease or elevated airways resistance of the chronic airway obstruction which may accompany chronic bronchitis.[177,178] For reasons described in Chapter 3, frequency dependence of compliance is most readily explained by patchy changes in resistance to airflow in small peripheral airways, rather than central bronchi and trachea. In chronic bronchitis with severe airway obstruction, the degree of narrowing of the central airways due to mucous gland thickening would not appear adequate to explain the physiologic aberration. Neither does obstruction due to the secretions themselves appear to be an entirely satisfactory explanation. Small airways obstruction due to goblet cell proliferation or other manifestations of bronchiolitis would be an attractive explanation. Therefore, the attention of investigators has recently been directed toward changes in small peripheral airways in chronic bronchitis.

A study of young smokers dying of causes other than respiratory failure has shown a characteristic respiratory bronchiolitis with associated collections of pigmented macrophages.[125] This lesion may explain the subtle physiologic abnormalities shown by others in similar subjects,[126,127] and might be a precursor of severe obstruction of small peripheral airways with respiratory failure. Matsuba and Thurlbeck[128] have shown organic narrowing and mucus plugging of airways less than 2 mm in diameter in a group of subjects with chronic bronchitis and airways obstruction. Karpick and associates have shown an association of goblet cell metaplasia with death from respiratory failure.[179] More recently, Thurlbeck and associates have demonstrated goblet cell metaplasia in the bronchioles of patients with chronic bronchitis, emphysema, and airflow obstruction, but not in subjects with bronchitis and no emphysema.[180]

Currently available evidence, therefore, would suggest that the chronic productive cough which characterizes chronic bronchitis is related to an increase in volume of bronchial mucous glands, especially involving large central airways. The obstruction to air flow which produces subtle physiologic abnormalities in smokers, and which is often seen in advanced chronic bronchitis with respiratory insufficiency, appears more closely related to goblet cell metaplasia and other morphologic changes involving small peripheral airways. Better understanding of these relationships will surely accompany future investigation.

Other morphologic changes accompanying the goblet cell and bronchial gland abnormalities of chronic bronchitis include fragmentation and destruction of cilia, inflammatory cell infiltration of the epithelium and subepithelium, and basal cell hyperplasia and squamous metaplasia of columnar epithelium.[181]

GENERALIZED OBSTRUCTIVE PULMONARY EMPHYSEMA

Pulmonary emphysema is generally defined as an abnormal morphologic condition characterized by enlargement of the alveoli accompanied by destructive changes in the alveolar walls.[135,136,173,181,182] There are two forms of this disorder which are relatively common. They are progressive, and involve the lungs diffusely so as to result in severely disturbed respiratory function and disability. These forms, *centrilobular* (or centriacinar) and *panlobular* (or panacinar) *emphysema*, are discussed together in the following section. The less common forms of alveolar enlargement and disruption and occurrence of abnormal air-containing spaces in the lung will be discussed separately.

The two major forms of generalized emphysema take their morphologic terminology from the distribution within lung units of the morphologic changes which they produce. The lobule (secondary lobule of Miller) is a macroscopic lung unit, and emphysema which can be seen macroscopically on whole-lung sections to involve chiefly the central portions of the lobules is referred to as centrilobular emphysema. Disease which involves the lobule diffusely is called panlobular emphysema. Corresponding terminology based upon a microscopic lung unit, the acinus (primary lobule of Miller), refers to centriacinar and panacinar emphysema. It is widely believed that centrilobular or centriacinar emphysema is a complication of chronic bronchitis or other disease involving conducting airways, while panlobular or panacinar emphysema is a primary disorder of lung parenchyma (see detailed presentation in Chap. 3).

The morphologic distinction between these two forms is less straightforward than these definitions imply, however, and pathologists may not agree upon the classification of an individual case. The distinction is of critical importance to investigators attempting to classify chronic lung diseases with the aim of identifying causative factors; however, for clinical purposes, the distinction is less important. It is evident from the foregoing discussion, however, that patients with relatively pure emphysema and little or no chronic bronchitis would be expected to have panacinar emphysema. Although the definition of this disorder is an anatomic one, such patients are generally agreed to demonstrate an identifiable clinical picture, as described below. The clinical presentation of patients with homozygous α_1 antitrypsin deficiency is usually that of primary emphysema, and morphologically these patients tend to have panacinar emphysema.

Clinical Presentation

The classic patient with primary emphysema, presenting clinically as Dornhorst's *pink puffer*,[141] Burrow's *type A*,[142,143] or Filley's comparable *pp*[144–147] is expected to exhibit the morphologic changes of panacinar emphysema when the lungs undergo anatomic examination. Patients with α_1 antitrypsin deficiency often present with primary emphysema as described under *Pathogenesis*.

The predominant symptom, and certainly the earliest to appear in the patient with primary emphysema, is shortness of breath on exertion. It is a nonspecific enough symptom, to be sure, but often somewhat distinctive in its manifestations if carefully explored. The appearance and progression are slower and more insidious than in most infiltrative diseases of the interstitium, such as idiopathic diffuse interstitial fibrosis. Several years may elapse between the first awareness of dyspnea on heavy exertion and the point when disability restricts normal activities. There is an absence of the cough characteristic of chronic bronchitis and many other respiratory disorders. The exacerbations and remissions of bronchial asthma are notably absent. The orthopnea and paroxysmal nocturnal dyspnea of pulmonary edema are absent as well.

Occasionally, the insidious, slowly progressive nature of this symptom is not elicited and the patient describes a rather abrupt onset of respiratory disability. Often this represents a failure to observe early exertional dyspnea in a sedentary patient who seldom engages in heavy exertion. Such a patient may become aware of his disability only when it becomes so severe as to limit even mild activity.

Weight loss is commonly observed in the pink puffer for unclear reasons. Commonly, its onset coincides with exertional dyspnea noticed by the patient. The reason for this is baffling, since a chronic bronchitic with a similar degree of disability is more characteristically normal in body weight, or even obese.

As primary emphysema progresses, activity becomes severely limited and the patient's subjective awareness of dyspnea becomes intense. Seemingly, he is characterized by a drive to maintain normal or increased minute ventilation and normal blood gases even at considerable cost in terms of work of breathing. The chronic bronchitic with comparable ventilatory abnormality more characteristically tolerates hypoxemia and hypercapnia with relatively less subjective distress. In addition to maintaining total ventilation, the primary emphysema patient is protected against hypoxemia by the destruction of capillaries in emphysematous areas of lung, thus decreasing perfusion effectively in areas of impaired ventilation, preventing physiologic shunting. The bronchitic has areas of lung in which secretions obstruct ventilation, but blood flow is maintained, resulting in shunting, hypoxemia and cyanosis.

Perhaps in part because of this tendency to maintain normal values for arterial P_{O_2} and P_{CO_2}, the patient with primary emphysema develops the peripheral edema of overt right heart failure only during the terminal stages of his disease. Similarly, secondary polycythemia is uncommon. When these complications do occur, they have grave prognostic significance, and respond poorly to treatment. Chronic productive cough and recurrent bronchopulmonary infections may also occur late in the course of primary emphysema, although they are conspicuously absent during the earlier stages.

The conspicuous classic features of the emphysemic, then, are those of an emaciated individual struggling to maintain labored breathing, but acyanotic and without obvious evidence of peripheral edema. Closer examination reveals a fixed, hyperinflated chest with minimal movement of the rib cage or of the low-lying diaphragm. Retraction of the intercostal spaces and supraclavicular fossae during inspiration are accompanied by contraction of accessory muscles of respiration. Expiration is prolonged and carried out against pursed lips. The patient exhibits a preference for a posture in which he sits bent forward at the waist, with elbows propped upon a table near shoulder height. This position tends to give mechanical advantage to accessory respiratory muscles and presses abdominal contents upward towards the diaphragm, arching it for better movement during inspiration and expressing air during expiration. Breath sounds are suppressed, and rales and rhonchi tend to be minimal or absent. The chest is hyperresonant and silent, so much so as to simulate pneumothorax, or to make the latter diagnosis difficult by physical examination in a patient with emphysema. Dry, crackling inspiratory rales are occasionally present in such a patient and may bear some resemblance to the rales of pulmonary edema.

Examining the heart of a patient with emphysema is often difficult. The overinflated lungs interpose air between the heart and chest wall obscuring findings which otherwise could be elicited by palpation, percussion, and auscultation. The heart sounds may be nearly inaudible over the anterior chest, but may be heard in the epigastrium as a result of the low-lying diaphragm on which the heart rests. A loud pulmonic component of the second sound and an audible fourth sound may accompany pulmonary hypertension; and a third sound, louder during inspiration, may signify right ventricular failure.

Roentgenography

An abnormal chest roentgenogram, properly interpreted, can be a reliable predictor of the presence of moderately or severely advanced, generalized emphysema (Fig. 14-6). Inclusion of both anteroposterior (AP) and lateral views increases reliability. A normal roentgenogram does not exclude the presence of emphysema, and no single finding or combination of findings has been described which serves especially well to detect early asymptomatic disease. Roentgenographic findings of emphysema can be grouped in two major classes: those indicative of lung hyperinflation, and those representative of vascular changes accompanying emphysema.

The findings of lung hyperinflation are several. Among the less helpful are generalized lucency of the lung fields, along with increased distance between ribs, low diaphragms, and increased AP diameter as seen on a lateral view. Lucency of the lung fields is of limited value because of its dependence on factors other than lung volume, such as thickness of chest wall and technique of exposure and development of the roentgenogram. Dimensions of the thorax can be used reliably to calculate lung volume; but there is a wide normal range for lung volume, and in addition, air trapping in an acute asthmatic attack may produce all the findings described above.

The depth of the retrosternal air space as viewed from the lateral projection has been shown to be somewhat reliable and specific when observed along with other findings of emphysema. The upper limit of normal for this distance from the posterior surface of sternum to the anterior border of aorta is around 2.5[183] to 3 cm.[184,185]

Simon[184,185] has suggested that the diaphragm may be considered low if the center of the right dome on inspiration lies at or below the level of the 7th rib anteriorly; and flat if the maximum curvature of the right dome is less than 1.5 cm. Flatness of the diaphragms, or even concavity upwards, has greater diagnostic usefulness than level as judged by counting ribs. The level of the diaphragm may vary normally; but flattening of the contour on both AP and lateral views does not occur normally and is usually transient in severe attacks of asthma.

The pulmonary vascular changes of emphysema as interpreted by an experienced observer may be quite reliable. The central pulmonary

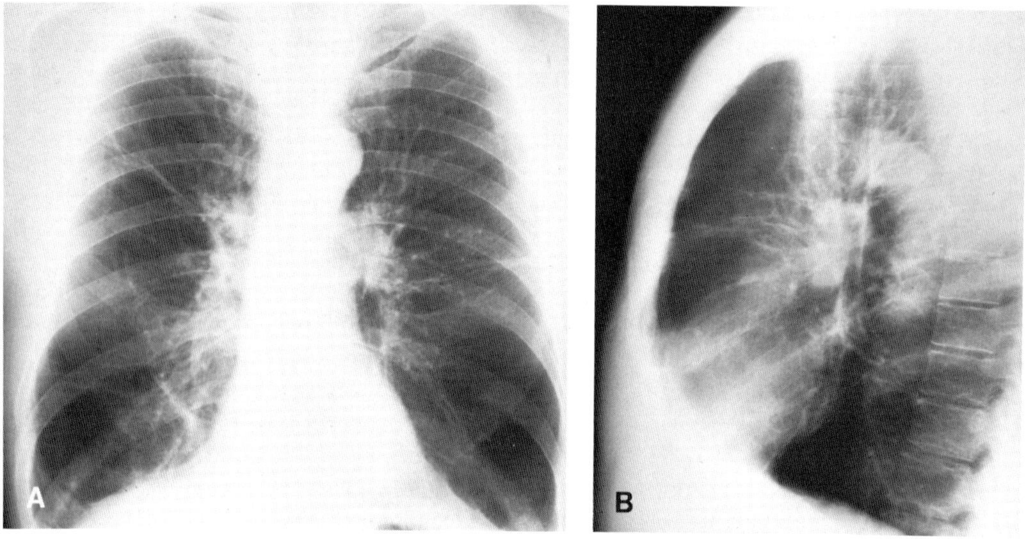

FIG. 14-6. Chest roentgenogram of patient with diffuse obstructive emphysema. Note flattened diaphragms, narrow, vertical heart, and patchy areas of hyperlucency. **A.** Posteroanterior view; **B.** lateral view.

arteries attain prominence, but because of dilation and change of position relative to their origins, the peripheral vessels become attenuated and develop a pruned appearance, with loss of fine distal arborization. Accompanying cardiac findings more difficult to quantitate are a long, narrow cardiac contour on AP view (related to lowering of the diaphragm supporting the heart) and an increase in the volume of the right ventricle (related to pulmonary hypertension of long standing).

Patchy areas of hyperlucency and of increased lung markings, even in the absence of roentgenographically definable walls of bullae, are indicative of emphysematous changes. Such patchy alterations are often more readily recognized than are uniform, diffuse changes in radiodensity. Interpreted with caution and taken in conjunction with other indicators of emphysema, they provide valuable supportive evidence of its presence. Bullae may sometimes be clearly recognized in patients with generalized emphysema but may also exist in subjects with otherwise normal lungs.

Several investigators have evaluated the accuracy of the roentgenographic diagnosis of emphysema by correlation with morphologic findings at autopsy.[183–188] They have used various combinations of the criteria described above, and most of these criteria are subject to substantial difference in interpretation by individual observers. The roentgenographic evaluation of emphysema has not yet become an exact science.

Laws and Heard (1962)[186] reported results of a study of 100 cases and attempted to evaluate virtually all the roentgenographic criteria described above. They concluded that very severe emphysema could usually be detected radiologically and that a reduction in the caliber and number of the peripheral pulmonary arteries was the most helpful sign. Similarly, Simon and coworkers (1973)[185] concluded that the roentgenographic diagnosis of emphysema could be made with confidence only when attenuation of vasculature was present as well as signs of overinflation.

Thurlbeck (1963)[187] described a morphologic evaluation of the criteria, not precisely defined, in use by radiologists at Massachusetts General Hospital. He found, in a study of 159 cases, that 71% of subjects with severe emphysema had been correctly identified roentgenographically.

Emphysema of lesser severity was much less often recognized and 6 of 61 patients with normal lungs were incorrectly diagnosed as emphysematous.

Reid (1964),[188] in a correlation of radiographic and morphologic indicators of emphysema, found that subjects with roentgenographic evidence of both overinflation and vascular changes of emphysema virtually always had moderate or severe morphologic emphysema, but that mild morphologic emphysema never produced convincing radiologic manifestations. Her study employed the criteria of Simon.[184]

Sutinen and associates (1965)[189] evaluated four roentgenographic signs: flattening of diaphragms on AP projection; irregular areas of radiolucency; increased retrosternal air space; and flattening of diaphragms on lateral projection. They found that all of their subjects with two or more of these signs had morphologic evidence of emphysema; and that of 19 asymptomatic subjects with morphologic emphysema 13 could be diagnosed by applying these radiographic criteria.

Nicklaus and co-workers (1966)[183] reexamined the four criteria described above, and found that, using more than one of these criteria, 93% of subjects with moderate to severe emphysema could be correctly diagnosed. Only 32% of patients with mild emphysema were correctly identified, and 10% of those with normal lungs were incorrectly diagnosed as having emphysema. This group of workers also reevaluated the sign found most useful by Laws and Heard (reduction in caliber and number of the peripheral branches of the pulmonary artery). In the hands of Nicklaus and co-workers, this sign was less helpful and subject to more variation of interpretation than the criteria of Sutinen.

Although the investigators described above disagree upon certain points, there is general agreement that severe morphologic emphysema is usually recognizable on chest roentgenogram. A recent paper by McCarthy and associates[190] suggests that even severe emphysema as assessed by pulmonary function abnormalities, particularly a maximum elastic recoil of less than 10 cm H_2O, may be missed on chest roentgenogram.

It is important to note Fraser's observation[153] that a substantial group of bronchitics with accompanying emphysema fail to demonstrate the usual *arterial deficiency* (*AD*) pattern of vascular changes described above. These patients may exhibit a pattern of increased bronchovascular markings, probably related to their bronchitis and incidental to the severe emphysema which may accompany it. They have referred to this pattern as that of *increased markings* (*IM*).

Electrocardiogram

The electrocardiographic abnormalities which occur in chronic obstructive lung disease have already been discussed (see Fig. 14-5). Shmock and associates[155,191] have presented evidence that morphologic emphysema with severe airway obstruction may produce low voltage and *pseudo-left-axis*.[191] These investigators also found *P. pulmonale* to be associated with emphysema rather than bronchitis with airway obstruction.[155] Both atrial and ventricular arrythmias are common in patients with respiratory insufficiency caused by chronic bronchitis and emphysema.

Other Laboratory Studies

Sputum smears and cultures may be useful in guiding antibiotic therapy in patients with bronchitis complicating emphysema. Often, cultures of sputum grow an assortment of bacteria of uncertain significance. Treatment is probably best guided by clinical evidence of infection (fever, leukocytosis, purulent sputum), and antibiotic choice influenced by cultures and sensitivities only when there is clinical infection accompanied by a predominant or pure culture of a pathogen.

Hematologic studies may be useful when complicating infection produces leukocytosis or when advanced respiratory failure is accompanied by erythrocytosis. Serologic studies to identify α_1-antitrypsin deficiency are indicated in young persons with primary emphysema, especially in the presence of a positive family history or the absence of a smoking history. (See section on Pathogenesis.)

Pulmonary Function Evaluation

Both chronic bronchitis and emphysema may produce a decrease in vital capacity, with increased residual volume and reduced maximum expiratory flow rates. Maximum voluntary ventilation is reduced in both. Total lung capacity tends to be increased in emphysema, and severe increases in residual volume, functional residual capacity, and the RV:TLC ratio appear to be more characteristic of emphysema than of bronchitis.[192,193] Although bronchodilator administration may improve reduced flow rates in asthma and bronchitis, there will be no improvement in emphysema alone.

The tendency for expiratory flow rates to be impaired to a greater extent than vital capacity was observed by early investigators, and was emphasized by a study which identified 10 subjects with clinically manifest emphysema who had greater than normal vital capacity.[194]

The earliest studies providing a correlation between functional and morphologic abnormalities sought, with some success, to use residual volume, total lung capacity, and the ratio of these measurements to predict emphysema.[195–197] In spite of some discrepancies among these studies, it appears that each of these parameters possesses some value for identification of diffuse pulmonary emphysema. The predictive value of total lung capacity appears to be improved when measurement is carried out by roentgenographic and plethysmographic techniques. Methods utilizing inert gas dilution or washout may underestimate lung volume in patients with unequal distribution of inspired gas, as is the case in emphysema.

Measurement of mechanical properties of the lung is of great help in identifying emphysema, as well as in understanding its pathophysiology. Loss of elastic recoil of lung in emphysema was documented as early as 1934 by Christie.[198] The usefulness of this observation in identifying emphysema has since been repeatedly documented.[199–203] Reduction in recoil pressure at a defined inflation volume or the more sensitive analysis of the slope of the pressure volume curve[204] have come to be recognized as the most specific physiologic measurements available for identifying advanced emphysema.

Measurements of airways resistance in emphysema have not produced such consistent data, however. Subclinical emphysema has been shown in one study to be associated with a detectable decrease in maximum expiratory flow rates at low lung volumes, but normal or near normal airways resistance.[205] Another study has suggested that decreased elastic recoil alone is capable of severely limiting expiratory flow.[201] The relative importance of intrinsic changes in the airways, and the loss of radial traction as causes of reduced flow, remains under discussion[169,200–207] (see also Chap. 3, Fig. 3-14).

Frequency dependence of dynamic compliance has been shown to occur in emphysema,[199] and theoretically might be caused by this disorder alone. However, it may more often be due to associated obstructive disease of small airways. Alterations in compliance of the chest wall have been demonstrated in emphysema,[208–210] but are probably a result rather than a cause of this disease.

Ventilation and respiratory gas exchange are altered in emphysema, with nonuniformity of distribution of ventilation and perfusion. Increased total ventilation[192] tends to preserve effective ventilation in the face of ventilation-perfusion inequality and subnormal cardiac output tends to modify hypoxemia.[146] Therefore, although hypoxemia is common in emphysema, and hypercarbia occurs in advanced obstructive lung disease of the emphysematous type, these abnormalities are less striking than in chronic bronchitis with a similar degree of ventilatory impairment. Hypoxemia may worsen with exercise in patients who clinically appear emphysematous, and improve with exercise in clinical chronic bronchitis,[211] though the correlations reported between exercise response and type of disease have not been consistent.[146]

Diffusing capacity is widely regarded as highly predictive of the presence of morphologic emphysema.[153,203–205,212,213] The reduction in alveolocapillary surface area for diffusion which must occur provides a logical explanation for this observed correlation. A failure to increase the diffusing capacity with exercise is characteristic of emphysema as well.[214]

Pathology

Pulmonary emphysema has been defined by the American Thoracic Society (ATS) as "an anatomic alteration of the lung characterized by an abnormal enlargement of air spaces distal to the terminal, nonrespiratory bronchiole, accompanied by destructive changes of the alveolar walls."[135] Even this simple, straightforward definition has its critics, some of whom object to restricting the diagnosis by demanding that alveolar wall destruction be included. The definition is complicated by difficulty in defining the normal size of an alveolus. It is further confused by common use of the term "emphysema" to describe abnormal air collections in the lungs originating from developmental anomalies, or occurring in a subpleural location displacing but not destroying alveolar walls. The ATS definition is useful, however, in discussion of the common forms of diffuse pulmonary emphysema accompanied by decreases in expiratory flow rates and abnormalities of respiratory gas transfer. Other forms of "emphysema" and related conditions will be discussed separately.

The two major forms of diffuse *obstructive* emphysema are classified according to the distribution within the lung of the abnormal changes of alveolar enlargement and destruction. A brief description of macroscopic and microscopic lung anatomy is necessary in order to understand this classification.[182,215]

The lung is divided by invaginations of connective tissue continuous with the visceral pleura into macroscopic units called lobules (secondary lobules of Miller). Distribution of emphysematous changes within these lobules can be seen on examination of whole-lung slices. Categorization of emphysema into panlobular and centrilobular forms on the basis of whether it is distributed evenly throughout the lobules or primarily at the center of the lobules has been proposed.[181,216–218]

A corresponding classification based on microscopic anatomy refers to distribution of emphysema within the functional unit called the acinus. Each acinus is composed of the branching series of air-containing and gas-exchanging chambers distal to a terminal bronchiole. Panacinar emphysema involves all portions of the acinus, while centriacinar emphysema destroys preferentially the proximal, central portions of the acinus closest to the terminal bronchiole.[136,173]

Conveniently, the acini within a lobule are so arranged spatially that terminal bronchioles are grouped near the center of the lobule. Emphysematous disease classified grossly as panlobular will then be seen microscopically as panacinar in distribution, while centrilobular emphysema will correspond to centriacinar disease. The two classifications are therefore often used interchangeably. (See also Chap. 3.)

The importance of this classification lies in the possibility that these two forms of emphysema may have different causes. There is widespread belief that centrilobular and panlobular emphysema are both morphologically and etiologically distinct, in spite of evidence that expert observers often disagree about classification of individual cases.[219] A well-recognized form of centrilobular emphysema is seen in soft-coal miners, in whom pigment collections in the vicinity of dilated terminal bronchioles accompany dilated air spaces.[220] It is postulated that the centrilobular deposition of inhaled carbon particles produces mechanical distortion or inflammatory weakening of surrounding alveolar walls. A more common but less clearly defined form of destructive centrilobular emphysema accompanies chronic bronchitis.[153,217] The infection and inflammation accompanying this disorder would be well calculated to produce proteolytic damage to alveolar walls as bacteria, leukocytes, and macrophages invade the area, and then die and release lysosomal enzymes. The destruction would be expected to be most severe near the center of the acinus, nearest the infected and inflamed tracheobronchial tree. Panlobular emphysema, distributed evenly throughout the acinus and the lobule, would be more easily explained by an intrinsic defect in the structure of the lung parenchyma or by a blood-borne agent of injury. The observation that the emphysema occurring in homozygous inheritance of α_1-antitrypsin deficiency is often panlobular, supports this concept.

The distribution within the lungs of panlobular and centrilobular emphysema appears to be somewhat distinctive as well, with panlobular changes characteristically involving the lower and centrilobular, the upper zones preferentially.[221,222]

The importance of quantitation of emphysema has recently gained attention, as attempts to correlate its occurrence with various possible etiologic factors have become more refined. Weibel[223] pioneered attempts at quantitation, and Dunnill[172] recently summarized the importance of these efforts. Since both increased size of alveoli and disappearance of alveolar walls define emphysema, it is apparent that this pathologic diagnosis is inevitably a quantitative one. Such matters as variation in normal alveolar size from the top to the bottom of the lung and the degree of inflation must be taken into account by the pathologist attempting to identify pulmonary emphysema. Current techniques necessitate fixation of specimens during inflation, under uniform inflation pressures. Lung macrosections are then studied by comparison with standard sections which are graded for severity, or by superimposition of grids which permit estimation of alveolar wall integrity by counting of dots or lines upon the grid which fall upon or intersect with alveolar walls.

Certain morphologic changes accompanying emphysema have provided clues to its pathogenesis as well as to its pathophysiology. The frequent association of emphysema with chronic bronchitis has been well documented.[224] Organic narrowing and mucus plugging of bronchioles have been described[128] and increased resistance of airways smaller than 2 mm in diameter has been observed in emphysematous lungs.[124] Macrophages laden with pigment have been described in normal lung parenchyma adjacent to areas of emphysematous destruction and in the sputum of smokers.[225] Most recently, a characteristic respiratory bronchiolitis associated with collections of pigment-laden macrophages has been described in the lungs of young asymptomatic smokers dead of nonrespiratory causes.[125]

It is possible that this respiratory bronchiolitis may be the lesion which produces uneven distribution of ventilation in smokers and severe impairment of airflow in advanced emphysema. It is likewise possible that these collections of macrophages, through their death and release of lysosomal enzymes, may be directly responsible for the production of emphysema in some cases.

The loss of lung elasticity that occurs in lower lung zones with age and in accelerated forms in α_1-antitrypsin deficiency may result from circulating leukocytes.[92]

COMPLICATIONS OF COPD: COR PULMONALE AND SECONDARY POLYCYTHEMIA

CHRONIC COR PULMONALE DUE TO OBSTRUCTIVE LUNG DISEASE

Use of the term *cor pulmonale* varies, and may refer to increased pulmonary vascular resistance or pulmonary artery pressure due to primary disease of the lungs, to the right ventricular hypertrophy which results from longstanding pulmonary hypertension, or to the clinical syndrome of congestive failure of the right ventricle which occurs subsequent to the previously mentioned changes. The clinician often employs the last usage, since pulmonary hypertension and right ventricular hypertrophy without signs of failure may be difficult to recognize. The World Health Organization has defined cor pulmonale as "hypertrophy of the right ventricle resulting from diseases affecting the function and/or structure of the lung, except when the pulmonary alterations are the result of diseases that primarily affect the left side of the heart, or of congenital heart disease."[226]

The pathogenesis of cor pulmonale[227] can most simply be understood in terms of increased pulmonary vascular resistance due to irreversible anatomic destruction or restriction of pulmonary vessels,[228] or to reversible spasm of the pulmonary arterioles resulting from hypoxemia[229–237] or from acidosis.[238] One or more of these mechanisms appears to be operative in each of the clinical conditions which commonly produce chronic cor pulmonale. There is little doubt that other mechanisms are sometimes contributory, however. These include multiple small pulmonary emboli,[228,239] increased alveolar pressure during expiration in obstructive lung disease,[240] increased blood viscosity contributing to flow resistance in secondary polycythemia, increased blood volume, intrapulmonary shunts contributing to volume overload of the right ventricles,[241] and reduced myocardial contractility from acidosis and hypoxemia.[242,243] In addition, it is probable that prolonged vasospasm and elevated pulmonary vascular pressure result, in some cases, in a component of elevated resistance due to smooth muscle hypertrophy and other morphologic changes in pulmonary vessels. This component may be reversible with time.

The degree to which functional and anatomic mechanisms are operative is of considerable importance, since the former would be expected to be the more responsive to therapy. Hypoxemia is recognized as being capable of producing pulmonary hypertension by increasing pulmonary vascular resistance. The amount of reversibility of pulmonary hypertension achieved by correction of hypoxemia, acutely and chronically, has varied in the studies reported. In one study carried out in Denver, where the barometric pressure and hence the ambient oxygen tension is less than at sea level, there was a significant fall in pulmonary arteriolar resistance related to a month of supplemental oxygen administration in patients with chronic obstructive lung disease.[234] A subsequent study at sea level failed to demonstrate improvement in pulmonary hypertension, but cardiac output was not successfully measured in this study, and pulmonary vascular resistance therefore not calculated.[237] This difference in results might easily be explained by the difference in ambient oxygen tension in the two studies. Differences in patient selection might also have affected the results observed.

Acidosis has also been shown to produce a pulmonary vasospastic response which is enhanced by hypoxemia.[238] Therefore, normalization of arterial blood gases should be a goal of therapy in patients with cor pulmonale who have hypoxemia and respiratory acidosis. The effectiveness of this therapy in reversing pulmonary hypertension and right ventricular failure varies from one patient to another, depending upon the combination of factors producing these manifestations.

Differences in the pathophysiology of cor pulmonale have been observed between patients with emphysematous and bronchial types of chronic obstructive pulmonary disease and these differences may provide some guidelines for predicting the results of therapy.[244] Patients with clinical disease suggesting predominant emphysema tend to have high pulmonary vascular resistance and low cardiac output, with preservation of relatively normal arterial blood gases. Those with predominant chronic bronchitis have normal cardiac output, producing high pulmonary artery pressures as well as elevated pulmonary vascular resistance. Hypoxemia and hypercarbia are more frequent and more severe in the latter groups of patients, who also exhibit clinical signs of congestive heart failure at an early, more reversible stage of their obstructive lung disease. These patients are believed to respond more often to correction of abnormal gas exchange, and to other therapeutic measures, with improvement in the florid clinical manifestations of cor pulmonale.

Left ventricular function has been studied extensively in patients with cor pulmonale, with variable results. Studies utilizing different techniques have reported abnormal left ventricular function to be absent, or usual in severe COPD.[245–253] Currently, the predominant evidence would suggest that when left ventricular performance is abnormal in patients with COPD, the cause is usually arteriosclerotic or hypertensive heart disease. Certainly, to the clinician, pulmonary edema does not appear to be a usual sequela of COPD, nor does left ventricular enlargement detectable on physical examination or chest roentgenogram. Bass has pointed out[254] that COPD and left heart failure tend to mutually conceal characteristic findings when they do co-exist.

Pathology

Wagenvoort, Heath, and Edwards[239] have summarized the vascular changes which occur in patients with pulmonary emphysema, as well as those which occur in exposure to the hypoxemia of altitude or of hypoventilation. The former group of patients might be expected to exhibit alterations caused by the disease process itself, with superimposed lesions secondary to hypoxemia.

Surprisingly, the medial hypertrophy of small muscular pulmonary arteries which characterizes the changes resulting from hypoxemia is not prominent in pulmonary emphysema. Even in emphysema severe enough to produce substantial hypertrophy of the right ventricle, medial thickness of muscular pulmonary arteries may remain normal. Abnormalities which are characteristic of emphysema include atheromata of elastic pulmonary arteries, intimal fibrosis of muscular pulmonary arteries, tortuosity of arteries and arterioles, and loss of pulmonary capillary bed.

The quantitative roles of each of these changes in the production of elevated pulmonary vascular resistance is uncertain. Dunnill[228] has suggested that vascular deformity and pressure upon vessels from emphysematous air spaces are of primary importance.

Autopsy studies of right ventricular size in chronic obstructive lung disease have not provided an answer to this question. Thurlbeck and associates[153] have summarized the seemingly discrepant reports of positive, negative, and absent correlation between severity of emphysema and right ventricular size. They have pointed out the ways in which case selection may have brought about these varying results.

Clinical Manifestations

The classic presentation of patients with right ventricular failure from COPD includes signs and symptoms resulting from the lung disease causing it.

Shortness of breath and productive cough are worse during episodes of right ventricular failure, though it is seldom clear whether the failure is a cause, an effect, or both.

Venous distention and dependent peripheral edema may be dramatic in advanced cardiac failure. There may be mild neck vein distention during expiration and pedal edema in severe obstructive lung disease without failure, however. High intrathoracic pressure resulting from airways obstruction impedes venous return to the heart, producing venous distention and sometimes increased paradoxic pulse. Poor nutrition and many hours in the sitting position presumably may lead to pedal edema in severe COPD. Low, flat diaphragms in pulmonary emphysema may cause the liver edge to be palpable below the right costal margin in the absence of hepatomegaly. An actual increase in liver size with tenderness may occur when right ventricular failure supervenes.

Plethora and cyanosis and warm moist skin often accompany cor pulmonale, due in part to secondary erythrocytosis, desaturation of arterial, and therefore capillary blood, peripheral vasodilation from hypercarbia, and elevated venous pressure. Engorgement of retinal veins may be seen, and papilledema has been reported.[255,256] Drowsiness and altered consciousness are frequent when severe hypercarbia is present. Asterixis occurs, especially during periods of worsening or improvement of hypoventilation and hypercarbia.

Examination of the heart itself may be surprising for its lack of helpful findings. Evidence of right ventricular enlargement may be obscured by a large retrosternal air space.

Auscultatory evidence of pulmonary hypertension, in the form of a loud pulmonic component of the second heart sound, may be muffled as well. A ventricular gallop indicates ventricular failure if present and increased intensity during inspiration will identify the right ventricle as its origin. However, increased volume of air-containing lung between the stethoscope and the heart may obscure this finding, along with the murmur of tricuspid insufficiency which occasionally results from dilation of the valve ring in right heart failure.

Electrocardiographic findings have already been described and include evidence of right ventricular hypertrophy and right atrial enlargement and atrial and ventricular arrythmias. The high incidence of false-positive and false-negative results obtained with current electrocardiographic criteria for right ventricular hypertrophy have been summarized.

Chest roentgenograms provide another imperfect method for identifying cor pulmonale, since right ventricular hypertrophy is seen only on lateral views, if at all. Enlargement of central pulmonary arteries may be easily visualized on PA or lateral views. Enlargement of the heart in transverse diameter is seen only when left ventricular failure supervenes, and this roentgenographic finding is by no means an inevitable accompaniment even of severe cor pulmonale.

Secondary polycythemia, a relatively uncommon sequel of obstructive lung disease, often accompanies clinical findings of right ventricular failure. An elevation in hemoglobin and hematocrit may suggest polycythemia. These findings may be misleading since elevated plasma volume may accompany cor pulmonale and mask an elevated red blood cell mass or diuretic therapy may lower plasma volume.

Although right ventricular decompensation

has traditionally been viewed as a poor prognostic sign in COPD, some recent studies indicate that the evolution of hemodynamic changes in cor pulmonale is slow.[257-259] There is even encouraging evidence that survival for several years is possible after an episode of right ventricular failure.[259,260] Hopefully, improved management based on physiologic principles can be credited with improved survival.

Treatment of cor pulmonale and associated secondary polycythemia is discussed in the section on Management of COPD.

SECONDARY POLYCYTHEMIA

Arterial hypoxemia is well recognized as a stimulus of bone marrow production of red blood cells. Patients with COPD may develop arterial hypoxemia as a result of abnormal gas exchange in the lungs or carboxyhemoglobin in smokers. The arterial hypoxemia is frequently worse during sleep. Cardiac output may be reduced relative to tissue demands further reducing tissue oxygen availability. These factors, and the classification of polycythemic disorders are considered in Chapter 5 under Oxygen Transport.

It is somewhat surprising that the arterial hypoxemia of obstructive lung disease produces a less constant and predictable response of hematocrit and hemoglobin, and generally a quantitatively smaller response. A portion of this discrepancy between the response of normal subjects and COPD patients to hypoxemia is related to variations in plasma volume in the latter group.[261-265] Cor pulmonale and diuretic therapy produce increases and decreases in plasma volume which obscure or exaggerate the red blood cell response respectively as assessed by measurement of peripheral blood hematocrit or hemoglobin concentration. Measurement of total red blood cell mass by isotopic techniques, and of serum and urine erythropoietin, has suggested that the bone marrow response to hypoxemia is often blunted in COPD, however[265] and that this is the result of a relative decrease in marrow responsiveness rather than a deficiency in erythropoietin release.[266]

The usefulness of a polycythemic response as an adaptive mechanism to hypoxemia in COPD is a matter of some uncertainty. Other adaptive mechanisms which enable the body to tolerate hypoxemia may be activated and these mechanisms have been discussed in the section of this book which discusses normal adaptation to high altitude. These circulatory and tissue mechanisms, along with changes in hemoglobin function, may minimize the importance of erythrocytosis to the patient. In addition, it may be that an unfettered increase in red blood cell production can be a physiologic disadvantage. Some experimental evidence suggests that at a hematocrit above 50% an increase in blood viscosity overcomes any advantages to the organism of increased oxygen carrying capacity.[267,268]

This evidence, along with studies which show hemodynamic improvement following phlebotomy in polycythemic subjects with cor pulmonale and high blood volumes, has been used to justify therapeutic phlebotomy as an adjunct to therapy in such acutely ill patients. Studies of cerebral blood flow in patients with high normal hematocrits (50%) have demonstrated marked improvement in cerebral blood flow with reduction of hematocrit to 45% or less. Neuropsychologic function appears to improve when hematocrits are reduced below 45%, suggesting this is the desirable level.[270-271b]

Long-term management of cor pulmonale and COPD should optimally not include repeated phlebotomy, however. Adequate management should have as its goal maintenance of an arterial oxygen tension high enough to control hematocrit below 45%. Oxygen supplementation of inspired air on a long-term basis may be required in order to accomplish this goal. The use of long-term oxygen therapy is further discussed in the section dealing with management of COPD.

PRINCIPLES OF MANAGEMENT OF COPD

The management of bronchial asthma has been discussed separately because the prognosis and response to therapy, and hence the goals of asthma therapy, are somewhat different in this disorder than in chronic bronchitis, emphysema, or mixed COPD. Death from asthma is unusual, and a realistic therapeutic goal is often complete control of symptoms. Chronic bronchitis and emphysema more characteristically do progress, however, producing an irreversible loss of lung function. Goals of management take three forms, all of which are commonly faced by physicians caring for these patients: prevention of irreversible deterioration of lung function; control of symptoms and of disability, seldom with complete success in advanced cases; and prevention of death from respiratory insufficiency.

Prevention

Prevention of lung destruction due to COPD should ideally begin early in the course of the disease, before the onset of symptoms. Commonly, patients delay in seeking medical help until symptoms have been present for many years and have progressed to the point where respiratory insufficiency has led to disability. The problems inherent in screening asymptomatic subjects for mild, early COPD have been discussed above: current techniques for detecting asymptomatic abnormalities of pulmonary function have not yet been proven to correctly identify those subjects who will progress to clinically manifest COPD. Moreover, prevention of progression is limited chiefly to avoidance of cigarette smoking. Our techniques for motivating smokers to discontinue this habit are primitive and commonly ineffective.

Nevertheless, cigarette smoking has been shown to be the major cause of COPD; it is highly probable that cessation will abort the progression of pulmonary dysfunction and that mild abnormalities of pulmonary function do identify subjects at high risk for development of more severe dysfunction. Therefore it is clear that physicians have an obligation to discourage the use of cigarettes in all cases, with particular emphasis on persons shown to have abnormal tests of ventilatory function which might indicate early COPD.

The desirability of extensive use of screening programs, except as part of investigational efforts, is controversial, however. A universally applicable approach to the problem of urban air pollution as it may contribute to the pathogenesis of COPD is likewise unavailable to the individual physician. Measures directed at improving antiprotease activity in the lungs remain experimental, as discussed under Etiologic Considerations.

Management of Mild and Moderate Symptomatic COPD

Preventing progression of pulmonary dysfunction over an extended period of time in patients with clinical COPD is probably limited to their not smoking. The numerous treatment modalities to be described below are of great help in treatment of life-threatening complications and in modification of symptoms, but have not been convincingly shown to modify the course of the underlying disease process.[272–275] Management of COPD, therefore, should be an individualized program designed to control symptoms of cough, bronchopulmonary infection, and respiratory insufficiency; to avoid complications; and to maintain life during periods when reversible exacerbations or complications are life-threatening.

The mainstays of therapy in most symptomatic but ambulatory patients include avoidance of cigarettes and of industrial or other pollutants recognized to produce symptoms in the individual patient; prophylaxis against influenza and pneumococcal infection by immunization; and the use of oral bronchodilators and antibiotics.

Bronchodilators, discussed in detail under *Asthma*, may be used on a regular basis to reduce bronchospasm or to prevent exacerbations during cough or exercise. The degree of bronchospasm contributing to symptoms is highly variable in patients with COPD and aggressiveness of treatment must be individualized. Response of pulmonary function abnormalities to bronchodilator is a useful guide to the degree of reversibility but symptomatic response should not be discounted. A relatively modest objective response may produce useful subjective improvement. Some patients with primary emphysema may have little or no bronchitis or bronchospasm and derive no objective or subjective benefit from bronchodilators and thus should not be treated with them. Dosage of oral bronchodilator must always be individualized and observation for toxic side-effects carried out.

Antibiotics should be used in treatment of exacerbations of bronchial infection, and prophylactically as needed in patients troubled by frequent infections throughout the year or during winter months. Patients should be educated in the administration of antibiotics at the onset of exacerbations, and a prescription or a supply of drug made available for use when needed. Specific treatment of bacterial organisms demonstrated by smear or culture to be predominant, is often impractical, since a mixed flora is commonly demonstrated, for which tetracyline or ampicillin, used empirically, are usually helpful. *Pneumococcus* and *Hemophilus influenzae* are frequently associated with exacerbations of bronchitis, and are generally sensitive to these drugs. The occurrence of pneumonia, on the other hand, is an important indication for sputum smear and culture, as well as blood culture, in an attempt to facilitate specific antibiotic therapy.

Aerosolization of saline and mucolytics is often unnecessary in stable patients with mild or moderate disease. Aerosolized saline and mucolytics along with postural drainage and percussion may be of help in selected patients with voluminous or viscid secretions. Detergents are not of demonstrable usefulness. Intermittent positive pressure breathing is probably not in itself of major benefit in this group of patients, and should be regarded as an effective means of delivering bronchodilator in patients unable to use other devices effectively because of severe ventilatory insufficiency, impaired manual dexterity, or other problems.

Oral administration of expectorants, especially potassium iodide and glyceryl guaiacollate, is popular and generally harmless. These agents have not been convincingly demonstrated to be helpful, and should not be relied upon as major measures in treatment of viscid sputum. Combination preparations which include antihistamines, which dry the tracheobronchial muscosa, should be avoided.

Outpatient Management of Severe COPD

Patients with COPD producing respiratory insufficiency severe enough to limit activities essential to gainful employment, or even self-care, may require additional therapy. These measures are aimed at limiting disability due to respiratory insufficiency and at controlling manifestations of cor pulmonale. Maximum effective use of the measures described for treatment of mild or moderate symptoms should be achieved before more expensive modalities and those with greater side-effects are instituted.

Corticosteroids are of limited usefulness in selected patients with prominent bronchospasm or bronchitis. Their long-term use may be attended by a host of metabolic side-effects which these individuals can ill afford, and they should be avoided if possible. Prophylactic isoniazid should accompany use of steroids in order to prevent activation of tuberculosis in tuberculin reactors.

Oxygen supplementation has demonstrable usefulness in certain hypoxemic patients. However, at present, major indications for long-term oxygen therapy remain limited and are discussed in detail under *Other Treatment Measures.*

Although improving ventilation and oxygenation is basic to treating cor pulmonale, diuretics and digitalis, used with caution, are helpful in some cases. These drugs are less effective and more often toxic in cor pulmonale than in left ventricular failure from other causes.

Physical measures sometimes helpful in limiting disability from COPD include general conditioning exercises and breathing-retraining, consisting of controlled, slow deep breaths with expiration against pursed lips. Postural drainage and percussion are increasingly important in severe disability particularly when combined with bronchodilator therapy and nebulization of saline, in patients with copious secretions.

Hospital Management of Acute Exacerbations

Patients with COPD are prone to episodes of increased shortness of breath and cough. These episodes may lead to acute respiratory failure, depending upon the severity of the underlying disease and of the precipitating event, and often require hospitalization for adequate management. The causes of such exacerbations include bronchopulmonary infection, congestive heart failure, depression of ventilation due to sedatives or uncontrolled oxygen administration, and fail ure to continue maintenance medications. The first two causes accounted for by far the greatest number of episodes of acute respiratory failure requiring hospitalization over a four-year period in a recent study.[276]

With few exceptions, inhospital administration of a treatment program identical to that prescribed for home use results in improvement in a deteriorating patient. It is not surprising that a complex and difficult management plan should be more effectively carried out by trained personnel than by a disabled patient and his harried family. Appropriate alterations in treatment can also be accomplished more readily in the hospital, and intravenous administration of fluids and of some medications may be advantageous. The essential treatment modalities remain the same, however: antibiotics, bronchodilation, liquification and evacuation of secretions, and controlled oxygen supplementation.

Hospital care becomes most clearly essential when acute respiratory failure supervenes or is imminent. Monitoring by trained personnel and institution of mechanically assisted ventilation when needed is clearly a hospital function, requiring a high level of technical expertise. Treatment of acute respiratory failure is discussed in detail in Chapter 7. It is noteworthy, however, that home-care programs directed at early detection and management of exacerbations of illness have dramatically reduced the duration of hospitalization required by such patients.

TREATMENT MEASURES DESIGNED TO IMPROVE VENTILATION AND DECREASE WORK OF BREATHING

Bronchodilators

The use of sympathomimetic bronchodilator drugs, by aerosol and oral routes, and of oral and intravenous methylxanthines is discussed in the section on Management of Bronchial Asthma. Principles of use of these agents in chronic bronchitis and emphysema are not substantially different, although the degree of benefit to be anticipated is less than in asthma. Most patients with COPD have some degree of complicating bronchospasm, although the significance varies widely and the benefits to be anticipated from use of bronchodilator drugs include modification of dyspnea and improved clearance of secretions from narrowed airways.

Reduction in airways resistance of about 40% of initial values has been shown to occur in COPD following nebulized bronchodilator administration,[277] although there is considerable individual variation in response.[278] In one series, the decrease was greatest when initial values were highest.[277] Reduction in functional residual capacity appears to be modest (5%) and regional distribution of ventilation is in fact altered adversely with respect to gas exchange, in most cases.[279]

Since it is probable that no long-term benefit accrues from the use of bronchodilators in COPD, it seems advisable to evaluate the results and side-effects both objectively and subjectively in individual patients, and to consider symptomatic improvement the goal of therapy. Route of administration and sustained or intermittent use should depend upon the individual patient's needs.

Hydration, Humidification and Bland Aerosols

Methods of modifying the composition of sputum and facilitating its evacuation should be considered major therapeutic objectives in COPD.[280] However, useful recent reviews point out that our fundamental knowledge of this area is very limited.[281–283,284a]

Adequate systemic hydration has favorable implications for the patient's general welfare and is believed by most clinicians to facilitate evacuation of tracheobronchial secretions. Therefore, this principle provokes little debate in spite of limited data with which to defend it.[284,284a]

Humidification of inspired gas, that is, addition of water vapor, is likewise a well-accepted principle of physiologic management, as contrasted with pharmacologic therapy. The atmosphere of modern heated buildings is often dry, and addition of supplemental oxygen further reduces the water vapor content of inspired air, since stored compressed gas has very low relative humidity when it returns to atmospheric pressure. Dry inspired gas produces discomfort, cracking and bleeding of the nasal and oropharyngeal mucosa, and has been shown to reduce mucociliary clearance.[281] The latter effect is more likely to produce a problem if the warming and humidifying function of the nose is bypassed by mouthbreathing, or especially by a tracheostomy or endotracheal tube. Humidification modifies these harmful effects. Commonly used humidifiers, such as devices which bubble oxygen through water at room temperature, fail to achieve full humidification of inspired air as it reaches body temperature. Heaters and nebulizers, or aerosol generators, are commonly used to increase the water content of inspired air, and particles of water in liquid form may or may not reach the pulmonary airways when such devices are used. Transformation of water from aerosol to vapor state takes place at a variable rate as air is moved from nebulizer to patient, until full humidification is achieved. Humidification is a desirable goal even in administration of oxygen to patients without airways disease, and simply attempts to minimize drying of nasal, pharyngeal and tracheobronchial mucosa.

Nebulization therapy or *aerosol therapy* attempts to add water to sputum and to decrease its viscosity, and hence to facilitate evacuation of sputum. Deposition of water particles in the tracheobronchial tree is a goal of therapy which should be viewed somewhat apart from the physiologic management aim of full humidification of inspired gas. Clinically, these aims do appear to be met when efficient aerosol generators are employed. Delivery of a few milliliters of water from the medication nebulizer of an IPPB apparatus is ineffective for this purpose, as are attempts to fill a room with nebulized particles. Delivery of visible clouds of aerosol from a nebulizer to facemask or "face-tent" through large bore tubing is essential, and continual delivery for 15 minutes to several hours, if tolerated, is desirable. The goal is a clinical response.

Much has been made of the problem of generating aerosols with a particle size small enough to result in deposition deep within the tracheobronchial tree. It is known that large particles (greater than 10μ in diameter) are deposited high in the mouth, pharynx, and large airways and that smaller particles (1–10μ) are more likely to reach small airways and alveoli. Most investigations studying optimal particle size have used stable, nonhygrophilic particles.[281] Liquid aerosols are nonstable. Therefore our knowledge of the exact site of deposition of therapeutic aerosols is really quite limited.[282,284a,285–288] The clinician must depend heavily on judgmental decisions based on observation of the patient and his response to therapy. Since knowledge about deposition of aerosols in the lung has great significance to public health as it relates to exposure to atmospheric pollutants, research in this area is likely to provide useful information in the future.

In the meantime, the ultrasonic nebulizer may be viewed as a prototype of a device which provides a high density of particles of small size. Especially when using less efficient nebulizers, addition of solute to the water administered may be helpful. Miller has pointed out that slower absorption of solute-containing solutions may make them locally more effective, and notes that increased density of aerosol particles enhances their deposition.[280] Saline and propylene glycol are commonly used for this purpose.

Side-effects of aerosol therapy can be controlled but are of substantial importance. Bronchospasm may be produced even by inert aerosols and hypoxemia may be worsened by this effect.[289] Bronchospasm can be modified by concurrent or prophylactic use of bronchodilator drugs, and oxygen supplementation may be wise in hypoxemic subjects. Some dyspneic patients with hyperreactive airways may be unable or unwilling to tolerate prolonged or intense aerosol therapy. Since reservoirs of liquid, especially if heated, may provide an excellent medium for proliferation of bacteria, aerosol therapy is a potential cause of bronchopulmonary infection. Cross-infection, as well as instillation of overwhelming numbers of bacteria which originated in the patient's own tracheobronchial tree, can produce devastating consequences. Frequent cleaning of nebulization equipment and use of sterile liquid for aerosolization are essential.[290]

Detergents and Mucolytics

Barton[291] recently reviewed evidence for the usefulness of aerosolized detergents in COPD.

These agents are used with the aim of wetting viscid sputum to facilitate its evacuation. Barton referred to studies indicating that detergents are or are not superior to water alone for this purpose. He pointed out that these agents have little mucolytic action but that they might facilitate deposition of aerosol by stabilizing particles.

The summary report of the conference at which Barton presented this review did not find adequate evidence to support the use of nebulized detergents.[281]

The evidence supporting the usefulness of certain mucolytic agents, however, has been somewhat more convincing.[291,292] The major agents available in this class are acetylcysteine and pancreatic dornase. Acetylcysteine is a sulfhydryl compound which can be shown to alter the physical characteristics of sputum *in vitro* and *in vivo.* It has not been convincingly shown that this effect is clinically beneficial when acetylcysteine is administered in nebulized form to patients with COPD. It appears clinically that selected patients with viscid mucoid or purulent sputum do benefit from this form of treatment. Direct intratracheal instillation appears useful in some cases of mucus plugging as well.

Foul odor and production of bronchospasm in some patients are disadvantages of the use of acetylcysteine. The latter side-effect can be modified by routinely administering this agent along with a bronchodilator. Acetylcysteine is known to inhibit the antibacterial action of penicillins, an effect which would contraindicate its use with these drugs given in aerosol form.

Pancreatic dornase (deoxyribonuclease) decreases the viscosity of purulent sputum, apparently by its depolymerizing action on leukocyte DNA. As with acetylcysteine, clinical benefit has not been shown as convincingly as has the effect on the physical characteristics of sputum. As a foreign protein, this agent might be expected to be capable of producing adverse immunologic reactions. As a protease, it has been pointed out that an emphysema-producing effect could be a side-effect, especially in subjects with deficiency of antiproteases.[292] Although this has not been demonstrated to be a side-effect of dornase, the theoretic objection to its use remains.

Expectorants

Oral expectorant agents are widely used in an attempt to improve clearance of secretions in COPD. Many patients are convinced of their usefulness, but scientific evidence to support this impression is scant, and authorities are divided in opinion.[293–301] The agents most commonly used for their expectorant action are ammonium chloride, potassium iodide, and glyceryl guaiacolate.

The agents have been shown by animal research to be capable of increasing the volume of tracheobronchial secretions and are believed to decrease viscosity, effects which might be expected to facilitate evacuation. These effects are at least partially dependent upon reflexes stimulated by gastric irritation and mediated by the vagus.[293,294] Perhaps this observation has a clinical counterpart in the benefit reported by many patients from drinking hot liquids to stimulate sputum evacuation.

Therefore, there is some evidence to support the use of expectorants in patients who claim symptomatic benefit, although clinical research proving benefit is lacking. Certain precautions should be kept in mind in prescribing these agents. Iodides cause hypersensitivity reactions in some patients and may even depress thyroid function when given over prolonged periods. Some commercial cough preparations containing expectorants also contain antihistamines which are drying to the respiratory mucosa and are relatively contraindicated in COPD. Finally, these agents should not be used to the exclusion of therapeutic methods of proven value.

Intermittent Positive Pressure Breathing

Sustained use of intermittent positive pressure breathing as mechanical ventilatory support in respiratory failure is a well recognized medical technique. It clearly sustains life when used appropriately; indications and methods are described elsewhere. Periodic use of intermittent positive pressure breathing (IPPB) as a treatment modality in a variety of bronchopulmonary diseases is currently popular, but proper indications are a subject of debate.[284a,302–315]

Probably the most popular regimen for IPPB

treatment employs a pressure-cycled ventilator, triggered by patient effort, which augments tidal volume by inflating the lungs to a preset pressure, often 20 to 25 cm water. Administration of aerosolized bronchodilator from a nebulizer during each augmented tidal breath is usual practice. Treatments are customarily given over a period of 10 to 20 minutes, four times each day. Benefit is ascribed to the bronchodilator or other aerosol administered; less certain benefit is thought by some to be due to mechanical effects of the pressure-assisted and augmented ventilation itself. Documented effects of IPPB itself include increased tidal volume and minute ventilation, decreased work of breathing, and increased arterial oxygen tension with decreased carbon dioxide tension. These effects have potential value in chronic obstructive lung disease, for which IPPB is often prescribed; but the demonstrable effects are transient. More sustained effects may result from aerosolized medications given by IPPB. The use of bland aerosols, bronchodilator, mucolytic and antibiotic aerosols, and nebulized steroids is described elsewhere in this chapter.

In my view, in most cases, the usefulness of periodic IPPB is limited to that of the aerosol delivered. The superiority of this mode of administration over hand bulb, *freon*-propelled or motorized nebulizers has not been proven; but experience would suggest that patients with severely limited inspiratory capacity, and some with impaired coordination may more conveniently be given aerosol medication by IPPB. Administration of bland aerosols by IPPB is not practical, however. The volume of water or saline which can be delivered to the tracheobronchial tree from the medication nebulizer of an IPPB machine is miniscule. This method should be reserved for the administration of pharmacologically active agents effective with delivery of small volumes, and bland aerosols should be given by a nebulizer capable of delivery of larger amounts.

Periodic IPPB may in itself be of use in three circumstances:

1. Temporary support of ventilation in rapidly advancing respiratory failure.
2. Augmentation of inspired volume to maintain lung inflation when monotonous small tidal volumes occur as a result of central nervous system depression, neuromuscular impairment or splinting due to pain on deep breathing.
3. Pulmonary edema.

When rapidly progressive deterioration of ventilatory function occurs in chronic lung disease with respiratory insufficiency, improvement from drugs, and measures to clear secretions may reverse the downward course in a matter of hours. Frequent use of IPPB via a conventional mouthpiece may forestall the need for intubation and total ventilatory support in such a patient. Fifteen minute treatments every hour or two, or even continual support for hours, may be required. Patient cooperation and skilled and attentive nursing and respiratory therapy staff are necessary in such circumstances. Adequate humidification of inspired air and oxygen is essential.

There is evidence that a program of augmented ventilation and bronchodilation and other measures to assist in clearance of tracheobronchial secretions can prevent and reverse atelectasis in postoperative patients with chronic bronchitis. The role of IPPB itself in such combined therapy programs is not entirely certain. This modality is probably not useful in preoperative preparation of patients with normal lungs and it is probably not superior to other measures which augment tidal volume in postoperative patients with splinting due to pain. Individuals with small, monotonous tidal volumes due to CNS depression and neuromuscular chest-wall disease may benefit from periodic IPPB, but overinflation must be employed several times each hour in order to be effective and should be accompanied by frequent position changes, postural drainage, percussion, and removal of secretions by suctioning as needed. This sort of regimen lends itself to short-term acute problems rather than to chronic illness.

In simple pulmonary edema, IPPB has long been considered a useful adjunct to other therapeutic measures. Increased alveolar pressure achieved with IPPB is believed to reduce the ingress of fluid into the alveoli, although it is uncertain whether this mechanism really operates to the patient's advantage. Temporary assisted ventilation may reduce the work of breathing and relieve dyspnea in some patients, provided that apprehension and inability to cooperate with use of the machine are not excessive. Mechanical and pharmacologic bronchodilation are useful, since bronchospasm may accompany pulmonary edema. Hypotension accompanying pulmonary edema is a relative contraindication to the use of IPPB, which sometimes worsens the reduction in cardiac output. Availability of potent diuretic agents has improved treatment of acute pulmonary edema to the extent that the role of IPPB is usually one of minor importance.

As is suggested by the foregoing discussion, there is little reason to believe that IPPB in itself is an important treatment modality in long-term management of chronic obstructive lung disease. Its role is chiefly as a method of administering bronchodilators and other aerosols, and the frequency of its use should be governed by the duration of action of the medication used. Daily or weekly treatments, then, have little usefulness, and outpatient use of IPPB is impractical. The duration of each treatment should be that needed for delivery of an appropriate dose of aerosol and diluent, usually a total of 5 ml given over about 15 minutes. Pressure used should be adequate to produce a tidal volume about 1.5 times the patients usual tidal volume. IPPB should be chosen over other methods of administration of aerosol medications when severe reduction of inspiratory capacity or impairment of motor ability suggests that it is needed for patient comfort and convenience.

OTHER TREATMENT MEASURES IN COPD

Physical Measures

Physical measures employed in the management of COPD include those directed at clearing secretions from the tracheobronchial tree, improving efficiency of ventilation, and improving the general physical fitness of the patient. These measures are relatively expensive in terms of the time and effort. They are simple in concept, however, and there is reasonable evidence to suggest that they do play a useful role in symptomatic management. As with other types of treatment used in COPD, the overall course of the disorder does not appear to be altered by the use of physical measures.[274,284a]

Measures Directed Toward Clearance of Secretions. Postural drainage, chest vibration, and percussion are widely used methods aimed at clearing secretions from the airways of patients with an assortment of lung diseases, including COPD.[316–325] These techniques may be employed from one to four times daily, depending on the degree of sputum production. The early morning treatment is especially likely to yield a substantial quantity of sputum, with symptomatic benefit, since secretions commonly accumulate in central airways during the night in bronchitic patients.

Administration of a therapeutic dose of bronchodilator, followed by bland aerosol therapy for 15 to 30 minutes, is often beneficial prior to postural drainage and percussion therapy. Fifteen to 30 minutes in a prone, head-downward position on a tilt table or hospital bed, is perhaps adequate as a postural drainage maneuver aimed at draining lower lobes. Alternatively, the patient may lie prone on a bed or couch, with his head resting on folded arms on the floor and his trunk directed downward above the waist. If drainage of the middle lobe or lingula is desired, a supine, head-downward position should be assumed, with the side of the thorax to be drained, raised on a pillow. A discussion of postural drainage positions directed at specific lobes and segments is provided in the useful *Brompton Hospital Guide to Chest Physiotherapy*.[326] Rapid, gentle vibration or chest percussion may be performed manually or with the aid of mechanical devices.

Short-term benefits include an increased rate of mucus clearance,[321,324] improved expiratory flow rates, improved conductance, and in some patients, improved arterial oxygenation.[317] Long-term benefits have not been so clearly shown.

Measures Directed Toward Improvement in Breathing Efficiency. A variety of measures have been advocated in attempts to favorably alter breathing patterns in COPD.[284a,327–330]

Slow, deep breaths, emphasizing abdominal (diaphragmatic) breathing have been advocated, with increase or decrease in functional residual capacity, and with expiration carried out against the resistance of pursed lips.

Grimby[327] reviewed some evidence relevant to the usefulness of breathing retraining. There is general agreement that a slow, deep ventilatory pattern, facilitated by exhalation against pursed lips, is advantageous in achieving relaxed breathing and in increasing the ratio of alveolar to deadspace ventilation. Improved ventilation distribution does not apparently occur. Maintenance of an optimal ventilatory pattern may be difficult for a patient, especially under stress, but training programs appear to facilitate achievement of this goal.

Breathing exercises directed at conditioning respiratory muscles have not been adequately evaluated in stable COPD.

General Physical Conditioning. It has been well demonstrated that a program of physical conditioning can be useful in increasing exercise tolerance in patients whose activity is limited by chronic obstructive lung disease.[331–336] Most regimens studied have consisted of treadmill walking at speeds one-half to three-quarters of the maximum tolerated. Exercise sessions from 5 to 15 minutes each, for a total of 30 to 60 minutes each day, appear to be satisfactorily tolerated and are effective. Patients who are severely hypoxemic or who become more hypoxemic with exercise are often unable to tolerate such training programs without supplemental oxygen, but do well breathing 30 to 40% oxygen while exercising. A training program aimed at achieving maximum benefit should be based on principles of physiologic conditioning. Exercise must be regular, increased until performance plateaus and then maintained. These programs generally require three to twelve weeks.

Conventional tests of ventilatory function are not consistently altered by physical conditioning, but maximum intensity and duration of tolerated exercise is increased. Heart rate, respiratory rate, minute ventilation, and oxygen consumption required for a given level of exercise are decreased, reflecting an improvement in musculoskeletal and cardiorespiratory efficiency. Improvement in these measurable parameters of the order of 20 to 25% is a reasonable goal. Since a portion of this improvement is specific for the exercise utilized in training, treadmill walking is especially practical, improving the patient's skill and tolerance in the activities of daily living.

Patients requiring oxygen supplementation during training sessions also improve their tolerance to exercise carried out breathing room air. Planning for long-term use of oxygen is therefore not necessarily needed.

The time, effort, and expense required to carry out an effective training program in these patients is considerable, and realistic goals are somewhat limited. The benefits of such a program have been more clearly proven than is the case with many other modalities of management in COPD, however; and an increase of 25% in maximum exercise tolerance may have a great effect upon the independence, productivity, and happiness of a severely disabled patient.

Prevention of Infection: Vaccination

It would seem prudent to use vaccinations routinely to protect against pneumococcal pneumonia and influenza in patients with chronic bronchitis who would be expected to suffer a high mortality from these illnesses. Chemoprophylaxis with amantadine may have a role during an epidemic illness known to be due to Influenza A virus.[336a] Details are discussed in Chapter 8.

Treatment of Infection: Antibiotics

The role of antibiotic agents in treatment, as well as prophylaxis, of acute purulent exacerbations of chronic bronchitis is established in common clinical practice. A somewhat empirical approach to the use of wide-spectrum antibiotics, with minimal attention to sputum smear and culture results, is rather widely accepted and has some basis in objective data.

Evidence was collected in the 1950s that *Hemophilus influenzae* and *Streptococcus pneumoniae* are often associated with exacerbations of purulent sputum in chronic bronchitis.[111] A good deal of evidence has since been collected indicating that treatment and prophylaxis with agents effective against these organisms is of clinical benefit,[102,338,339] and it is the common experience of clinicians that benefit does not depend upon prior demonstration of the presence of these organisms or of their antibiotic sensitivity.

The drugs most often recommended for use in the prophylaxis of exacerbations in chronic bronchitis are tetracyclines, erythromycin, and ampicillin, all of which have been found effective for this purpose. Tetracycline, 1 g daily, divided in two or four doses, has the advantages of low cost, broad spectrum, and modest side-effects. Regular treatment, either year-round or during the winter months, with intermittent schedules, such as daily for a week, or 10 days each month, is a popular prophylactic regimen. The optimal approach, combining effectiveness with low cost and minimal side-effects, differs among individual patients. Many persons can readily be educated to self-administer such antibiotic regimens at the earliest evidence of sputum purulence, with satisfactory results.

A decrease in overall morbidity during the course of a year can be anticipated as a result of prophylaxis in bronchitic patients troubled by exacerbations. The benefit can more clearly be seen in terms of decreased duration than incidence of respiratory illness, a finding which has led some observers to believe that viral illness most often precipitates, while bacterial superinfection complicates and prolongs, these episodes.

Treatment of exacerbations of sputum purulence with antibiotics is likewise often carried out empirically, without examination or culture of sputum.[340] The relation of specific organisms to symptoms is so often obscure that Burrows[339] has suggested empiric use of tetracycline for mild exacerbations and ampicillin, cephalothin or, less often, chloramphenicol for severely ill patients. He comments that "if a prompt therapeutic response is not obtained, it seems reasonable to modify therapy on the basis of results of sputum culture and sensitivity." Recognition of the occurrence of bronchopneumonia in a severely ill patient with systemic symptoms should prompt early recourse to sputum examination and sputum and blood cultures, although treatment should certainly not await results of cultures (see Chap. 8).

Well-referenced analytic reviews of the evidence supporting the use of antibiotics in COPD have recently appeared.[338,339] An exhaustive analysis of current knowledge concerning the role of infection in chronic bronchitis is also available.[101] The latter review rightly points out many flaws and contradictions in the evidence supporting the current widespread use of antibiotics in this disease. A major change in accepted practice is unlikely to be forthcoming, however, since the weight of evidence and clinical experience is rather heavily in favor of both antibiotic treatment and prophylaxis.

Antibiotic aerosols have been used alone and in combination with systemic antibiotics in an attempt to treat bronchopulmonary infections with a minimum of systemic side-effects.[341,342] The usefulness of such an approach is as yet uncertain.

Oxygen Supplementation

Certain hypoxemic patients with COPD benefit from long-term outpatient use of oxygen-enriched inspired air.[343–359c] However, the financial cost and inconvenience attendant upon long-term oxygen therapy are substantial. In addition, the possible toxic effects of long-term, low-dose oxygen supplementation are not entirely clear. Therefore, this therapeutic modality ought not be prescribed unless the indications and anticipated benefits are well-defined for an individual patient. At present, major clear indications are hypoxemia (arterial P_{O_2} less than 55 mm Hg) with clinically manifest cor pulmonale and secondary erythrocytosis not well managed with simpler measures; and hypoxemia with exercise intolerance which can be shown to be modified by oxygen supplementation. Therapy should be given continually, or throughout the night, for the first indication, and during exercise for the latter.

Treatment of cor pulmonale with oxygen-enriched air is based upon the knowledge that hypoxemia can produce pulmonary vasospasm and hypertension; that this effect is responsible for pulmonary hypertension in patients with COPD, to an extent which varies a great deal from one patient to another; and that chronic relief of hypoxemia can reverse the pulmonary hypertension and manifestations of cor pulmonale to a variable extent in such patients. (See section on *Cor Pulmonale.*) Important recent studies indicate improvement in survival of patients with hypoxemic COPD attendant upon long-term oxygen therapy. The British Medical Research Council has shown a survival benefit of oxygen supplementation for 15 hours each day,[359b] while a study group sponsored by the US National Institutes of Health indicates improved survival with continuous therapy as compared with 12-hour nocturnal therapy.[359a] As data continue to be analyzed and reported, we can expect further refinement of our understanding of the indications for long-term oxygen use.

Secondary erythrocytosis is commonly associated with the clinical manifestations of cor pulmonale. Both the resultant increase in blood viscosity and the elevation of blood volume may be contributing factors. The decrease in hematocrit which occurs in response to oxygen supplementation is therefore probably beneficial in itself. It is not effective in those who continue to smoke.[360] Limitation of exercise tolerance in COPD is chiefly due to mechanical factors producing dyspnea and ventilatory limitation. Hypoxemia is usually not a major factor. Occasionally, hypoxemia is worsened by exercise, and appears to play a major role in exercise intolerance. In such cases, a trial of oxygen supplementation during exercise is clearly indicated. The level and duration of exercise should be documented, and the pulmonary function laboratory with a treadmill or bicycle ergometer is an appropriate place to carry out such evaluation. Clinical observation, monitoring of the pulse, electrocardiography, and measurement of blood gases are desirable. Hypoxemic patients in whom arterial oxygen tension does not drop with exercise may also benefit from oxygen during exercise. The increase in activity tolerance, both in level and duration, is usually modest, but a 10 to 20% change for the better may substantially improve the quality of life in severely handicapped patients.

Home oxygen therapy is occasionally indicated in individual cases for reasons other than those specified above. When oxygen can be shown to reverse certain signs or symptoms which may be due to tissue hypoxia, its use may be justified. Cardiac arrhythmias, congestive failure of the left ventricle, and central nervous system symptoms are examples. Oxygen therapy for the latter indication has received support from the studies of Block, which demonstrate objective improvement in certain psychometric tests with oxygen supplementation.[337,355,358] Until advances are made in oxygen delivery systems and in knowledge of the benefits and side-effects of oxygen therapy, long-term use for these indications should be limited and carefully individualized.

The use of oxygen by COPD patients at home for the purpose of modifying dyspnea during attacks of anxiety and shortness of breath should particularly be discouraged. Hypoxemia, for all its adverse effects, is not normally a potent respiratory stimulant, nor does it contribute much to dyspnea. Mechanical abnormalities of lungs, airways, and chest wall are the major causes of shortness of breath in COPD. The patient who is taught to equate oxygen inhalation with relief of dyspnea is prone to overdose. He tends to increase inspired oxygen concentration in an attempt to gain relief, and relief is forthcoming only as carbon dioxide narcosis ensues.

A final statement of general principle in prescribing chronic oxygen therapy concerns the use of arterial oxygen tension alone in making the decision to treat. Many patients with chronic hypoxemia tolerate this physiologic abnormality very well, compensating in a number of ways involving bone marrow, hemoglobin function, circulation, and tissue transport and utilization of oxygen. Other patients with anemia and circulatory insufficiency tolerate hypoxemia poorly. Therefore, arterial hypoxemia alone may not be an indication for chronic oxygen therapy, and some patients with rather mild hypoxemia may benefit from its use. It has been suggested that venous oxygen tension might reflect tissue oxygenation better than arterial sampling, but sampling of venous blood draining critical organs is generally impractical, and mixed venous sampling provides a poor index of critical organ oxygenation.

Recognizing the theoretic and actual limitation of arterial oxygen tension as an index of tissue oxygenation, it is a useful generalization to state that patients with arterial Po_2 less than 45 mm Hg will usually benefit from oxygen therapy, while those with values above 60 mm Hg, seldom will.

Certain precautions are essential when oxygen supplementation is prescribed. In most cases, an in-hospital evaluation of clinical and blood gas response to therapy should be carried out. Most COPD patients will achieve an adequate (above 50 mm Hg) but not excessive (not above 70 mm Hg) arterial oxygen tension with an inspired concentration between 24 and 30%. In most cases, carbon dioxide retention will not worsen greatly if these guidelines are followed. Regular measurement of arterial blood gases is advisable in order to ensure that oxygen enrichment at a given concentration does not produce progressive hypoventilation over a period of hours, however. A 10 or even 20 mm Hg rise in Pco_2 may be tolerated if a stable value is reached and the level of consciousness is not impaired. Once a satisfactory inspired concentration is determined, careful patient education is essential to avoid future overdose. In some cases, administration by venturi mask, at a fixed concentration, is a wise precaution. (At oxygen flow rates above 4 L/min concentration, these devices provide a constant, predictable concentration. At lower flow rates, they may be inaccurate.) If nasal prongs are preferred, flow meters may be modified to prevent delivery of flows above a predetermined rate (see also Chap. 7, Acute Respiratory Failure).

Humidification of added oxygen is desirable since compressed gas is very dry and will dehydrate nasopharyngeal mucous membranes, with consequent discomfort, cracking, and bleeding. Proper cleaning of humidification equipment should be taught the patient or his family, although the problem of contamination is much more critical when nebulizers rather than simple humidifiers are used.

Some evidence has been presented suggesting that oxygen supplementation over a period of many months may produce a histologically demonstrable reaction of lung tissue. Clinical experience has not identified clinically important toxicity at the concentrations usually required in patients with stable COPD, but until further data are obtained, this therapeutic modality cannot be considered entirely free of potential ill-effects.[346]

Long-term oxygen therapy continues to be expensive and inconvenient, although significant advances in technology have improved cost and availability. Conventional oxygen supply in the form of compressed gas sold in heavy containers of limited capacity and portability has been supplanted to some extent by liquid oxygen[361] and by oxygen concentrators.[362,363] Liquid oxygen, though expensive, has a major advantage for some patients in that it is supplied in a large stationary container from which a small, lightweight, portable cannister can be readily refilled. The benefit of this system for a patient who needs oxygen at work or when leaving his home for other purposes is evident. The oxygen concentrator, while not portable, is less expensive. This equipment can be purchased or leased and provides inspired air of increased oxygen concentration in a manner which is acceptable for a patient who needs supplementation only at night, or who is not able to leave his home in any event.

Management of Cor Pulmonale

The definition, clinical recognition, and pathogenesis of cor pulmonale have been discussed elsewhere. Management of this disorder has a rational basis in the knowledge collected concerning its pathogenesis.

Treatment measures are aimed primarily at reducing those components of elevated pulmonary vascular resistance which are reversible. Improvement in myocardial contractility and control of blood volume and viscosity are less successful, but often important measures.[364]

Since hypoxemia and respiratory acidosis are important causes of pulmonary vasospasm in some patients with cor pulmonale, improvement in respiratory gas exchange is central to the management of the disorder. Virtually every effective treatment measure for respiratory insufficiency is indirectly a useful mode of therapy for cor pulmonale.

Oxygen supplementation of inspired air has specifically been well shown to have a beneficial effect both acutely and chronically in cor pulmonale. Controlled oxygen therapy should be part of the treatment program for all acutely decompensated patients with COPD, hypoxemia, and cor pulmonale. Long-term oxygen therapy should be considered when cor pulmonale is a recurrent problem in a patient in whom hypoxemia is persistently severe and other measures inadequate. The subject of long-term oxygen therapy for COPD is discussed above. It seems likely that an acute beneficial effect, over hours to days, is the result of reversal of vasospasm; and that a second slow phase of improvement over weeks or months may result in reduction of medial smooth muscle hypertrophy.

Reduction in pulmonary vascular tone and increase in cardiac output are secondary effects of methylxanthine drugs used in COPD primarily for their bronchodilator action. These effects may be of benefit in cor pulmonale and occur even in patients with predominant emphysema.[73]

Improved myocardial contractibility may be a side-effect of methylxanthine as well as sympathomimetic drugs which also increase oxygen consumption. The relative benefits and debits of these effects in cor pulmonale are not entirely clear. Digitalis is often used primarily for its inotropic effect, and the beneficial effects are subject to disagreement. Certainly cor pulmonale seems to respond less favorably to digitalis than do other forms of heart disease, especially left heart failure which is not due to outflow obstruction. In addition, patients with cor pulmonale seem to be unusually sensitive to digitalis toxicity,[365,366] perhaps partly because of hypoxemia[367] and electrolyte and acid-base disturbances. A reasonable approach to the use of digitalis preparations in cor pulmonale is the use of a conservative maintenance dose, such as 0.125 to 0.250 mg digoxin daily, without a loading dose.[368]

Reduction of blood volume may produce hemodynamic improvement in patients with manifestations of cor pulmonale and volume overload. This can be accomplished by phlebotomy or by the use of diuretics.[269,369,370] The clinical importance of elevated blood viscosity in impairing oxygen transport in a given patient with erythrocytosis and cor pulmonale is difficult to assess because of complex interactions of volume and viscosity on cardiac output, and the effect of hematocrit and of hemoglobin function on oxygen transport and delivery. There is experimental evidence to suggest that a hematocrit above 45% should be reduced, and phlebotomy of no more than 500 cc per day is a reasonable method in an acutely ill subject (see Secondary Polycythemia, above). Over the long-term, control of erythrocytosis should be achieved by maintaining adequate arterial oxygenation, and of edema, by diuretic therapy, if needed. Adequate intake of potassium and chloride is especially important when diuretics which deplete the body of these substances are used.

Corticosteroids

Corticosteroids have a substantially more limited usefulness in treatment of mixed COPD than in bronchial asthma.[371–376a] Studies have shown a relatively consistent subjective response, which can be supported by objective measurement of improvement in only a few cases. Any improvement is usually modest. The mechanism of action of corticosteroids is generally believed to be an antiinflammatory response in bronchitis and "antiallergic" when atopy plays a role in mixed disease. Patients most likely to respond favorably are those with a prominent bronchitic or bronchospastic component, sputum eosinophilia, or a history suggesting allergy; and those with acute exacerbations of bronchitis with respiratory insufficiency.[376a]

A trial of corticosteroid therapy may be warranted in patients in these categories when other measures, used maximally, have not given a satisfactory response. Intravenous therapy may be indicated in acutely ill hospitalized patients. In ambulatory subjects, the equivalent of 40 mg of prednisone daily for 2 weeks provides a reasonable clinical trial, and subjective as well as objective evaluation in the pulmonary function laboratory should be carried out. In patients showing favorable responses, an attempt should be made, after maximum benefit appears to be reached, to reduce the dose to 10 to 15 mg per day in decrements of 2.5 to 5.0 mg weekly, and to utilize an alternate day dosage regimen if possible. INH prophylaxis should be given to tuberculin reactors receiving steroids, and antacid prophylaxis of peptic ulcer disease is often wise. When a patient fails to benefit from steroids, the medication should be withdrawn in 5 mg weekly decrements. Regrettably, some patients failing to benefit greatly seem to show worsening on withdrawal. Because of this, even a trial of steroid therapy should be undertaken only in carefully selected patients, since the undesirable side-effects of long-term corticosteroid therapy may be of great consequence, as is well recognized and described in textbooks of medicine and endocrinology.[376]

The possible role of nonabsorbable steroid aerosols in COPD remains to be defined. It is reasonable to hope that these agents will provide a useful adjunct to current methods of therapy without the adverse metabolic effects of systemic corticosteroids.[342]

Respiratory Stimulants

The notion that increasing ventilation by pharmacologic stimulation of neurologic respiratory control might be useful in COPD has long been attractive. Reversal of the respiratory depression which occurs in severe or chronic carbon dioxide retention would seem to have great potential value. Stimulation of increased ventilation, even in patients without carbon dioxide retention, would have the effect of increasing alveolar and hence arterial oxygen tension, and could be helpful.

However, the primary problem in the hypoventilation of COPD is one of lung mechanics, and treatment aimed at respiratory stimulation has generally had modest and brief success.[377–379]

Prolonged oral use of respiratory stimulants has limited, if any, use in COPD management. Intravenous administration of respiratory stimulants in acute respiratory failure may have real benefit for short periods of time when hypoventilation is aggravated by sedatives or by oxygen administration.

Moser and co-workers have shown that during an initial 2-hour period of controlled oxygen supplementation in patients with hypoxemia and acute worsening of COPD, doxapram infusion can modify or prevent an increase in carbon dioxide tension attendant upon the oxygen therapy.[380] This might make it unnecessary to resort to mechanical ventilation in a few such patients.

The mild respiratory stimulation which aminophylline produces may be a desirable side-effect of this popular bronchodilator, and the metabolic acidosis produced by diuretics which are carbonic anhydrase inhibitors causes a mild stimulation of ventilation. The latter drugs may occasionally be a useful adjunct when metabolic alkalosis contributes to respiratory depression and responds poorly to potassium and chloride replacement.[376]

Surgery

The role of surgery in long-term management of chronic obstructive lung disease is very limited, as Laforet has commented in a recent review.[381] Acute complications, such as pneumothorax, may require surgical intervention, and tracheostomy may sometimes be indicated for purposes of facilitating tracheal suction and mechanical ventilation in respiratory failure. Resection of well-defined bullous lesions is the only procedure of major importance in restoring lung function in disabled patients, and proper indications for this procedure are rarely found. Severe symptoms may be relieved in the occasional patient with a bulla occupying most of a hemithorax in whom potentially functional atelectatic lung is displaced by the lesion, and can be reexpanded after bullectomy. Selection of patients who may benefit from this procedure is further discussed in the section on Bullous Emphysema. Resection of bronchiectatic lung for control of symptoms of infection is discussed in the chapter dealing with that disorder.

Surgical measures which have been advocated for COPD in the past have included "tailoring" of lung (trimming it to fit the chest), pleurodesis to improve blood supply, and an assortment of denervation procedures, including glomectomy, to control symptoms. These measures have no proper place in current management.

Lung transplantation has received considerable attention and is discussed in Chapter 11, under Lung Transplantation.

Agents to be Avoided or Used Only with Caution

Three classes of therapeutic agents are commonly sought for use by patients with COPD, but should generally be avoided: cough suppressants, antihistamines, and sedatives. Another group of drugs, beta adrenergic blocking agents, are not infrequently needed for treatment of hypertension, angina pectoris, or arrhythmias in patients with COPD. They are relatively contraindicated because they interfere with the therapeutic effect of adrenergic bronchodilators. Occasionally the clinical benefits of beta blockers may outweigh this relative contraindication, especially in stable patients without much bronchospasm. The bronchodilation produced by theophylline is not prevented by these agents; and beta blockers with cardiovascular selectivity are becoming available and probably do have an advantage in COPD patients.[376]

An irritating, nonproductive cough in acute respiratory tract infections in patients with normal lungs can safely be suppressed, but the cough of chronic bronchitis is often productive and essential for adequate clearance of secretions, and in this event should not be suppressed. Antihistamines are an ingredient of many commercial cough syrups, and tend to dry mucous membranes and impact secretions in COPD; hence, these agents should be avoided as well.

Sedatives are very commonly requested by fatigued, irritable, depressed, and sleepless patients with COPD, and denying such requests is difficult. Nevertheless, such agents are clearly contraindicated in patients with hypercarbia, since they are often exquisitely sensitive to small doses of sedatives and carbon dioxide narcosis is a common sequela. Even patients without hypercarbia but with severely compromised ventilatory function may suffer ill-effects from such drugs, commonly gaining little symptomatic benefit from small doses and increasing consumption until deep sedation and respiratory acidosis ensues rather abruptly and unexpectedly. Anxiety and sleeplessness resulting from breathlessness and deranged respiratory gas exchange should be treated by adequate management of the primary disease process and the temptation to employ tranquilizers and sedatives should be resisted.

ASTHMA

Asthma is a term which has been used clinically for centuries to refer to disorders characterized by shortness of breath. Currently used by most physicians as well as by lay persons, it refers to a particular presentation of obstructive lung disease with episodic wheezing and dyspnea. However, a clear definition of asthma, as the term is generally used, is difficult to arrive at.

A CIBA Symposium published in 1959[382] addressed itself to the classification of COPD and arrived at a useful clinical definition of chronic bronchitis, as well as a morphologic definition of emphysema. With somewhat more caution, the symposium offered a physiologic definition of asthma, as follows: "Asthma refers to the condition of subjects with widespread narrowing of the bronchial airways, which changes its severity over short periods of time either spontaneously or under treatment, and is not due to cardiovascular disease." (Similarly, the American Thoracic Society[383] states: "Asthma is a disease characterized by an increased responsiveness of the trachea and bronchi to various stimuli and manifested by a widespread narrowing of the airways that changes in severity either spontaneously or as a result of therapy.")

The definitions of chronic bronchitis and emphysema which were offered have been useful, in that clinical, physiologic, and morphologic correlates of both disorders have evolved and communication among investigators has been facilitated. The definition of asthma still presents problems, however. It is generally agreed that this definition suffers from the fact that it fails to cover some patients with obstructive pulmonary disease whose obstruction is irreversible, yet who have certain features that many clinicians associate with asthma. In addition, it includes many subjects who have chronic bronchitis, by its current clinical definition and pathologic correlates. However, a subsequent CIBA Foundation Symposium addressed specifically to better defining this term failed to arrive at a consensus.[384]

Nevertheless, there are many patients with a clinical disorder that most clinicians and investigators would call asthma; and much is known about its presentation, physiology, and morphology, and even biochemistry and etiology. This chapter will analyze the disorder in two different ways in order to best display what is known about it in a useful way: first, as a discussion of the extrinsic and intrinsic types; then, as a discussion of bronchial reactivity as a hyperactive response. The reader seeking a more detailed discussion of various aspects of bronchial asthma is referred to the comprehensive textbook edited by Weiss and Segal, which is entirely devoted to this disorder.[385]

PREVALENCE

In view of the considerable disagreement about the identification of asthma, some uncertainty about its prevalence is not surprising. Overall, it appears that about 1 to 5% of the population has, or has had, asthma. Men and children appear to be more often affected, and certain studies have estimated that as many as 5% of men and 10% of children or more have had the disorder.[385,386]

Of all children with asthma, well over half become asymptomatic by the time they reach adulthood.[387,388] However, in over half of all asthmatics, the onset of disease occurs after age 15.[389] In general, asthma with onset during childhood is more often intermittent, being associated with specific allergens, and has a better prognosis. Wheezing during very early childhood (i.e., before the age of three years) is often not a symptom of asthma, but viral bronchiolitis, or "wheezy bronchitis,"[106,108,387] and may not recur; however, the onset of asthma with an episode of bronchiolitis does not seem to be rare.

There is little doubt that heredity plays a role in the development of asthma. The hereditary relationship between different forms of asthma and various other "allergic" diseases is unclear, however. Many studies have demonstrated an increased prevalence of asthma in families with hay fever, eczema, and asthma. The prevalence is highest when a family member has extrinsic asthma.[87] There is no simple genetic factor to explain the inheritance; studies of lymphocyte histocompatibility types have produced conflicting results.[34]

Despite being a disease which is so often capable of causing severe disability, asthma is a relatively uncommon cause of death. In the United States, the death rate from asthma has fallen from 3 to 0.8 per 100,000 population between 1960 and 1976.[386] This rather low overall mortality rate should not encourage a casual attitude towards treatment of severe asthmatics, since the risk of death may be considerably higher in certain subgroups. A substantial increase in the frequency of death from asthma in young people occurred during the 1960s in England and Wales,[390] perhaps due to the marketing of an especially potent isoproterenol nebulizer. Those with severe, frequent attacks of poorly responsive bronchospasm certainly appear to have a risk greater than that in the overall population of asthmatics; and the risk in the elderly is greater than in young adults[390] (see below, Management of Severe Asthma).

EXTRINSIC AND INTRINSIC ASTHMA

A conventional classification of asthma divides the disorder into two forms: extrinsic and intrinsic. This classification in an 1864 textbook by Salter was popularized in the United States by Rackemann in the 1940s and 1950s.[388] An oversimplified but clinically useful view of this classification would regard extrinsic asthma as that form of the disease in which attacks can clearly be attributed to an immunologic response of the patient to exposure to an allergen, a substance to which he has a specific hypersensitivity. According to the original usage, extrinsic asthma is that which occurs in atopic subjects, and which has been found to be due to a Type I allergic reaction (immediate hypersensitivity, anaphylaxis) according to the classification of Coombs and Gell (Table 14-7). This form is mediated by immunoglobulin E. It has more recently been suggested that asthma can result from a specific hypersensitivity response in nonatopic subjects. Therefore it is appropriate that both atopic and nonatopic forms of extrinsic asthma be recognized. Intrinsic asthma is that form of the disease in which an inciting cause extrinsic to the patient cannot clearly be identified. The cause is therefore not identifiable, but presumably is within the patient. Table 14-6 summarizes features of the two classic forms of the disorder.[385]

Extrinsic asthma is the form which is most easily recognized as a discrete entity. It is most easily diagnosed, with little disagreement among

TABLE 14-6. Characteristics of Extrinsic and Intrinsic Asthma

Characteristics	Extrinsic (Atopic)	Intrinsic
Genetic influence	Present	Variable
Age of onset	< 35	< 5, > 35
Hay fever	Frequent	Infrequent
Skin sensitizing antibody	Usually present	Absent
Sputum	Eosinophils	Eosinophils PMN leukocytes Bacteria
Associated infection	Secondary	Primary
Intractable asthma	Uncommon	Common
Death	Rare	More frequent

clinicians or investigators. It occurs in subjects who can be demonstrated to be *atopic*, that is those with a propensity to develop immediate wheal and flare reactions to skin tests with a battery of allergens. These subjects often have a family history of allergic manifestations of various sorts (asthma, hay fever and urticarial eruptions) and may themselves exhibit allergic symptoms other than asthma. They have increased serum levels of immunoglobulin E, and there is considerable evidence that this immunoglobulin class contains antibodies which develop in response to extrinsic allergens, and play a role in producing the clinical manifestations of the disorder. The mechanism by which this sequence takes place is described in more detail below. Extrinsic (atopic) asthma often appears in childhood and abates at adolescence. Clinical manifestations include cough, wheezing, and shortness of breath, which may occur promptly following exposure to a recognized allergen. Anxiety, exertion, and inhalation of irritants may also precipitate attacks. Attacks may be life-threatening, but most often the course of the disorder is benign and the patient is most often clinically well between attacks. Sputum and blood eosinophilia are characteristic features. A subject with all the features described above would readily be diagnosed as an extrinsic asthmatic by most clinicians and there would be little disagreement among allergists or chest physicians, pediatricians or internists about the classification.

Recent work summarized by Pepys[391] suggests that there are at least four other identifiable forms of extrinsic allergic asthmatic reaction, distinct from the atopic form. Sequential measurements of ventilatory function after inhalation challenge have contributed substantially to this categorization. An immediate asthmatic reaction mediated by IgG antibody appears to occur in nonatopic subjects,[392,39] and three forms of nonimmediate, or "late" reactions have been described. A poorly understood reaction can occur beginning at 1 hr and lasting 2 to 3 hr; a more common and better defined Type III precipitating-antibody immune-complex reaction begins at 3 to 4 hr, peaks at 5 to 8 hr and lasts 24 to 36 hr; and a recurrent early morning reaction may occur for a few days after inhalation challenge.[394]

Intrinsic asthma is a much greater nosologic and diagnostic problem, since this class is made up of those patients in whom an extrinsic allergen cannot be identified as a cause of symptoms. It includes a group of subjects with onset often after age 35 or 40 years, in whom a personal or family history of allergy is absent. Skin tests show absence of immediate hypersensitivity to common allergens, and blood levels of immunoglobulin E are not abnormally elevated. These subjects are more often refractory to treatment than is the case in extrinsic asthma. Purulent sputum is more frequent, and this has resulted in an impression that tracheobronchial or other infection, with hypersensitivity to infecting organisms, plays an etiologic role. Diagnostic overlap with chronic bronchitis occurs in this group of patients.

Attempts have been made to further subdivide patients with extrinsic and intrinsic asthma. These include aspirin-induced asthma and occupational asthma caused by a variety of substances (to be discussed), and a number of forms which are not sufficiently well developed to be helpful to the clinician.

A CLINICIAN'S VIEW OF ASTHMA: A STATE OF BRONCHIAL HYPERREACTIVITY

A pragmatic approach to the clinical classification, described by Howell,[395] considers asthma to be a disorder or group of disorders in which the common factor is bronchial hyperreactivity which is manifested by symptoms in a wide range of circumstances. The background of bronchial hyperreactivity in asthma is complex in itself and the cause no doubt varies among subjects exhibiting the phenomenon.

Circumstances in which Asthma Occurs
Acute exposure to antigen
Precipitated by drugs and diagnostic procedures
For no apparent reason in either atopic or nonatopic subjects
In response to infection
Exposure to air pollution
Occupational asthma
Coughing or laughing
In response to emotional stress
Nocturnal asthma
Exercise-induced asthma

Bronchial smooth muscle in normal subjects can be demonstrated to respond to a variety of stimuli and the degree of response is greater in asthmatics. Slowing of maximal expiratory flow rates in response to a histamine aerosol has been a well studied method of demonstrating normal and exaggerated reactivity of the airways. The control of bronchial smooth muscle has been extensively reviewed.[396–403]

The Role of Autonomic Influences in Bronchial Reactivity

The state of tonus of the bronchial smooth muscle is affected by both parasympathetic influences mediated by the vagus, tending to increase tonus, and sympathetic influences which tend to decrease tonus. Normally, a mild degree of parasympathetic preponderance exists, so that vagal section in animals, or atropine administration in humans, results in an increase in diameter of the airways. This being the case, it is not surprising that autonomic imbalance has attracted a great deal of attention as a possible basis for the pathophysiology of asthma. Gold and co-workers[399] have provided evidence for involvement of the vagus in the early phase of allergic bronchospasm, but parasympathetic influences are less directly involved in later stages when chemical mediators have appeared. Vagal blockade studies suggest that the vagus has a greater influence on central than on peripheral airways.[404] The sympathetic nervous system influences the lungs chiefly through circulating catecholamines rather than through direct innervation, and beta antagonists chiefly influence peripheral rather than central airways.[404] There is evidence that asthma is the result of decreased responsiveness of tissue to beta-adrenergic stimuli,[400] or increased response to alpha-adrenergic stimuli.[405] The role of the autonomic nervous system in the production of asthma remains in doubt, although it is clear that certain therapeutic manipulations based on neuropharmacology are useful.

Bronchoconstriction in response to histamine aerosols and in response to pharmacologically inactive irritant aerosols occurs in healthy subjects and is more marked in asthmatics. This response can be modified in animals by vagal section, and in healthy and asthmatic human subjects by atropine and by sympathomimetic drugs. Sympathetic blocking agents and vagal stimulation, on the other hand, may produce an increase in bronchial smooth muscle tonus or in the bronchoconstrictor response to aerosol stimulation.

The bronchoconstrictor response to inert aerosols is at least partially dependent upon superficial irritant receptors in the tracheobronchial tree. Histamine may also have a local pharmacologic effect upon smooth muscle when administered as an aerosol, and intravenous or intraarterial injection of histamine has a constrictor action upon smooth muscle. There has been intense investigative interest of late in the role of cyclic nucleotides in mediating and in

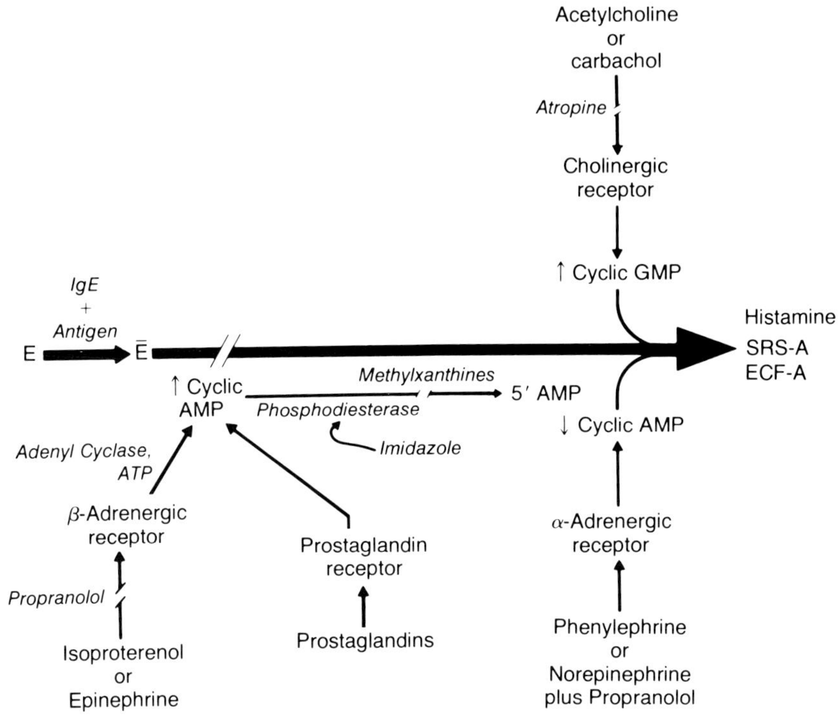

FIG. 14-7. Control of cyclic nucleotides which influence bronchial reactivity. (Austen, KF: Reaction mechanisms in the release of mediators of immediate hypersensitivity from human lung tissue. Fed Proc, 33:256, 1974)

modifying smooth muscle activity (to be discussed).

Surgical attempts to alter autonomic balance favorably in asthma have included carotid body resection (glomectomy)[406–408] and pulmonary denervation (these are discussed under Management, Miscellaneous Treatment Measures).

Although atropine would seem to be a promising agent for use in blocking the vagal stimulation of bronchial smooth muscle tonus,[396] its use has been limited, partially because of its inhibitory effect on mucus production and the potential danger of causing inspissation of the viscid secretions which result.

Sympathomimetic drugs have an important place in the treatment of bronchospasm and their use and attendant risks are discussed elsewhere. The danger of drugs which produce both β-1 and β-2 blockade in patients with bronchospasm is recognized, and propranolol should be avoided or used with caution when indicated for treatment of cardiovascular disease in patients who also have asthma.[409] Beta blockers with more selectivity for the cardiac β-1 receptors may provide a solution to this problem.

The Role of Cyclic Nucleotides in Bronchial Reactivity

Without doubt the possibilities for effectively controlling any disorder are enhanced by understanding the basic mechanisms which produce its manifestations. Therefore, it is of interest to clinicians that great strides are being made in understanding the biochemistry of bronchial smooth muscle function[410] (Fig. 14-7).

Evidence is accumulating that smooth muscle contraction is enhanced by depletion of tissue concentration of adenosine 3′5′ phosphate (cyclic AMP), and that relaxation is associated with

TABLE 14-7. Classification of Allergic Reactions

Coombs and Gell classification	Other terms	Some examples in man
Type I	Anaphylactic Reagin-dependent	Anaphylactic shock
Type II	Cytotoxic	Transfusion reaction Hemolytic disease of the newborn
Type III	Damage by toxic complexes	Arthus reaction Serum sickness Allergic alveolitis Bronchopulmonary aspergillosis
Type IV	Delayed Tuberculin-type Cell-mediated	Tuberculin skin reaction

Adapted from Coombs RRA, Gell PGH: Classification of allergic reactions responsible for clinical hypersensitivity and disease. In Gell PGH, Coombs RRA: Clinical Aspects of Immunology (3rd ed). Oxford, Blackwell, 1975

increased concentrations. Bronchospasm and bronchodilation, which occur in a host of normal circumstances and disease states as well as in response to administration of drugs, are mediated by alterations in cyclic AMP. A similar but opposite effect on smooth muscle is seen with guanosine 3′5′ phosphate (cyclic GMP).[411,412]

Of clearest interest to the clinician is evidence that catecholamines produce their relaxant effect on bronchial smooth muscle by stimulating the production of cyclic AMP from ATP under the influence of adenylate cyclase.[411] This effect is blocked, as might be expected, by β-adrenergic blocking agents. Theophylline, on the other hand, may produce bronchodilation by inhibiting the phosphodiesterase enzymes which inactivate cyclic AMP. Hence the action of theophylline is also mediated by cyclic AMP but its effect is not influenced by adrenergic blocking drugs.

Suggestions that cholinergic agents may produce an increase in cyclic GMP in smooth muscle and by this mechanism produce bronchoconstriction have similar potential importance to clinical medicine.[397,413]

In addition to directly suppressing smooth muscle contractility, there is evidence that cyclic AMP inhibits release of mediators of smooth muscle contraction in anaphylaxis.

These fascinating developments both have some immediate relevance to therapy of asthma and hold great promise for future therapeutic advances.

Asthma in Response to Acute Exposure to Antigen

Immediate Asthmatic Reactions. A great deal is known about the mechanisms of asthma as it occurs in clear association with exposure to an antigen. This form of asthmatic reaction can be demonstrated by observing a prompt decrease in expiratory flow rates following inhalation of the antigen to be studied. Such attacks of asthma are believed to be predominately a manifestation of a Type I allergic reaction (*immediate* hypersensitivity, *anaphylaxis*) according to the classification of Coombs and Gell (Table 14-7).[414] The Type I reaction lends itself relatively well to study in the intact patient, in an intact animal model, and in a number of *in vitro* preparations.

An early landmark in the study of the mechanisms of this phenomenon was the observation by Prausnitz and Kustner that passive transfer of specific hypersensitivity could be accomplished in humans.[415] The classic experiment was carried out with serum from Kustner himself, then a 24-year-old man, who was sensitive to fish, exhibiting rhinorrhea, dyspnea, and generalized urticaria within half-an-hour of ingesting small amounts. Intradermal injection of small amounts of fish antigen produced a local wheal and flare reaction. This skin sensitivity could be transferred to other persons by intradermal injection of small amounts of this serum and subsequently demonstrated by injection of fish antigen into the same site.

The antibody mediating this skin sensitivity has long been known as *reagin*, and the reaction occurring after passive transfer is commonly referred to as the Prausnitz-Kustner, or P-K reaction. Reaginic antibodies appear to be responsible for a group of manifestations of the Type I, or immediate hypersensitivity reaction, including generalized responses such as extrinsic allergic asthma, hay fever, and urticaria. The ability to become fixed to cell surfaces appears to be an important property which enables reaginic antibody to produce the manifestations of immediate hypersensitivity.

Discovery of immunoglobulin E (IgE) by Ishizaka and Ishizaka (1966) was another milestone in the study of immediate hypersensitivity, since this immunoglobulin class appears to be at least partially responsible for reagin-mediated hypersensitivity. IgE can be demonstrated to combine with tissue mast cells and basophil granulocytes and to trigger the release of chemical substances which presumably mediate the clinical manifestations of hypersensitivity. Little doubt remains of the importance of IgE as a reaginic antibody; but the possibility remains that other immunoglobulins, especially IgG may also have reaginic properties.[391,392,416]

Antigen-induced asthma is of particular interest because inhaled foreign material must impinge on the wall of the tracheobronchial tree and in some fashion, cause bronchoconstriction. Hogg has demonstrated that in experimental asthma, the respiratory effects become demonstrable within seconds of inhalation of the antigen. He has suggested that antigen-antibody reactions with surface mast cells in the bronchial lumen may cause early release of mediators, stimulation of mucosal irritant receptors, and increased mucosal permeability. Following these initial effects of the antigen, the airways are more permeable to additional antigen and more responsive to nonspecific irritants and mediators such as histamine.[417,418]

Chemical Mediators. There has been much investigative interest in recent years in a number of chemical substances which have been suspected to mediate the clinical response to the reaction between antigen and reaginic antibody fixed to cell surfaces.[419–421] Acetylcholine has been studied with interest because of its demonstrated potential to produce bronchoconstriction, vasodilation, and stimulation of mucous glands. It has not clearly been assigned a role in human asthma, however. Serotonin (5-hydroxytryptamine), plasma kallikrein and bradykinin, rabbit aorta contracting substance (RCS) and its releasing factor (RCS-RF), certain prostaglandins, eosinophil chemotactic factor, and platelet activating factor have all received attention because of their pharmacologic properties and because they have been shown to be present following antigen-antibody reactions in certain animal systems used to study anaphylaxis. None has clearly been shown to play a role in human asthma, however.

The two substances most extensively studied, and currently appearing most likely to play important roles in human asthma, are histamine and slow-reacting substance of anaphylaxis (SRS-A). These two substances, and a third called eosinophil chemotactic factor of anaphylaxis (ECF-A) have been detected in diffusates of human lung fragments sensitized with IgE antibody and challenged with ragweed antigen.[422]

Histamine, an extensively studied and pharmacologically active substance, was the first mediator found to be associated with allergic reactions, in 1910, by Dale and Laidlaw. Histamine exists in high concentration in granules of tissue mast cells and circulating basophils, and is released in response to the reaction between antigen and antibody on the surface of these cells. Mast cells are abundant in the tracheobronchial tree, underneath the mucosa, and histamine produces vasodilation and edema and bronchiolar spasm. Therefore, histamine released from mast cells would appear to be a logical substance to be implicated as an important mediator of allergic bronchial asthma. However, the role of histamine is somewhat clouded by the clinical ineffectiveness of antihistaminic drugs in the treatment of asthma; it has been suggested that the reason for this clinical observation is that the drugs of this class currently available do not achieve sufficient concentration at an appropriate site to effectively block the large amounts of histamine released.[423]

The mediator known as SRS-A[424] was first observed in 1940, when perfusates from guinea pig lungs subjected to anaphylaxis were noted to produce a smooth muscle contraction more sustained than that caused by histamine. SRS-A has subsequently been studied extensively.

The substance ECF-A produces an attraction for eosinophils across a millipore membrane. Its structure is not defined, and its role in human asthma is not yet clear.[422]

"Late" or "Non-immediate" Asthmatic Reactions. Asthmatic reactions to specific substances can be provoked by inhalation challenge and then studied by measurement of expiratory flow rates at sequential time intervals. In addition to the immediate reactions already discussed, there are at least three distinctive forms of late or non-immediate reactions.[391] The most common and best defined is that beginning at 3 to 4 hr, peaking at 5 to 8 hr, and lasting 24 to 36 hr. This form is considered to be a manifestation of Type III hypersensitivity. A less common and less well understood earlier reaction appears at about 1 hr and lasts 2 to 3 hr. A recurrent early morning reaction occurring for a few days following inhalation challenge has also been demonstrated.[392,425,426]

The role of the Type III allergic response, or Arthus reaction, in asthma and other pulmonary diseases has been attracting increasing attention. This type of reaction is delayed for several hours following exposure to antigen, and is mediated by the formation of precipitin which forms as a product of antigen-antibody combination and results in an inflammatory response. The Type III response may be clinically manifest as a delayed skin reaction following intradermal injection of antigen, as a delayed asthmatic attack after inhalation, or may be recognized as *allergic alveolitis*, with fever, leukocytosis, and pulmonary infiltrates accompanying dyspnea. Precipitating antibodies to the provoking antigen may be demonstrated in serum. There is evidence that the occurrence of a delayed Type III reaction is somehow dependent on the occurrence of a preceding immediate Type I reaction, which may or may not be clinically evident. In some subjects, a single antigenic substance may be capable of provoking a dual response to inhalation challenge, a dual skin test reaction, and serum precipitating antibodies.

Depending upon the particular antigen involved, and the prominence of various manifestations of the response, a Type III reaction may be recognized as one of several clinical syndromes: as simple asthma, allergic aspergillosis, or Farmer's lung; or as the syndrome of pulmonary infiltrates with eosinophilia or allergic alveolitis with or without a recognizable inciting allergen.

Aspergillus fumigatus provokes a range of clinical disorders which make allergic bronchopulmonary aspergillosis a useful prototype of immunologic lung diseases.[391] In atopic subjects, the fungus may provoke a Type I reaction producing simple asthma. In some atopic subjects, the production of precipitating antibody may result in a Type III asthmatic reaction as well, along with pulmonary eosinophilia. These subjects may exhibit episodes of fever, malaise, wheezing, and transitory infiltrates as seen on chest radiograph. Sputum plugs may contain eosinophils and branching fungal hyphae. These plugs, when not expectorated, may produce segmental or subsegmental atelectasis; and the antigenic material diffusing from hyphae is believed to cause proximal bronchietasis by a destructive Type III reaction.

These patients may have dual skin test and inhalation challenge reactions; serum precipitating antibodies against *Aspergillus fumigatus;* and specific IgE antibody and elevated total IgE concentration. Cromolyn sodium, bronchodilators and corticosteroids are therapeutically useful.

The extrinsic allergic alveolitis which *A. fumigatus* may cause in nonatopic subjects is discussed elsewhere.

The fungus may grow as a saprophyte in pulmonary cavities left by other destructive lung diseases (fungus ball, aspergilloma). It may produce invasive, even disseminated disease in immunologically incompetent patients.

Asthma Precipitated by Drugs and Diagnostic Procedures

Numerous drugs may precipitate bronchospasm.[427] Aspirin and other analgesics are discussed below. Additives such as tartrazine, a dye commonly used for food coloring, produce bronchospasm through unknown mechanisms. Inhaled or instilled topical lidocaine causes bronchoconstriction in most asthmatics. This side-effect must be considered and can be prevented by the use of bronchodilators in asthmatics who need bronchoscopy.[428,429] Iodinated contrast material may act as an irritant in some persons when instilled intratracheally, but severe reactions, which most commonly occur during angiography, are generally anaphylactic in nature.[427] Beta adrenergic blocking drugs, generally prescribed for hypertension or angina pectoris, may aggravate bronchospasm in a previously known asthmatic, or cause asthma to be symptomatic for the first time.[427,376] Many medications used in the treatment of asthma may cause bronchospasm in certain persons. These rare reactions are discussed in relation to each medication.

Asthma with Aspirin Intolerance and Nasal Polyposis. There exists a subset of adult perennial asthmatics, more often women, in whom severe exacerbations are precipitated by aspirin ingestion, and in whom nasal polyps are common.[430,431] This group made up 3.8% of one series of adult asthmatics.[432] Familial occurrence has been reported,[433] but is not the rule; and these patients are not generally atopic.

The mechanism of bronchospasm in them is not entirely clear. There is evidence suggesting immunologically induced mast cell degranulation,[434] and other evidence suggesting an abnormality of prostaglandin synthesis.[435–437] Salicylates other than acetylsalicylic acid appear to be well tolerated in patients with this syndrome but other drugs, chiefly analgesics, have been reported to precipitate bronchospasm and include indomethacin, fenamates, phenylbutazone, aminopyrine, ibuprofen, and fenoprofen.[433–436] Some of these drugs share an ability to suppress synthesis of prostaglandin E2, a bronchodilator, but not prostaglandin $F_2\alpha$, a bronchoconstrictor, suggesting a possible mechanism of their action. The asthma in these patients is characteristically difficult to control, even if provoking drugs are avoided, and they may need long-term corticosteroid therapy. Some degree of protection from acute attacks[434] and improvement of chronic asthma[438] has been reported from cromolyn sodium. It has been suggested that nasal polypectomy may exacerbate symptoms, but if this occurs it is apparently in a minority of cases.[439]

Asthma Occurring for No Apparent Reason in Either Atopic or Nonatopic Subjects

This probably represents the largest group seen in hospital practice. Some patients are undoubtedly relegated to this group because of the individual physician's failure to recognize one of the commonly known precipitating events. A larger number probably represent those with asthma of an unknown cause.

Asthma in Response to Infection

Bronchospasm in association with sputum purulence is common, but the significance and therapeutic implications of the association may not be entirely clear in the individual patient. Bronchiolitis in children may mimic asthma. Viral infections may cause bronchial hyperreactivity in healthy persons and apparently can precipitate attacks in asthmatic children and adults.[440–443] Bacterial infections may complicate asthma and must be treated appropriately when present. Demonstrable infection only accounts for exacerbations in about 10% of such episodes, and more than half are viral.[443,444] The important role of *Aspergillus* infection in some patients is discussed under Late Asthmatic Reactions.

Asthma on Exposure to Air Pollution

Geographical displacement of large numbers of people to areas of heavy air pollution might be expected to result in development of asthmatic symptoms in some previously asymptomatic subjects with hyperreactive bronchi. This sequence of events has occurred during movement of troops for military purposes, and terms such as Tokyo and Yokohama Asthma have resulted. These entities are not generally regarded as sufficiently distinctive to warrant a new diagnostic classification.

There is little doubt that atmospheric pollutants play a major role in the exacerbation of symptoms in some asthmatics, however. The specific agents at fault, the mechanisms by which they produce bronchospasm, and the needed concentrations to produce this effect are not well defined. Oxides of nitrogen and sulfur, hydrocarbons, and ozone are among the better-known irritant gases which are components of the atmosphere of modern industrial cities, along with particulate matter of a wide range of size and composition. The problem of adverse effects of atmospheric pollutants is reviewed in Chapter 1.

Occupational Asthma

Exposure to certain dusts and fumes in the course of employment may precipitate bronchospasm in sensitive persons. Bronchial provocation tests have been used increasingly to clarify the cause and to characterize the time course of reactions to particular inhalants. Substances recognized to have a particular tendency to provoke asthma include complex salts of platinum; piperazine hydrochloride used in drug manufacture; antimicrobial drugs; toluene diisocyanate (TDI); cotton, grain, and wood dusts; pyrolysis products of polyvinyl chloride wrapping material; and soldering fluxes and resins.[20a,445–447] Many inhaled substances are now recognized to produce nonspecific bronchial reactivity in previously healthy persons.[402] This increased reactivity remains poorly explained, but can be readily demonstrated during methacholine inhalation[448] and gradually disappears after removal from the exposure.

Optimal methods for identifying those with increased airway reactivity related to specific environmental hazards have not been established. Some combination of immunologic methods (skin tests, antigen-specific antibody assays), inhalation tests, and assessment of nonspecific reactivity may prove useful, particularly when assessing previously unsuspected industries.[447–450] (See also Bronchial Provocation Tests, below.)

Asthma Precipitated by Coughing or Laughing

Wheezing precipitated by coughing or laughing often occurs in various forms of asthma. Mechanical stimuli would appear to be an adequate explanation.[451] It has recently been shown that coughing may be the only clinical manifestation of asthma in those with hyperreactive airways,[452] and the onset of wheezing in such patients might provide a mistaken impression that the cough was the inciting event.

Asthmatic Attacks in Response to Emotional Stress

So common is the clinical observation of an emotional trigger producing asthmatic attacks, that a psychological basis for the cause and treatment of asthma is often sought. Seldom is a definitive solution for an individual patient to be found by an approach grounded only in psychodynamics, however. A recent study[453] suggests that overt neurotic disorders are not disproportionately high in asthmatics, an observation which fails to support the idea that emotion is a common basic cause of this disorder. Another study of the personality profiles of asthmatics demonstrated patterns which have been called characteristic of psychosomatic disease, but these patterns correlated with the severity of functional impairment rather than with the presence or absence of asthma, and were also noted in subjects with emphysema.[454] This study could be interpreted as suggesting that emotional disturbance is usually a result rather than a cause of asthma. In planning a treatment program, simple supportive psychotherapy as an adjunct to other forms of treatment is most often appropriate.

Such a supportive approach may be exceedingly helpful in management. The patient should be well informed about his disease, and the importance of emotional triggers should be discussed and brought to his awareness. Avoidance of situations which produce anxiety and wheezing is usually the most practical means of dealing with them. There have been intriguing reports of successful attempts at behavior therapy, aimed at modification of the emotional and physiologic responses to stressful situations,[455,456] and of the beneficial effects of suggestion.[457]

Nocturnal Asthma

Patients with allergic asthma are not infrequently awakened by attacks of wheezing and dyspnea in the early morning hours. A cause for this phenomenon which can be widely applied has not been identified.[458] A diurnal rhythm of airway obstruction has been demonstrated in bronchitis and asthma, with the nocturnal flow rates as low as 30 to 50% of mid-day rates. Asthmatics have the greatest deterioration and may have evening as well as morning "dips" in flow rate.[459] Patients with sleep deprivation continue to demonstrate increased nocturnal obstruction, and pretreatment with bronchodilators or corticosteroids provides only modest improvement.[459,460] The effects of prolonged reversal of diurnal sleep activity patterns have not been studied. The demonstrable nocturnal asthma which occurs for several nights following provocation tests may permit more detailed studies of the mechanisms.[394,461] The nocturnal deterioration varies greatly between patients and when severe, may identify those at particular risk for sudden asthmatic death.[462]

Exercise-Induced Asthma

The phenomenon of exercise-induced bronchospasm in asthmatic subjects has received increased interest in the past few years, with a number of studies being addressed to the mechanisms involved.[463–470a] The therapeutic implications are evident, since it is this very phenomenon which surely must produce the most troublesome aspect of the disease in many children and young adults, hampering participation in sports and in certain vocational efforts.

Discrepancies in the data so far collected suggest that more than one mechanism is probably involved in exercise-induced bronchospasm and that the dominant mechanism may not be the same in every patient. There are some areas of consensus, however. Decrease in maximal expiratory flow rates and increase in airways resistance appear to develop a few minutes after exercise has ceased; in fact, some data[465] suggest that bronchodilation occurs during exercise. Atropine seems not to inhibit it,[463,466] suggesting that autonomic reflexes mediated by the vagus are not the major mechanisms inducing bronchodilation. Isoproterenol is effective in its prevention,[463] suggesting that smooth muscle contraction is involved; and a protective effect of disodium cromoglycate has also been shown.[464,467,468]

Voluntary hyperventilation is recognized as being capable of increasing airways resistance through hypocapnia and this is probably significant in some patients. The reported effects of CO_2 inhalation in preventing or reversing exercise-induced bronchospasm have, however, varied among investigators,[466,469] making it difficult to assess the role of hypocapnia in this phenomenon. Some[464,465] but not all[463] studies have shown evidence of bronchospasm in nonasthmatic subjects following exercise, so the response is not limited to asthmatic subjects, though this is the area of chief importance.

A series of ingenious studies[470,470a] by Deal and associates in Boston may resolve some of the conflicting data on this subject. Their studies indicate that the occurrence and severity of exercise-induced asthma is related to heat loss from the airways attendant upon the hyperpnea of exercise, and that this heat flux is a result of both convective and evaporative cooling.

The clinically observed usefulness of bronchodilator administration prior to exercise in asthmatics has objective support.

CLINICAL EVALUATION

In the current state of imperfect knowledge of the nature of asthma, the disorder is most often recognized as such by the patient, from its presentation in the form of attacks of wheezing and shortness of breath. The suspected diagnosis is confirmed by the physician when he observes an attack and hears wheezing with or without a stethoscope, and elicits a history of asymptomatic intervals and well-recognized precipitating events. Cardiac and other pulmonary causes for wheezing and dyspnea must be excluded, and a chest roentgenogram is usually taken for the purpose of excluding other disorders, since the diagnosis of asthma is clearly not a roentgenographic one. An experienced physician will usually be correct in his impression based on this minimal data. Blood and sputum eosinophilia, skin test evidence of atopy, and characteristic pulmonary function findings should be sought if there is doubt about the diagnosis, and will usually be helpful in planning therapy if such information can be readily obtained, even in a straightforward case.

History

Intermittent attacks of wheezing and shortness of breath are well known as the cornerstone of a diagnosis of asthma, although they may occur in association with a number of other disorders. Especially characteristic of asthma are the features of onset within minutes of a precipitating event, rapid (minutes) increase in severity, and persistence, if untreated, for hours. Great variation in this pattern is possible, however. Response to bronchodilator drugs administered either by aerosol or parenterally is characteristically prompt and dramatic. Complete absence of symptoms between attacks is supportive of asthma as a cause, and certain of the precipitating events which were discussed in detail are so typical of asthma that their association with attacks is diagnostic.

A family history of asthma or a personal or family history of other manifestations of asthma is suggestive specifically of extrinsic asthma.

Cough is frequently the only symptom of asthma, generally worse at night, and it may act as a trigger for more severe attacks with wheezing and dyspnea.[452] The cough may be dry or productive and sputum is most characteristically mucoid and tenacious. Purulence suggests tracheobronchial infection. Cough and dyspnea may be worse in the recumbent posture, mimicking symptoms of pulmonary edema, or orthopnea may be absent, simplifying exclusion of the latter disorder. Chronic bronchitis must be considered whenever productive cough is prominent and persistent, thus obscuring precise diagnostic classification.

In some extrinsic asthmatics, rhinorrhea, urticaria, and conjunctivitis may accompany asthmatic attacks and clarify the cause. A history of allergic rhinitis or nasal polyps should raise suspicion of asthma.[471]

Physical Examination

Contrary to common teaching, the physical findings in patients with asthma tend to be misleading and inconsistent. Mild to moderate degrees of airway obstruction are commonly present without any objective physical signs; the physical findings with severe attacks serve to alert the physician but do not quantitate the problem. The routine use of a portable device to measure the expiratory flow rate ($FEV_{1.0}$, peak flow, and so forth) is essential as part of the routine examination and follow up of patients with asthma.[472]

The musical rhonchi, or wheezes of asthma may be audible without a stethoscope, or may be heard only with its use on tidal breathing or forced expiration. Expiratory wheezes and expiratory prolongation are most marked but labored inspiration accompanied by wheezing is not uncommon. Wheezing may sometimes be mild though the asthmatic attack is severe, indicating that there is almost no flow of air through the obstructed airways.

Other physical findings generally indicate rather severe bronchospasm. These findings include use of the accessory muscles of respiration, an overinflated, hyperresonant thorax, and pulsus paradoxus. Asymmetrical overinflation with decreased breath sounds and evidence of mediastinal shift should cause suspicion of complicating pneumothorax, and crepitation of mediastinal and subcutaneous emphysema. In children, a chronic barrel chest deformity correlates well with sustained hyperinflation.[473] Tachycardia is common but an increased pulmonic component of the second sound as evidence of pulmonary hypertension is not and is suggestive of a severe attack. The absence of cyanosis is not a reliable sign that hypoxemia is absent, but central cyanosis suggests that it is present and severe. Peripheral cyanosis may be due to vasoconstriction if α-adrenergic drugs have been used, or to coincident decrease in cardiac output.

Disturbances of consciousness are uncommon in asthma and provide evidence of severe blood gas derangement (to be discussed).

The Chest Roentgenogram

There are no specific roentgenographic signs of asthma, and the chest roentgenogram is commonly normal during and between attacks.

The air trapping which occurs may be visible on a roentgenogram taken during an attack (Fig. 14-8). An increased retrosternal air space and flattening of the diaphragms may occur, and normal distribution and tapering of vessels may suggest that emphysema is not the cause. With the use of planimetry of anterior and lateral views, lung volume may be calculated and the degree of overinflation quantitated.[474]

Roentgenographic evidence of bronchial wall thickening has been described in asthma and has been related to chronic infection in the patients in whom it occurs[475] (Fig. 14-9). Pathologic confirmation of this interpretation is not definitive.

Segmental and subsegmental infiltrates and atelectasis attributed to mucus plugging of bronchi are not rare in asthmatics.[476–478] It is believed that this phenomenon sometimes results in bronchiectasis. The presence of this type of bronchiectasis is not an indication for treatment modification and bronchograms are seldom if ever recommended for its detection.

Laboratory Studies

Demonstration and quantitation of blood eosinophilia is useful in diagnosing and in planning therapy in asthma. Eosinophilia in itself is profoundly nonspecific, but in the patient with wheezing in whom the role of chronic bronchitis as opposed to asthma is in question, eosinophilia may suggest the latter diagnosis, with appropriate modifications in therapy.

Specifically, it has been suggested that the total eosinophil count may be useful as a guide to steroid usage in asthma.[479] A study of adult patients with active intrinsic asthma showed elevated total eosinophil counts in most, and there was correlation between the degree of eosinophilia and the activity of the disease. Steroid treatment decreased counts in both healthy subjects and asthmatics. Average counts per mm^3 were 122 ± 74(SD) in untreated and 43 ± 22(SD) in prednisone-treated healthy subjects. Patients with active bronchial asthma had counts above 350 if untreated, and above 85 on steroids. Mild degrees of eosinophilia sometimes co-existed with mild abnormalities of pulmonary function in asymptomatic asthmatics, suggesting that the eosinophil count may prove to be useful in the early detection of attacks.

Skin testing for immediate hypersensitivity to common antigens plays a useful role in the diagnostic workup and management of some asthmatics. Positive tests may identify the subject

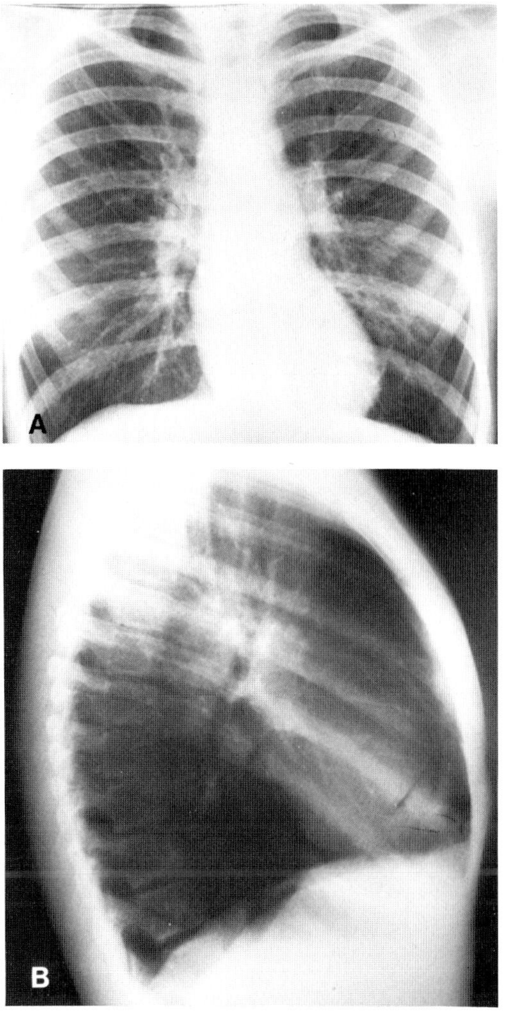

FIG. 14-8. Chest roentgenogram of a child with asthma during acute attack, demonstrating hyperinflation. **A.** Posteroanterior view; **B.** lateral view.

with atopy, but a positive test to a specific antigen may not necessarily indicate that antigen is playing a clinically important role in causing exacerbations. However, if a suggestive history of symptoms on clinical exposure to a substance is supported by a positive skin test to that antigen, then avoidance or immunotherapy should be considered. In case of doubt, challenge by inhalation of antigen may be carried out.

Microscopic examination of sputum can be of great value in asthma, demonstrating eosino-

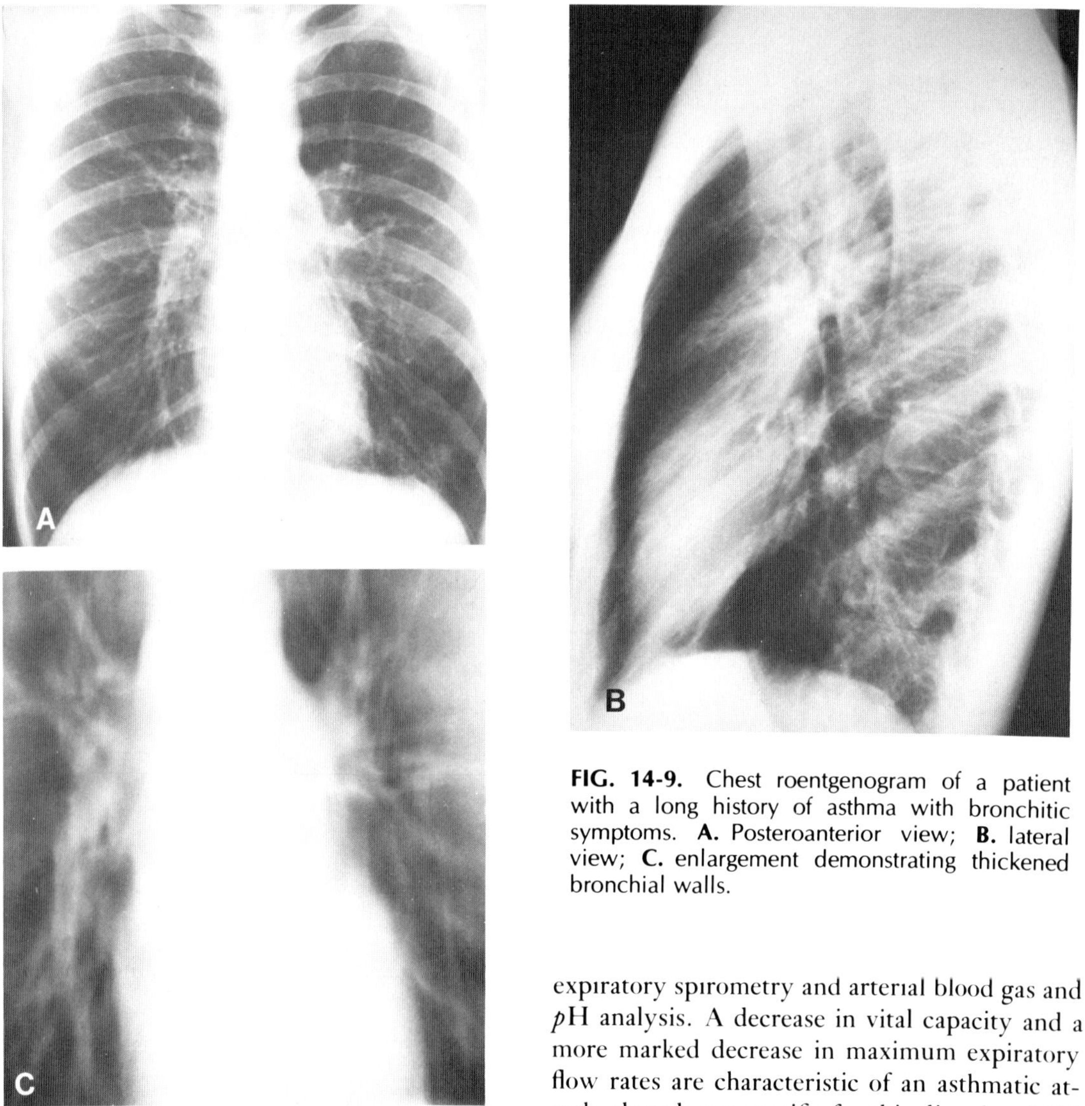

FIG. 14-9. Chest roentgenogram of a patient with a long history of asthma with bronchitic symptoms. **A.** Posteroanterior view; **B.** lateral view; **C.** enlargement demonstrating thickened bronchial walls.

phils, Charcot-Leyden crystals, Curschmann's spirals and Creola bodies. However, sputum eosinophilia is also common in chronic bronchitis.[480] This topic will be discussed further with a description of material found in the bronchial lumina in asthmatics. The occurrence of bacteria and neutrophilic leukocytes in sputum indicates infection.

Pulmonary Function Evaluation

Satisfactory evaluation and management of asthma patients can be carried out with simple expiratory spirometry and arterial blood gas and *p*H analysis. A decrease in vital capacity and a more marked decrease in maximum expiratory flow rates are characteristic of an asthmatic attack, though not specific for this disorder. Mild to moderate hypoxemia and hypocarbia characterize the usual blood gas abnormalities, and in the unusual, very severe attack, hypoxemia may be severe, and may be accompanied by acute elevation of carbon dioxide tension and acidosis.

Measurement of lung volumes including residual volume, diffusing capacity, compliance, and airways resistance are helpful especially when differentiation of asthma and emphysema is a problem. If a patient is asymptomatic and pulmonary function tests are normal, inhalation of histamine or methacholine may be used to confirm or exclude the presence of hyperreactivity of the airways. Asthmatic subjects will nearly always have demonstrable hyperreactivity. Under carefully controlled conditions, inhalation of specific antigens or irritants will produce measurable bronchospasm. This provides definitive information regarding the cause and dose, which may be responsible for asthma in a given patient.[481,482] Further discussion of this, along with a description of the mechanisms producing the functional alterations in asthma, may be found under the heading Pathophysiology.

Electrocardiogram

Ordinarily, only sinus tachycardia is seen electrocardiographically during asthmatic attacks. Severe asthma may result in ventricular or atrial arrhythmias, which are probably the cause of most unexplained deaths in these patients.[483–485] Electrocardiographic changes include right axis deviation, clockwise rotation, evidence of right ventricular and right atrial enlargement (p pulmonale), and evidence of S-T segment and T-wave abnormalities.[483–485] These changes are presumably due to high pulmonary vascular resistance and disappear as the asthma attack dissipates.

Severe asthma may result in signs of acute obstruction to right ventricular outflow. Presumably, hypoxemia and acidosis or alkalosis may produce direct effects upon the myocardium. Arteriolar constriction due to hypoxemia and acidosis, and mechanical obstruction related to high alveolar pressure may cause acute cor pulmonale.

Problems in Differential Diagnosis

Perhaps the most common and most difficult diagnostic problem in asthma is its differentiation from other chronic obstructive lung diseases, since other conditions may present with intermittent wheezing and shortness of breath.

Congestive heart failure, particularly predominant left-ventricular failure or mitral stenosis may occasionally present with episodic shortness of breath accompanied by wheezing. This symptom complex is sufficiently widely recognized to have been labeled *cardiac asthma*. An association of attacks with the recumbent posture should prompt consideration of this diagnosis; and in fact the history, physical examination, and laboratory workup of any asthmatic should be designed to exclude heart disease as a cause. Ronchi may be a result of peribronchial edema with reduced size of the airways. Cardiomegaly, a ventricular gallop, crackling inspiratory rales at the posterior lung bases, and roentgenographic evidence of pulmonary edema are especially common signs of heart failure to be excluded.

Recurrent small pulmonary emboli may be manifested by attacks of shortness of breath and wheezing heard on careful auscultation. In practice, this syndrome is probably seldom accompanied by wheezing of enough intensity to cause confusion.

Laryngotracheal obstruction due to any of a number of causes may produce shortness of breath and wheezing. An impression of intermittency may be created by obstruction to the degree that symptoms occur only during exercise, when minute ventilation, and hence airflow through the obstructed segment, is increased. Inspiratory stridor is characteristic of this form of airway obstruction. Soft-tissue roentgenograms may be used to identify narrowing of the pharyngeal and tracheobronchial air passages, and laryngoscopy or bronchoscopy may be diagnostic. Ventilatory testing may reveal characteristic findings, with flow volume loops being virtually diagnostic in some cases.

The carcinoid syndrome is an uncommon cause of episodic wheezing and its association with flushing of the skin and diarrhea should prompt consideration of this entity. Gastroesophageal reflux with recurrent aspiration of gastric contents may precipitate bronchospasm in previously healthy subjects or may aggravate asthma.[486]

Assessment of Severity of Asthma

Asthma of Mild to Moderate Severity. Between attacks, the asthmatic individual may be entirely normal, both subjectively, and in tests of respiratory function. The intensity of an asthmatic attack ranges from asymptomatic, detectable only on painstaking physical examination or pulmonary function testing, to bronchospasm of a terrifying and truly life-threatening degree.

The onset of an attack may vary greatly in its abruptness, as well as intensity. A severe attack may clear rapidly, either spontaneously or in response to treatment with bronchodilator. Remissions may last for years, or even for a lifetime, especially following childhood asthma. At the other extreme, wheezing and dyspnea may be perennial and incapacitating, and poorly responsive to treatment. There is no consistent relation between duration and intensity of bronchospasm. A very severe attack may be brief and self-limited, and perennial asthma is occasionally mild enough to permit a reasonably tolerable and productive existence.

One series of asthmatic subjects studied by McFadden and co-workers[487] revealed expiratory flow rates reduced well below 40% of normal values when the patient presented with symptoms. During recovery, function was between 40 and 50% of normal when symptoms abated, and between 60 and 70% when wheezing as an objective sign cleared. Objective wheezing in fact correlated poorly with dyspnea and with tests of ventilatory function. Retraction of the sternocleidomastoid muscles did correlate with severe symptoms, however, and with severe reduction in the forced expiratory volume at 1 second to less than 1 liter.

Severe Asthma. The early recognition of a severe attack of asthma is equivalent to identifying a patient at high risk of death. Detailed attention to the criteria of severity permits treatment with appropriate aggressiveness. Patients should be considered with particular care when they have a history of previous severe attacks, recent repetitive treatment which has been partially effective, deterioration in spite of a good medical program, or home conditions which are inadequate to provide support. Lack of detailed records regarding the clinical condition, failure to measure lung function (peak flow or 1 second vital capacity at the bedside), and delayed administration of medications are conspicuous features of deaths due to asthma.[462,488–491] Shim and Williams have pointed out that patients may be better judges of severity of attack than their physicians. These investigators encourage attention to the history and to measurement of flow rates in assessing severity.[491a] Rebuck and Read[483] and Rebuck[492] have described a useful approach to the assessment and management of severe asthma, based on their experience with a series of well studied and generally successfully managed patients (Table 14-8). These patients required hospital admission, and therefore as a group were by definition somewhat resistant to usual bronchodilator therapy. Some observers might use the term *status asthmaticus* to describe this clinical state. The term suffers from lack of precise agreement among those who use it, but in general refers to an attack of bronchospasm which is severe in intensity, prolonged, and relatively resistant to treatment.

Rebuck and Read[483] suggested that within this group of patients, three subgroups could be identified with therapeutic and prognostic significance, and that progress toward improvement would take place through these stages from most to least severe. The most severe group could be identified by the presence of one or more *danger signs* which will be described below. Patients without these signs can be divided into less severe groups which are *nonresponsive* and *responsive* to bronchodilator drugs. Since lack of response to bronchodilators is a frequent reason for hospital admission, most hospitalized asthmatics will enter in a danger or nonresponsive phase and will pass through a responsive phase during recovery.

Assuming reduction in vital capacity and expiratory flow rates, and some degree of unresponsiveness to bronchodilators, the features indicating a *dangerous* degree of severity of an asthmatic attack included disturbance of consciousness, cyanosis, arterial oxygen tension below 60 mm Hg, and carbon dioxide tension above 45 mm Hg, obvious hyperinflation on chest roentgenogram, electrocardiographic abnormalities, pulsus paradoxus, and pneumothorax or pneumomediastinum.

Disturbance of consciousness was unusual in this series, and was a manifestation of severe blood gas derangement and therefore clearly an ominous sign.

Central cyanosis was also rather uncommon, and its absence did not exclude the presence of severe arterial hypoxemia. In fact, a reduced ar-

TABLE 14-8. Severity of Asthmatic Attack

Severity	Criteria	Therapeutic implications
Responsive	Prompt improvement with bronchodilator	Outpatient treatment adequate
Non-responsive		
Without danger signs	See below	Hospitalization usually indicated
With danger signs	Disturbance of consciousness Cyanosis Use of accessory muscles Arterial O_2 tension below 60 mm. Hg Arterial CO_2 tension above 45 mm. Hg Hyperinflation on chest roentgenogram Abnormal electrocardiogram Pulsus paradoxus >10 mm. Hg Pneumothorax or pneumomediastinum	Hospitalization, continual observation, availability of intubation and mechanical ventilation indicated

Adapted from Rebuck AS, Read J: Assessment and management of severe asthma. Am J Med 51:788, 1971

terial oxygen tension to between 60 and 80 mm Hg was usual, even in mild attacks, and most often did not cause cyanosis. Respiratory alkalosis resulting in increased oxygen affinity for hemoglobin often prevented cyanosis. The presence of cyanosis was a reliable indicator of severe hypoxemia, however, and was more consistently present in those patients with acidemia.

The presence of pulsus paradoxus correlated well with severity of impairment of expiratory flow rates and indicated that the FEV_1 was reduced to 1.25 liters or below. Its disappearance signaled improvement.

The most common pattern of blood gas derangement was mild or moderate hypoxemia with a reduced arterial carbon dioxide tension. Hypercarbia was unusual, and signaled loss of ventilatory reserve.

Roentgenographic evidence of thoracic overinflation was common in this series and did not always correlate with the presence of other danger signals. It was always present in patients judged most severely ill according to other criteria.

Electrocardiographic abnormalities other than sinus tachycardia were common in severe attacks and disappeared with improvement. Those suggesting pulmonary hypertension in particular were considered secondary to asthma. Other varieties of electrocardiographic abnormalities may be a manifestation of coronary artery disease co-existing with asthma in older patients.

PATHOPHYSIOLOGY

In simple terms, the pathophysiology of asthma consists of obstruction to air flow, particularly expiratory air flow, associated with hypoxemia resulting from ventilation-perfusion mismatching, and carbon dioxide retention only during attacks severe enough to be life-threatening (Table 14-9). The mechanisms producing these abnormalities cannot be described so simply, however, and do need to be understood in order to plan effective therapy for asthma.[493]

Ventilatory Abnormalities

The characteristic spirogram in asthma presents as a relatively nonspecific *obstructive pattern*, with decreases in maximum expiratory flow rates, whether measured as forced expiratory volume, timed, or as average or instantaneous flow rates. The vital capacity is decreased, as is the maximum voluntary ventilation. A dramatic improvement in an abnormal spirogram of the obstructive sort may be strongly suggestive of asthma. A return to normal in such a spirogram may be virtually diagnostic. Failure of the spirogram to improve with bronchodilator does not exclude a diagnosis of asthma, since spasmodic

TABLE 14-9. Lung Function Abnormalities in Asthma in Exacerbation

Ventilatory Abnormalities	Change
Forced expiratory volume	↓
Expiratory flow rate	↓
Airways resistance	↑
Vital capacity	↓
Residual volume	↑
Functional residual capacity	↑
Total lung capacity	⟷ (or minimal increase during attack)
Improvement with bronchodilator	Marked
Respiratory Gas Exchange	**Change**
Diffusing capacity	⟷
Arterial oxygen tension	↓
Arterial carbon dioxide tension	↓ (Increased during severe attack—carries ominous prognosis)

asthma may at times be refractory, even to substantial doses of conventional drugs. Occasionally, clinical and arterial blood gas improvement may accompany an increase in vital capacity and a decrease in residual volume without improved maximal expiratory flow rates.[494] This phenomenon probably reflects airway caliber which is reduced at lower lung volumes. In spasmodic asthma, as in bronchitis, the decrease in maximum expiratory flow is truly due to an increase in flow resistance[495] rather than to a decrease in elastic recoil which may be the cause in some subjects with pulmonary emphysema. Measuring the ventilatory changes after inhalation challenge is becoming increasingly important in the assessment of patients with asthma. These procedures are described under Bronchial Provocation Tests.

The decrease in vital capacity in asthma is due to an increased residual volume, again a nonspecific finding seen also in other obstructive diseases. Measurement of other compartments of lung volume usually reveals an increase in functional residual capacity, and a normal or near normal total lung capacity, although some studies of asthmatics during severe exacerbations have shown an increase in total lung capacity which is reversible.[496,497] It is widely considered, however, that an increased total lung capacity favors the diagnosis of emphysema. This interpretation is in general valid, especially when the finding is demonstrated in a clinically stable patient. Static compliance is in general normal in asthma, and increased compliance favors a diagnosis of emphysema in a patient with an obstructive spirogram; but, again, a reversible increase in compliance has been described in severe asthmatics during exacerbation.[498] This increase in compliance is seen in association with increased total lung capacity. The mechanisms involved in these changes are unclear, but the characteristics of the elastic properties of the alveolar lining, or changes in tone of alveolar duct smooth muscle, are intriguing possibilities for future investigation.

Inspiratory stridor is common during severe asthma, and measurements of airway resistance suggest inspiratory obstruction at the level of the extrathoracic trachea and larynx.[495a]

The site and nature of expiratory flow obstruction in asthma have been subject to debate. Smooth muscle constriction and hypertrophy, mucosal edema, and plugging of airways with secretions and cellular debris all play a part, the contribution of each depending on the patient and circumstances. The route of entry of a substance provoking bronchospasm undoubtedly influences the site of response, as shown by studies which demonstrate that intravenous histamine produces constriction mainly of peripheral airways, while histamine introduced into the bronchial arteries causes chiefly constriction of central airways.[402] The site of effect of inhaled bronchodilator substances likewise is probably influenced by the site of their deposition.[402] Vagally mediated changes in airway caliber influence more central airways, while beta adrenergic stimulants have a greater effect on peripheral airways, at least under certain conditions.[404] Bronchiolar or even more peripheral obstruction must be invoked in order to explain the frequency dependence of compliance, uneven distribution of ventilation, and hypoxemia in asthmatics under some circumstances,[499–502] while evidence has been presented that some patients experience large airway constriction or collapse during severe attacks.[503,504] Both central and peripheral airways have been shown to be affected in some studies.[505–507] Mucociliary transport is impaired in asthma; whether this is a result of mediators or other factors has not been determined. Mucus plugs and secondary infection may relate to reduced clearance.[508]

Perfusion Abnormalities

There is no doubt that in asthmatic attacks, poorly ventilated areas of the lung receive less than normal blood flow.[503] This regional reduction of perfusion is reversible in remissions, and may be reversed pharmacologically as well. It may be viewed as a protective response, in that it modifies the hypoxemia which results from mismatching of ventilation and perfusion. Recognition of this phenomenon may be of diagnostic importance, since an abnormal radioisotope perfusion scan in an asthmatic could easily be misinterpreted as evidence for pulmonary embolization. A ventilation scan in such a case of asthma would demonstrate decreased ventilation corresponding to areas of decreased perfusion. The ventilation scan in pulmonary embolization, especially in the absence of infarction, might be entirely normal.

The hemodynamic effects of bronchial asthma are particularly interesting. Increased pulmonary vascular resistance probably results from hypoxemia, perfusion at high lung volumes, and in severe cases, acidemia. The pulmonary artery pressure as measured is frequently within normal range, however. This is a result of the strikingly low intrapleural pressure which occurs while breathing at high lung volumes. Hemodynamic studies must therefore take intrathoracic pressure rather than atmospheric pressure as the reference pressure, in assessing right atrial, right ventricular, and pulmonary artery transvascular pressure.[484] These negative intrapleural pressures have been implicated as a cause for developing, or becoming susceptible to, pulmonary edema.[509]

Pulsus paradoxus greater than 10 mm Hg is commonly seen in severe asthma. Although it is not a completely reliable sign of severe obstruction, the correlation in large series is remarkably good.[483,510] Most patients with this sign will have an $FEV_{1.0}$ or a peak flow of less than 35% predicted. The mechanism of pulsus paradoxus has not been firmly established but the most persuasive evidence relates to the excessive negative intrathoracic pressure swings, with high left ventricular afterload during inspiration.[511]

Hypoxemia

Widespread availability of arterial blood gas analysis in recent years has led to recognition that arterial hypoxemia is a very common occurrence during asthmatic attacks, even those of rather moderate severity.[512] The degree of hypoxemia may not correlate especially well with symptoms; in fact, hypoxemia may worsen in response to bronchodilator therapy while airways obstruction improves and relief of dyspnea is experienced.[513] The reason for this phenomenon is that common bronchodilator drugs also dilate pulmonary vessels and increase cardiac output. This cardiovascular response may exceed the bronchodilator effect of these drugs, resulting in increased shunting and hypoxemia. Therefore, oxygen supplementation is often a useful, even essential supplement to bronchodilator therapy in severe asthmatic attacks.

Arterial Carbon Dioxide Tension

Hypocarbia is usual in mild or moderate exacerbations of asthma. Hypercarbia is an indicator of a precarious condition, and should be regarded as one of the medical emergencies in which prompt management truly may be lifesaving.[512]

Chronic, stable hypercarbia, on the other hand, is common in chronic bronchitis and emphysema, and may be present for months or even years, associated with a blunted ventilatory response to carbon dioxide and a near normal blood *p*H. In such cases, it is well recognized that uncontrolled oxygen administration may be dangerous, leading to further carbon dioxide accumulation and acidosis. The reluctance to administer uncontrolled oxygen in the presence of carbon dioxide retention in this latter situation should not be extended to a hypoxemic asthmatic during a severe acute attack. Since hypercarbia is acute in asthmatics, blunting of the respiratory response to carbon dioxide is not common unless respiratory acidosis is severe. The danger of acute hypoxemia in such a case may be greater than the danger from oxygen administration on a short-term basis.

Range of Severity of Physiologic Abnormality

The severity of this disorder ranges from complete absence of symptoms and demonstrable physiologic abnormalities during remission on the one hand to death from a severe attack on the other.

Subtle physiologic abnormalities can be demonstrated in some asthmatics during symptom-free periods, however.[500,514,515] McFadden[516] has pointed out that symptoms accompanying episodes of physiologic exacerbation may sometimes take an atypical form, such as cough and exertional dyspnea without wheezing. Bronchial hyperreactivity in response to histamine or methacholine aerosol can be demonstrated. Frequency dependence of compliance can be shown in some asthmatics in clinical remission,[500] and even less sensitive ventilatory tests may lag behind clinical symptoms as improvement takes place following an exacerbation of asthma.[487] Perhaps the feature most clinically significant is the severity of abnormalities which may be present when symptoms suggest that obstruction is mild.[517]

Pulmonary Diffusing Capacity

In patients with asthma, the diffusing capacity for carbon monoxide is not clinically helpful. In general, results demonstrate decreased values in exacerbation by a steady-state technique, with a change toward normal in remission, but elevated values by a single breath method, decreasing toward normal in remission.[518,519] Clearly, results of this test must be interpreted with caution when the patient has airways obstruction.

Bronchial Provocation Tests

The wide range of activities, medications, chemicals in foods, and inhalants which may precipitate asthma make definitive diagnosis of an inciting agent most difficult. Where there is a clear history relating to a single or numerous precipitating factors no further diagnostic measures are indicated. Occasionally, the symptoms and clinical features are absent when the patient is seen by the physician, and attempts to provoke an attack may be suitable. More frequently, provocation tests are used in attempts to elucidate specific causes. These tests are potentially dangerous and should only be carried out by experienced personnel in well-equipped laboratories. Severe asthmatic attacks with respiratory failure and life-threatening arrhythmias are readily provoked when doses of antigen or inhaled medications are not carefully controlled. An ideal, simple, safe, definitive, and widely applicable test has yet to be developed.[520]

In 1978, the Bronchoprovocation Committee of the American Academy of Allergy held a workshop to consider the status of bronchial provocation testing. The subsequent report summarizes the current state of this field.[447] This approach to diagnosis of airways disease is used in order to assess four major clinical situations:

Nonspecific Airways Reactivity. Most patients with asthma or hay fever and many without clinically apparent asthma can be shown to develop expiratory flow obstruction at lower doses of inhaled methacholine or histamine than are needed in healthy persons. These patients generally also experience postexercise and posthyperventilation bronchoconstriction.[521] Failure to demonstrate hyperreactivity to methacholine or histamine on inhalation of cold (subfreezing) dry air is strong evidence against the diagnosis of asthma. False-positive results do occur. Nonspecific hyperreactivity has been demonstrated to occur after viral respiratory tract infections, inhalation of ozone, and in grain dust workers,[402,448,522] and their relationship to clinical asthma remains unclear.

Antigen Inhalation Tests. Specific antigens, inhaled chemicals, or dusts may be evaluated by inhalation of carefully prepared materials with graded doses. Some laboratories use complex, naturally occurring substances such as grain dust and cedar while others attempt to use the chemical constituent most likely to cause bronchospasm.[445,447] Individual responses are particularly difficult to predict when testing with organic dusts.

Occupational Asthma. Every month new industries, chemicals, and dusts are incriminated as the cause of bronchospasm. The usefulness of a search for occupational causes often relates to the extent of risk to a population rather than to a specific patient. If more than the expected number of persons develop symptoms of airways disease, the entire population may warrant careful and detailed studies. Provocation with suspect materials or increased prevalence of nonspecific hyperreactivity will require careful interpretation. When patients with known asthma regularly get increased bronchospasm at work (immediate response) or within 12 hours (nonimmediate response), their expiratory flow rates should be monitored with a portable device, 4 times per day, and for 5 to 7 days after removal from their work environment. Specific inhalation challenge may be redundant if work-related bronchospasm is demonstrated.

Drug Challenge. Perhaps the most hazardous and least controlled is the provocation test related to medications. When an anaphylactic reaction has been experienced, the medication should be avoided. If suspicion regarding an important therapeutic drug causes concern, carefully controlled drug challenge can be conducted.[447]

PATHOLOGICAL CHANGES ASSOCIATED WITH ASTHMA

Two very basic problems hamper a discussion of the morphologic correlates of asthma. First and most obvious, a clear definition of the disorder is not agreed upon, and the term is used in various ways by various investigators. Second, much of the data available from autopsy studies concern patients who have died of asthma and represent a rather small and perhaps morphologically and etiologically distinctive subset of patients with reversible airways disease. Nevertheless, a substantial amount of interesting and useful information has been accumulated.

The Bronchial Lumina

Material occupying the lumina of the airways has been studied at autopsy as well as in the expectorated sputum of patients with asthma.

In patients dying of status asthmaticus, there is generally a remarkable degree of obstruction of airways by viscid secretions. This observation has caused some consternation among clinicians seeking correlation between physiologic and pathologic changes. The abrupt onset and resolution of many asthmatic attacks is more readily explained if bronchial smooth muscle contraction is the cause of obstruction than if thick secretions must be implicated. Furthermore, the production of expectorated sputum is a rather minor aspect of the clinical syndrome in many, if not most, asthmatics.

A reasonable explanation, of course, would be that smooth muscle spasm, secretions and mucosal edema may all contribute to airway obstruction in asthmatics and that the predominance of each may vary among patients and in the same patient during different phases of illness.

Pathologic sections of lungs from patients with fatal asthma show extensive plugging with dense mucoid material from segmental bronchi as far distally as the respiratory bronchioles.[523] The noncellular component of this material stains nonhomogenously with hematoxylin and eosin, and probably is made up both of mucus produced by deep glands and goblet cells and of a protein-laden transudate from dilated submucosal capillaries. Eosinophilic polymorphonuclear leukocytes and shed mucosal epithelial cells are present in abundance; neutrophilic leukocytes are few.

Expectorated sputum from asthmatics, when examined for structural elements, shows qualitatively similar findings.[524,525] Eosinophilic rather than neutrophilic leukocytes are characteristic,[526–528] and associated crystalline structures known as "Charcot Leyden crystals" are thought to represent coalescence of free eosinophilic granules. Stained sputum smears[525] or unstained wet preparations[524] may be employed in looking for these elements.

Mucosal cells are shed in large numbers in asthma and may be identified in large, compact clusters recently referred to as "Creola bodies."[527] Bronchiolar casts composed of strips and laminae of sputum components assume a characteristic appearance in asthma and have long been known as "Curschmann's spirals."[524]

The Bronchial Wall

The shedding of ciliated bronchial mucosal cells observed in the lumina of bronchi from patients

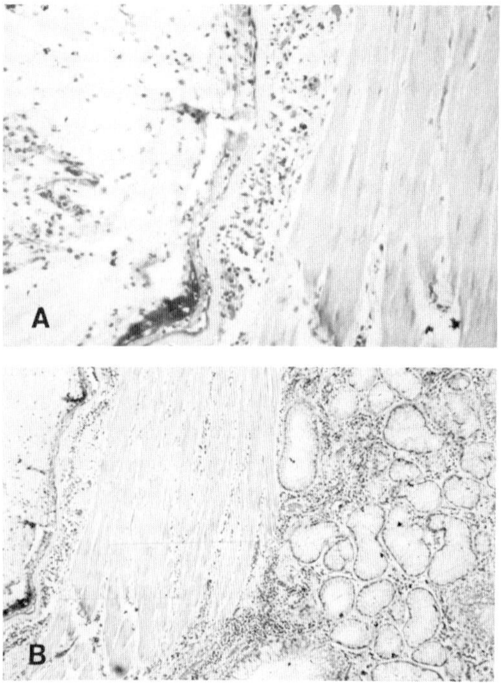

FIG. 14-10. Bronchial wall from patient dying of asthma. Note especially (A) thickened basement membrane and (B) hypertrophied smooth muscle and hyperplastic mucous glands.

who have died of asthma has been attributed to transudation of edema fluid from capillaries of the submucosa.[523] Areas of regeneration sometimes occur in the form of simple stratified epithelium. Thickening of the basement membrane (Fig. 14-10) and tissue infiltration with eosinophilic leukocytes have been described in both autopsy[523] and biopsy[524] material. Mucous glands have been reported to be increased in volume[530] and goblet cells increased in number.[529,530] Bronchial smooth muscle has been reported to be increased,[530–532] and one investigator has reported that this increase is due chiefly to hyperplasia rather than to hypertrophy of smooth muscle cells.[533] Mast cells are reportedly decreased in number and degranulated in asthma,[529] an especially interesting finding which supports the hypothesis that the release of chemical mediators from mast cells plays an important role in producing clinical manifestations of asthma.

Areas of cystic bronchiectasis occur in asthmatics, as often in upper as in lower lobes, perhaps occurring secondary to focal atelectasis.[523]

The Lung Parenchyma

Focal areas of atelectasis have been well documented in asthma,[523] and have a logical explanation in mucous plugging of bronchi.

Emphysema, if defined only as distention of lung, undoubtedly occurs in severe asthmatic attacks.[534] Destructive changes in alveolar walls probably do not occur as a consequence of asthma, even of long standing.[523,534–537] A long-held clinical belief that asthma is an important cause of emphysema presumably was a result of a broader application of the term asthma than is currently common.

MANAGEMENT

General Principles

Since the range of severity of asthma, as well as the cause, is varied, a rational approach to management must also vary from one patient to another (Table 14-10). The assortment of therapeutic measures which have been recommended in the medical literature over the years ranges far beyond rational flexibility. Perusal of the Index Medicus alone permits the inference that asthma must indeed sometimes remit in response to virtually any therapeutic intervention, or in response to none. This being the case, the critical clinician attempting to assess the role of any old or new therapeutic intervention in asthma should look carefully for well-controlled, preferably double-blind studies as evidence of real efficacy. Regrettably, such evidence is scanty or lacking, even for some of the relatively well accepted management measures described below.

Management of Mild Symptoms. In many asthmatic patients, precipitating factors cannot readily be identified or easily avoided, but symptoms are mild and infrequent. Treatment is needed only when symptoms occur or can be anticipated. In this group, inhaled sympathomimetic bronchodilators may provide adequate treatment with little inconvenience, and side-effects

TABLE 14-10. Drug Therapy of Asthma

Severity	Mode of therapy	Route of administration
Mild, intermittent symptoms	Sympathomimetic bronchodilators	Inhalation
Frequent or persistent symptoms	Sympathomimetic bronchodilators	Inhalation, oral, subcutaneous
	Methylxanthines	Oral
	Disodium cromoglycate	Inhalation
	Corticosteroids	Inhalation, oral
Severe asthma	Sympathomimetic bronchodilators	Inhalation
	Methylxanthines	Intravenous
	Corticosteroids	Intravenous, oral
	Oxygen	Inhalation
	Water	Oral, intravenous, inhalation
	Antibiotics	Oral, parenteral
	Mechanical ventilation—if all else fails	

which can be controlled and tolerated.[537a] Administration with a handbulb nebulizer or pressurized nebulizer is satisfactory, and these devices can be carried about easily for use when symptoms develop. Satisfactory relief within 10 to 20 minutes is usual, and the duration of effect is often greater than 2 hr. Administration prior to a recognized, unavoidable precipitating event may prevent or modify symptoms. The patient should be instructed about cardiac side-effects so that overuse may be avoided. Lack of response, or the need for repeated administrations at intervals of less than 2 or 3 hr should prompt a call for medical advice.

Oral theophylline or sympathomimetic preparations may play a role in treatment of mild, intermittent attacks in some patients, but the longer delay of onset of relief will usually prove to be an inconvenience. Occasionally, oral theophylline is a useful supplement to inhaled sympathomimetics, since the mode of bronchodilator action is different, and the two drugs are additive. Theophylline by rectal administration and epinephrine given subcutaneously are likewise inconvenient, and have no substantial advantages for most individuals.

Management of Frequent or Persistent Symptoms. In this group, continuous administration of oral or inhaled bronchodilators at 4- to 6-hr intervals is indicated. Pulmonary function abnormalities may be detectable in asthmatics even when symptoms and abnormal physical findings have resolved, and this residual abnormality is associated with increased responsiveness to asthmogenic stimuli. On the basis of this observation it may be desirable to place asthmatics on continuous therapy for as long as they have alterations in lung function.[538]

The benefits of inhaled agents for this purpose have been recently reviewed, and it can be argued that they represent a safe and effective approach.[539] Although a substantial amount of inhaled bronchodilator is absorbed and has a systemic effect, there appears to be some local effect with enhanced proportion of bronchodilation relative to cardiovascular effect. Another advantage of the inhaled route of administration of a B_2 agonist is that protection against exercise-induced asthma is far greater than can be achieved with oral administration.

When oral agents are used, there is evidence to suggest that many patients can be managed with doses of adrenergic agents or theophylline low enough to produce minimal or no side-effects.[540] It has been suggested[541] that therapy be started with a low dose of sympathomimetic (terbutaline, 2.5 mg or metaproterenol, 10 mg) or theophylline (aminophylline, 200 mg). If side-effects are troublesome, the first drug may be stopped and the other instituted. If symptoms are not controlled, the two types of drugs may be combined at low doses. Only when symptoms continue with the combination in low dose need higher doses with more potential for side-effects be instituted.

Another approach to combination therapy preferred by some clinicians is the use of a B_2 agonist in aerosol form together with oral theophylline. The advantage of the aerosol route of administration of B_2 agonists has been presented above.

Disodium cromoglycate may be added when bronchodilator therapy is inadequate to control symptoms. Its usefulness is sometimes substantial, but seems to vary from one patient to another. It has the disadvantage of high cost but the advantage of remarkably low toxicity.

The addition of corticosteroids must be considered when the above measures are inadequate for control. Nonabsorbable steroid aerosols have been shown to have an important role here, and to control symptoms in most patients at a dose which produces no systemic effects.[542] Side-effects are limited to local irritation with hoarseness, and a tendency to oral candidiasis which can be controlled with local antifungal medication. Systemic steroid therapy, given orally, may be necessary in some patients but the side-effects of long-term administration are well known to be a major drawback. Furthermore, the long-term management of persistent asthma is not so clearly benefited by steroids as is management of acute exacerbations. It is not unusual for dependence upon these agents to develop even though symptoms continue with their use. Alternate-day steroid therapy clearly is associated with less toxicity than a daily regimen, but asthmatic symptoms on the days off steroids are often intolerable.

Because of these considerations, systemic steroids should be reserved for exacerbations and withdrawn if possible; they should be continued chronically only when unavoidable.

Management of Severe Symptoms. Therapy in severe asthma accompanied by the danger signals described by Rebuck and Read[483] and described above should take place in a hospital, if possible in an intensive care unit under continual observation. Capability of intubation and mechanical ventilation is essential, should conservative measures fail. Intubation is clearly indicated when the patient is unconscious or in the event of cardiorespiratory arrest. Rebuck[483] has suggested that persistence of an arterial carbon dioxide tension above 70 mm Hg during therapy is another indication. Clinical judgment may suggest that mechanical ventilation should be instituted in an exhausted patient whose poor response to treatment falls short of these specific indications.

Therapy should include intravenous aminophylline as a continual infusion in a dose approximate to 1 mg/kg/hr in an adult; inhalation every 2 hours of a sympathomimetic bronchodilator; controlled oxygen, systemic hydration, and inhaled nebulized saline as indicated and tolerated. Antibiotics should be instituted if bronchial infection is suspected and chest physiotherapy should be considered if secretions are profuse or inspissated.

Corticosteroids should be used in substantial dosage. High doses are most clearly indicated if the patient has been maintained chronically on steroids. There is no clear scientific guide to minimal adequate dose. Rebuck and Read[483] have suggested 200 mg of hydrocortisone intravenously every 2 hours until danger signs have cleared, with concurrent commencement of 30 to 60 mg of prednisone daily by mouth.

Disappearance of some or all of the danger signs in this series usually occurred in a matter of hours, while the time to achieve the responsive phase required an average of 5 days, with substantial variation. Responsiveness was defined as the ability of inhaled bronchodilator to return the $FEV_{1.0}$ to near the patient's predicted normal.

Absence of danger signals permits some relaxation of degree of nursing supervision of the patient, and reliance upon oral rather than high-dose intravenous corticosteroids. Prolongation of the interval between inhalations of bronchodilator may be possible. Corticosteroids should not be reduced below a dose of 30 mg prednisone daily until a responsive phase is entered.

During the responsive phase of an attack, oral rather than intravenous theophylline is often satisfactory and 4-hr intervals between bronchodilator inhalations are usually satisfactory. Steroids need not be instituted, and may be carefully tapered.

It should be noted that disodium cromoglycate has no place in the acute management of an attack in asthma. This drug modifies the response to certain precipitating events subsequent to its administration. It is not an effective bronchodilator when given during an attack, and in fact the inhalation of the particulate-dosage form may stimulate bronchospasm acutely.

Management of Asthma with Associated Disease. Because it is so common, asthma is frequently symptomatic but undiagnosed in patients with other chronic disease. Patients with associated disease may need particularly understanding management of their asthma. Renal failure, inflammatory bowel disease, and innumerable nonpulmonary diseases provide no immunity from asthma, and therefore can result in mismanagement unless the possibility of coexistent asthma is considered. This diagnosis becomes even more difficult in patients with chronic bronchitis, emphysema, cystic fibrosis, diffuse parenchymal infiltrative diseases or heart failure, who may have co-existent asthma. In these patients a trial of therapy may be warranted.

Pregnancy is known to be associated with changes in symptoms in the asthmatic; however, about a third improve, a third deteriorate, and a third remain unchanged. Treatment is similar to that for nonpregnant patients except for avoidance of medications contraindicated in pregnancy (tetracycline, prostaglandins, iodine preparations), and diagnostic radiation.[543]

Hyperthyroidism has long been a recognized factor which aggravates asthma, which is conversely improved by hypothyroidism. Recent studies have demonstrated the improvement of nonspecific reactivity in a patient with asthma after treatment for hyperthyroidism.[544]

Avoidance of Precipitating Factors

A patient and thorough history should be taken to enable precipitating events to be identified to the greatest possible extent in each patient. Whether these events are emotionally stressful, or represent exposure to a specific allergen or to tracheobronchial irritants or physical exertion, their identification may be of greater importance in management of some patients than any pharmacologic maneuvers. If a thorough, conventional history is unrevealing, a search for subconscious conflicts by psychoanalysis or specific unsuspected allergens by skin-testing is much less likely to be rewarding.

Avoidance of precipitating factors may or may not be practical in an individual patient, and this sort of judgment can only be based on common sense, and participated in by both the patient and his physician. Avoidance of animal danders is often practical, while avoidance of seasonal pollens is more often not feasible. A move to another geographic location may achieve the latter goal, but at great cost to most patients, without assurance of a desirable response. Emotionally stressful situations may sometimes be avoidable, but certain minor stresses are part and parcel of a normal social existence and are necessary for gainful employment. Physical exertion may sometimes be easily modified, yet may be of such great importance to the happiness of a child or to the employment of an adult that drug management is more desirable than avoidance of exercise.

Psychotherapy

In some patients, emotional factors are so clearly associated with asthmatic attacks that the disorder seems truly to be a psychosomatic disease. In many others, anxiety, if not a trigger for, is a prominent symptom of bronchospasm. Not surprisingly, then, psychiatric interventions such as hypnosis[457] or behavioral modification[455,456] have been reported to produce a favorable response in some subjects with asthma. Physicians experienced in the treatment of the disorder would not rely solely upon such an approach or upon indepth psychotherapy or analysis in most patients, however. They would agree that attention to the possibility of emotional causes and complications in asthma is fundamental to good management, and that good rapport, counseling, and superficial psychotherapy may be of great help in many subjects.

Sedatives and Tranquilizers

Since anxiety is so commonly a complaint in patients with asthma, and so frequently seems to trigger attacks, the use of sedative or tranquilizer drugs has great and sometimes dangerous attraction for the physician and the patient. These agents may be used regularly by oral prescription in anxious patients, or parenterally in acute attacks of bronchospasm, in which case their use may occasionally be associated with dramatic relief of symptoms.

The use of sedatives and tranquilizers in asthmatics is controversial at best, however, and in some situations can be extremely hazardous. Experience suggests that a placebo effect may be operative in many cases of an apparently good response to these agents. And potentially undesirable side-effects include worsened bronchospasm due to histamine release in response to morphine; mucosal drying as a result of an atropine-like effect in phenothiazines; and respiratory center depression with virtually any central nervous system depressant.

Therefore, a reliance upon these agents in management of asthma should be discouraged. And, more importantly, parenteral use in severe asthmatic attacks should be resorted to in spontaneously breathing patients only if subsequent careful bedside observation is possible, and the physician has immediate access to resuscitative equipment.

If intubation and mechanical ventilatory assistance are imminent, or have been instituted in status asthmaticus, then heavy sedation is usually necessary, and does not affect the basic disease process adversely.

Immunotherapy

Immunotherapy refers to modification of the allergic response to an antigen by its parenteral administration in small but increasing doses. The discovery of immunotherapy was empiric, and the rationale for its use and evidence of its effectiveness were poorly documented for many years. Investigation over the last 20 years has provided reasonable support for its use in selected circumstances. Excellent recent reviews summarize this information.[545,546]

The asthmatic in whom immunotherapy can most convincingly be shown to be useful would appear to be the pollen-allergic extrinsic asthmatic in whom immediate, IgE-mediated allergy is operative. In this patient, the presence of atopy can be demonstrated by skin testing and the clinical importance of a specific allergen identified by clinical history or even by inhalation challenge. A preparation of the allergen suitable for injection can be made up and standardized. Controlled clinical trials have thus been possible in this type of patient, and the usefulness of immunotherapy has been documented.

The mechanism of action of immunotherapy in this type of situation is not entirely clear. Repetitive injections of antigen are associated with the development of an antigen-specific IgG antibody (blocking antibody) which combines with subsequently administered antigen and may play a role in preventing the interaction of IgE and antigen. Immunotherapy is furthermore associated with decreased levels of IgE, blunted seasonal increase in IgE, and reduced release of histamine from basophils. Results of recent studies suggest the generation of antigen-specific suppressor cells during allergy desensitization, a mechanism which could have broad implications.[547]

It is not surprising that the usefulness of immunotherapy in other forms of asthma is in doubt. One would not logically expect immunotherapy to be useful unless an antigen-antibody reaction is a cause of the disorder, and in fact, application of the therapy is not even possible unless a causative antigen can be identified and prepared in pure enough form for injection. Evaluation of immunotherapy in suspected allergy to bacterial substances and housedust has been hampered by difficulty in preparing satisfactory antigen for standardization.

Because of these considerations, the selection of a patient for immunotherapy should be made with discrimination. In particular, a positive skin test to a specific antigen should not alone be taken as an indication for hyposensitization. Atopic persons may demonstrate skin test reactivity to a number of antigens which have little or no clinical role in producing symptoms. The ability of an antigen to produce symptoms depends upon its presence in the environment, and upon the route and intensity of exposure. Bronchospasm generally results from inhalation rather than from ingestion or injection of an antigen. A history of symptoms upon inhalant exposure to a particular antigen should first be sought, and then skin-test reactivity to that antigen demonstrated as evidence that the symptoms are due to allergy, rather than a nonspecific irritant response. Such a combination of findings would provide good evidence that a trial of immunotherapy might be warranted. Further evidence for the role of a specific antigen in producing asthma can be obtained by inhalation challenge with the antigen, thus simulating exposure by the route which presumably is operative in the clinical setting.

In the absence of a history of symptoms on exposure to an identifiable antigen, application of a battery of skin test antigens may nevertheless be somewhat useful. Identification of the atopic state by demonstration of a number of positive tests will in itself clarify the diagnosis, and specific positive tests may guide further history taking and identification of a clinically important antigen.

Immunotherapy, once undertaken, is expensive and time-consuming. Injection of gradually increasing dosages of antigen over a period of weeks must be carried out. The degree of protection is correlated with the size of antigen dose reached. Duration of protection, once achieved, probably does not continue beyond a few months following discontinuation of treatment. Better clarification of optimum duration of treatment and duration of protection will be possible when a satisfactory measure of protection becomes available.

Sympathomimetic and Methylxanthine Bronchodilators

Sympathomimetic and methylxanthine bronchodilator drugs are the major agents available for treatment of symptomatic asthma, regardless of cause. A comprehensive and lucid review of these drugs[548] is strongly recommended to the reader interested in acquiring a fuller understanding of their clinical pharmacology. These agents are widely available in an assortment of analogues and dosage forms and are potent not only as therapeutic agents but in the production of side-effects as well, especially upon the cardiovascular system. In choosing a specific sympathomimetic agent, it should be considered that β- rather than α-adrenergic effects are sought for bronchodilation; and further, that some recently released drugs have a preferential β-2 (bronchial smooth muscle) rather than β-1 (cardiovascular) effect (Table 14-11,[376,549–560]). It is fortuitous that the alterations in cathechol nucleus and side chains which have produced β-2 selectivity also have produced drugs with other advantages. The newer drugs are resistant to monoamine oxidase (MAO) in the gastrointestinal tract, and therefore are effective when taken orally. They are also resistant to catechol-O-methyl transferase (COMT) in tissues and to MAO at nerve endings and therefore their action is prolonged. The methylxanthine drugs used for bronchodilation are all theophylline analogues,[561] and differ chiefly in theophylline content (Table 14-12)[562] and in rate of absorption (Table 14-13)[563] from the gastrointestinal tract. Slow absorption may be an advantage in providing constant blood levels, but enteric-coated preparations are sometimes so well coated as not to be absorbed at all.

The bronchodilator action of both these groups of drugs is thought to be mediated by production of increased tissue levels of cyclic AMP. Adrenergic agents achieve this increase by stimulating cyclic AMP synthesis by the enzymic action of adenylcyclase, while methylxanthines inhibit conversion of cyclic AMP to a noncyclic compound by phosphodiestrase. Increase in cyclic AMP, in turn, influences bronchial smooth muscle in two ways. It inhibits release of mediators of bronchoconstriction following antigen exposure, and it influences smooth muscle directly as well, favoring relaxation.[411] This dual effect of cyclic AMP supports the use of agents producing an increase in its tissue levels in cases of asthma produced by allergic responses.

In addition to bronchodilation, there is some evidence that both the adrenergic agents and the methylxanthines enhance mucociliary clearance. The clinical significance of this is not yet entirely clear, but a beneficial effect would be expected.[548] The evidence that adrenergic agents and methylxanthines influence cyclic AMP by different routes suggests that these agents might be useful in combination, and many clinicians

TABLE 14-11. Sympathomimetic Bronchodilator Drugs

Type	Drug	Usual route of administration	Average adult dose (mg.)	Approximate duration of action (hrs.)
Mixed α and β adrenergic	Ephedrine	Oral	25	3–4
	Epinephrine	Subcutaneous	0.1–0.5	4
		Intramuscular (suspension)	0.5–1.5	4
		Inhalation	0.25–0.6	2–3
Mixed β_1 and β_2	Isoproterenol	Inhalation	0.25–0.6	1–1.5
Predominant β_2	Isoetharine (available in combination with phenylephrine)	Inhalation	0.25–1.0	3–4 (in combination with phenylephrine)
	Orciprenaline (metaproterenol)	Inhalation	1.3–2.0	1–5
		Oral	20	4+
	Terbutaline	Subcutaneous	0.25	4+
		Oral	2.5–5.0	4+
	Salbutamol (albuterol)	Inhalation	0.1–0.2	4+
		Oral	2.0–5.0	4+
	Feneterol	Inhalation	0.1–0.4	up to 8
		Oral	5–10	6
	Carbuterol	Inhalation	0.1–0.2	4
		Oral	2–4	4+

TABLE 14-12. Content of Anhydrous Theophylline in Theophylline Formulations

Formulation	Percent anhydrous theophylline
Aminophylline (theophylline ethylenediamine)	85
Oxtriphylline (choline theophyllinate)	64.4
Theophylline NF (monohydrate)	91
Theophylline calcium salicylate	48
Theophylline sodium glycinate	50

Ellis EF, Eddy ED: Anhydrous theophylline equivalence of commercial theophylline formulations. J Allergy Clin Immunol 53:116, 1974

believe that this indeed true. However, if the therapeutic effects of these two groups are additive, it must be kept in mind that certain of their undesirable side-effects are additive, as well.

In mild or moderate symptomatic asthma, bronchodilators are generally used in oral and aerosol forms, since these routes are most practical for self-administration. They may be used on a regular basis, to provide as near continuous bronchodilation as possible; to treat symptoms as they occur; or immediately prior to events known to precipitate symptoms in the individual patient. The most appropriate regimen for a particular patient should be designed to his own needs, of course. In some patients the bronchodilator regimen may facilitate raising viscid secretions. In other cases, bronchodilator administration may facilitate subsequent administration of other agents by inhalation, including saline aerosol for liquification of sputum. The use of combined therapy with an oral or inhaled B_2 agonist together with a methylxanthine has been discussed above under Management of Frequent or Persistent Symptoms.

Ephedrine, terbutaline, metaproterenol, salbutamol, feneterol, carbuterol (Table 14-11), and a number of methylxanthine preparations (Tables 14-12, 13) are suitable for oral use in asthma, as well as in other obstructive diseases. Disadvantages of ephedrine, a mixed α- and β agonist, include a tendency to mucosal drying, and to produce urinary retention, the

TABLE 14-13. Peak Blood Levels after Oral Administration of Theophylline Preparations

Theophylline preparation	Time of maximum blood level (hrs.)
Alcohol-water solution of theophylline	1
Uncoated aminophylline tablets	2
Coated tablets of oxtriphylline (choline theophyllinate)	>4

Schluger J, McGinn JT, Hennessy DJ: Comparative theophylline blood levels following the oral administration of three different theophylline preparations. Am J Med Sci 233:296, 1957

latter primarily in elderly men. Methylxanthines produce nausea, anorexia, and vomiting primarily by a central effect which is related to blood levels of the drugs, and may produce seizures at very high blood levels, especially in children. A dosage equivalent to 1200 mg of aminophylline (theophylline ethylenediamine) over 24 hr, in divided doses at 4- to 6-hr intervals will produce a satisfactory serum level of 10 to 20 μg/ml in most adults, although considerable variation has been observed. A lower dose of 800 mg of aminophylline over 24 hours has been suggested as a starting dose in patients with mild symptoms. If a satisfactory therapeutic effect occurs, this regimen can usually be continued without the need for measurement of serum theophylline levels. Recently developed sustained release capsules may permit ingestion every 12 hours, with improved patient compliance. Both groups of drugs produce tachycardia, nervousness and insomnia, and tremulousness, all of which are dose-related. Terbutaline, fenterol, metaproterenol, and salbutamol are preferential β-2 agonists with longer action and less marked cardiovascular side-effects than ephedrine, but may produce a fine motor tremor by a peripheral effect on muscle. Most patients can achieve excellent therapeutic results with only minor, acceptable side-effects from the use of these drugs at appropriate dose levels, alone or in some combination.

The most commonly available proprietary combinations of bronchodilator drugs have certain disadvantages, although they are effective and have excellent patient acceptance. Most of these combinations contain ephedrine sulfate in an adequate therapeutic dose of 25 mg. Theophylline is usually present in a dose of about 100 mg, which is insufficient to produce a clinically useful effect in most patients. Therefore a usual dosage schedule, such as one capsule or tablet every 4 to 6 hr in an adult, will provide a satisfactory dose of ephedrine, but a suboptimal dose of methylxanthine. A dosage schedule of one of these combinations which would provide a good therapeutic blood level of theophylline will be prevented by ephedrine toxicity. The third component of most popular combination oral bronchodilators is a sedative, provided to modify the unpleasant effects of ephedrine. The sedative dose is a safe, conservative one in most combinations, and respiratory depression does not seem to be a problem when such a small dose is administered along with ephedrine. It should be kept in mind, however, that phenobarbital has been reported to induce hepatic enzyme systems to metabolize certain corticosteroids more rapidly.[564] Therefore, steroid dose adjustment may be indicated in asthmatic patients receiving both phenobarbital and corticosteroids.

Aerosol administration of sympathomimetic bronchodilator agents is convenient and popular. Motorized nebulizers, hand-bulb nebulizers and pressurized nebulizers are commercially available.

Fluorocarbon propelled nebulizers have aroused anxiety because of the increase in asthma mortality which accompanied their introduction in Europe and Great Britain, and because of studies suggesting a cardiotoxic property of certain fluorocarbons.[565,566] Recent analyses have suggested that this unfortunate effect may have been due to a specific nebulizer providing a very high dose of bronchodilator drug. This high-dose product was never marketed in the United States, where a rise in asthma mortality has not been observed. Recent reviews of data concerning these problems are reassuring about the safety of these nebulizers.[539,540]

Sympathomimetic drugs do, of course, have the potential for dangerous toxic effects. They produce cardiovascular responses which may include atrial and ventricular arrhythmias, and also may worsen hypoxemia by increasing pulmonary blood flow to poorly ventilated areas of lung in asthmatics. This latter effect is noted in a small but significant percentage of patients, and may be produced by aminophylline as well. Administration of supplemental oxygen is wise, therefore, when bronchodilator drugs are being used aggressively in the treatment of severe asthmatic attacks.[513] There is debatable evidence that overuse of aerosolized bronchodilators may lead to resistance to their therapeutic effect, or even a paradoxical worsening of bronchospasm.[567–571] Resistance and paradoxic response to isoproterenol has been most clearly demonstrated, and may in some cases be due to its rapid local metabolism by catechol-o-methyl transferase, and conversion to a compound which is a β-blocker. Other studies with terbutaline have shown no resistance or reduced bronchodilation with long-term use.[572,573]

Parenteral administration of bronchodilator drugs in asthma most often involves intravenous use of aminophylline or subcutaneous use of epinephrine in severe attacks in hospitalized patients. Intravenous aminophylline is especially valuable in this situation. Recent reviews of dosage schedules provide a useful guide.[574–582] An initial loading dose of 350 mg (about 5 mg/kg) followed by a continuous infusion of 800 to 1000 mg per 24 hr (about 0.5 mg/kg/hr) will achieve a safe therapeutic serum level (10 to 20 μg/ml) in most adults, although considerable variation in clearance of theophylline among patients has been demonstrated.[578–582] Earlier recommendations for a higher maintenance dose had been based on data which probably included many cigarette smokers, who have been recognized to eliminate theophylline more rapidly than nonsmokers.[580] Furthermore, recent data indicate that acutely ill patients, especially those with congestive heart failure or severe liver disease, eliminate theophylline still more slowly, and should be maintained with dosages of as low as 0.2 mg/kg/hr. Observation of the patient for therapeutic and toxic effects is essential and theophylline blood levels are useful if available.

Cardiac monitoring is desirable in severely ill patients receiving high doses of bronchodilator drugs since arrhythmias are important side-effects of both adrenergic and methylxanthine bronchodilators. Nausea and vomiting are troublesome side-effects of high blood levels of theophylline as well; and very high doses of this drug may produce seizures, especially in children.

It may be anticipated that further improvement in selective β-2 adrenergic drugs will be forthcoming, and that other classes of bronchodilator drugs will become available. Among promising possibilities are prostaglandin E, a potent smooth muscle relaxant, which is in the early stages of investigation[583] and nifedipine, a calcium antagonist.[583a]

Anticholinergic Bronchodilators

Although atropine has been used clinically for centuries, and vagal blocking agents are recognized to have an antiasthmatic effect, these drugs have not been greatly used by physicians to treat bronchospasm in recent decades. Some of this lack of popularity has been due to concern about side-effects, including possible drying of airway secretions.

Recently, there has been a revival of interest in atropine and in ipratropium bromide as bronchodilators[548,584–589] The effectiveness of these drugs appears greatest when given by the inhaled aerosol route and they have been shown to have a significant effect on bronchial smooth muscle in normal, asthmatic, and bronchitic subjects, with an acceptable duration of action. The effect is chiefly on the central, vagally innervated airways. The influence of these agents on histamine-induced bronchospasm is small compared with that of a β agonist, and they provide little protection against antigen challenge. Nevertheless, the mode of action on smooth muscle, which is to decrease the concentration of cyclic GMP, would be expected to complement the action of β agonists and methylxanthines and the future appears promising for anticholinergic bronchodilators. Their role in the treatment of asthma has not yet been well defined, however.

Disodium Cromoglycate (DSCG)

Disodium Cromoglycate (DSCG) was synthesized in 1965, in the course of a research program investigating analogs of the ancient antispasmodic drug, khellin. It has since been found that DSCG inhibits release of mediators of anaphylaxis from mast cells.[590–592]

In keeping with this mode of action, it can be shown that DSCG prevents bronchospasm if administered prior to specific antigen challenge in sensitized subjects, but that it is not effective in reversing bronchospasm produced in this way. It is of interest that the drug, when given prophylactically, also inhibits delayed Type III hypersensitivity, the occurrence of which seems to be dependent in some way upon a prior Type I reaction. DSCG has also been shown to inhibit postexercise bronchospasm, suggesting that mediator release from mast cells may be a mechanism in this phenomenon.[593] The drug provides protection against occupational asthma caused by a variety of agents including complex salts of platinum, piperazine, wood dusts, soldering fluxes, enzymes, and toluene diisocyanate.[594] It has also been shown to provide modest benefit in long-term therapy of aspirin-sensitive asthmatics.[595]

DSCG is administered by inhalation of the particulate drug from a specially designed device 4 times each day. Except for an occasional irritative response to the particulate aerosol, the drug is remarkably free of side-effects, and has rapidly gained acceptance as a useful adjunct to other asthma therapy. The bronchospasm induced by the aerosol in some patients can be prevented by administration of aerosolized bronchodilator 20 to 30 minutes before DSCG.

Although experimentally the inhibitory effect on the response to antigen challenge is prompt, and a 20% effect is still demonstrable after 18 hr, clinical improvement in established asthma may be delayed from 2 to 4 weeks. Because of the expense and inconvenience, DSCG is usually reserved for use in moderately severe asthma, not easily controlled with bronchodilators. The agent clearly has a useful role in decreasing or eliminating the need for steroids in difficult-to-manage patients. Although clear cut extrinsic asthma would logically be expected to be most responsive to DSCG, its usefulness does not seem to be limited to such subjects.[593–599]

Systemic Corticosteroids

The role of systemic corticosteroids in asthma is well established in clinical practice, although the mechanisms of their action in the disorder remain unclear, optimum dose is disputed, and limitations not well defined.[376]

Best supported by solid data is the use of steroids in the severely ill hospitalized patient with status asthmaticus. An early, well-controlled study by the British Medical Research Council showed an advantage of cortisone acetate over placebo in such a group.[600] A chronically ill group of asthmatic patients studied by the BMRC[601] also showed some benefit from cortisone acetate as compared with placebo, but this benefit was lost after 8 weeks of treatment. Nevertheless, difficulty was encountered in withdrawing steroid therapy or placebo in a substantial number of subjects!

The fascinating results of this 20-year-old study continue today to illustrate the extent of our practical knowledge of the usefulness of steroids in asthma, and the clinician continues to grapple with the problems it illustrates. Subjective and objective improvement is frequently dramatic when steroids are first used in acute and chronic asthma; withdrawal of steroids, or tapering to a dose below the equivalent of 10 mg per day of prednisone, is often met with exacerbations in patients with chronic, perennial bronchospasm. Long-term steroid therapy in these patients is often less than satisfying, with undesirable side-effects more apparent than remission of symptoms.

Steroid resistance is not uncommon,[564,602,603] and this phenomenon is partially explained by altered steroid metabolism. Whatever the mechanism, some clinicians strongly believe that high doses are frequently beneficial when lower doses fail. There is, however, no objective evidence as yet that a dosage higher than the equivalent of

60 to 80 mg of prednisone per 24 hr is advantageous in asthma.

Clinical debate about the relative advantages of various steroid preparations is not clearly resolved by objective data either, although differences in metabolic pathway and rate of degradation merit further study.

A reasonable approach, based upon present knowledge, would encourage the use of high doses of parenteral or oral steroids acutely in the severely ill patient. Chronic steroid use should be minimized and avoided whenever possible, making optimum use of other modes of therapy in attempts to obviate long-term corticoid treatment.

Intravenous or intramuscular corticosteroid in a dose equivalent to at least 20 mg prednisone, every 4 hours or less, is appropriate in treating a critically ill patient with status asthmaticus. Other investigators have suggested 200 mg hydrocortisone every 2 hr.[483,492] Continuous infusions may permit better control with less side-effects.[376] Oral steroid preparations are well absorbed, and may be initiated along with parenteral agents. In a severely, but not critically ill patient able to retain oral medications, 60 to 80 mg of prednisone or prednisolone per day is appropriate. Whenever steroids are used in asthma, optimum benefit should be sought early in the course, by intensive treatment, and tapering attempted after maximum improvement is achieved. Objective improvement is delayed, beginning 6 to 12 hr after initiation of the drug.[376,603a]

If a complete remission is achieved, as documented by symptomatic and spirometric evidence, after a brief (2 to 3 days) steroid burst, rapid taper or even abrupt discontinuance may be possible. Tapering should not be attempted unless at least a stable chronic level of bronchospasm has been achieved, and if this sort of result is deemed the best hoped for in a refractory patient, rapid taper to about 10 mg per day of prednisone is usually possible. Reduction to a lower maintenance dose in a refractory patient is usually difficult, and should be carried out in small decrements with close observation, in a hospital if at all practical. The lowest possible maintenance dose should be sought, and an alternate-day dose adopted if possible, since such a regimen clearly minimizes steroid side-effects. Alternate day steroid therapy is often unsatisfactory in asthmatics because of exacerbation of symptoms on days off the drug, however.

Precautions related to steroid toxic effects are important in asthma as well as in any other disorder in which chronic steroid therapy is adopted. Details of these toxic effects are beyond the scope of this discussion.[376]

Steroid Aerosols

Aerosol administration of corticosteroids in asthma has previously not offered great advantage over oral use, because most aerosol forms are well absorbed and are capable of producing systemic side-effects. The recent development of aerosol steroid agents (beclamethasone dipropionate and triamcinolone acetonide) which are not systemically absorbed is encouraging, and these agents are preferred in any asthmatic in whom chronic steroids are unavoidable.[542,604–606] The possibility of systemic steroid withdrawal effects must be taken into account when nonabsorbable aerosol steroid is substituted for an oral preparation in a chronic steroid user. In general, it appears that aerosolized steroids can be substituted for systemic steroids in most patients needing less than 10 mg of prednisone daily; and that substantial dose reduction is possible in those needing higher doses. Inhaled beclamethasone may be supplemented by systemic steroids during exacerbations, as it is more effective in preventing attacks than in treating acute episodes. Patients with general atopy may have recurrent allergic rhinitis when administration by inhalation replaces systemic steroids. The major undesirable side-effect is oropharyngeal moniliasis.

A frequent dosage schedule is two puffs of an aerosol (50 μg/puff) 4 times a day. One investigator has suggested that when this dose is ineffective, larger doses are often no more beneficial.[606] Some patients do benefit from higher doses, and some evidence suggests that up to 1600 μg per day can be used without systemic toxicity.[542]

Oxygen

Since hypoxemia is usual in asthma, and may be life-threatening in severe attacks, oxygen supplementation is an important treatment modality. The usual caution should be employed to avoid unnecessary risk of oxygen overdose, but in case of inability to obtain arterial blood gas determinations, and doubt as to appropriate dose, oxygen should be given to increase inspired concentration to 25 or 30%. Respiratory depression because of unresponsiveness to carbon dioxide as a ventilatory stimulus is not the rule in an acute attack of asthma, although it is frequent in an acute exacerbation in a patient with chronic bronchitis and emphysema. Hypoxemia is a greater acute risk in an asthmatic patient than is respiratory depression, and it is wise to err on the side of oxygen administration in case of doubt.

Liquefaction of Sputum

Adequate hydration is a basic need in severe asthma, when secretions may be tenacious and difficult to clear. Parenteral fluids should be used if oral intake is limited.

Inspired air or oxygen should always be humidified and nebulization of particles of saline may be useful. Unfortunately, nebulized aerosols may stimulate bronchospasm in some asthmatics. Concurrent use of bronchodilators may permit aggressive use of saline aerosols.

Addition of detergents to aerosolized fluids is of little use, and mucolytic enzymes are usually impractical because they stimulate bronchospasm in asthmatics.

The value of expectorants such as iodides and glyceryl guaiacolate is uncertain in asthmatics, as in other patients. This topic is discussed under Management of COPD. Bronchopulmonary lavage has been reported as a useful adjunct in severe asthma but cannot currently be considered widely applicable since its use requires special expertise.

Physical Measures

Postural drainage and percussion appear to be of benefit for some severe asthmatics in whom clearance of secretions is a problem. Breathing exercises seem to be of relatively little value for this group of patients. Adherence to a slow, deep ventilatory pattern, and expiration against pursed lips is sometimes useful during an acute attack, and may be of use in long-term management of an occasional severe perennial asthmatic.

A formal program of general conditioning exercises is occasionally useful, and may be facilitated by prophylactic use of bronchodilators in patients with postexercise bronchospasm.

Mechanical Ventilation

Mechanical ventilatory support is a last resort in management of status asthmaticus. Aggressive medical therapy early in the course of the disease will reduce the need for ventilation to a small number of exceptionally resistant patients.[488–491] The complications of mechanical ventilation occur much more frequently in asthmatic patients. Pneumothorax, pneumonia, inadequate ventilation, tube malfunction, and machine failure occurred 3 to 8 times more frequently than in patients ventilated for other diseases in one series [606a] and 8 of the 19 patients died.

This observation should not, however, cause undue reluctance to use this form of treatment, when acute respiratory acidosis due to asthma is unresponsive to more conservative measures. Without doubt, mechanical ventilation can occasionally preserve life in an asthmatic patient until the attack has resolved, either spontaneously or as a result of treatment.

The principles of mechanical ventilatory support are discussed under Acute Respiratory Failure. Certain special problems associated with asthma require comment, however. Intubation is often especially difficult in asthmatic subjects who are fearful and severely dyspneic, and who may respond to attempts at endotracheal tube placement by struggling and by worsening of bronchospasm. Sedation in such a situation may be life-threatening unless a bag and mask are available to sustain life until an endotracheal tube is in place. An anesthetist or other physician skilled in such techniques should be available if possible.

Once a tube is placed, its presence sometimes tends to maintain bronchospasm by irritation of laryngeal and other superficial sensory receptors. Heavy sedation is then indicated.

High inspiratory pressures are often needed in order to overcome high airways resistance, and a slow respiratory rate is usually necessary because expiration is slow. Large tidal volumes usually permit adequate ventilation in spite of these problems.

Miscellaneous Treatment Measures

Among the many measures which have been proposed for treatment of asthma over the centuries, a few of limited, occasional, or uncertain value have sufficient current interest to require mention. Asthmatics have been especially subject to the claims of various forms of quackery over the years; and even the "scientific" literature is laden with reports of uncontrolled trials of bizarre forms of therapy, usually said to be successful. The need for blinded control studies before a final conclusion about the usefulness of a new form of treatment is reached, is nowhere more evident than in the case of asthma, because of the strong placebo response in patients with the disorder. The well controlled British Medical Research Council study[601] of the use of cortisone acetate in asthma reflects this observation. Of 49 patients begun on this drug, 33 remained on the drug at the end of 12 weeks in spite of efforts to stop; and of 47 patients treated with placebo, in 27 cases the placebo could not be discontinued.

The experience of the past few years with glomectomy is likewise an example of the pitfalls of uncontrolled evaluation of a therapeutic measure in asthma. For a short time, unilateral cervical glomectomy enjoyed great popularity based on uncontrolled observations of its benefits. Blinded control studies, when finally carried out, quickly dampened enthusiasm for its use,[407,408] but not before thousands of patients had been operated upon.[406] Subsequently, bilateral glomectomy appeared with adherents showing enthusiasm similar to that previously reserved for the unilateral procedure, and debate about the merits of the procedure continue.[607,608] An especially thorough review of this and other surgical procedures which have been used in asthma is available.[609] It would appear that the bilateral procedure produces ablation of the ventilatory response to hypoxia and decreased exercise hyperpnea which might explain a decrease in dyspnea in some patients.[610,611] Some danger might be attendant upon ablation of the hypoxic ventilatory response, however.

Antihistamines once appeared to have great promise as a pharmacologically specific group of agents for treatment of allergic disease. Regrettably, antihistamines have proven of virtually no use in asthma, perhaps because of insufficient concentrations achieved, or because of mediators of bronchospasm other than histamine which are operative.[424] These drugs have the adverse effect of drying the mucosa and their use should be avoided in asthmatics, especially those in whom viscid sputum is a clinically observable problem.

Antibiotics should be used when evidence of bronchopulmonary infection accompanies an asthmatic attack. No valid generalization is possible about the role of *bacterial* infection as a causative factor in asthma. Purulent sputum containing neutrophilic rather than eosinophilic leukocytes should be considered evidence of infection which must be treated as a possible contributory factor to an asthmatic attack.

An assortment of anesthetic agents have been occasionally helpful in breaking asthmatic attacks. Among these, ether has received frequent mention, and rectal administration of this agent has sometimes been effective. The bronchorrhea produced may explain its reported success in status asthmaticus.

Sodium bicarbonate has been suggested as an occasionally life-saving agent when refractory asthma is accompanied by acidosis. This mode of therapy has a rational basis, in that acidosis interferes with the action of catecholamines. Since the advent of mechanical ventilation, it is perhaps wiser in most cases to correct respiratory acidosis by this means, as an alternative to imposing a bicarbonate load which will result in metabolic alkalosis once the bronchospasm is relieved.

A variety of less commonly used modalities have been recently reviewed.[376]

BRONCHIECTASIS

Bronchiectasis is, by definition, a morphologic change consisting of the persistent abnormal dilatation of bronchi. It may occur diffusely throughout the tracheobronchial tree or it may be localized to a segment or a lobe. It may be associated with troublesome symptoms of chronic productive cough, recurrent pneumonia, or intermittent hemoptysis, or may be asymptomatic, and have no clinical importance.

Several specific causes of bronchiectasis are recognized but the condition may also be extensive and symptomatic in patients in whom a specific cause cannot be identified. Prior to about 1940, these patients were commonly seen in the practice of chest medicine, and generally faced a poor prognosis with chronic debilitating illness. Surgical resection of localized ectatic disease provided the only possibility of cure, and medical management was unsatisfactory at best. This "syndrome" of idiopathic, symptomatic bronchiectasis has become less common and much more easily managed since the advent of antibiotic chemotherapy. In many patients, in fact, control of symptoms is readily achieved with management similar to that of chronic bronchitis, and the differentiation of these two conditions is of little importance. Occasionally, however, localized bronchiectasis amenable to surgical resection produces clinical problems of a magnitude justifying this approach, and a thorough diagnostic evaluation becomes important.

Roentgenographic examination of the tracheobronchial tree, after instillation of a radiopaque medium, is a definitive part of the diagnostic evaluation of bronchiectasis, although this procedure need not be performed in every patient in whom the diagnosis is entertained. If symptoms are mild and easily controlled by conservative therapy, bronchography will not influence management of an individual patient, though localized or diffuse ectatic changes may be present. If symptoms are severe, and history, chest roentgenographs, and pulmonary-function evaluation indicate diffuse bronchiectasis in a patient with respiratory insufficiency, bronchography would add little to management since surgical resection is clearly impractical. Occasional cases are seen in which chronic productive cough, recurrent pneumonia, or hemoptysis are significant and poorly responsive to medical therapy, and in which respiratory reserve and general medical condition warrant consideration of surgery. In such cases, bronchography should be carried out to prove the presence of bronchiectasis and to demonstrate that it is localized and amenable to resection.

CLASSIFICATION

A simple and useful morphologic classification of bronchiectasis is that of Reid,[612] who describes *cylindrical* dilatation, *saccular* dilatation, and an intermediate, irregular form of ectatic change referred to as *varicose* (Figs. 14-11, 14-12, 14-13, 14-14). Reid's description of these forms includes correlation of bronchographic findings with the results of gross and microscopic pathologic examination, and provides a review of other more cumbersome systems of classification. Since the information concerning etiology provided by more complex classifications is rather limited and not widely agreed upon, other terminology will not be discussed. The reader interested in pursuing this topic further is referred to the paper by Whitwell[613] whose classification is employed in the pathology text by Spencer,[614] and in the paper by Reid.

Of major interest to the clinician is the observation that cylindrical dilatation of the bronchi may occur transiently following episodes of pneumonia; this has been referred to as *reversible* bronchiectasis,[615–617] since saccular, or *true* bronchiectasis is generally not reversible. A decision to surgically remove a bronchiectatic lobe or segment should not be based on cylindrical changes seen on bronchograms done during the first four months following an episode of pneumonia. Morphology, as defined by bronchography, does not provide an absolute means of

(*Text continues on P. 747*)

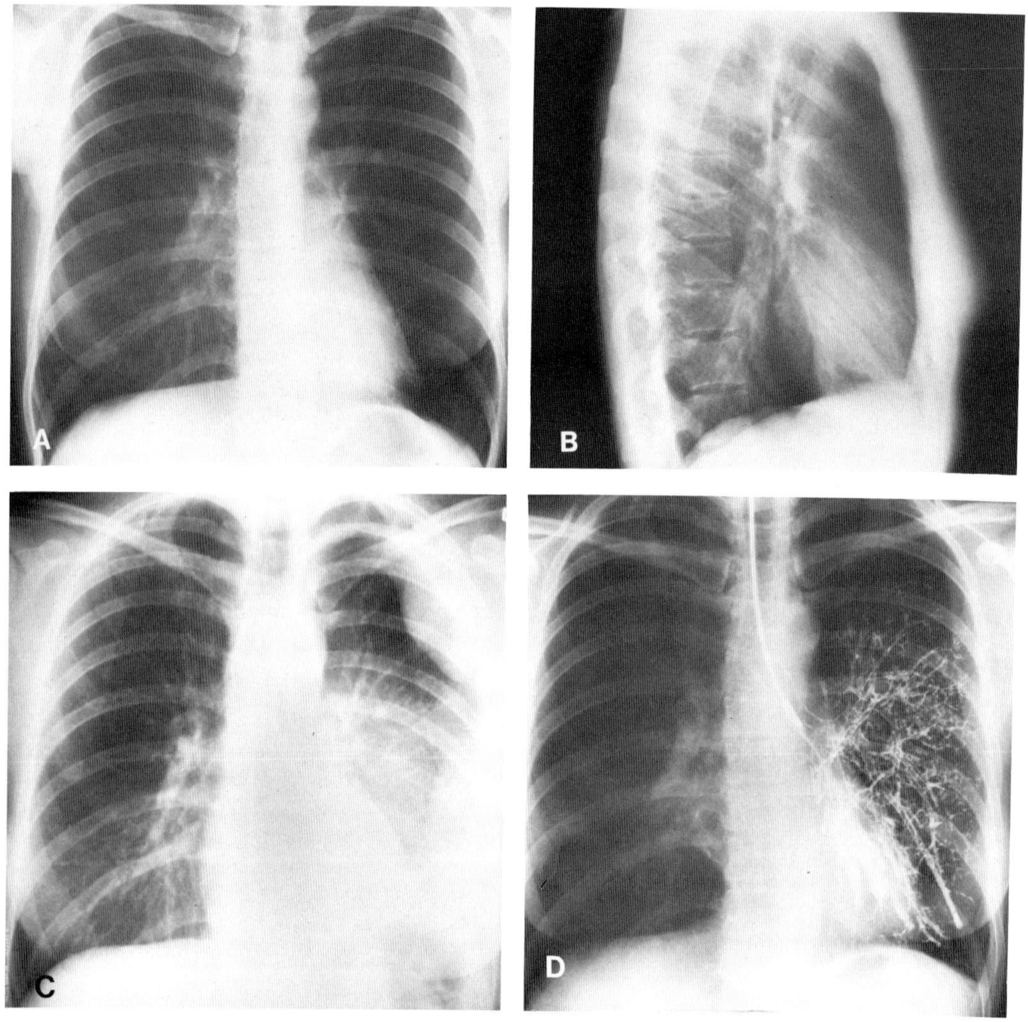

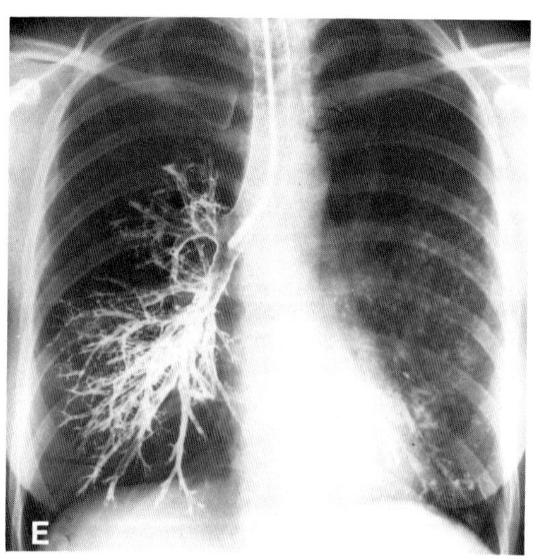

FIG. 14-11. Localized bronchiectasis of left lower lobe complicated by pneumonia and empyema. (**A**) Posteroanterior and (**B**) lateral roentgenograms of the chest during a clinically stable period show increased bronchial markings in retrocardiac area suggestive of bronchiectasis. **C.** Posteroanterior roentgenogram during an episode of bronchopulmonary sepsis shows complicating pneumonia and empyema. **D.** Bronchograms demonstrate crowding and ectasia, with advanced cylindrical and early cystic changes, localized to the left lower lobe. The remainder of the tracheobronchial tree is normal (**E**).

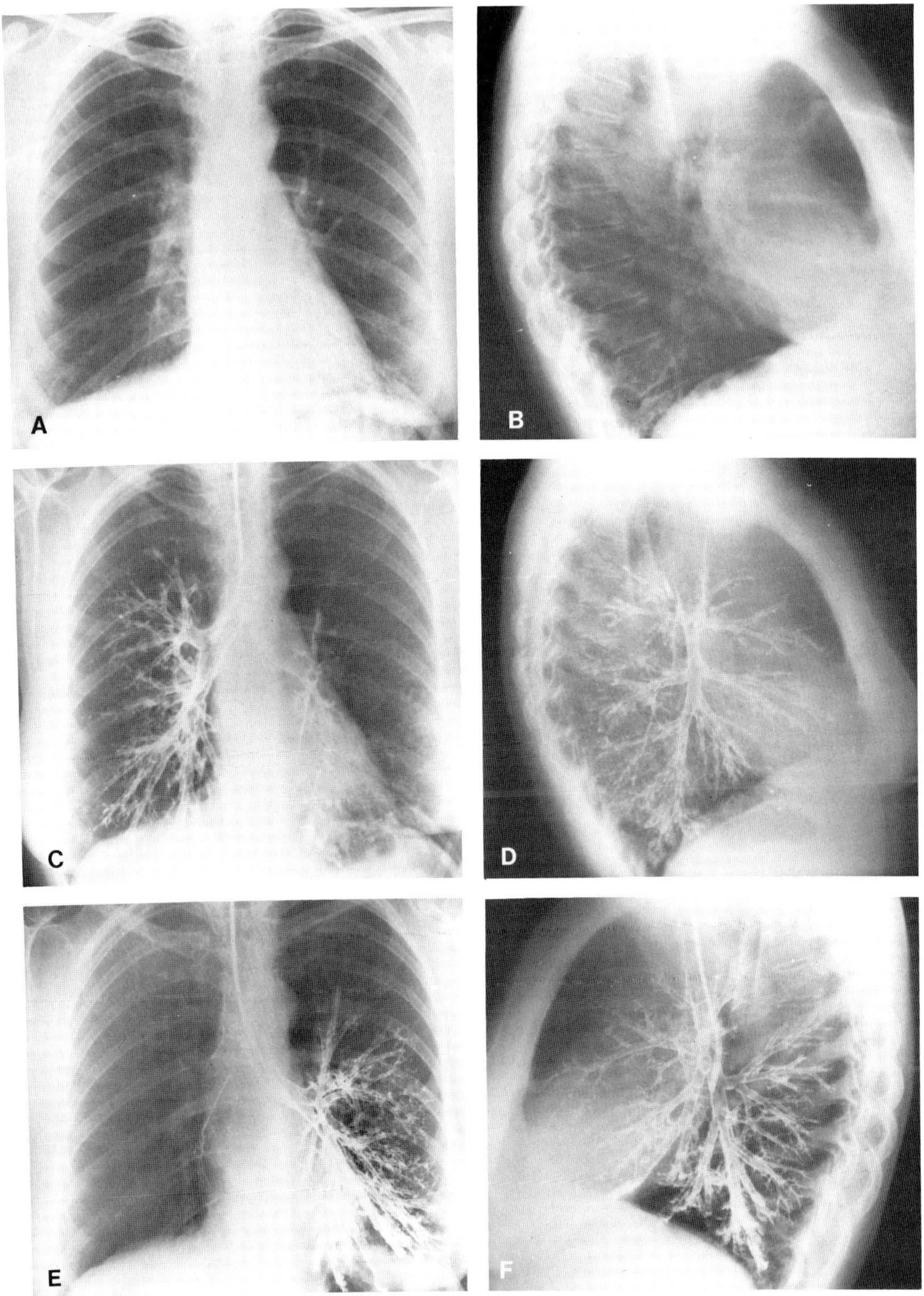

FIG. 14-12. Bilateral cylindrical bronchiectasis. Plain chest roentgenograms show increased peribronchial markings to posterior portions of lower lobes. Bronchograms confirm presence of cylindrical bronchiectatic changes in basilar segments of lower lobes. **A.** Posteroanterior plain film. **B.** Lateral plain film. **C,D,E,F.** Bronchograms.

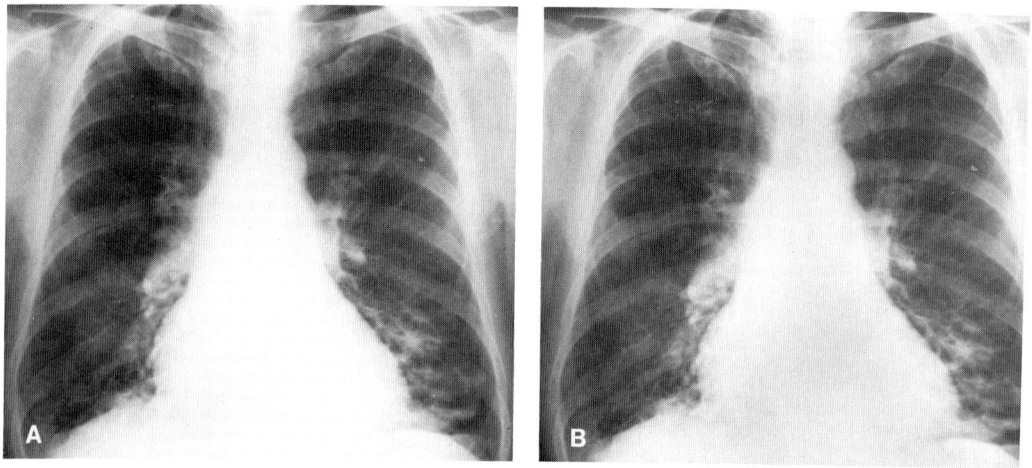

FIG. 14-13. Bilateral cystic bronchiectasis. This sequence of plain chest roentgenograms shows changes which, in combination with a compatible clinical history, are virtually diagnostic of bronchiectasis. The cystic areas in the lower zones are accompanied by air-fluid interfaces which appear and disappear repeatedly as effective antibiotic therapy and postural drainage produce changes in chronic sputum production. **A.** Exacerbation with presence of interfaces; **B.** clinical improvement with disappearance of air-fluid interface.

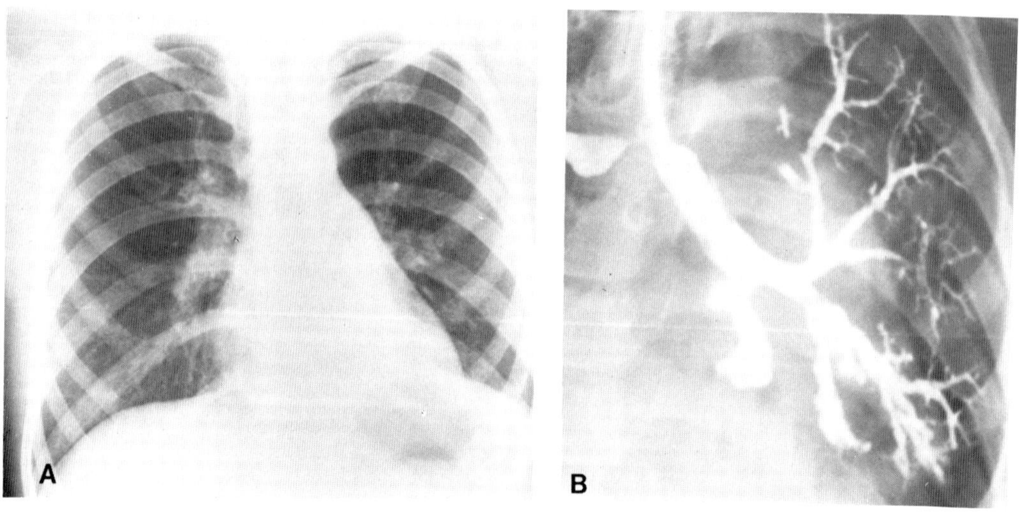

FIG. 14-14. Cylindrical, varicose, and cystic bronchiectasis. **A.** Plain chest roentgenogram in posteroanterior projection shows increased bronchovascular markings and a retrocardiac density suggestive of left lower lobe atelectasis in this child with a history of recurrent pneumonia. **B.** Enlargement of bronchogram of tracheobronchial tree on the left shows cystic dilatation of lower lobar bronchus without filling of basilar segmental bronchi. Cylindrical and varicose changes are present in the segmental bronchi of the lingula, and minimal cylindrical changes in the segmental bronchi of the upper lobe.

determining reversibility, since cylindrical change may persist, and early saccular change has been shown capable of reversal.[618]

Bronchograms in cylindrical bronchiectasis demonstrate failure of the lumina to taper normally; but there is no increase in diameter peripherally. The walls are in general regular, the bronchi end squarely and abruptly, and finer bronchi and bronchioles may not be visible. Mucus plugging and edema of walls of the airways are partially responsible for the failure of smaller branches to fill with radiopaque medium. The number of generations of branching present is reduced from the normal of about 17 to an average of 7, according to Reid.[612]

In varicose bronchiectasis, irregularity of the bronchial shadows is produced by constrictions and dilatations which deform the air passages. In Reid's series, still fewer subdivisions could be seen by bronchography, and obliteration by fibrous tissue supported this finding, as shown by correlative microscopic study.

Saccular bronchiectasis was seen bronchographically as termination of the bronchi in large ballooned structures beneath the pleural surface. No more than 5 subdivisions could be identified on bronchograms.

Etiologic Factors in Bronchiectasis

Congenital anomalies
Defects of cilia
Cystic fibrosis
Immunologic deficiency
Infection: Measles
Pertussis
Tuberculosis
Obstruction
Atelectasis
Corrosive gases

ETIOLOGIC CONSIDERATIONS

Bronchiectasis has a number of well-recognized causes and predisposing factors. It also occurs commonly in localized or diffuse, symptomatic or asymptomatic form, without discernible cause, and in this circumstance is presumed to have arisen from an unrecognized episode of bronchopulmonary infection, perhaps occurring coincidentally in a patient with a structurally weak tracheobronchial tree.

Congenital Anomalies

Localized or diffuse idiopathic bronchiectasis first recognized later in life may occasionally date from birth, although this can usually not be proved or disproved. Pulmonary sequestration is a localized congenital anomaly which may be associated with bronchiectasis.

A syndrome has been described in which bronchiectasis co-exists with lymphedema and yellow nails.[619] The cause is unknown, and onset has not been observed prior to age 10 years, but a congenital origin is a possibility. The Williams-Campbell syndrome is a congenital defect of cartilage in which bronchiectasis is a result.[620,621]

Immotile Cilia Syndrome

The significant association of bronchiectasis with sinusitis and situs inversus has been recognized at least since a description by Kartagener (1933),[622] and the combination of findings is usually referred to as *Kartagener's syndrome*, or triad. The first reported case of bronchiectasis associated with situs inversus has been attributed to Siewert, in 1903.[623]

Subsequent studies have indicated that bronchiectasis occurs in 15 to 25% of patients with situs inversus, strongly suggesting a congenital etiology for the bronchiectasis in these subjects.[623–627] The studies of Holmes and associates[625] suggest that the syndrome is inherited as an autosomal recessive trait.

Recent studies have demonstrated immotile cilia in the bronchial mucosa in such patients, presumably causing recurrent infection through impaired clearance mechanisms.[628,629] Clearance of inhaled radioactive particles is impaired, and ciliated cells in the nasal and bronchial mucosa, and spermatazoa demonstrate structural defects of cilia. Viewed by electron microscopy, the abnormalities include absent dynein arms, defective radial spokes, and clumping of fibrils. The diagnostic characteristics, range of patients affected, and clinical presentation of this "immotile cilia syndrome" will be of great interest during coming years. Although patients with Kartagener's syndrome are probably all affected, many patients without situs inversus have now been identified.[630–633]

Male patients are infertile, although fertility is normal or nearly so in female patients. Sinusitis, otitis, and recurrent lower respiratory tract infections are all related to the impaired clearance of respiratory epithelium. At present, no specific treatment is known (see also Chap. 8).

Cystic Fibrosis

Another hereditary disorder associated with bronchiectasis is cystic fibrosis of the pancreas, or mucoviscidosis. This disorder was first reported by Fanconi in 1936,[634] and was later extensively studied by Andersen.[635,636] Increasing awareness of this primarily pediatric problem in adolescents and adults has prompted discussions of manifestations in these older age groups.[637–642] Although the basic defect is unknown, mucoviscidosis affects exocrine glands, and most of its clinical manifestations can be explained by secretions which obstruct secretory ducts and organ passages. Studies attempting to define specific defects in mucins and glycoproteins in these patients have not been entirely convincing, however.[642] Pancreatic exocrine insufficiency and COPD frequently dominate the clinical presentation, and glucose intolerance occurs but is less frequent and severe: Intestinal obstruction and biliary cirrhosis may also occur.

Mucoviscidosis is inherited as an autosomal recessive trait, and presents no identifiable clinical or laboratory manifestations in heterozygotes, who make up about 5% of the white population. The disease occurs in only about one in 2000 white births, and once in 17,000 births in the black population.[641] Although the incidence is the same for males and females at birth, females have a higher mortality rate, and in some series of older patients there is a significant preponderance of men. The secretory abnormality which most readily provides a laboratory means of confirming a clinical diagnosis is one of relatively little clinical consequence: a high concentration of sodium and chloride in sweat.[642] A sweat chloride concentration greater than 60m Eq/L is generally considered diagnostic, although there is some increase in normal values with age, and interpretation of a borderline value may be difficult in an adult. It has been pointed out, however, that most patients with the disorder have values which clearly separate them from normal; and the chief hindrance to interpretation of the test is imprecision in its performance.[644,645] Proper induction of sweating, collection, and measurement of electrolyte concentrations have several pitfalls. It is recommended that sweating be induced by iontophoresis of pilocarpine into the skin by the technique of Gibson and Cooke,[646] and that sweat be collected by placing filter paper covered by plastic over the area of skin containing pilocarpine. The filter paper is quickly placed into a glass jar to prevent evaporation and the quantity of sweat assessed by weight. The sweat is then leached into distilled water, and the sodium or chloride concentration measured by an accurate technique. The entire test should be carried out in duplicate, on separate days, on at least 100 mg of sweat, by a laboratory experienced in its performance.

The diagnosis of mucoviscidosis is generally made by an abnormal sweat chloride concentration in the presence of clinical evidence of malabsorption from pancreatic exocrine insufficiency, or chronic obstructive pulmonary disease, or a family history of the disorder. Occasionally it may be desirable to confirm the presence of pancreatic insufficiency by collecting duodenal fluid and measuring the volume and concentration of proteolytic enzymes and bicarbonate.

The phenomenon of high electrolyte concentration in sweat appears to be due to the presence of a substance referred to as *sodium reabsorption inhibitory factor.*[647] It is of little clinical importance unless prolonged exposure to high temperature results in sodium chloride depletion. Measuring this factor requires a complex bioassay and is not practical for clinical diagnostic purposes. Likewise, serum and saliva from mucoviscidosis patients contain a substance which inhibits ciliary function in some experimental preparations, but the possible diagnostic and pathogenetic significance of this *ciliary dyskinesia factor* (CDF) is not clear.[642,644,651,651a]

Clinical manifestations of mucoviscidosis may commence with intestinal obstruction present at birth due to meconium plugs in the small intestine. Treatment of this condition may require surgical intervention, but instillation into the bowel of radiographic contrast material of high osmolarity has been reported to be therapeutic as well as diagnostic.[648] Rectal prolapse is also common in early life. A recent review of 75 adults with mucoviscidosis reported 48 episodes of intestinal obstruction in 21 patients.[641] This obstruction was due to intussusception, or "meconium ileus equivalent," and was often relieved following enemas of diatrizoate sodium. The need for surgery was not uncommon, however.

The development of malnutrition due to pancreatic insufficiency and malabsorption may be delayed, as may the onset of chronic pulmonary disease. Diagnosis and early treatment is of considerable importance and may further delay the onset of chronic illness. Pancreatic enzyme replacement therapy, physical measures to improve clearance of tracheobronchial secretions, and prompt treatment of respiratory infections are the major measures to be instituted. Although some patients with cystic fibrosis die in infancy or childhood, the prognosis is improved substantially with treatment. Di Sant 'Agnese recently estimated a mean survival age of 15 to 20 years, and reported his oldest surviving patient to be 42 years of age. Genetic counseling of heterozygotes is not usually possible until mating has produced an affected child, since screening has not been perfected. Sweat chlorides are normal in heterozygotes, and attempts to identify them by various techniques including studies of metabolism of skin fibroblasts have not been entirely successful,[642] although attempts continue.[642a,b] The risk of disease in offspring of two heterozygotes is one in four. Fertility in homozygous men and women is greatly reduced, but fertility in men and pregnancy in women have been observed.[649,650]

The pulmonary disease of cystic fibrosis has generally been considered the result of inadequate clearance of tracheobronchial secretions due to their increased viscosity and the result of the presence of a substance in serum which is capable of interfering with normal ciliary function.[651] Infection, particularly with *Staphylococcus aureus* and *Pseudomonas aeruginosa*, is often seen, presumably mostly facilitated by this poor clearance. Resistance to extrapulmonary infection is normal in these patients. Recent studies actually demonstrating normal rates of clearance of particles from the tracheobronchial tree raise questions about this theory of pathogenesis.[642,652,653]

Nevertheless, mucus plugging and infection do occur, and subsegmental bronchiectasis and bronchiolectasis characterize the pulmonary disease in mucoviscidosis.[654] Involvement of the upper lobes is characteristic in this disease[655,656] (Fig. 14-15), unlike usual idiopathic bronchiectasis, which preferentially affects the lower lobes. Pulmonary pathophysiology is that of bronchiectasis, with an obstructive ventilatory pattern, poor compliance, and elevated flow resistance. Residual volume is variably increased, generally without increase in total lung capacity.[657–660] Impaired intrapulmonary gas mixing is seen[661] with increased closing volume[662] and frequency dependence of compliance,[663] and regional abnormalities of lung function are demonstrable with xenon techniques even when routine tests of pulmonary function are normal.[664] Hypoxemia and sometimes hypercarbia occur, eventually complicated by cor pulmonale.[665–668]

A closer examination of manifestations of mucoviscidosis in adults seems appropriate, since internists are caring for increasing numbers of these patients. This trend is probably due both to longer survival of pediatric patients, who often died before the age of 5 or 10 years before early and aggressive treatment was emphasized; and to increasing recognition that some patients have delayed onset of symptoms and may not be diagnosed until late adolescence or early adulthood. A recent review of 30 adult patients in the literature pointed out that many had survived into the third decade of life and some into the fourth, and that a few patients were asymptomatic when diagnosed in adulthood.[611]

Important observations from this review are that in older patients with mucoviscidosis, the predominant symptoms were related to pulmo-

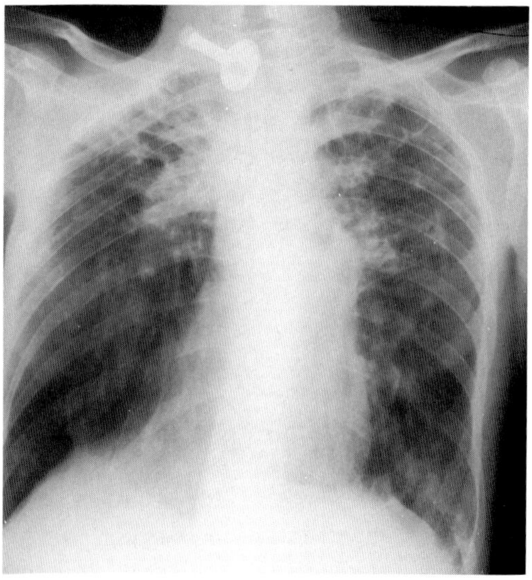

FIG. 14-15. Cystic fibrosis. This plain chest roentgenogram taken in the posteroanterior view shows extensive post-inflammatory changes in the predominant upper zone distribution characteristic of the bronchiectasis associated with cystic fibrosis.

nary disease rather than to malabsorption, and that the parents might be tall, well developed, and well nourished in appearance. When weight loss occurred it was related to severity of lung disease rather than to malabsorption. There was usually laboratory evidence of pancreatic exocrine insufficiency (95%), however, and the occasional occurrence of intestinal obstruction with intussusception has already been pointed out. It seems reasonable to consider that adequate replacement therapy with pancreatic enzymes might prevent recurrence of this complication. Pancreatic extracts also appear to be effective in reducing fecal bile losses and the lithogenic effect of bile. Since they are only partially effective in reducing steatorrhea, supplementation with fat-soluble vitamins is indicated as well.

Biliary cirrhosis of distinctive histologic appearance was common but usually not symptomatic. Cholelithiasis was relatively common. Glucose intolerance was usually mild, with glycosuria in 8% of adolescents and adults. Since both alpha and beta cell function was disrupted by the pancreatic fibrosis, both insulin and glucagon levels were low.

Most adults with mucoviscidosis (97%) had pulmonary disease, which was usually the cause of death (47 of 48). Chest radiographs showed that hyperinflation was less common than in children but an upper lobe preponderance of parenchymal abnormalities was noted as in children, and included increased interstitial markings, cystic bronchiectasis, mucus plugging, and lobar aletectasis which had a predilection for the right upper lobe.[668a] Pulmonary function tests most often showed predominantly obstructive spirometry but mixed or predominantly restrictive patterns were occasionally seen. The diffusing capacity remained relatively normal. Atelectasis was frequent.

The pulmonary disease had a much greater suppurative component than is seen in usual adult COPD. Sputum cultures showed a predominance of *S. aureus* early, and *P. aeruginosa* late in the course. The psuedomonas was often mucoid (an unusual finding in patients without mucoviscidosis) and often of serotype Homma 8.

Complications of the pulmonary disease were common. Clubbing of digits was usual,[669] hypertrophic pulmonary osteoarthropathy was occasionally quite troublesome, and minor and major hemoptysis,[670] pneumothorax, and a syndrome of inappropriate secretion of antidiuretic hormone occurred. Cor pulmonale occurred late in the course of disease and had a poor prognosis, but secondary erythrocytosis was not common. Radiographic evidence of paranasal sinusitis was almost universal, although the disorder was usually not symptomatic. Nasal polyposis was often troublesome and often required surgery. Interestingly, it did not appear to be related to atopy.

The pulmonary disease of mucoviscidosis appears to progress somewhat more rapidly and inexorably than that of usual adult COPD. A series which included but was not limited to adult patients suggests that when these persons progress to respiratory failure, assisted ventilation does not add greatly to prognosis. Only 3 of 46 patients treated with this modality survived longer than a year.[671]

Immunologic Deficiency

The lung is the site of infection by a wide variety of organisms in immunologic deficiency diseases. Bronchiectasis is especially characteristic of humoral immunity disorders, both congenital and acquired.[672–675] Deficient synthesis of all three major groups of immunoglobulins, IgA, IgM, and IgG, is referred to as "agammaglobulinemia," or perhaps more accurately, "hypogammaglobulinemia," and occurs in congenital sex-linked and acquired forms. Pulmonary infections are very prominent in these disorders, and various mixed disorders of cellular and humoral immunity may present similar pulmonary manifestations. Isolated IgA deficiency, more recently recognized, has a significant association with respiratory infections, but in a much milder form.[676–681] Although not rare, it does not seem to account for a large proportion of the adult COPD population.[682–684] A review of this interesting phenomenon[678] defines its patients as those presenting with: (1) less than 0.05 mg/ml serum of IgA; (2) no deficiency of other immunoglobulins; (3) normal cellular immunity; and (4) normal humoral antibody production. So defined, selective deficiency of IgA occurs in one in 700 live births and sometimes seems to be only an incidental finding; but its association with a variety of autoimmune and other disorders as well as respiratory infections is becoming increasingly recognized. Most, if not all individuals with serum IgA deficiency lack secretory IgA. At least one case has been reported in which serum IgA was normal but lack of secretory piece was associated with a deficiency of secretory IgA.[680] Associated disorders reported include allergies, malabsorption, malignancies, and autoimmune disorders of which rheumatoid arthritis, systemic lupus erythematosis, pernicious anemia, and thyroiditis have been most common.

Disordered humoral immunity predisposes especially to pyogenic bacterial infections, while resistance to viral, mycobacterial, and fungal infections may be normal. Recurrent pneumonia due to *Streptococcus pneumoniae* is common, and *Streptococcus pyogenes*, *P. aeruginosa* and *Hemophilus influenzae* are also characteristic invaders. Bronchiectasis is presumably a result of repeated inflammatory injury to the tracheobronchial tree resulting from infection with these organisms.

Treatment of acute infections with appropriate antibiotics may be life-saving, and prophylaxis with administration of immunoglobulin preparations is useful in hypogammaglobulinemia. The latter approach is less effective in preventing infection of the tracheobronchial tree than of other sites, perhaps because the deficiency of secretory IgA from respiratory mucosa in these subjects is not corrected by parenteral immunoglobulin administration. The use of prophylactic antibiotics is of debatable benefit.

Infection, Obstruction, and Atelectasis

It is believed that many cases of bronchiectasis have been acquired during childhood following an episode of pneumonia, especially subsequent to measles or pertussis. Other cases appear to have their origin in pneumonia or bronchial obstruction in adults.[685–691] Atelectasis and bronchiectasis often co-exist, but when these two conditions follow infection of the lung parenchyma, the role of airway obstruction by secretions is often unclear. However, whether by foreign body, tumor, or stenosis, the capacity of bronchial obstruction to produce distal bronchiectasis is clearly recognized.

Tuberculosis may be associated with bronchiectatic changes which persist after the disease is inactive, and which may be asymptomatic or give rise to hemoptysis.[692]

With the exception of tuberculosis, the specific organisms cultured from sputum of patients with established bronchiectasis are usually regarded as secondary invaders rather than having played an important role in the pathogenesis of the disorder.[693–695] As secondary invaders, they do contribute in a major way to symptoms. Localized bronchiectatic changes may be seen in asthmatics and are associated with mucus plugging and atelectasis.[523] *Aspergillus fumigatus* can sometimes be cultured from mucus plugs in these patients, and may be seen in hyphal form invading bronchial walls in some cases. In such cases, a destructive immunologic reaction to the organism may play a part in producing bronchiectasis.[391]

Corrosive Gases

Exposure to corrosive gas is an uncommon cause of bronchiectasis, and in patients subjected to inhalation of various irritant gases, such as oxides of sulfur and nitrogen, more characteristic late sequelae are obliterative bronchiolitis and interstitial fibrosis in severe cases, or simply chronic bronchitis in less intense exposures. Bronchiectasis is an occasional result, however, and mustard gas was adjudged the cause of 5% of the cases reported by Wynn-Williams.[686]

In most of the above circumstances, as well as in diffuse bronchiectasis of unknown cause with heavy sputum production, the pathogenesis of bronchiectasis is unclear. Constitutional weakness of bronchial walls, mechanical distortion, and inflammatory destruction are possible factors.[613]

CLINICAL PRESENTATION

Bronchiectasis is by definition a morphologic entity and may exist without producing clinical manifestations. It is not truly a discrete disease entity but rather a disorder with many causes.

Nevertheless, a clinical presentation of recurrent bronchopulmonary infection and voluminous purulent sputum production is commonly associated with the term *bronchiectasis*, and it is to this clinically manifest form of the disorder that this discussion is primarily addressed.[696]

Characteristically, the history of symptoms of bronchiectasis dates to childhood, sometimes to an episode of pneumonia, especially following measles or pertussis. As prophylaxis and treatment of these disorders has advanced, bronchiectasis has become less common, and the cases now seen are more often related to an underlying disorder such as hypogammaglobulinemia or mucoviscidosis.

Productive cough may be perennial, although exacerbations with febrile illness, and sometimes with pneumonia, are characteristic. In contrast to chronic bronchitis, sputum in bronchiectasis is usually purulent, giving rise to the traditional description of three-layered sputum containing pus which settles to the bottom, saliva above it, and mucus on the top. The quantity may be measured in cupfuls. Prior to the use of antibiotics, anaerobic superinfection was common and resulted in a putrid odor which in itself was a major social and occupational handicap in patients with bronchiectasis.

Diffuse bronchiectasis, or localized bronchiectasis associated with chronic bronchitis, may be associated with respiratory insufficiency of a primarily obstructive type. Cor pulmonale is a frequent complication, along with nonspecific systemic symptoms of chronic illness.

Hemoptysis is not uncommon, and may take the form of blood-streaking of the sputum or of intermittent massive hemoptysis. It may accompany other symptoms of clinical bronchiectasis or it may occur as an unexpected event in an otherwise asymptomatic patient with previously unrecognized bronchiectasis, especially involving upper lobes. This form of the disorder has been referred to as *dry* bronchiectasis and in some cases may be a result of previous tuberculosis. The lack of symptoms of infection is perhaps due to a tendency of upper lobe segments to clear secretions with the help of gravity.

The most characteristic physical finding referable to bronchiectasis is the detection of crepitant rales over the affected lobe or segment. Diffuse bronchiectasis with accompanying bronchitis, emphysema, and respiratory insufficiency may present findings referable to these disorders. Clubbing of the fingers is relatively common in bronchiectasis.[697]

ROENTGENOGRAPHIC FINDINGS

Routine chest roentgenograms in bronchiectasis are seldom normal, yet seldom diagnostic. The often quoted study of Gudberg reviewed roentgenographic findings in 112 cases of bronchiectasis.[698] He found increased lung markings in 85%, honeycombing in 43%, atelectasis in 31%, and pleural changes in 47% of his subjects. Only 7.1% of this series had films which were interpreted as normal. None of the findings listed above can be considered specific for bronchiectasis, of course, but the combination of characteristic clinical symptoms with a compatible chest roentgenogram is often adequate for a presumptive diagnosis, and more definitive evidence may not be necessary for satisfactory management (Figs. 14-11 to 14-15).

Bronchography provides a morphologic diagnosis of bronchiectasis, as well as localization (Figs. 14-14, 14-15). This technique consists of instilling radiopaque medium into the tracheobronchial tree and roentgenograms being taken, usually in fluoroscopically selected views. Bronchography is useful in the evaluation of bronchiectasis, chiefly when surgical resection is contemplated, in order to verify the diagnosis and to establish that the process is limited to the area of contemplated resection. Asymptomatic bronchiectasis need not be identified by bronchograms, and disease which is believed clinically, and by conventional roentgenography to be so diffuse as to be unresectable often need not be studied further. Sometimes in such a case, bronchography may be helpful in directing postural drainage, however.

Bronchography is generally carried out by instilling liquid radiopaque contrast medium into the tracheobronchial tree through a catheter introduced into the trachea through the nose or mouth, after topical anesthesia has been administered.[699,700] The contrast material is directed into the desired site by appropriately positioning the patient. In the past, liquid materials used have included oily iodine compounds and iodine-oil mixtures which acutely produce dyspnea and reduce pulmonary function, and which may also be retained in the tracheobronchial tree and produce lipoid pneumonia and granulomata.[699] Aqueous iodinated compounds prevent the latter problem but may cause febrile reactions and bronchial obstruction and of course, any iodine-containing substance may prompt allergic reactions in sensitive persons.[427,699] Since unilateral bronchograms reduce pulmonary function parameters by about 20% acutely, and bilateral studies produce 30 to 50% reduction, certain precautions are indicated in carrying out bronchography.[701,702] Patients with pulmonary insufficiency should not have bilateral examinations at the same sitting, and chest surgery or sequential unilateral bronchograms should be delayed for 72 hours following the initial examination. Postural drainage should be carried out in order to evacuate contrast material from the tracheobronchial tree following bronchography.

Powdered barium compounds and powdered tantalum have been used as inhalates to outline the tracheobronchial tree.[703–706] Barium compounds may produce granulomatous reactions and late fibrosis. Tantalum is not as yet available for general use.

Since pneumonia may produce reversible cylindrical bronchiectatic changes, a diagnosis of irreversible bronchiectasis should not be made from demonstration of such changes during the first 4 months following an episode of pneumonia.[615–617] In order to avoid such misinterpretation, bronchography is usually not carried out during this interval.

The bronchographic abnormalities seen in cylindrical, varicose, and saccular bronchiectasis have been described in the portion of this chapter entitled Classification (Figs. 14-11, 14-12, 14-14).

PATHOPHYSIOLOGY

It might be anticipated that bronchial dilatation in itself would have relatively little effect upon pulmonary function. However, bronchiectasis is associated with an assortment of abnormalities which profoundly affect respiration, including atelectasis, obliteration of the smaller branches of the tracheobronchial tree, and diffuse bronchitis.

Respiratory insufficiency is therefore common in patients with bronchiectasis and the pattern of physiologic abnormalities generally resembles that of chronic bronchitis and emphysema.[707–710] Decreased vital capacity with more severely decreased expiratory flow, decreased maximum voluntary ventilation, increased ratio of residual volume to total lung capacity, and impaired mixing of inspired gas characterize the ventilatory defect. Pulmonary resistance is increased, and dynamic compliance decreased. Increase in venous admixture may produce hypoxemia, along with a decrease in diffusing capacity, and arterial carbon dioxide tension may be increased in severe cases.

Functional Abnormalities in Bronchiectasis

↓ vital capacity
↓ expiratory flow
↓ maximum voluntary ventilation
↑ ventilation-perfusion imbalance with hypoxemia

In general, the severity of functional abnormality correlates with the extent of bronchiectasis,[708] but this correlation is imperfect, presumably because of the frequency of associated diffuse bronchitis in these patients. Deterioration has been shown to be slow,[708] and worsening of function tests in Cherniack's series of 18 patients studied for 7 years was so slight as to be statistically insignificant. Repeated lower respiratory infections appear to hasten the decline of respiratory function, however, and patients with certain underlying disorders such as mucoviscidosis have an accelerated decline.

Cor pulmonale may accompany severe respiratory insufficiency in patients with bronchiectasis, as it does in those with chronic bronchitis and emphysema.

PATHOLOGY

Bronchiectasis consists of dilatation of the lumina of the bronchi accompanied by substantial inflammatory and destructive changes.[153,612–614] Whether these latter changes are secondary or cause the dilatation may not always be entirely clear in any given case. A preexisting structural weakness of the bronchial wall may sometimes predispose to ectatic changes.

The classification proposed by Reid[612] has already been discussed, and describes the dilated lumina of ectatic bronchi as cylindrical, varicose, and saccular. The primary importance of this classification is related to the observation that cylindrical dilatation may follow pyogenic pneumonia and may be reversible within a few months, while more advanced ectasia, with irregular distortion giving rise to a varicose or saccular appearance of the bronchi on bronchographic or direct anatomic examination, is usually (though not invariably) irreversible. More detailed classifications, attempting to attribute specific etiologic factors to different morphologic appearances, have not been met with wide enough acceptance to be adoptable by the clinician.

Columnar epithelium may be ulcerated, and is often replaced by hyperplastic squamous epithelium. All layers of the bronchial wall may be infiltrated with inflammatory cells and fibrous tissue, and destroyed by abscess formation. Lymphoid tissue is hyperplastic. Smaller bronchial subdivisions are plugged with secretions or are obliterated by fibrous tissue. The parenchyma supplied by diseased airways may be extensively atelectatic.

Vascular changes in bronchiectasis may be extensive, and are of clinical significance.[697] Large anastomotic channels between bronchial and pulmonary circulations develop, and an increase in bronchial arterial blood flow results. The frequency of hemoptysis in patients with chronic bronchiectasis is presumably a result of this phenomenon. Turner-Warwick has found an association between finger-clubbing and the enlargement of bronchial arteries in lung diseases.[697]

PROGNOSIS

Asymptomatic, localized bronchiectasis may be an incidental finding of no clinical consequence and may have no effect on life expectancy. In the past bronchiectasis producing the classical symptoms of bronchopulmonary sepsis had a very gloomy prognosis; however, this has been brightened by advances in medical and surgical therapy during the past half-century.

Wynn-Williams[686,710] has reviewed the subject of prognosis in this disorder. Prior to antibiotic therapy, the average duration of symptoms prior to death was 5 years, and the average time from diagnosis until death was less than 2 years. In Wynn-Williams' own series of patients, survival after the onset of symptoms appeared to be greater than 14 years, probably reflecting not only improved medical management with availability of antibiotic agents, but sample selection as well. The influence of case selection upon estimated survival time is difficult to assess. Some subjects with mild symptoms, well-controlled with medical measures, appear to incur little if any decrease in life expectancy; and localized bronchiectasis may be cured by resectional surgery. On the other hand, diffuse bronchiectasis with underlying mucoviscidosis or immunologic deficiency may have a poor prognosis.

MEDICAL MANAGEMENT

Medical management consists chiefly of measures to improve drainage of secretions from involved areas, and of antibiotic treatment of infection.[712] Surgical management involves resection of localized bronchiectasis for the control of symptoms, although prevention of spread of the disorder has, in previous years, been considered a goal.

Since bronchiectasis is both a result and a cause of impaired bronchial clearance, physical measures to aid in evacuation of pooled secretions are indicated. Postural drainage is the major technique available and consists of positioning the patient so that bronchi-draining-involved areas are made dependent.[324,326] Upper lobe bronchi are normally well-drained by gravity in upright humans. The lower lobes drain best with the patient in a prone posture with the head and upper thorax dependent. This position is readily achieved by having the patient lie supine with his lower trunk and legs on a low bed or couch and his head supported by arms folded and resting upon the floor. An effective modified position may be facilitated in an elderly or debilitated subject by the use of an adjustable hospital bed or tilt table. Middle lobe and lingula are drained in the supine position with head dependent and a pillow under the affected hemithorax. Stable patients should assume the appropriate drainage positions for at least 10 or 20 minutes, morning and evening. Increased duration and frequency are appropriate when conditions warrant. Rapid chest percussion with cupped hands over involved areas may facilitate drainage.

Adequate hydration with oral or parenteral fluids is essential, and nebulization of normal saline is often helpful. Nebulization of acetylcysteine is useful when secretions are viscid.[292] Prominent bronchospasm sometimes contraindicates use of this latter substance which is irritating to the tracheobronchial tree and should always be used in combination with a bronchodilator.

Aerosolized, oral, or parenteral bronchodilators frequently improve expiratory flow rates[711] and facilitate evacuation of secretions even when bronchospasm is not clinically prominent. They may be administered prior to postural drainage and chest percussion. The usefulness of expectorants is a matter of debate and these agents should not be relied upon as a major part of therapy.

Antibiotic treatment of exacerbations of bronchopulmonary infection is indicated, and should be guided by sensitivity of the offending organism if it can be identified by sputum smear and culture. If not, tetracycline or ampicillin may be employed, since these agents are relatively low in toxic side-effects, and are usually clinically helpful. In at least some cases, their usefulness is perhaps related to their activity against *H. influenzae*,[694] a common organism in the sputum of patients with bronchiectasis. Penicillin and its analogs are especially effective when the fetid odor of sputum suggests anaerobic infection. The odor itself is now seldom a major problem for patients with bronchiectasis because of the advent of antibiotics. Previously, it often represented a major social handicap.

Antibiotic administration for prophylaxis of exacerbations has been demonstrated to be of benefit.[713] In 1957, a report by the British Medical Research Council described a reduction in morbidity from bronchiectasis during a one year trial of penicillin, oxytetracycline, and a placebo, each given 2 days a week in a dose of 500 mg, 4 times a day. Subsequent experience with chemoprophylaxis in bronchiectasis and in bronchitis suggests that emergence of resistant organisms is not a prohibitive problem, and that continuous or intermittent chemoprophylaxis with tetracycline or ampicillin in dosages from 500 mg to 1 g daily may be tailored to the needs of individual patients, with symptomatic benefit.

The management of hemoptysis in bronchiectasis relies primarily on the exclusion of other causes by sputum examination for malignant cells and tubercle bacilli, chest radiography, and sometimes bronchoscopy. Treatment of any exacerbation of bronchopulmonary infection is indicated. Monitoring of pulse and blood pressure, hemoglobin and hematocrit, and respiratory status may be required if bleeding is brisk. Identification of the bleeding site at bronchoscopy or angiography[714] should be carried out when bleeding is brisk or persistent, and resection of the segment or lobe considered if life is threatened.[715] Since death is most commonly due to asphyxiation, tracheal intubation with a double-lumen Carlens tube may be performed under emergency conditions, occluding the main bronchus on the affected side and maintaining ventilation to the opposite lung. Other methods of endobronchial tamponade may be devised, according to the devices and skills available.[716] In a less urgent situation, the patient may be placed at bedrest with the affected side dependent to minimize aspiration of blood to the opposite side. Cough suppressants may be useful and parenteral blood replacement is occasionally a requirement.

The treatment of associated bronchitis, respiratory insufficiency, and cor pulmonale is similar to that appropriate for patients with chronic bronchitis without bronchiectasis.

SURGICAL MANAGEMENT

Surgical treatment of bronchiectasis by excision was once viewed as the only available hope of modifying a very gloomy prognosis in this disorder. Excisional therapy reached its peak of popularity soon after World War II, and then began to decline as antibiotic usage resulted in the decreased incidence and more satisfactory medical management of bronchiectasis.[717–719] A series of leading articles in *The Lancet* in the late 1950s[720–722] expressed the prevailing conservative viewpoint, suggesting that medical management utilizing postural drainage and antibiotic therapy was sufficiently rewarding that cases appropriate for surgical intervention were now unusual. This viewpoint was expressed with acknowledgment that antibiotic therapy, along with improvement in surgical and anesthetic techniques, had greatly reduced the risks of surgery. The experience of Lindskog and Hubbell,[687] reporting an operative mortality of 2.4% in a series of 165 resections, was considered representative.

Even those espousing the conservative approach would recognize the usefulness of surgical resection in certain selected cases of bronchiectasis, however.[723,723a] The aim of such therapy is primarily to control the symptoms of bronchopulmonary infection and hemoptysis,

Factors Favoring Surgery in Management of Bronchiectasis

Significant symptoms of bronchopulmonary infection, poorly controlled for a year or longer by conservative management.
Bronchiectasis sufficiently localized to permit complete resection.
Absence of a generalized disorder favoring development of further bronchiectatic changes (mucoviscidosis, immunologic defect).
Absence of diffuse bronchitis and emphysema.

since the notion that bronchiectasis, if unresected, tends to spread is not well supported.[724–726] The ideal candidate for surgical treatment would be a young adult or adolescent, without underlying mucoviscidosis or immunologic deficiency, but with significant problems from persistent productive cough and recurrent bronchopulmonary infection, or perhaps hemoptysis, caused by bronchiectasis. Failure of medical management to control symptoms over the course of a year or two would warrant consideration of surgery. Bronchiectasis ought to be proven at bronchography before resection is undertaken and it should be recalled that cylindrical bronchiectasis may be present for 3 or 4 months after pneumonia and may be reversible. Saccular changes are generally irreversible. The demonstration at bronchography that the bronchiectasis was well enough localized to permit complete resection would be required by the conservative internist or surgeon; and absence of bronchitis elsewhere in the tracheobronchial tree would be desirable. Pulmonary function testing would help in determining the latter, as well as in demonstrating the patient's potential ability to tolerate surgery (see also Respiratory Effects of Resectional Surgery, Chap. 11).

Failure to adhere to these principles in selecting subjects for surgery will increase the possibility of an occasional surgical or anesthetic accident in a patient operated upon for trivial symptoms; and inevitably result in imperfect relief of symptoms in patients with diffuse disease treated by incomplete resection. The most distressing case is the occasional patient rendered pulmonary-insufficient by overly aggressive resection, and this without the relief of the symptoms of bronchopulmonary infection.

Nevertheless, some observers believe that surgical resection is justified in occasional mild cases and that incomplete resection is beneficial in some patients in whom complete removal of bronchiectatic lung is not possible.[689,689a727]

Borrie and Lichter[689] reported results of operation on 125 patients between 1952 and 1962. Of the 91 who had unilateral resection, 84 were alive and well up to 10 years later; 97% of these had excellent or good results. Of 34 patients who had bilateral surgery, 32 were alive and well at follow up, up to 10 years after surgery, and 84% had excellent or good results. The authors of this series believe that "incomplete but worthwhile relief of symptoms can be obtained even in the presence of known bronchitis and minimal bronchiectasis in the remaining lung tissue." There was no operative mortality in this series, but half the patients had complications which included lobar collapse, pneumothorax, fistula, infection, and hemothorax.

Sanderson and co-workers[727] have reported results of a series of patients managed surgically and medically, and also provide a defense for the extended use of surgical resection. Of their series of 393 cases, two-thirds were managed surgically and one-third medically. Of the 242 patients treated in this series, there were 81 early complications, 1 intraoperative death, and 4 later deaths due to bronchiectasis. This 2% death-rate from the disease in the surgical group was compared to a 9% deathrate due to bronchiectasis in the nonsurgical group, of whom a number had severe disease initially. Eighty-one complications were observed in the 272 operations on 242 patients; surgical complications are frequent in most series of patients operated on for bronchiectasis.

Nevertheless, Sanderson and associates believe that their results from surgical treatment of a wide range of severity and extent of bronchiectasis support the use of resection in certain cases in which mildness of symptoms or severity and diffuseness of disease would rule out its employment by other practitioners. They suggest that mild cases may be treated surgically and that severely symptomatic poor risk cases may be ameliorated by partial resection.

CONGENITAL AND MISCELLANEOUS ACQUIRED DISORDERS OF THE LUNGS AND AIRWAYS

Congenital anomalies of the lungs and tracheobronchial tree are most commonly manifested in early life and are within the province of the neonatologist and pediatrician. For more complete discussions of these disorders, the reader is referred elsewhere.[728–730] The section which follows emphasizes those disorders most likely to be seen by the physician dealing primarily with adult patients, and includes some conditions of uncertain origin, and a few miscellaneous ones which are clearly acquired.

Congenital Anomalies Involving Pulmonary Parenchyma

- Agenesis of lung(s)
- Hypoplasia of lung(s)
- Absence of lobes
- Herniation of the lungs
- Horseshoe lung
- Variants of emphysema
  - Bullous emphysema
  - Unilateral and lobar emphysema
  - Congenital (infantile) lobar emphysema
- Idiopathic pulmonary microlithiasis
- Pulmonary lymphangiomyomatosis
- Congenital pulmonary lymphangiectasis
- Bronchopulmonary dysplasia and Wilson-Mikity syndrome
- Congenital cystic adenomatoid malformation
- Pulmonary blastomas and hamartomas

AGENESIS, HYPOPLASIA, AND ECTOPIA OF THE LUNGS

A variety of major anomalies of lung are evident at birth, are frequently incompatible with life, and are components of syndromes of multiple anomalies. Agenesis (absence) of one or both lungs; absence of lobes, and hypoplasia (decreased size with normal number of lobes) may occur. Unilateral agenesis is a malformation which may be compatible with the patient's having prolonged survival in relatively good health. Frequent infections may occur, with pooling of secretions in a blind bronchial stump and "spillage pneumonitis." This group of anomalies, along with several syndromes in which they may occur is discussed by Landing.[728]

Herniation of lungs into the neck, through the diaphragm, and through an intercostal space has been described. Horseshoe lung is a rare disorder in which the lungs are fused between the esophagus and heart, and may be associated with other anomalies.[731]

VARIANTS OF PULMONARY EMPHYSEMA

Terminology

The most common form of pulmonary emphysema which presents to the physician as a clinical problem is the diffuse form, characterized by both enlargement of normal air spaces and destruction of their walls, and is associated with obstruction to expiratory flow. The panlobular and centrilobular forms of diffuse obstructive emphysema have been discussed. Several other forms of abnormal air spaces may occur within the lung in more localized form, and are discussed below.

Certain of these forms of abnormal air spaces are very discrete and have walls which are visible roentgenographically or upon direct examination. Three terms are commonly used to refer to these well-demarcated air spaces: *cysts*, *blebs*, and *bullae*. Usage of these three terms is not widely consistent.[136,173,732]

A *lung cyst*, when this term is used to refer to an air rather than fluid-containing structure, usually connotes an abnormal air space with a thin wall which has an epithelial lining. A congenital or infectious origin is implied.

A *bleb*, as defined by Miller,[732] is an air space within the layers of the visceral pleura, and does not affect the lung parenchyma itself, except by displacement. Reid[173] believes that the lesions termed *blebs* by Miller are in fact intraparenchymal, and equates them with paraseptal emphysema.

A *bulla* is an air-containing structure within the lung parenchyma itself. It presumably arises from disruption of alveolar walls and compression of alveoli at its periphery, and may be seen as a sequela of diffuse obstructive emphysema. The walls of a bulla are composed of connective tissue remnants of interlobular and interlobar septa, and compressed remnants of disrupted and destroyed lung tissue. Bullae may be multiloculated and have many communications with surrounding lung. Remnants of blood vessels may be seen within them.

Short of surgery or autopsy, the cause of abnormal air spaces and the characteristics of their walls often cannot be determined other than by inference. It is therefore not surprising that the terms defined above are used rather loosely by clinicians and radiologists. Indeed, etiology may very often not be determined even from morphologic examination, especially when a differentiation is sought between a postinfectious and a congenital cause of an epithelium-lined cyst. The descriptive terminology the clinician uses may thus depend upon size of the abnormal air space: *cyst* and *bleb* generally refer to small structures, and those described as *bullae* are more often large. A 1959 Ciba Symposium[136] suggested that an abnormal air space greater than 1 cm in diameter can be considered a bulla; and Fraser and Pare[733] have suggested that the term *pneumatocele* be employed to describe those occupying a third or more of a hemithorax. To others, the latter term is reserved for the abnormal air spaces which characteristically occur acutely in staphylococcal pneumonia, especially in infants.

Bullous Emphysema

Abnormal air spaces in the lung have clinical importance when they are associated with recurrent spontaneous pneumothorax, when their roentgenologic appearance suggests lung abscess or granulomatous infection, and when they are so large that respiratory function is compromised. The term *bullous emphysema* is generally employed to describe the roentgenographic appearance of discrete abnormal air spaces large enough to suggest that respiratory function may be impaired by their presence (Fig. 14-16).[734–736]

Although solitary or multiple bullae may occur in association with any form of localized or diffuse emphysema, the large, roentgenographically discrete lesions to which the term *bullous emphysema* is attached fall loosely into two categories. Progressively enlarging upper lobe bullae in young adults with otherwise normal lungs probably arise most often from localized paraseptal emphysema. Patients in this group most often benefit from surgical resection of the lesions, if these are large enough to compromise respiratory function by the compression of adjacent normal lung. Bullae in older persons with diffuse emphysema, especially of the panacinar variety, tend to be associated with respiratory insufficiency which is due to the diffuse disease process rather than to space occupation by the bullae themselves. Patients in this category are less likely to benefit from surgical removal of the lesions. Unfortunately, these two groups are not so discrete as to permit confident preoperative identification of those patients who will benefit from bullectomy.

The manner in which bullous lesions compromise pulmonary function appears to be based chiefly on space occupation. The lesions are generally poorly ventilated as well as poorly perfused, and therefore do not contribute greatly toward either shunting or dead space ventilation. Adjacent lung may be compressed, or at least collapsed; the pressure relationships between bullae and adjacent lung are not clearly understood.

It has been suggested that the volume occupied by bullae might be estimated as the discrepancy between lung volume measured by plethysmography and by inert gas techniques, which tend to underestimate volume, since ventilation to the lesions is poor.

The abnormalities of pulmonary function produced by bullae resemble the abnormalities of diffuse obstructive emphysema. Therefore, the laboratory's ability to help predict the outcome of bullectomy is limited. Laurenzi and associates[736] have studied patients with bullous lesions with and without co-existent diffuse obstructive disease, and have found increased residual volume and functional residual capacity and reduced vital capacity in both groups. The patients without diffuse disease had a tendency toward increased expiratory reserve volume and relatively normal diffusing capacity, however.

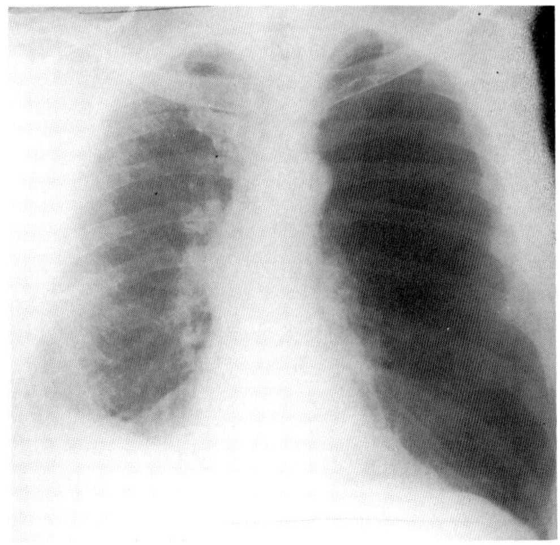

FIG. 14-16. Bullous emphysema. The absence of lung markings and hyperlucency in the left upper lung zone represent a large bulla which has enlarged slowly during the past 10 years. Severe reduction of expiratory flow and patchy perfusion and ventilation defects shown on lung scan indicate diffuse obstructive disease involving both lungs, and precluding a satisfactory result from bullectomy. Pleural changes on the right are the result of a previous episode of empyema.

Slowing of expiratory flow rates can result from bullous lesions alone as well as from diffuse obstructive disease; and decreased elastic recoil can occur in both situations. Gelb and associates[737] have demonstrated that loss of elastic recoil in one group of patients with bullous disease was quantitatively sufficient to account for the abnormalities in airways resistance and expiratory airflow observed. This sort of painstaking quantitative approach may prove clinically useful in the future in predicting improvement following the surgical resection of bullae.

Current knowledge provides only rough guidelines for selecting those patients with bullous emphysema who are likely to benefit from surgery.[738–746] Certainly symptoms should be sufficient to justify some possible benefit in return for the risks of thoracotomy. Exertional dyspnea severe enough to limit the patient's ordinary daily activities warrants consideration of surgery.

Most authors consider the roentgenographic size of the lesions to be resected to be of some importance. In order for a bulla to contribute significantly to dysfunction, it has been suggested that it must occupy a fourth to a third or more of a hemithorax.[740] One group has reported most consistent benefit from the removal of large lesions occupying most of the volume of a hemithorax.[742] Davies and associates differ from most other authors in suggesting that the size of a lesion is not a reliable predictor of results of removal.[741]

Evaluation of the integrity of the lung apart from the bulla is obviously important, since it is generally agreed that severe generalized disease is a relative contraindication to surgery. In surgery, the risk is high in patients with diffuse disease and very severe functional impairment, and surgical cure is not possible. Some authors have even suggested that significant ventilatory impairment is in itself evidence of diffuse disease. Nevertheless, symptomatic and functional improvement following surgery is possible, even in respiratory cripples and in the presence of diffuse disease, though a well-established method of quantitating the degree of impairment due to the bullous lesion is not available. Therefore, angiography and radioisotope studies of regional ventilation and perfusion should be used in combination with the other more routine tests of overall respiratory function in an attempt to evaluate the integrity of underlying lung prior to selection of patients for bullectomy. It has been very convincingly argued that angiographic evidence of intact lobar vessels displaced and crowded by the bullous lesions is the single most reliable piece of evidence that surgery may be of benefit.[745,746] The final decision must be a highly individualized, educated guess, based on as much information as can be collected about the patient under consideration.

Unilateral and Lobar Emphysema

The physician is occasionally presented with the problem of differential diagnosis of the roentgenologic appearance of unilateral lung hyperlucency in a patient who may be asymptomatic or may have nonspecific symptoms of cough or shortness of breath. Weg and associates[747] have presented a classification of entities which may present as unilateral hyperlucent lung. Among these is the *unilateral hyperlucent lung syndrome*, described by Swyer and James,[748] and later by MacLeod.[749] Review of the reported cases of this syndrome suggests that it represents a localized form of the acquired emphysema associated with obliterative bronchiolitis,[750] probably most often subsequent to a viral or mycoplasmal pulmonary infection in childhood.[751–754] The syndrome may be recognized by roentgenographically demonstrating failure of the hyperlucent hemithorax to empty on expiration. During inspiration, the hyperlucent lung may be normal in size or smaller than normal. On expiration, the hyperlucent hemithorax remains inflated and the mediastinum shifts toward the normal side, which empties normally. Bronchograms characteristically demonstrate a "broken bough" appearance, representing the failure of peripheral bronchi and bronchioles to fill with contrast material.[755] Pulmonary arterial blood flow may be so reduced that demonstration of a morphologically normal vascular tree may be difficult, but autopsy studies have shown sufficiently normal vessels to indicate that this group of patients is distinct from those in which congenital hypoplasia or aplasia of the pulmonary artery presents the roentgenographic picture of unilateral hyperlucent lung.

Many of the patients with this syndrome are asymptomatic, having adequate respiratory function provided by the normal lung; and the abnormal lung is not necessarily a focus of recurrent infection.[756–759] In such cases, specific treatment is not usually necessary.

Physiologic studies have shown that overinflation of the lung is characteristic, but that de-

Classification of Entities That May Present as a Unilateral Hyperlucent Lung

Chest Wall
- Absence of pectoral muscle
- Absence of breast
- Scoliosis

Parenchymal
- Compensatory emphysema
  - Atelectasis
  - Aplasia or hypoplasia of a segment or lobe
  - Surgical excision of lung tissue
- Obstructive emphysema
  - Bleb or bulla formation
- Central obstruction with ball-valve mechanism
  - Tumor
  - Foreign body
  - Congenital bronchial defect

Vascular
- Congenital cardiac and great vessel anomaly
- Pulmonary embolus or thrombosis

Unilateral Hyperlucent Lung Syndrome
- Nonvisualization of the pulmonary artery ("absence") with airway obstruction on the affected side
- Poor visualization of the pulmonary artery ("small") with airway obstruction ("bronchitis") on the affected side
- Poor visualization of the pulmonary artery ("small") with airway obstruction ("bronchitis") and bronchiectasis on the affected side

Weg JG, Krumholz RA, Hackleroad LE: Unilateral hyperlucent lung. Ann Intern Med 62:675, 1965

structive emphysema is not a regular feature. Obliteration of bronchi and bronchioles with fibrous tissue is seen. Major pulmonary vessels are intact, though perhaps reduced in size, while alveolar walls are avascular.

Lobar emphysema in adults presumably represents a more localized form of the syndrome described above, and is not to be confused with congenital or infantile lobar emphysema.

Congenital (Infantile) Lobar Emphysema

Congenital lobar emphysema usually comes to the attention of the physician because of respiratory distress during the first few weeks after birth,[760–764] but in milder cases, the functional disturbance may not be recognized until later in childhood, when infection produces respiratory distress. The presence of lobar emphysema is recognized roentgenologically as overinflation of a lobe, most dramatically seen during expiration, when it fails to empty, and mediastinal displacement occurs toward the opposite side.

In most cases, the cause appears to be underdevelopment of cartilaginous support of an upper lobe bronchus with consequent collapse causing obstruction during expiration. Bronchial obstruction due to vascular anomalies may also occur. Unlike lobar emphysema in adults, this condition often requires surgical removal of the involved lobe,[765,766] the presence of which impairs ventilation to the remainder of the infant's lungs.

Senile Emphysema

The term *senile emphysema* was once applied to the changes in shape which sometimes occur in the thorax in association with kyphosis in elderly persons. These changes are not properly referred to as emphysema, and are not associated with the morphologic or physiologic features of true pulmonary emphysema.[767]

After age 20 to 25 years, vital capacity and maximum expiratory flow rates fall, while residual volume increases. Distribution of ventilation is less uniform, closing volume increases, and arterial oxygen tension drops from an average of 95 mm Hg in the third decade of life to 75 mm Hg[768] in the seventh.

Paraseptal Emphysema

In *paraseptal emphysema*, dilatation of alveoli and disruption of alveolar walls in areas adjacent to pleural surfaces or septae is a common finding at autopsy, and is not usually associated with recognizable causative factors, symptoms, or functional disturbance.[769,770] Miller considered these lesions to be between pleural surfaces, and called them blebs,[732,771] while Reid believed that they were subpleural and intraparenchymal.[173] Their location adjacent to septae places them at the periphery of lobules or acini, hence the terms *paraseptal* or *periacinar*. The most common sites of this form of emphysema are the sharp edges of the periphery of lobes, adjacent to fissures, and at the cardiodiaphragmatic rim.

Although these lesions are ordinarily benign, it appears that they are sometimes the site of lung rupture with spontaneous pneumothorax. It is probable that in some cases they may also give rise to radiologically visible air spaces with thin, hair-like rims, occasionally large enough to be referred to as *giant bullae* and to produce functional disturbances by space occupation.

Compensatory Emphysema

In compensatory emphysema, overinflation, probably without resultant disruption of alveoli, occurs in remaining lung after resection, or in adjacent lung following atelectasis. In general, the function of the overdistended lung is increased rather than decreased, as it accommodates blood which previously flowed through the collapsed or resected pulmonary vessels, occupying additional space and accommodating additional airflow as well. Bates, Macklem, and Christie have summarized data concerning the functional effect of resection.[768]

Miscellaneous Forms Associated with Other Lung Injury

Overdistention and disruption of alveoli inevitably develops in areas of lung adjacent to the fibrosis which can result from a wide range of causes of lung injury.[173] When the injury and fibrosis are limited in extent, emphysema (presumably due to traction and distortion from scarring) is also limited in extent and significance. One form of centrilobular emphysema, which develops in early coalworkers' pneumoconiosis in relation to traction and distortion from dust deposition, is widespread in extent, but produces relatively mild functional disturbance. Alveolar-arterial oxygen tension difference is widened, residual volume is increased, and diffusing capacity and forced expiratory volumes are slightly reduced.

Diffuse parenchymal infiltrative lung disease of any sort, especially diffuse interstitial fibrosis, is eventually complicated by extensive emphysematous changes which may have a great deal of functional significance. Lung volumes may increase above the abnormally low values caused by fibrosis and airflow obstruction may become apparent. Clear quantitative assessment of the pathologic correlates of functional abnormalities are impossible in such a mixed disorder.

Emphysematous changes distal to large or small airways obstruction from an assortment of causes may occur. Infantile lobar emphysema with bronchial collapse, described above, is only one example of emphysema distal to large airway obstruction.

Diffuse bronchiolar obstruction from obliterative bronchiolitis may give rise to the rapid development of diffuse emphysema, and the resulting respiratory disability is clinically and pathophysiologically similar to that of severe diffuse obstructive emphysema of the more usual sort. Viral infections and inhalation of irritant gases are the causes of the acute bronchiolitis which may give rise to irreversible fibrotic changes of obliterative bronchiolitis.

IDIOPATHIC PULMONARY MICROLITHIASIS

Idiopathic pulmonary microlithiasis, a peculiar disease discussed in Chapter 12, is considered by some to be congenital since it may occur in premature infants and has a familial occurrence.

PULMONARY LYMPHANGIOMYOMATOSIS

Also called muscular cirrhosis of the lung,[772] pulmonary muscular hyperplasia, and bronchiolar emphysema, pulmonary lymphangiomyomatosis consists of a proliferation of smooth muscle in the lung which tends to cause progressive respiratory insufficiency with an obstructive, restrictive, or mixed ventilatory defect. It apparently occurs only in women. It is identical pathologically to the pulmonary lesion of tuberous sclerosis, and although the latter disease is inherited as an autosomal dominant, the pulmonary manifestations occur chiefly in women. It has been suggested that when the pulmonary lesions occur alone, they represent a "forme fruste" of tuberous sclerosis. Radiologically, lymphangiomyomatosis presents linear and nodular densities in the lung bases and progresses to cause bullous change or honeycombing. The course varies but progression to death over a course of about 10 years is characteristic. Pneumothorax, chylous pleural effusion, and hemoptysis are frequent complications. Improvement has been reported following progesterone administration.[772a]

CONGENITAL PULMONARY LYMPHANGIECTASIS

Neonatal respiratory distress may occur with diffuse dilatation of pulmonary lymphatics.[773] This phenomenon occurs especially in association with obstruction to pulmonary venous drainage, including total anomalous pulmonary venous return. Whether it occurs in primary, isolated form is not entirely clear. The lungs are diffusely mottled on x-ray and firm and heavy at morphologic examination. Treatment is unsatisfactory and prognosis is poor.

BRONCHOPULMONARY DYSPLASIA AND WILSON–MIKITY SYNDROME

Chronic respiratory distress in premature infants is characterized radiologically in Wilson–Mikity syndrome by diffuse interstitial infiltrate with cystic areas at the lung bases.[774,775] Pathologically, there are areas of immature, atelectatic parenchyma with adjacent areas of hyperaeration. The process may resolve, passing through a stage of resolution of infiltrates and coalescence of cystic foci with overexpansion and hyperlucency, and the chest radiograph may eventually become normal.

The initial reports of the Wilson–Mikity syndrome and bronchopulmonary dysplasia were distinctive, but it is likely that oxygen toxicity, mechanical ventilation, and atelectasis and pulmonary edema contribute to both. Obstructive pulmonary disease persisting to adolescence, with linear or cystic radiographic infiltrates, is relatively common.[108a,776]

CONGENITAL CYSTIC ADENOMATOID MALFORMATION

Replacement of a lobe or lobes by enlarging cysts interspersed with normal lung and overgrowth of bronchiolar and alveolar duct tissue characterizes congenital cystic adenomatoid malformation, an uncommon disorder.[777] The malformed cystic tissue may produce respiratory distress in a newborn by displacement of normal lung and lobectomy may be curative. Secondary infection may be a less urgent indication for resection in later life.[766,778]

PULMONARY BLASTOMAS AND HAMARTOMAS

Pulmonary blastomas and hamartomas, tumors of importance to physicians caring primarily for adult patients, are discussed in Chapter 15.

CONGENITAL ANOMALIES OF THE TRACHEOBRONCHIAL TREE

Agenesis of the Trachea or Bronchi

Tracheal agenesis is usually associated with a fistulous communication between the esophagus and the airway just distal to the atretic segment. A classification has been proposed which describes three types. In Type I, the fistula occurs at the level of the distal trachea; in Type II, at the level of the carina; and in Type III, there are two communications, one each between the main bronchi and the esophagus. An infant with tracheal agenesis may survive and surgical correction may thus be possible.[728]

Bronchial atresia is compatible with normal growth and development, and may present as an incidental radiographic abnormality in an asymptomatic adult. Characteristic is a mass near the hilum with hyperlucency of the lung distal to the mass. At surgery, the mass is found to be a dilated, fluid-filled segment of bronchus (mucocele) distal to the atretic segment.[779,780]

Constrictions of the Trachea and Bronchi

Webs and fibrous stenoses may involve the trachea or bronchi. When bronchi are involved, the lung distal to the obstruction may be atelectatic and infected, or occasionally overinflated and

Congenital Anomalies of the Tracheobronchial Tree

Agenesis or Atresia

Constriction
Webs
Fibrous stenosis of tracheal or bronchial segments

Abnormalities of Cartilage
Tracheomalacia, bronchomalacia
Compression due to vascular anomalies
Tracheopathea osteoplastica

Tracheal, Bronchial Enlargement
Mounier-Kuhn syndrome

Evaginations or Outgrowths
Tracheoceles, bronchoceles, diverticula, cysts
Fistulas: tracheo-esophageal, tracheobiliary, bronchobiliary

Abnormal Bifurcation
Subnumerary and supernumerary bronchi, lobes, fissures
Bronchial isomerism syndromes

Bronchopulmonary Sequestrations
Intrapulmonary
Extrapulmonary

Scimitar Syndrome

emphysematous.[728,729] Membranous webs can sometimes be treated simply by dilatation. Fibrous strictures may require extensive surgical procedures for correction.

Tracheobronchomalacia

Inadequate cartilaginous support of portions of the trachea and large bronchi may be congenital or acquired.[781–788] Acquired forms include dilatation and softening of the trachea due to prolonged intubation and mechanical ventilation through a cuffed endotracheal tube,[786–788] and tracheal involvement by a disorder of cartilage known as relapsing polychondritis.[783–785] The latter disorder may respond to treatment with corticosteroids. Other forms may lend themselves to excision of involved segments if the condition is localized and if expiratory collapse produces clinical problems.

Compression Due to Vascular Anomalies

A variety of vascular malformations can cause narrowing of the trachea or the right or left main bronchi.[728,729] Aortic arch anomalies are the most frequent causes of airway obstruction, but the subclavian, innominate, and carotid arteries may be involved, as may the left pulmonary artery. Stridorous respiration and recurrent infections may occur.

Tracheopathia Osteoplastica (Tracheobronchopathia Osteochondroplastica)

Tracheopathia osteoplastica is an unusual disease of uncertain cause, characterized by outgrowth of cartilaginous and bony spicules into the lumina of the trachea and major bronchi from the cartilaginous rings of their anterior and lateral aspects.[789–795] The disorder is recognized chiefly in men and may produce symptoms of infection distal to obstruction, hemoptysis, or respiratory distress. It may also be an incidental finding at necropsy in a patient in whom it produced no apparent symptoms. Roentgenographically, it may be recognized as multiple, small, partially calcified projections into the tracheal or bronchial lumina, best seen on laminograms. At bronchoscopy, the spicules are noted to be covered by intact respiratory mucosa.

Clinical manifestations depend upon the degree of involvement and of obstruction produced. Treatment is symptomatic.

Tracheobronchomegaly

Tracheobronchomegaly is an unusual disorder first described by Mounier-Kuhn in 1932,[796] and his name has been used to refer to it. Several useful reviews are available.[797–799] The syndrome consists of dilatation of the trachea and main bronchi, with chronic respiratory tract infection. The cause is believed to be a congenital defect of the supporting tissue of the tracheobronchial tree, perhaps inherited as an autosomal recessive trait.

The spectrum of clinical manifestations associated with tracheobronchomegaly ranges from absence of symptoms to severe respiratory insufficiency, suggesting that chronic infection, when it occurs, is a result rather than a cause. Onset of chronic cough and airways obstruction in adulthood are characteristic, and presumably result from expiratory collapse of the poorly supported large airways.

The roentgenographic signs include deep corrugations produced by redundant tissue between cartilaginous rings and an increase in the size of the trachea and bronchi. The normal size of the trachea has been defined by Katz and coworkers as 20.2 mm (SD ± 3.4 mm); of the right main bronchus, 16.0 mm (SD, 2.6 mm); and of the left main bronchus, 14.5 mm (SD ± 2.8 mm). Patients with tracheobronchomegaly have airways which exceed normal diameter by more than three standard deviations, according to these observers.

Treatment is that of chronic respiratory tract infection.

Tracheal Diverticuli

Outpouchings from the tracheobronchial tree have been categorized by Suprenant and O'Loughlin[800] into four classes: 1) rudimentary bronchus, most often arising from the lower right lateral aspect of the trachea; 2) cystic dilatation of mucous gland ducts; 3) tracheocele, or acquired outpouching from the right lower posterior trachea, in an area of weak structural support; and 4) acquired diverticuli associated with the congenital tracheal wall weakness of tracheobronchomegaly. These diverticuli are ordinarily of minimal or no clinical significance in themselves.

Bronchogenic Cysts

Bronchogenic cysts are congenital malformations, in which portions of lung have anomalous arterial supply, abnormal venous drainage, investment with visceral pleura, and discontinuity of the bronchial tree with cystic changes. These four anomalies occur in a variety of combinations and a range of extent of involvement. Within this variety of vascular and cystic anomalies, certain syndromes have been described which can be recognized by roentgenographic techniques, and which have therapeutic significance.

Congenital cystic abnormalities of lung without associated vascular anomalies may be single or multiple, large or small, and unilateral or bilateral. They may be asymptomatic and recognized roentgenographically as small lesions in the pulmonary parenchyma or mediastinum (see Chap. 15), or may present with recurrent infection or hemoptysis; or less often may be multiple, and associated with respiratory insufficiency. Congenital bronchiectasis is a form of cystic abnormality of the air passages. The symptoms which might bring this disorder to medical attention were described earlier in this chapter.

Several attempts have been made to classify congenital cystic disease of the lungs,[801–803] but difficulty is often encountered even in separating congenital lesions from acquired cysts in which inflammatory disease had produced cavities which become epithelialized in the process of healing. Therefore, the classification of an individual case may be impossible, the cause may remain obscure, and treatment must be individualized. Conservative treatment of infection may be indicated, or surgical resection may be necessitated when differential diagnosis includes neoplasm or when infection or hemoptysis are poorly controlled.[804]

Although a congenital or inflammatory origin may be impossible to infer even from morphologic examination of resected cystic lesions, there is little doubt that a congenital form of cystic disease exists.[805–807] Boyden[805] has found cystic changes in the lungs of infants, and the studies of Hinds[808] among Maori natives and of Baum and co-workers[809] in Israel have established a hereditofamilial factor in at least some cases.

Tracheoesophageal and Bronchoesophageal Fistula

Communications between the esophagus and various parts of the tracheobronchial tree may be congenital or may be acquired as a result of neoplasm, infection, or trauma.[810–814] An iatrogenic form of traumatic tracheoesophageal fistula may be produced by prolonged endotracheal intubation with a cuffed tube. Formation of a fistula is favored by inflation of the cuff under high pressure, constant movement of the cuff as in prolonged mechanical ventilation, and the presence of a semirigid tube in the esophagus behind and adjacent to the trachea.

Clinical manifestations of tracheoesophageal fistula are those of recurrent aspiration during swallowing. Diagnosis is made by demonstration of contrast material in the fistulous tract, introduced through the esophagus. The possibility of satisfactory surgical correction depends upon the location and the cause of the fistulous communication.

Congenital bronchobiliary fistula has been reported, and is manifested by production of bile-stained sputum in infancy, with focal atelectasis and pneumonitis. The fistulous tract most often connects the biliary tree with the right main bronchus.[728]

Subnumerary and Supranumerary Bronchi, Lobes, and Fissures

Landing[728] has discussed bronchial isomerism syndromes in which bilateral branching patterns characteristic of normal right or left lung anatomy occur. These syndromes include anomalies of other thoracic and abdominal viscera. Among the many other variants of bronchial anatomy which may occur, additive anomalies are by far more common than subtractive ones.

Incomplete development of intralobar fissures is common but is usually not clinically apparent except at surgery. Accessory fissures may be radiologically apparent. Commonly observed accessory fissures include those which demarcate the superior segments of the lower lobes, and those which produce the azygous lobe. The latter may be easily seen on an AP chest radiograph on which a dense parasagittal fissure separates the medial portion of the upper lobe from the remainder of that lobe. The fissure has its lower and medial termination at the azygous vein on the right, or hemiazygous on the left. Its chief importance lies in its occasionally being mistaken for a disease process since it is so readily seen on chest radiograph.

Bronchopulmonary Sequestration

When a congenitally cystic mass of bronchopulmonary tissue is supplied by an aberrant systemic, rather than a pulmonary artery, the condition is referred to as bronchopulmonary sequestration.[815–818,819,819a] It usually occurs in the posterior portion of the lower lobes and more often in the left than right. Recurrent infection of the sequestered portion of lung is the usual presenting manifestation and surgical resection is often indicated. Preoperative diagnosis and angiographic definition of the aberrant vascular supply is of great clinical importance because of the hazard of intraoperative hemorrhage through inadvertent transection of a vessel.

The reviews of Pryce[815] and of Smith[816] classified sequestration as intralobar and extralobar, depending upon the investment by visceral pleura which occurs in the latter form, separating the sequestered portion of lung into an accessory lobe. These investigators believed that the two forms were different entities, both clinically and etiologically, considering extralobar sequestration to have anomalous venous drainage into the azygos system and to be occasionally associated with other malformations, especially esophageal communications.

Subsequent studies have suggested that the two forms are not distinct and that associated anomalies may occur with intralobar sequestration. A recent review suggests that both intralobar and extralobar sequestrations arise from an accessory bronchopulmonary bud on the foregut.[817]

A diagnosis of sequestration is suggested when there is recurrent pulmonary infection in association with a persistent radio-opacity in the posterior portion of the left lower lobe. Surgical resection is usually indicated and preoperative evaluation should include a thoracic aortogram and contrast study of the upper gastrointestinal tract.[766]

Scimitar Syndrome

An anomaly of vascular supply to the lung known as the *scimitar syndrome* has usually been reported to occur without associated cystic changes of the lung,[820] but at least 1 case has been reported in which sequestration accompanied this malformation.[818]

The usual full syndrome consists of: 1) hypoplasia of the right lung with dextroposition of the heart; 2) hypoplasia of the right pulmonary artery; 3) anomalous arterial supply from the abdominal aorta to the right lower lobe; and 4) anomalous venous drainage of the right lung into the inferior vena cava.

It is the appearance of the large, scimitar-shaped anomalous vein coursing from the hilum to the inferior vena cava near the diaphragm which gives the syndrome its name.

Affected patients tend to develop repeated

respiratory infections associated with the hypoplasia of the right lung.

MISCELLANEOUS DISORDERS OF AIRWAYS

Small Airways Disease

Involvement of the small peripheral airways in chronic bronchitis and emphysema has been discussed above and in Chapter 4.

Bronchiolectasis

Buckley and co-workers have described a clinical syndrome associated with bronchographic demonstration of ectatic changes in bronchioles.[821] This roentgengographic lesion is not unusual in patients with ordinary chronic bronchitis but the patients described by Buckley were notable for having histories of prolonged exposure to irritant gases and purulent sputum and hemoptysis.

Bronchiolitis Obliterans

Acute bronchiolitis caused by viral infection is discussed in Chapter 8, and possible reasons for the respiratory distress this disorder is capable of producing in children, as opposed to adults, are discussed in Chapter 3.

An irreversible fibrosing disorder of small airways, bronchiolitis obliterans appears to be a sequela of acute viral infection,[108a,752,753] as well as a late complication of inhalation of irritant gases.[822] Emphysematous destruction of lung distal to the small-airways-obstructive lesions is usual, and a generalized form of this disorder may produce severe respiratory insufficiency similar in pathophysiology and clinical picture to advanced chronic bronchitis and emphysema of the usual sort; treatment is the same. It is believed that the unilateral hyperlucent lung syndrome and lobar emphysema in the adult are localized forms of bronchiolitis obliterans. These localized forms may be asymptomatic if the uninvolved portions of lung are functionally intact.

Mucoid Impaction

Obstruction of lobar or segmental bronchi, especially of upper lobes, with tenacious mucoid plug, can present a radiologic and clinical picture which strongly suggests neoplastic endobronchial obstruction.[476–478,823,824,824a] This phenomenon occurs especially in patients with episodic asthma and sometimes in chronic bronchitis, and has been reported to be a not uncommon complication of mucoviscidosis. The occasional finding of septate, branching hyphae in these plugs, or culturing of aspergillus, raises the question of a possible etiologic role of this organism in some patients. Bronchial casts may require removal by bronchoscopy.[824a]

Roentgenologically, segmental or lobar atelectasis is the most frequent sign of mucoid impaction. A "cluster of grapes" appearance of the plugs themselves visible on chest roentgenograms is more specific when it occurs in large central impactions. Bronchoscopy or bronchography may confirm bronchial obstruction but may not exclude endobronchial tumor unless the obstruction can be removed endoscopically with a forceps or suction tip, or with the aid of instilled acetylcysteine. Surgical resection may be necessary for diagnosis or expectant treatment of possible tumor, and less often for removal of a persistently infected lobe or segment.

Broncholithiasis

Calcified hilar lymph nodes are ordinarily benign sequelae of tuberculosis and histoplasmosis which give rise to no symptoms, but are readily visualized on chest roentgenograph. Occasionally, these nodes produce symptoms of bronchial obstruction by extrinsic pressure, by producing inflammatory bronchostenosis, or by eroding into the lumen of a bronchus. The last event may give rise to an episode of hemoptysis or of coughing up a "rock," in which instance a diagnosis may be supported by the roentgenographic disappearance of a previously visible hilar node. Bronchoesophageal fistula is an uncommon but clinically significant and surgically correctable complication of broncholithiasis. Arrigoni and co-workers have presented an interesting review of the experience of the Mayo Clinic with this phenomenon over a 30-year period.[825]

Hemoptysis

Coughing up of blood occurs in a wide range of lung diseases and coagulopathies. Massive hemoptysis is readily diagnosed by the cough, gurgling tracheal sounds, and frothy associated sputum. Less severe hemoptysis can be confused with hematemesis or with bleeding from the nasal passages or larynx. Hematemesis, however, is commonly associated with nausea and vomiting, dark red blood, food particles in the blood, and associated gastrointestinal symptoms.[826]

As emphasized throughout this text, hemoptysis may be associated with acute or chronic parasitic, fungal or bacterial infections of the lung; pulmonary vascular diseases; neoplastic diseases; diffuse hemorrhagic lung disease; bronchitis; bronchiectasis; and broncholithiasis. When hemoptysis first occurs in a previously healthy person, a complete evaluation for specific causes is mandatory. When it is first seen in a patient with well known acute or chronic bronchitis, bronchiectasis, or inflammatory disease, a period of observation to characterize the course is warranted. An appropriate evaluation for significant hemoptysis includes a chest roentgenogram, sputum and skin tests for tuberculosis, bronchoscopy, and careful follow up.

When minor and due to known disease, hemoptysis is generally self-limiting and requires no further intervention. When more than 20 ml of blood has been coughed up, the patient should be hospitalized and placed on bedrest, clotting factors should be assayed, and the patient observed closely. Aggravating cough should be suppressed but not eliminated by use of codeine. Bronchoscopy should be carried out early in order to determine the site of bleeding. Massive hemoptysis (more than 200 ml per day) is life-threatening. Definitions vary widely, but there is general agreement that if bleeding persists for 24 to 48 hours, the prognosis is ominous. Some studies have indicated a 50 to 75% mortality while others claim better than 80% survival.[826–829] Unless the site of bleeding is known, the patient should undergo fiberoptic bronchoscopy if bleeding slows sufficiently to enable visualization of the tracheobronchial tree. Selective pulmonary or bronchial angiography may help to localize the site of active bleeding.[719] Clotting defects should be corrected. Supportive care should include bedrest, oxygen, antibiotics if indicated, and, if necessary, an endotracheal tube to maintain the airway. If the site of bleeding is known and resectable, surgery should be considered for continuing or recurrent massive hemoptysis or when bleeding is sufficient to necessitate transfusion.[715] Alternative forms of treatment include bronchial artery embolization in bronchiectasis and tuberculosis[826,829] and pulmonary artery embolization in pulmonary arteriovenous fistulae. Tamponade of the bleeding lobe or lung may be accomplished by passing a cuffed Carlen's tube and ventilating the nonbleeding bronchus or by packing the bleeding bronchus with gauze through a fiberoptic bronchoscope.[716]

Upper Airway Obstruction

Noninvasive diagnostic techniques, and renewed interest in the oropharyngeal muscles, have resulted in more frequent recognition of upper airway obstruction.[830–840]

Causes of Upper Airway Obstruction

Oropharynx
Enlarged tonsils, adenoids
Epiglottitis
Cricopharyngeal muscle weakness

Larynx
Bilateral vocal cord paralysis
Edema
- Angioedema
- Infection (diphtheria)
- Postintubation

Tumors
Trauma

Trachea
Tumors of trachea
Extratracheal tumors
Tumors of mediastinum
Thyroid enlargement
Tracheomalacia
- Postintubation
- Trauma
- Relapsing polychondritis

Tracheal Strictures

The clinical manifestations in severe upper airway obstruction include inspiratory stridor (at least on exercise), dyspnea, hoarseness, and clinical evidence of respiratory failure. As summarized in Chapter 4, under Flow-Volume Relations, fixed obstruction produces characteristic changes in the flow volume loop. Obstruction may, however, only be apparent during sleep. (See Chap. 6.) Structural lesions may be clearly delineated by tantalum cine laryngo-tracheography.

Since upper airway obstruction may cause acute or chronic respiratory failure, and may be confused with asthma or with right ventricular failure due to other causes, the physician should be well familiar with the predisposing causes. Treatment is generally that for the underlying disease, but intrinsic disease of the trachea (tracheomalacia, stenosis or tumors) may necessitate surgical intervention.

REFERENCES

1. AYRES SM: Cigarette smoking and lung disease: An update. Basics of R D 3(5). American Thoracic Society, 1975
2. US Public Health Service: Smoking and Health: A Report of the Surgeon General. Part I. The health consequences of smoking. US Department of Health & Welfare, No. 79–500 66, 1979
3. WILSON RW: Cigarette smoking, disability days and respiratory conditions. J Occup Med 15:236, 1973
4. US Public Health Service: Smoking and Health: A Report of the Surgeon General. Chapter 3: Morbidity. US Department of Health & Welfare, No. 79–500 66, 1979
5. HAMMARSTEN JF et al: An epidemiological approach to chronic obstructive pulmonary disease and alpha$_1$ antitrypsin in hospital patients: A triracial study. Trans Am Clin Climatol Assoc 82:124, 1970
6. KRUTE A, BURDETTE ME: 1972 Survey of disabled and nondisabled adults: Chronic disease, injury and work disability. Social Security Bulletin 41(4):3–17, 1978
7. US Public Health Service: Smoking and Health: Report of the Advisory Committee to the Surgeon General of the Public Health Service. Washington, DC, US Department of HEW, Public Health Service Publication No. 1103, 1964
8. US Public Health Service: The Health Consequences of Smoking, a Public Health Service review: 1967. Washington, DC, US Department of HEW, Public Health Service Publication No. 1696
9. US Public Health Service: The Health Consequences of Smoking, 1968. Supplement to the 1967 PHS Review. Washington, DC, US Department of HEW, Public Health Service Publication, 1969
10. US Public Health Service: The Health Consequences of Smoking, 1969. Supplement to the 1967 PHS Review. Washington, DC, US Department of HEW, Public Health Service Publication No. 1696–2, 1969
11. US Public Health Service: The Health Consequences of Smoking, a Report of the Surgeon General: 1971. Washington, DC, US Department of HEW, DHEW Publication No. (HSM) 71–7513, 1971
12. US Public Health Service: The Health Consequences of Smoking, a Report of the Surgeon General: 1972. Washington, DC, US Department of HEW, DHEW Publication No. (HSM) 72–6515, 1972
13. US Public Health Service: The Health Consequences of Smoking: 1973. Washington, DC, US Department of HEW, DHEW Publication No. (HSM) 73–8704, 1973
14. US Public Health Service: The Health Consequences of Smoking: 1974. Washington, DC, US Department of HEW, DHEW Publication No. (CDC) 74–8704, 1974
15. US Public Health Service: The Health Consequences of Smoking: 1975. US Dept of HEW, Public Health Service, Health Services and Mental Health Administration DHEW Publication No. (CDC) 76–8704, 1975

15a. FRIEDMAN GD, PETITTI DB, BAWOL RD, SIEGELAUB AB: Mortality in cigarette smokers and quitters. N Engl J Med 304:1407, 1981

15b. KIMBEL P, KUEPPERS F: The biochemical basis of emphysema: The oxidant effect of cigarette smoke? Ann Intern Med 92:564, 1980

16. SHY CM, GOLDSMITH JR, HACKNEY JD et al: Health Effects of Air Pollution. New York, American Thoracic Society, 1975

16a. EBERT RV: Coal smoke and cigarette smoke. N Engl J Med 304:1486, 1981

17. DYSINGER PW, LEMON FR, CRENSHAW GI et al: Pulmonary emphysema in a non-smoking population. Dis Chest 43:17, 1963
18. HOLLAND WW, REID DD: The urban factor in chronic bronchitis. Lancet 1:445, 1965
19. SPEIZER FE, FERRIS BG JR: Exposure to automobile exhaust. I. Prevalence of respiratory symptoms and disease. Arch Environ Health 26:313, 1973
20. SPEIZER FE, FERRIS BG JR: Exposure to automobile exhaust. II. Pulmonary function measurement Arch Environ Health 26:319, 1973

20a. DOSMAN JA et al: Chronic bronchitis and decreased forced expiratory flow rates in lifetime nonsmoking grain workers. Am Rev Respir Dis 121:11, 1980

21. DAWSON SV, SCHENKER MB: Health effects of inhalation of ambient nitrogen dioxide. Am Rev Respir Dis 120:281, 1979
22. FERRIS BG JR, CHEU H, PUELO S et al: Chronic nonspecific respiratory disease in Berlin, New Hampshire, 1967–73. A further follow-up study. Am Rev Respir Dis 113:475, 1976
23. MANFREDA J, NELSON N, CHERNIACK RM: Prevalence of respiratory abnormalities in a rural and an urban community. Am Rev Respir Dis 117:215, 1978
24. FERRIS BG JR, SPEIZER FE, SPENGLER JD et al: Effects of sulfur oxides and respirable particles on human health, methodology and demography of populations in study. Am Rev Respir Dis 120:767, 1979
25. LINN WS, HACKNEY JD, PEDERSEN EE et al: Respiratory function and symptoms in urban office workers in relation to oxidant air pollution exposure. Am Rev Respir Dis 114:477, 1976
26. LEVY D, GENT M, NEWHOUSE M: Relationship between acute respiratory illness and air pollution levels in an industrial city. Am Rev Respir Dis 116:167, 1977
27. KURT TL, MOGIELNICKI RP, CHANDLER JE: Association of the frequency of acute cardiorespiratory complaints with ambient levels of carbon monoxide. Chest 74:10, 1978
28. KURT TL, MOGIELNICKI RP, CHANDLER JE et al: Ambient carbon monoxide levels and acute cardiorespiratory complaints; an exploratory study. Am J Public Health 69:360, 1979
29. BECKER WH, SCHILLING FJ, VERMA MP: The effect on health of the 1966 Eastern seaboard air pollution episode. Arch Environ Health 16:414, 1968
30. BURROWS B, KELLOGG AL, BUSKEY J: Relationship of symptoms of chronic bronchitis and emphysema to weather and air pollution. Arch Environ Health 16:406, 1968
31. GLASSER M, GREENBERG L, FIELD F: Mortality and morbidity during a period of high levels of air pollution. Arch Environ Health 15:684, 1967
32. LEBOWITZ MD et al: The effects of air pollution and weather on lung function in exercising children and adolescents. Am Rev Respir Dis 109:262, 1974
33. MCKUSICK VA, GOODMAN RM, DANKS DM: Genetic aspects of respiratory disease. Arch Environ Health 6:25, 1963
34. LITWIN SD (ed): Genetic Determinants of Pulmonary Disease. New York, Marcel-Dekker, 1979
35. LAURELL CB, ERIKSSON S: The electrophoretic α_1 globulin pattern of serum in α_1 antitrypsin deficiency. Scand J Clin Lab Invest 15:132, 1963
36. ERIKSSON S: Pulmonary emphysema and alpha$_1$-antitrypsin deficiency. Acta Med Scand 175:197, 1964
37. JACOBSSON K: Studies on the trypsin and plasmin inhibitors in human blood serum. Scand J Clin Lab Invest 7[Suppl 14]:55, 1955
38. SCHULTZE HE, HEIDE K, HAUPT H: α_1-antitrypsin and human serum. Klin Wochenschr 40:427, 1962
39. ERIKSSON S: Studies in alpha$_1$ antitrypsin deficiency. Acta Med Scand 177[Suppl 432]:1, 1965
40. GUENTER CA, WELCH MH, HAMMARSTEN JF: Alpha$_1$ antitryspin deficiency and pulmonary emphysema. Annu Rev Med 22:283, 1971
41. KUEPPERS F: Inherited differences in alpha$_1$ antitryspin. Litwin SD (ed): In Genetic Determinants of Pulmonary Disease. New York, Marcel-Dekker, 1978
42. MITTMAN C: Alpha$_1$ antitrypsin deficiency and other genetic factors in lung disease. In Litwin SD(ed): Genetic Determinants of Pulmonary disease, Chap 10. New York, Marcel-Dekker, 1979
43. KUHNL P, and SPIELMANN W: P_i^T: A new allele in the alpha$_1$ antitrypsin system. Hum Genet 50:221, 1979

43a. COX DW, JOHNSON AM, FAGERHOL MK: Report of nomenclature meeting for α_1 antitrypsin. Human Genetics 53:429, 1980

43b. TALAMO RC, BRUCE RM, LANGLEY CE et al: Alpha$_1$ Antitrypsin Laboratory Manual. US Department of Health, Education and Welfare, Publ. No. (NIH) 78–1420, 129 pp. 1978

44. MORSE JO: Alpha$_1$ antitrypsin deficiency. N Engl J Med 299:1045, 1099, 1978
45. LIEBERMAN J: Heterozygous and homozygous alpha$_1$-antitrypsin deficiency in patients with pulmonary emphysema. N Engl J Med 281:279, 1969
46. KUEPPERS F, FALLAT R, LARSON RK: Obstructive lung disease and α_1 antitrypsin deficiency gene heterozygosity. Science 165:899, 1969
47. LIEBERMAN J, MITTMAN C, SCHNEIDER AS: Screening for homozygous and heterozygous α_1 antitrypsin deficiency. JAMA 210:2055, 1969
48. WELCH MH, REINECKE ME, HAMMARSTEN JF et al: Antitrypsin deficiency in pulmonary disease; the significance of intermediate levels. Ann Intern Med 71:533, 1969
49. LARSON RK, BARMAN ML, KUEPPERS F et al: Genetic and environmental determinants of chronic obstructive pulmonary disease. Ann Intern Med 72:627, 1970
50. STEVENS PM, HNILLICA V, JOHNSON PC: Pathophysiology of hereditary emphysema. Am Rev Respir Dis 101:1012, 1970
51. FALLAT R et al: Chronic obstructive lung disease with intermediate alpha$_1$ antitrypsin deficiency. Proceedings of 13th Annual Aspen Conference on Research in Emphysema. Chest 59 [Suppl]:20s, 1971
52. RESNICK H, LAPP NL, MORGAN WKC: Serum trypsin

inhibitor concentrations in coal miners with respiratory symptoms. JAMA 215:1101, 1971

53. KUEPPERS F, DONHARDT A: Obstructive lung disease in heterozygotes for alpha$_1$ antitrypsin deficiency. Ann Intern Med 80:209, 1974
54. OSTROW DN, CHERNIACK RM: The mechanical properties of the lungs in intermediate deficiency of alpha$_1$ antitrypsin. Am Rev Respir Dis 106:377, 1972
55. KANNER RE et al: Pathologic patterns of chronic obstructive pulmonary disease in patients with normal and deficient levels of alpha$_1$ antitrypsin. Am J Med 54:706, 1973
56. WEBB DR et al: Serum antitrypsin variants: Prevalence and clinical spirometry. Am Rev Respir Dis 108:918, 1973
57. MORSE JA, LEBOWITZ MD, KNUDSON RJ et al: A community study of the relation of alpha$_1$ antitrypsin levels to obstructive lung diseases. N Engl J Med 292:278, 1975
58. BLACK LE: Alpha$_1$ antitrypsin deficiency. Chest 70:449, 1976
59. SIGEOKA JW, HALL WJ, HYDE RW et al: The prevalence of alpha$_1$ antitrypsin heterozygotes (PiMZ) in patients with obstructive pulmonary disease. Am Rev Respir Dis 114:1077, 1976
60. COX DW, HOEPPNER VH, LEVISON H: Protease inhibitors in patients with chronic obstructive pulmonary disease: The alpha$_1$ antitrypsin heterozygote controversy. Am Rev Respir Dis 113:601, 1976
61. MORSE JO, LEBOWITZ MD, KNUDSON RJ et al: Relation of protease inhibitor phenotypes to obstructive lung diseases in a community. N Engl J Med 296:1190, 1977
62. MITTMAN C: The PiMZ phenotype: Is it a significant risk factor for the development of chronic obstructive lung disease. Am Rev Respir Dis 118:649, 1978
63. KOZAREVIC D, LABAN M, BUDIMIR M et al: Intermediate alpha$_1$ antitrypsin deficiency and chronic obstructive pulmonary disease in Yugoslavia. Am Rev Respir Dis 117:1039, 1978
64. CHAN-YEUNG M, ASHLEY MJ, COREY P et al: Pi phenotypes and the prevalence of chest symptoms and lung function abnormalities in workers employed in dusty industries. Am Rev Respir Dis 117:239, 1978
65. LEBOWITZ MD, KNUDSON RJ, MORSE JO et al: Closing volume and flow volume abnormalities in alpha$_1$ antitrypsin phenotype groups in a community population. Am Rev Respir Dis 117:179, 1978
66. BUIST AS, SEXTON GJ, AZZAM AH et al: Pulmonary function in heterozygotes for alpha$_1$ antitrypsin deficiency: A case-control study. Am Rev Respir Dis 120:759, 1979
67. TATTERSHALL SF et al: Lung distensibility and airway function in intermediate alpha$_1$ antitrypsin deficiency (PiMZ). Thorax 34:637, 1979
68. MCDONAGH DJ, NATHAN SP, KNUDSON RJ et al: Assessment of alpha$_1$ antitrypsin deficiency heterozygosity as a risk factor in the etiology of emphysema. J Clin Invest 63:299, 1979

68a. COCKCROFT DW, TENNENT RK, HORNE SL: Pulmonary emphysema associated with the FZα_1 antitrypsin phenotype. CMAJ 124:737, 1981

68b. BENCZE K, SABATKE L, FRUHMANN G: Alpha$_1$ antitrypsin: The PiMM subtypes. Chest 77:761, 1980.

68c. MITTMAN C, TAYLOR JC: PiM subtypes and lung disease: A cautionary note. Chest 77:721, 1980

68d. HORNE SL, TENNENT RK, COCKCROFT DW: A new anodal alpha$_1$ antitrypsin variant associated with emphysema. Am Rev Respir Dis 123-2S:108, 1981

69. GUENTER CA et al: The pattern of lung disease associated with alpha$_1$ antitrypsin deficiency. Arch Intern Med 122:254, 1968
70. BELL RS: The radiographic manifestations of alpha$_1$ antitrypsin deficiency. Radiology 95:19, 1970
71. ROSEN RA et al: The roentgenographic findings in alpha$_1$ antitrypsin deficiency. Radiology 95:25, 1970
72. WELCH MH et al.: The lung scan in α_1-antitrypsin deficiency. J. Nucl Med 10:687, 1969
73. STEIN PD, LFU JD, WELCH MH et al: Pathophysiology of the pulmonary circulation in emphysema assocated with alpha$_1$ antitrypsin deficiency. Circulation 43:227, 1971
74. TALAMO RC, ALLEN JD, KAHAN MG et al: Hereditary alpha$_1$ antitrypsin deficiency. N Engl J Med 278:345, 1968
75. FAGERHOL MK: Quantitative studies on the inherited variants of serum α_1 antitrypsin. Scand J Clin Lab Invest 23:97, 1969
76. FAGERHOL MK: The pi-system; genetic variants of serum α_1 antitrypsin. Series Haematol 1:153, 1968
77. MATHIS RK et al: Alpha$_1$ antitrypsin in the respiratory distress syndrome. N Engl J Med 288:59, 1973
78. SHARP HL, BRIDGES RA, KRIVIT W et al: Cirrhosis associated with alpha$_1$ antitrypsin deficiency: A previously unrecognized inherited disorder. J Lab Clin Med 73:934, 1969
79. GHERADRI GJ: Alpha$_1$ antitrypsin deficiency and its effect on the liver. Hum Pathol 2:173, 1971
80. BERG NO, ERIKSSON S: Liver disease in adults with alpha$_1$ antitrypsin deficiency. N Engl J Med 287:1264, 1972
81. ERIKSSON S, LARSSON C: PAS-positive inclusion bodies from the liver in alpha$_1$ antitrypsin deficiency. N Engl J Med 292:176, 1975
82. TRIGER DR et al: Alpha$_1$ antitrypsin deficiency and liver disease in adults. Q J Med 45:351, 1976

82a. HODGES JR, MILLWARD–SADLER GH, BARBATIS C, WRIGHT R: Heterozygous MZ alpha$_1$ antitrypsin deficiency in adults with chronic active hepatitis and cryptogenic cirrhosis. N Engl J Med 304:557, 1981
83. KUEPPERS F, BEARN AG: A possible experimental approach to the association of hereditary alpha$_1$ antitrypsin deficiency and pulmonary emphysema. Proc Soc Exp Biol Med 121:1207, 1966
84. LAURELL CB, KULLANDER S, THORELL J: Effect of administration of a combined estrogen–progestin contraceptive on the level of individual plasma proteins. Scand J Clin Lab Invest 21:337, 1968
85. KUEPPERS F: Genetically determined differences in the response of alpha$_1$ antitrypsin levels in human serum to typhoid vaccine. Hum Genet 6:207, 1968
86. LIEBERMAN J: The use of diethylstilbestrol for confirming heterozygosity in alpha$_1$ antitrypsin deficiency. Am Rev Respir Dis 101:1011, 1970
87. SIBBALD B, TURNER-WARWICK M: Factors influencing the prevalence of asthma among first degree relatives of extrinsic and intrinsic asthmatics. Thorax 34:332, 1979
88. LEM S, ABBOUD RT, CHAN-YEUNG M et al: Neutrophil elastase and pulmonary function in subjects with intermediate alpha$_1$ antitrypsin deficiency. Am Rev Respir Dis 119:941, 1979
89. COHEN AB: Opportunities for the development of specific therapeutic agents to treat emphysema. Am Rev Respir Dis 120:723, 1979
90. KIMBEL P: Proteolytic lung damage. Chest (Suppl) 77:2:274, 1980
91. JANOFF A et al: Lung injury induced by leucocyte proteases. Am J Pathol 97:111, 1979
92. GUENTER CA, COALSON JJ, JACQUES J: Emphysema associated with intravascular leucocyte sequestration: Comparison with papain induced emphysema. Am Rev Respir Dis 123:79, 1981
93. HOOD JM et al: Liver transplantation for advanced liver disease with alpha$_1$ antitrypsin deficiency. N Engl J Med 302:272, 1980
94. GADEK J et al: Danazol-induced elevation of serum alpha$_1$ antitrypsin in individuals with severe deficiency of this antiprotease. Chest (Suppl) 77:2:279, 1980
95. JANOFF A, DEARING R: Prevention of elastase-induced experimental emphysema by oral administration of a synthetic elastase inhibitor. Am Rev Respir Dis 121:1025, 1980
96. LEIGH D, MARLEY E: Bronchial Asthma. A Genetic, Population, and Psychiatric Study. Oxford, Pergamon Press, 1967
97. TAGER IB, ROSNER B, TISHLER PV et al: Household aggregation of pulmonary function and chronic bronchitis. Am Rev Respir Dis 114:485, 1976
98. KAZAZIAN HH JR: A geneticist's view of lung disease. Am Rev Respir Dis 113:261, 1976
99. COHEN BN, CHASE GA: Familial aggregation of chronic obstructive pulmonary disease. In Litwin SD (ed): Genetic Determinants of Pulmonary Disease, Chap 7. New York, Marcel-Dekker, 1978
100. GRAVES CG et al: Patterns of forced expiratory flows in groups at risk for chronic obstructive pulmonary disease. Johns Hopkins Med J 146:41, 1980
101. TAGER I, SPEIZER FE: Role of infection in chronic bronchitis. N Engl J Med 292:563, 1975
102. British Medical Research Council: Value of chemoprophylaxis and chemotherapy in early chronic bronchitis. Br Med J 1:1317, 1966
103. SMITH CB, GOLDEN C, KLAUBER MR et al: Interactions between viruses and bacteria in patients with chronic bronchitis. J Infect Dis 134:552, 1976
104. OSWALD NC, HAROLD JT, MARTIN WJ: Clinical pattern of chronic bronchitis. Lancet 2:639, 1953
105. REID DD, FAIRBAIRN AS: The natural history of chronic bronchitis. Lancet 1:1147, 1958
106. LARAYA-CUASAYZ LR, DEFOREST A, HUFF D et al: Chronic pulmonary complications of early influenza virus infection in children. Am Rev Respir Dis 116:617, 1977
107. HAAS H, MORRIS JF, SAMSON S et al: Bacterial flora of the respiratory tract in chronic bronchitis: Comparison of transtracheal, fiberbronchoscopic and oropharyngeal sampling methods. Am Rev Respir Dis 116:41, 1977
108. BURROWS B, KNUDSON RJ, LEBOWITZ MD: The relationship of childhood respiratory illness to adult obstructive airway disease. Am Rev Respir Dis 115:751, 1977
108a. KATTAN M: Long-term sequelae of respiratory illness of infancy and childhood. Pediatr Clin North Am 26:525, 1979
109. WOOLCOCK AJ, LEEDER SR, PEAT JK et al: The influence of lower respiratory illness in infancy and childhood and subsequent cigarette smoking on lung function in Sydney school children. Am Rev Respir Dis 120:5, 1979
110. HALL WJ, HALL CB: Alterations in pulmonary function following respiratory viral infection. Chest 76:458, 1979
111. MAY JR: The bacteriology of chronic bronchitis. Lancet 2:534, 1953
112. ASMUNDSSON T, KILBURN KH: Survival of respiratory failure. Ann Intern Med 70:471, 1969
113. BURROWS B, EARLE RH: Prediction of survival in patients with chronic airway obstruction. Am Rev Respir Dis 99:865, 1969
114. BURROWS B and EARLE RH: Course and prognosis of chronic obstructive lung disease. N Engl J Med 280:397, 1969

115. TRAVER GA, CLINE MG, BURROWS B: Predictors of mortality in chronic obstructive pulmonary disease. A 15 year follow-up study. Am Rev Respir Dis 119:895, 1979
116. POSTMA DS, BUREMA J, GIMENO F et al: Prognosis in severe chronic obstructive pulmonary disease. Am Rev Respir Dis 119:357, 1979
117. BATES DV: The fate of the chronic bronchitic: A report of the ten year follow-up in the Canadian Department of Veterans Affairs Coordinated Study of Chronic Bronchitis. Am Rev Respir Dis 108:1043, 1973
118. FLETCHER CM: Recent clinical and epidemiological studies of chronic bronchitis. Scand J Respir Dis 48:285, 1967
119. FLETCHER CM, TINKER CM, HILL ID et al: A five year prospective field study of early obstructive airway disease. Eleventh Aspen Conference. USPHS Publ 1879:249, 1968
120. FLETCHER C, PETO R, TINKER C et al: The Natural History of Chronic Bronchitis and Emphysema. London, Oxford University Press, 1976
121. FLETCHER C, PETO R: The natural history of chronic airflow obstruction. Br Med J 1:1645, 1977
122. BURROWS B: Early detection of airways obstruction. Chest 65:239, 1974
123. BATES DV: The prevention of emphysema. Chest 65:437, 1974
124. HOGG JC, MACKLEM PT, THURLBOCK WM: Site and nature of airway obstruction in chronic obstructive lung disease. N Engl J Med 278:1355, 1968
125. NIEWOEHNER DE, KLEINERMAN J, RICE DB: Pathologic changes in the peripheral airways of young cigarette smokers. N Engl J Med 291:755, 1974
126. COSIO M et al: The relations between structural changes in small airways and pulmonary function tests. N Engl J Med 298:1277, 1978
127. MACKLEM PT: Obstruction in small airways. A challenge to medicine. Am J Med 52:721, 1972
128. MATSUBA K, THURLBECK WM: Disease of the small airways in chronic bronchitis. Am Rev Respir Dis 107:552, 1973
129. MCLEAN KH: The pathogenesis of pulmonary emphysema. Am J Med 25:62, 1958
130. TURINO GM, RODRIQUEZ JR, GREENBAUM LM et al: Mechanisms of pulmonary injury. Am J Med 57:493, 1974
131. GROSS PM, BABYAK MA, TOLKER E et al: Enzymatically produced pulmonary emphysema. J Occup Med 6:481, 1964
132. JOHANSON WG JR, REYNOLDS RC, SCOTT TC et al: Connective tissue damage in emphysema. An electron microscopic study of papain-induced emphysema in rats. Am Rev Respir Dis 107:589, 1973
133. WITTELS EH, COALSON JJ, WELCH MH et al: Pulmonary intravascular leukocyte sequestration: A potential mechanism of lung injury. Am Rev Respir Dis 109:502, 1974
134. KARLINSKY JB, SNIDER GL: Animal models of emphysema. Am Rev Respir Dis 117:1109, 1978
135. MENEELY GR et al: Definition and classification of chronic bronchitis, asthma and pulmonary emphysema. Am Rev Respir Dis 85:762, 1962
136. Terminology, definitions and classification of chronic pulmonary emphysema and related conditions: A report of the conclusions of the CIBA Guest Symposium. Thorax 14:286, 1959
137. Definition and classification of chronic bronchitis for clinical and epidemiological purposes: A report of the medical research council by their committee on the aetiology of chronic bronchitis. Lancet 1:775, 1965
138. FLETCHER CM, JONES NL, BURROWS B et al: American emphysema and British bronchitis: A standardized comparative study. Am Rev Respir Dis 90:1, 1964
139. BURROWS B, NIDEN AJ, FLETCHER CM et al: Clinical types of chronic obstructive lung disease in London and Chicago. Am Rev Respir Dis 90:14, 1964
140. BURROWS B et al: The emphysematous and bronchial types of chronic airways obstruction: A clinicopathological study of patients in London and Chicago. Lancet 1:830, 1966
141. DORNHORST AC: Respiratory insufficiency. Lancet 1:1185, 1955
142. BURROWS B, NIDEN AH, BARCLAY WR et al: Chronic obstructive lung disease: Clinical and physiologic findings in 175 patients and their relationship to age and sex. Am Rev Respir Dis 91:521, 1965
143. BURROWS B, STRAUSS RH, NIDEN AH: Chronic obstructive lung disease: Interrelationships of pulmonary function data. Am Rev Respir Dis 91:861, 1965
144. MITCHELL RS, FILLEY GF: Chronic obstructive bronchopulmonary disease. I. Clinical features. Am Rev Respir Dis 89:360, 1964
145. MITCHELL RS et al: Clinical and morphological correlations in chronic airway obstruction. Am Rev Respir Dis 97:54, 1968
146. FILLEY GF, BECKWITT HJ, REEVES JT et al: Chronic obstructive bronchopulmonary disease: Oxygen transport in two clinical types. Am J Med 44:26, 1968
147. FILLEY GT: Emphysema and chronic bronchitis: Clinical manifestations and their physiologic significance. Med Clin North Am 51:283, 1967
148. PAROT S et al: Breathing pattern and hypercapnea in patients with obstructive pulmonary disease. Am Rev Respir Dis 121:985, 1980
149. BOYSEN PG et al: Nocturnal pulmonary hypertension in patients with chronic obstructive pulmonary disease. Chest 76:536, 1979

150. BATES DV et al: Report on the third and fourth stages of the co-ordinated study of chronic bronchitis in the Department of Veterans Affairs, Canada. Med Services J Can 22:5, 1966
151. SIMON G: Radiological changes in chronic bronchitis. Br J Radiol 32:292, 1959
152. SIMON G, GALBRAITH HJB: Radiology of chronic bronchitis. Lancet 2:850, 1953
153. THURLBECK WM, HENDERSON JA, FRASER RG et al: Chronic obstructive lung disease: A comparison between clinical, roentgenologic, functional and morphologic criteria in chronic bronchitis, emphysema, asthma and bronchiectasis. Medicine 49:81, 1970
154. MILLARD FJ: The electrocardiogram in chronic lung disease. Br Heart J 29:43, 1967
155. SHMOCK CL et al: The electrocardiogram in chronic airways obstruction. The role of bronchitis and emphysema. Chest 60:335, 1971
156. TAHA RA et al: The electrocardiogram in chronic obstructive pulmonary disease. Am Rev Respir Dis 107:1067, 1973
157. CARILLI AD, DENSON J, TIMMAPURI MD: Electrocardiographic estimation of pulmonary impairment in chronic obstructive lung disease. Chest 63:483, 1973
158. MURPHY ML, HUTCHESON F: The electrocardiographic diagnosis of right ventricular hypertrophy in chronic obstructive pulmonary disease. Chest 65:622, 1974
159. CORAZZA LJ, PASTOR BH: Cardiac arrhythmias in chronic cor pulmonale. N Engl J Med 259:862, 1958
160. HUDSON LD, KURT TL, PETTY TL et al: Arrythmias associated with acute respiratory failure in patients with chronic airway obstruction. Chest 63:661, 1973
161. HOLFORD FD, MITHOEFER JC: Cardiac arrythmias in hospitalized patients with chronic obstructive pulmonary disease. Am Rev Respir Dis 108:879, 1973
162. KLEIGER RE, SENIOR RM: Longterm electrocardiographic monitoring of ambulatory patients with chronic airways obstruction. Chest 65:483, 1974
163. SIDERIS DA, KATSADOROS DP, VALIANOS G et al: A type of cardiac dysrhythmias in respiratory failure. Am Heart J 89:32, 1975
164. KENNEDY HL, CARALIS DG: Ambulatory electrocardiography: A clinical perspective. Ann Intern Med 87:729, 1977
165. FLICK MR, BLOCK AJ: Nocturnal vs diurnal cardiac arrhythmias in patients with chronic obstructive pulmonary disease. Chest 75:8, 1979
166. SENIOR RM, LEFRAK SS, KLEIGER RE: The heart in chronic obstructive pulmonary disease; arrhythmias. Chest 75:1, 1979
167. SHINE KI, KASTOR JA, YURCHAK PM: Multifocal atrial tachycardia. N Engl J Med 279:344, 1968
168. BECKLAKE MR, PERMUTT S: Evaluation of tests of lung function for "screening" for early detection of chronic obstructive lung disease. In Macklem PT, Permutt S (eds): The Lung in Transition Between Health and Disease, Chap 12. New York, Marcel-Dekker, 1979
169. PENMAN RWB, O'NEILL RP, BEGLEY L: Lung elastic recoil and airway resistance as factors limiting expiratory flow. Am Rev Respir Dis 101:528, 1970
170. PENMAN RWB, O'NEILL RP, BEGLEY L: The progress of chronic airway obstruction in relation to measurements of airway resistance and lung elastic recoil. Am Rev Respir Dis 101:536, 1970
171. DUFFELL GM, MARCUS JH, INGRAM RH JR: Limitation of expiratory flow in chronic obstructive pulmonary disease. Relation of clinical characteristics, pathophysiological type, and mechanisms. Ann Intern Med 73:365, 1970
172. DUNNILL MD: The contribution of morphology to the study of chronic obstructive lung disease. Am J Med 57:506, 1974
173. REID L: The Pathology of Emphysema. Chicago, Year Book Medical Publishers, 1967
174. REID L: Measurement of the bronchial mucous gland layer: a diagnostic yardstick in chronic bronchitis. Thorax 15:132, 1960
175. THURLBECK WM, ANGUS GE: A distribution curve for chronic bronchitis. Thorax 19:436, 1964
176. DULFANO MJ, ADLER K, PHILIPPOFF W: Sputum viscoelasticity in chronic bronchitis. Am Rev Respir Dis 104:88, 1971
177. MARTIN CJ, KATSURA S, COCHRAN TH: The relationship of chronic bronchitis to the diffuse obstructive pulmonary syndrome. Am Rev Respir Dis 102:362, 1970
178. THURLBECK WM: Aspects of chronic airflow obstruction. Chest 72:341, 1977
179. KARPICK RJ, PRATT PC, ASMUNDSSON T et al: Pathologic findings in respiratory failure: Goblet cell metaplasia, alveolar damage, and myocardial infarction. Am Rev Respir Dis 101:451, 1970
180. THURLBECK WM, MALAKA D, MURPHY K: Goblet cells in the peripheral airways in chronic bronchitis. Am Rev Respir Dis 112:65, 1975
181. HEARD BE: Pathology of Chronic Bronchitis and Emphysema. Baltimore, Williams & Wilkins, 1969
182. RODMAN T, STERLING FH: Pulmonary Emphysema and Related Lung Diseases. St. Louis, CV Mosby, 1969
183. NICKLAUS TM, STOWELL DW, CHRISTIANSEN WR et al: The accuracy of the roentgenologic diagnosis of chronic pulmonary emphysema. Am Rev Respir Dis 93:889, 1966
184. SIMON G: Radiology and emphysema. Clin Radiol 15:293, 1964
185. SIMON G, PRIDE NB, JONES NL et al: Relation between abnormalities in the chest radiograph and

changes in pulmonary function in chronic bronchitis and emphysema. Thorax 28:15, 1973

186. LAWS JW, HEARD BE: Emphysema and the chest film: A retrospective radiological and pathological study. Br J Radiol 35:750, 1962

187. THURLBECK WM: A clinico-pathological study of emphysema in an American hospital. Thorax 18:59, 1963

188. REID L, MILLARD FJC: Correlation between radiologic diagnosis and structural lung changes in emphysema. Clin Radiol 15:307, 1964

189. SUTINEN S, CHRISTOFORIDIS AJ, KLUGH GA et al: Roentgenologic criteria for the recognition of nonsymptomatic pulmonary emphysema. Correlation between roentgenologic findings and pulmonary pathology. Am Rev Respir Dis 91:69, 1965

190. MCCARTHY DS, ROBERTSON M, SIMON G: Diagnosis of emphysema. Chest 68:46, 1975

191. SHMOCK CL et al: The electrocardiogram in emphysema with and without chronic airways obstruction. Chest 60:328, 1971

192. BALDWIN E DE F, COURNAND A, RICHARDS DW JR: Pulmonary insufficiency. III. A study of 122 cases of chronic pulmonary emphysema. Medicine 28:201, 1949

193. WILLIAMS MH JR, ZOHMAN LR: Cardiopulmonary function in chronic obstructive emphysema. Am Rev Respir Dis 80:689, 1959

194. LEINER GC, ABRAMOWITZ S, SMALL MJ: The vital capacity in pulmonary emphysema. Ann Intern Med 60:61, 1964

195. SWEET HC, WYATT JP, KINSELLA PW: Correlation of lung macrosections with pulmonary function in emphysema. Am J Med 29:277, 1960

196. WATANABE S, MITCHELL M, RENZETTI AD JR: Correlation of structure and function in chronic pulmonary emphysema. Am Rev Respir Dis 92:221, 1965

197. NICKLAUS TM, WATANABE S, MITCHELL MM et al: Roentgenologic, physiologic, and structural estimations of the total lung capacity in normal and emphysematous subjects. Am J Med 42:547, 1967

198. CHRISTIE RV: The elastic properties of the emphysematous lung and their clinical significance. J Clin Invest 13:295, 1934

199. CHERNIACK RM: The physical properties of the lung in chronic obstructive pulmonary emphysema. J Clin Invest 35:394, 1956

200. MACKLEM PT, BECKLAKE MR: The relationship between the mechanical and diffusing properties of the lung in health and disease. Am Rev Respir Dis 87:47, 1963

201. STEVENS PM, ORMAN BF, GRAVES G JR: Contributions of lung recoil and airway resistance to forced expiratory flow limitation. Am Rev Respir Dis 100:54, 1969

202. PARK SS, JANIS M, SHIM CS et al: Relationship of bronchitis and emphysema to altered pulmonary function. Am Rev Respir Dis 102:927, 1970

203. BOUSHY SF, ABOUMRAD MH, NORTH LB et al: Lung recoil pressure, airway resistance, and forced flows related to morphologic emphysema. Am Rev Respir Dis 104:551, 1971

204. GREAVES IA, COLEBATCH HJH: Elastic behaviour and structure of normal and emphysematous lungs post mortem. Am Rev Respir Dis 121:127, 1980

205. GELB AF et al: Physiologic diagnosis of subclinical emphysema. Am Rev Respir Dis 107:50, 1973

206. BOUSHY SF, NORTH LB, FAGAN TJ: The role of parenchymal and airway disease in limiting forced expired flows in chronic obstructive pulmonary disease. Am Rev Respir Dis 108:870, 1973

207. MACKLEM PT: Changes in lung mechanics. In Macklem PT, Permutt S (eds): Changes in the Lung in Transition Between Health and Disease, Chap 4. New York, Marcel-Dekker, 1979

208. TING EY, LYONS HA: Pressure–volume relations of the lung and thoracic cage in pulmonary emphysema. J Appl Physiol 16:517, 1961

209. CHERNIACK RM, HODSON A: Compliance of the chest wall in chronic bronchitis and emphysema. J Appl Physiol 18:707, 1963

210. KRUMHOLZ RA, ALBRIGHT CD: The compliance of the chest wall and thorax in emphysema. Am Rev Respir Dis 97:827, 1968

211. JONES NL: Pulmonary gas exchange during exercise in patients with chronic airway obstruction. Clin Sci 31:39, 1966

212. JENKINS DE et al: Correlation of morphologic emphysema with pulmonary function parameters. Trans Assoc Am Physician 78:215, 1965

213. SYMONDS G, RENZETTI AD, MITCHELL MM: The diffusing capacity in pulmonary emphysema. Am Rev Respir Dis 109:391, 1974

214. MARCUS JH, MCLEAN RL, DUFFELL GM et al: Exercise performance in relation to the pathophysiologic type of chronic obstructive pulmonary disease. Am J Med 49:14, 1970

215. MILLER WS: The Lung. Springfield, Charles C Thomas, 1937

216. GOUGH J: The pathological diagnosis of emphysema. Proc R Soc Med 45:576, 1952

217. LEOPOLD JG, GOUGH J: The centrilobular form of hypertrophic emphysema and its relation to chronic bronchitis. Thorax 12:219, 1957

218. WYATT JP, FISCHER VW, SWEET HC: Panlobular emphysema: Anatomy and pathodynamics. Dis Chest 41:239, 1962

219. THURLBECK WM et al: A cooperative study of certain measurements of emphysema. Am Rev Respir Dis 98:217, 1968

220. HEPPLESTON AG: The pathological anatomy of simple pneumokoniosis in coal workers. J Pathol Bacteriol 66:235, 1953

221. SNIDER GL, BRODY JS, DOCTOR L: Subclinical pulmonary emphysema: Incidence and anatomic patterns. Am Rev Respir Dis 85:666, 1962
222. THURLBECK WM: The incidence of pulmonary emphysema, with observations on the relative incidence and spatial distribution of various types of emphysema. Am Rev Respir Dis 87:206, 1963
223. WEIBEL ER: Principles and methods for the morphometric study of the lung and other organs. Lab Invest 12:131, 1963
224. THURLBECK WM, ANGUS GE: The relationship between emphysema and chronic bronchitis as assessed morphologically. Am Rev Respir Dis 87:815, 1963
225. MCLAUGHLIN RF, TUELLER EE: Anatomic and histologic changes of early emphysema. Chest 59:592, 1971
226. Chronic cor pulmonale: Report of an expert committee of the World Health Organization. Circulation 27:594, 1963
227. FISHMAN AP: Chronic cor pulmonale. Am Rev Respir Dis 114:775, 1976
228. DUNNILL MS: An assessment of the anatomical factor in cor pulmonale in emphysema. J Clin Pathol 14:246, 1961
229. COURNAND A: Some aspects of the pulmonary circulation in normal man and in chronic cardiopulmonary diseases. Circulation 2:641, 1950
230. WESTCOTT RN et al: Anoxia and human pulmonary vascular resistance. J Clin Invest 30:957, 1951
231. FISHMAN AP, MCCLEMENT J, HIMMELSTEIN A et al: Effects of acute anoxia on the circulation and respiration in patients with chronic pulmonary disease studied during the "steady state." J Clin Invest 31:770, 1952
232. WILSON RH, HOSETH W, DEMPSEY MF: The effects of breathing 99.6% oxygen on pulmonary vascular resistance and cardiac output in patients with pulmonary emphysema and chronic hypoxia. Ann Intern Med 42:629, 1955
233. HOLT JH, BRANSCOMB BV: Hemodynamic responses to controlled 100% oxygen breathing in emphysema. J Appl Physiol 20:215, 1965
234. LEVINE BE et al: The role of long-term continuous oxygen administration in patients with chronic airway obstruction with hypoxemia. Ann Intern Med 66:639, 1967
235. HORSFIELD K, SEGEL N, BISHOP JM: The pulmonary circulation in chronic bronchitis at rest and during exercise breathing air and 80% oxygen. Clin Sci 34:473, 1968
236. ABRAHAM AS, COLE RB, BISHOP JM: Reversal of pulmonary hypertension by prolonged oxygen administration to patients with chronic bronchitis. Circ Res 23:147, 1968
237. BLOCK AJ, CASTLE JR, KEITT AS: Chronic oxygen therapy: Treatment of chronic obstructive pulmonary disease at sea level. Chest 65:279, 1974
238. HARVEY RM et al: Further observations on the effect of hydrogen ion on the pulmonary circulation. Circulation 35:1019, 1967
239. WAGENVOORT CA, HEATH D, EDWARDS JE: The Pathology of the Pulmonary Vasculature. Springfield, Charles C Thomas, 1964
240. HARRIS P, SEGEL N, GREEN I et al: The influence of the airways resistance and alveolar pressure on the pulmonary vascular resistance in chronic bronchitis. Cardiovasc Res 2:84, 1968
241. SEGEL N, BISHOP JM: The circulation in patients with chronic bronchitis and emphysema at rest and during exercise, with special reference to the influence of changes in blood viscosity and blood volume on the pulmonary circulation. J Clin Invest 45:1555, 1966
242. BONIFACE KJ, BROWN JM: Effect of carbon dioxide excess in contractile force of the heart in situ. Am J Physiol 172:753, 1953
243. DARBY TD, ALDINGER EE, GADSDEN RH et al: Effects of metabolic acidosis on ventricular isometric systolic tension and the response to epinephrine and levarterenol. Circ Res 8:1242, 1960
244. BURROWS B et al: Patterns of cardiovascular dysfunction in chronic obstructive lung disease. N Engl J Med 286:912, 1972
245. RAO BS, COHN KE, ELDRIDGE FL et al: Left ventricular failure secondary to chronic pulmonary disease. Am J Med 45:229, 1968
246. WILLIAMS JF JR et al: Left ventricular function in patients with chronic obstructive pulmonary disease. J Clin Invest 47:1143, 1968
247. DAVIES H, OVERY HR: Left ventricular function in cor pulmonale. Chest 58:8, 1970
248. BAUM GL, SCHWARTZ A, LLAMAS R et al: Left ventricular function in chronic obstructive lung disease. N Engl J Med 285:361, 1971
249. HOOPER RG, WHITCOMB ME: Systolic time intervals in chronic obstructive pulmonary disease. Circulation 50:1205, 1974
250. MURPHY ML, ADAMSON J, HUTCHESON F: Left ventricular hypertrophy in patients with chronic bronchitis and emphysema. Ann Intern Med 81:307, 1974
251. STEELE P, ELLIS JH JR, VANDYKE D et al.: Left ventricular ejection fraction in severe chronic obstructive airways disease. Am J Med 59:21, 1975
252. KLINE LF, CRAWFORD MH, MACDONALD WJ JR et al: Noninvasive assessment of left ventricular performance in patients with chronic obstructive pulmonary disease. Chest 72:558, 1977
253. KACHEL RG: Left ventricular function in chronic obstructive pulmonary disease. Chest 74:286, 1978
254. BASS H: Lung function in chronic obstructive lung disease and coexistent left heart failure. Am J Med 48:413, 1970

255. SIMPSON T: Papilledema in emphysema. Br Med J 2:639, 1948
256. KNOWLES JH: Prognostic significance of papilledema in the course of respiratory insufficiency. JAMA 183:161, 1963
257. BOUSHY SF, NORTH LB: Hemodynamic changes in chronic obstructive pulmonary disease. Chest 72:565, 1977
258. SCHRIJEN F, UFFHOLTZ H, POLU JM et al: Pulmonary and systemic hemodynamic evolution in chronic bronchitis. Am Rev Respir Dis 117:25, 1978
259. WEITZENBLUM F, LOISEAU A, HIRTH C et al: Course of pulmonary hemodynamics in patients with chronic obstructive pulmonary disease. Chest 75:651, 1979
260. ALPERT JS: Pulmonary hypertension and cardiac function in chronic obstructive pulmonary disease. Chest 75:651, 1979
261. LERTZMAN M, ISRAELS LG, CHERNIACK RM: Erythropoiesis and ferrokinetics in chronic respiratory disease. Ann Intern Med 56:821, 1962
262. VANIER T, DULFANO MJ, WU C, DESFORCES JF: Emphysema, hypoxia and the polycythemic response. N Engl J Med 269:169, 1963
263. GALLO RC, FRAIMOW W, CATHCART RT et al: Erythropoietic response in chronic pulmonary disease. Arch Intern Med 113:559, 1964
264. HUME R, GOLDBERG A: Acute and predicted-normal red-cell and plasma volumes in primary and secondary polycythemia. Clin Sci 26:499, 1964
265. MASSARO D, CUSICK AM, KATZ S: Erythropoiesis in subjects with chronic bronchitis. Am Rev Respir Dis 91:541, 1965
266. WHITCOMB WH et al: The erythropoietic factor in hypoxic patients with emphysema without secondary polycythemia. Arch Intern Med 103:871, 1959
267. CASTLE WB, JANDL JH: Blood viscosity and blood volume: Opposing influences upon oxygen transport in polycythemia. Semin Hematol 3:193, 1966
268. THORLING EB, ERSLEV AJ: The tissue tension of oxygen and its relation to hematocrit and erythropoiesis. Blood 31:332, 1968
269. RAKITA L, GILLESPIE DG, SANCETTA SM: The acute and chronic effects of phlebotomy on general hemodynamics and pulmonary functions of patients with secondary polycythemia associated with pulmonary emphysema. Am Heart J 70:466, 1965
270. THOMAS DJ et al: Effect of hematocrit on cerebral blood flow in man. Lancet ii:941, 1977
271. HUMPHREY PRD et al: Cerebral blood flow and viscosity in relative polycythemia. Lancet ii:873, 1979
271a. MENON D et al: Optimal hematocrit and blood viscosity in secondary polycythemia as determined from cerebral blood flow. Clin Invest Med 4:117, 1981
271b. YORK EL et al: Effects of secondary polycythemia on cerebral blood flow in COPD. Am Rev Respir Dis 121:813, 1980
272. PETTY TL et al: A comprehensive care program for chronic airway obstruction. Ann Intern Med 70:1109, 1969
273. EMIRGIL C et al: A study of the long-term effect of therapy in chronic obstructive pulmonary disease. Am J Med 47:367, 1969
274. LEFCOE NM, PATERSON NAM: Adjunct therapy in chronic obstructive pulmonary disease. Am J Med 54:343, 1973
275. PETTY TL: Does treatment for severe emphysema and chronic bronchitis really help? (A response.) Chest 65:124, 1974
276. BURK RH, GEORGE RB: Acute respiratory failure in chronic obstructive pulmonary disease. Arch Intern Med 132:865, 1973
277. ISHIKAWA S, CHERNIACK RM: The effect of nebulized bronchodilators on air flow resistance in chronic airways obstruction. Am Rev Respir Dis 99:703, 1969
278. LIGHT RW, SUMMER WR, LUCHSINGER PC: Response of patients with chronic obstructive lung disease to the regular administration of nebulized isoproterenol. Chest 67:634, 1975
279. WATANABE S, RENZETTI AD JR, BIGLER A: Bronchodilator and corticosteroid effects on regional and total airway resistance in patients with asthma, chronic bronchitis and chronic pulmonary emphysema. Am Rev Respir Dis 106:392, 1972
280. MILLER WF: Aerosol therapy in acute and chronic respiratory disease. Arch Intern Med 131:148, 1973
281. LOURENCO RV: Aerosol therapy: Introduction (Conference on the Scientific Basis of Respiratory Therapy). Am Rev Respir Dis 110[Part 2]:85, 1974
282. MORROW RE: Aerosol characterization and deposition. Am Rev Respir Dis 110[Part 2]:88, 1974
283. GIBSON LE: Use of water vapor in the treatment of lower respiratory disease. Am Rev Respir Dis 110[Part 2]:100, 1974
284. CHOPRA SK, TAPLIN GV, SIMMONS DH et al: Effects of hydration and physical therapy on tracheal transport velocity. Am Rev Respir Dis 115:1009, 1977
284a. PIERCE AK (chairman): Proceedings of conference on the scientific basis of in-hospital respiratory therapy. Am Rev Respir Dis 122 (2):1–161, 1980
285. STUART BO: Deposition of inhaled aerosols. Arch Intern Med 131:60, 1973
286. GOLDBERG IS, LOURENCO RV: Deposition of aerosols in pulmonary disease. Arch Intern Med 131:88, 1973
287. BARTON AD, LOURENCO RV: Bronchial secretions

and mucociliary clearance. Arch Intern Med 131:140, 1973
288. BRAIN JD, VALBERG PA: Deposition of aerosol in the respiratory tract. Am Rev Respir Dis 120:1325, 1979
289. TAGUCHI JT: Effect of ultrasonic nebulization in blood gas tensions in chronic obstructive lung disease. Chest 60:356, 1971
290. PIERCE AK, SANFORD JP: Bacterial contamination of aerosols. Arch Intern Med 131:156, 1973
291. BARTON AD: Aerosolized detergents and mucolytic agents in the treatment of stable chronic obstructive pulmonary disease. Am Rev Respir Dis 110[Part 2]:104, 1974
292. LIEBERMAN J: The appropriate use of mucolytic agents. Am J Med 49:1, 1970
293. BOYD EM: Expectorants and respiratory tract fluid. Pharmacol Rev 6:521, 1954
294. BECKMAN H: Expectorants. JAMA 167:1638, 1958
295. HIRSCH SR, VIERNES PF, KORY RC: The expectorant effect of glyceryl guaiacolate in patients with chronic bronchitis. Chest 63:9, 1973
296. CHODOSH S, MEDICI TC: Letter: Expectorant effect of glyceryl guaiacolate. Chest 64:543, 1973
297. HIRSCH SR, KORY RC: Letter: Expectorant effect of glyceryl guaiacolate. Chest 64:544, 1973
298. LANGLANDS JHM: Double-blind clinical trial of bromhexine as mucolytic drug in chronic bronchitis. Lancet 1:448, 1970
299. THOMSON ML, PAVIA D, JONES CJ et al: No demonstrable effect of S-carboxymethylcysteine on clearance of secretions from the human lung. Thorax 30:669, 1975
300. EDWARDS GF, STEEL AE, SCOTT JK et al: S-carboxymethylcysteine in the fluidation of sputum and treatment of chronic airway obstruction. Chest 70:506, 1976
301. GOODMAN RM, YERGIN BM, SACKNER MA: Effects of S-carboxymethylcysteine on tracheal mucus velocity. Chest 74:615, 1978
302. ZIMENT I: Why are they saying bad things about IPPB? Respir Care 18:677, 1973
303. BAKER JP: Magnitude of usage of intermittent positive pressure breathing. Am Rev Respir Dis 110[Part 2]:170, 1974
304. LOKE J, ANTHONISEN NR: Effect of intermittent positive pressure breathing on steady state chronic obstructive pulmonary disease. Am Rev Respir Dis 110[Part 2]:178, 1974
305. CHENEY FW, NELSON EJ, HORTON WG: The function of intermittent positive pressure breathing related to breathing patterns. Am Rev Respir Dis 110[Part 2]:183, 1974
306. CHERNIACK RM: Intermittent positive pressure breathing in management of chronic obstructive pulmonary disease: Current state of the art. Am Rev Respir Dis 110[Part 2]:188, 1974
307. MURRAY JF: Review of the state of the art in intermittent positive pressure breathing therapy. Am Rev Respir Dis 110[Part 2]:193, 1974
308. PETTY TL: A critical look at IPPB. Chest 66:1, 1974
309. YANDA RL: Quality control of inhalation therapy. Chest 66:1, 1974
310. GOLD MI: The present status of IPPB therapy. Chest 67:469, 1975
311. NOEHREN TH: IPPB therapy—where do we go from here? Chest 67:471, 1975
312. CHERNIACK RM, SVANHILL E: Long-term use of intermittent positive-pressure breathing (IPPB) in chronic obstructive pulmonary disease. Am Rev Respir Dis 113:721, 1976
313. SHIM C, BAJWA S, WILLIAMS MH JR: The effect of inhalation therapy on ventilatory function and expectoration. Chest 73:798, 1978
314. NOEHREN TH, KLAUBER MR: Controversy over intermittent positive pressure breathing. Chest 73:782, 1978
315. O'DONOHUE WJ JR: Maximum volume IPPB for the management of pulmonary atelectasis. Chest 76:683, 1979
316. PETTY TL: Physical therapy: Introduction. Am Rev Respir Dis 110[Part 2]:129, 1974
317. JONES NL: Physical therapy—present state of the art. Am Rev Respir Dis 110[Part 2]:132, 1974
318. COCHRANE GM, WEBBER BA, CLARKE SW: Effects of sputum on pulmonary function. Br Med J 2:1181, 1977
319. NEWTON DAG, BEAVANS HG: Physiotherapy and intermittent positive-pressure ventilation of chronic bronchitis. Br Med J 2:1525, 1978
320. NEWTON DAG, STEPHENSON A: Effect of physiotherapy on pulmonary function. Lancet 2:228, 1978
321. OLDENBURG FA JR, DOLOVICH MD, MONTGOMERY JM et al: Effects of postural drainage, exercise and cough on mucus clearance in chronic bronchitis. Am Res Respir Dis 120:739, 1979
322. FELDMAN J, TRAVER GA, TAUSSIG LM: Maximal expiratory flows after postural drainage. Am Rev Respir Dis 119:239, 1979
323. MAY DB, MUNT PW: Physiologic effects of chest percussion and postural drainage in patients with stable chronic bronchitis. Chest 75:29, 1979
324. MURRAY JF: The ketchup-bottle method. N Engl J Med 300:1155, 1979
325. BATEMAN JRM et al: Regional lung clearance of excessive bronchial secretions during chest physiotherapy in patients with stable chronic airways obstruction. Lancet i:294, 1979
326. GASKELL DV, WEBBER BA: The Bromptom Hospital Guide to Chest Physiotherapy, 2nd ed. Oxford, Blackwell Scientific Publications, 1974

327. GRIMBY G: Aspects of lung expansion in relation to pulmonary physiotherapy. Am Rev Respir Dis 110[Part 2]:145, 1974

328. SHARP JT et al: Respiratory muscle function in patients with chronic obstructive pulmonary disease: Its relationship to disability and to respiratory therapy. Am Rev Respir Dis 110[Part 2]:154, 1974

329. BRACH BB, CHAO RP, SGROI VL et al: ^{133}Xenon washout patterns during diaphragmatic breathing: studies in normal subjects and patients with chronic obstructive pulmonary disease. Chest 71:735, 1977

330. HUGHES RL: Does abdominal breathing affect regional gas exchange? Chest 76:288, 1979

331. PIERCE AK, TAYLOR HF, ARCHER RK et al: Response to exercise training in patients with emphysema. Arch Intern Med 113:28, 1964

332. PIERCE AK, PAEZ PN, MILLER WF: Exercise training with the aid of a portable oxygen supply in patients with emphysema. Am Rev Respir Dis 91:653, 1965

333. PAEZ PN, PHILLIPSON EA, MASANGKAY M et al: The physiologic basis of training patients with emphysema. Am Rev Respir Dis 95:944, 1967

334. CHRISTIE D: Physical training in chronic obstructive lung disease. Br Med J 2:150, 1968

335. BASS H, WHITCOMB JF, FORMAN R: Exercise training therapy for patients with chronic obstructive pulmonary disease. Chest 57:116, 1970

336. NICHOLAS JJ, GILBERT R, GALF R et al: Evaluation of an exercise therapy program for patients with chronic obstructive pulmonary disease. Am Rev Respir Dis 102:1, 1970

336a. DELKER LL, MOSER RH, NELSON JD et al: Amantadine: Does it have a role in the prevention and treatment of influenza? Ann Intern Med 92:256, 1980

337. ALPERT JS, BASS H, SZUCS MM et al: Effects of physical training on hemodynamics and pulmonary function at rest and during exercise in patients with chronic obstructive pulmonary disease. Chest 66:647, 1974

338. BRUMMER DL (Chairman): Chemoprophylaxis of chronic bronchitis. A statement of the Committee on Therapy. Am Rev Respir Dis 104:776, 1971

339. BURROWS B, NEVIN W: Antibiotic management in patients with chronic bronchitis and emphysema. Ann Intern Med 77:993, 1972

340. PATERSON IC, PETRIE GR, CRAMPTON GK et al: Chronic bronchitis: Is bacteriological examination of sputum necessary? Br Med J 2:537, 1978

341. LAKE KB, VANDYKE JJ, RUMSFELD JA: Combined topical pulmonary and systemic gentamycin. Chest 68:62, 1975

342. WILLIAMS MH: Steroid and antibiotic aerosols. Am Rev Respir Dis 110[Part 2]:122, 1974

343. ELDRIDGE F, GHERMAN C: Studies of oxygen administration in respiratory failure. Ann Intern Med 68:569, 1968

344. SWAIN BK, PARK SS, WILLIAMS MH JR: The effect of 30 percent and 100 percent oxygen breathing in patients with chronic obstructive pulmonary disease. Am Rev Respir Dis 98:22, 1968

345. NEFF TA, PETTY TL: Long-term continuous oxygen therapy in chronic airway obstruction. Ann Intern Med 72:621, 1970

346. PETTY TL, STANFORD RE, NEFF TA: Continuous oxygen therapy in chronic airway obstruction. Observation on possible oxygen toxicity and survival. Ann Intern Med 75:361, 1971

347. LONGO AM, MOSER KM, LUCHSINGER PC: The role of oxygen therapy in the rehabilitation of patients with chronic obstructive pulmonary disease. Am Rev Respir Dis 103:690, 1971

348. STARK RD, FINNEGAN P, BISHOP JM: Daily requirement of oxygen to reverse pulmonary hypertension in patients with chronic bronchitis. Br Med J 3:724, 1972

349. STARK RD, FINNEGAN P, BISHOP JM: Long-term domiciliary oxygen in chronic bronchitis with pulmonary hypertension. Br Med J 3:467, 1973

350. KETTEL LJ, BIGELOW DB, LEVINE BE: Recommendations for continuous O_2 therapy in chronic obstructive lung disease. Report of the Committee on Emphysema, American College of Chest Physicians. Chest 64:505, 1973

351. SACKNER MA: A history of oxygen usage in chronic obstructive pulmonary disease. Am Rev Respir Dis 110[Part 2]:25, 1974

352. BURROWS B: Arterial oxygenation and pulmonary hemodynamics in patients with chronic airways obstruction. Am Rev Respir Dis 110[Part 2]:64, 1974

353. BLOCK AJ: Low flow oxygen therapy: Treatment of the ambulant outpatient. Am Rev Respir Dis 110[Part 2]:71, 1974

354. NEFF TA: Selection of patients for oxygen therapy. Chest 68:481, 1975

355. STEWART BN, HOOD CI, BLOCK AJ: Long-term results of continuous oxygen therapy at sea level. Chest 68:486, 1975

356. FLENLEY DC: Clinical hypoxia; causes, consequences and correction. Lancet 1:542, 1978

357. BRADLEY BL, GARNER AE, BILLIU D et al: Oxygen-assisted exercise in chronic obstructive lung disease. The effect on exercise capacity and arterial blood gas tensions. Am Rev Respir Dis 118:239, 1978

358. KROP HD, BLOCK AJ, COHEN E et al: Neuropsychologic effects of continuous oxygen therapy in the aged. Chest 72:737, 1977

359. FLICK MR, BLOCK AJ: Continuous in-vivo monitoring of arterial oxygenation in chronic obstructive lung disease. Ann Intern Med 86:725, 1977

359a. Nocturnal Oxygen Therapy Trial Group: Continuous or nocturnal oxygen therapy in hypoxemic chronic obstructive lung disease. Ann Intern Med 93:391, 1980

359b. STUART–HARRIS C, FLENLEY DC, BISHOP JM et al: Long-term domiciliary oxygen therapy in chronic hypoxic cor pulmonale complicating chronic bronchitis and emphysema. Lancet 1:681, 1981

359c. TIMMS RM, KVALE PA, ANTHONISEN NR: Selection of patients with chronic obstructive pulmonary disease for long-term oxygen therapy. JAMA 245:2514, 1981

360. FOSTER LJ, CORRIGAN K, GOLDMAN AL: Effectiveness of oxygen therapy in hypoxic polycythemic smokers. Chest 73:572, 1978

361. GESSNER DM: New developments in oxygen-therapy equipment for home use. Respiratory Therapy 8:29, 1978

362. BROWN HV, ZIMENT I: Evaluation of an oxygen concentrator in patients with COPD. Respiratory Therapy 8:55, 1978

363. CHUSID EL, LIBROT M, UTZURRUM F et al: Treatment of hypoxemia with an oxygen enricher. Chest 76:278, 1979

364. HARRIS P: Principles of management of cor pulmonale. Chest [Suppl 2] 58:437, 1970

365. BAUM GL et al: Factors involved in digitalis sensitivity in chronic pulmonary insufficiency. Am Heart J 57:460, 1969

366. GREEN LH, SMITH TW: The use of digitalis in patients with pulmonary disease. Ann Intern Med 87:459, 1977

367. HARRISON DC, ROBINSON MD, KLEIGER RE: Role of hypoxia in digitalis toxicity. Am J Med Sci 256:352, 1968

368. OGILVIE RT, RUEDY J: An educational program in digitalis therapy. JAMA 222:50, 1972

369. HEINEMANN HO: Right sided heart failure and the use of diuretics. Am J Med 64:367, 1978

370. GERTZ I, HEDENSTIERNA G, WEBSTER PO: Improvement in pulmonary function with diuretic therapy in the hypervolemic and polycythemic patient with chronic obstructive pulmonary disease. Chest 75:146, 1979

371. KLEIN RC, SALVAGGIO JE, KUNDUR VG: The response of patients with "idiopathic" obstructive pulmonary disease and "allergic" obstructive bronchitis to prednisone. Ann Intern Med 71:711, 1969

372. BEEREL FR, VANCE JW: Prednisone treatment for stable pulmonary emphysema. Am Rev Respir Dis 104:264, 1971

373. WATANABE S, RENZETTI AD JR, BIGLER A: Bronchodilator and corticosteroid effects on regional and total airway resistance in patients with asthma, chronic bronchitis, and chronic pulmonary emphysema. Am Rev Respir Dis 106:392, 1972

374. SAHN SA: Corticosteroids in chronic bronchitis and pulmonary emphysema. Chest 73:389, 1978

375. SHIM C, STOVER DE, WILLIAMS MH: Response to corticosteroids in chronic bronchitis. J Allergy Clin Immunol 62:563, 1978

376. ZIMENT I: Respiratory Pharmacology and Therapeutics. Philadelphia, WB Saunders, 1978

376a. ALBERT RK, MARTIN TR, LEWIS SW: Controlled clinical trial of methylprednisolone in patients with chronic bronchitis and acute respiratory insufficiency. Ann Intern Med 92:753, 1980

377. BADER ME, BADER RA: Respiratory stimulants in obstructive lung disease. Am J Med 38:165, 1965

378. WOOLF CR: The use of "respiratory stimulant" drugs. Chest 58:49, 1970

379. BICKERMAN HA, CHUSID EL: The case against the use of respiratory stimulants. Chest 58:53, 1970

380. MOSER KM et al: Respiratory stimulation with intravenous doxapram in respiratory failure. N Engl J Med 288:427, 1973

381. LAFORET EG: Surgical management of chronic obstructive lung disease. N Engl J Med 287:175, 1972

382. FLETCHER CM, GILSON JG, HUGH-JONES P et al: Terminology, definitions and classification of chronic pulmonary emphysema and related conditions. A report of the conclusions of a CIBA guest symposium. Thorax 14:286, 1959

383. MENEELY GR et al: Definitions and classification of chronic bronchitis, asthma and pulmonary emphysema. A statement by the American Thoracic Society, Committee on Diagnostic Standards for Nontuberculous Respiratory Diseases. Am Rev Respir Dis 85:762, 1962

384. PORTER R, BIRCH J (eds): Identification of Asthma. CIBA Foundation Study Group no 38. London, Churchill Livingstone, 1971

385. WEISS EB, SEGAL MS: Bronchial Asthma. Boston, Little, Brown & Co, 1976

386. US Bureau of the Census, Statistical Abstracts of the United States: 1978 (99th edition). Washington, DC, 1978

387. WILLIAMS H, MCNICOL KN: Prevalence, natural history and relationship of wheezy bronchitis and asthma in children. An epidemiological study. Br Med J 4:321, 1969

388. RACKEMANN FM, EDWARDS MC: Asthma in children: A follow-up study of 688 patients after an interval of twenty years. N Engl Med 246:815, 858, 1952

389. Editorial: Age of onset of asthma. Lancet, 2:477, 1971

390. SPEIZER FE, DOLL R: A century of asthma deaths in young people. Br Med J 3:245, 1968

391. PEPYS J: Clinical and therapeutic significance of patterns of allergic reactions of the lungs to extrinsic agents. Am Rev Respir Dis 116:573, 1977

392. PARISH WE: Skin sensitizing non-IgE antibodies. Prog Immunol 4:19, 1974

393. BRYANT DH, BURNS MW, LAZARUS L: Identification of IgG antibody as a carrier of reaginic activity in asthmatic patients. J Allergy Clin Immunol 56:417, 1975

394. DAVIES RJ, GREEN M, SCHOFIELD NM: Recurrent nocturnal asthma after exposure to graindust. Am Rev Respir Dis 114:1011, 1976

395. HOWELL JBL: Asthma: A clinical view. In Porter R, and Birch J (eds): Identification of Asthma. London, Churchill Livingstone, 1971

396. NADEL JA: Neurophysiologic aspects of asthma. In Austen KF, Lichtenstein LM (eds): Asthma: Physiology, Immunopharmacology, and Treatment. New York, Academic Press, 1973

397. SCHULTZ G, HARDMAN JG, SUTHERLAND EW: Cyclic nucleotides and smooth muscle function. In Austen KF, and Lichtenstein LM (eds): Asthma: Physiology, Immunopharmacology and Treatment. New York, Academic Press, 1973

398. FLEISCH JH, KENT KM, COOPER T: Drug receptors in smooth muscle. In Austin KF, Lichtenstein LM (eds): Asthma: Physiology, Immunopharmacology, and Treatment. New York, Academic Press, 1973

399. GOLD WM: Cholinergic pharmacology in asthma. In Austen KF, Lichtenstein LM (eds): Asthma: Physiology, Immunopharmacology, and Treatment. New York, Academic Press, 1973

400. PARKER CW· Adrenergic responsiveness in asthma. In Austen KF, and Lichtenstein LM (eds): Asthma: Physiology, Immunopharmacology, and Treatment. New York, Academic Press, 1973

401. MIDDLETON E JR: Anatomical and biochemical basis of bronchial obstruction in asthma. Ann Intern Med 63:695, 1965

402. BOUSHY HA, HOLTZMAN MJ, SHELLER JR et al: Bronchial hyperreactivity. Am Rev Respir Dis 121:389, 1980

403. BROCKLEHURST WE: Pharmacodynamics and Mechanisms of Asthma. In Weiss EB, Segal MS (eds): Bronchial Asthma, Chap 9. Boston, Little, Brown & Co, 1976

404. HENSLEY MJ, O'CAIN CF, MCFADDEN ER JR et al: Distribution of bronchodilation in normal subjects: Beta agonist versus atropine. J App Physiol 45:778, 1978

405. HENDERSON WF et al: Alpha adrenergic hyper-responsiveness in asthma. N Engl J Med 300:642, 1979

406. NAKAYAMA K: Surgical removal of the carotid body from bronchial asthma. Dis Chest 40:595, 1961

407. O'ROURKE DA, O'ROURKE HM: Removal of the carotid body for asthma. An appraisal of results. Med J Aust 2:869, 1964

408. CURRAN WS et al: Glomectomy for severe bronchial asthma: A double-blind study. Am Rev Respir Dis 93:84, 1966

409. NORDSTROM LA, MACDONALD F, GOBEL FL: Effect of propranolol on respiratory function and exercise tolerance in patients with chronic obstructive lung disease. Chest 67:287, 1975

410. AUSTEN KF: Reaction mechanisms in the release of mediators of immediate hypersensitivity from human lung tissue. Fed Proc 33:256, 1974

411. MURAD F: Mechanism of action of some bronchodilators: Cyclic nucleotide metabolism in tracheal preparations. Am Rev Respir Dis 110:[Part 2]:111, 1974

412. PLATSHON LF, KALINER M: The effects of the immunologic release of histamine upon human lung cyclic nucleotide levels and prostaglandin generation. Clin Invest 62:1113, 1978

413. AUSTEN KF, ORANGE RP: Bronchial asthma: The possible role of the chemical mediators of immediate hypersensitivity in the pathogenesis of subacute chronic disease. Am Rev Respir Dis 112:423, 1975

414. COOMBS RRA, GELL PGH: Classification of allergic reactions responsible for clinical hypersensitivity and disease. In Gel PGH, Coombs RRA (eds): Clinical Aspects of Immunology, 3rd ed. Oxford, Blackwell Scientific Publications, 1975 Press, 1973

415. PRAUSNITZ C, KÜSTNER H: Studies on supersensitivity (trans from the original German). In Gell PGH, and Coombs RRA (eds): Clinical Aspects of Immunology. Oxford, Blackwell Scientific Publications, 1968

416. ISHIZAKA K, ISHIZAKA T: Role of IgE and IgG antibodies in reaginic hypersensitivity in the respiratory tract. In Austen KF, Lichtenstein Km (eds): Asthma: Physiology, Immunopharmacology, and Treatment. New York, Academic Press, 1973

417. HOGG JC, PARE PD, BOUCHER RC: Bronchial mucosal permeability. Fed Proc 38:197, 1979

418. HOGG JC, PARE PD, BOUCHER RC et al: The pathophysiology of asthma. Can Med Assoc J 121:409, 1979

419. VALENTINE MD: Chemical Mediators in Asthma. In Weiss EB, and Segal MS (eds): Bronchial Asthma. Boston, Little, Brown & Co, 1976

420. NAKANO J, RODGERS RL: The prostaglandins. In Weiss EB, and Segal MS (eds): Bronchial Asthma. Boston, Little, Brown & Co, 1976

421. KELLERMEYER RW, SCHWARTZ HJ: The kinins. In Weiss EB, and Segal MS (eds): Bronchial Asthma. Boston, Little, Brown & Co, 1976

422. AUSTEN KF: A review of immunological, biochemical and pharmacological factors in the release of chemical mediators from human lung. In Austen KF, Lichtenstein LM (eds): Asthma:

Physiology, Immunopharmacology, and Treatment. New York, Academic Press, 1973

423. LICHTENSTEIN LM: The control of IgE mediated histamine release: Implications for the study of asthma. In Austen KF, Lichtenstein LM (eds): Asthma: Physiology, Immunopharmacology, and Treatment. New York, Academic Press, 1973
424. BROCKLEHURST WE: Pharmacological mediators of hypersensitivity reactions. In Gell PGH, Coombs RRA (eds): Clinical Aspects of Immunology, 3rd ed. Oxford, Blackwell Scientific Publications, 1975
425. PARISH WE, PEPYS J: The lung in allergic disease. In Gell PGH, and Coombs RRA: In Gell PGH, Coombs RRA (eds): Clinical Aspects of Immunology. Oxford, Blackwell Scientific Publications, 1975
426. PEPYS J: Immunochemical mechanisms in asthma. In Porter R, and Birch J (eds): Identification of Asthma. London, Churchill Livingstone, 1971
427. RIBON A, PARIKH S: Drug-induced asthma: a review. Ann Allergy 44:220, 1980
428. WEISS EB, PATHWARDHAN AV: The response to lidocaine in bronchial asthma. Chest 72:429, 1977
429. FISH JE, PETERMAN VI: Effects of inhaled lidocaine on airway function in asthmatic subjects. Respiration 37:201, 1979
430. SAMTER M, BEERS RF JR: Intolerance to aspirin: Clinical studies and consideration of its pathogenesis. Ann Intern Med 68:975, 1968
431. GIRALDO B, BLUMENTHAL MN, SPINK WW: Aspirin intolerance and asthma: A clinical and immunological study. Ann Intern Med 71:479, 1969
432. SETTIPANE GA, CHAFFEE FH, KLEIN DE: Aspirin intolerance: A prospective study in an atopic and normal population. J Allergy Clin Immunol 53:200, 1974
433. LOCKEY RF, RUCKNAGEL DL, VANSELOW NA: Familial occurrence of asthma, nasal polyps and aspirin intolerance. Ann Intern Med 78:57, 1973
434. NESTOR AM: Bronchial and intravenous provocation tests with indomethacin in aspirin-sensitive asthmatics. Am Rev Respir Dis 120:1073, 1979
435. SZCZEKLIK A, GRYGLEWSKI RJ, CZERNIAWSKA-MYSIK G: Relationship of inhibition of prostaglandin biosynthesis by analgesics to asthma attacks in aspirin sensitive patients. Br Med J 1:67, 1975
436. SZCZEKLIK A, GRYGLEWSKI PJ, CZERNIAWSKA-MYSIK G et al: Aspirin-induced asthma. J Allergy Clin Immunol 58:10, 1976
437. TOOGOOD JH: Aspirin intolerance, asthma, prostaglandins and cromolyn sodium. Chest 72:135, 1977
438. GWIN E, KERBY GR, RUTH WE: Cromolyn sodium in the treatment of asthma associated with aspirin hypersensitivity and nasal polyps. Chest 72:148, 1977
439. SCHENCK NL: Nasal polypectomy in the aspirin sensitive asthmatic. Trans Am Acad Ophthalmol, Otolaryngol 78:109, 1974
440. BERKOVICH S, MILLIAN SJ, SNYDER RO: The association of viral and mycoplasma infections with recurrence of wheezing in the asthmatic child. Ann Allergy 28:43, 1970
441. EMPEY DH, LAITINEN LA, JACOBS L et al: Mechanisms of bronchial hyperreactivity in normal subjects after upper respiratory tract infection. Am Rev Respir Dis 113:131, 1976
442. MINOR TE, DICK EC, BAKER JW et al: Rhinovirus and influenze type A infections as precipitants of asthma. Am Rev Respir Dis 113:149, 1976
443. CLARKE CW: Relationships of bacterial and viral infections to exacerbations of asthma. Thorax 34:544, 1979
444. NUDGEL DW, LANGSTON L, SELNOR JC et al: Viral and bacterial infections in adults with chronic asthma. Am Rev Respir Dis 120:393, 1979
445. PEPYS J, HUTCHCROFT BJ: Bronchial provocation tests in etiological diagnosis and analysis of asthma. Am Rev Respir Dis 112:829, 1975
446. SLAVIN RG: Asthma in adults: Occupational asthma. Hosp Pract 13:6, 133, 1978
447. ROSENTHAL RR et al: Bronchoprovocation tests in asthma, report of 1978 workshop. J Allergy Clin Immunol 64:563–692, 1979
448. LAM S, WONG R, YEUNG M: Nonspecific bronchial reactivity in occupational asthma. J Allergy Clin Immunol 63:28, 1979
449. NOVEY HS, MARCHIOLI LE, SOKOL WN et al: Papain induced asthma—physiological and immunological features. J Allergy Clin Immunol 63:98, 1979
450. KARR RM, LEHRER SB, BUTCHER BT et al: Coffee workers' asthma: A clinical appraisal using the radioallergosorbent test. J Allergy Clin Immunol 62:143, 1978
451. SIMONSSON BG, JACOBS FM, NADEL JA: Role of autonomic nervous system and the cough reflex in the increased responsiveness of airways in patients with obstructive airway disease. J Clin Invest 46:1812, 1967
452. CORRO WM, BRAMAN SS, IRWIN PS: Chronic cough as the sole presenting manifestation of bronchial asthma. N Engl J Med 300:633, 1979
453. AITKIN RCB, ZEALLEY AK, ROSENTHAL SV: Some psychological and physiological considerations of breathlessness. In Porter R (ed): Breathing: Hering–Breuer Centenary Symposium. London, J & A Churchill, 1970
454. HEISKELL CL, RHODES JM, THAYER KH: Some psychosomatic aspects of asthma. JAMA 170:1764, 1959
455. MOORE N: Behaviour therapy in bronchial

asthma: A controlled study. J Psychosom Res 9:257, 1965
456. SERGEANT HGS, YORKSTON NJ: Verbal desensitization in the treatment of bronchial asthma. Lancet 2:1321, 1969
457. LUPARELLO T, LYONS HA, BLEECKER ER et al: Influences of suggestion in airway reactivity in asthmatic subjects. J Psychosom Med 30:819, 1968
458. KALES A et al: Sleep studies in asthmatic adults: Relationship of attacks to sleep stage and time of night. J Allergy Clin Immunol 41:164, 1968
459. CONNOLLY CK: Diurnal rhythms in airway obstruction. Br J Dis Chest 73:357, 1979
460. NEWMAN TAYLOR AJ, DAVIES RJ, HENDRICK DJ et al: Recurrent nocturnal asthmatic reactions to bronchial provocation tests. Clin Allergy 9:213, 1979
461. HETZEL MR, CLARK TJH: Does sleep cause nocturnal asthma? Thorax 34:749, 1979
462. HETZEL MR, CLARK TJH, BRATHWAITE MA: Asthma: Analysis of sudden deaths and ventilatory arrests in hospital. Br Med J 1:808, 1977
463. MOIRA MW, CHAN-YEUNG VYAS MN, GRZYBOWSKI S: Exercise-induced asthma. Am Rev Respir Dis 104:915, 1971
464. ANDERSON SD, MCEVOY JDS, BIANCO S: Changes in lung volumes and airways resistance after exercise in asthmatic subjects. Am Rev Respir Dis 106:30, 1972
465. LEFCOE NM, CARTER RP, DILDAR A: Postexercise bronchoconstriction in normal subjects and asthmatics. Am Rev Respir Dis 104:562, 1971
466. REBUCK AS, READ J: Exercise-induced asthma. Lancet 2:429, 1968
467. POPPIUS H et al: Exercise asthma and disodium cromoglycate. Br Med J 4:337, 1970
468. DAVIES SE: Effect of disodium cromoglycate on exercise-induced asthma. Br Med J 3:593, 1968
469. ALLEN TW, CUGELL DW, ADDINGTON WW et al: Postexercise bronchospasm. Chest 59:557, 1971
470. DEAL EC, MCFADDEN ER JR, INGRAM RH JR et al: Role of respiratory heat exchange in production of exercise-induced asthma. J Appl Physiol 46:467, 1979
470a. MCFADDEN ER JR: Exercise-induced asthma. Am J Med 68:471, 1980
471. SETTIPANE GA, CHAFEE FH: Nasal polyps in asthma and rhinitis. J Allergy Clin Immunol 59:17, 1977
472. KELSEN SG et al: Emergency room assessment and treatment of patients with acute asthma. Am J Med 64:622, 1978
473. GILLAM GL, MCNICOL KN, WILLIAMS NE: Chest deformity, residual airways obstruction and hyperinflation, and growth in children with asthma. Arch Dis Child 45:789, 1970
474. MARMORSTEIN BL, CIANCULLI FD: Planimetric measurement of total lung capacity in asthma. Chest 66:378, 1974
475. HODSON CJ, TRICKEY SE: Bronchial wall thickening in asthma. Clin Radiol 11:183, 1960
476. SHAW R: Mucoid impaction of the bronchi. J Thorac Surg 22:149, 1951
477. GREER AE: Mucoid impaction of the bronchi. Ann Intern Med 46:506, 1957
478. BRAMAN S, WHITCOMB M: Mucoid impaction of the bronchus. JAMA 223:641, 1973
479. HORN BR, ROBIN ED, THEODORE J et al: Total eosinophil counts in the management of bronchial asthma. N Engl J Med 292:1152, 1975
480. O'CONNEL JM, BAIRD LJ, CAMPBELL AM: Sputum eosinophila in chronic bronchitis and asthma. Respiration 35:65, 1972
481. CADE JF, WOOLCOCK AJ, REBUCK AS: Lung mechanics during provocation of asthma. Clin Sci 40:381, 1971
482. PEPYS J: Inhalation challenge tests in asthma. N Engl J Med 293:758, 1975
483. REBUCK AS, READ J: Assessment and management of severe asthma. Am J Med 51:788, 1971
484. GELB AF et al: P pulmonale in status asthmaticus. J Allergy Clin Immunol 64:18, 1979
485. SIEGLER D: Reversible electrocardiographic changes in severe acute asthma. Thorax 32:328, 1977
486. MAYS EE: Intrinsic asthma in adults. JAMA 236:2626, 1976
487. MCFADDEN ER, KISER R, DEGROOT WJ: Acute bronchial asthma: Relations between clinical and physiologic manifestations. N Engl J Med 288:221, 1973
488. WESTERMAN DE, BENATOR SR, POLGIETER PD et al: Identification of the high risk asthmatic patient. Am J Med 66:565, 1979
489. BATEMAN JRM, CLARKE SW: Sudden death in asthma. Thorax 34:40, 1979
490. COCHRANE GM, CLARK TJH: A survey of asthma mortality in patients between ages 35 and 64 in the Greater London hospitals in 1971. Thorax 30:300, 1979
491. MACDONALD JB, MACDONALD ET, SEATON A et al: Asthma deaths in Cardiff 1963–74. Br Med J 2:721, 1976
491a. SHIM CS, WILLIAMS MH JR: Evaluation of the severity of asthma: Patients vs. physicians. Am J Med 68:14, 1980
492. REBUCK AS: The clinical picture of asthma. Can Med Assoc J 110:409, 1974
493. MCFADDEN ER, FELDMAN NT: Asthma Pathophysiology and clinical correlates. Med Clin North Am 61:1229, 1977
494. WOOLCOCK AJ, READ J: Improvement in bronchial asthma not reflected in forced expiratory volume. Lancet 2:1323, 1965
495. OLIVE JT JR, HYATT RE: Maximal expiratory flow

and total respiratory resistance during induced bronchoconstriction in asthmatic subjects. Am Rev Respir Dis 106:366, 1972

496. WOOLCOCK AJ, REBUCK AS, CADE JF et al: Lung volume changes in asthma measured concurrently by two methods. Am Rev Respir Dis 104:703, 1971

497. BROWN R, INGRAM RH JR, MCFADDEN ER: Problems in the plethysmographic assessment of changes in total lung capacity in asthma. Am Rev Respir Dis 118:685, 1978

498. WOOLCOCK AJ, READ J: The static elastic properties of the lungs in asthma. Am Rev Respir Dis 98:788, 1968

498a. LISBOA C, et al: Is extrathoracic airway obstruction important in asthma? Am Rev Respir Dis 122:115, 1980

499. WILSON AF et al: The significance of regional pulmonary function changes in bronchial asthma. Am J Med 48:416, 1970

500. HILL DJ, LANDAU LI, PHELAN PD: Small airway disease in asymptomatic asthmatic adolescents. Am Rev Respir Dis 106:873, 1972

501. RILEY DJ, FISHER AB, HANSELL JR et al: Regional bronchoconstriction in asthma; ^{133}Xenon washout scans following parenteral methacholine. Chest 70:715, 1976

502. WAGNER PD, DANTZKER DR, IACOVONI VE et al: Ventilation–perfusion inequality in asymptomatic asthma. Am Rev Respir Dis 118:511, 1978

503. MACKLEM PJ, DESPAS PJ, LEROUX MD: Site of airway obstruction in asthma. Chest (Suppl) 63:28S, 1973

504. CHAN-YEUNG M, ABBOUD R, TSAO MS et al: Effect of helium on maximal expiratory flow in patients with asthma before and during induced bronchoconstriction. Am Rev Respir Dis 113.433, 1976

505. FISHER HK, HANSEN TA: Site of action of inhaled 6% carbon dioxide in the lungs of asthmatic subjects before and after exercise. Am Rev Respir Dis 114:861, 1976

506. FISH JF, ROSENTHAL RR, BATRA G et al: Airway responses to methacholine in allergic and nonallergic subjects. Am Rev Respir Dis 113:579, 1976

507. ANTIC R, MACKLEM PT: The influence of clinical factors on site of airway obstruction in asthma. Am Rev Respir Dis 114:851, 1976

508. WANNER A: The role of mucociliary dysfunction in bronchial asthma. Am J Med 67:477, 1979

509. STALCUP SA, MELLINS RB: Mechanical forces producing pulmonary edema in acute asthma. N Engl J Med 297:592, 1977

510. SHIM C, WILLIAMS MH JR: Pulsus paradoxus in asthma. Lancet ii:530, 1978

511. PARSONS GH, GREEN JF: Mechanisms of pulsus paradoxus in upper airway obstruction. J Appl Physiol 45:598, 1978

512. MCFADDEN ER JR, LYONS HA: Arterial blood gas tension in asthma. N Engl J Med 278:1027, 1968

513. GAZIOGLU K, CONDEMI JJ, HYDE RW et al: Effect of isoproterenol on gas exchange during air and oxygen breathing in patients with asthma. Am J Med 50:185, 1971

514. COOPER DM et al: The relative sensitivity of closing volume in children with asthma and cystic fibrosis. Am Rev Respir Dis 109:519, 1974

515. MCCARTHY D, MILIC-EMILI J: Closing volume in asymptomatic asthma. Am Rev Respir Dis 107:559, 1973

516. MCFADDEN ER: Extertional dyspnea and cough as preludes to attacks of asthma. N Engl J Med 292:555, 1975

517. RUBINFELD AR, PAIN MCF: How mild is mild asthma? Thorax 32:177, 1977

518. OHMAN JL JR et al: The diffusing capacity in asthma. Am Rev Respir Dis 107:932, 1973

519. KERNS TG et al: Evaluation of the single breath diffusing capacity in asthma and cystic fibrosis. Chest 76:41, 1979

520. MENKES HA: Airways reactivity and the need for a simple test. Am Rev Respir Dis 121:619, 1980

521. DEAL EC et al: Airway responsiveness to cold air and hyperpnea in normal subjects and in those with hay fever and asthma. Am Rev Respir Dis 121:621, 1980

522. CHAN-YEUNG M, WONG R, MACLEAN L: Respiratory abnormalities among grain elevator workers. Chest 75:461, 1979

523. DUNNILL MS: The pathology of asthma, with special reference to changes in the bronchial mucosa. J Clin Pathol 13:27, 1960

524. EPSTEIN RL: Constituents of sputum: A simple method. Ann Intern Med 77:259, 1972

525. CHODOSH S: Examination of sputum cells. N Engl J Med 282:854, 1970

526. WILLIAMS DA: Asthma and bronchitis with emphysema. Acta Allergol (Kbh) 16:400, 1961

527. NAYLOR B: The shedding of the mucosa of the bronchial tree in asthma. Thorax 17:69, 1962

528. SANERKIN NG, EVANS DMD: The sputum in bronchial asthma; Pathognomonic patterns. J Pathol Bacteriol 89:535, 1965

529. SALVATO G: Some histological changes in chronic bronchitis and asthma. Thorax 23:168, 1968

530. DUNNILL MS, MASSARELLA GR, ANDERSON JA: A comparison of the quantitative anatomy of the bronchi in normal subjects, in status asthmaticus, in chronic bronchitis, and in emphysema. Thorax 24:176, 1969

531. GLYNN AA, MICHAELS L: Bronchial biopsy in chronic bronchitis and asthma. Thorax 15:142, 1960

532. TAKIZAWA T, THURLBECK WM: Muscle and mucous gland size in the major bronchi of patients

with chronic bronchitis, asthma, and asthmatic bronchitis. Am Rev Respir Dis 104:331, 1971
533. HOUSSAIN S: Quantitative measurement of bronchial muscle in men with asthma. Am Rev Respir Dis 107:99, 1973
534. GOUGH J: Correlation of radiological and pathological changes in some diseases of the lung. Lancet 1:161, 1955
535. WILLIAMS DA, LEOPOLD JG: Death from bronchial asthma. Acta Allergol (Kbh) 14:83, 1959
536. LOWELL FC: The relationship of allergy to emphysema. In Symposium on emphysema and the chronic bronchitis syndrome, Aspen, Colorado, 1958. Am Rev Respir Dis 80:181 (Part 2), 1959
537. CARDELL BS, PEARSON RSB: Death in asthmatics. Thorax 14:341, 1959
537a. SHIM C, WILLIAMS MH: Bronchial response to oral versus aerosol metaproterenol in asthma. Ann Intern Med 93:428, 1980
538. MCFADDEN ER JR: The chronicity of acute attacks of asthma-mechanical and therapeutic implications. J Allergy Clin Immunol 56:18, 1975
539. WOOLCOCK AJ: Inhaled drugs in the prevention of asthma. Am Rev Respir Dis 115:191, 1977
540. WOLFE JD, TASHKIN DP, CALVARESE B et al: Bronchodilator effects of terbutaline and aminophylline alone and in combination in asthmatic patients. N Engl J Med 298:363, 1978
541. SNIDER GL: The treatment of asthma. N Engl J Med 298:397, 1978
542. WILLIAMS MH: Steroid aerosols for asthma. Ann Intern Med 86:650, 1977
543. WEINSTEIN AM et al: Asthma and pregnancy. JAMA 241:1161, 1979
544. COCKCROFT DW, SILVERBERG JDH, DOSMAN JA: Decrease in non-specific bronchial reactivity in an asthmatic following treatment of hyperthyroidism. Ann Allergy 41:160, 1978
545. PATTERSON R: Clinical efficacy of allergen immunotherapy. J Allergy Clin Immunol 64:155, 1979
546. LICHTENSTEIN LM: An evaluation of the role of immunotherapy in asthma. Am Rev Respir Dis 117:191, 1978
547. ROCKLIN RE, SHAFFER AL, GREINEDER DK et al: Generation of antigen-specific suppressor cells during allergy desensitization. N Engl J Med 302:1213, 1980
548. PATERSON JW, WOOLCOCK AJ, SHENFIELD GM: Bronchodilator drugs. Am Rev Respir Dis 120:1149, 1979
549. LANDS AM et al: Differentiation of receptor systems activated by sympathomimetic amines. Nature 214:597, 1967
550. MILLER WF: Aerosol therapy in acute and chronic respiratory disease. Arch Intern Med 131:148, 1973
551. TATTERSFIELD AE, MCNICOL MW: Salbutamol and isoproterenol: bronchodilator and cardiovascular activity. N Engl J Med 281:1323, 1969
552. CHOO-KANG YFJ, PARKER SS, GRANT IWB: Response of asthmatics to isoprenaline and salbutamol aerosols administered by intermittent positive pressure ventilation. Br Med J 4:465, 1970
553. CHOO-KANG YFJ, SIMPSON WT, GRANT IWB: Controlled comparison of the bronchodilator effects of three β-adrenergic stimulant drugs administered by inhalation to patients with asthma. Br Med J 2:287, 1969
554. TASHKIN DP, METH R, SIMMONS DH et al: Double-blind comparison of acute bronchial and cardiovascular effects of oral terbutaline and ephedrine. Chest 68:133, 1975
555. RHOADES RB, LEIFER KN, BLOOM FL et al: Spirometric comparison of carbuterol and isoproterenol aerosol therapy in bronchial asthma: A double-blind, matched pair study of 28 adults and a double-blind crossover study of 28 children. Am Rev Respir Dis 114:79, 1976
556. FUNAHASHI A, HAMILTON LH: A study of a new bronchodilator: Carbuterol. Am Rev Respir Dis 113:398, 1976
557. STEEN SN, SMITH R, KUO J et al: Comparison of the bronchodilator effects of aerosol fenoterol and isoproterenol. Chest 72:724, 1977
558. GEUMEI AM, MILLER WF, MILLER J et al: Bronchodilator effect of a new oral beta-adrenoreceptor stimulant: Thll65a. Chest 70:460, 1976
559. PENNOCK BE, ROGERS RM, RYAN BR et al: Aerosol administration of fenoterol hydrobromide (Thll65a) in subjects with reversible obstructive airway disease. Chest 72:731, 1977
560. HUHTI E, POUKKULA A: Clinical comparison of fenoterol and albuterol administered by inhalation. Chest 73:348, 1978
561. Oral theophylline drugs for asthma. Med Lett Drugs Ther 17:9, 1975
562. ELLIS EF, EDDY ED: Anhydrous theophylline equivalence of commercial theophylline formulations. J Allergy Clin Immunol 53:116, 1974
563. SCHLUGER J, MCGINN JT, HENNESSY DJ: Comparative theophylline blood levels following the oral administration of three different theophylline preparations. Am J Med Sci 233:296, 1957
564. BROOKS SM et al: Adverse effects of phenobarbital on corticosteroid metabolism in patients with bronchial asthma. N Engl J Med 286:1125, 1972
565. AVIADO DM: Toxicity of aerosols. J Clin Pharmacol 15:86, 1975
566. CONOLLY ME: Acquired resistance to beta stimulants: a possible explanation for the rise in the asthma death rate in Britain. Chest (Suppl) 63:16S, 1973
567. REISMAN RE: Asthma induced by adrenergic aerosols. Chest (Suppl) 63:16S, 1973

568. KEIGHLEY JF: Iatrogenic asthma associated with adrenergic aerosols. Ann Intern Med 65:985, 1966
569. STANESCU DC, VANDE WOESTIJNE KP: Asthma attack induced by isoprenaline aerosols. Respiration 29:532 1972
570. TRAUTLEIN J, ALLEGRA J, FIELD J et al: Paradoxic bronchospasm after inhalation of isoproterenol. Chest 70:711, 1976
571. JENNE JW, CHICK TW: "Unresponsiveness" to isoproterenol. Chest 70:691, 1976
572. WILSON AF et al: Cardiopulmonary effects of long-term bronchodilator administration. J Allergy Clin Immunol 58:204, 1976
573. LARSSAN S, SVEDMYR N, THIRINGER G: Lack of bronchial beta adrenoceptor resistance in asthmatics during long term treatment with terbutaline. J Allergy Clin Immunol 59:93, 1977
574. NICHOLSON DP, CHICK TW: A re-evaluation of parenteral aminophylline. Am Rev Respir Dis 108:241, 1973
575. WAGNER JG: A safe method for rapidly achieving plasma concentration plateaus. Clin Pharmacol Ther 16:691, 1974
576. PIAFSKY KM, OGILVIE RI: Drug therapy: dosage of theophylline in bronchial asthma. N Engl J Med 292:1218, 1975
577. JENNE JW, WYZE E, ROOD FS et al: Pharmacokinetics of theophylline. Application to adjustment of the clinical dose of aminophylline. Clin Pharmacol Ther 13:349, 1972
578. JUSKO WJ, KOUP JR, VANCE JW et al: Intravenous theophylline therapy; nomogram guidelines. Ann Intern Med 86:400, 1977
579. HENDELES L, WEINBERGER M, BIGHLEY L: Disposition of theophylline after a single intravenous infusion of aminophylline. Am Rev Respir Dis 118:97, 1978
580. POWELL JR, VOZEK S, HOPEWELL P et al: Theophylline disposition in acutely ill hospitalized patients. The effect of smoking, heart failure, severe airway obstruction and pneumonia. Am Rev Respir Dis 118:229, 1978
581. MANGIONE A, IMHOFF TE, LEE RV et al: Pharmacokinetics of theophylline in hepatic disease. Chest 73:616, 1978
582. VAN DELLEN RG: Intravenous aminophylline. Chest 76:2, 1979
583. ADOLPHSON RL, TOWNLEY RG: Comparison of the bronchodilator activities of isoproterenol and of prostaglandin E_1 aerosols. Chest (Suppl) 63:5S 1973
583a. CERRINA J, DENJEAU A, ALEXANDRE G et al: Inhibition of exercise-induced asthma by a calcium antagonist, nifedipine. Am Rev Respir Dis 123:156, 1981
584. CAVANAUGH MJ, COOPER DM: Inhaled atropine sulfate: Dose response characteristics. Am Rev Respir Dis 114:517, 1976
585. FISH JF, ROSENTHAL RR, SUMMER WR et al: The effect of atropine on acute antigen-mediated airway constriction in subjects with allergic asthma. Am Rev Respir Dis 115:371, 1977
586. LARSEN GL, BARROW RJ, COTTON EK et al: A comparative study of inhaled atropine sulfate and isoproterenol hydrochloride in cystic fibrosis. Am Rev Respir Dis 119:399, 1979
587. CHICK TW, JENNE JW: Comparative bronchodilator responses to atropine and terbutaline in asthma and chronic bronchitis. Chest 72:719, 1977
588. CHAN-YEUNG M: The effect of SCH 1000 and disodium cromoglycate on exercise-induced asthma. Chest 71:320, 1977
589. BAIGELMAN W, CHODOSH S: Bronchodilator action of the anticholinergic drug, ipratropium bromide (SCH 1000) as an aerosol in chronic bronchitis and asthma. Chest 71:324, 1977
590. COX JSG et al: Disodium cromoglycate (Intal). Adv Drug Res 5:115, 1970
591. PEPYS J: Disodium cromoglycate in clinical and experimental asthma. In Austen KF, Lichtenstein LM (eds): Asthma: Physiology, Immunopharmacology, and Treatment. New York, Academic Press, 1973
592. INTAL (CROMOLYN SODIUM): A Monograph. Bedford, Fisons Corporation, 1973
593. BERNSTEIN DL, JOHNSON CL, TED TSE CS: Therapy with cromolyn sodium. Ann Intern Med 89:228, 1978
594. PEPYS J, HUTCHCROFT BJ: Bronchial provocation tests in etiologic diagnosis and analysis of asthma. Am Rev Respir Dis 112:829, 1975
595. GWIN E, KERBY GR, RUTH WE: Cromolyn sodium in the treatment of asthma associated with aspirin sensitivity and nasal polyps. Chest 72:148, 1977
596. TOOGOOD JH, LEFOE NM, ROSE DK et al: A double-blind study of disodium cromoglycate for prophylaxis of bronchial asthma. Am Rev Respir Dis 104:323, 1971
597. IRANI FA, JONES NL, GENT M et al: Evaluation of disodium cromoglycate in intrinsic and extrinsic asthma. Am Rev Respir Dis 106:179, 1972
598. HYDE JS, ISENBERG P, FLORO LD: Short- and long-term prophylaxis with cromolyn sodium in chronic asthma. Chest 63:875, 1973
599. TOOGOOD JH, LEFCOE NM, BUCK D et al: A clinical index of disability due to chronic asthma tested during a trial of cromolyn sodium treatment. Chest 63:881, 1973
600. BRITISH MEDICAL RESEARCH COUNCIL: Cortisone acetate in status asthmaticus. Lancet 2:803, 1956
601. BRITISH MEDICAL RESEARCH COUNCIL: Cortisone acetate in chronic asthma. Lancet 2:798, 1956
602. SCHWARTZ HJ, LOWELL FC, MELBY JC: Steroid resistance in bronchial asthma. Ann Intern Med 69:493, 1968

603. DWYER J, LAZARUS L, HICKIE JB: A study of cortisol metabolism in patients with chronic asthma. Aust Ann Med 16:297, 1967
603a. COLLINS JV et al: The use of corticosteroids in the treatment of acute asthma. Q J Med 44:259, 1975
604. HODSON ME, BATTEN JC, CLARKE SW et al: Beclomethasone dipropionate aerosol in asthma. Am Rev Respir Dis 110:403, 1974
605. WILLIAMS MH JR: Steroid and antibiotic aerosols. Am Rev Respir Dis 110(Part 2):122, 1974
606. KASS I, NAIR SV, PATIL KD: Beclomethasone dipropionate aerosol in the treatment of steroid-dependent asthma; an assessment of 18 months of therapy. Chest 71:703, 1977
606a. SCOGGIN CH, SAHN SA, PETTY TL: Status asthmaticus. JAMA 238:1158, 1977
607. WINTER B: Bilateral carotid body resection in children with severe asthma. Chest 75:532, 1979
608. WASSERMAN K: The carotid bodies; pathologic or physiologic? Chest 73:564, 1978
609. DOS SJ, JACOBSON MJ, SOROFF HS: The role of surgery in the management of chronic bronchial asthma. In Weiss EB, and Segal MS (eds): Bronchial Asthma. Boston, Little, Brown & Co, 1976
610. CHANG KC, MORRILL CG, CHAI H: Impaired response to hypoxia after bilateral carotid body resection for treatment of bronchial asthma. Chest 73:667, 1978
611. HONDA Y, MYOJO S, HASEGAWA S et al: Decreased exercise hyperpnea in patients with bilateral carotid chemoreceptor resection. J Appl Physiol 46:908, 1979
612. REID LM: Reduction in bronchial subdivision in bronchiectasis. Thorax 5:233, 1950
613. WHITWELL F: A study of the pathology and pathogenesis of bronchiectasis. Thorax 7:213, 1952
614. SPENCER H: Pathology of the Lung. Oxford, Pergamon Press, 1978
615. BACHMAN AL, HEWITT WR, BEEKLEY HC: Bronchiectasis. A bronchographic study of 60 cases of pneumonia. Arch Intern Med 91:78, 1953
616. PONTIUS JR, JACOBS LG: The reversal of advanced bronchiectasis. Radiology 68:204, 1957
617. NELSON SW, CHRISTOFORIDIS A: Reversible bronchiectasis. Radiology 71:375, 1958
618. DRAPANAS T, SIEWERS R, FIEST JH: Reversible poststenotic bronchiectasis. N Engl J Med 275:917, 1966
619. BOWERS D: Unequal breasts, yellow nails, bronchiectasis, and lymphedema. Can Med Assoc J 100:437, 1969
620. WILLIAMS H, CAMPBELL P: Generalized bronchiectasis associated with deficiency of cartilage in the bronchial tree. Arch Dis Child 35:182, 1960
621. WAYNE KS, TAUSSIG LM: Probably familial congenital bronchiectasis due to cartilage deficiency (Williams–Campbell Syndrome). Am Rev Respir Dis 114:15, 1976
622. KARTAGENER M: Zur pathogenese, der bronkiektasien. Bronkiektasien bei situs viscerum inversus. Beitr Klin Tuberk 83:489, 1933
623. SIEWERT AK: Ueber einen Fall von bronchiectasie bein einen Patienten mit Situs inversis viscerum. Berl Klin Wochenschr 139, 1903
624. KARTAGENER M, STUCKI P: Bronchiectasis with situs inversus. Arch Pediatr 79:193, 1962
625. HOLMES LB, BLENNERHASSETT JB, AUSTEN JF: A reappraisal of Kartagener's syndrome. Am J Med Sci 255:13, 1968
626. KATSUHARA J, KAWAMOTO S, WAKABAYASHI T et al: Situs inversus totalis and Kartagener's syndrome in a Japanese population. Chest 61:56, 1972
627. MILLER RD, DIVERTIE MD: Kartagener's syndrome. Chest 62:130, 1972
628. AFZELIUS BA: A human syndrome caused by immotile cilia. Science 193:317, 1976
629. ELIASSON R, MOSSBERG B, CAMNER P et al: The immotile cilia syndrome: A congenital ciliary abnormality as an etiologic factor in chronic airway infections and male sterility. N Engl J Med 297:1, 1977
630. WAKEFIELD ST JOHN, WAITE D: Abnormal cilia in Polynesians with bronchiectasis. Am Rev Respir Dis 121:1003, 1980
631. VEERMAN AJP, VAN DELDEN L, FEENSTRA L: The immotile cilia syndrome. Pediatrics 65:698, 1980
632. COX DW, TALAMO RC: Genetic aspects of pediatric lung disease. Pediatr Clin North Am 26:467, 1979
633. ROSSMAN CM, FORREST JB, RUFFIN RE et al: Immotile cilia syndrome in persons with and without Kartagner's syndrome. Am Rev Respir Dis 121:1011, 1980
634. FANCONI G, UEHLINGER E, KNAUER C: Das Coeliakiesyndrom bei angeborener zystischer Pancrease fibromatose under Bronkiektasien. Wien Med Wochenschr 86:753, 1936
635. ANDERSEN DH: Cystic fibrosis of pancreas and its relation to celiac disease: Clinical and pathological study. Am J Dis Child 56:344, 1938
636. ANDERSEN DH: Cystic fibrosis of the pancreas. J Chronic Dis 7:58, 1958
637. MITCHELL-HEGGS P, MEAENS M, BATTEN JC: Cystic fibrosis in adolescents and adults. Q J Med 45:479, 1976
638. STERN RC, BOAT TF, DOERSHUK CF et al: Cystic fibrosis diagnosed after age 13. Ann Intern Med 87:188, 1977
639. SHWACHMAN H, KAWALSKI M, KHAW KT: Cystic fibrosis: A new outlook. Medicine 56:129, 1977
640. FINK RJ, DOERSHUK CF, TUCKER AS et al: Pulmonary function and morbidity in 40 adult patients with cystic fibrosis. Chest 74:643, 1978
641. DISANT'AGNESE P, DAVIS PB: Cystic fibrosis in

adults. 75 cases and a review of 232 cases in the literature. Am J Med 66:121, 1979

642. DAVIS PB, DISANT' AGNESE PA: A review. Cystic fibrosis at forty—quo vadis? Pediatr Res 14:83, 1980

642a. BRESLOW JL, MCPHERSON J, EPSTEIN J: Distinguishing homozygous and heterozygous cystic fibrosis fibroblasts from normal cells by differences in sodium transport. N Engl J Med 304:1, 1981

642b. LITTLEFIELD JW: Research on cystic fibrosis. N Engl J Med 304:44, 1981

643. HANDWERGER S et al: Glucose intolerance in cystic fibrosis. N Engl J Med 281:451, 1969

644. HOWELL DA et al: Report of the committee for a study for evaluation of testing for cystic fibrosis. J Pediatr 88:711, 1976

645. SHWACHMAN H, MOHMOODIAN A: Quality of sweat test performance in the diagnosis of cystic fibrosis. Clin Chem 1:158, 1979

646. GIBSON LE, COOKE RE: A test for concentration of electrolytes in sweat in cystic fibrosis of the pancreas utilizing pilocarpine by iontophoresis. Pediatrics 23:545, 1959

647. MANGOS JA, MCSHERRY NR: Sodium transport: Inhibitory factor in sweat of patients with cystic fibrosis. Science 158:135, 1967

648. MCPARTLIN JR, DICKSON JAS, SWAIN VA: The use of gastrographin in the relief of residual and late bowel obstruction in cystic fibrosis. Br J Surg 60:707, 1973

649. GRAND RJ, TALAMO RC, DISANT'AGNESE PA et al: Pregnancy in cystic fibrosis of pancreas. JAMA 195:993, 1966

650. TAUSSIG LM, LOBECK CC, DISANT'AGNESE PA et al: Fertility in males with cystic fibrosis. N Engl J Med 287:586, 1972

651. SPOCK A, HEICK HMC, CRESS H et al: Abnormal serum factor in patients with cystic fibrosis of pancreas. Pediatr Res 1:173, 1967

651a. WILSON GB et al: Cystic fibrosis ciliary dyskinesia substances and pulmonary disease. J Clin Invest 68:171, 1981

652. SANCHIS J et al: Pulmonary mucociliary clearance in cystic fibrosis. N Engl J Med 288:651, 1973

653. WARING WW: Cilia and cystic fibrosis. N Engl J Med 288:681, 1973

654. ANDERSEN DH: Pathology of cystic fibrosis. Ann NY Acad Sci 93:500, 1962

655. TOMASHEFSKI JF, CHRISTOFORIDIS AJ, ABDULLAH AK: Cystic fibrosis in young adults. Chest 57:28, 1970

656. SCHWARTZ EE, HOLSCLAW DS: Pulmonary involvement in adults with cystic fibrosis. Am J Roentgenol Radium Ther Nucl Med 122:708, 1974

657. WEST JR, LEVIN SM, DISANT'AGNESE PA: Pulmonary function in cystic fibrosis of pancreas. Pediatrics 13:155, 1954

658. COOK CD et al: Studies of respiratory physiology in children II. Lung volumes and mechanics of respiration in 64 patients with cystic fibrosis of pancreas. Pediatrics 24:181, 1959

659. BEIER FR, RENZETTI AD JR, MITCHELL M et al: Pulmonary pathophysiology in cystic fibrosis. Am Rev Respir Dis 94:430, 1966

660. FEATHERBY EA et al: Dynamic and static lung volumes, blood gas tension and diffusing capacity in patients with cystic fibrosis. Am Rev Respir Dis 102:737, 1970

661. DEMUTH GR, HOWATT WF, TALNER NS: Intrapulmonary gas distribution in children with cystic fibrosis. Am J Dis Child 103:129, 1962

662. COOPER DM et al: The relative sensitivity of closing volume in children with asthma and cystic fibrosis. Am Rev Respir Dis 109:519, 1974

663. LANDAU LI, PHELAN PD: The spectrum of cystic fibrosis. A study of pulmonary mechanics in 46 patients. Am Rev Respir Dis 108:593, 1973

664. TAM CH et al: Dynamic regional lung function studies in patients with asthma and cystic fibrosis. Am Rev Respir Dis 108:283, 1973

665. GOLDRING RM et al: Pulmonary hypertension and cor pulmonale in cystic fibrosis of pancreas. J Pediatr 65:501, 1964

666. BOWDEN DH, FISCHER VW, WYATT JP: Cor pulmonale in cystic fibrosis: Morphometric analysis. Am J Med 38:226, 1965

667. MOSS AJ et al: Cor pulmonale in cystic fibrosis of pancreas. J Pediatr 67:797, 1965

668. KELMINSON LL, COTTON EK, VOGEL JHK: Reversibility of pulmonary hypertension in patients with cystic fibrosis. Pediatrics 39:24, 1967

668a. FRIEDMAN PJ, HARWOOD ER, ELLENBOGEN PH: Pulmonary cystic fibrosis in the adult. Am J Roentgen 136:1131, 1981

669. LEMEN RJ, GATES AJ, MATHE AA et al: Relationship among digital clubbing, disease severity and serum protaglandin F_2 alpha and E concentration in cystic fibrosis patients. Am Rev Respir Dis 117:639, 1978

670. STERN RC, WOOD RE, BOAT TF et al: Treatment and prognosis of massive hemoptysis in cystic fibrosis. Am Rev Respir Dis 117:825, 1978

671. DAVIS PB, DISANT'AGNESE PA: Assisted ventilation for patients with cystic fibrosis. JAMA 239:1851, 1978

672. GOOD RA, MAZZITELLO WF: Chest disease in patients with agammaglobulinemia. Dis Chest 29:9, 1956

673. FUDENBERG HH, SPITLER LE, LEVIN AS: Treatment of immune deficiency. Am J Pathol 69:529, 1972

674. BODE FR, PARE JAP, FRASER RG: Pulmonary diseases in the compromised host. Medicine 53:255, 1974

675. SOOTHILL JF: Immunity deficiency states. In Gell PGH, Coombs RRA, Lachmann PJ: Clinical

Aspects of Immunology. Oxford, Blackwell Scientific Publications, 1975

676. SOUTH MA, COOPER MD, WOLHEIM EA et al: The IgA system: II Clinical significance of IgA deficiency. Am J Med 44:168, 1968

677. VASSALLO CL, ZAWADZKI ZA, SIMONS JR: Recurrent respiratory infections in a family with immunoglobulin A deficiency. Am Rev Respir Dis 101:245, 1970

678. AMMANN AS, HONG R: Selective IgA deficiency: Presentation of 30 cases and review of the literature. Medicine 50:223, 1971

679. CHIPPS BE, TALAMO RC, WINKELSTEIN JA: IgA deficiency, recurrent pneumonias and bronchiectasis. Chest 73:519, 1978

680. STROBER W, KRAKAUER R, KLAEVEMAN HL et al: Secretory component deficiency: A disorder of the IgA system. N Engl J Med 294:351, 1976

681. DUKES RJ, ROSENOW EC, HERMANS PE: Pulmonary manifestations of hypogammaglobulinemia. Thorax 33:603, 1978

682. FALK GA, OKINAKA AJ, SISKIND GW: Immunoglobulins in the bronchial washings of patients with chronic obstructive pulmonary disease. Am Rev Respir Dis 105:14, 1972

683. ORFANAKIS MG et al: Factors related to serum and secretory immunoglobulin concentrations in patients with chronic obstructive pulmonary disease. Am Rev Respir Dis 107:728, 1973

684. KAGAN E et al: Immunologic studies in patients with recurrent bronchopulmonary infections. Am Rev Respir Dis 111:441, 1975

685. WILLIAMS H, O'REILLY RN: Bronchiectasis in children: its multiple clinical and pathological aspects. Arch Dis Child 34:192, 1959

686. WYNN-WILLIAMS N: Bronchiectasis: A study centered on Bedford and its environs. Br Med J 1:1194, 1953

687. LINDSKOG GE, HUBBELL DS: An analysis of 215 cases of bronchiectasis. Surg Gynecol Obstet 100:643, 1955

688. AVERY ME, RILEY MC, WEISS A: The course of bronchiectasis in childhood. Bull Johns Hopkins Hosp 109:20, 1961

689. BORRIE J, LICHTER J: Surgical treatment of bronchiectasis: Ten year survey. Br Med J 2:908, 1965

689a. GEORGE SA, LEONARDI HK, OVERHOLT RA: Bilateral pulmonary resection for bronchiectasis: A 40 year experience. Ann Thorac Surg 28:48, 1979

690. CLARK NS: Bronchiectasis in childhood. Br Med J 1:80, 1963

691. GLAUSER EM, COOK CD, HARRIS GBC: Bronchiectasis: A review of cases in children with follow-up pulmonary function studies in 1958. Acta Paediatr Scand [Suppl] 165:1, 1966

692. SHEK JL, COPE JA: Bronchiectatic sequelae of pulmonary tuberculosis and its subsequent complication. Dis Chest 30:566, 1956

693. SMITH CE, RUSK GY: Pulmonary spirochetosis. Am J Pathol 3:225, 1927

694. ALLIBONE EC, ALLISON PR, ZINNEMANN K: Significance of H. influenzae in bronchiectasis of children. Br Med J 1:1457, 1956

695. RYTEL MW et al: Infectious agents associated with cylindrical bronchiectasis. Dis Chest 46:23, 1964

696. CROFTON J: Diagnosis and treatment of bronchiectasis. I. Diagnosis. Br Med J 1:721, 1966

697. TURNER-WARWICK M: Systemic arterial patterns in the lung and clubbing of the fingers. Thorax 18:238, 1963

698. GUDBJERG CE: Radiological diagnosis of bronchiectasis and prognosis after operative treatment. Acta Radiol (Stockh) 143 [Suppl], 1957

699. BRUMMER CL: Bronchography. A statement by the committee on therapy, American Thoracic Society. Am Rev Respir Dis 101:815, 1970

700. WILSON JF, PETERS GN, FLESHMAN K: A technique for bronchography in children. Am Rev Respir Dis 105:564, 1972

701. BHARGAVA RK, WOOLF CR: Changes in diffusing capacity after bronchography. Am Rev Respir Dis 96:827, 1967

702. CHRISTOFORIDIS AJ, NELSON SW, TOMASHEFSKI JF: Effects of bronchography on pulmonary function. Am Rev Respir Dis 85:127, 1962

703. SHOOK CD, FELSON B: Inhalation bronchography. Chest 58:333, 1970

704. NADEL JA, WOLFE WG, GRAF PD: Powdered tantalum as a medium for bronchography in canine and human lungs. Invest Radiol 3:229, 1968

705. HINCHCLIFFE WA et al: Roentgenographic study of the human trachea with powdered tantalum. Radiology 97:327, 1970

706. NADEL JA et al: Powdered tantalum. A new contrast medium for roentgenographic examination of human airways. N Engl J Med 283:281, 1970

707. CHERNIACK N et al: Pulmonary function tests in fifty patients with bronchiectasis. J Lab Clin Med 53:693, 1959

708. CHERNIACK NS, CARTON RW: Factors associated with respiratory insufficiency in bronchiectasis. Am J Med 41:562, 1966

709. CHERNIACK NS, DOWLING HF, CARTON RW et al: The role of acute lower respiratory infection in causing pulmonary insufficiency in bronchiectasis. Ann Intern Med 66:489, 1967

710. WYNN-WILLIAMS N: Observations on the treatment of bronchiectasis and its relation to prognosis. Tubercle 38:133, 1957

711. NOGRADY SG, EVANS WV, DAVIES BH: Reversibility of airway obstruction in bronchiectasis. Thorax 33:635, 1978

712. CROFTON J: Bronchiectasis-II. Treatment and prevention. Br Med J 1:783, 1966
713. MEDICAL RESEARCH COUNCIL: Prolonged antibiotic treatment of severe bronchiectasis. Br Med J 2:255, 1957
714. WAGNER RB, BAEZA OR, STEWART JE: Active pulmonary hemorrhage localized by selective pulmonary angiography. Chest 67:121, 1975
715. MCCOLLUM WB, MATLOX KL, GUINN GA et al: Immediate operative treatment for massive hemoptysis. Chest 67:152, 1975
716. GOTTLIEB LS, HILLBERG R: Endobronchial tamponade therapy for intractable hemoptysis. Chest 67:482, 1975
717. CHESTERMAN JT: Recurrence after resection for bronchiectasis. Br J Surg 45:155, 1957
718. HELM WH, THOMPSON VC: The long-term results of resection for bronchiectasis. Q J Med 27:353, 1958
719. DAVIS MB, HOPKINS WA, WANSKER WC: The present status of the treatment of bronchiectasis. Am Rev Respir Dis 85:816, 1962
720. BRONCHIECTASIS. Lancet 2:489, 1955
721. LUNG RESECTION FOR BRONCHIECTASIS. Lancet 1:631, 1958
722. SURGERY FOR BRONCHIECTASIS. Lancet 2:734, 1958
723. GEORGE SA, LEONARD HK, OVERHOLT RH: Bilateral pulmonary resection for bronchiectasis. Ann Thorac Surg 28:48, 1979
723a. BOLMAN RM III, WOLFE WG: Bronchiectasis and bronchopulmonary sequestration. Surg Clin North Am 60:867, 1980
724. PERRY KMA, KING DS: Bronchiectasis. A study of prognosis based on a follow-up of 400 patients. Am Rev Tuberculosis 41:531, 1940
725. STRANG C: The fate of children with bronchiectasis. Ann Intern Med 44:630, 1956
726. FIELD CE: Bronchiectasis: A long-term follow-up of medical and surgical cases from childhood. Arch Dis Child 36:587, 1961
727. SANDERSON JM, KENNEDY MCS, JOHNSON MF et al: Bronchiectasis: Results of surgical and conservative management. A review of 393 cases. Thorax 29:407, 1974
728. LANDING BH: Congenital malformations and genetic disorders of the respiratory tract (larynx, trachea, bronchi and lungs). Am Rev Respir Dis 120:151, 1979
729. HOLINGER PH: Congenital anomalies of the tracheobronchial tree. Postgrad Med 36:151, 1964
730. SALZBERG AM: Congenital malformations of the lower respiratory tract. In Kendig EL Jr (ed): Pulmonary Disorders, Vol I of Disorders of the Respiratory Tract in Children. Philadelphia, WB Saunders, 1972
731. ORZAN F et al: Horseshoe lung. Am Heart J 93:501, 1977
732. MILLER WS: A study of the human pleura pulmonalis: Its relation to the blebs and bullae of emphysema. Am J Roentgenol 15:399, 1926
733. FRASER RG, PARE JAP: Diagnosis of Diseases of the Chest, 2nd ed. Philadelphia, WB Saunders, 1979
734. BALDWIN E DEF et al: Pulmonary insufficiency: IV. A study of 16 cases of large pulmonary air cysts or bullae. Medicine 29:169, 1950
735. OGILVIE C, CATTERALL M: Patterns of disturbed lung function in patients with emphysematous bullae. Thorax 14:216, 1959
736. LAURENZI GA, TURINO GM, FISHMAN AP: Bullous disease of the lung. Am J Med 32:361, 1962
737. GELB AF, GOLD WM, NADEL JA: Mechanisms limiting airflow in bullous lung disease. Am Rev Respir Dis 107:571, 1973
738. CAPEL LH, BELCHER JR: Surgical treatment of large air cysts of the lung. Lancet 1:759, 1957
739. STONE DJ, SCHWARTZ A, FELTMAN JA: Bullous emphysema. A long-term study of the natural history and the effects of therapy. Am Rev Respir Dis 82:493, 1960
740. WOO-MING M, CAPEL LH, BLECHER JR: The results of surgical treatment of large air cysts of the lung. Br J Dis Chest 57:79, 1963
741. DAVIES GM, SIMON G, REID L: Pre- and post-operative assessment of emphysematous bullae. Br J Dis Chest 60:120, 1966
742. BOUSHY SF, BILLIG DM, KOHEN R: Changes in pulmonary function after bullectomy. Am J Med 47:916, 1969
743. LOPEZ-MAJANO V: Pulmonary resection in bullous disease. Am Rev Respir Dis 99:554, 1969
744. PRIDE NB, BARTER CE, HUGH-JONES P: The ventilation of bullae and the effect of their removal on thoracic gas volumes and tests of overall pulmonary function. Am Rev Respir Dis 107:83, 1973
745. HARRIS J: Severe bullous emphysema; successful surgical management despite poor preoperative blood gas levels and marked pulmonary hypertension. Chest 70:658, 1976
746. BILLIG DM: Surgery for bullous emphysema. Chest 70:572, 1976
747. WEG JG, KRUMHOLZ RA, HACKLE ROAD LE: Unilateral hyperlucent lung. Ann Intern Med 62:675, 1965
748. SWYER PR, JAMES GCW: A case of unilateral pulmonary emphysema. Thorax 8:133, 1953
749. MACLEOD WM: Abnormal transradiancy of one lung. Thorax 9:147, 1954
750. PROWSE CM, FUCHS JE, KAUFMAN SA et al: Chronic obstructive pseudoemphysema. A rare cause of unilateral hyperlucent lung. N Engl J Med 271:127, 1964
751. REID L, SIMON G, ZORAB PA et al: The development of unilateral hypertransradiancy of the lung. Br J Dis Chest 61:190, 1967
752. GOLD R, WILT JC, ADHIKARI PK et al: Adenoviral

pneumonia and its complications in infancy and childhood. J Can Assoc Radiol 20:218, 1969

753. MACPHERSON RI, CUMMING GR, CHERNICK V: Unilateral hyperlucent lung: a complication of viral pneumonia. J Can Assoc Radiol 20:225, 1969

754. STOKES D, SIGLER A, KHOURI NF et al: Unilateral hyperlucent lung (Swyer–James Syndrome) after severe mycoplasma pneumoniae infection. Am Rev Respir Dis 117:145, 1978

755. REID L, SIMON G: Unilateral lung transradiancy. Thorax 17:230, 1962

756. KENT DC: Physiologic aspects of idiopathic hyperlucent lung with a review of the literature. Am Rev Respir Dis 90:202, 1964

757. DRAKE CS, CHRISPIN AR, SNOWDEN BS: Unilateral lung transradiancy: A physiological study. Thorax 15:74, 1960

758. HOUK VN, KENT DC, FORSBURG RG: Unilateral hyperlucent lung: A study in pathophysiology and etiology. Am J Med Sci 253:406, 1967

759. NAIRN JR, PRIME FJ: A physiological study of MacLeod's syndrome. Thorax 22:148, 1967

760. COTTOM DG, MYERS NA: Congenital lobar emphysema. Br Med J 1:1394, 1957

761. STOVIN PGI: Congenital lobar emphysema. Thorax 14:254, 1959

762. MANDELBAUM I, HEIMBURGER I, BATTERSBY JS: Congenital lobar obstructive emphysema: Report of eight cases and literature review. Ann Surg 162:1075, 1965

763. HENDREN WH, MCKEE DM: Lobar emphysema of infancy. J Pediatr Surg 1:24, 1966

764. REID JM, BARCLAY RS, STEVENSON JG et al: Congenital obstructive lobar emphysema. Dis Chest 49:359, 1966

765. EIGEN H, LEMEN RJ, WARING WW: Congenital lobar emphysema: Long-term evaluation of surgically and conservatively treated children. Am Rev Respir Dis 113:823, 1976

766. HALLER JA et al: Surgical management of lung bud anomalies: Lobar emphysema, bronchogenic cyst, cystic adenomatoid malformation and intralobar pulmonary sequestration. Ann Thorac Surg 28:33, 1979

767. PIERCE JA, EBERT RV: The barrel deformity of the chest, the senile lung and obstructive pulmonary emphysema. Am J Med 25:13, 1958

768. BATES DV, MACKLEM PT, CHRISTIE RV: Respiratory Function in Disease. Philadelphia, WB Saunders, 1971

769. HEARD BE: A pathological study of emphysema of the lungs with chronic bronchitis. Thorax 13:136, 1958

770. EDGE J, SIMON G, REID L: Periacinar (paraseptal) emphysema: Its clinical, radiological and physiological features. Br J Dis Chest 60:10, 1966

771. MILLER WS: The Lung. Springfield, Charles C Thomas, 1947

772. CORRIN B, LIEBOW AA, FRIEDMAN PJ: Pulmonary lymphangiomyomatosis: A review. Am J Pathol 79:348, 1975

772a. MCCARTY KS JR, MOSSLER JA, MCLELLAND R, SIEKER HO: Pulmonary lymphangiomyomatosis responsive to progesterone. N Engl J Med 303:1461, 1981

773. FRANCE NE, BROWN RJK: Congenital pulmonary lymphangiectasis: Report of 11 examples with special reference to cardiovascular findings. Arch Dis Child 46:528, 1971

774. WILSON MG, MIKITY VG: A new form of respiratory disease in premature infants. J Dis Child 99:489, 1960

775. MIKITY VG: Chronic respiratory distress in the premature infant (Wilson–Mikity Syndrome). In Kendig EL Jr (ed): Pulmonary Disorders, Vol I of Disorders of the Respiratory Tract in Children. Philadelphia, WB Saunders, 1972

776. EDWARDS DK, WAYNE ME, NORTHWAY WH: Twelve years experience with bronchopulmonary dysplasia. Pediatrics 59:839, 1977

777. STOCKER JT, DRAKE RM, MADWELL JE: Cystic and congenital lung disease in the newborn. In Rosenberg H, and Bolande R (eds): Perspectives in Pediatric Pathology, Vol 4. Chicago, Year Book Medical Publishers, 1978

778. OSTOR AG, FORTUNE DW: Congenital cystic adenomatoid malformation of the lung. Am J Clin Pathol 70:595, 1978

779. MONTAGUE NT, SHAW RR: Bronchial atresia. Ann Thorac Surg 18:337, 1974

780. MENG RL, JENSIK RJ, FABER LP et al: Bronchial atresia. Ann Thorac Surg 25:184, 1978

781. WILLIAMS H, CAMPBELL P: Generalized bronchiectasis associated with deficiency of cartilage in the bronchial tree. Arch Dis Child 35:182, 1960

782. BAXTER JD, DUNBAR JS: Tracheomalacia. Ann Otol Rhinol Laryngol 72:1012, 1963

783. HORNS JW, O'LOUGHLIN BJ: Tracheal collapse in polychondritis. Am J Roentgenol 87:844, 1962

784. BEAN WB, DREVETS CC, CHAPMAN JS: Chronic atrophic polychondritis. Medicine 37:353, 1958

785. PEARSON CM, KLINE HM, NEWCOMER VD: Relapsing polychondritis. N Engl J Med 263:51, 1960

786. KING K, MANDAVA B, KAMEN JM: Tracheal tube cuffs and tracheal dilation. Chest 67:458, 1975

787. DANE TCB, KING EG: A prospective study of complications after tracheostomy for assisted ventilation. Chest 67:398, 1975

788. HEDDEN M, ERSOZ CJ, DONNELY WH: Laryngotracheal damage after prolonged use of orotracheal tubes in adults. JAMA 207:703, 1969

789. DALGAARD JB: Tracheopathia chondroosteoplastica. A case elucidating the problems concerning development and ossification of elastic cartilage. Acta Pathol Microbiol Scand 24:118, 1947

790. BOWEN DAL: Tracheopathia osteoplastica. J Clin Pathol 12:435, 1959

791. CARR DT, OLSEN AM: Tracheopathia osteoplastica. JAMA 155:1563, 1954
792. HOWLAND W JR, GOOD CA: The radiographic features of tracheopathia osteoplastica. Radiology 71:847, 1958
793. BAIRD RB, MCCARTNEY JN: Tracheopathia osteoplastica. Thorax 21:321, 1966
794. MARTIN CJ: Tracheobronchopathia osteochondroplastica. Arch Otolaryngol 100:290, 1974
795. BERGERON D, CORMIER Y, DESMEULES M: Tracheobronchopathia osteochondroplastica. Am Rev Respir Dis 114:803, 1976
796. MOUNIER-KUHN P: Dilatation de la trachée: Constations radiographiques et bronchoscopiques. Lyon Med 150:106, 1932
797. KATZ I, LEVINE M, HERMAN P: Tracheobronchomegaly. The Mounier–Kuhn syndrome. Am J Roentgenol 88:1084, 1962
798. JOHNSTON RF, GREEN RA: Tracheobronchomegaly. Report of five cases and demonstration of familial occurrence. Am Rev Respir Dis 91:35, 1965
799. HIMALSTEIN MR, GALLAGHER JC: Tracheobronchomegaly. Ann Otol Rhinol Laryngol 82:223, 1973
800. SURPRENANT EL, O'LOUGHLIN BJ: Tracheal diverticula and tracheobronchomegaly. Dis Chest 49:345, 1966
801. KOONTZ AR: Congenital cysts of the lung. Bull Johns Hopkins Hosp 37:340, 1925
802. COOKE FN, BLADES B: Cystic disease of the lungs. J Thorac Surg 23:546, 1952
803. MOFFAT AD: Congenital cystic disease of the lungs and its classification. J Pathol Bacteriol 79:361, 1960
804. SCHMIDT FE, DRAPANAS T: Congenital cystic lesions of the bronchi and lungs. Ann Thorac Surg 14:650, 1972
805. BOYDEN EA: Bronchogenic cysts and the theory of intralobar sequestration: New embryologic data. J Thorac Surg 35:604, 1958
806. SCHENCK SG: Congenital cystic disease of lung, a clinicopathological study. Am J Roentgenol 35:604, 1936
807. SCHENCK SG: Diagnosis of congenital cystic disease of lung. Arch Intern Med 60:1, 1937
808. HINDS JR: Bronchiectasis in the Maori. NZ Med J 57:328, 1958
809. BAUM GL et al: Cystic disease of the lung, report of eighty-eight cases, with an ethnologic relationship. Am J Med 40:578, 1966
810. WARE GW, HALL A: Congenital tracheoesophageal fistula in the adult. J Thorac Surg 36:58, 1958
811. WYCHULIS AR, ELLIS FH JR, ANDERSON HA: Acquired nonmalignant esophagotracheobronchial fistula. Report of 36 cases. JAMA 196:117, 1966
812. SACKS RP, DUBOIS JJ, GERGER JP et al: The esophagobronchial fistula. Case report and review of the literature. Am J Roentgenol 99:204, 1967
813. JUDD DR, DUBUQUE T JR: Acquired benign esophagotracheobronchial fistula. Dis Chest 54:237, 1968
814. HEDDEN M, ERSOZ CJ, SAFAR P: Tracheoesophageal fistulas following prolonged artificial ventilation via cuffed tracheostomy tubes. Anesthesiology 31:281, 1969
815. PRYCE DM: Lower accessory pulmonary artery with intralobar sequestration of the lung. A report of seven cases. J Pathol Bacteriol 58:457, 1946
816. SMITH RA: A theory of the origin of intralobar sequestration of the lung. Thorax 11:10, 1956
817. IWAI K et al: Intralobar pulmonary sequestration with special reference to developmental pathology. Am Rev Respir Dis 107:911, 1973
818. SAEGESSER F, BESSON A: Extralobar and intralobar pulmonary sequestrations of the upper and lower lobes. Report of eleven cases, including one case of the scimitar syndrome. Chest 63:69, 1973
819. HOLSTEIN P, HJELMS E: Bronchopulmonary sequestration. J Thorac Cardiovasc Surg 65:462, 1973
819a. SAVIC B et al: Lung sequestration: A report of seven cases and review of 540 published cases. Thorax 34:96, 1979
820. ROEHM JOF, JUE KL, AMPLATZ K: Radiographic features of the scimitar syndrome. Radiology 86:856, 1966
821. BUCKLEY CE III, TUCKER DH, THORNE NA et al: Bronchiolectasis. The clinical syndrome and its relationship to chronic lung disease. Am J Med 38:190, 1965
822. BAAR HS, GALINDO J: Bronchiolitis fibrosa obliterans. Thorax 21:209, 1966
823. IRWIN RS, THOMAS HM III: Mucoid impaction of the bronchus. Diagnosis and treatment. Am Rev Respir Dis 108:955, 1973
824. WARING WW, BRUNT CH, HILMAN BC: Mucoid impaction of the bronchi in cystic fibrosis. Pediatrics 39:166, 1967
824a. FAIRSHTER RD, RILEY CA, HEWLETT RJ: Large bronchial casts. Arch Intern Med 139:522, 1979
825. ARRIGONI MG, BERNATZ PE, DONOGHUE FD: Broncholithiasis. J Thorac Cardiovasc Surg 62:231, 1971
826. LYONS HA: Differential diagnosis of hemoptysis and its treatment. Basics of RD 5, No. 2, 1976
827. BREDIN CP et al: Treatment of massive hemoptysis by combined occlusion of pulmonary and bronchial arteries. Am Rev Respir Dis 117:969, 1978
828. YANG CT, BERGER HW: Conservative management of life threatening hemoptysis. Mount Sinai J Med 45:329, 1978
829. STERN RC et al: Treatment and prognosis of massive hemoptysis in cystic fibrosis. Am Rev Respir Dis 117:825, 1978

830. PROCTOR DF: The upper airways. Am Rev Respir Dis 115:97, 315, 1977

831. HANNALLAH R, ROSALES JK: Acute epiglottitis. Canad Anaesth Soc J 25:84, 1978

832. GELFAND JA et al: Acquired C_1 esterase inhibitor deficiency and angioedema: A review. Medicine 58:321, 1979

833. HARRISON BDW: Upper airway obstruction, a report of 16 patients and review of the literature. Quarterly J Med 45:625, 1976

834. MCADAM LP et al: Relapsing polychondritis. Medicine 55:193, 1976

835. DOBIE RA, TOBEY DM: Clinical features of diphtheria in the respiratory tract, JAMA 242:2197, 1979

836. JAUREGUI R, LILKER ES, BAYLEY A: Upper airway obstruction in euthyroid goiter. JAMA 238:2163, 1977

837. WARREN CPW: Acute respiratory failure and tracheal obstruction in the elderly with benign goiters. Canad Med Assoc J 121:191, 1979

838. WHITED RE: Laryngeal fracture in the multiple trauma patient. Am J Surg 136:354, 1978

839. GAMSU G, BORSEN DE, WEBB WR et al: Structure and function in tracheal stenosis. Am Rev Respir Dis 121:519, 1980

840. STITIK FP, BARTLET D, JAMES AE et al: Tantalum tracheography in upper airway obstruction: 100 experiences in adults. Am J Roentgenol 130:35, 1978

Chapter 15

Neoplastic Disease and Mediastinal Disorders

JAY J. ROHWEDDER

LUNG CANCER

INCIDENCE, MORTALITY, AND SURVIVAL

"Women who smoke like men die like men who smoke." Joseph A. Califano's pithy summary of new data in the 1979 Report of the Surgeon General emphasizes that lung cancer, the leading cause of death from cancer in American men, will become the leading cause of death in women by 1990.[1] Lung cancer deaths in women are then expected to exceed deaths from breast cancer. In 1950, 19.9 male deaths per 100,000 population were caused by lung cancer; this increased to 63 deaths per 100,000 in 1976. Among women, the increase was from 4.5 to 19.5 deaths per 100,000 in the same period. The increases are not explained by aging of the population. Improved diagnosis likely had a minor effect on these figures because the techniques which permit eventual recognition of lung cancer have changed little since 1950. Table 15-1 shows the epidemic proportions of this disease, which in 1978 killed 280 persons each day in the United States.

The male to female death-rate ratio for lung cancer among whites reached a peak of 6.8:1 in 1960. In 1969, the male to female ratio had fallen to 4.3:1, not because male deaths declined, but because female deaths rose more rapidly—the delayed consequence of the increased social acceptance of cigarette smoking among women which began after World War I.[1] Mortality rates for nonwhite men and women have risen even faster, although the white male lung cancer mortality rate, while still rising, has begun to level off because of a downward trend in smoking among men (and in the tar and nicotine content of the cigarettes smoked). When men born between 1910 and 1919 were surveyed in 1955, when they were thus between the ages of 35 and 45 years, 62% were cigarette smokers. Ten years later, the number of smokers had fallen to 53%. In 1970, 4 years later, only 37% smoked cigarettes. Patterns for other cohorts are similar.[3] The incidence of lung cancer among women is expected to continue to increase but to fall short of that in men today, in part because women smoke fewer cigarettes and tend to smoke those with lower tar yields. The percentage of the teenage population smoking cigarettes regularly has reached 16% and continues to increase. Equal numbers of teenage boys and girls now smoke.[1]

TABLE 15-1. Mortality from Selected Leading Causes of Death in the United States

Disease	Year	Deaths
Lung cancer	1950	18,313
	1964	45,838
	1979	112,000
Emphysema	1979	17,796
Digestive organ cancer (combined)	1979	105,150
Breast cancer	1979	34,500
Leukemia	1979	15,400
All accidents	1979	100,761
US Vietnam War Dead*	1961–1973	46,163

* Statistical Abstracts of the United States, 1974.

(Derived from National Cancer Institute's Surveillance, Epidemiology and End Results (SEER) Program, and US Public Health Service. Smoking and Health: A Report of the Surgeon General. Washington, US Department of Health, Education and Welfare, 1979)

The End Results Group reported that less than a quarter of lung cancers are classified as localized at diagnosis, a proportion that has remained nearly constant since 1940.[4] Although the improvement in overall 3-year survival rates for both sexes was modest (6%, 1940 to 1949; 11%, 1965 to 1969), the 3-year survival rate for males with localized disease from 1965 through 1969 was 35%; for females, 55%. These favorable results apply to only 11% of lung cancer patients: those with localized disease whose general health permits successful surgical resection.[3] There has been little or no improvement in the 10% overall 5-year survival rate in the last decade.[1]

ETIOLOGY

Tobacco Smoking

The overwhelming evidence establishing a causative relationship between tobacco smoking and lung cancer summarized in the epochal 1964 Report to the Surgeon General has been supplemented by additional US Public Health Service reports on the health consequences of smoking.[1,5,6] Past epidemiologic studies, as well as nine current studies indicate: (1) a dose-response relationship exists between smoking, especially of cigarettes, and lung cancer; (2) the demographic distribution of lung cancer correlates with smoking habits; (3) reduced lung cancer rates are found among ex-smokers; and (4) lung cancer has been induced with the administration of tar or inhaled cigarette smoke in experimental animals.[1,5-7] For both men and women, the risk of developing lung cancer is directly related to total exposure to cigarette smoke as measured by the number of cigarettes smoked per day, the total lifetime number of cigarettes smoked, the duration of smoking in years, the age at initiation of smoking, the depth of inhalation, and the tar and nicotine levels in the cigarettes smoked.[6] Worldwide prospective epidemiologic studies confirm these associations and indicate that in comparison with nonsmokers, average smokers of cigarettes have approximately a 9- to 10-fold increased risk of developing lung cancer and heavy smokers at least a 20-fold risk-increase. According to a recent study done in Japan, even nonsmoking wives of heavy smokers have an increased risk of lung cancer, a finding of considerable public health significance.[6a]

Most major studies carried out in the United States have also associated cigar and pipe smoking with lung cancer. The association has been less strong than that observed in some European countries, the varying risks being explained by differences in degree of exposure to smoke.[8] The overall mortality ratios of pipe and cigar smokers in the United States are slightly higher than that of nonsmokers. (The mortality ratio is the ratio of the death-rate of smokers to that of nonsmokers, the mortality rate of nonsmokers, by definition always being one.) That of cigar smokers is higher than that of pipe smokers. As with cigarettes, a dose-response relationship may exist between the number of cigars and pipefuls smoked and overall mortality. Heavy smoking and inhalation of small cigars has been shown to result in a risk of lung cancer that is similar to that run by cigarette smokers.[8] The condensate of pipe and cigar smoke is generally found to be alkaline, more irritating to the respiratory tract, and less likely to be inhaled than the slightly acidic condensate of cigarette smoke. Once a smoker has learned to inhale cigarettes, there is a tendency to inhale the smoke of other tobacco products which contain many of the same chemical constituents, including nicotine, other alkaloids, phenols, and polycylic aromatic hydrocarbons (see also Chap. 1, Air Pollution).

Hammond's study on exsmokers aged 50 to 69 yr who had smoked 20 or more cigarettes daily showed that, after 10 yr of not smoking, exsmokers have a death rate from lung cancer similar to nonsmokers.[6,9] Exsmokers who had been light smokers (1–19 cigarettes per day) had a reduced lung-cancer risk 1 to 4 yr after stopping. Manufacturing changes have reduced the tar content of nonfilter as well as filter cigarettes in recent years and this may account for the fact that current lung cancer patients have been shown to have smoked more cigarettes than did lung cancer patients in the period from 1948 to 1950.[10] Although filter cigarette smokers with high exposure have a risk of lung cancer which is still 5 times as great as the risk for nonsmokers, there is convincing evidence that the risk of lung cancer is significantly lower among those who smoke filter cigarettes exclusively.[10,11] The magnitude of the reduction in cancer mortality among filter smokers as compared to nonfilter smokers (40–60%) is similar whether one considers population groups that smoke 1 to 19 cigarettes or 40 or more cigarettes per day. A significant reduction in lung cancer mortality has also been demonstrated among middle-aged nonfilter smokers who switch to filter cigarettes; however, no change can be expected among heavy smokers aged 50 to 69 yr who shift to filter cigarettes for less than 5 years.[10] Available filters do not selectively remove carcinogenic agents from particulate material in cigarette smoke, and, on a gram-to-gram basis, the tar from existing filter cigarettes has the same carcinogenic activity as does nonfiltered smoke.[10] The common cellulose acetate fiber filter likewise fails to selectively remove gas-phase components such as hydrogen cyanide and volatile aldehydes which are toxic to cilia.

Large-scale educational efforts against smoking should be encouraged but can be expected to fall short of complete success. It is naive to anticipate a total legislative ban on cigarettes in the foreseeable future. Therefore, deliberate managerial measures directed toward the development of a safer cigarette, having quantitative or qualitative changes in tar yield, seem to offer the best chance of reducing tobacco-related disease.[12]

Aryl Hydrocarbon Hydroxylase

Lung cancer has been epidemiologically linked to exposure to polycyclic aromatic hydrocarbons (PAH) in cigarette smoke. Aryl hydrocarbon hydroxylase (AHH) is one of the enzymes which metabolize PAH into carcinogens. The enzyme is membrane-bound and inducible *in situ* in alveolar macrophages and in peripheral lymphocytes. Investigators disagree as to whether more lung cancer patients (as compared with noncancer patients) have high AHH inducibility.[1] The validity of these studies has been questioned because the levels of AHH measured and reported in individual lung cancer patients' lymphocytes do not reflect levels of the enzyme in freshly excised lung tissue.

Influence of Sex and Genetics

The sex ratio of bronchogenic carcinoma (the ratio of affected men to affected women) varies widely in different parts of the world, and in people of different racial origin in the same part of the world.[13] The major dissimilarity in the national sex-ratios is due to differences in the incidence of lung cancer among men, in turn a reflection of differences in smoking habits. On the other hand, bronchial carcinoma represents a much more constant proportion of all malignant disease among women of widely differing ethnic groups, despite widely varying tobacco consumption. That variation which occurs among women is randomly spread throughout the world, regardless of race. These data suggest that a sex-linked genetic factor may have some influence on the differing incidence between the sexes.

The proportions of various cell types and the location of tumors, whether central or peripheral, are also different among different peoples: the incidence of bronchial carcinoma in Japan has risen threefold in the last 10 years and the proportion of adenocarcinomas is almost 40%. Adenocarcinomas represent less than 10% of bronchial malignancies in Iceland, a country with an overall incidence of lung cancer similar to that in Japan. Lung cancer is said to be very uncommon among North American Indians.[13] Differences in life-expectancy and in the sizes of age cohorts for different ethnic groups do not seem to adequately explain such differences, which may result, in part, from genetic factors. Experiments on different genetically defined strains of mice clearly show that genetic factors influence susceptibility to both spontaneous and induced neoplasms. It would be surprising if the same were not true for man. Were genetic factors anything like as important as carcinogen exposure in the development of lung cancer, one would expect this to show up in identical-twin studies. To date, there is no indication of an excess in cancer of any site in the twins of lung cancer patients.

Influence of Carcinogen Exposure on Cell Type

Nonsmokers rarely have squamous or oat cell carcinomas. They more often develop adenocarcinoma, bronchiolar carcinoma, or carcinoid tumors. The increase in lung cancer among smokers appeared to center around squamous and oat cell cancers until the last 10 years when adenocarcinoma became progressively more prevalent relative to the other cell types. The increase affects men as well as women.[14,15] Adenocarcinoma accounted for 34% of 300 consecutive autopsies on recent VA Lung Group patients, and thereby displaced squamous cell carcinoma as the most common histologic type.[14] This suggests an absolute increase in the prevalence of adenocarcinoma because the data are from men alone, and the review panel has not changed its histopathologic criteria in 20 years.

The epidemiologic link between adenocarcinoma (bronchiolar cancer is a subtype) and smoking is longstanding but often unrecognized.[16,17] One large study representative of earlier data found that 87% of patients with lung cancer smoked.[18] Among 1682 recent cases, 81% of the women and 98% of the men smoked.[15] Adeno- or bronchiolar carcinomas were found in two-thirds of the nonsmoking women and in nearly half of the nonsmoking men; nevertheless, 89% of patients with adenocarcinoma smoked, as did 98% with squamous and oat cell cancer.

In summary, squamous and oat cell carcinomas display epidemiologic differences when compared with adenocarcinomas. The former have a greater male to female sex ratio, the victims smoke significantly more, and there are fewer nonsmokers. Men with squamous cell cancer tend to be older. Multiple primary lung cancers and individually occurring cancers associated with exposure to asbestos, chromates, chloromethyl methyl ether, and radioactivity in uranium mining have been predominantly squamous and oat cell tumors.[19]

Industrial Factors

A thoroughly documented association exists between lung cancer and exposure to irradiation among uranium miners. A similar relationship exists for asbestos workers. In both occupations, there is a more-than-additive interaction between smoking and industrial exposure for, after taking into account the age distributions of smokers and nonsmokers, there is a very large difference in lung cancer death rates in the two groups, more than expected from a summation of smoking and work exposure.[20] Death rates from lung cancer in New York insulation workers are 7 times those expected. No correlation between cigarette smoking and malignant mesotheliomas of the pleura has been noted. There is no clear evidence to implicate a particular type of asbestos fiber in carcinoma of the lung: chrysotile, crocidolite, and amosite asbestos may all be of importance. Present evidence implicates crocidolite in the development of mesotheliomas (see Chap. 12, Pleural Disease).

Workers engaged in the production of chromates from the raw material, chrome iron ore, have an increased mortality from lung cancer. There is usually a long latent period before the appearance of the cancer, similar to the 20 years that commonly elapse following asbestos exposure.[21] Nickel refinery workers were once found to have a 3- to 5-fold increase in lung cancer mortality and a 150-fold increase in risk for nasal cancer.[21] Nickel dust was the likely responsible carcinogen, although generally adopted changes in the refinery process made before the Second World War not only drastically reduced dust levels, but also reduced worker-exposure to arsenic. Arsenic is a known carcinogen which has been implicated in the development of lung cancer in those exposed through arsenical therapy or the manufacture and use of pesticides. An unusually high incidence of bronchogenic carcinoma has also been reported for workers engaged in the operation of coal and gas retorts and the manufacture of mustard gas for military use.[20]

Hematite (iron oxide) mining is associated with an increased risk of lung cancer. In addition, a number of industries in which there is a common exposure to iron and silica may be responsible for a poorly quantitated but increased risk. These include the mining of various metals, metal grinding, sand blasting, and iron and steel foundry work. Although some studies found the autopsy incidence of bronchogenic carcinoma to be increased with anthrasilicosis, this has not been a uniform finding.[22] Haloethers, including chloromethyl methyl ether widely used by industry in organic synthesis and in the preparation of ion-exchange resins, produced an eight-fold increase in the incidence of lung cancer among exposed workers. Some had never smoked. There was a striking predominance of oat cell carcinomas.[22a]

Occupations which repeatedly stand out when studying lung cancer in nonsmoking populations include those in which workers are exposed to paint fumes and hot metal dust, and carpentry.[18] The dilemma presented by risk of carcinogenicity in the face of useful industrial development has become a major concern.[22b]

The Urban Factor: Air Pollution

Investigators have differed as to whether the incidence of lung cancer differs significantly between urban and rural areas after populations are standarized for tobacco usage; however, the existence of a small urban factor in lung-cancer incidence now seems firmly established.[1,5,7] The influence of greater numbers of occupational exposures and more available diagnostic facilities on this urban excess is less clear. Roe feels that taking the epidemiologic evidence as a whole, nonsmokers exposed to heavy air pollution, and heavy smokers living in truly rural areas, have a lower expectation of lung cancer than their calculated intake of carcinogens would indicate as likely. This suggests an element of synergism between tobacco smoke and air pollution. Experimental evidence has been presented showing that when extracts of filtered air pollutants are mixed with tobacco smoke condensate and applied to mouse skin, the carcinogenicity of the two is at least additive. Others feel that epidemiologic patterns are not those expected were there any interaction between smoking and air pollution.[20]

The Association of Lung Cancer and Other Pulmonary Diseases

The extensive literature emphasizing the association between lung scars and lung cancer has been summarized in a number of reviews.[18,23,24,25] Tuberculosis, bronchiectasis, pulmonary infarcts, anthracosis, and diffuse interstitial fibrotic diseases of the lung may lead to atypical metaplasias, both squamous and adenomatous in type, explaining some lung carcinomas as similar in genesis to the origin of hepatocellular carcinoma in the cirrhotic liver.

When lung cancer occurs with diseases which cause atypical acinar proliferation as part of a diffuse fibrotic pattern characterized by honeycombing of the lung (*e.g.*, idiopathic diffuse interstitial fibrosis and sclerodema), bronchiolo-alveolar cell carcinoma and adenocarcinoma represent approximately 25% of the cases, about twice as many as when honeycombing is not present.[25,26] That the epithelium of the acini may also undergo squamous metaplasia explains the relatively common occurrence of epidermoid tumors in these patients.

Coexistence of tuberculosis and bronchogenic carcinoma is common and lung cancers can cause activation of dormant tuberculous foci or the shedding of *Mycobacterium tuberculosis* or atypical mycobacteria into the sputum in the absence of an apparent granulomatous residual on the chest roentgenogram. For this reason, bronchogenic carcinoma patients who have positive tuberculin skin tests are often given isoniazid chemoprophylaxis. Opinion as to whether tuberculous scarring of the lung appreciably increases the risk of developing lung cancer is divided, and the evidence is less than convincing.[23] The frequency with which they are associated in some population groups is probably related to co-existing socioeconomic and cultural risk factors (primarily alcoholism and cigarette use) because local factors resulting from tuberculosis involvement of the lung do not play a significant role in localizing the carcinoma. Moreover, the few reports of adenocarcinomas occurring in a tuberculosis scar are offset by data indicating there is no difference in the types of cancer in patients with and without tuberculosis. Response to antituberculous chemotherapy is satisfactory, despite the debilitating effect of cancer and its treatment.

The possible relationship between preexisting chronic bronchitis and lung cancer is difficult to evaluate because the available data have, as with tuberculosis and cancer, produced conflicting conclusions from retrospective rather than prospective studies.[1,23] Chronic obstructive lung disease is clearly associated with an increased incidence of bronchogenic carcinoma[27] which may extend to first-degree relatives.[28]

PATHOLOGY

Revised World Health Organization Classification

The revised nomenclature for malignant tumors of the lung adopted by the World Health Organization (WHO) Expert Committee on Lung Cancer in October 1977 appears in the list on p. 802. This scheme differs in important respects from the widely used classifications the committee originated in 1958 and 1965. The new classification is consistent with a unified theory of origin for lung cancers shown in Yesner's Y construct in Figure 15-1. This diagram demonstrates that all lung cancers are thought to arise from the primitive foregut endoderm and places a homogeneous small cell (oat cell) carcinoma at the base.[29] Transitions occur chiefly between adjacent types but also between histologic extremes. The observations that led to this classification were made by means of both light and electron microscopy. Table 15-2 gives the malignant counterparts of cells normally found in the bronchial epithelium. The Y construct recognizes that the histologic appearance of tumors at adjacent points tend to overlap. Occasional tumors have sufficient overlap so that more than one arm of the Y is expressed, and a carcinoma with combined histology results. The most common combination is differentiated squamous and mucin-producing adenocarcinoma. Transitions between small cell carcinoma and squamous cell or adenocarcinoma also are relatively common.

The uniform small cell carcinoma that undergoes transition to the polygonal small cell carcinoma often forms giant cells, making it difficult to distinguish it from some large cell carcinomas. In the revised classification, the intermediate small cell carcinoma has replaced the po-

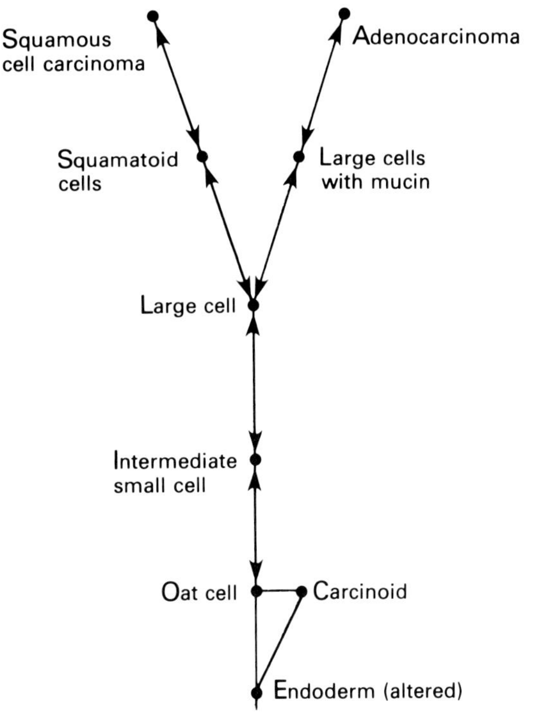

FIG. 15-1. Derivation of bronchogenic carcinomas. (Y construct courtesy of Dr. Raymond Yesner, Chairman, WHO Expert Committee on Lung Cancer)

TABLE 15-2. Bronchogenic Carcinomas: Cell of Origin

Bronchial Cell Type	Cancer Cell Type
Basal layer cell	Oat cell
Intermediate basal layer	Intermediate small cell
Ciliated cell	Squamous
Kultschitzky (K) cell	Carcinoid adenoma
Goblet cell	Adenocarcinoma
Bronchiolar mucous cell	Bronchiolar cancer*
Bronchiolar stem	Bronchiolar cancer*
cell {Clara cell, Ciliated cell}	
Type II alveolar pneumocyte	Alveolar cell cancer*

* Ultrastructural studies suggest that most bronchiolo-alveolar cell carcinomas arise from a bronchiolar stem cell; nevertheless, bronchiolo-alveolar cell carcinoma is used in the text as a generic term for any malignancy arising from one of these three cells.

Revised WHO Histologic Classification of Lung Tumors (October 1977)

Epithelial Tumors
- Benign
  - Papillomas
    - Squamous cell papilloma
    - "Transitional" papilloma
  - Adenomas
    - Pleomorphic adenoma ("mixed" tumor)
    - Monomorphic adenomas
    - Others
- Dysplasia and carcinoma *in situ*
- Malignant
  - Squamous cell carcinoma (epidermoid carcinoma)
  - Variant: spindle cell (squamous) carcinoma
  - Small cell carcinoma
    - Oat cell carcinoma
    - Intermediate cell type
    - Combined oat cell carcinomas
  - Adenocarcinoma
    - Acinar adenocarcinoma
    - Papillary adenocarcinoma
    - Bronchiolo–alveolar carcinoma
    - Solid carcinoma with mucus formation
  - Large cell carcinoma
  - Variants:
    - Giant cell carcinoma
    - Clear cell carcinoma
  - Adenosquamous carcinoma
  - Carcinoid tumor
  - Bronchial gland carcinomas
    - Adenoid cystic carcinoma
    - Mucoepidermoid carcinoma
    - Others
  - Others

Soft Tissue Tumors

Mesothelial Tumors
- Benign mesothelioma
- Malignant mesothelioma
  - Epithelial
  - Fibrous (spindle cell)
  - Biphasic

Miscellaneous Tumors
- Benign
- Malignant
  - Carcinosarcoma
  - Pulmonary blastoma
  - Malignant melanoma
  - Malignant lymphomas
  - Others

Secondary Tumors

Unclassified Tumors

Tumorlike lesions
- Hamartoma
- Lymphoproliferative lesions
- Tumorlet
- Eosinophilic granuloma
- "Sclerosing hemangioma"
- Inflammatory pseudotumor
- Others

Classification courtesy of Dr. Raymond Yesner, Chairman, WHO Expert Committee on Lung Cancer, West Haven, Connecticut

lygonal small cell tumor in recognition of its intermediate position. In addition, the spindle cell variant in the old small cell category has been eliminated and a combined type (with squamous cell or adenocarcinoma) has been introduced. Large cell carcinomas with significant intracellular mucin have been moved into the adenocarcinoma category.

The pleomorphism of bronchial carcinomas has caused pathologists classifying poorly differentiated squamous and adenocarcinomas to disagree in as many as 40% of their observations.[30] Large cell carcinomas and polygonal small cell carcinomas can be particularly difficult to classify. Some feel that oat cell cancers are the malignant counterpart of carcinoid tumors and that both derive from the Kulchitsky cell of the neuroectoderm.[32] Electron microscopy does show that both contain dense-core granules of the neurosecretory type. Also, both appear capable of amine precursor uptake and decarboxylation (APUD) and polypeptide hormone secretion. APUD cells from the neurocrest include pancreatic alpha and beta cells, thyroid C cells, and enterochromaffin cells throughout the gastrointestinal tract. Tumors derived from these cells are called apudomas.

Other investigators emphasize that the transition between small cell carcinomas and differentiated squamous and adenocarcinomas must signify that small cell carcinomas and carcinoids are like siblings: their biologic behavior is quite dissimilar despite their minor cytochemical resemblance. Small cell carcinomas differ from carcinoids in that they contain few dense-core granules, are much more common, and increase among workers exposed to radioactivity, chloro-

TABLE 15-3. Representative Roentgenographic Patterns in Carcinomas of Different Cell Types

Roentgenographic Observation	Squamous Carcinoma	Adenocarcinoma	Alveolar Cell Carcinoma	Small Cell Undifferentiated Carcinoma	Large Cell Carcinoma
Most common location	Central	Mid-lung to peripheral	Peripheral: pneumonic; diffuse nodular pattern	Central	Central, mid-lung, or peripheral
Frequency of volume loss	Common	Uncommon	Rare	Common	Less common
Hilar mass	Common	Rare	Rare	Common	Uncommon
Cavitation	Common	Common	Uncommon	No	Common
Wide mediastinum	Less common	Less common	Rare	Most common cell type	Uncommon
Superior sulcus tumor	Most common cell type	Uncommon	Rare	Rare	Common

methyl methyl ether, and cigarette smoke. They are notoriously malignant in contrast to the slow-growing apudomas. Thus, it seems likely that the gene that accounts for the production of dense-core granules in carcinoids is partly expressed in "oat cells," but less so as these develop characteristics of more differentiated tumors.

Difficulties in classification have led many authors to use a simplified, practical division that includes five cell types: squamous carcinoma, adenocarcinoma, large cell carcinoma, small cell carcinoma, and undifferentiated carcinoma other than small cell cancer.

The diverse clinical findings and roentgenographic features that tend to be associated with bronchogenic carcinomas of specific cell type largely result from their development in different anatomic locations within the lung. The anatomic location of the primary cancer often determines the clinical presentation. Minor statistical differences in the method or distribution of metastases from cancers of differing cell type are of less importance, because no one cell type is dominant when lymphangitic or hematogenous patterns of metastases are considered, and all may invade pleura, pericardium, heart, mediastinum, and chest wall by direct extension. Even when metastases appear in organs that are less commonly involved by bronchogenic cancer (*e.g.*, lung-to-lung spread), one cell type is about as likely to be responsible as another. Exceptions to this statement, the clinical features or roentgenologic patterns that are peculiar to specific cell types, are discussed below. Table 15-3 categorizes some of the more common roentgenographic findings. Paraneoplastic neurologic and endocrine syndromes also are more common with specific types of tumors.

The proportion of lung cancers reported to be represented by individual cell types varies widely in different studies because it is influenced by case selection in autopsy or surgical series and by the histologic criteria used in diagnosis.

Squamous Cell Carcinoma

Squamous cell carcinomas comprise 30 to 45% of bronchogenic carcinomas.[14,15,33] Four criteria are used in their diagnosis: (1) the presence of intracellular bridges; (2) cell nest formation; (3) the presence of keratin pearls; and (4) polarization or whorling arrangement of cells (Fig. 15-2). Squamous carcinomas occur mainly in the large bronchi and are the most common tumors originating in mainstem, lobar, and segmental bronchi. About a third originate in the periphery of the lung where they occasionally arise in relation to scars. Cavitation with or without an air fluid interface is seen in 10 to 20% of these tumors in either location (Fig. 15-3). The roentgenographic appearance of cavitation within a bron-

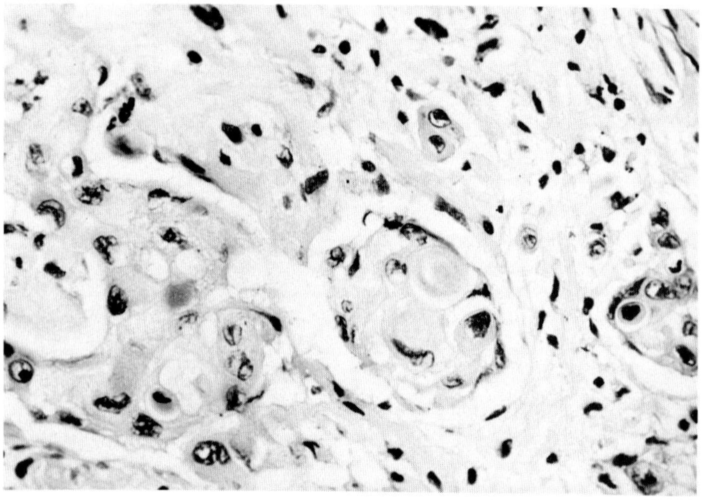

FIG. 15-2. Squamous carcinoma. In the center of this section there is a suggestion of the formation of a keratin pearl. The darker-staining round formations are keratinized cells with complete nuclear loss. The very dark pyknotic nuclei with keratinized cytoplasms are characteristic. Intercellular bridges are difficult to see in this section. (Histologic section courtesy of Dr. Lee Weatherbee, Ann Arbor, Michigan)

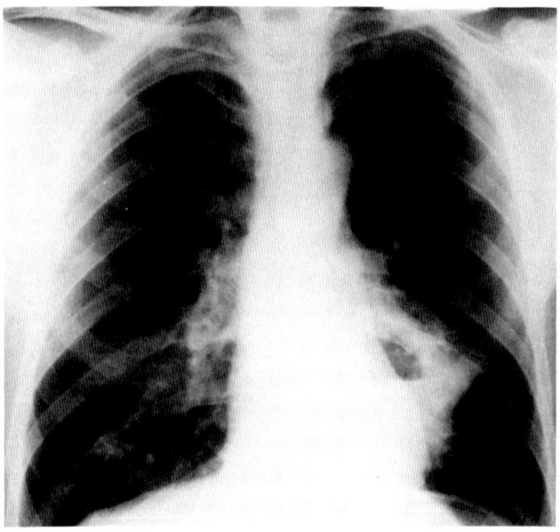

FIG. 15-3. Squamous carcinoma. Spontaneous cavitation within the tumor resulted in a thick wall with an irregular inner border and a fluid level which was formed by liquefied necrotic debris. Autopsy proven.

chogenic carcinoma is similar, regardless of cell type; the majority of these excavations are thick-walled with shaggy inner margins. The presence of a mural nodule, which is usually fixed to the internal margin of the excavation, suggests neoplasm. Occasionally, the nodule moves with positioning of the patient and therefore resembles a mycetoma or fungus ball within a parenchymal excavation of nonneoplastic origin. Cavitation due to necrotizing pneumonia distal to a neoplastic endobronchial obstruction is surprisingly uncommon, much less common than excavation of the tumor itself. The most common roentgenographic presentation of squamous carcinoma is that of volume loss involving a single lobe or an individual segment within a lobe (Fig. 15-4). Disproportionate radiolucency produced by hyperinflation of lung parenchyma distal to a check valve mechanism produced by an endobronchial carcinoma is uncommon. This finding would probably be recognized more frequently with squamous carcinomas if chest roentgenograms were taken in expiration whenever minor degrees of asymmetry were noted in the radiopacity of the lung fields. Because of their relative frequency and central location, squamous carcinomas are the most common tumors to produce a hilar mass (Fig. 15-5). Rarely, squamous tumors produce an infiltrative pattern on the chest x-ray film (Fig. 15-6), a roentgenographic appearance more commonly associated with bronchiolo-alveolar cell carcinoma. The linear-reticular pattern of lymphangitic spread within the lung parenchyma is also relatively uncommon in squamous carcinoma (Fig. 15-7).

A prominent feature in the spread of squamous carcinomas is their extension in the extracartilaginous part of the bronchial wall with direct invasion of adjacent lymph glands. Despite

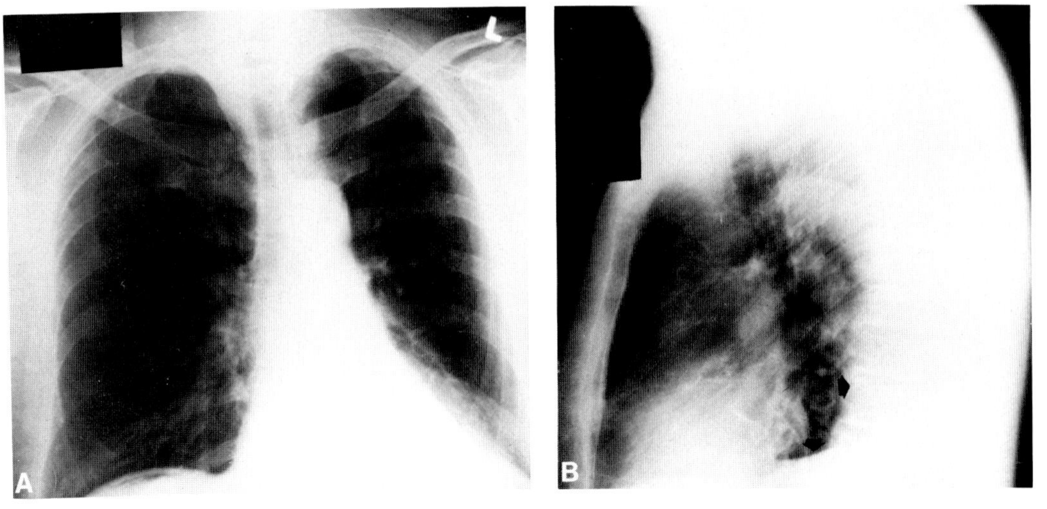

FIG. 15-4. Squamous carcinoma. **A.** Because of its endobronchial location, the tumor is not visible, but the left lower lobe projects as a triangular increase in density behind the heart. Collapse of the lobe occurred following abdominal surgery for peptic ulcer disease, and air is present below the right hemidiaphragm. **B.** In the lateral view collapsed lobe overlies the spine (*horizontal arrow*), producing uniform density of the thoracic vertebral bodies which normally appear to become progressively more lucent from the lung apex to the diaphragm. The only segment of left diaphragm visible is that portion which lies between the silhouette produced by the heart anteriorly and that caused by the collapsed lobe posteriorly (*vertical arrow*). The diagnosis was made by fiberoptic bronchoscopy.

this propensity for direct local extension, clinical and postmortem evidence of distant lymphatic and hematogenous dissemination is not rare. Squamous carcinomas do, however, have the lowest overall incidence of metastases and the highest incidence of solitary extrathoracic metastasis; at postmortem examination, approximately half are limited to the hemithorax in which they originated. The majority of pulmonary cancers which invade the chest wall by direct extension are squamous tumors, but this cell type infrequently sheds cells into pleural effusions, and so is less likely to be diagnosed by cytologic examination of pleural fluid than is adenocarcinoma.

Unlike adenocarcinomas, the biologic behavior of well-differentiated and poorly differentiated squamous carcinomas appears to be similar, the rates of nonmetastatic presentation being 60 to 70% for both types. Surgical survival rates and duration of survival among inoperable lung cancer patients have generally been found to be greatest in patients with squamous cell tumors.[31]

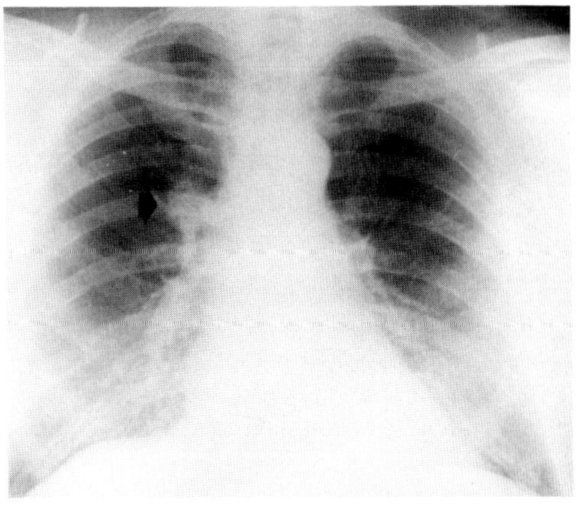

FIG. 15-5. Squamous carcinoma. These tumors usually originate in a proximal bronchus and are the most common pulmonary neoplasm to produce a hilar mass.

Because these tumors are centrally located, they are more likely to be visualized during bronchoscopy and to present with primary pulmonary symptoms, including change in cough pattern,

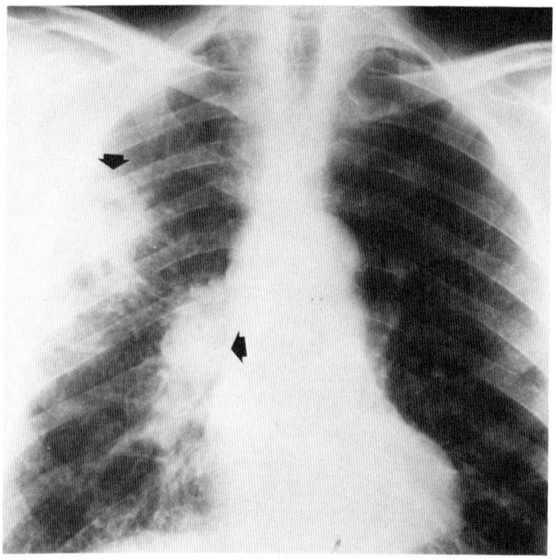

FIG. 15-6. Squamous carcinoma. The primary neoplasm appears as an unusual infiltrative pattern in the right upper lobe (*vertical arrow*) and has metastasized to the bronchopulmonary lymph nodes in the right lung root, producing a mass lesion (*horizontal arrow*). Autopsy proven.

FIG. 15-7. Squamous carcinoma. This neoplasm originated in the superior segment of the left lower lobe and is just visible behind the heart. The diffuse linear-reticular pattern of lymphangitic spread, more visible in the right lung, is relatively uncommon with tumors of this cell type. Autopsy proven.

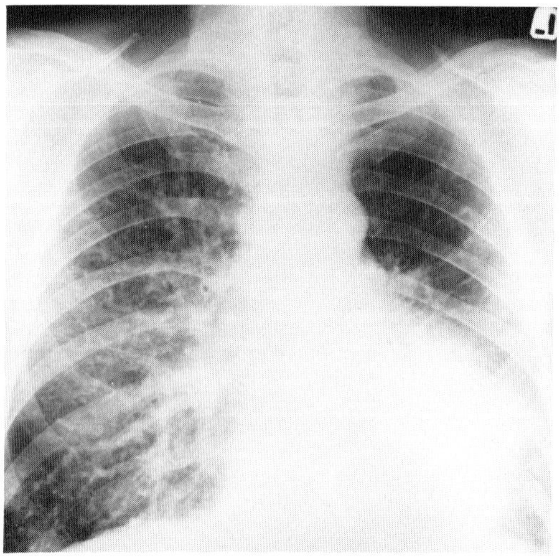

hemoptysis, dyspnea, localized wheezing or chest "tightness," and recurrent infection distal to an obstructed bronchus.

Adenocarcinoma

Adenocarcinoma accounts for 30 to 40% of lung cancers in the United States and has become the most common type in some studies.[14,15] The increase is due in part to changes in histopathologic criteria and in part to the increased incidence of lung cancer in women who more frequently have adenocarcinoma. However, the VA Lung Group data support an unexplained absolute increase in adenocarcinoma in men.[14] These tumors may arise from mucous glands in the walls of large bronchi but the majority arise in the peripheral lung fields where they present as solitary nodules which often remain clinically silent until metastatic symptoms develop. Some histologic studies suggest that peripheral adenocarcinomas develop from bronchiolo-alveolar epithelium; many occur in relation to preexisting pulmonary scars.[25,34] Adenocarcinoma of the lung is diagnosed when the tumor forms definite acinar and papillary structures (Fig. 15-8). True glandular formation with mucin secretion is not a constant finding. When undifferentiated tumors show abundant mucin production, they are labeled adenocarcinomas. The 1977 WHO classification places large cell carcinomas with significant intracellular mucin with adenocarcinomas. Bronchiolo-alveolar cell carcinomas are an adenocarcinoma variant and also produce mucus. The neoplastic cells at the margin of an adenocarcinoma may grow on unaltered alveolar walls and thereby further resemble a bronchioloalveolar cell carcinoma.

Approximately three-quarters of adenocarcinomas are located in the mid- and outer thirds of the lung fields compared with figures of a third and a fifth for squamous and oat cell carcinomas. Cavitation is common, but less so than with squamous or large cell carcinomas. Because of their peripheral location, bronchial obstruction with distal secondary infection is less common with adenocarcinomas than with squamous carcinomas; change in cough, hemoptysis, dyspnea, and localized physical findings of endobronchial obstruction are therefore also less

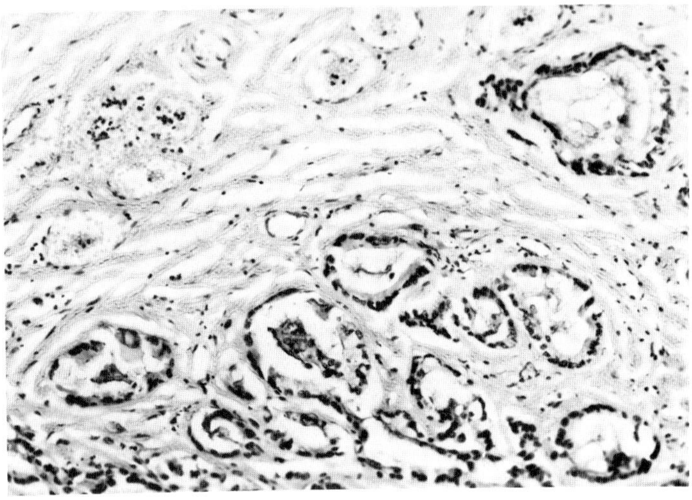

FIG. 15-8. Adenocarcinoma. Well-formed glandlike spaces are seen in a densely fibrous stroma. The cells are malignant but well-differentiated, and mucin is seen in the spaces. (Histologic section courtesy of Dr. Lee Weatherbee, Ann Arbor, Michigan)

common. The degree of differentiation may have some prognostic significance for patients with adenocarcinoma. Well-differentiated tumors of this type in asymptomatic patients, or in patients with primary pulmonary symptoms, result in a survival frequency similar to that for patients with squamous carcinoma. Patients with poorly differentiated adenocarcinomas appear to have substantially poorer prognoses, whether or not the disease is operable at the time of diagnosis.[31]

Bronchiolo-Alveolar Cell Carcinoma

Bronchiolo-alveolar cell carcinomas comprise less than 10% of lung cancers. It is becoming apparent from electron microscopic studies that alveolar cell carcinoma must be rare. Two cell types appear to be responsible for the tumors which have been called bronchiolo-alveolar carcinomas. Both are of bronchial origin. One cell is a metaplastic bronchiolar mucous cell and the other is a bronchiolar stem cell with ultrastructural features of both the respiratory ciliated and the respiratory nonciliated ("Clara") cell. Hyperplastic Type II alveolar epithilial cells may be found at the margins of these tumors and may have been mistaken for the neoplastic cells.[25,31,34,35,36]

Liebow defines this tumor as "a generally well-differentiated adenocarcinoma in the periphery of the lung beyond a grossly recognizable bronchus, with a tendency to spread chiefly within the confines of the lung by aerogenous and lymphatic routes, the walls of the distal air spaces often acting as supporting stroma for the neoplastic cells."[25] As do other adenocarcinomas, the bronchiolo-alveolar cell carcinoma may arise in relation to localized pulmonary scars or from the widespread atypical regenerative proliferation seen in the acini of "honeycomb" lung. It is possible that the diffuse or multinodular forms of this disease result from tumors having multicentric origin, but it is more likely that the majority of these cases represent aerogenous (endobronchial) spread from a single focus, since the postoperative prognosis is favorable for anatomically localized forms of this cancer. The histologic appearance of alveolar cell carcinoma may closely resemble metastatic adenocarcinoma from an extrathoracic primary. The alveoli are lined, or may be filled by papillary formations of columnar or low cuboidal cells with eosinophilic cytoplasm and basal nuclei (Fig. 15-9). Mucin is produced by about 80% of these tumors, a figure similar to that for other adenocarcinomas.

Alveolar cell carcinoma has been called a great imitator because its growth rate, natural history, roentgenographic appearance, and clinical presentation are the most varied of the lung cancers.

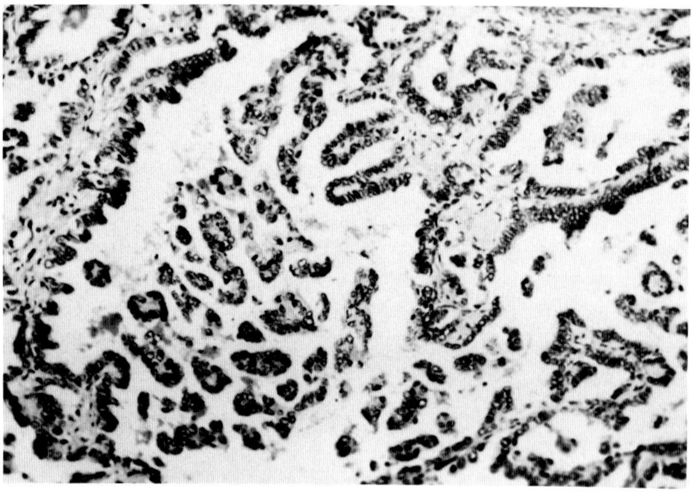

FIG. 15-9. Alveolar cell carcinoma. Note the typical papillary configuration of the carcinoma. This neoplasm tends to line the alveolar spaces in a single layer and is characteristically well-differentiated. The cytoplasm is usually more abundant than in this particular neoplasm (Histologic section courtesy of Dr. Lee Weatherbee, Ann Arbor, Michigan)

The average age of patients with this tumor is not much different from that of other lung cancers, and the sex distribution is about equal.

The most common roentgenographic pattern is an indolent, ill-defined patch of disease at first localized to one segment or lobe that is often mistaken for tuberculosis or other granulomatous disease (Fig. 15-10).[37] Diffuse disease is often bilateral and ranges from multiple, well-circumscribed nodules to extensive diffuse consolidation. Pleural effusion occurs but cavitation is uncommon. As progression occurs, these abnormalities coalesce into pneumonia-like consolidations, often without evidence of volume loss (Fig. 15-11). The physical findings can also mimic pneumonia: rales, bronchial breath sounds, and increased fremitus are sometimes present over the involved segment(s). In advanced cases, a characteristic bronchographic pattern consisting of a uniform threadlike narrowing, elongation, and rigidity of smaller bronchi produces a leafless tree appearance.[38] The diagnosis of alveolar cell carcinoma can be made by cytologic examinations of the sputum with about the same frequency as with tumors of other cell types.

Cough and chest pain occur as with other lung cancers. Dyspnea may be profound in the diffuse form; nevertheless, many patients maintain a good nutritional status until the lungs are extensively involved. Voluminous, foamy, mucoid sputum typical of mucin-producing tumors is seen in 10% of patients. This finding usually appears late, and is more common in patients with diffuse disease.[38a] Massive intrapulmonary venoarterial shunting is sometimes responsible for severe hypoxemia and widespread disease may produce a restrictive ventilatory defect with rapidly deteriorating pulmonary diffusing capacity for carbon monoxide.[39,40] Osteoarthropathy has been described.[39]

The prognosis of patients with alveolar cell carcinoma is similar to that of patients with other bronchogenic carcinomas.[39,41] Although a few of these tumors remain localized for years, about half are considered inoperable at the time of diagnosis. Patients with multinodular, diffuse, and pneumonic forms seldom survive more than 3 years, even when the process is confined to a single lobe.[39]

Small Cell Undifferentiated (Oat Cell) Carcinoma

Small cell undifferentiated tumors represent approximately 20% of lung cancers. The cells have dense, hyperchromatic nuclei with very little surrounding cytoplasm, and may be fusiform or polygonal, or may closely resemble lymphocytes (Fig. 15-12). The 1977 WHO classification recognizes gradations between these forms and

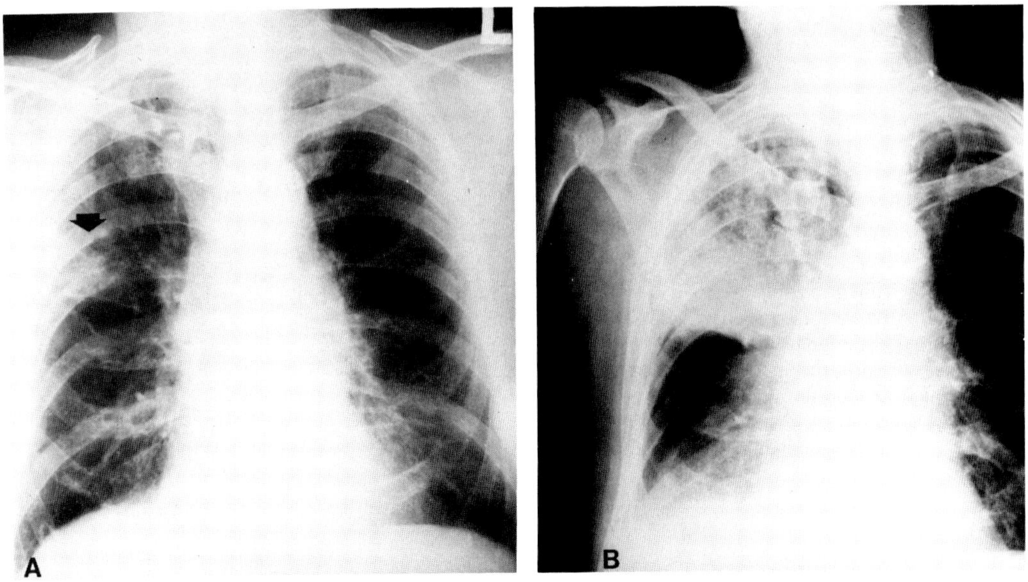

FIG. 15-10. Alveolar cell carcinoma. **A.** The small infiltrate in the posterior segment of the right upper lobe just above the minor fissure was thought to represent tuberculosis because of the patient's positive tuberculin skin test and the presence of calcified granulomatous disease in the extreme apex of the right lung. **B.** Progression of this infiltrative carcinoma resulted in copious mucoid sputum production. The physical findings mimicked those of pneumonic consolidation, with rales, and increased breath sounds and vocal fremitus. A bronchogram might have suggested the diagnosis by showing a "leafless tree" appearance.

introduces a combined small cell category while eliminating the spindle cell variant. In this scheme, an intermediate small cell category replaces the polygonal cell subgroup (see p. 802). Opinions differ as to whether small cell cancers with differing histologic appearances respond differently to treatment. It is therefore likely that the differences are minor and are related to selection and interpretation.[42]

In scalene lymph node or other biopsy specimens, oat cell carcinomas may be mistaken for lymphosarcomas. This delayed their recognition until 1926. Oat cell carcinomas and bronchial carcinoid tumors are closely related (see sections on Revised WHO Classifications, Bronchogenic Carcinoma and Ectopic Hormone Production, and Bronchial Adenomas).

The majority of these highly malignant tumors arise centrally. Mediastinal invasion and thoracic and extrathoracic metastases occur early, sometimes from very small tumors that

FIG. 15-11. Alveolar cell carcinoma. This tumor produced a combined pattern with a mass in the left upper lobe (*arrow*) and widespread "pneumonic" infiltrates without significant volume loss. Sputum production was scanty.

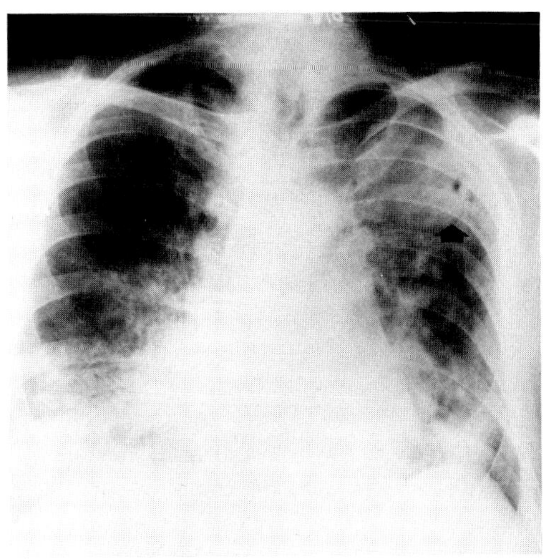

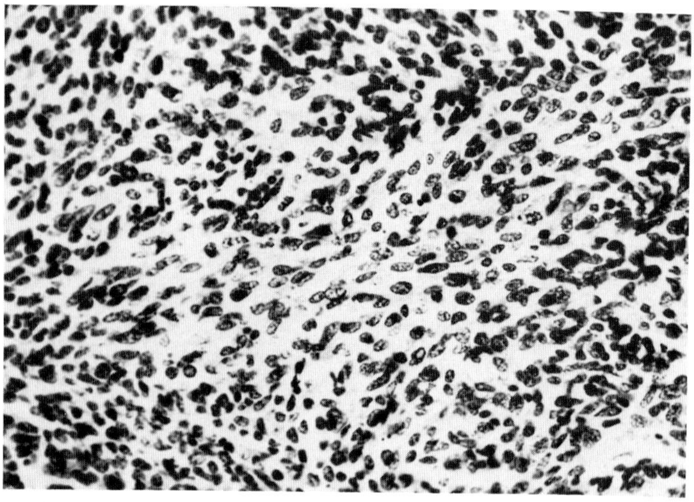

FIG. 15-12. Oat cell carcinoma. Note the small, dark, oval nuclei of relatively uniform size. The cytoplasm is poorly defined or even absent in some areas. (Histologic section courtesy of Dr. Lee Weatherbee, Ann Arbor, Michigan)

escape both roentgenographic and bronchoscopic detection. Bone marrow biopsy frequently demonstrates tumor invasion at the time of initial evaluation. The majority of patients with superior vena caval obstruction have undifferentiated small cell carcinomas originating in one of the more proximal bronchi of the right upper lobe. Obstructive jaundice is found in approximately 5% of patients with lung cancer; almost without exception, these patients are found to have oat cell carcinoma metastatic to lymph nodes in the hepatic portal.

Oat cell carcinomas so rarely show roentgenographic evidence of excavation that cavitation within a tumor mass virtually excludes this cell type. With the exceptions noted, the pulmonary roentgenographic manifestations of oat cell carcinomas resemble those of squamous carcinomas because of their common central location.

The prognosis of small cell carcinomas is the poorest among the lung cancers; however, recent chemotherapeutic gains made against this type of tumor are more substantial than those against cancers of other cell types.[42,43] The median survival time has increased from 2 months in the untreated patient to 6 to 12 months, with 25% living at 2 years. Radiotherapy is the treatment of choice in patients with this tumor who, were it not for the histology of their neoplasm, would appear to be candidates for surgery. The 5-year survival for this favorable group is about 4%.

Large Cell Carcinomas

Polygonal and undifferentiated large cell carcinomas consist of large clear cells that resemble less differentiated adenocarcinomas as well as the cells that line alveolar cavities during fetal development (Fig. 15-13). While some may represent anaplastic squamous tumors in which the characteristic features of squamous cells are lost, their ultrastructural characteristics, peripheral location, and lack of obvious connection to bronchi suggest a common origin with adenocarcinomas.[35,44] Some carcinomas with periodic acid-Schiff (PAS) positive mucin-staining material were once called large cell cancers. The 1977 WHO Classification places these among the adenocarcinomas. Large cell tumors often grow to a large size before diagnosis, and both lymphangitic and hematogenous metastases occur. Cavitation is common.

CLINICAL MANIFESTATIONS

The symptoms and physical findings produced by lung cancer can be classified into one of four groups: (1) local disturbances from the primary tumor (hemoptysis); (2) effects from regional or distant metastases (pericardial effusion, bone pain); (3) nonspecific systemic findings (weight loss); and (4) nonmetastatic endocrine, neurologic, and connective tissue disorders (ectopic ACTH production, neuromyopathy, os-

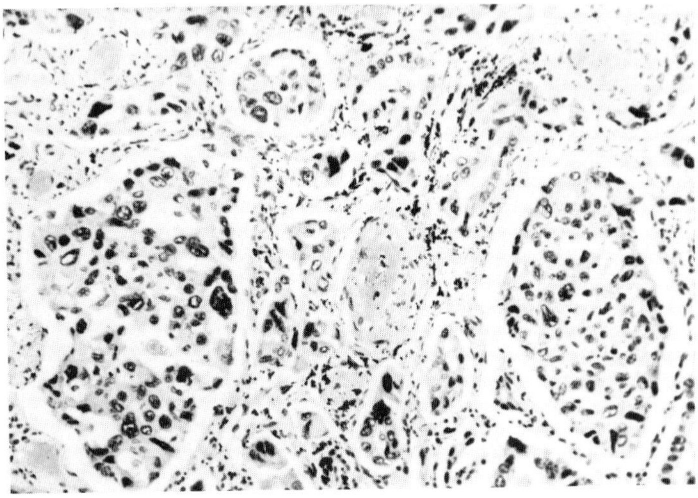

FIG. 15-13. Large cell carcinoma. The carcinoma nuclei vary greatly in size and often have abundant cytoplasm. There is insufficient differentiation to place this carcinoma in either the squamous cell carcinoma or adenocarcinoma group. (Histologic section courtesy of Dr. Lee Weatherbee, Ann Arbor, Michigan)

teoarthropathy). The important influence of the location of the primary cancer on thoracic symptoms has been stressed in the discussion of individual cell types. The approximate frequencies are: main bronchus, 25%; lobar bronchus, primary or segmental division, 50%; mid-lung zone, 13%; and subpleural location, 12%. The symptoms and physical findings among 2000 lung cancer patients studied prospectively by the VA Lung Group are given in Table 15-4. Because sputum production, dyspnea, hemoptysis, cough, and chest pain (cough fracture, intercostal muscle tenderness) may be related to preexisting bronchitis or emphysema, the significance of these symptoms cannot be accurately interpreted without a chest roentgenogram. This study is essential to the complete physical examination of the chest.

TABLE 15-4. Initial Symptoms of 2000 Patients with Bronchogenic Carcinoma: VA Lung Cancer Group, 1969–1972

Initial Symptom	% of Patients
Cough	74
Weight loss	68
Dypsnea	58
Chest pain	49
Hemoptysis	29
Lymphadenopathy	23
Bone pain	25
Hepatomegaly	21
Clubbing	20
Intracranial	12
Superior vena cava	4
Hoarseness	18

(Adapted from Hyde L, Hyde CI: Clinical manifestations of lung cancer. Chest 65:299–306, 1974)

Findings Associated With Cancers of the Main Bronchus

Tumors that arise in or adjacent to a main bronchus commonly produce findings related to irritation and mediastinal invasion before bronchial occlusion is complete enough to cause volume loss with attendant dyspnea and suppuration. Chronic nonproductive cough may appear for the first time. A preexisting productive bronchitic cough may acquire unusual severity and persistence. Blood-streaked sputum produced by tumor erosion is more common than expectoration of larger quantities of the partially clotted blood that originates from the bronchial circulation that supplies primary lung cancers. (The pathogenesis and management of massive hemoptysis is considered in Chap. 14.) Tumors in this location may cause a localized expiratory or inspiratory wheeze, or "honk," which is sometimes reproduced only when the patient lies on the affected side. Uncomplicated chronic bronchitis, however, is the most common cause of wheezing, which at first appears to be localized; careful repeated auscultation after deep breathing and coughing demonstrates that, in this disease, the wheezes are neither localized nor persistent.

When tumors from a main bronchus invade the mediastinum, hoarseness and dysphagia usually indicate paralysis of the left recurrent laryngeal nerve and compression of the esophagus by lymph node metastases. Dyspnea may result from a variety of insults: encroachment on the phrenic nerve with diaphragmatic paralysis; malignant pericardial effusion; obstruction of the superior vena cava with large secondary pleural effusion(s); invasion or thrombosis of the pulmonary circulation; or unilateral total ventilatory obstruction. Pain receptors within the chest are limited to the parietal pleura, mediastinum, larger blood vessels, and peribronchial afferent vagal fibers. Dull, intermittent, poorly localized, retrosternal chest pain is commonly present with central tumors. Persistent, severe, localized pain suggests metastases to the parietal pleura or bone. Pleural pain may respond to antibiotics when pleural inflammation results from infection distal to an obstructing neoplasm. Nonspecific electrocardiographic changes, arrhythmias, and congestive heart failure usually reflect direct extension to pericardium; occasionally, multiple discrete myocardial metastases are responsible. Nonbacterial, verrucal (marantic) endocarditis may be associated with lung cancer; the majority of patients with this complication have had adenocarcinomas.

Superior Vena Cava Syndrome. Obstruction of the superior vena cava is an uncommon clinical problem resulting from benign causes in about 20% of cases and malignant neoplasms in the remaining 80%.[45] The benign causes include mediastinal fibrosis (see p. 882) and venous thrombosis generally related to indwelling catheters or pacemaker wires.[45a]

Of malignant tumors that produce obstruction, 70 to 80% are bronchogenic carcinomas. Others include lymphomas, metastatic carcinomas, and other primary mediastinal tumors. The cell type of bronchogenic carcinoma is not as important as the location; Approximately 80% of these cases are caused by neoplasms arising in proximal bronchi on the right.[46] Interruption of flow usually results from compression by the primary tumor or involved lymph nodes; intraluminal extension and thrombosis are less common. The speed with which the obstruction develops and the adequacy of the collateral circulation determine the severity of the symptoms. The main tributary of the superior vena cava is the azygos vein which arises at the level of the renal veins and ascends in the posterior mediastinum to join the superior vena cava at the level of the take-off of the right upper lobe bronchus (second costal cartilage).

When obstruction to the superior vena cava occurs distal to (above) its junction with the azygos vein, venous drainage from the head and neck proceeds to the heart through the external jugular vein, the superficial plexus on the anterior chest wall, and the perforating branches of the intercostal and mammary veins which finally enter the azygos system. Less commonly, the obstruction occurs proximal to (below) the entrance of the azygos vein into the superior vena cava. This produces symptoms of greater severity. In this circumstance, the blood in the dilated veins of the chest wall flows toward the abdomen, and superficial veins in the back and groin carry blood to the inferior vena cava.

The symptoms produced include dyspnea and cough which are greatly aggravated by recumbancy. Headache, vertigo, psychotic behavior, stupor, and coma may be mistakenly ascribed to hypercalcemia or cerebral metastases. Death in this wet-brain syndrome results from cerebral anoxia and failure of the respiratory centers, or from edema of the glottis. In fully developed cases, a reddish to dusky cyanosis accompanies edema of the face, neck, upper extremities, and thorax. The prominence of the collateral venous pattern correlates poorly with the severity of symptoms. Patients may experience great distress and have evidence of large pleural effusion(s) when venous engorgement appears limited to the retinal veins and right external jugular vein. A doubtful diagnosis is reliably confirmed by phlebography or by measurement of venous pressure in the anticubital veins, using a spinal fluid manometer or central venous pressure catheter. Pressures of 15 to 30 cm of saline are common.[47] Deep scalene lymph node biopsy and mediastinoscopy are hazardous procedures in patients with superior vena caval obstruction.

Diuretics often cause immediate and pronounced relief of symptoms and intensive therapy should be started as soon as the diagnosis is made, although the notion that this syndrome represents a medical emergency has been questioned.[47a] Patients are more comfortable in a semi-upright position. The effectiveness of antiagulants in preventing further compromise from venous thrombosis is unproven. Dexamethasone is sometimes given with large doses of furosemide to decrease cerebral edema. Irradiation therapy or antineoplastic chemotherapy must follow promptly. A slow, low-dose irradiation schedule (a daily dose of 100 rad gradually increased to 250 rad as the patient improves) is often used because of fear of aggravating the patient's symptoms with radiation edema. With this schedule, symptomatic improvement may be delayed 10 days or more, and more rapid relief can often be achieved with the use of a single dose of intravenous cyclophosphamide (1100 mg/m^2 body area) or nitrogen mustard (0.4 mg/kg body weight). Rapid high-dose irradiation with a daily dose of 400 rad has also been used. This dose is reduced to 150 to 200 rad after 2000 rad has been given or as soon as edema regresses. The effectiveness and safety of the latter regime compares favorably with one in which low dose irradiation is combined with chemotherapy.[48,49] Immediate and conscientious treatment is important because many of the anaplastic tumors responsible for the syndrome respond dramatically. In some series, a sizeable majority of patients have complete relief of symptoms, and survival is comparable to that of other patients receiving palliative therapy.[48,49] Prolonged survival is unusual but does occur.[49a]

Findings Associated With Carcinoma of the Lobar Bronchus

The common initial events in the largest group of lung cancers, those that arise in the lobar bronchus, are symptoms, physical findings, and roentgenologic patterns related to bronchial obstruction with distal pulmonary infection. Cough, hemoptysis, a localized wheeze, and sputum production occur early. Diagnosis of these tumors often is preceded by one or more episodes of *sentinel* pneumonia in which roentgenographic resolution is slow or incomplete. The area of parenchymal infiltration is limited to the segment or lobe normally ventilated by the obstructed bronchus. The physical findings, therefore, are quite different from those found over an uncomplicated pneumonia in which the bronchus serving the diseased area is open. With pneumonia, rales, increased breath sounds (bronchial or bronchovesicular), and increased fremitus are present because sound transmission is increased through partially solidified lung. With local bronchial obstruction from bronchial carcinomas, adenomas, or foreign bodies, sound transmission through the bronchus is interrupted, causing decreased or absent breath sounds and fremitus. Rales are not heard.

When radiopacity is limited to one of the upper lobes or their segments, and is produced by neoplastic obstruction of the bronchus, increased transmission of the normal tracheal breath sounds and fremitus may be mistaken for the bronchial breathing and increased fremitus characteristic of an uncomplicated upper lobe pneumonia. The obstructing neoplasm causes volume loss and ipsilateral displacement of the trachea. The tracheal deviation contributes to pronounced transmission of tracheal sounds. "Transmitted tracheal sounds [and obstruction] . . . are probably present if the sounds are not heard in the axilla, if they are quite harsh, without a pause between inspiratory and expiratory phases, or if an area of [broncho] vesicular breathing seems to be interposed between the trachea and the abnormal breath sounds."[50] Vocal fremitus (blue-moon, ninety-nine) transmitted from the trachea through such an obstructed lobe will also be found to have a peculiar nasal or bleating sound if care is taken to compare one side of the chest with the other. In contrast, the presence of rales over the upper lobe in question strongly favors true bronchial breathing, in which case the rales and bronchial breathing are evidence against neoplastic obstruction and support a diagnosis of uncomplicated pneumonia (Fig. 15-14).

These physical findings are distinct, repro-

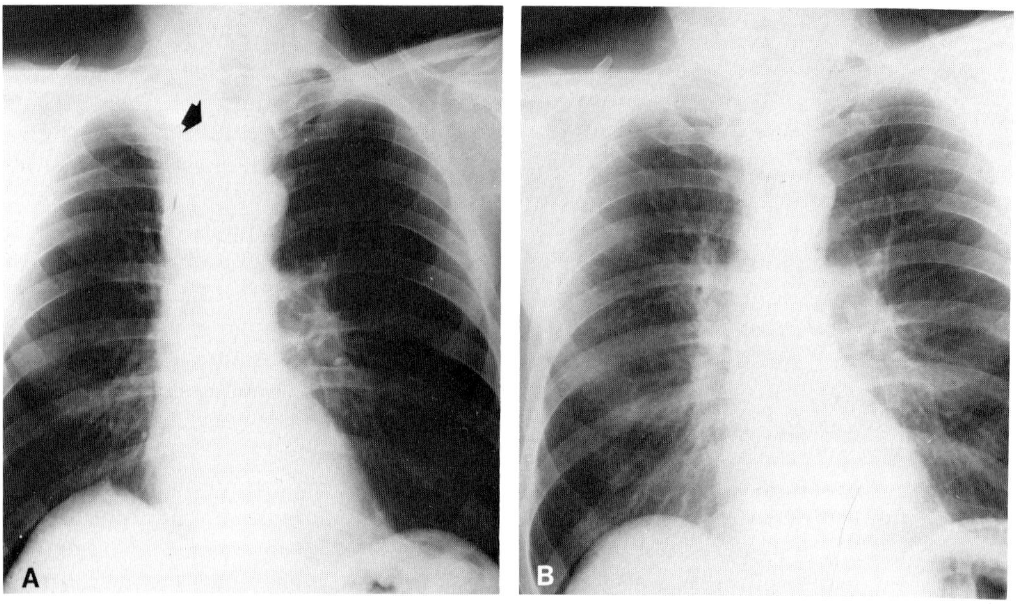

FIG. 15-14. Squamous carcinoma. **A.** This endobronchial tumor in the anterior segmental bronchus of the right upper lobe is not visible, but has caused the affected segment to become pancaked against the mediastinum anteriorly. The trachea is deviated to the right and the arrow points to its lateral wall. Increased transmission of tracheal breath sounds and fremitus heard in a narrow band adjacent to the sternum on the right were mistaken by the resident physician for the bronchial breathing and increased vocal fremitus characteristic of uncomplicated upper lobe pneumonia. Rales were not present. See text for discussion of the significance of these physical findings. **B.** Reexpansion of the segment following radiotherapy.

ducible, and of great importance if pneumonia is to be distinguished from lung cancer originating in a lobar bronchus. Even partial neoplastic bronchial obstruction usually presents with the findings of complete obstruction.

While it is true that neoplastic obstruction is suggested by the complete absence of air bronchograms within an anatomically localized infiltrate, the reverse is not true. That is, the presence of an air bronchogram does not exclude complete endobronchial obstruction, because the pleural surfaces which make up the fissures separating individual lobes are incomplete in many patients, allowing cross-ventilation between lobes as well as segments (Fig. 15-15).

At first, these physical findings are best appreciated if time is taken to reexamine those patients whose chest roentgenograms or bronchoscopic examinations are known to show endobronchial lobar obstruction with partial volume loss. With practice, the appearance of the chest roentgenogram often can be predicted from the physical examination. Examination for deviation of the trachea should never be omitted because minor evidence of tracheal shift helps prompt the careful ausculation necessary to the recognition of these useful but localized findings.

On the chest roentgenogram, tumors obstructing a lobar or segmental bronchus are seen to cause parenchymal infiltrates and volume loss within uni-anatomic subdivisions of lung. Thus, a bronchial adenoma or carcinoma in the bronchus intermedius may collapse the middle and lower lobes, but would be unlikely to present with some combination of middle lobe disease with disease in any one isolated segment of the ipsilateral upper lobe. Review of a bronchial

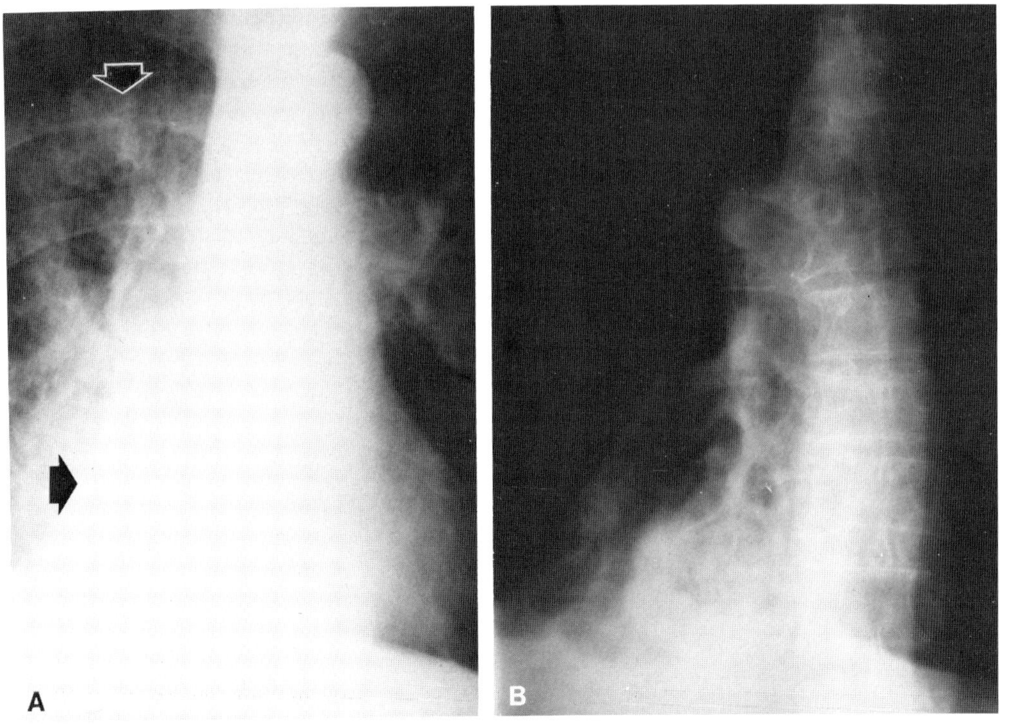

FIG. 15-15. Squamous carcinoma. **A.** The right lower lobe collapse (*horizontal arrow*) caused by this cavitary carcinoma (*vertical arrow*) had been present untreated for one year. **B.** On the overpenetrated x-ray film, air within dilated bronchi destroyed by suppuration may be the result of cross-ventilation from the middle lobe across an incomplete oblique fissure, since the endobronchial tumor completely obstructed the right lower lobe bronchus. Autopsy proven.

anatomy diagram will illustrate why most roentgenographic abnormalities are uni-anatomic when produced by endobronchial obstruction.

Findings Associated With Tumors of the Mid-Lung Field

The small minority of lung cancer patients who are truly asymptomatic is usually found among the group with tumors of the mid-lung field, in which there is no roentgenologic evidence of involvement of the hilus, pleura, or regional lymph nodes. These patients have the highest rate of resectability and the best survival. The differential diagnosis and management of such tumors is discussed in the section on the solitary pulmonary nodule.

Findings Associated With Subpleural Carcinomas, Including Pleural Effusion

The visceral pleura is essentially without sensation, and patients with lung cancers originating in a subpleural location often experience little or no pain until late in their disease, when tumor extension to the parietal pleura, intercostal nerves, and ribs has occurred.[51–54] Tumors immediately adjacent to the visceral pleura often cause early, insidious formation of pleural effusion which is responsible for the initial complaint of dyspnea. Cough occurs late and is usually not a prominent symptom. Hemoptysis is uncommon. Most pleural effusions caused by lung cancer are not associated with fever; pleural friction rubs are also less common than when inflammatory disease causes pleural fluid formation.

Lung cancer can cause pleural effusion in one or a combination of the following ways: (1) direct invasion, irritation, and interference with the venous and lymphatic drainage of the pleura; (2) increased hydrostatic pressure produced by central obstruction of veins and lymphatics; and (3) bronchial obstruction and distal suppuration with resulting pleural inflammation. It is uncommon for the third mechanism to operate alone, and this is difficult to document. It is the only one which does not preclude surgical treatment.[55] When pleural fluid protein and specific gravity measurement are used to distinguish transudates and exudates, nearly a fifth of malignant effusions are incorrectly classified as transudates. Pleural effusions caused by lung cancer are almost invariably classified as exudates if the criteria used for an exudate are: (1) a pleural fluid-to-serum protein ratio greater than 0.5; (2) a pleural fluid LDH greater than 200 IU; and (3) a pleural fluid-to-serum LDH ratio greater than 0.6.[52]

Lung cancer is the most common cause of hemorrhagic pleural effusion in middle-aged and elderly male smokers. Other causes of bloody effusions (trauma, tuberculosis, spontaneous pneumothorax, and congestive heart failure with pulmonary embolus) can often be excluded without difficulty. In approximately half of the lung cancer patients with pleural effusion, the fluid is serous. A serous fluid which later becomes sanguineous suggests neoplasm. Lymphocytes and mesothelial cells usually predominate in serous effusions caused by direct pleural invasion by cancer. A leukocyte count greater than 2500/mm^3 suggests a fluid is an exudate; nevertheless, 40% of exudates have a leukocyte count of less than 2500 cells/mm^3; most exudates produced by lung cancer have leukocyte counts between 500 and 2500/mm^3. The eosinophil count in a pleural fluid may be high whenever blood is present. Although mediastinal lymphoma and metastatic cancer are the most common nontraumatic causes of chylothorax, a fistula between the thoracic duct and the pleural space is an uncommon complication of lung cancer.

Pneumothorax and its sequela, bronchopleural fistula, seldom result from neoplastic invasion of the pleura unless produced during diagnostic thoracentesis and pleural biopsy.[51,51a] When a tear in diseased visceral pleural is inadvertently produced during these procedures, the resulting bronchopleural communication is usually permanent, despite efforts to reexpand the lung by chest-tube drainage and suction. Often, the neoplastic invasion of pleura which leads to this complication represents distal extension of a more proximal cancer which has already compromised ventilation and perfusion in the underlying subdivision of lung. In this circumstance, the fistula is usually well-tolerated, although the likelihood of a secondary infection of the pleural space is increased. Needle biopsy of the parietal pleura and cytologic examination of the pleural fluid provides a diagnosis in approximately half of the patients with malignant effusions.

Total radiographic opacification of one hemithorax in a middle-age smoker is most commonly caused by lung cancer, and gray scale (B-mode) echograms of the lung and pleural space sometimes gives precise localization of fluid collections for diagnostic thoracentesis and pleural biopsy.[56]

Management of Recurrent Pleural Effusions. Many pleural effusions caused by lung cancer require no specific treatment. When pleural effusion occurs with endobronchial obstruction and marked volume loss or massive intraparenchymal replacement with neoplasm, thoracentesis often fails to produce symptomatic improvement. Not all pleural effusions caused by malignancy recur, and intrapleural therapy or pleural irradiation to control malignant effusion should be limited to those symptomatic patients in whom the pleural effusion has recurred after one or more aspirations. There must be some expectation that the lung displaced by the effusion will be capable of reexpansion and gas exchange.

Tetracycline, nitrogen mustard, quinacrine (Atabrine) and radioactive isotopes have been used with success as intrapleural therapy to control recurrent effusions. Tetracycline is the sclerosing agent of choice because it can be given as a single dose and has a lower incidence of fever and severe pleuritic pain than quinacrine. Tetracycline is given as a single dose of 500 mg dissolved in 30 ml of saline injected and flushed through the chest tube with an additional 50 ml of saline. Direct cytotoxic effects are observed with the rest of these agents, but all are effective largely because they produce a pleuritis that causes symphysis of the visceral and parietal pleura. The complete removal of pleural fluid before and shortly after instillation of chemotherapy is important, and improves objective results.[57,58] This is accomplished with the least discomfort to the patient by use of a large indwelling polyethylene intravenous catheter connected to a suction device. The catheter is removed after the intrapleural injection and the patient's position is changed frequently. Chest roentgenograms in the lateral decubitus positions are repeated after 24 hours. If there has been a significant reaccumulation of fluid, the pleural space is evacuated with a second polyethylene intravenous catheter. Radioactive colloidal gold (^{198}Au) and chrome phosphate (^{32}P) are unwieldly and lack the immediate effectiveness of tetracycline, nitrogen mustard, or quinacrine. Many physicians prefer to use an indwelling chest tube, providing continuous drainage except for a 12-hour period immediately after instillation of the drug. The intrapleural dose of nitrogen mustard is 0.4 mg/kg body weight dissolved in 50 to 100 ml of isotonic saline. Quinacrine, in 200-mg ampules, is dissolved in 20 ml of isotonic saline and a total dose of 600 to 800 mg is injected over 2 to 3 days. The total dose of quinacrine may be given in a single injection, but then the incidence of transient side-effects including fever, pain, nausea, vomiting, and rarely hypotension or hallucination, probably increases. Intrapleural instillation of nitrogen mustard may cause fever, pleuritic pain, nausea, and bone marrow depression. Premedication with an antipyretic analgesic and an antiemetic is useful with either quinacrine or nitrogen mustard.

Pleurectomy is rarely indicated for recurrent pleural effusions related to lung cancer although pleurectomy may be done prophylactically at the time of thoracotomy when a tumor is found to be unresectable.

Subpleural Tumors of the Superior Sulcus (Pancoast Tumors). Bronchogenic carcinomas developing in a subpleural location at the extreme apex of the lung produce a misleading complex of symptoms that is often responsible for delayed diagnosis. Direct extension of these tumors to the intercostal nerves, brachial plexus, stellate ganglion, sympathetic chain, adjacent ribs, and vertebrae produce pain in the shoulder and down the ulnar distribution of the forearm (nerve roots C8 and T1). Motor weakness follows. Horner's syndrome with contraction of the pupil, ptosis of the eyelid, and ipsilateral absence of sweating of the face may be present. The pain is often mistaken for that of calcific tendinitis, bursitis, or shoulder-hand syndrome until metastatic rarefaction appears in the upper thoracic vertebral bodies or their posterior ribs. A spinal cord tumor may be suspected.

A superior sulcus tumor should be considered early in the differential diagnosis of persistent shoulder pain.[53] Helpful roentgenographic studies include a chest x-ray film in the apical lordotic projection and thoracic spine films with posterior rib detail. On the routine posterioanterior chest roentgenogram, these tumors produce minimal clouding in the area circumscribed by the clavicle and first rib; these subtle changes are frequently overlooked or mistaken for pleural thickening (Fig. 15-16).

The peripheral location of these tumors greatly reduces the diagnostic yield from cytologic examination of the sputum, and fiberoptic bronchoscopic examination is unavailing unless the lesion is very far advanced. Despite the location of these neoplasms, scalene node biopsy is often negative: two-thirds of the tumors are squamous cell carcinomas which invade primarily by direct extension. Most of the remaining tumors are large cell carcinomas which in this location metastasize via the subpleural lymphatics rather than by the usual paratracheal–scalene–lymph-node sequence. Because of these features, early cytologic confirmation is best obtained by means of needle aspiration under fluoroscopic control.

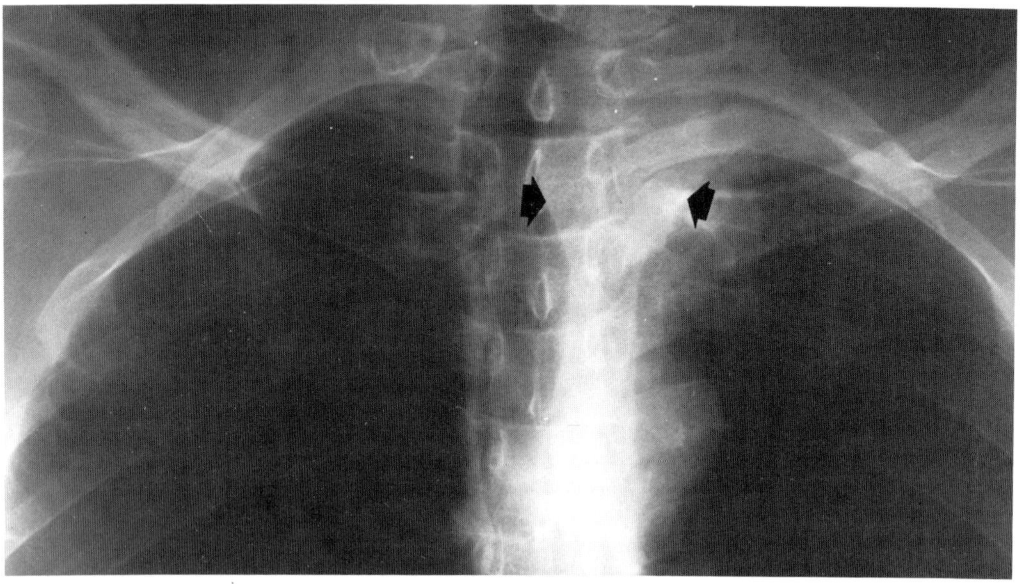

FIG. 15-16. Squamous carcinoma, superior sulcus or Pancoast tumor. This overexposed film demonstrates an increase in the density and width of the left superior mediastinum with a convex curvilinear lateral margin (*lateral arrow*). This posteriorly located neoplasm had invaded the mediastinum and posterior intercostal nerves, producing a right shift of the trachea (*medial arrow*) and severe pain in the shoulder. The tumor was dismissed as "apical pleural thickening," and for six months the pain was diagnosed as bursitis.

Paulson has reported a 35% 5-year survival for a selected group of patients with Pancoast tumors treated with preoperative irradiation, lobectomy or segmentectomy, and *en bloc* resection of the chest wall, including portions of the upper thoracic vertebrae.[54] His results have been confirmed by the experience of thoracic surgeons at Emory University in Atlanta, Memorial Hospital in New York, and the University of Maryland in Baltimore.[59,60] Avoidance of meddlesome preoperative invasive studies appears important to these results. Mediastinoscopy and computerized tomography are used. Preoperative irradiation consists of a tumor dose of 3000 rad given in 10 fractions over 12 days. Resection is done 3 weeks after irradiation is complete. Inoperable patients are usually treated with palliative doses of irradiation. Severe pain often persists despite x-ray treatment, and neurosurgical consultation may be needed in order to help with management.

Non-Metastatic Neuromyopathic Disorders and Lung Cancer

A variety of malignant neoplasms produce disorders of the nervous and muscular systems which are unrelated to invasion or metastases; no tumor produces such disabilities more frequently than does lung cancer, in which 5 to 10% of patients are affected.[61,62] Immunologic and toxic (metabolic) mechanisms are suspected of being the cause of some of these syndromes. Infection with neurotropic *slow viruses* (DNA-virus of the papova type and simian vacuolating virus) has been documented in patients with progressive multifocal leukoencephalopathy, one of the non-metastatic neurologic disorders largely limited to patients in the lymphoma and leukemia group. Differences in the histopathologic findings among the neurologic syndromes linked to lung cancer suggest that viruses may also be responsible for subacute carcinomatous

Non-Metastatic Neuromyopathic Disorders and Lung Cancer

Neuromyopathy

Peripheral Neuropathies
- Mixed sensorimotor
- Sensory (may occur with encephalomyelitis)

Spinal Cord Disease
- Motor neuron type (subacute carcinomatous poliomyelitis)
- Myelopathy

Subacute Cerebral Degeneration

Myopathy
- With myasthenia
- Without myasthenia
- Polymyositis or dermatomyositis

myelitis and sensory neuropathy with encephalomyelitis.[63]

Neurologic or muscular symptoms develop 6 months to 4 years before discovery of the pulmonary neoplasm in approximately half of the lung cancer patients affected by the diseases listed below. When the cerebellum, cerebrum, or spinal cord is involved, the neurologic deficit frequently evolves over days to weeks and then stabilizes. Control of the neoplasm or glucocorticoid therapy seldom, if ever, causes improvement when the central nervous system is involved. The onset and progression of the peripheral neuropathies and myopathies are more variable and improvement sometimes occurs with such treatment. In either circumstance, the progression appears unrelated to the patient's sex, age, or state of nutrition or to the tumor duration, growth rate, or size.

Neuromyopathy is the most common nonmetastatic neurologic disorder associated with lung cancer. This term is used to describe about half of the affected patients because it is not always possible to distinguish minor signs of lower motor neuron disease from mild muscle disease.[64] Weakness and wasting of the proximal muscles in the pelvic and shoulder girdle occurs with decreased deep tendon reflexes but without sensory change. Electrophysiologic studies show signs of denervation, but slowing of motor conduction velocity, an indication of peripheral nerve demyelinization seen with sensorimotor neuropathy, is uncommon. Most cases of neuromyopathy are mild and of little importance to the patient.

The frequency of mixed or sensorimotor peripheral neuropathy ranks third behind metastatic neurologic disease and neuromyopathy in lung cancer patients.[65] In this condition, the legs are usually more severely involved than the arms and bulbar palsy is uncommon. The cell count in the cerebral spinal fluid is not elevated but the protein is often raised. Once developed, neurologic signs may show little change; nevertheless, neurologic deterioration occurs in more than one-half of patients. Many of these neurologic and myopathic disorders have occurred in combination in individual patients, making classification difficult. Relapsing neuropathy, however, is distinctly uncommon among lung cancer patients.

In addition to myositis, whether combined with a skin rash in the form of dermatomyositis, or without a skin rash, as polymositis, a few lung cancer patients display abnormalities of neuromuscular transmission reminiscent of myasthenia gravis.[66] This disability differs from myasthenia gravis in several important respects and is referred to as the Eaton-Lambert syndrome, after the authors who drew attention to its association with oat cell carcinoma. Unlike the ordinary patient with myasthenia gravis, ocular and bulbar involvement is uncommon, deep tendon reflexes are decreased or absent, there is a poor response to neostigmine, and the proximal muscles of the extremities are weak at the beginning of contraction but may reach normal strength after repeated or sustained effort. Upon maximal stimulation of a peripheral nerve to such a muscle at 10 times per sec, a facilitation of the action potential is usually seen, rather than the decrease in action potential characteristic of myasthenia gravis. Occasional patients with oat cell carcinoma and a myasthenic syndrome, however, have electromyographic changes identical to those of myasthenia gravis. Increased sensitivity to neuromuscular blockade with curarelike drugs occurs in both conditions but the failure with Eaton-Lambert syndrome to improve on anticholinesterase drugs such as neostigmine and the response to guanidine at 35 mg/kg body weight suggests a defect in the release of acetycholine, as postulated for botulism.[66,67] In contrast to patients with carcinomatous dermatomyositis or polymyositis, muscle biopsy specimens and muscle enzyme determinations in serum are normal. The bedside diagnosis of this condition is aided by the demonstration that deep tendon reflexes are facilitated after strong voluntary contraction of a muscle against resistance. The occurrence of this myasthenic syndrome in sarcoidosis and in occasional patients with hypothyroidism, thyroiditis, and pernicious anemia, with hyperthyroidism, and with Sjögren's syndrome suggests that an autoimmune phenomenon may occur in some.[68] Improvement is sometimes seen after effective treatment of the neoplasm and in one case, strength was noted to improve with glucocorticoid therapy. Muscle relaxants should be avoided.

Nonmetastatic autonomic neuropathy may be associated with bronchogenic carcinoma causing hypotension, loss of sweating, nonobstructive urinary retention, and impotence.[69,70]

Cerebral Metastases From Lung Cancer

A fourth or more of lung cancer patients have cerebral metastases demonstrated at post-mortem examination, although only about a third of the metastatic lesions give rise to clinical manifestations. One in 10 is a solitary brain implant unassociated with other brain or systemic tumor deposits.[71,72] Typically, the patient develops a mild, diffuse, early morning headache before rising, which disappears whether or not analgesics are taken. Over several days to weeks, the morning headache recurs and becomes gradually worse until mental changes and seizures lead to medical examination, where abnormalities of cognitive function, motor deficit, pathologic reflexes, and papilledema are the most common findings. In the great majority of patients, the cerebral symptoms are of less than 2 months duration. Since the life-span of untreated patients with cerebral symptoms is approximately 3 months, investigation is warranted in selected patients: those who show little evidence of cachexia and whose physical examination and routine laboratory studies would seem to exclude additional metastases.

The first diagnostic efforts should be directed at determining the histology of the primary lung cancer. If the tumor is a small cell carcinoma, treatment may be somewhat more aggressive despite widespread metastases and will be more likely to include brain irradiation. The cerebral spinal fluid, often abnormal in patients with cerebral metastases, rarely yields evidence of significant diagnostic value since the abnormalities are nonspecific. Malignant cells are not found in the fluid when only parenchymal metastases are present. If the results of the initial noninvasive tests (*i.e.*, brain scan and electroencephalogram) and the later arteriogram are such that a decision is made to treat the cerebral disease by surgery, lumbar puncture may be performed to determine if leptomeningeal carcinomatosis is also indicated by the presence of malignant cells. This finding would exclude surgical therapy.

No controlled studies comparing surgery and irradiation therapy in a randomly selected group are available, and comparisons between several authors are complicated by selection of patients in better condition for surgery. In general, however, the results appear similar: the 1-month surgical mortality is 40 to 60%, and with either modality, the median survival is 3.5 to 6 months with 10% or less surviving 1 year.[71,72,73] In unstable patients, the initial treatment is directed toward decreasing cerebral edema with dexamethasone, 10 mg intravenously followed by 4 mg every 6 hours. Symptomatic improvement is evident within 48 hours in two-thirds of patients, and drug administration is gradually tapered to an individualized maintenance dose. Patients treated with irradiation also often receive dexamethasone. This steroid used alone may produce dramatic and surprisingly long-lived improvement in neurologic symptoms. Despite the general reluctance to withhold radiotherapy in patients with brain metastases, there is no evidence that patients who demonstrate improvement with dexamethasone are ill-served by a decision to withhold radiotherapy until symptoms recur.[74] There is little evidence that systemic chemotherapy is efficacious in the treatment of cerebral metastases, although lipid-soluble drugs which cross the blood-brain barrier (CCNU, Methyl-CCNU, hydroxyurea) may be tried.

Patients with small cell carcinoma with normal neurologic function and normal radionuclide brain scans given prophylactic brain irradiation with 3000 rad in 10 fractions develop fewer symptomatic brain metastases. Patient survival has not been lengthened by this policy; moreover, these data do not support a policy of giving every patient with small cell carcinoma brain irradiation: the patient's disease extent, age, general condition, and response to chemotherapy also must be considered. Similar approaches are now under study for adenocarcinoma.

Epidural Metastases

Epidural metastases from bronchogenic carcinomas, like brain metastases, should be managed after thought has been given to the patient's general situation and to the histology of the tumor. Irradiation and chemotherapy may produce rapid reduction in the size of an oat cell carcinoma before permanent neurologic damage occurs. Tumor sterilization is not required and 3000 rad in 2 weeks or 2000 rad in 1 week are most commonly used. High doses of dexamethasone are sometimes useful. Surgical treatment of epidural metastases from lung cancer rarely benefits the patient unless the physical and laboratory examination suggest that a solitary metastasis is present.[75]

Bronchogenic Carcinoma and Ectopic Hormone Production

A number of the manifestations of serious illness produced by bronchogenic carcinomas are secondary to the production of hormones not usually associated with the bronchial mucous membrane cell (Table 15 5). The production of similar and as yet unrecognized tumor products may be responsible in part for the commonly witnessed phenomenon of clinical deterioration and death occurring without adequate explanation at the post-mortem examination. One current and widely accepted view is that neoplastic and undifferentiated cells lose specific depressors of genetic material which ordinarily prevent some functions of the primordial totipotential cell from developing (*e.g.*, although the bronchial mucous membrane cell does not produce ACTH, its embryonic precursors had the DNA necessary for ACTH synthesis). If ACTH depressors are lost as a consequence of malignant change, ectoptic ACTH production may develop, causing a disease resembling Cushing's syndrome. Recent demonstration that parathormone, ACTH, melanocyte stimulating hormone, and chorionic gonadotropin produced by tumors each vary immunochemically from their normal counterparts casts some doubt on the depressor theory.

Regardless of the mechanism by which the endocrine abnormalities are produced, evidence of ectopic hormone production can be found in approximately 10% of patients with bronchogenic carcinoma.[76] Four considerations make these hormone-mediated syndromes important to the clinician:

1. The metabolic abnormalities may antedate discovery of the neoplasm; the symptoms and physical findings produced serve as the harbinger of the malignancy. Clubbing of the nails with hypertrophic pulmonary osteoarthropathy is such a finding (see Fig. 15-17). It is included here although proof that it results from an endocrine imbalance is lacking. Tumor-related serologic abnormalities may eventually serve as tumor markers.

2. Some endocrine syndromes are commonly or even exclusively associated with bronchogenic neoplasms of specific cell types; their recognition may suggest an appropriate order and type of diagnostic study. Since oat cell carcinoma and bronchial carcinoid adenoma are the pulmonary tumors usually responsible for ectopic ACTH production, evaluation of the patient with a lung mass and Cushing's syndrome should include bone marrow biopsy. Bone marrow metastases have been demonstrated in up to 46% of patients with advanced oat cell carcinoma.[77]

3. Clinical findings that result from tumor hormone production may cause unwarranted prognostic and therapeutic pessimism if they are confused with similar findings commonly caused by metastatic disease. For example, hypercalcemia caused by tumor elaboration of a parathormonelike polypeptide may be mistakenly ascribed to skeletal metastases.

4. Effective therapeutic management of the severe symptoms sometimes produced by ectopic hormones can materially add to the patient's comfort.

Bronchogenic Carcinoma With Hypercalcemia. There are two distinct types of hypercalcemia seen with malignancy. A hypophosphatemic type is produced by tumor elaboration of a bogus hormone having parathormonelike activity; the tubular reabsorption of phosphorus is also low as it would be in primary hyperparathyroidism. In the absence of liver metastases, the alkaline phosphatase is usually normal. The second variety of hypercalcemia is associated with a normal or elevated serum phosphorus and normal tubular reabsorption of phosphate.[78] There are two causes of this second type of hypercalcemia: the most common is skeletal metastases where even in the absence of liver metastases the alkaline phosphatase may be elevated; the second is tumor elaboration of osteolytic phytosteryl esters and/or prostaglandins with vitamin D-like action. This mechanism is important in breast carcinoma.[79,80] Immobilization causes hypercalciuria at all ages but the hypercalcemia which results from inactivity is so slight as to be of importance only in children. Decisions as to which mechanism is producing hypercalcemia must include consideration of factors which affect phosphorus metabolism. Glucose infusions, corticosteroids, cytotoxic agents and sex hormones may lower the serum phosphorus regardless of the cause of hypercalcemia. Phosphorus abnormalities associated with excess parathormone (PTH) production tend to be invalidated by coexisting renal impairment.

The most common overall cause of hypercalcemia in malignancy is bone metastases. These may not be accompanied by bone pain and radiographic evidence of bone destruction until late in the course of the hypercalcemia. Bone scans with ^{99m}Tc-polyphosphate may demonstrate bone metastases before bone roentgenograms become abnormal. The ratio of urinary hydroxyproline to creatinine can also be of value because it increases several months before defects appear on bone roentgenograms.[81]

PTH activity in the serum is heterogenous. A pro-PTH molecule is cleaved into active C- and N-terminal fragments.[82] The latter is short-lived. The recommended initial test for hypercalcemic disorders is the C-terminal PTH which is elevated in 95% of patients with primary or ectopic hyperparathyroidism. Most patients with ectopic PTH production have a lower immunoreactive PTH value for a given serum calcium concentration than do those with primary hyperparathyroidism. Serum concentrations of PTH must be evaluated in relation to the serum calcium: hypercalcemia normally causes a reduction in endogenous parathormone. A normal parathormone value may be abnormal when considered with an elevated serum calcium.

It must be emphasized that half of cancer patients with hypercalcemia and hypophosphatemia (and no bone metastases) have no detectable PTH. Some humoral substance other than PTH is thought to mediate the hypercalcemia in these patients. In some who respond to aspirin or indomethacin, the hypercalcemia may be caused by a prostaglandin.[80] Increased PTH-like polypeptides can be demonstrated in the serum of some patients with bronchogenic carcinoma, even in the absence of hypercalcemia. There is reason to believe that these cancers may elaborate both a normal PTH similar to the circulating product of the parathyroid gland and abnormal tumor hormone(s) recognizable immunologically but having less calcium increasing activity.[80] Squamous cell carcinoma of the lung and renal carcinoma are the tumors most frequently implicated in PTH production. Hypercalcemia from PTH is less common with large cell carcinomas, adenocarcinomas, and oat cell carcinomas of the bronchus. There is no definite relationship between the degree of differentiation of a lung cancer and its ability to produce

PTH, although undifferentiated squamous cell carcinomas may be responsible more often than well-differentiated tumors of the same cell type. As indicated in Table 15-5, hypercalcemia may be produced by ectopic hormone production in up to 16% of patients with bronchogenic carcinoma.

Postmortem examination of patients with PTH-producing bronchogenic carcinomas have shown the majority to have normal or hypoplastic parathyroid glands. Although occasional reports of parathyroid gland hyperplasia are found, the diagnosis has depended on a reduction of the adipose tissue in the glands as a criterion of hyperplasia. This criterion is useful when evaluating hypercalcemia resulting from primary hyperparathyroidism but may be invalid in the diagnosis of parathyroid hyperplasia in a patient wasted by malignant disease.

Clinical Manifestations. The hypercalcemic syndrome produced by PTH excess is of greater clinical importance than that of ectopic ACTH production with Cushing's syndrome because it is more common and more amenable to treatment. Hypercalcemia, regardless of cause, produces its deleterious effects on the kidney, the central nervous system, and the gastrointestinal tract. Hypercalcemia reduces the renal tubular reabsorption of water by interfering with the action of ADH on the distal tubule. The resulting inability to concentrate the urine causes nocturia, polydipsia, polyuria, and dehydration, the severity of which may be reminiscent of diabetes insipidus. When hypercalcemia develops rapidly, modest elevations of the serum calcium to 12–13 mg per 100 ml may produce confusion, weakness, and somnolence; more dramatic hypercalcemia results in psychosis and coma. Deep tendon reflexes remain intact. These central nervous system symptoms are frequently mistaken for brain metastases. Marked hypoproteinemia, sometimes seen in malnourished cancer patients, is associated with a decrease in calcium proteinate which lowers the total serum calcium. This may mask an increase in the diffusible ionized calcium, the fraction responsible for the patient's symptoms. The reduced contractility of smooth muscle produced by the elevated serum calcium causes anorexia, nausea, vomiting, and in some cases, adynamic ileus. The electrocardiogram may show a short QT interval, loss of the isoelectric component of the ST segment, and prolongation of the T wave. Hypokalemic alkalosis is often present and is related to the hypercalcemia; this must not be confused with the hypokalemic alkalosis that results from ectopic ACTH production by oat cell rather than squamous carcinomas.[82]

Management. Truly effective control of bronchogenic carcinomas by resection, irradiation, or chemotherapy will correct hypercalcemia caused by osseous metastases or PTH excess. Since such control is seldom achieved in patients already hypercalcemic, the majority of these patients require specific calcium-lowering therapy. In most, the treatment is simple, rapidly effective, and gratifying. Mild asymptomatic hypercalcemia is managed by hydration and low calcium intake. Salt supplements will promote urinary calcium excretion. Corticosteroids (the equivalent of 30 to 60 mg prednisone daily) will lower serum calcium over a period of 2 weeks in most patients with malignancy. These agents have an adverse effect on survival in bronchogenic carcinoma and are best avoided, except when dexamethasone is used to reduce cerebral edema in patients with intracranial metastases.

The dehydration resulting from increased renal excretion of salt and water in hypercalcemia is often aggravated by poor oral intake which accompanies confusion and vomiting and intravenous saline may produce dramatic clinical improvement resulting largely from correction of the dehydration. The cardinal requirement for intravenous fluid replacement is saline, not dextrose solution. Renal tubular reabsorption of calcium and sodium are interdependent processes and in many patients, an increase in urinary calcium excretion can be induced by augmenting sodium intake. In addition, most of the water administered during rehydration will eventually enter the intracellular space, making glucose solutions a poor choice unless hypercalcemia is accompanied by hypernatremia.

Acutely ill patients with severe hypercalcemic symptoms are best treated by forced saline

TABLE 15-5. Endocrine–Metabolic Syndromes Produced by Bronchogenic Carcinomas

Endocrine Abnormality	Hormones Associated	Frequency	Predominant Cell Type(s) Associated
Hypercalcemia	Parathormone ? Prostaglandin E_2 ? Vitamin D ? Osteoclast activating factor	Common	Squamous cell
Inappropriate ADH	ADH/Oxytocin/Neurophysin	Common	Small cell Large cell Adenocarcinoma
Pulmonary osteoarthropathy	Endocrine etiology unproven; growth hormone, growth hormone releasing factor, estrogen	Common	Adenocarcinoma Squamous cell
Cushing's syndrome, excessive pigmentation	ACTH/MSH	Common	Small cell Large cell Adenocarcinoma Squamous
Gynecomastia	Chorionic gonadotropin stimulates estrogen release from testes, adrenals	Common	Large cell
Hypoglycemia	Insulin	Rare	Squamous Small cell Carcinoid
Acromegaly	Growth hormone and growth hormone releasing factor	Rare	Carcinoid
Watery diarrhea with hypokalemia	Vasoactive polypeptide	Rare	Squamous
Hyperamylasemia	Amylase	Rare	Adenocarcinoma
Malignant hypertension and hypokalemia	Renin	Rare	Adenocarcinoma
Carcinoid Syndrome	5-hydroxytryptamine (serotonin) 5-hydroxytryptophan Kallikrein Prostaglandins Histamine	Rare	Carcinoids Small cell
Increased urine and serum calcitonin Hypocalcemia ?	Calcitonin	Common	Oat cell All cell types
Increased serum alkaline phosphatase without metastases	Alkaline phosphatase	Common	Large cell

diuresis using intravenous isotonic saline and furosemide in doses up to 40 to 80 mg every 4 to 6 hr.[82–87] Care must be taken to avoid depletion of sodium, potassium, and magnesium. The furosemide causes calcium diuresis by blocking tubular reabsorption. Thiazide diuretics decrease urinary excretion of calcium and should not be used. The diuresis will worsen the preexisting contraction of the extracellular fluid volume unless that volume deficit is corrected by isotonic saline administration before furosemide or ethacrynic acid is given. The urine volume, sodium, and potassium are measured in pooled 4-hr specimens during the diuresis. Urinary losses are accurately replaced by intravenous isotonic saline containing potassium and magnesium supplements and careful weights are obtained using a bed scale when necessary. Approximately 15 mg of magnesium per hour is required to compensate for the magnesium diuresis.[85] The reduction in the serum calcium produced by these two techniques lasts from 1 to 14 days. Sodium sulfate infusions using 0.12 M isotonic sodium sulfate (38.9 g of sodium sulfate decahydrate per l) utilizes sodium to produce calciuresis and has a theoretic advantage because a relatively soluble, nonresorbable calcium sulfate complex is formed that should augment calcium excretion. In practice, sodium sulfate has no advantage over isotonic saline used with furosemide.[76]

The maintenance of an acceptable serum calcium concentration can often be achieved by oral administration of inorganic phosphate as Na_2HPO_4 and KH_2PO_4 (Hyper-Phos) or Na_2HPO_4 and NaH_2PO_4 (*Fleets' Phospho-Soda*) once intravenous fluid therapy has reduced the serum calcium to nearly normal values. Intravenous phosphate (In-Phos) is also effective in an acute hypercalcemia crisis, but must be given with great caution to patients with impaired renal function. The calcium lowering effect of phosphate is poorly understood but is not due to increased urinary excretion of calcium. Development of soft tissue, renal, and myocardial calcification following phosphate administration has been reported but not well established. This may only be a problem when large doses of phosphate are given intravenously before the plasma calcium has been reduced to normal levels.[86] Isotonic saline with furosemide diuresis followed by oral phosphate therapy appears to be the treatment of choice in severe hypercalcemia until there is more evidence concerning the development of metastatic calcification with intravenous phosphate.

Bronchogenic carcinoma is occasionally responsible for hypercalcemia which cannot be controlled by intravenous fluid therapy; hypercalcemic symptoms initially controlled by intravenous fluid therapy may rapidly recur in some patients unable to tolerate oral phosphate therapy because of severe diarrhea, which is occasionally seen as a side-effect of this treatment. Mithramycin is the treatment of choice in these two circumstances. This cytostatic antibiotic lowers the serum calcium within 1 to 4 days when given in doses one-tenth of those required for antitumor effect. The mechanism of action is not well established, but may involve a "turning off" of bone cells, since a reduction of serum calcium occurs in normal patients as well as in those with PTH excess or osseous metastases.[87] A single dose of 25 μg given intravenously is repeated in 24 to 48 hr if there has been no decline in the serum calcium or if the previously lowered calcium has returned to symptomatic hypercalcemic levels. When single doses fail to lower the serum calcium, daily doses are given until the desired effect is seen or continous intravenous infusions may be used. The doses required to lower the serum calcium for up to one month are small, and when hypercalcemic patients have received other antitumor agents without improvement, mithramycin can usually be added to their regimens without producing significant additional bone marrow depression. Metastatic calcification is not a problem with mithramycin.

Bronchogenic Carcinoma and the Syndrome of Inappropriate Antidiuretic Hormone: SIADH or the Schwartz–Bartter Syndrome. The second most common paraendocrine syndrome associated with bronchogenic carcinoma results from tumor production of antidiuretic hormone (ADH, vasopressin). Oat cell carcinoma is found in nearly all lung cancer patients with the syndrome of inappropriate antidiuretic hormone (SIADH) but the syndrome has been described with adenocarcinomas, bronchial carcinoids, and possibly with squamous and large cell carcinomas.[30] Asymptomatic IADH is recognized by the failure of water-loading to produce a diuresis or to suppress arginine vasopressin. Patients with oat cell carcinoma have these findings much more commonly than do those with the complete syndrome.[88] Other malignancies including Hodgkin's disease, thymoma, and carcinomas of the pancreas and duodenum have been responsible for SIADH; the condition is also seen with a variety of other diseases of the lung, central nervous system, and endocrine glands (see below).[89–92] Approximately 50% of the reported cases of SIADH have been associated with tumors; with the exception of oat cell carcinomas, most nonpulmonary neoplasms have been shown to produce ADH in 1 or 2 patients. Oat cell carcinomas are responsible for the SIADH about a third as often as are all the central nervous system diseases combined.[92] Patients with these tumors have been found to have inappropriately elevated levels of ADH-like activity in tumor, serum, and urine as shown by radioimmuno- and bioassay.

A syndrome closely resembling the SIADH is occasionally seen with pituitary or adrenal metastases and with cyclophosphamide or vincristine therapy. When pituitary or extensive adrenal metastases are responsible, this hypervolemic, hyponatremic syndrome results from cortisol deficiency; or in the case of hypopituitarism caused by metastatic disease, ACTH deficiency and, in turn, cortisol deficiency. Since cortisol is needed for normal water excretion, either by tonic inhibition of ADH release or through a permissive renal mechanism independent of ADH, replacement doses of glucocorticoid will correct the hyponatremia in these patients with metastatic cancer.

Vincristine and large-dose intravenous cyclophosphamide commonly cause impairment of water excretion, hyponatremia, and inappropriately concentrated urine in patients otherwise without evidence of inappropriate antidiuresis. The active hepatic metabolite of cyclophosphamide appears to be responsible for the hyponatremia which peaks 10 to 14 hr after the drug is administered. The mechanism by which the drug produces the syndrome is unknown and its action through increased hormone release from tumor has not been established.[93,94] Whatever the means by which the drug-induced dilutional syndromes occur, they appear to be self-limited. There is no good evidence that they contribute significantly to the nausea and vomiting experienced by some patients following drug treatment or that they pose the therapeutic difficulties seen with fully developed water intoxication as produced by the tumor ADH elaboration now described.

Conditions Associated with Inappropriate Antidiuretic Hormone Secretion

Malignancies
- Oat cell carcinoma of the bronchus
- Adenocarcinoma, bronchial carcinoid
- ? Squamous cell and large cell bronchial cancers
- Carcinoma of the pancreas and duodenum
- Hodgkin's disease
- Thymoma
- Carcinoma of the colon
- Carcinoma of the nasopharynx
- Carcinoma of the alveolar ridge

CNS Disease
- Brain metastases
- Head injury (*basilar skull fracture*)
- Meningitis
- Brain abscess, tumor, hemorrhage
- Acute intermittent porphyria

Pulmonary Disease
- Tuberculosis
- Lung abscess
- Pneumonia

Endocrine Disease
- Myxedema
- Addison's disease
- Hypopituitarism

Clinical Manifestations. The SIADH produced by oat cell carcinoma includes: hyponatremia with proportionate hypochloremia; hyposmolality of the serum and extracellular fluid; urine osmolality inappropriately high for the observed plasma osmolality; absence of significant edema with normal skin turgor and blood pressure; normal renal and adrenal function. Expansion of the extracellular fluid volume increases the glomerular filtration rate (GFR) and the blood urea nitrogen (BUN) is typically below 20 mg/dl. A BUN below 10 mg/dl is frequent enough to be a helpful diagnostic clue in a hyponatremic patient.

It appears that the persistent naturesis and absence of edema in inappropriate ADH secretion is caused by inhibition of proximal tubular reabsorption of sodium secondary to extracellular fluid expansion. There is evidence indicating that renal salt loss is not a consequence of decreased aldosterone secretion; neither is it due to the high GFR with its increase in filtered sodium. The expanded extracellular fluid volume does inhibit the renin-angiotensin system. The renin is appropriately low but, surprisingly, aldosterone secretion rate and excretion are normal.[90,92] The hyponatremia results, then, both from dilution of body fluids by excess water retention and from increased renal sodium loss.

It is important to note that while many patients with SIADH have urine which is persistently hypertonic to plasma, such urine hypertonicity is not necessary in order that the tonicity of the serum be maintained at subnormal values. The urine may be hypotonic to plasma so long as it is less than maximally diluted in the presence of an already hypotonic plasma. The urine will also become hypotonic to plasma if the extracellular fluid volume is further expanded by rapid infusion of isotonic saline. This therapeutic misadventure will cause only a transient escape from the existing antidiuresis.

The signs and symptoms encountered reflect the degree of hyponatremia. The seriously ill cancer patient may have voluntarily restricted fluid intake and the initial serum sodium determination may be near normal. Anorexia is often the only finding when the serum sodium is above 120 mEq/l. Nausea and vomiting may first appear when the patient seeks to augment the patient's fluid intake. Neurologic abnormalities appear when the serum sodium concentration reaches 110 to 115 mEq/l. Muscular weakness, loss of deep tendon reflexes, confusion, positive Babinski sign, and bulbar palsy may be present. Convulsions, coma, and death are seen as the serum sodium falls below 100 mEq/l.

The differential diagnosis of SIADH is not difficult because other causes of hyponatremia caused by salt depletion show contraction of the extracellular volume with dehydration indicated by poor skin turgor, hypotension, and an elevated BUN as a consequence of prerenal azotemia. These findings are characteristic of patients hyponatremic from vomiting, diarrhea, diuretic excess, and renal failure. The elevated serum potassium, reduced serum bicarbonate, low blood sugar, and arterial hypotension seen with hyponatremia from adrenal insufficiency are not found in SIADH. A BUN of 10 mg/dl or below is uncommon in adults; when such a value is seen in a hyponatremic patient, SIADH should be considered.

Management. Life-threatening water intoxication occurs more often when the SIADH is a complication of bronchogenic carcinoma than when the syndrome is associated with other pulmonary diseases where there is a tendency for a new steady state to be reached with serum sodium concentrations somewhere above 110 mEq/l. Treatment of these nonmalignant diseases usually results in spontaneous correction of the hyponatremia. Surgical resection of oat cell carcinomas, or, more appropriately, treatment with irradiation with or without alkylating agents has occasionally been responsible for improvement or disappearance of the syndrome; however, additional specific therapy is usually needed for water intoxication in cancer patients.

Most patients with SIADH are treated successfully by restricting fluid intake to 500 to 700 ml per day. This restores the renal capacity to conserve sodium because the faulty proximal tubular reabsorption of sodium that occurs in response to an expanded extracellular volume is eliminated. These seriously ill anorexic patients usually have very poor oral sodium intakes and if a low sodium intake accompanies stringent water restriction, dehydration may supervene while the serum sodium remains low. Water restriction will always cause an increase in the serum solute conconcentration in SIADH, unless the patient also has Addison's disease with low aldosterone secretion or a salt wasting renal disease. Superimposition of these conditions on the syndrome caused by bronchogenic carcinoma is rare and if fluid restriction fails to cause an increase in the serum sodium, the more likely explanation is a continuing excess of water or deficient salt intake.

Infusion of hypertonic saline is occasionally necessary when treating the severely water intoxicated patient until vomiting and convulsions can be controlled. The sodium load administered is rapidly excreted in the urine unless fluid intake is also simultaneously reduced. Hypertonic saline produces additional volume expansion which can precipitate congestive heart failure in older patients. Therefore, the best method of treatment for patients with severe symptoms is rapid correction of the serum osmolality by induction of an ethacrynic acid or furosemide diuresis (1 mg/kg body weight intravenously). A negative water balance is achieved while urinary sodium and potassium losses are measured hourly, and replaced by administration of a 3% hypertonic sodium chloride solution to which appropriate amounts of potassium chloride are added.[95] Since urinary sodium and potassium, but not water, losses are made up during the diuresis, the water losses result in a rise in plasma sodium concentration within 6 to 8 hr. Diuretic agents administered alone have a deleterious effect on the serum sodium and may cause an abrupt worsening of water intoxication.[96]

Demeclocycline (600 to 1200 mg daily) and lithium carbonate have been effective in the long-term treatment of SIADH caused by neoplasms.[97] Both act through inhibition of ADH in the collecting and distal tubules of the kidney. Phenytoin inhibits release of ADH in the collecting and distal tubules of the kidney. Phenytoin inhibits release of ADH from the hypophysis, is used in SIADH not caused by tumors, and may be used to distinguish patients with SIADH from central nervous system disease (responders) from those with SIADH from autonomously secreting tumors (nonresponders).

Salt-retaining steroids given in amounts sufficient to maintain sodium balance in patients with adrenal insufficiency (desoxycorticosterone acetate, 5 mg per day or 9 α-fluorohydrocortisone, 0.2 mg per day) do not produce significant sodium retention, in SIADH. However, these same agents given in doses of 20 mg and 3 to 8 mg per day, respectively, will reduce sodium excretion in patients with SIADH. The sodium retention induced by these large doses of mineralocorticoids is usually accompanied by an increase in the serum sodium unless a large fluid intake is continued. These agents do not correct the underlying problem of overhydration and if used chronically may result in hypertension and congestive heart failure.

Bronchogenic Carcinoma and ACTH Production. Oat cell bronchogenic carcinomas, bronchial carcinoid adenomas, epithelial thymomas, pancreatic islet cell tumors, gastrointestinal carcinoid tumors, pheochromocytomas, malignant melanoma, and some ovarian tumors may ectopically produce ACTH and cause Cushing's syndrome.[98] Approximately 25% of all patients evaluated for Cushing's syndrome have an ectopic source for ACTH prodution and oat cell carcinoma is the tumor by far the most often responsible.[98] Among male smokers, oat cell carcinoma causes the syndrome more commonly than does disease of the hypothalamic-pituitary-adrenal system. If careful testing is done, at least 10% of patients with oat cell carcinoma have evidence of hyperadrenocortisolism.[99] The biologic activity, chromatographic mobility, physical, and chemical characteristics of the ACTH produced by some oat cells carcinomas closely resemble those normally produced by the pituitary.

The majority of lung cancers of other cell types produce immunoreactive "big" ACTH (as distinguished from the 39 amino-acid pituitary peptide). The biologic activity of big ACTH is less than 4% of its immunologic potency, so Cushing's syndrome results only when it is produced in large quantities by oat cell carcinoma. The finding of a predominance of this form of ACTH in most samples of lung cancer tissue is consistent with a defect in conversion, since big ACTH is converted by the normal pituitary to "little" ACTH. The concentrations of big ACTH found in bronchogenic carcinomas vary inversely with their differentiation on the Y construct (Fig. 15-1), a finding that supports the unified concept of histologic types of lung cancer.[30] The value of big ACTH as a marker for lung cancer[100] is reduced because about a third of patients with COPD have elevated plasma levels as compared with only 6% of nonsmokers. Likewise, immunoreactive ACTH does not have prognostic value for remission or for long-term survival, probably because the tumor is not the sole source of the elevated blood levels.[101]

Another group of patients have bronchial carcinomas of histologic types other than oat cell carcinoma, and these patients have adrenocortical hyperplasia, hyperfunction, and hyperresponsiveness. In these, Cushing's syndrome or hypokalemic alkalosis is absent. In contrast to the low pituitary levels of ACTH found in patients with ACTH-secreting oat cell carcinomas, the levels in these patients are high. They may also show elevated plasma ACTH, lack of diurnal rhythm, hyperresponsiveness to exogenous ACTH and metyrapone (Metopirone) administration, elevated plasma corticoids, and simultaneously decreased urinary excretion of conjugated 17-OH-CS with normal excretion of free 17-OH-CS. These cancer patients will show suppression of plasma ACTH with low-dose dexamethasone (2 mg every 6 hr for 3 days). They therefore resemble patients with Cushing's syndrome caused by benign bilateral adrenal hyperplasia in their hyperresponsiveness to intravenous ACTH and metyrapone as well as suppression with low-dose dexamethasone. However, they show no clinical evidence of hypercorticoidism. Their plasma 17-OH-CS half-life is normal, indicating that the elevated plasma corticoids are not due to failure of hepatic conjugation as has been described in some terminally ill patients.[102] It therefore seems likely that the increased plasma cortisol levels in many patients with lung cancer are the consequence of an increase in the protein-bound fraction of hydrocortisol which is physiologically inactive.[103]

When Cushing's syndrome is caused by ectopic ACTH from oat cell carcinoma, the increased plasma ACTH, increased plasma corticoids, and increased urinary corticoids are not suppressed, even by large doses of dexamethasone (8 mg every 6 hr). In the patient with lung cancer with adrenal hyperresponsiveness but without Cushing's syndrome, elevation of the plasma ACTH and cortisol will be suppressed by a 3 mg dexamethasone regimen. The plasma ACTH is low or absent when an autonomous adrenal tumor is present. In untreated Cushing's syndrome due to pituitary ACTH excess and benign adrenal hyperplasia, the plasma ACTH is usually in the normal range, despite elevation of the plasma cortisol. The plasma ACTH and its response to attempts at suppression with varying dexamethasone doses is therefore a reliable method of obtaining an antemortem diagnosis of "nonendocrine" Cushing's syndrome; however, the diagnosis of tumor ACTH production is most secure when tumor extracts show ACTH activity with radioimmunoassay. Plasma levels of ACTH above 200 μg/ml are strongly suggestive. The adrenals are more enlarged than in classic Cushing's disease.

A second tumor peptide with corticotropin-releasing factor (CRF)-like activity contributes to the development of Cushing's syndrome in some patients with oat cell carcinoma.[104] This peptide is devoid of ACTH activity but has been produced by cancers which simultaneously elaborate an ACTH-like hormone. The presence of ectopic CRF continues to promote synthesis and release of pituitary ACTH despite the presence of high circulating levels of tumor ACTH and cortisol from the hyperfunctioning adrenals.

Patients whose carcinomas produce CRF show a positive response to metyrapone and partial dexamethasone suppression not seen when adrenal hyperplasia is caused by ectopic ACTH alone. The metyrapone-induced increase in urinary 17-OH-CS in patients with ectopic CRF indicates some retention of adrenal-pituitary reserve: the feedback mechanism by which depressed plasma cortisol normally stimulates the hypothalmic-pituitary system is partially intact. However, the set point for the feedback is at a level higher than normal because high-dose dexamethasone only partially suppresses steroid production. These responses have therapeutic implications because the patient with ectopic CRF may experience a partial correction of elevated plasma cortisol and remission of hypokalemic with metyrapone or dexamethasone.[104]

Clinical Manifestations. There are important clinical differences between the classic Cushing's syndrome caused by excess pituitary ACTH with bilateral benign adrenal hyperplasia and that seen with ectopic ACTH from oat cell carcinoma of the lung. These are summarized in Table 15-6. The findings in patients with excess pituitary ACTH are related to the duration rather than to the level of cortisol excess and are predominantly those of changes in bodily appearance including moon facies, dorsal and supraclavicular fat pads, plethora, central obesity, and purple abdominal striae. In con-

TABLE 15-6. Clinical Findings in True Cushing's Syndrome vs. Ectopic ACTH Production by Bronchogenic Carcinoma

Excess Pituitary ACTH with Bilateral Adrenal Hyperplasia	Oat Cell Carcinoma
Females predominate 5:1	Males over 45 yr predominate
History of symptoms > 1 yr	History of symptoms < 6 months
Presentation dominated by physical appearance	Presentation dominated by biochemical abnormalities
Obvious muscle wasting 50%	Often dominates clinical picture
Increased pigmentation 10%	Common
Thirst, polyuria, edema uncommon	Present in one-third
Fasting hyperglycemia 10%	Hyperglycemia and glycosuria > 50%
Dexamethasone suppression (2 mg every 6 hr)	No suppression (even with 8 mg every 6 hr)
Hyperresponsiveness to ACTH	No hyperresponsiveness to ACTH
Hyperresponse to metyrapone	No response unless ectopic CRF also present
Plasma ACTH normal	Plasma ACTH very high

trast, adrenocortical hyperfunction due to oat cell carcinoma has an acute onset with much higher plasma ACTH and cortisol levels.[105] Biochemical abnormalities predominate in these patients. Among the more reliable indicators suggesting ectopic ACTH from oat cell carcinoma are the presence of hypokalemic alkalosis, hyperglycemia, glycosuria, and deep pigmentation with extreme muscle wasting in the absence of other Cushingoid body features. Excessive adrenal androgen production may cause masculinization in females. Emotional instability, acne, osteoporosis, and hypertension may also be present.

Bronchial adenomas, pancreatic islet cell tumors, thymomas, and other mediastinal malignancies cause the majority of cases of ectopic ACTH syndrome not attributable to oat cell carcinomas. The syndrome resulting from the more indolent pancreatic and thymic tumors more closely resembles true Cushing's disease. When bronchial carcinoid adenomas produce hyperadrenocortisolism, the clinical presentation shares characteristics of both classic Cushing's syndrome and ectopic ACTH as produced by oat cell carcinomas. The hypokalemic alkalosis, hyperglycemia, weight loss, and peripheral edema seen in patients with ACTH-producing oat cell carcinomas may also be present when ectopic ACTH originates in bronchial adenomas. However, the patient with an ACTH-producing bronchial carcinoid adenoma is usually more Cushingoid than the patient with oat cell carcinoma. In true Cushing's disease, the adrenals are not under maximal stimulation and steroid secretion can be greatly augmented by exogenous ACTH. Likewise, the hypothalamic-pituitary-adrenal servomechanism is disordered but will respond to 2 mg dexamethasone suppression and metyrapone stimulation. Half of the patients with bronchial carcinoid adenoma with ectopic ACTH production will show the same suppression with dexamethasone and a third are likewise hyperresponsive to metyrapone.[106] The failure of hyperadrenocortisolism to respond to these manipulations when caused by ACTH from oat cell carcinomas has been discussed. The presence of significant hypokalemic alkalosis, hyperglycemia, and peripheral edema should therefore suggest bronchial adenoma in the frankly Cushingoid patient whose other biochemical tests are consistent with classic Cushing's syndrome. Recognition of this dichotomous presentation is important because over 60% of bronchial carcinoid adenomas are not detected by routine chest roentgenograms at the time of diagnosis of hyperadrenocortisolism.[106] Functioning carcinoid tumors are rare. In one series, only 3 of 203 patients with carcinoid tumors presented with the carcinoid syndrome.[107] Pulmonary tumorlets have also been associated with Cushing's syndrome, lending support to the concept that they are small, peripheral, carcinoid tumors.[108]

Management. Treatment of Cushing's syndrome resulting from ectopic ACTH production is of limited effectiveness. In one cooperative study, only 11 of 105 patients with various types of neoplasms responsible for the syndrome appeared to be cured of their tumors.[109] It is well established that the majority of patients with oat cell carcinoma live less than 8 months. Radiotherapy or cyclophosphamide is used in most patients with ACTH-producing oat cell carcinomas because palliative surgery for the typically widely metastatic pulmonary cancer is ineffective. A British Medical Research Council cooperative, randomized, prospective study has shown that even in the apparent absence of metastatic disease, radiotherapy is preferred to surgery for treating oat cell carcinoma.[110] Control of the debilitating effects of hypercortisolism by bilateral adrenalectomy is impractical because of the patient's poor general condition, short prognosis, and the dangers of wound infection or dehiscence. The hypokalemic alkalosis may in itself be life-threatening as a result of profound muscular weakness, cardiac abnormalities, and hypotension. Clinical improvement may follow potassium supplementation, salt restriction, and diuresis with spironolactone.

The rapidly acting inhibitors of adrenocorticoid synthesis, aminoglutethimide and metyrapone, are sometimes successful in reducing the hypercortisolism of ectopic ACTH syndrome.[111,112] Aminoglutethimide given in a dose of 1 g daily is a potent inhibitor of aldosterone and the sodium diuresis produced may result in loss of edema before any significant reduction in plasma or urinary steroids occurs. Salt supplementation may be required. Aminoglutethimide causes marked lethargy and somnolence; thyroid function declines and thyroid replacement may be necessary. The adrenocorticolytic drug O,p'-DDD, 3 to 6g given daily in divided doses, can also be useful but several weeks must pass before its full effects are seen. Side-effects include ataxia, anorexia, nausea, lethargy, and mental confusion.

Either aminoglutethimide or metyrapone may effectively diminish cortisol secretion and improve the patient's physical condition when the adrenals are stimulated by ACTH from a bronchial adenoma. Such treatment may make a seriously ill patient a candidate for thoracic exploration.

Bronchogenic Carcinoma, Digital Clubbing, and Secondary Hypertrophic Osteoarthropathy (Pierre Marie–Bamberger Syndrome)

Digital clubbing, Hippocratic fingers, or acropachy (from the Greek, *akro* meaning extremity and *pachus* meaning thick) refer to a bulbous enlargement of the fingers and toes due chiefly to overgrowth and inflammatory changes in the soft tissue of the terminal phalanges (Fig. 15-17). Increased mobility of the nail on the nail bed produces the impression of a spongy cuticle and the curvature of the nail is increased; however, the most reliable characteristic of true clubbing is the "profile sign." When only exaggerated curving of the nail is present, the 160° obtuse angle seen in profile between the skin of the dorsum of this phalanx and the nails is undisturbed. When acropachy is present, this angle is obliterated (*i.e.*, becomes greater than 180°). Because of the increase in the peripheral blood flow, the tips of the fingers may feel warm with mild burning paresthesia but pain is unusual. The skin at the base of the nail is often reddened. The bony structure of the terminal phalanges usually shows no changes.[113] Clubbing is probably diagnosed more frequently than it should be because too little attention is paid to the profile sign; nevertheless, it is a common finding, now most often associated with bronchogenic carcinoma. Clubbing has been found in patients with bacterial endocarditis, cyanotic congenital heart disease, bronchiectasis, lung abscess, thoracic cysts, empyema, tuberculosis, regional enteritis, ulcerative colitis, neoplasms of the gastrointestinal tract, thyrotoxicosis, varying types of cirrhosis, and benign or malignant, primary or metastatic pleural, thoracic, and mediastinal tumors. Unilateral clubbing may be seen in patients with aneurysms of the great thoracic vessels. Clubbing has been loosely identified with hypertrophic osteoarthropathy, and it is important to

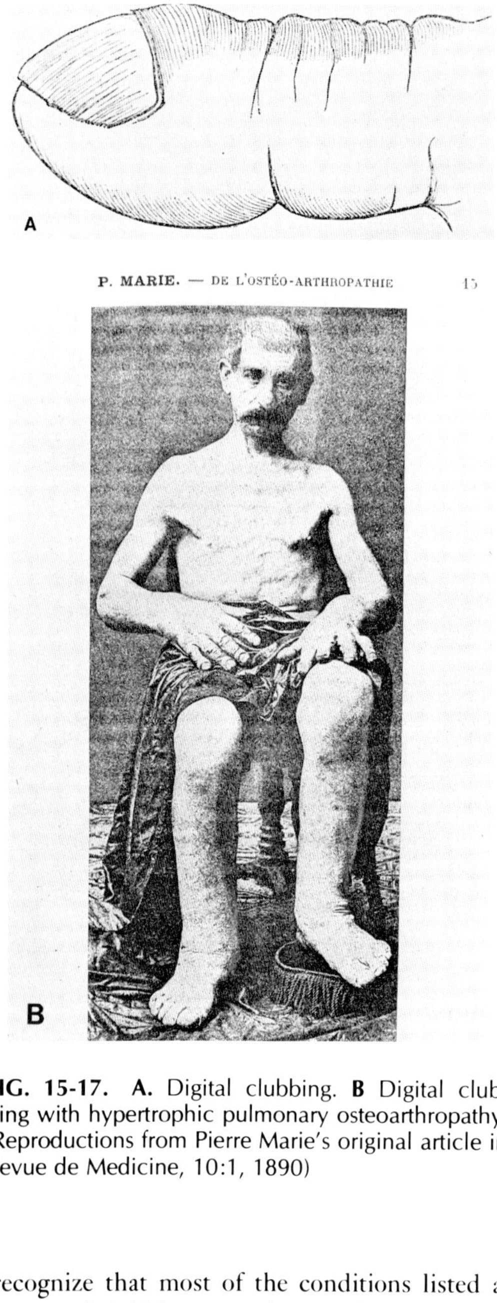

FIG. 15-17. A. Digital clubbing. **B** Digital clubbing with hypertrophic pulmonary osteoarthropathy. (Reproductions from Pierre Marie's original article in Revue de Medicine, 10:1, 1890)

recognize that most of the conditions listed as causes of clubbing are only occasionally accompanied by the more extensive bony changes of secondary hypertrophic osteoarthropathy.[114] Cirrhosis, pregnancy, thyroid disease, rheumatoid arthritis, and a variety of benign tumors have been associated with occasional reports of hypertrophic osteoarthropathy.[114,115] Although like clubbing, hypertrophic osteoarthropathy is most often associated with bronchogenic carcinoma, clubbing is not an essential feature of osteoarthropathy; the frequent association of the two conditions in the same patients should not be interpreted to mean that clubbing is but an early manifestation of full-blown hypertrophic osteoarthropathy.[114]

The most characteristic finding in secondary hypertrophic osteoarthropathy is a proliferative periostitis beginning in the distal thirds of the tibia, fibula, radius, and ulna (Fig. 15-18). The process originates and is more marked on the dorsal and medial aspects of the bone. The periosteal changes diminish near the expanded ends of the diaphyses and are rarely seen in areas covered by the articular capsules although accompanying joint symptoms may mimic rheumatoid arthritis with morning stiffness, painful, warm joints, limitation of motion, and in very rare cases, deformity and ankylosis.[113] Because joint symptoms may be present in the absence of roentgenographic changes in the joints themselves, it is important to specifically request "long bone films for periosteal reaction" rather than routine views of the elbows, wrists, knees, and ankles. Many patients complain of "arthritis," but on closer questioning have aching in the extremities unrelated to any joint findings. Marked periosteal tenderness may then be demonstrated by squeezing the arm or leg well above what is often a well-functioning and painless joint. Periarticular tenderness may be present for several months before typical periosteal changes are seen on x-ray. Radionuclide bone scans may be positive in such early cases. Striking linear accumulation of the isotope is seen along the periosteum of affected bones.[116] In the occasional patient with a joint effusion, the joint fluid resembles that seen in traumatic effusions except that it clots on standing. The average leukocyte count in the fluid is under 2000 cells/mm^3, about 15% being polymorphonuclear. The mucin clot is good to fair.[117,118] Synovial biopsy shows minimal infiltration of the synovium with chronic inflammatory cells and moderate hyperplasia of synovial cells with fibrosis. Electron microscopic studies show microvascular injury with electron-dense vascular deposits in synovial biopsies from patients with

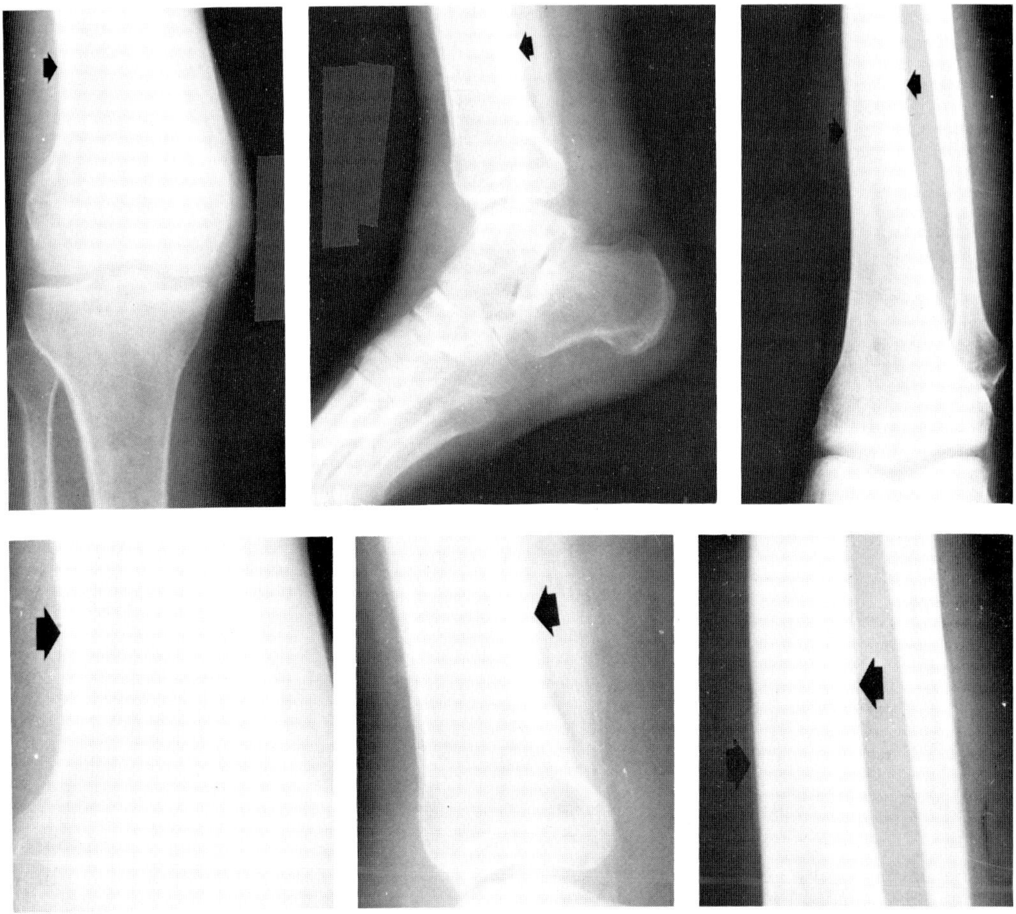

FIG. 15-18. Hypertrophic pulmonary osteoarthropathy. The proliferative periostitis produced by this lung cancer is seen as a dense irregular line separated from the cortex of the femur and tibia by a narrow band of radiolucency.

painful joint effusions. The deposits resemble those caused by immune complex deposition in renal glomeruli in systemic lupus erythematosus.[119] The subcutaneous tissue about the affected bones becomes edematous and in far-advanced cases the skin is warm and dusky red. The skin of the face and scalp may occasionally become thickened and furrowed; hyperhidrosis and palmar and plantar hyperkeratosis may be prominent.

Secondary or acquired clubbing and hypertrophic osteoarthropathy are common and are unrelated to two rare conditions which they closely resemble: pachydermoperiostosis (or idiopathic hypertrophic osteoarthropathy) and hereditary clubbing [120] There are approximately 60 case-reports of pachydermoperiostosis. A fourth of the cases have been familial and the clubbed digits, coarsened facial features, and bone changes usually begin at puberty, have an insidious onset, and are painless. Hereditary clubbing without hypertrophic osteoarthropathy has been reported in some 18 families and occurs as a sex-limited, Mendelian dominant condition with low expression in females. The onset is in the first or second decade. Neither of these conditions has been associated with underlying disease; the general health of involved persons is good, and little or no disability results.

A welter of hypotheses have been advanced to

explain clubbing and secondary hypertrophic osteoarthropathy. None is entirely satisfactory and an exhaustive review of their relative complexities and merits is unnecessary. Venous occlusion plethysmography has established the presence of increased blood flow to the affected extremities which is persistently reduced following section of vagal afferent nerve fibers. Prompt regression of vascular connective tissue overgrowth then occurs and arthralgias disappear immediately postoperatively. Other manifestations of osteoarthropathy rapidly clear with 4 out of 5 patients becoming symptom-free in a week to a month. Clubbing regresses more slowly. Three to 8 months are usually necessary before substantial change is seen.[118] The type of operation performed has little bearing on the relief obtained, and dramatic improvement has followed exploratory thoracotomy with vagal section even without tumor removal; segmentectomy, lobectomy, and pneumonectomy provide equal relief when the vagus nerve is sacrificed. The efferent pathway in this neuro- or neuroendocrine reflex arc is unknown. Selective blockade of vagal efferent motor fibers with atropine has no effect. The efferent path of the reflex does not appear to be neural because denervation of the limb or high spinal anesthesia has no effect on the increased blood flow. Even section of the vagus nerve does not consistently reduce blood flow in dogs with osteoarthropathy.[114]

Evidence that various endocrine imbalances occur with some frequency in a minority of patients with clubbing and hypertrophic osteoarthropathy has prompted a search for a responsible humoral factor. Ginsburg and Brown found increased urinary excretion of estrogen in males with osteoarthropathy.[121] Bronchogenic carcinoma, gynecomastia, and osteoarthropathy have been reported frequently enough so as to merit distinction as a "classic triad" by some authors. Urinary excretion of gonadotropic activity has been elevated in some patients with osteoarthropathy although this has been a common finding in lung cancer patients without bony and soft tissue changes.[122] Autonomous tumor secretion of growth hormone (HGH) has been suggested by findings in a few patients with carcinoma of the bronchus and hypertrophic osteoarthropathy. High levels of pituitary HGH-releasing activity have also been associated with some bronchogenic carcinomas. Other patients with these skeletal changes have shown no abnormality in HGH levels with or without hypo- or hyperglycemic testing, and despite some similarities between this condition and acromegaly, it seems unlikely that HGH is important in the pathogenesis of either clubbing or hypertrophic osteoarthropathy.[123] Cross-perfusion experiments between normal dogs and those with hypertrophic osteoarthropathy produced no changes in extremity blood flow in either, but do not conclusively exclude a humoral origin.[114]

Alkylating agents and irradiation have produced partial or complete remission of symptoms, but improvement in objective signs of clubbing and hypertrophic osteoarthropathy are less consistently produced by such therapy. Spontaneous remission has been reported and in rare cases arthritic symptoms have reappeared with the development of metastases or local tumor recurrence. In a retrospective review of 1879 patients who underwent thoracotomy for lung lesions at the Mayo Clinic, Stenseth, Clagett, and Woolner found the 10% of those with primary tumors of the lung exhibited evidence of osteoarthropathy. Among the 231 patients having thoracotomies for disease metastatic to the chest, 3% had hypertrophic osteoarthropathy.[118] In contrast, Semple, emphasizing the difference between simple clubbing and generalized osteoarthropathy, placed the incidence of the latter at a more familiar 1 to 2%.[124] Histologic analysis of the primary lung tumors in the Mayo Clinic Study indicated that osteoarthropathy was seen with all cell types but was least common (5%) with oat cell carcinoma. Osteoarthropathy occurred predominantly among patients with adenocarcinoma in the large experience of the VA Lung Group.[30] There is remarkably little information concerning the prognosis of patients with lung cancer and osteoarthropathy; the extensive Mayo Clinic Study found the condition to have no influence on the rate of tumor resectability or patient survival.[118]

Other Endocrine Abnormalities Associated with Bronchogenic Carcinoma

Gynecomastia with and without hypertrophic osteoarthropathy is a relatively common early physical finding in male patients with bronchogenic carcinoma and has been recognized one year before clinical identification of a pulmonary cancer. One early report limited the association of gynecomastia to gonadotropin (HCG)-producing large cell carcinomas of the lung but other cell types are now known to be occasionally involved.[126–133] The predominance of large cell carcinomas, many with bizarre giant cells, suggests a relationship between HCG production and choriocarcinomas. It is reason to maintain the large cell carcinoma, giant cell type, as a separate category in the revised WHO classification.[130] The only other nontrophoblastic tumors known to produce gonadotropin are the hepatoblastoma, adrenocortical carcinoma, and some undifferentiated retroperitoneal tumors; therefore, lung cancer appears to be easily the most common extragonadal tumor producing gonadotropins, and the presence of gynecomastia in a male smoker should prompt endocrine and pulmonary investigation. Occasionally, patients with lung cancer have titers of urinary gonadotropins equivalent to those seen in human pregnancy or choriocarcinoma. The commonly used commercial agglutination-inhibition slide test for pregnancy (Gravidiex, Ortho Labs) identifies such patients as having abnormal LH-HCG production. However, the failure of this test to detect gonadotropins in unconcentrated urine does not exclude lung cancer as the cause of gynecomastia. Urine specimens concentrated with a tungstic acid precipitation method may be reliably examined by the agglutination-inhibition slide test.[129] Radioimmunoassay of whole or concentrated plasma or the more cumbersome mouse uterine bioassay may also be used.[130,131]

The relation seen in some cases of increased gonadotropin secretion and gynecomastia with bronchogenic carcinoma has been assumed to result from a gonadotropin-stimulated increase in estrogen secretion by the Leydig cells of the testis or by the adrenal gland. While an increase in at least one estrogen fraction has been demonstrated in many lung cancer patients having gynecomastia with excessive gonadotropins, there are reports of these phenomena occurring in the absence of Leydig cell hyperplasia or estrogen elevation.[129] It would appear that the gynecomastia is not simply related to estrogen production but may depend on other factors. It is somewhat paradoxic that increased estrogen production has been more consistently associated with generalized hypertrophic osteoarthropathy than with gynecomastia.[121] Testicular biopsy appears to be of little value in the evaluation of these patients because there is no uniform histologic appearance of the testes in patients with gynecomastia due to gonadotropin-producing tumors.[132]

Bronchogenic carcinomas and other neoplasms have been the site for the ectopic production of two additional placental hormones: human chorionic somatomammotropin (HCS) and placental alkaline phosphatase (PAP). Unlike other ectopic hormones, HCG, HCS, and PAP may serve as specific markers for neoplasms since they are not detected in normal males or nonpregnant females. Weintraub and Rosen used radioimmunoassay to study 64 patients with bronchogenic carcinoma for HCS. Positive assays were obtained in 7 of the 13 patients who exhibited gynecomastia.[126]

Regression of gynecomastia has followed treatment of bronchogenic carcinoma with pulmonary resection, irradiation, or alkylating agents.

This progress in hormone research makes it clear that a male smoker with breast enlargement who is not receiving digitalis, chlorpromazine, reserpine, or spironolactones, all of which can produce gynecomastia, deserves further investigation.

Other Biologic Markers. Lung cancer occasionally produces insulin, glucagon, calcitonin, renin, vasoactive intestinal polypeptide, prostaglandins, prolactin, and serotonin.[133–140] Insulin and insulinlike activity have been isolated from oat cell carcinomas, squamous carcinomas, and carcinoid adenomas.[133] Patients with tumors producing these hormones may also have hypoglycemia. Glucagon has also been found in some patients with oat cell carcinoma. It is not clear whether the large stores of glucagon in some oat cell carcinomas influence blood glucose homeostasis in the direction of hyperglycemia.[134] Ectopic secretion of calcitonin, the hypocalcemic hormone normally produced by the C cells of the thyroid, has been elaborated by lung cancers of various cell types. The urinary calcitonin was increased in two-thirds or more of 41 patients studied by Becker and associates.[136] The increased calcitonin values in serum and urine are not diagnostic but also occur with inflammatory disease of the lung. No clinical abnormalities were attributed to the hypercalcitonemia; the patients remained normocalcemic with a normal serum phosphate. Reinin produced by an adenocarcinoma caused malignant hypertension and hypokalemia.[137] Squamous cell carcinomas of the lung rarely elaborate vasoactive intestinal polypeptide causing one or more elements of the watery diarrhea syndrome: peripheral vasodilation, elevated serum calcium, watery diarrhea, hypokalemia, and achlorhydria.[138] Both bronchial carcinoid adenomas and oat cell carcinomas are very occasionally associated with the carcinoid syndrome more frequently produced by malignant intestinal carcinoid tumors. The syndrome is discussed in the section dealing with bronchial adenomas.

Two-thirds of patients with lung cancer have an elevated carcinoembryonic antigen (CEA) regardless of cell type. The CEA, which is most useful when following patients with carcinoma of the colon who have undergone curative therapy, is not selective or specific enough for screening purposes in lung cancer. In one large series, 40% of patients whose lung tumors could be treated with surgery had normal CEA concentrations. Moreover, in an assay in which the upper limit of normal was 2.5 ng/ml or less, levels in many lung cancer patients ranged between 2.5 ng/ml and 8 ng/ml; similar levels have been found in a variety of diseases, including benign pulmonary disease.[141] However, the investigators felt a CEA level persistently greater than 8 ng/ml increased suspicion in a patient being investigated for lung cancer and a value greater than 15 ng/ml made successful resection doubtful. In these patients, the CEA level frequently dropped within 2 months after surgery. In many patients who had not had successful surgery, the antigen rose again after 6 to 15 months. Other workers have found this expensive radioimmunoassay useful in very few patients.[142] It did not help to distinguish those patients with mediastinal metastases.

Alpha-fetoprotein is elevated in few patients with lung cancer.[143]

THE SOLITARY PULMONARY NODULE

General Characteristics

Routine chest roentgen examination of asymptomatic patients is largely responsible for identifying the problematic solitary pulmonary nodule. The rounded abnormality is commonly but inappropriately termed a coin lesion because of its appearance in a single radiographic projection. Many reported series of resected solitary nodules have stressed the importance of early thoracotomy because the lesions are frequently malignant.

Solitary nodules are usually defined as those abnormalities in asymptomatic patients that are as follows: (1) round, ovoid, or slightly lobulated; (2) located in the lung parenchyma and surrounded by aerated lung; (3) at least moderately well circumscribed; (4) uncalcified; and (5) without associated pneumonitis, volume loss, lymphadenopathy, or significant satellite lesions (Fig. 15-19). Because areas of radiolucency can be demonstrated in some lesions that are partially filled with semi-solid or liquid caseous granuloma or necrotic tumor material, some investigators have also included nodules which have the appearance of cavitation. The percentage of nodules found to be malignant varies greatly with age and sex distribution, geographic location, and selection from thoracic surgery referral clinics, routine hospital admission roentgenograms, or community roentgen surveys. In the largest series of nodules recognized by routine hospital admission roentgenograms on male patients, malignant nodules comprised 35.6% of 1034 solitary nodules which came to resection. It must be recognized that many other benign nodules were identified

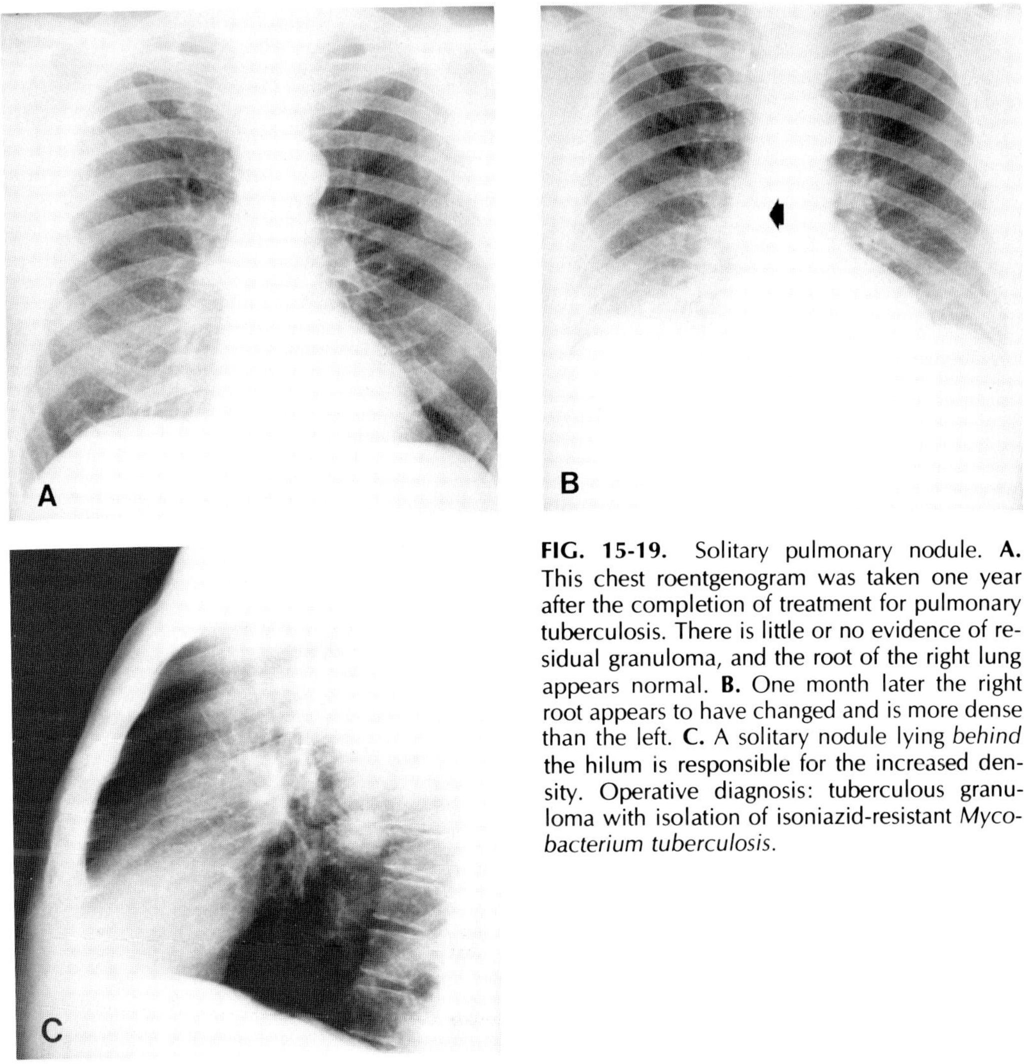

FIG. 15-19. Solitary pulmonary nodule. **A.** This chest roentgenogram was taken one year after the completion of treatment for pulmonary tuberculosis. There is little or no evidence of residual granuloma, and the root of the right lung appears normal. **B.** One month later the right root appears to have changed and is more dense than the left. **C.** A solitary nodule lying *behind* the hilum is responsible for the increased density. Operative diagnosis: tuberculous granuloma with isolation of isoniazid-resistant *Mycobacterium tuberculosis.*

among patients in this same population. These benign lesions are not represented in the final figures because concern over their possible malignant nature was not sufficient to cause them to come to operation. When the operated patients were stratified by age, the incidence of carcinoma was as follows: 25 to 29 years, 2%; 35 to 39 years, 13% 45 to 49 years, 26%; and 60 to 69% years, 50%. These figures and the manner in which they were obtained are representative of many studies in which malignancy has been found in a third to half of resected lesions. The larger figure is more characteristic of highly selected thoracic surgery referral collections, which sometimes inappropriately include symptomatic patients.[147]

In contrast, malignancy is uncommon among patients with solitary nodules discovered by community mass chest roentgenogram surveys. In these studies, the solitary nodule has an approximate overall prevalence rate of 1 per 1000 persons examined, and 3 to 6% are malignant. The number of malignant nodules does not increase significantly with advancing age in this group, being 4.5% for those 45 to 64 years or older.[148–151] There are few better examples of the importance of disease definition and patient preselection than this wide variation in the incidence of malignancy among studies of the solitary pulmonary nodule.

A variety of diagnostic techniques can be used to assess the likelihood of malignancy in a solitary nodule. The number of studies performed on a routine basis is limited but includes a chest roentgenogram in the posterioranterior and lateral projections; serologic tests for fungi; skin tests and sputum smears and cultures for tuberculosis and fungi; efforts to obtain earlier chest roentgenograms; and, depending on the size and location of the nodule, cytologic examination of three or four sputum specimens for cancer cells. Because these studies often fail to provide a definitive diagnosis short of surgical exploration, two equally unfortunate attitudes tend to develop. In the first, the absence of proof of malignancy is too often used to justify an unwarranted period of observation in a high-risk patient. A second overly aggressive attitude ignores the fact that, even in operated series, two-thirds of solitary nodules are benign; this approach allows simple, rapidly available information which would occasionally establish a preoperative diagnosis to go uncollected.

The patient's age, sex, areas of residence, occupation, disease exposure, and previous medical or smoking history serve as guidelines for selecting the specific diagnostic studies which should be repeated or stressed. In the patient who has received treatment for an earlier granulomatous disease, special emphasis may be placed on the number and quality of sputum specimens examined by smear and culture. History of a previous operation for cancer may point to the need for diagnostic studies such as bronchoscopy or full-chest laminography which would establish local recurrence or indicate multiple parenchymal metastases. One common association is that of bronchogenic carcinoma appearing as a solitary nodule in a patient treated for laryngeal or oral carcinoma. A new lung lesion in such a patient is often a second primary carcinoma rather than a metastasis from the upper respiratory tract cancer.

Metastatic malignancy rarely presents as a solitary nodule in the totally asymptomatic patient. In one series in which 26 metastatic lesions were found among 306 malignant solitary nodules, all but 3 patients had previous histories of malignancy.[146] In the absence of a positive review of systems or of a physical examination that suggests a primary site of neoplasm from which the solitary metastasis may have arisen, a prolonged, fruitless, multisystem evaluation should be avoided. In the patient free of gastrointestinal symptoms, a thorough physical examination, stool guaiac tests, and hemoglobin determination can be safely substituted for the barium enema and upper gastrointestinal series. Similarly, the intravenous pyelogram will rarely be of value in the patient with a solitary pulmonary nodule when the urinalysis is normal and the patient is free of genitourinary tract complaints.

Diagnostic Approaches

The patient's earlier chest roentgenograms are critically important because if they show a nodule to be unchanged in size for 2 years or longer, malignancy is excluded. If this rule is to be applied, the nodule must be sufficiently well circumscribed to permit accurate measurement and there must be no increase in size. When earlier films are known to exist, a short delay imposed while efforts are made to acquire them is fully justified, and surgery should be postponed until they have been reviewed. These roentgenograms are of such importance that early telephone and mail requests to another hospital's director or the patient's union steward may be necessary to prompt an otherwise recalcitrant radiology department or employer to make them available.

The presence of calcification in a solitary nodule may sometimes allow malignancy to be excluded with a high degree of confidence.[152] Despite occasional reports of calcification within a malignant lesion, it does not occur in circumscribed bronchogenic carcinomas except in the rarest of circumstances in which a cancer develops around a preexisting calcified parenchymal focus.[153] While overpenetrated films or laminograms (tomograms) may be of value in establishing the presence of calcification in occasional cases, a nodule is either calcified and calcified in a pattern which effectively excludes malignancy or it must be considered noncalcified. The expression, "probably calcified," cannot be used to support a therapeutic decision not to operate or to "wait and see." Patterns of calcification which indicate a benign lesion are laminated, diffuse stippling, popcorn (hamartoma), or dense central calcifications occupying a significant proportion of the volume of the nodule and shown on at least two views to be within the nodule rather than in a position approximate to the nodule. When calcification is carefully defined, the general experience is similar to that of the Mayo Clinic Group who found that in 156 resected cases, calcium was found in 28% of the hamartomas and in 32% of the granulomas, but in no other lesion.[154–158]

The absence of calcification does not prove that the nodule is malignant, and embarrassing mistakes can be avoided by excluding, through careful physical examination, chest wall lesions such as chondromas, moles, or soft tissue tumors which may project as a solitary lung nodule in a single roentgen view.

Skin tests for tuberculosis, histoplasmosis, and coccidioidomycosis offer no definitive diagnosis in the patient with a solitary lung nodule; when negative they are useful because they add to the suspicion of malignancy. However, even in the patients whose resected nodules were proven to be specific granulomas, skin tests were negative for 11% of the tuberculomas, 19% of the histoplasmomas, and 30% of the coccidioidomas.[159] Patients should be given isoniazid prophylaxis if the resected nodule is shown to be tuberculous, and some believe that any tuberculin-positive patient undergoing thoracotomy for pulmonary resection should receive such prophylaxis. The skin tests serve to focus attention on adequate sputum collection and thoracotomy will occasionally be avoided when a patient with an ominous roentgen abnormality but positive skin test is promptly shown to have smears positive for acid-fast bacilli or fungi. When a resected nodule proves to be a granuloma, knowledge of the skin tests helps to direct the efforts of the pathology laboratory in isolating the causative organism.

Roentgenographic studies including overpenetrated films,laminograms, and oblique, apical lordotic, and kyphotic projections may demonstrate calcification or identify other closely associated but unsuspected abnormalities. They are also useful in localizing the lesion for the surgeon. Computerized tomography may prove exceedingly helpful as greater experience with it is accumulated.[159a] Additional parenchymal disease, particularly disease in a different segment of the same lobe as the solitary nodule, increases the likelihood of inflammatory disease and granulomas constitute the majority of lesions abutting on the lobar pleural surfaces. These roentgenographic findings in a nonsmoking female patient under age 40 with positive skin tests would justify the 2- to 6-week delay necessary to obtain complement fixation studies for fungi and cultures for mycobacterial and fungal disease. The same findings in a smoking male patient of the same age with the additional history of previous active granulomatous disease represent a greater challenge but should stimulate the most aggressive effort to obtain earlier roentgenograms.

An individual nodule first recognized because of its coexistence with known active granulomatous disease is commonly a more circumscribed manifestation of that same disease, and the nodule may undergo a definite reduction in size within a few weeks of the institution of appropriate drug treatment. If the lesion remains unchanged or grows larger, it should be resected while therapy for the granulomatous disease is continued. When a well circumscribed, isolated nodule strongly suggests neoplasm by its large size and lobulated appearance in a patient with active tuberculosis, surgery can be safely performed soon after antituberculous chemotherapy is begun.

Cytologic examination of the sputum may be of value in some patients with isolated lung nodules. The percent of positive smears in patients with these small peripheral tumors varies with the experience of the cytologist and with the size and location of the lesion but has been reported to range from 31 to 79%, with 50% being the average number reported by 10 investigators.[159] However, Hattori found sputum cytology to be positive in only 37.5% of patients with peripheral tumors less than 3 cm in diameter, even when small brushes were advanced to the lesions using a Métras catheter under television fluoroscopic control.[160] Those studies reporting success for sputum examination in tumors above 4 to 5 cm in diameter are not representative of most series of solitary nodules where the majority of lesions are less than 3 cm. In Steele's work, cytologic preparations of the sputum and bronchial washings were positive in only 5 of the 500 patients having these examinations.[161]

Little inconvenience or expense is added if a limited number of cytologic examinations are done with the recognition that negative results cannot be used to exclude cancer or justify delay. Others feel these studies have limited value in the small peripheral lesion because positive or negative results lead to thoracotomy unless the cytologist can unequivocally label an occasional preparation as being one from an oat cell carcinoma. In this circumstance, irradiation is the treatment of choice.

Similar objection can be made to efforts to obtain cytology by aspiration through a small gauge needle with an outer diameter of 0.9 to 1.1 mm under fluorscopic control, or from bronchial brush cytology obtained through mobile catheters directed by a television fluoroscope system. The cytologic material obtained with these techniques is often insufficient to allow a definite diagnosis of a specific granuloma or benign neoplasm. Reports that chronic inflammatory cells are seen on the smear do not exclude cancer unless time-consuming cultures from the specimen are positive for a granulomatous disease. Although those brush biopsy and small-needle aspiration specimens interpreted as being cytologically positive for malignancy provide a conclusive diagnosis of cancer, the 10 to 25% false-negative rate is high enough that surgical exploration must be considered almost without regard to the result.[162–165]

Adenocarcinomas are the most common malignancies to present as solitary peripheral nodules. In one series of 1223 patients undergoing needle aspiration biopsy, there was a conspicuous 50% failure rate with adenocarcinomas. Among 82 patients later shown to have adenocarcinoma, 42 had a false-negative aspiration with an 18 gauge needle. The false-negative rate was 13% with squamous carcinomas. The contention that needle aspiration of solitary nodules is indicated because a diagnosis of small cell carcinoma avoids ill-advised surgery is not convincing, because small cell cancers are not usually peripheral tumors likely to be subject to aspiration. Small cell carcinoma presenting as a solitary pulmonary nodule in an asymptomatic patient is rare indeed.

Cutting-needle biopsy using the Franklin modification of the Vim-Silverman needle, or trephrine biopsy by high-speed drill from which a small core of lung tissue is obtained, are most satisfactory.[166,167] These procedures are most applicable for disease within 3 cm of the pleural surface, but require good patient cooperation, absence of cysts or bullae in the area to be biopsied, and absence of clinical evidence of significant pulmonary hypertension. Fluoroscopy is used to direct the cutting needle into the lesion; this cannot be done with the high-speed drill, limiting its usefulness to fluoroscopically visualized large peripheral lesions or diffuse lung disease. Review of the risk of these biopsies indicates a mortality rate of 0.5% in 792 patients compared with 0.9 to 2.6% for open lung biopsy.[164] Needle tract implantation of tumor after percutaneous lung or pleural biopsy is so rare that it should not create skepticism for the procedures.[167]

Scalene lymph node biopsy and mediastinoscopy have little place in the preoperative evaluation of the smaller, peripheral, solitary pulmonary nodule because these structures are seldom invaded by tumor in totally asymptomatic patients with otherwise normal roentgenograms. Bronchoscopy with a rigid bronchoscope rarely aids in the diagnosis. Bronchoscopy with the flexible fiberoptic bronchoscope, which can be advanced into segmental and subsegmental bronchi so as to obtain cytologic specimens by brushing, may be of value if isolated nodules are examined under fluoroscopic control.[168] The fiberscopic yield is influenced by the size of the tumor and by its distance from the hilum. A tissue diagnosis is obtained in only about a quarter of the cases in which the nodule is 2 cm or less in diameter or more than 6 cm from the hilum.[169] Larger tumors, and those between 2 and 6 cm from the hilum, may be diagnosed in two-thirds of cases.

Predictive Criteria

Some characteristics of individual nodules have been widely discussed but are of marginal usefulness when diagnostic decisions are made. The first of these characteristics is the size of the nodule. Larger nodules are more often malignant. One community mass roentgen survey found only 3% of 666 solitary nodules to be malignant; among the 43 largest nodules (4 cm and more in diameter) 23% were malignant.[148] While the majority of granulomas are 2 cm or less in diameter, 25% or more of primary carcinomas are also under 2 cm.[146] No minimum dimension is recognized below which a nodule can be followed, in contrast to colonic polyps which may be followed safely if they are less than 1 cm in diameter.

Predictions about a nodule's character based on its location are also of limited value. There is a prevalent concept that primary carcinomas are more likely to be located in the anterior segments of the upper lobes than granulomas, but in Steel's experience, only 15% of 280 primary carcinomas were located in the anterior segments, while 37% were in the apical and posterior segments. Histoplasmal and coccidioidal granulomas were equally distributed among the segments of upper lobes, and only tuberculosis was uncommon in the anterior segment. In the tuberculin-positive smoker, a solitary nodule cannot be assumed to be a tuberculous residual because it lies in an apical-posterior segment of an upper lobe or a superior segment of a lower lobe, despite the fact that these segments are the ones most often involved in adult tuberculosis.

Hazy, indistinct, lobulated margins and umbilication support a diagnosis of malignancy, but the sharply marginated sphere may also be cancer. Lesions of medium and light density are more often malignant, but no conclusions can be drawn unless a nodule is so dense as to assure that it is calcified, and therefore benign.

A biomathematic approach can be used to evaluate the solitary nodule's growth rate whereby the volume-doubling time of a lesion can be calculated if serial roentgenograms permit accurate measurement of successive increases in tumor diameter.[170,171] If it is assumed that a neoplasm originates with one or a few cells 10 μ in diameter, 20 doublings are required to produce a mass of 1-mm diameter and 30 doublings produced a 1-cm nodule at the limit of radiographic recognition. After 10 additional doublings, or 40 in all, the tumor would be 10 cm in diameter, would weigh approximately 1 kg, and would presumably cause death. The distribution of estimated doubling times for bronchogenic carcinomas ranges from approximately 30 days for some undifferentiated cancers to 500 days for some adenocarcinomas. The mean is 120 days.[172,173] Therefore, if the doubling time of a solitary nodule is less than 1 month or more than 16 months, it is unlikely to be malignant. It should be noted that these figures refer to volume doublings which must be calculated from changes in measured diameters plotted on a chart prepared on cube-root graph paper.[170] Because such studies require serial films and show a 15-fold difference in the doubling times of different bronchogenic carcinomas, the technique has seldom been used to exclude cancer.

In all age groups, pulmonary nodules which grow so rapidly that the doubling time is less than 30 days are far more likely to be benign than malignant. Nathan recommends that the growth of all nodules which remain undiagnosed after needle and brush biopsy be followed with serial roentgenograms, so that only nodules with doubling times at least consistent with a diagnosis of cancer are resected.[174] This policy is theoretically attractive, but unproven, and accepts additional growth before removal of some nodules which would be proven neoplastic after some delay. This may be unacceptable when Steel's data and conclusions are considered: the effect of primary tumor size on survival was as strong or stronger than the effect of tumor doubling time[144] (see also the section on neoplasms metastatic to the lung).

Despite the number of large surgical series emphasizing the malignant solitary nodule, relatively little information is available concerning the overall prognosis for unselected patients with such lesions. Three studies have provided overall health and mortality data for asymptomatic patients unselected except by factors which induced them to accept chest roentgen examination.[148–151] Holin and associates found that among 576 persons with solitary nodules whose health status could be established 5 or more years after diagnosis, 7.1% were ill or had died because of the nodules.[148] Only 2.6% of the deaths within the study population were directly or indirectly related to the nodules. The deaths were all caused by malignant nodules. Reactivation tuberculosis was responsible for the illness occurring in the majority of the small remaining number of patients who experienced symptoms. In a smaller group of 88 solitary nodules identified from a mass roentgen survey, Comstock identified 5 deaths directly associated with the nodules.[151] Three patients died from carcinoma of the lung and 2 had reactivation tuberculosis. He concluded that neither routine observation nor indiscriminate excision could be recommended, and that careful application of diagnostic leads be made in patients selected for surgery. These cases in studies by Holin and Comstock were obtained from *prevalence studies* in which unfavorable cases with short survival times are always underrepresented.[148,151] The Philadelphia Pulmonary Neoplasm Research Project followed 121 *incident cases* in which malignant solitary pulmonary nodules were found after initially negative chest roentgenograms. The resection rate of only 33% and the 8% 5-year survival rate emphasize the difference between hospital or clinic prevalence studies and the Philadelphia Project's incidence data.[149,150]

The prognosis for the patient with a malignant solitary nodule occurring among those in a selected surgical series is well documented and is outlined in Table 15-7. The observed survival rates which show approximately a third of the patients to be alive at 3 and 5 years are remarkably consistent when interstudy variations in nodule size, histopathology, patient age, and presence of symptoms are considered. There have been no wide differences in survival related to cell type. Jackman found the 3-year survival rate for 17 alveolar cell carcinomas to be 94%. Ten of these tumors were under 2 cm in diameter and their small size may have materially affected survival; Steel found the survival for 17 patients with alveolar cell carcinoma to be no different from that for patients with other types of adenocarcinomas.[179,180] Oat cell carcinomas represent a very small percentage of malignant solitary nodules and only 10 oat cell carcinomas were found among the 585 primary bronchogenic carcinomas in these two studies. Occasional long-term survivals have occurred after the resection of solitary nodules shown to be oat cell carcinomas; however, when such diagnoses are established before surgery, irradiation is the treatment of choice.[110]

There is some difference of opinion as to how much the prognosis is altered when bronchogenic carcinomas are resected as solitary nodules. Vance and Bateson independently concluded that the survival of patients operated upon for a solitary circumscribed lesion of the lung resulting from bronchogenic carcinoma was no better than that for a composite group of patients in which all types of resectable bronchogenic carcinoma were represented.[175,178] In contrast, O'Connor, in a study of 46 patients with malignant solitary nodules, found the resectability rate to be 100%. The observed 5-year survival rate in this group was 93%.[177] In a second composite group of 453 patients with bronchogenic carcinoma having a resectability rate of 23%, he found the 5-year survival to be 7%. The difference in the findings of these three studies appears to be in the larger number of symptomatic patients treated by Vance and Bateson. The resectability rate or the number of patients in whom all apparent carcinoma is removed does increase when operations are done for asymptomatic solitary nodules.

Some authors stress the survival achieved when only those patients who appear to have undergone "curative resection" and who survive operation and hospitalization are counted. This derivative figure may also be statistically treated by life-table analysis so as to give relative survival: what survival would be after subtracting the mortality expected in a normal population of the same age. This method of determining outcome yields 5-year survivals of approximately 50% but is difficult to compare with studies reporting observed survival (Table 15-7). Relative survival rates are useful when analyzing survival

TABLE 15-7. Survival of Patients with Malignant Pulmonary Nodules

Author	Year	Cases	Percent Unre-sectable	Percent Resected Total	Percent Resected For Cure	Percent Operative Mortality	Percent Survival 3 Yr	Percent Survival 5 Yr
Vance[175]	1959	94	10	90	87	5.3	36.6*	
Tala[176]	1960	97		100		6.2	34*‡	26.5*‡
O'Connor[177]	1963	46						93*
Bateson[178]	1964	100	12	88		10	37.5*	
Steel[179]	1966	392	5.6	94	79	6.4		38* (45.4)†
Jackman[180]	1969	193	5.7		94.3	7.3		45.3†

* Observed survival.
† Relative survival rate statistically calculated by life table analysis (*i.e.*, what survival would be after correction for mortality expected to occur in a normal population of the same age).
‡ Excludes operative mortality.

by histologic type, because the incidence of different cell types varies with age. A calculated survival rate which also excludes unresectable cases and operative mortalities is of less obvious value.[180] Regardless of how the survival figures are statistically treated, approximately 4 patients in 10 can be expected to be alive 5 years after operation for a solitary malignant nodule. Those who die from their malignancy are about evenly divided between those with local recurrence and those with distant metastases. Three factors: patient age, tumor doubling time, and primary tumor size, have marked and independent influences on survival. Poor prognosis is associated with age over 65 years, fast-growing tumors with doubling times less than 120 days, and tumor diameter greater than 2.5 cm. There appears to be a real advantage in the resection of smaller nodules since tumor-free long-term survivors differ from those who die of their malignant nodules, not in having slower growth rates, but in having smaller tumors at resection.[144,150]

Common Nonmalignant Lesions Presenting as Solitary Pulmonary Nodules

Very Common
- Granulomas
  - Histoplasmoma, tuberculoma, coccidioidoma
  - Cryptococcosis, blastomycosis, actinomycosis
- Unidentified granulomas

Common
- Lung abscess before evacuation into a bronchus
- Slowly resolving circumscribed pneumonia
- Lipoid pneumonia
- Hamartoma

Less Common
- Bronchogenic cyst
- Pulmonary infarct
- Bronchial adenoma
- A-V fistula
- Enlarged pulmonary artery
- Infected, fluid-filled bulla
- Rheumatoid nodule

Differential Diagnosis

The more common nonmalignant lesions which may assume a solitary nodular configuration are listed at right. The granulomas and hamartomas make up 50–60% of all solitary nodules and represent 90% of the nonmalignant nodules. Hamartomas alone comprise approximately 10% of nonmalignant nodules. In the Mississippi and Ohio River valleys of the north and central United States, histoplasmomas are more numerous than tuberculomas. Solitary coccidioidal granulomas are so common in the southwestern and western states that they reduce the incidence of malignant solitary nodules from 30 to 5% in some surgical series.[181,182] The miscellaneous granulomas listed above are responsible for only a small percentage of benign isolated lesions.

The solitary lesions produced by tuberculosis, histoplasmosis, and coccidioidomycosis include: the blocked cavity; circumscribed, rounded, necrotic infiltrates developing centrifugally from a small central focus; and the histoplasmoma (tuberculoma, coccidioidoma) in which a thick layer of concentrically oriented fibrous tissue is found to surround a small necrotic center. The necrotic zone often contains a small number of viable organisms which can be demonstrated by special stains. The histoplasmoma (tuberculoma, coccidioidoma) is the most common benign lesion mistaken for carcinoma and slow concentric enlargement may occur in all three diseases. If unequivocal dense central or laminated calcification is demonstrated, surgical resection can be safely avoided even though enlargement occurs.[183] The blocked cavity may show a dense calcific deposit characteristically eccentrically located along one margin.

When surgery is done to exclude carcinoma and granulomatous disease is found, direct smears with special stains should be done in addition to cultures. The value of Gomori's methenamine silver, Gridley, and periodic acid-Schiff stains over cultures is particularly apparent in the recognition of histoplasmomas and coccidioidomas.[144] The mucicarmine stain may be of use in cryptococcosis. Amphotericin B is not used in conjunction with surgical resection of histoplasmomas or most coccidioidomas.[181,184] However, preoperative amphotericin may be obligatory when contemplating resection of a solitary nodule which may represent a blocked coccidioidal cavity adjacent to the pleural surface, or when an undiagnosed nodule is to be removed from an area in which an earlier coccidioidal pneumonia is known to have existed.[181] Wedge resection is preferred to segmental resection for most granulomas in the peripheral lung field; segmental resection is done only for more central lesions that are difficult to remove with a wedge technique. A portion of the specimen is submitted for pathologic examination, and more extensive resection is performed if the lesion proves to be carcinoma. There is no evidence that initial lobectomy without first ascertaining the benign or malignant nature of the nodule improves survival in those patients proven to have malignancy.

The hamartoma of the lung is a benign growth occurring in an intrapulmonary or, rarely, endobronchial location. Generally considered a tumor resulting from a developmental malformation, the hamartoma is often composed predominantly of cartilage with clefts of bronchial epithelium, fat, smooth muscle and fibrous tissue. Both the intrapulmonary and endobronchial forms have their highest incidence in the sixth decade, an unusual presentation for a developmental lesion. Few cases have been reported in childhood and no cell rests from which hamartomas might develop are recognized in infancy. Given these features, Bateson has persuasively suggested that the lesions are true acquired connective tissue tumors originating in bronchial walls.[185,186] Other concepts of this common tumor are reviewed by Koutras.[186] Malignant change, if it occurs at all, is very rare and although the uncommon endobronchial form may produce obstructive symptoms, the usual peripheral hamartoma is asymptomatic even if located beneath the pleural surface. Since the majority of the tumors are less than 3 cm in diameter, are peripheral, and are within the parenchyma, there is no bronchial obstruction and no abnormal physical finding.

The roentgenographic appearance is that of a nodule having either a hairline sharp margin or the hazy, indistinct margin typical of many carcinomas. The latter appearance is more common because hamartomas have no surrounding capsule. However, in constrast to the lobulated border more characteristic of carcinoma, the border of the hamartoma is usually smooth. Laminograms may demonstrate radiolucencies produced by necrosis or the tumor's fat content.[187] There is no predisposition for any lobe or segment. A popcorn pattern of calcification so strongly suggests hamartoma as to be diagnostic, but calcification of any type is described in only 5 to 25% of cases[188] (Fig. 15-20). Hamartomas may enlarge slowly but occasionally more rapid growth occurs causing a new nodule to appear when recent roentgenograms in adult life have been normal. When the typical popcorn pattern of calcification is recognized, surgery can be withheld even if there is modest growth.

A circumscribed area of unresolved pneumo-

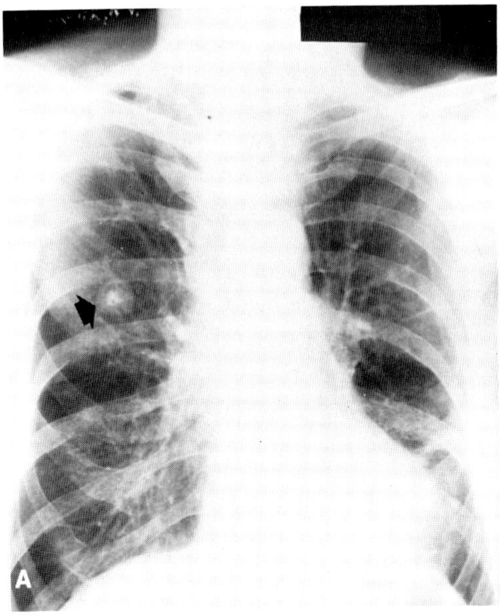

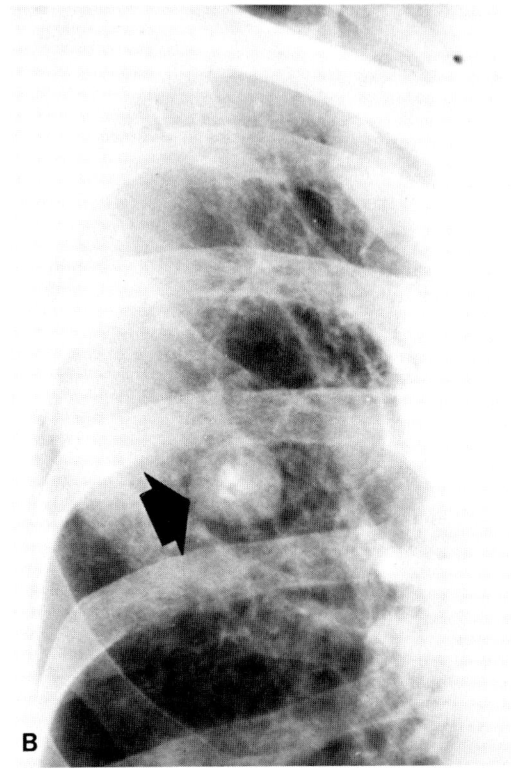

FIG. 15-20. Pulmonary hamartoma. **A.** Pulmonary hamartoma with "popcorn" calcification. **B.** Enlarged photograph. (Chest roentgenogram courtesy of Dr. Robert A. Green, Ann Arbor, Michigan)

nia or an early lung abscess may appear as a solitary pulmonary nodule. The lung abscess presents as a homogeneously dense, roughly spherical abnormality until bronchial communication is established. Evacuation of the liquid contents in the necrotic center into a bronchus then produces an air-fluid interface similar to that seen in some carcinomas. The history and physical examination are critical if these conditions requiring prompt treatment are to be differentiated from malignancy. Superficially, the history may suggest a subacute or chronic disease process consistent with malignancy. Unless carefully questioned as to the symptoms experienced in the first day or two of illness then several weeks past, the patient often fails to relate the initial acuteness of the onset when fever, rigor, emesis, productive cough, chest pain, and prostration typical of pyogenic disease were present. Persistence of fever and leukocytosis may be helpful. Careful auscultation over the involved segment often demonstrates rales, increased vocal fremitus, and bronchial breathing, findings not associated with malignant solitary nodules.

Lipoid pneumonia may also present as a solitary pulmonary nodule. The diagnosis is infrequently made short of thoracotomy because the history fails to include questions concerning the use of mineral oil or oil-containing nose drops. Pulmonary emboli with infarction infrequently masquerade as asymptomatic solitary nodules. A history of peripheral phlebitis followed by an acute insult with pleuritic chest pain, dyspnea, and hemoptysis may or may not be obtained. Infarction of the lung may be suggested by a vaguely wedge-shaped rather than nodular or spheroidal density on the roentgenogram. The base of the wedge occurs on a pleural surface with the apex directed toward the hilum. An isolated parenchymal density is nearly as common as a small unilateral pleural effusion.[100] Arterial blood gases show changes not expected with other solitary pulmonary nodules. Hypoxia is often present. In the absence of hypoxia, the P_{CO_2} may be depressed, indicating that the normal P_{O_2} is maintained by an increase in ventilation. The correctly timed electrocardiogram supports the diagnosis in a minority of cases but may show right axis deviation, right bundle branch block, and acute right heart strain. The abnormality on the chest roentgenogram may persist unchanged or may undergo involution over days to weeks. Ventilation-perfusion scans or pulmonary arteriograms may be diagnostic (see also Chap. 10).

Arteriovenous fistulas may have the roentgenographical appearance of solitary and somewhat lobulated pulmonary nodules.[190] These may be acquired, but are more commonly congenital, and are part of Osler–Weber–Rendu disease (hereditary hemorrhagic telangiectasia) in which arteriovenous communications occur in the lung, skin, mucous membranes, and other organs. In the lung, the fistula or aneurysm is fed and drained by single or multiple pulmonary arteries and veins which may be faintly visualized on the standard chest roentgenogram as serpentine vascular shadows originating from the hilum and directed toward the left atrium. These vessels are best seen on laminograms or pulmonary arteriograms. Larger pulmonary lesions may be associated with dyspnea, clubbing of the fingers, polycythemia, and a continuous thoracic murmur accentuated by inspiration. At fluoroscopy, the fistula can sometimes be shown to decrease in size during the Valsalva maneuver and to increase in size with the Mueller maneuver. In a third of the cases, the pulmonary lesions are multiple; arteriograms are often required to demonstrate more than one lesion (see also Chap. 10).

Enlarged pulmonary arteries may occasionally be mistaken for solitary pulmonary nodules when the chest roentgenograms of patients in congestive heart failure are interpreted. This error most commonly involves lower lobe vessels as they project behind the heart shadow in the lateral projection; it is best avoided by reserving judgement as to the presence of parenchymal lung disease until clinical and roentgenographic evidence of congestive heart failure is resolved by therapy.

Surgical Management

When deciding whether surgery is needed for treating a solitary pulmonary nodule, a simple, somewhat artificial mental maneuver is useful; the assumption is made that there can be no follow-up roentgenogram at 1, 2, or 3 months. An attempt is then made to place the nodule in one of three risk groups:

1. The nodule is probably malignant: little or no clinical information is available to suggest an alternative diagnosis.
2. The nodule may be benign but must be resected now: the clinical information supporting its benign nature is not totally convincing.
3. The nodule is benign: the clinical information is such that there is no reason to explore the problem further.

If the nodule remains unclassified after all available clinical information has been conscientiously collected and weighed, the lesion is placed in the second group and resected. This artifice seeks to force a decision as to whether to resect the nodule at the time it is first recognized. In order to avoid procrastination, one thus deliberately, but only momentarily for the sake of decision-making, ignores the need for additional roentgenograms in the few patients with uncalcified nodules which are to be left in place because they are known not to have changed in size for two years or longer. For example, earlier roentgenograms may indicate that a nodule almost certainly represents a tuberculoma: the isolated, unchanging residual of an inadequately or remotely treated tuberculous pneumonia in a patient now sputum-negative. Such a patient should receive one year of isoniazid chemoprophylaxis because 20% of these lesions result in reactivation of disease. Additional roentgen examination would then be appropriate at 3, 6, and 12 months to document whether involution occurred. When a decision is made not to resect other nodules which have remained unchanged for 2 or more years, the possibility that a lesion may be an adenoma with potential for late growth and metastasis must also be considered. Again, additional periodic roentgenograms would be required to document that such an uncalcified, unchanging, presumably benign, but unresected and undiagnosed nodule remains unchanged. Should subsequent roentgenograms demonstrate enlargement, the lesion might well be resected with adenoma in mind.

The unchanging character of the nodule must be convincingly demonstrated; any doubt on the part of the observer should be resolved by surgery.

SCREENING AND EARLY DIAGNOSIS

In 1971, the Cooperative Early Lung Cancer Group (Mayo Clinic, John Hopkins University, Sloan-Kettering Cancer Center) began a program to determine whether obtaining chest x-ray films annually and sputum cytology every 4 months would lead to a significant reduction in the death rate from lung cancer among men 45 years of age or older who smoked. A periodic health questionnaire was also used.

Early data suggest the program may benefit high-risk patients.[191,192] Men with normal chest roentgenograms and positive sputum cytologies are examined by fiberoptic bronchoscopy under general anesthesia. If initial localizing attempts are unsuccessful, reexamination is done at 1 month and at 2-month intervals thereafter until the cancer is found.[192] If no lesion is visualized, localization is confirmed by bronchial brushing of a segmental orifice on two occasions before surgery is recommended. Chest x-ray films and sputum examinations are complementary because patients with positive sputum cytology usually have central squamous or oat cell carcinomas, while most tumors found with x-ray films are peripheral adenocarcinomas. Ten percent of the patients in the positive cytology–negative chest-x-ray-film category have had cancer in the mouth, pharynx, and larynx. Approximately half the patients with negative chest x-ray films and positive cytologies have had lesions that are seen easily with fiberoptic bronchoscopy. Unfortunately, half have also had cancer invading submucosa. Additional diagnostic yield may be possible by visualizing hematoporphyrin-induced tumor fluorescence through the fiberoptic bronchoscope. Unfortunately, the costs and the photosensitivity induced by the hematoporphyrin may limit the use of this technique.[193,194]

In the Mayo Clinic experience, 86 of 9313 men were found to have lung cancer when they entered the study. Half had occult or otherwise surgically manageable neoplasms. A third of the total were still considered to have a good prognosis after surgery.[191] Fewer rapidly growing tumors and a better overall prognosis would be expected for these prevalence cases. Cancers found at 4-month rescreenings are incidence cases; 59% have been good candidates for surgery. Without this surveillance program, less than a fourth would be expected to be good candidates for exploration.

It is still too early to recommend specific screening programs, or the population most likely to benefit.

THERAPEUTIC PLANNING FOR PATIENTS WITH BRONCHOGENIC CARCINOMA

Long-term survival following radiotherapy or chemotherapy for bronchogenic carcinoma is rare, and only few patients survive 5 years without surgical treatment. Surgical removal of the tumor remains the best hope for all but small cell carcinoma. The best surgical procedure is the one that removes all the tumor with the least possible amount of lung tissue. Lobectomy and pneumonectomy are equally curative, and the use of wedge resections is increasingly being considered for treating small peripheral tumors. Unfortunately, about four-fifths of these patients are beyond surgical salvage when the diagnosis is made. Curative resection in which all the tumor is removed is possible in approximately a quarter of all cases, and only a third of this favorable group lives 5 years.[195] Weiss' detailed analysis of 9 reports appearing between 1960 and 1967 encompassing 6810 operated patients provides an overview of these grim statistics.[196] He has concluded that better selection of patients for exploration rather than more aggressive surgery was responsible for the higher resection rates and improved 5-year survivals among more recently operated patients. Nevertheless, when survivals were calculated so as to include operative deaths, the best individually published 5-year survival rates were 17 and 18%. These figures reflect a national salvage rate which approximates 8%.[197] Publications with data obtained after 1966 confirm that Weiss' conclusions are still valid.[197a,198] Furthermore, the rate of additional primary tumors is high. In one series of 10-year survivers, 20% developed second primaries, half of which were in the lung.[198a]

The Fruitless Thoracotomy

There is evidence that avoidance of the fruitless thoracotomy by appropriately thorough preoperative evaluation directly benefits patients who cannot, or should not, be offered surgical treatment. The operative mortality for right pneumonectomy in men over 60 was 30% in 12 Philadelphia teaching hospitals. Left pneumonectomy was associated with a 10% mortality rate.[199] The surgical mortality for patients who have exploration without resection is commonly overlooked; it was 9.3% in one 1966–1970 study.[198] Several investigators believe that thoracotomy without resection or thoracotomy with inappropriate radical interference with the regional lymphatic filter hastens cancer dissemination, reducing survival time.[200,201] Between 1950 and 1959, Lawrence and his associates investigated extended pneumonectomy with intrapericardial ligation of the pulmonary vessels and removal of gross tumor where there was extension to the mediastinum, heart, pleura, and trachea. In his and other series, this procedure produced an operative mortality 2 to 4 times that seen with conventional lobectomy or pneumonectomy done as curative operations for more conservatively selected patients. Extended pneumonectomy was associated with an average operative mortality of 19%; average 5-year survival rates were less than 7%. Only 22% of Lawrence's patients lived longer than 8 months, and 16% survived 1 year.[202] Palliative pneumonectomies performed when the cancer proves to be unresectable at thoracotomy have been even less rewarding. All 22 patients in Dillon and Postlethwait's series were dead within a year.[203] Delarue and Strasberg reported that none of their patients having palliative pneumonectomy survived 2 years, despite postoperative irradiation.[197] Guttmann's data indicated that the survival of patients irradiated following incomplete resection was inferior to that of patients irradiated after exploratory thoractomy in which no attempt was made to perform a palliative operation for surgically incurable disease.[204]

These and similar figures developed over the last 20 years suggest that the term "palliative operation" is sometimes used euphemistically when surgically incurable cancer is first diagnosed at thoracotomy; they support Harken's early (1954) conclusion that palliative surgery should be reserved for patients having life-threatening hemorrhage or infection.[205] Paulson succinctly summarized this accumulated experience: "Too often the decision to operate is justified on the basis of giving the patient his only chance. More often the patients's best interests as to length and quality of survival are best served by a decision *not* to operate."[200]

If it is important to recognize the shortcomings of the so-called palliative operation for lung cancer, it is critical that the use of thoracotomy as an investigative tool not be so limited as to overlook potentially resectable and curable disease.[206–209]

The Importance of Symptoms and Biologic Predeterminism

Feinstein emphasized that therapeutic decisions for lung cancer patients were generally based on estimates of prognosis arrived at through a staging system which was called clinical, but was really morphologic: the tumor's histology, location, size, and metastatic distribution were considered but its clinical effects in terms of the patient's symptoms were assigned little prognostic or therapeutic significance unless they suggested the presence of obvious, distant, extrathoracic metastases.[210,211] When patients classified into symptom groups (Table 15-8 A) were combined into three clinical stages (Table 15-8 B), Feinstein found a survival gradient that persisted even after the same patients were divided into the conventional morphologic (*i.e.*, anatomic and histologic groups based on a similar extent of tumor spread. Failure to carefully develop

TABLE 15-8. Clinical Classification Including Symptoms: Influence on Survival in Lung Cancer

A. Symptomatic Group	Definition	
Indolent	Asymptomatic	
	Long primary:	Pulmonary symptoms only for > 6 months
Obtrusive	Short primary:	Pulmonary symptoms only for < 6 months
	Systemic:	Anorexia, fatigue, weight loss, osteoarthropathy, and endocrine syndromes caused by the tumor in the absence of metastatic symptoms, with or without primary symptoms.
Deleterious	Metastatic:	Bone pain, some neurologic symptoms

Five-year Survival Rates in Lung Cancer (regardless of type of therapy)

B. Clinical Group	Anatomic Group %)			
	Localized	Regional	Distant	Totals (%)
Indolent	24	10	4	17
Obtrusive	15	5	1	7
Deleterious	0	0	0	0

(Adapted from Feinstein AR: A new staging system for cancer and reappraisal of "early" treatment and "cure" by radical surgery. N Engl J Med 279:747–754, 1968)

and record the presence and duration of local and systemic (nonmetastatic) symptoms was thus shown to introduce serious error in the stratification of patients into treatment groups whose members ideally should closely resemble one another so far as the functional consequences of their cancers are concerned. Because the response of such supposedly homogeneous groups determines the apparent value of various methods of treatment, major differences in therapies may be missed if tumors rather than patients are grouped together for comparison. For example, since slow-growing tumors produce symptoms slowly, it is not surprising that patients who are asymptomatic or who have protracted local symptoms before diagnosis have a higher survival rate than do those whose symptoms are systemic or pulmonary but of short duration.

The importance of this classification was further documented when Senior and Adamson applied Feinstein's system of patient stratification by symptoms to 646 patients with cancer of the lung.[212] Half the patients with *nonspecific* symptoms of excessive fatigue, weight loss, and anorexia had extrathoracic metastases. Whereas 45% of patients with pulmonary symptoms for longer than 6 months were candidates for surgical treatment, only 20 to 28% of patients having either pulmonary symptoms of short duration or systemic but nonmetastatic symptoms could be surgically treated with any expectation of cure. When plotted against duration of symptoms, survival rates followed the same curve.

The differences in survival relative to the symptoms experienced by the group of patients whose tumors all appear localized, are pertinent when deciding how thorough the preoperative evaluation should be in an individual patient. For example, it is difficult to justify routine exploratory laparotomy in all patients shown to have roentgenologically localized, apparently resectable, peripheral, lower lobe neoplasms even though postmortem studies show abdominal lymph node involvement to be more common than involvement of supraclavicular and cervical glands with all bronchogenic neoplasms.[213] On the other hand, when such a cancer occurs in a patient with weakness, anorexia, marked weight loss, and vague gastrointestinal symptoms, laparotomy might be considered before thoracotomy even if the mediastinal lymph nodes examined by mediastinoscopy are negative.

The survival distinction between symptomatic stages appears most significant in the anatomically less extensive tumors that are often treated surgically; therefore, analysis of treatment results among various groups of operated patients would be more profitable if there were some assurance that morphologically similar groups had the same initial performance status with comparable symptoms. In developing the hypothesis of neoplastic "biologic predeterminism," Ian Macdonald stressed that many cancers with similar morphology show different rates of growth and invasiveness.[214] Consequently, the traditional doctrine that curability is directly related to the "earliness" of treatment applies to relatively few cancers such as squamous carcinomas of the skin. The favorably directed bronchogenic carcinoma amenable to surgical cure is more difficult to identify but Feinstein's work makes it clear that it is best to begin with a history and physical examination which carefully document the patient's symptoms.

Contraindications to Surgery in Bronchogenic Carcinoma

- Absolute Contraindications
  - Inadequate pulmonary function and associated cardiac disease
  - Extrathoracic metastases
  - Bronchoscopic observations
    - Widening and fixation of the carina at the tracheal bifurcation
    - Tracheal invasion
    - Advanced left mainstem bronchial involvement within 2 cm. of main carina
  - Persistent, recurrent, and/or bloody pleural effusion
  - Left recurrent laryngeal nerve paralysis secondary to a central neoplasm
  - Esophageal constriction or mucosal distortion by tumor
  - Roentgenographic evidence of bilateral mediastinal lymph node enlargement
  - Hemidiaphragmatic paralysis associated with a central tumor
  - Undifferentiated small or oat cell carcinoma
- Relative Contraindications
  - Advanced age (>70 years)
  - Chest wall invasion
  - Hemidiaphragmatic paralysis associated with a peripheral tumor
  - Superior sulcus tumor with Horner's syndrome or bone involvement
  - Roentgenographic evidence of hilar or mediastinal lymphadenopathy
  - Microscopic evidence of tumor in mediastinal lymph nodes
  - Esophageal displacement by tumor mass in the absence of rigidity, mucosal involvement, or loss of peristalsis
  - Pronounced systemic symptoms: anorexia, weight loss, excessive fatigue often accompanied by vague, unexplained thoracic or abdominal discomfort

In the majority of inoperable patients with bronchogenic carcinoma, surgical treatment is precluded by the anatomic location or extent of the cancer. The absolute and relative contraindications to surgery are given above. There is a growing consensus that patients known to have undifferentiated small cell or oat cell carcinoma should be treated with chemotherapy and radiotherapy. A controlled, prospective, randomized, cooperative study by the British Medical Research Council showed a statistically significant though small increase in mean patient survival when tumors of this type diagnosed by bronchoscopic biopsy were treated with radiation rather than surgery. The survival rates for 71 patients in the surgery series and 73 patients in the radiotherapy series were 4% and 10% at 24 months, 3% and 7% at 48 months, and 1% and 4% at 60 months.[110] Multiple-drug chemotherapy would now also be used in such cases.

TNM Classification

The American Joint Committee for Cancer Staging and End Results Reporting (AJC) encourages the methodical classification of lung cancer patients according to the tumor–nodal–metastasis (TNM) system. The letter T with ascending subscripts indicates the size and extension of the primary tumor, N the degree of regional lymph node disease, and M the presence or absence of distant metastases.[215,216] Table 15-9 gives the essential elements of the TNM system. The carcinomas represented by TNM combinations are grouped into three stages in such a way that those in a given stage have a sim-

TABLE 15-9. Tumor–Node–Metastasis (TNM) Classification of Bronchogenic Cancer

	T Primary Tumor
$T_xN_0M_0$	Positive cytology, negative chest roentgenogram and bronchoscopy
T_1	Tumor ≤ 3 cm, surrounded by lung without evidence of invasion proximal to lobar bronchus at bronchoscopy
T_2	Tumor > 3 cm or any size tumor invading visceral pleura or having associated obstructive atelectasis or pneumonia extending to hilum. Must be 2 cm distal to the carina. Atelectasis or pneumonia must involve less than entire lung. No pleural effusion.
T_3	Tumor of any size with direct extension to parietal pleura, chest wall, diaphragm, or mediastinum. Tumor otherwise more extensive than stage 2.
	N Regional Lymph Nodes
N_0	No lymph node metastases
N_1	Regional lymph node metastases excluding mediastinum
N_2	Mediastinal lymph node metastases
	M Distant Metastases
M_0	No distant metastases
M_1	Metastases outside the thorax or to the contralateral hilar lymph nodes or lung

TABLE 15-10. TNM Staging of Bronchogenic Cancer

Stage I	$T_1N_0M_0$ $T_1N_1M_0$ $T_2N_0M_0$
Stage II	$T_2N_1M_0$
Stage III	T_3 with any N or M N_2 with any T or M M_1 with any T or N

Five Year Survival Rates

	Stage		
Cell Type	*I(%)*	*II(%)*	*II(%)*
Squamous	38	16	9
Adenocarcinoma	32	7	3
Large cell	30	6	5
Small cell	0	0	0

ilar prognosis with comparable treatment. The TNM stages and 5-year survival rates for tumors of different cell types are given in Table 15-10.

Effective use of the TNM system also requires that the performance status of the host be recorded. This is indicated by the letter H and encompasses general condition, activity, and symptoms. The prognostic importance of performance status has been recognized for some time and the older Karnofsky Scale still is used to rank patients. Table 15-11 (p. 865) shows the Karnofsky scale with the equivalent Host Performance Status (H) for the AJC-TNM system. The percentile groups in the Karnofsky scale are collapsed into five H groups; for example, patients capable of normal activity (Karnofsky 90 to 100) are identified as H_0.

Correct definition of the T (tumor) subscript requires a chest roentgenogram and bronchoscopy. Lung and mediastinal tomograms, a gallium-67 radionuclide scan, and some method of mediastinal exploration may be used to place a patient in the proper N (node metastases) group. The patient's history, physical examination, admission laboratory panel with the liver function tests, and radionuclide scans all may be necessary when fixing the M (metastases) class for a patient with vague symptoms or pronounced weight loss. The TNM system promotes thorough examination and improves comparisons of different treatments by making patient groups more homogeneous.

The Preoperative Evaluation: Avoiding a Routine

Following the history, physical examination, and chest roentgenogram in the posteroanterior and lateral projections, the preoperative evaluation of any potentially operable patient with bronchogenic carcinoma should include pulmonary function tests, electrocardiogram, hemogram, serum calcium determination, liver and kidney function tests, and coagulation profile. The latter anticipates additional diagnostic studies such as bronchoscopic biopsy and is needed if surgery proves feasible. All other invasive or noninvasive investigations should be undertaken only after some thought is given to their potential diagnostic yield. Below is a list of studies which are done for diagnosis and therapeutic planning; the worth of each technique is largely dependent on the discrimination with which it is used.

Methods for Assessment of Operability for Bronchogenic Carcinoma

Clinical Evaluation
- Symptomatic stage
- Anatomic stage
- Biologic predeterminism of the tumor
  - Earlier roentgenograms may allow growth rate to be determined

Special Radiographic Techniques
- Laminograms (tomograms)
- Fluoroscopy
- Contrast studies
  - Barium swallow
  - Pulmonary arteriogram
  - Intraosseous azygour venography
- Bone survey (very low yield in absence of bone pain)

Radionuclide Studies
- Gallium scan of primary tumor and mediastinum
- Pulmonary ventilation-perfusion scan
- Liver, bone and brain scan
- Scintillation venocavogram
- Electroencephalography
- Bronchoscopy
- Bronchial brushing
- Bone marrow biopsy
- Percutaneous pleural or parenchymal needle biopsy
- Scalene lymph node biopsy
- Mediastinoscopy
- Limited cervico—or parasternal mediastinal exploration
- Transabdominal exploration
- Exploratory thoracotomy

Although more useful pulmonary function data are obtained after the smoking patient has received an adequate course of chest physiotherapy, antibiotics, and bronchodilators, these tests should not be long delayed in patients with bedside evidence of serious generalized respiratory disease. No patient should be subjected to a battery of uncomfortable and expensive preoperative investigations only to be denied surgery on the basis of respiratory or cardiac reserve so marginal as to demand documentation at the outset. (See detailed discussion, Pulmonary Effects of Surgical Procedures, Chap. 11.)

When there is pleural effusion, thoracentesis and pleural biopsy should be performed early. If the effusion is bloody, and the pleural fluid cell block or biopsy is shown to contain malignancy, there is little reason to examine the cytology of multiple sputum specimens; bronchoscopy is equally unnecessary because treatment will not be surgical. Similarly, sputum cytology and bronchoscopy with a rigid bronchoscope are unlikely to be helpful in evaluating small peripheral nodules (see The Solitary Pulmonary Nodule), and an early decision should be made as to how many cytologic specimens from sputum are to be processed. This will depend on the skill of the local cytologist and on the size and location of the nodule. Histologic confirmation and classification of late stage cancer is sometimes more easily obtained by aspiration or excisional biopsy of obvious rib, lymph node, or subcutaneous metastases than bronchoscopy. Subcutaneous nodules are commonly known to the patient who fears their significance, and so fails to volunteer their location. Enlarged, firm, superficial, supraclavicular and cervical lymph nodes should be carefully sought. Biopsy of these glands is not associated with the small but definite morbidity and mortality seen with scalene fat pad dissection, mediastinoscopy, or limited cervical-mediastinal exploration. Some patients with enlarged lymph nodes in these areas will have negative biopsies, emphasizing the importance of histologic confirmation before hope of surgical treatment is abandoned. In the absence of extensive chest wall invasion, lung cancer seldom involves the axillary lymph nodes, and enlargement of these glands is seldom an indication for biopsy. These lymph nodes are commonly enlarged in patients whose work causes repeated minor cuts and abrasions on the extremity.

When all efforts to obtain preoperative histologic confirmation of cancer fail in the patient with a circumscribed and apparently resectable mass lesion, efforts are sometimes made to obtain positive cytology by percutaneous aspiration through a small 20-21 gauge needle. This technique provides only aspirated cytologic material for study and produces a false-negative specimen in 10 to 25% of patients. The policy of confirming a cancer diagnosis by using this procedure as a last resort in operable patients who almost certainly harbor cancer seems unwarranted, because thoracotomy will be performed whether or not the cytology obtained is positive. Needle aspiration is of more value in the inoperable patient whose cancer proves difficult to verify prior to anticipated drug or irradiation therapy.

Specific Tests for Difficult Decisions

Patients with central tumors in close proximity to the mediastinal structures, and those with prominent systemic symptoms in whom pronounced weight loss is often accompanied by vague, unexplained thoracic, abdominal, or skeletal discomfort require a more comprehensive preoperative investigation to exclude surgically incurable metastatic disease. An esophagogram should be performed early in all patients with medially located tumors in whom spread to the posteroinferior mediastinal (paraesophageal) and/or carinal lymph nodes may have occurred. Neoplasms in the lower lobe of either the right or left lung may involve the paraesophageal nodes which lie adjacent to the lower half of the esophagus. Enlargement of these nodes produces an indentation on the right side of the esophagus several centimeters below the carina on the posterioranterior roentgenogram. The esophagogram may also demonstrate disease in the carinal nodes at the bifurcation of the trachea. Since the esophagus passes slightly to the left of the main carina, the left anterior oblique projection often shows carinal node enlargement to the best advantage. As indicated in the preceding list, enlargement of these nodal "sump" areas is a relative contraindication to surgery. Rigidity, fixation, or mucosal distortion seen during fluoroscopy or esophagoscopy are absolute contraindications to surgery.

Well-penetrated Bucky films and laminograms of the mediastinum in the anteroposterior and lateral views may also identify lymphadenopathy unsuspected on routine chest roentgenograms. Benign reactive hyperplasia and sarcoid reactions are very occasionally responsible for roentgenographic enlargement of lymph nodes draining tumor-bearing areas but there is good correlation between operative findings of malignant invasion of lymph nodes and laminographic demonstration of lymphadenopathy.[217,218] When assessing operability, these investigations complement and should precede the more invasive techniques of pulmonary angiography, azygous venography, mediastinoscopy, and bronchoscopy. The easily performed, inexpensive, risk-free laminogram and esophagogram are useful in selecting patients for mediastinoscopy; when grossly abnormal they may establish inoperability obviating the need for additional studies, including bronchoscopy.

Early regional metastases from tumors originating close to the mediastinum commonly cause phrenic nerve paralysis and the fluoroscopic examination performed with the esophagogram provides important information concerning movement of the diaphragm. When one hemidiaphragm appears fixed on physical examination or is shown to occupy an elevated position on the chest roentgenogram, chest fluoroscopy must include the sniff test. Complete fixation of the diaphragm is seen with adjacent suppurative processes such as subdiaphragmatic abscess, but can also occur in some cases of paralysis, eventration, and traumatic herniation. In the latter three conditions, the diaphragm shows paradoxic motion with the sniff test: the affected side rises on inspiration because the increased abdomino-thoracic pressure difference causes passive upward displacement of the involved hemidiaphragm. When a peripheral cancer, remote from the hilum, causes paralysis of the diaphragm by medial extension and infiltration of the phrenic nerve as it passes over the pericardium, resection is sometimes possible if a portion of the pericardium is excised. Paradoxical movement of the diaphragm associated with tumors originating in a more medial location indicates invasion of the phrenic nerve with the mediastinum at the lung root, an absolute indication of inoperability. Appreciation of the importance of the motion of the diaphragm as determined by physical examination and inspiratory-expiratory roentgenograms may therefore limit the preoperative evaluation to a single, noninvasive, inexpensive test: chest fluoroscopy with the sniff maneuver showing a paralyzed diaphragm. Ultrasound also can document abnormal motion of the diaphragm and gives a permanent record without exposure to irradiation.[56]

Direct central extension by the primary neoplasm and regional mediastinal lymphatic metastases may also be demonstrated by outlining the superior vena cava, main pulmonary vessels, and atrial silhouette by pulmonary angiography, a study used primarily to determine whether surgical resection is technically feasible. An angiogram may suggest that it is physically possible to resect the primary neoplasm when positive biopsies from mediastinal or scalene lymph nodes indicate surgical incurability. Angiography is defined as negative when the pulmonary vasculature is unaffected by tumor or when any change lies beyond the main pulmonary vessels and does not involve the superior vena cava. On the other hand, negative regional lymph node biopsies may encourage an unwarranted attempt at surgery when a pulmonary angiogram shows a technically unfavorable situation exists, the primary neoplasm involving the superior vena cava, pericardium, atrium, or pulmonary arteries within 2 cm of their origin.

The nonresectability rate in patients with a negative pulmonary angiogram approximates to 20%, but some patients with positive angiograms prove to be long-term surgical survivors.[208] The occasional long-term survivor and the high false-negative rate are probably responsible for the differences of opinion as to the value of the preoperative angiogram.[197,219]

Although the esophagogram and pulmonary angiogram evaluate somewhat similar areas for central extension, a positive angiogram is commonly associated with a negative esophagogram. A positive esophagogram usually indicates nonresectability, thus obviating the need for angiography; when angiograms are performed in such cases, they are nearly always positive.[197]

The intraosseous azygogram with or without superior vena cavography has also been used to evaluate the preoperative status of the mediastinum in patients with bronchogenic carcinoma. Contrast material is injected into the marrow cavity of the tenth rib in the mid or posterior axillary line using a 16-gauge bone marrow needle. Opacification of the azygous and hemiazygous veins occurs through their major tributaries, the intercostal veins, and overt blockage of flow, retrograde or collateral filling, and localized venous defects are considered indications of inoperability. Superior vena cavograms are then obtained with the same rapid-sequence film changer after 25 ml of Hypaque is simultaneously injected into the basilic veins in both antecubital fossae.[220] Frequent false-negative examinations make the normal azygogram of little value in ascertaining operability but an abnormal study is a strong indication of inoperability. Wolfel and his associates feel that these studies add little information as to the status of the mediastinum beyond what can be learned from simpler (esophagogram, laminogram) or more direct (angiogram) roentgenographic techniques.[221] Venacavography, aortography, azygograms, and pulmonary arteriograms are no longer used routinely because mediastinoscopy and cervico- or parasternal mediastinotomy are more reliable.

Patients with bronchogenic carcinoma who give histories or show evidence of change in voice should be examined by indirect or direct laryngoscopy. Second primary laryngeal carcinomas are not rare in these patients and involvement of the left superior tracheo-bronchial lymph nodes in the concavity of the aortic arch by bronchogenic carcinoma commonly causes infiltration of the recurrent laryngeal nerve with left vocal cord paralysis. A thorough oral and laryngeal examination should also be performed promptly whenever cytologic examination shows cancer cells in the sputum of a patient whose chest roentgenogram has demonstrated an undetermined abnormality or is interpreted as being negative. Paralysis of the left vocal cord from malignant invasion of the left recurrent laryngeal nerve is an absolute contraindication to surgical treatment.

Bronchoscopy

Bronchoscopic examination of the tracheobronchial tree is often a useful procedure for establishing a diagnosis of tumor and for providing additional information useful in planning therapy. Bronchoscopy for the latter indication may be carried out even in cases in which a diagnosis has already been established by sputum cytologic examination or biopsy of a metastatic lesion. Both the conventional, large, rigid bronchoscope popularized in 1904 and the smaller, flexible fiberoptic instrument introduced in the US in 1970 play important roles. There are specific indications for each.[222]

Technical aspects of the use of these instruments are discussed elsewhere.[222–225] The rigid instrument is introduced through the larynx via the open mouth, with the patient supine and the head extended, and its use requires excellent local or more commonly, general anesthesia. Mechanically assisted ventilation and oxygen supplementation can be maintained through a sidearm. The smaller-diameter flexible instrument can be introduced through the nares or the mouth, with or without prior placement of an endotracheal tube, with the patient sitting or supine. The small size and flexibility substantially reduce discomfort to the patient.

Bronchoscopy is most likely to provide a gross and histologic diagnosis of tumor in that group of patients whose presenting symptoms and signs are those described above under the headings Findings Associated with Cancers of the Main Bronchus and Findings with Carcinoma of the Lobar Bronchus. These include cough, hemoptysis, localized wheeze, and the physical and roentgenologic signs of bronchial obstruction with distal atelectasis or pneumonia. Such central tumors are generally accessible to the rigid bronchoscope and may be visualized and biopsied through this instrument. Preoperative assessment of the extent of necessary resection may be facilitated by direct observation of the degree of endobronchial extension. Deep biopsy of a normal-appearing carina occasionally provides microscopic evidence of submucosal spread. This technique may prevent fruitless thoracotomy in such a case of unresectable tumor.

Lesions which are more peripheral are accessible to the newer flexible fiberoptic bronchoscope. The field of vision of the rigid bronchoscope extends only to segmental orifices, while the flexible bronchofiberscope can readily be used to visualize subsegmental bronchi. In one early study by Ikeda[226] of 360 lung cancer cases, 159 lesions were seen with the rigid instrument, while another 140 tumors were accessible to the flexible bronchoscope. In addition, a certain number of visually inaccessible lesions still more peripheral in location can be brushed or biopsied with instruments passed beyond the tip of the bronchofiberscope under fluoroscopic control. In one series,[168] a 78% diagnostic yield was obtained in a series of peripheral tumors in which fluoroscopy confirmed entry of a brush into the lesion by this technique.

Review articles with excellent bibliographies give a history of bronchoscopy, explain the techniques, and state the indications and complications when the rigid and fiberoptic bronchoscopes are used.[222,223] The indications include unexplained cough, hemoptysis, localized wheeze, bronchial obstruction, atelectasis, abnormal chest roentgenograph, or sputum cytology, diaphragmatic or vocal cord paralysis, and diffuse parenchymal disease for transbronchial biopsy. Therapeutic bronchoscopy may be used to remove foreign bodies or tenacious secretions. Mechanical ventilation can be maintained through the side arm of the rigid bronchoscope, or a flexible instrument may be introduced through a T-tube adaptor while conventional mechanical ventilation is carried out with an endotracheal tube.

Rigid bronchoscopy is preferred for removal of foreign bodies and biopsy of vascular tumors, the latter since brisk hemorrhage may be more readily controlled by this method. Deeper biopsy of submucosal lesions is feasible with the larger forceps which can be passed through a rigid instrument.

Flexible fiberscopy generally causes less patient discomfort and is associated with fewer complications. It is clearly preferred for evaluations of peripheral or upper lobe lesions inaccessible to the rigid instrument, and in cases of mechanical hindrance such as stiff neck.

Complications of bronchoscopy include adverse reaction to medications, hemorrhage from brushing or biopsy, bronchospasm, breakage of the instrument inside the bronchus, laryngeal spasm edema and subglottic edema, hypoxemia, arrhythmias, sepsis and perforation with pneumothorax or pneumomediastinum. The latter two complications occur with rigid bronchoscopy. Air embolism has followed transbronchial biopsy of parenchymal abnormalities with the fiberscope.[227]

A recent survey of 25,000 bronchofiberscopies[228] found a very low incidence of complications. The incidence of minor complications was 0.2%; of major complications, 0.08%; and of death, 0.01%. Laryngospasm, bronchospasm, and side-effects of medications accounted for most of these problems.

Mediastinoscopy

The more closely a biopsy procedure approximates the primary cancer or its regional lymphatic filter, the better the surgical specimens obtained will reflect nonresectable extension of disease. Thus, in 1959 Carlens introduced the mediastinoscope which is used to visualize the superior mediastinum through a 3 to 4 cm transverse incision 2 cm above the suprasternal notch.[229] Under general anesthesia, a tissue cleavage plane is established by blunt dissection. Insertion of the instrument anterior to the trachea and posterior to the great vessels allows biopsy of the paratracheal, superior, and inferior tracheobronchial (subcarinal) lymph nodes on both sides of the mediastinum. Retrotracheal structures including the posterior inferior group of subcarinal nodes, as well as the anterior mediastinal nodes, and those lying adjacent to the inferolateral aspect of the aortic arch (subaortic nodes) are outside the field of the mediastinoscope and cannot be biopsied.[230] Mediastinoscopy has superseded scalene node biopsy in many centers because it allows examination of the ipsilateral high paratracheal and contralateral tracheobronchial lymph nodes. Involvement of these nodes by metastases is considered evidence of inoperability by many surgeons because the paratracheal nodes are one step removed from, and form the link between, the tracheobronchial nodes below and the inferior deep cervical (scalene) nodes above.

There is continuing controversy as to whether surgery should be performed on the relatively large and therefore important group of patients in which bronchial cancer has been identified in these superior mediastinal lymph nodes.[206–209, 230,231] Paulson's criteria for operability in this circumstance strike a reasonable compromise: to be operable, mediastinal node involvement should be ipsilateral; it should be low paratracheal or tracheobronchial (azygous, subcarinal, subaortic) in position; and it should be intranodal in type. Tumor which transgresses the capsule of these nodes is considered inoperable.[230] Pearson described 32 patients whose mediastinal examinations met these criteria.[230] Surgical treatment was given following preoperative irradiation with 4000 rad. The statistically projected 5-year survival of 26 of these 32 patients with squamous cell carcinoma was 20%. None of the patients with adenocarcinoma or small cell carcinoma survived a year after the combined therapy.

Kirsh and others have presented retrospective data suggesting that some cancers metastatic to the bronchopulmonary (interlobar and hilar), subcarinal, and superior mediastinal lymph nodes can be cured by surgery.[198,206,207] In Kirsh's work, success was limited to patients with squamous cell cancers with no tomographic evidence of mediastinal lymph node metastases.[206] Patients found to have mediastinal metastases at surgery were given postoperative irradiation. The 29.5% 5-year survival rate was achieved without preoperative mediastinoscopy, but was dependent on the most careful patient selection. It should be noted that other studies which were both prospective and controlled have shown neither pre- nor postoperative radiation to improve survival in patients resected with the expectation of surgical cure.[232,233]

Still other authors believe that mediastinoscopic demonstration of neoplasm in the superior mediastinal lymph nodes is an absolute contraindication to operation, since most series indicate less than 10% of patients in this group live 5 years.[234] Mediastinoscopy enthusiasts believe that the procedure should be routinely applied in the preoperative assessment of patients with presumably operable bronchial carcinoma and point out that the technique identifies metastases within the mediastinal lymph nodes in about 30% of patients otherwise considered operable.[200,230] False-negative results have been shown to be 5 to 20% and rates for "resection for cure" in patients with negative mediastinoscopic examination are generally above 80%, or more than double the usual figure.

Mediastinoscopy is least helpful in evaluating neoplasms of the left upper lobe and left hilum where metastases occur to the anterior mediastinal and subaortic lymph nodes which are inaccessible to the mediastinoscopist.[230] Parasternal anterior mediastinotomy therefore is employed as part of the evaluation of tumors of the left upper lobe.[205,235] When patients are considered inoperable following mediastinoscopy, the information obtained may be useful in planning radiotherapy.

The general anesthetic risk incurred with mediastinoscopy, lack of familiarity with the procedure, and significant differences in surgical salvage achieved among patients with mediastinal metastases all contribute to the reluctance of many to abandon the limited exploratory thoracotomy for otherwise operable patients who show no roentgenographic evidence of mediastinal disease. Carlens reviewed 5000 mediastinoscopies and found less than 3% complications and less than 1% mortality.[229]

Recently reports stress the high correlation of mediastinal tomograms and gallium-67 radionuclide scans with medastinoscopy results. This suggests a tendency to use mediastinoscopy more selectively. A 95% agreement between normal conventional mediastinal tomography and negative biopsy of mediastinal lymph nodes has been reported.[218,236,237]

Radionuclide Studies

Gallium-67 citrate has been used for imaging tumors and inflammatory foci, especially lung abscess. When other causes of ^{67}Ga uptake such as lymphoma, Hodgkin's disease, infection, and sarcoidosis are excluded, the procedure is helpful because the sensitivity in lung cancers is 85% or greater.[240] If the primary lung cancer and mediastinal lymph nodes take up ^{67}Ga, there is a 90% probability that the mediastinal lymph nodes contain tumor. Some would then stop the preoperative evaluation. That is, the patient would be denied surgery and mediastinoscopy would be done only if a histologic diagnosis of cancer was still needed. Occasional patients with false-positive scans would thereby be denied an operation with the potential for cure. In contrast, a third of the patients with ^{67}Ga concentration in the primary tumor but none in the mediastinum are false-negatives, that is metastatic neoplasm is present in lymph nodes.[240] Two disparate recommendations regarding gallium scans and mediastinoscopy have been published.[238–240] The more convincing suggests mediastinoscopy when the primary tumor concentrates gallium and the mediastinum does not; the more widely recognized says mediastinoscopy can be omitted in this situation but that it should be done when both the primary tumor and the mediastinum concentrate gallium. Both support mediastinoscopy when the primary tumor does not concentrate gallium.

The large number of false-negative ^{67}Ga mediastinal scans are most often caused by paramediastinal primary tumors obscuring ipsilateral lymph node metastases; the presence of lymph node metastases less than 2 cm in diameter (some intranodal); and metastases to supraclavicular nodes that appear to bypass the mediastinum.

Extrathoracic metastases also concentrate ^{67}Ga and a whole-body gallium scan makes it possible to restrict the number of specific organ scans.[208]

These conclusions seem warranted: patients with a perihilar mass confluent with mediastinal margins, or proximal to a lobar orifice at bronchoscopy are beyond surgical salvage if they have tomographic evidence of mediastinal adenopathy or laryngeal nerve palsy of recent onset. Those with normal tomograms but positive gallium scans in both primary and mediastinum should undergo mediastinal exploration if less invasive tests fail to confirm inoperability. If the tumor is in the upper lobe on the left, mediastinotomy is indicated. Patients with normal tomograms, gallium-positive peripheral lesions greater than 2 cm in diameter, and negative mediastinal gallium scans can be spared mediastinoscopy with 95% confidence. Those with ^{67}GA-positive central tumors and negative ^{67}GA scans of the mediastinum should undergo mediastinoscopy. If this is not planned, there is little point to doing the scan. Finally, "linear stranding toward the hilum" is more suggestive of granulomatous or other inflammatory disease than cancer and contributes nothing to discussions of operability.[236]

Studies in which radionuclide scans of the brain, liver, and bone have been routinely performed in patients with lung cancer indicate that there is a good probability of demonstrating metastatic disease only when the history, localized physical findings, or specific abnormalities in routine laboratory tests clearly focus clinical suspicion.[241] Without such directed suspicion, the diagnostic yield from radiopharmaceutical studies and roentgenographic bone surveys has ranged from 1 to 5%. Patients who experience pronounced weight loss, fatigue, or nondescript thoracic or abdominal discomfort without other clear-cut evidence of metastatic disease may warrant evaluation by abdominal exploration, biopsy of nonpalpable scalene lymph nodes, and radionuclide scans of the liver, bones, and brain.

Ventilation and perfusion scans of the lung are sometimes performed in patients with borderline pulmonary reserve in an effort to determine the proportion of the pulmonary function contributed by lung which is to be sacrificed at operation (see Pulmonary Effects of Surgical Procedures, Chap. 10). Lung scans are less useful in determining the anatomic extent and potential operability of neoplasms. Perfusion scans of the lung occasionally suggest the presence of a central tumor in the mediastinal area not noted on the roentgenograph, but peripheral tumors must be 3 cm in diameter to be depicted on perfusion scans. Benign and malignant lesions may produce similar perfusion defects regardless of location. Some perfusion abnormalities are the direct result of tumor compression or invasion of pulmonary vessels. Ventilation disorders caused by tumors indirectly may be responsible for perfusion defects. Increases in alveolar pressure produced by ball-valve mechanisms which interfere with expiration more than inspiration or decreases in alveolar oxygen tension caused by local neoplastic impediments to ventilation may cause corresponding reflex abnormalities of regional perfusion in some patients with lung cancer.[242] It is not uncommon for the perfusion defect to be much larger than the mass lesion on the chest roentgenogram. Whether the perfusion defects are the result of vessel invasion or of reflex vascular responses cannot be determined in individual cases. In general, patients with normal scans or with changes comparable to those on the chest roentgenogram have the best chance of resectability.[243] The correlation between the degree of functional perfusion defect and likelihood of successful resection is a relatively poor one, however, and the lung scan is seldom a major determinant in decisions about whether a patient should be operated on.[242,244]

Scalene Lymph Node Biopsy

Scalene lymph node biopsy has been used to determine operability in bronchial carcinoma since 1949 with the side for unilateral biopsy usually being selected on the basis of Rouviere's injection studies with newborns which suggested that the lymphatic drainage from the mid- and lower third of the left lung was mainly contralateral.[245] Mediastinoscopic studies in adults have improved understanding of the metastatic pathways taken by bronchial carcinomas in the lower lobe of the left lung, but confirm that contralateral spread with eventual involvement of the right scalene nodes occurs at least as frequently as does spread to the left scalene nodes. Left lower lobe tumors spread to the paratracheal nodes on the left less frequently than to the right paratracheal nodes. Nevertheless, the left scalene nodes often show metastatic disease from tumors in the left mid- and lower lung field. Upward spread is believed to occur through the chain of anterior mediastinal nodes lying on the inferior border of the left innominate vein rather than through the paratracheal group.

Tumors in the upper lobe of the left lung metastasize to the left and right scalene nodes with about equal frequency.[246,247] Lymphatic penetration by tumors in the whole of the right lung is predominantly ipsilateral but exceptions are sufficiently frequent as to allow Bramtigan to persuasively argue for bilateral scalene lymph node biopsy.[247]

Scalene node biopsy is indicated for patients who have palpable nodes but who appear otherwise potentially curable, and for incurable patients with palpable nodes in whom a tissue diagnosis cannot be made short of thoractomy. Poor-risk patients and those whose tumors are of questionable curability should be biopsied particularly when there is a suggestion of hilar or paratracheal extension. The overall yield of positive biopsies for patients who appear curable and who have no palpable adenopathy is less than 10%. Patients in this latter category who are known to harbor adenocarcinoma or undifferentiated carcinoma are often subjected to scalene biopsy because some series have shown that approximately 20% of biopsies are positive in the circumstance. Mediastinoscopy has replaced biopsy of nonpalpable scalene lymph nodes in many centers.

The major complications of scalene lymph node biopsy are insufficiently emphasized in the literature and include chylothorax, pneumothorax, hemorrhage, air embolism, and phrenic, axillary, and recurrent laryngeal nerve injury in perhaps 5% of patients. Deaths have resulted from the procedure.

Computed Tomography

Computed tomography (CT) is an important innovation in diagnostic radiology by which images of axial sections of the body 1 to 2 cm thick are viewed as if from below (Fig. 15–21-*B*). Many slices are needed in order to examine the thorax and each section must be examined through a range of window width and window level settings to show lung, soft tissue and bone.[248,249] A CT examination of the body results in an average skin radiation dose of about 3 rad. With the newer units, the radiation dose is smaller than that used for a gastrointestinal contrast examination.

The usefulness of CT in the management of thoracic neoplasms is still being determined. An outline of indications has been published.[250] Illustrated examples are helpful.[248,249] It is currently believed that CT should supplement conventional tomograms when lesions are partially or questionably hidden by the mediastinum, when the mediastinum is abnormal or questionably abnormal, and when studying the extent of parenchymal neoplasms close to the mediastinum.[251–253] It should not be used as a screening procedure for metastases from lung cancer. If a questionably abnormal hilum cannot be labeled confidently a pulmonary vessel after conventional tomograms, CT with intravenous injection of contrast material will identify the vascular shadow by contrast enhancement.

When fat or prominent great vessels are thought to be responsible for an abnormal mediastinum, CT should be the first approach because it is very useful in demonstrating mediastinal lipomatosis, a prominent pericardial fat pad, or an omental herniation through the foramen of Morgagni.

Underwood and associates showed that in a third of the cases, a CT scan of the thorax was inaccurate in predicting involvement of the middle mediastinum by metastatic lung cancer.[254] Most were false-negative scans, but one patient predicted to have mediastinal metastases had none. These findings combining CT and mediastinoscopy agree with the VA Surgical Adjuvant Group's data that about a third of patients dying within a 30-day postoperative period after a curative surgical procedure for lung cancer have persistent tumor.[255] Moreover, the 95% correlation said to exist between normal, conventional tomography and negative mediastinal biopsy in a retrospective analysis[236] is hard to reconcile with this prospective CT study and the VA autopsy data. If CT cannot replace mediastinal exploration in the staging of bronchogenic carcinoma, it will spare an occasional patient mediastinoscopy, and may play a role in guiding the mediastinoscopist.

CT has other limitations. Conventional 55° oblique tomograms may continue to be the procedure of choice for studying localized hilar adenopathy. Some feel that conventional tomograms better demonstrate minimal calcification in pulmonary nodules; CT makes it difficult to identify the concentric ring, target, and other

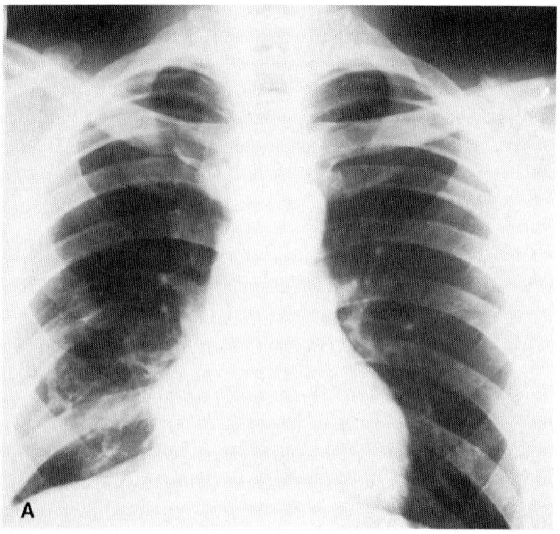

FIG. 15-21. **A.** The chest roentgenogram shows a density in the right hemithorax which x-ray films in the oblique projection showed was adjacent to the spine. There is destruction of the medial portion of the seventh rib, posteriorly. **B.** In this computerized tomogram, a soft tissue mass is seen in the right paraspinous area. The arrow indicates the right hemithorax. There is dissolution of the postero-lateral vertebral elements. Attenuation values indicated this was an abscess, not neoplasm. **C.** This is the normal vertebral anatomy lower in the thoracic spine, shown for comparison.

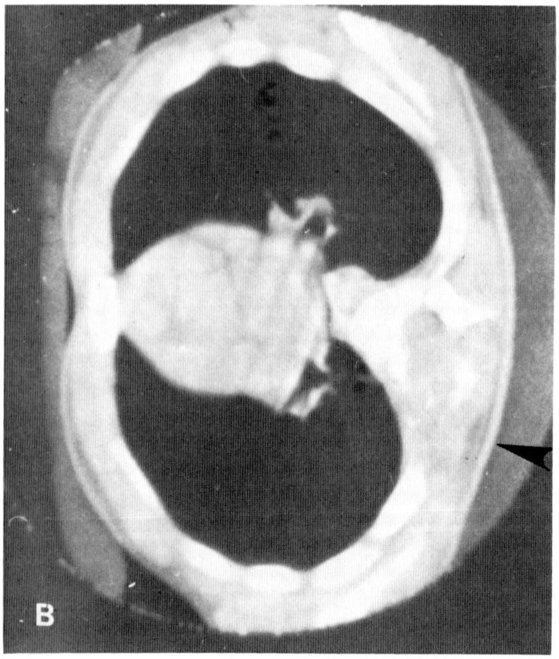

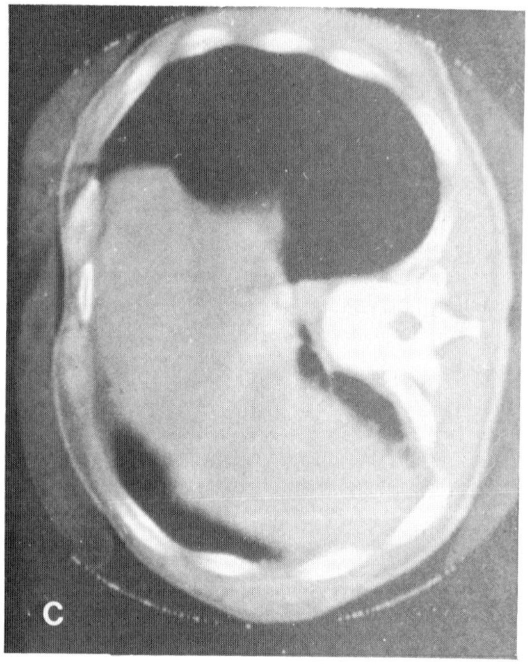

helpful patterns of calcification.[253] When used to evaluate metastatic disease, CT locates more metastatic nodules and pleural plaques than does linear tomography but it has not replaced it because small metastases cannot be distinguished from granuloma (see Neoplasms Metastatic to the Lungs).

There are problem areas in the thorax where CT may prove very helpful. Established uses in mediastinal disease have been mentioned. Mediastinal invasion by juxtaposed cancers and abdomino-thoracic tumor extension in lymph nodes at the aortic hiatus in the diaphragm can be seen as with no other technique. CT is very good at showing enlargement of subcarinal lymph nodes as they encroach on the lung in the upper part of the azygoesophageal recess inferior and posterior to the right mainstem bronchus. This may become important if Kirsh and Naruke's view that mediastinal lymph node deposits that are not seen on conventional tomograms are not a contraindication to surgery is generally accepted.[206,207] (Naruke has data suggesting that the poor prognosis for surgical patients with mediastinal metastases stems from the likelihood of contralateral mediastinal metastases in those with subcarinal lymph node disease.) CT is sometimes helpful in evaluating the patient with cancer cells in the sputum and with a normal chest x-ray film. It depicts differences between tissues of the chest wall more clearly than do conventional means. Therefore, extension of chest wall or sternal tumors into the pleural space is well seen. Abscesses may be distinguished from tumors and lipomas (Fig. 15-21). The extent of Pancoast tumors can be nicely demonstrated with CT. Patients who complain of pain after pneumonectomy can be evaluated for recurrence of tumor not seen on conventional tomograms because of the complete opacification of the operated hemithorax.

It is questionable whether routine cranial CT in neurologically intact patients with lung cancer being evaluated for surgery is cost-effective. CT will occasionally identify those metastases less than 2.5 cm in diameter or those in the midline and posterior fossa which are sometimes missed on radionuclide brain scanning.[256]

Abdominal Exploration

Reviews of necropsy series of bronchogenic carcinoma which demonstrate upper abdominal metastases in the liver and lymph nodes in 37 to 53% of patients have prompted the use of abdominal exploration as one adjunct in the evaluation of patients for thoracotomy. Laparotomy may be performed prior to thoracotomy under the same anesthesia or limited transdiaphragmatic abdominal exploration carried out after the customary posterolateral thoracotomy incision has allowed the operator to determine that the primary lesion is technically resectable. Approximately 15% of patients with normal liver chemistry studies whose bronchial neoplasms appeared otherwise resectable have been shown by these techniques to have liver metastases.[257,258] No well established guidelines exist to identify which patients should undergo abdominal exploration, there being little or no correlation between the histologic appearance or location of the primary tumor and the frequency of subphrenic metastases.[257] There is some evidence that abdominal exploration may be most appropriate for patients with undifferentiated carcinomas in whom other investigations suggest possible hilar or mediastinal lymph node metastases that might be expected to interfere with the normal cephalad lymphatic drainage.[258]

Peritoneoscopy was routinely performed in a research protocol for staging oat cell carcinoma.[259] Isolated hepatic metastases were found to be common in patients in good condition without other evidence of metastases and with normal liver function tests. These data underscore the need for systemic chemotherapy rather than relying on radiotherapy for treating small cell carcinoma which appears localized to the thorax. It does not support peritoneoscopy or laparatomy for staging all patients with small cell carcinoma.

PALLIATIVE THERAPY

Because an attempt at curative resection is possible in only 25% of all patients with bronchogenic carcinoma and only about 30% of this favorable group lives 5 years, palliative therapy becomes necessary even for the majority of operated patients. Cure is rare and prolonged survival an exception after radiotherapy and chemotherapy. It is surprising, then, that the maxim, "primum non nocere" (do no harm) is given so little weight even when the patient is to be treated outside the constraints of a research protocol. Drug combinations from a recently published research protocol are likely to be given whether or not they constitute an advance in treatment. The adage, "Diseases desperate grown, by desperate appliances are relieved, or not at all" (Shakespeare, Hamlet, IV, iii, 9) is a familiar one in radiotherapy articles even though it is inappropriate in discussions of palliation. Palliation implies that the patient is beyond cure *and also has symptoms which are distressing.* One then should not assess success or failure of a treatment by either survival-rate or by reduction of tumor volume alone. The intention is to improve the quality of life. Increased survival is an extra gain sometimes achieved by successful palliation.[260,261]

The decision to withhold therapy until the inoperable patient is significantly symptomatic is often reasonable. Indeed, the emphasis on guilt for withholding treatment for nonoperative disease should be changed to conscious justification for giving it.[260–264] As DesPrez has pointed out, "The tendency to put all cancer patients on protocols under the guise of patient treatment results in indifferent research and suboptimum (non-individualized) patient care."[265] Multihospital cooperative studies are more likely to avoid premature enthusiasm for ineffective regimens which first appear worthwhile in small groups of patients. Interhospital cooperatives large enough to evaluate promising regimens assigned at random are justified because their work represents the major clinical promise for better future treatment.

Two English studies that should be called into evidence more frequently suggest that clinical trials of palliative regimens should now include a no-immediate-treatment group as a reference. Durrant and associates randomly allocated 249 patients with inoperable bronchogenic carcinoma to 1 of 4 treatment policies. One policy was to wait for significant specific symptoms before beginning antitumor treatment, while the other 3 policies involved immediate treatment with irradiation, chemotherapy, or both. No difference was found in the quality of survival among the 4 groups. The mean survival for the wait-and-see group was 8.4 months; after irradiation, 8.3 months; after chemotherapy, 8.7 months; and after irradiation plus chemotherapy, 8.8 months.[260] Criticisms of the study included the fact that single-agent chemotherapy was used and the initial presence of symptoms in some patients in the wait-and-see group.

The design of a second study avoided these criticisms.[261] Patients were randomized into 3 sections—mandatory treatment and optional treatment. A patient was placed in the mandatory section if the physician felt that the symptoms demanded immediate anticancer treatment. The mandatory options were intermittent combination chemotherapy, continuous oral treatment with procarbazine, or radiotherapy. If the clinician was willing to draw a no-immediate-treatment policy, the patient was randomized into the optional section where the other optional treatments were the same combinations as in the mandatory section. It was anticipated that the latter would contain the patients with the more advanced disease and symptoms, but this was not so. That the groups were very similar was confirmed by the survival curves of the patients treated in a similar fashion in both groups. The conclusions are therefore likely to be applicable to all cases of inoperable lung cancer: In the no-immediate-treatment group, 30 of the 51 patients (59%) *never* needed specific anticancer therapy until their death. They did not need greater supportive therapy such as being given analgesics. The no-immediate-treatment group had better overall survival and fewer distressing symptoms than did the treated group. This clearly was the best policy for inoperable patients, particularly for those with minor symptoms.

Radiotherapy

Although some believe that selected patients with inoperable disease limited to one hemithorax must receive radical (curative) radiotherapy because even a few long-term survivors justify the interference in the lives of the majority, it is difficult to rationalize immediate, aggressive treatment for a majority of asymptomatic or moderately symptomatic patients if such a policy causes prolonged in hospital or outpatient treatment. When patients seem to have narrowly missed being operable and some strategic tumor extension removes hope for curative surgery, it is difficult to do nothing. Having failed to qualify for surgery, and often despite findings such as weight loss that indicate a poor prognosis, the otherwise minimally symptomatic patient is extended a so-called second chance through radical radiotherapy with "tumorcidal" doses approximating 6000 rad.

Tumor resolution (*i.e.*, radioresponsiveness) is most dramatic with rapidly growing tumors such as oat cell carcinoma but 1-year survival rates decrease as tumor growth rate increases (with or without radiotherapy). For this reason, tumor shrinkage correlates with the dose given but the survival rate does not. Claims for radiotherapy often include references to studies showing sterilization of the primary tumor and involved lymph nodes in 40% of selected patients who tolerate 4700 rad. A 6500 rad dosage is said to do the same for 95% of patients who complete the course. (That these data are from autopsies, the majority of which were done after death from lung cancer, also says something). Over the years, most radiotherapists have assumed that higher and higher doses of irradation are better. Review of the data is not convincing, and one is struck by the paucity of studies with a control group and random treatment assignment.[260,261,266,267]

The distressingly small statistical gain achieved by palliative radiotherapy is illustrated in one study by the VA Lung Group in which results obtained with moderate-dose orthovoltage radiation therapy (4,000 to 5,000 rad) were compared with those obtained with a placebo in 554 inoperable patients with disease limited to one hemithorax.[266] While the large number of patients studied made the small difference in survival significant, the 1 year survival rate for the treated group was only 18.2% as compared with 13.9% for the group given placebo. Larger doses (5000 to 6000 rad) did not materially change the outcome. There is little evidence that supervoltage therapy improves these results. In the widely quoted study showing the superiority of radiotherapy over surgery for treating small cell carcinoma, none of the radiotherapy patients who survived 5 years received more than 5200 rad.[110,268] Deeley, an enthusiast of radical radiotherapy, has summarized the results of the controlled trials which together suggest that more is not necessarily better.[267] Larger doses of irradiation may easily appear more effective when the tumors with the worst prognosis are given the smallest doses in uncontrolled trials.

The generally high performance status of patients accepted for aggressive x-ray therapy is not mentioned in most trials of radiotherapy. X-ray therapy causes side-effects, and this selection of the best patients acknowledges this toxicity. It also means that this group left untreated would be expected to have the longest and best quality of survival of any but those patients treated operatively. The median survival time for untreated high-performance patients with extensive disease—those with distant metastases or local extension that causes them to be rejected for x-ray treatment—is 8 months.[269] When patients with a similar high-performance status but limited disease—inoperable but encompassed in every portal for x-ray therapy—are given radiotherapy, the median survival time is but 11 months (and the treatment frequently takes nearly 2 of the best of these months).[270,271] These considerations have caused some radiotherapists to use a modified split-dose policy: When half of the treatments have been given, a rest period is allowed. If reassessment then shows no benefit, the treatments are discontinued. There is evidence that the incidence of radiation pneumonitis and fibrosis are the same, but that the reactions occur later and are milder. The treatment is more truly palliative, because as many as half of the patients in some studies do not resume the treatments after the rest period.[272]

Selection criteria which might relegate a patient to a treat-as-needed group were listed by a radiotherapist who supports early irradiation of asymptomatic patients.[271] The criteria which are associated with a significantly shorter survival time included supraclavicular adenopathy, mediastinal invasion, pleural effusion, low performance status, weight loss exceeding 12 lb (5.5 kg), involvement of both sides of the thorax, and distant metastases. If these surprisingly stringent exclusion criteria really were widely applied, many patients now receiving immediate radiotherapy for lung cancer would not be treated until symptomatic. Elderly patients whose onset of symptoms or earlier chest x-ray films indicate a slow-growing tumor may benefit from such individualized treatment. Experimental evidence that dosages of more than 4500 rad are advantageous has not been confirmed in a controlled clinical trial in which treatments were randomly assigned. Often, doses below 4000 rad are indicated for palliation of specific symptoms.

In sum, there is no evidence that given a minimally symptomatic inoperable patient, palliative radiotherapy results in fewer symptoms than the same treatment given when symptoms develop.[260,261,264] Most studies show only a marginal statistical extension of median survival; however, the figures do not accurately reflect the important benefit achieved for some patients with carefully planned and appropriately timed palliative irradiation or chemotherapy.[273]

Radiotherapy is more effective in a selected group of good-risk patients who are found to be unresectable only after exploratory thoracotomy. These patients are commonly treated with 5,000 to 6,000 rad over 5 to 6 weeks with the best reported survivals being 57% at 1 year and 8.7% at 5 years.[274] Such patients appear to be the best candidates for immediate treatment because the percentage surviving each time period approximates twice the national average for all patients given x-ray therapy for lung cancer.

There is little information about the effects of histology on survival after radiotherapy but the majority of reports show that squamous neoplasms have a better prognosis than do anaplastic or oat cell tumors.[233]

The place for radiotherapy in small cell cancer is controversial. The number of investigators who feel that chemotherapy should be the initial and principal treatment, and that radiotherapy is an adjunct, is increasing. Bronchoscopy done after x-ray therapy shows that radiation fibrosis obliterates an area on the chest x-ray film, falsely elevating the number of apparent complete responses. Past failure to recognize relapse in an irradiated area may have reflected the short survival of patients given what would now be considered inadequate chemotherapy for small cell carcinoma. It is therefore not surprising that in trials comparing marginal chemotherapy alone against marginal chemotherapy plus radiotherapy, thoracic relapse was recognized more often in the chemotherapy group. It seems clear, however, that modest doses of irradiation should be given any residual primary tumor confined to the thorax following initial polychemotherapy. Prophylactic brain irradiation with 3000 rad in 10 fractions reduced brain metastases in patients with small cell carcinoma. Patient survival, however was not affected.[225,276]

Controlled clinical trials have not demonstrated any advantage of routine pre- or postoperative irradiation for lung cancer, and the survival rate for at least one randomized preoperative treatment group was significantly less during the first postoperative year than in those patients treated with surgery alone.[232,233,277]

The palliative treatment of superior vena caval obstruction and brain metastases is discussed in the section on clinical manifestations of bronchogenic carcinoma. Radiotherapy also benefits a sizable percentage of patients experiencing pain from bone metastases, life-threatening hemoptysis, and intractable cough. Lung collapse can sometimes be avoided, or reexpansion made possible, by radiation of an obstructing endobronchial tumor. Vocal cord paralysis and the loss of lung function which occurs with complete atelectasis are seldom improved. Vigorous irradiation of late stump recurrences after lobectomy or pneumonectomy sometimes makes long survival possible.

Radiation therapy often produces anorexia. Patients also commonly develop dysphagia from esophagitis. Radiation pneumonitis, pulmonary fibrosis, pleuritis, pericarditis, and myelitis may also be seen. Rib fractures sometimes occur in the same vertical line. Brain irradiation causes alopecia (see also Chap. 13, Radiation Injury).

Chemotherapy

Placebo treatment is no longer used in organized trials, and the survival of modern inoperable patients of different performance status (Table 15-11) given true palliation—treated only when significant symptoms develop—is really unknown.

Buchberg found that half of 443 patients seen from 1932 to 1949 died within a year of the onset of striking symptoms and that a third had such symptoms 1 to 2 years before dying. It is impressive, moreover, that 15% lived for 2 to as long as 7.5 years; 4% lived 3 to 5 years; and 2% survived longer.

Prospective data from VA Lung Group studies performed 20 years ago with placebo-treated extensive disease patients found that those with

TABLE 15-11. Karnofsky and American Joint Commission (AJC) Performance Status Scales for the Clinical Evaluation of Lung Cancer Patients

Quality of Life		Performance Status	AJC
Able to carry on normal activity; no special care is needed	100	Normal, no complaints, no evidence of disease	H_0
	90	Able to carry on normal activity; minor signs or symptoms of disease	H_0
	80	Normal activity with effort; some signs or symptoms of disease	H_1
Unable to work; able to live at home, care for most personal needs; a varying amount of assistance is needed	70	Cares for self, unable to carry on normal activity or to do active work	H_1
	60	Requires occasional assistance but is able to care for most of his needs	H_2
	50	Requires considerable assistance and frequent medical care	H_2
Unable to care for self; requires equivalent of institutional or hospital care; disease may be progressing rapidly	40	Disabled; requires special care and assistance	H_3
	30	Severely disabled; hospitalization is indicated, although death not imminent	H_3
	20	Very sick; hospitalization necessary, active supportive treatment is necessary	H_4
	10	Moribund, fatal processes progressing rapidly	H_4
	0	Dead	

adenocarcinoma have the longest median survival (3 months). Untreated patients with small cell carcinoma had the shortest survival (1 to 2 months). The survival of those with squamous and large cell carcinoma was intermediate (2 to 3 months).[269] These figures include all the patients studied regardless of performance status; however, survival was directly related to performance status.

Patients with a performance status of 90% (Table 15-11) given only symptomatic nonspecific therapy had a survival of 5.5 months. Current patients in the same clinical condition have a median survival of 8 months when given cyclophosphamide (Cytoxan) plus doxorubicin hydrochloride (Adriamycin), a combination adopted by the VA Lung Group as the best control regimen against which new regimens were tested (see also Table 15-8).

In the older VA Lung Group studies, placebo-treated patients with a performance status of 40 had a median survival time of 1 month. The median survival of comparable modern patients given this combination chemotherapy is 2 months. Chemotherapy does not appear to benefit patients with non-small-cell carcinoma whose performance status is less than 40. Initial performance status is the dominant prognostic factor for survival in inoperable lung cancer. Extent of disease and recent weight loss rank second and third. They, too, have great strength relative to other patient characteristics. Age and tumor histology (other than small cell cancer) appear influential when considered alone, but hold little sway once correction is made for these three.[278]

In sum, today's patients with extensive non-oat-cell lung cancer treated with the best chemotherapy have a median survival of 2 to 8 months, depending on their performance status; similar untreated patients had median survival times of 1 to 5 months, 20 years ago. Palliative therapy should be neither prolonged nor distressing because the best current treatment is only slightly more effective than the others. Any inclination to use aggressive chemotherapy for non-small-cell cancers should be tempered by the admonition to do no harm.

One reasonable, conservative policy limits treatment to patients with significant symptoms or rapid tumor growth.[264] If improvement occurs in the first two courses of treatment, more treatment is given monthly for 6 months, and then at 2-month intervals. This approach is of benefit to some patients and usually is not harmful to those who fail to respond. Nearly all the chemotherapy responses occur within the first 6 to 9 weeks after 2 or 3 courses of chemotherapy. If the patient has continued to deteriorate, there is no point to continuing a failing regimen. Treatment should be stopped. Occasionally, different drugs then are tried if they are well tolerated by the patient. It is uncommon to see a cancer decrease in size and rare to see an improvement in performance status in this circumstance.

Response rates for chemotherapeutic agents used singly vary from zero to over 50%; average response rates of 36% for mechlorethamine (nitrogen mustard) and 23% for cyclophosphamide (Cytoxan) are representative.[278,279] Cyclophosphamide given intravenously in doses of 1100 mg/m^2/body area every 3 weeks produces a higher response rate than does the oral administration of 100-200 mg/m^2/day and is the standard against which other single or multiple drug regimens are measured. Cyclophosphamide is mainly activated and, to some extent, deactivated by microsomal enzymes in the liver and barbiturate stimulation of these enzymes may cause unexpected toxicity. Glucocorticoids and sex hormones inhibit these enzymes and close monitoring of the hemogram is indicated when doses of these steroids are being reduced.

Prospective randomized clinical trials of adjuvant chemotherapy and surgical resection versus surgical resection alone showed no beneficial effect when mechlorethamine, Cytoxan, or methotrexate was given intrapleurally at the completion of operation and for short- or long-term postoperative periods.[280,281] Only in one small subgroup in which oat cell tumors were diagnosed only at the time of operation was there any suggestion that the addition of cyclophosphamide was of any benefit.[280] Moreover, adjuvant chemotherapy was shown to have a harmful effect in at least one surgical study.[281]

In the treatment of malignant disease such as leukemia, lymphomas, and carcinoma of the breast, better results are achieved when several cytotoxic drugs are used simultaneously. Schabel has presented an elegant hypothesis which suggests that the rational chemotherapeutic approach to the treatment of malignant disease involves sequential therapy with cell-cycle-nonspecific drugs (*e.g.*, alkylating agents) followed by cell-cycle-specific anticancer agents (*e.g.*, anti-metabolities).[282]

Treatment of Small Cell Carcinoma

The gains made against small cell carcinoma are more substantial than those made against other types of lung cancer. Oat cell carcinoma is in this category. There are probably minor differences in response to treatment and prognosis among the subtypes of small cell carcinomas. That these differences are small is indicated by disagreement among investigators as to whether they exist at all. The median survival time has increased from 2 months in the untreated patient to 6 to 12 months for those given chemotherapy aggressive enough to cause approximately 10% to die from treatment.[275,276] Complete responses, in which all evidence of neoplasm disappears, have been reported in 42% of patients with disease limited to the thorax. These patients have a median survival time of 1 year, and 25% live 2 years. Complete response rates of 14% have been achieved in those with more extensive disease; they have a median survival of 6 months.[283] Again, most patients surviving more than 1 year come from the small number who present with limited disease. Such disease often would have been operated upon were it not for the cell type.

Patients with small cell carcinoma who achieve partial responses live only a few weeks longer than do untreated patients. The importance of obtaining a complete response in the first 6 weeks fully justifies early toxic therapy. If the initial tumor could be seen with a bronchoscope, bronchoscopy should be repeated before the patient is said to have achieved a complete response.

The patient who presents with systemic symptoms from metastatic small cell carcinoma and continues to show evidence of widespread disease after multiple drug chemotherapy will not live long. Management should reflect this fact. Enthusiasm for new treatments must not cause such patients' need for simple palliation to be superseded by what then becomes quixotic therapeutic aggressiveness. For example, nothing is gained from brain irradiation for a patient whose neurologic symptoms are controlled by dexamethasone when death is imminent from tumor replacement of bone marrow or liver.

Radiotherapy for small cell carcinoma is discussed above.

Immunotherapy

The dismal prognosis of patients with extensive lung cancer may be partially explained by tumor-induced suppression of cell-mediated host defense mechanisms. Marginally effective surgery, chemotherapy, and radiotherapy further suppress immune competence and may thereby contribute to the collapse-of-the-host phenomenon common among these patients. Nonspecific markers of cellular immunity are depressed in many lung cancer patients. They include decreased skin reactivity to tuberculin and other antimicrobial antigens, depressed sensitization to dinitrochlorobenzene (DNCB), reduced numbers of circulating T lymphocytes, lower absolute lymphocyte counts, and diminished lymphocyte reactivity to mitogen stimulation.[283] Studies which have tried to use these tests to predict operability or to determine prognosis have given conflicting results, as summarized by Liebler.[284]

Early reports that the complication of postoperative empyema after resection of lung cancer improved the prognosis from cancer prompted trials of immunotherapy in surgical patients.[285–287] Preliminary findings suggest that patients with Stage 1 bronchogenic cancer who receive intrapleural instillation of BCG vaccine at the time of thoracotomy are benefited. The mechanism is a nonspecific augmentation of regional and systemic immunity. Isoniazid is begun 2 weeks after the vaccine is placed in the pleural cavity at the completion of the pulmonary resection.[285,286]

Levamisole, an orally administered antihelminthic drug considered an immunoreconstituting agent rather than an immune stimulant, has produced mixed results when used in patients with bronchogenic carcinoma treated by surgery.[288,289] The drug has benefited some patients with advanced breast cancer and it has restored tumor-specific and nonspecific immunity among patients with a variety of solid tumors. Thymosin, a soluble product of calf thymus with immunologic properties, has been used with some effect in patients with small cell carcinoma.[290] How these agents work is not clear, but some data suggest that the number and function of lymphocytes and macrophages is augmented.

Most experience suggests that immunotherapy should follow maximum surgical or radiotherapeutic reduction of tumor burden. Although a few advanced metastatic tumors have been reported to regress with intravenous immunotherapy with *Corynebacterium parvum*[291], there has been no evidence that Levamisole benefits patients given Cytoxan and adriamycin for advanced bronchogenic carcinoma in one large VA Lung Group study. In controlled studies, Levamisole has produced uncontested improvement in survival only among breast cancer patients.[292] The impact of immunotherapy on lung cancer is wholly unknown at present. General reviews by Smith and Bast and associates are useful.[293–295]

BRONCHIAL ADENOMAS

Three histologically distinct bronchial tumors are classified as bronchial adenomas (see list p. 868). The carcinoid adenoma, cylindroma or adenoid cystic carcinoma, and mucoepidermoid bronchial tumors have little in common except a somewhat similar proximal endobronchial location which is responsible for their propensity to cause obstructive pneumonitis. These tumors were once classified as benign but are now known to be relatively indolent, locally invasive neoplasms which commonly metastasize to regional lymph nodes. Extrathoracic spread, particularly to liver, bone, and skin, does occur.

Adenomas make up 1 to 5% of all primary lung neoplasms, and are most often diagnosed later in the fourth decade.[296] Their occurrence in

Bronchial Adenomas

Carcinoids
- Nonfunctional
- Functional

Salivary Gland-Like Neoplasms
- Cylindromatous adenoma (or adenoid cystic carcinoma)
- Mucoepidermoid tumor

the second and third decade is not uncommon; they are least common in children and adolescents. There is a widely held misconception that these tumors are more common in women; tabulation of numerous small series of patients from the literature indicates an equal sex incidence. Peripheral bronchial adenomas have been said to occur in but 10% of affected individuals; 3 reports comprising 80 adenomas suggest peripheral lesions may be more accurately estimated at 25% of the total.[297–303] The majority of the tumors, however, occur in the main stem bronchi or in the proximal portions of lobar bronchi. Bronchial carcinoids comprise over 80% of the "adenomas"; they are somewhat less invasive than the adenoid cystic carcinomas. Mucoepidermoid tumors are the least common and most benign neoplasms in the group; however, regional lymph node metastases and local pleural implants do occur with this histologic type.

Adenoid cystic carcinomas comprise 12 to 15% and mucoepidermoid tumors, 2 to 3% of bronchial adenomas. These neoplasms are identical with those common to the salivary glands, nasal sinuses, and lacrimal glands. The adenoid cystic carcinoma and mucoepidermoid tumor arise from bronchial mucoid glands or ducts; the mucoepidermoid tumor may also originate from the surface of the bronchial epithelium. Adenoid cystic carcinomas are often located somewhat more proximally than carcinoids and involvement of the carina and trachea may occur.

Clinical Manifestations

Reviews of the symptoms produced by bronchial adenomas are so consistent as to be monotonous. Intermittent cough, hemoptysis, and pulmonary suppuration distal to the endobronchial obstructing lesion are often protracted for months to years before this classic symptom triad prompts bronchoscopic investigation. The most frequent physical finding is localized dullness with decreased or absent breath sounds and fremitus caused by bronchial obstruction, with its accompanying volume loss in the lung parenchyma. A localized wheeze most consistently demonstrated with the patient lying on the affected side is found in less than 20% of patients.[302] Clubbing may occur.

In the classical presentation, the chest roentgenogram confirms the physical findings by demonstrating volume loss involving a unianatomic division of consolidated lung parenchyma (Fig. 15-22). The findings here are similar to those seen with obstructing bronchogenic carcinomas; both differ from uncomplicated pneumonia where the breath sounds and fremitus are increased and are associated with rales, the consolidated parenchyma being ventilated through an open bronchus (see Clinical Manifestations of Lung Cancer; Findings in Carcinoma of the Lobar Bronchus). Pneumonia, abscess, or bronchiectasis may develop in the obstructed subdivisions of lung. The endobronchial tumor may be responsible for a ball-valve action which permits inspiration but interferes with expiration; an expiratory roentgenogram then demonstrates hyperlucency on the involved side: The hilus or mediastinum may also shift toward the side with the diseased bronchus when a rapid inspiratory movement or sniff is observed fluoroscopically. Because the diagnosis is usually made after considerable delay, approximately 25% of adenomas achieve sufficient size to project as a proximal mass in or near the hilum. Laminograms may be of value in demonstrating well-circumscribed, smoothly defined tumor encroachment on the air column within the trachea or major bronchi, and regional metastases to bronchopulmonary, subcarinal, tracheo-bronchial, or paraaortic lymph nodes may be evident with laminography (Fig. 15-23). Bronchography is only occasionally useful because the majority of these proximal endobronchial tumors may be visualized through fiberoptic bronchoscopy. Tumor calcification due to osseous metaplasia has been described but is uncommon. Bone

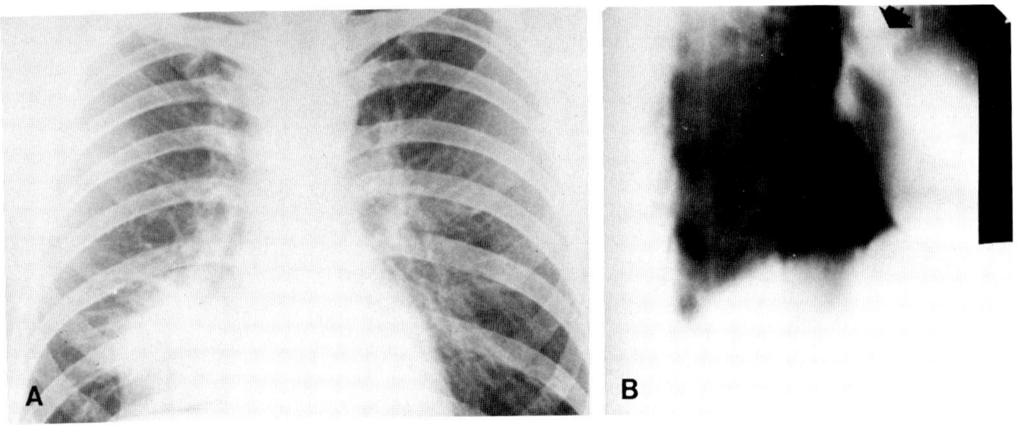

FIG. 15-22. Bronchial carcinoid adenoma. **A.** The adenoma caused obstruction of the right middle lobe bronchus. **B.** In this lateral laminogram, the adenoma is seen as a speroidal density (*arrow*) proximal to the oval infiltrate representing the middle lobe. (Chest roentgenogram courtesy of Dr. Robert A. Green, Ann Arbor, Michigan)

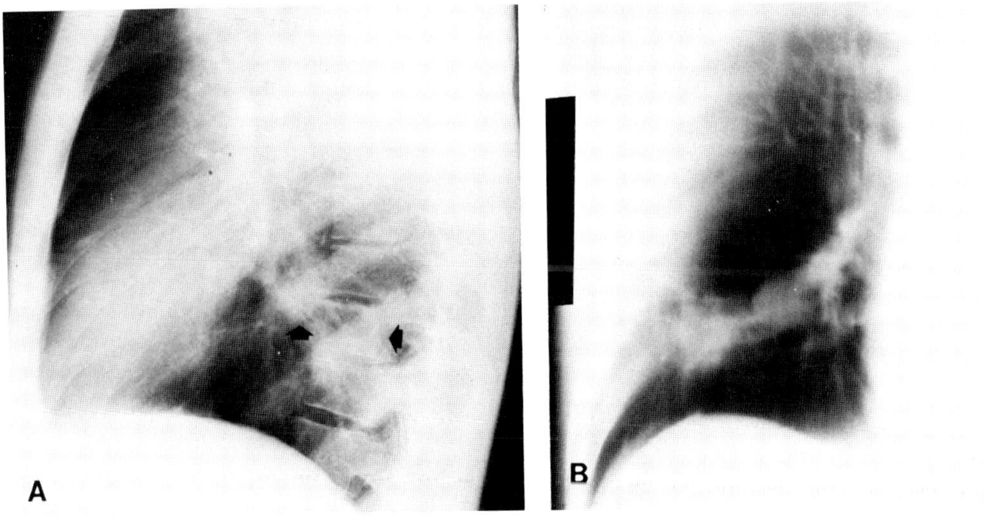

FIG. 15-23. Bronchial adenoma. **A.** The adenoma is seen as a rounded density in the superior segment of the right lower lobe (*vertical arrow*) just proximal to a pulmonary infiltrate containing a fluid level (*horizontal arrow*). **B.** This laminogram shows the well-circumscribed, sharply defined margins of the adenoma proximal to the secondary lung abscess. Cavitation and fluid within the abscess are not seen in this section (the films were taken with the patient supine). (Chest roentgenograms courtesy of Dr. Robert A. Green, Ann Arbor, Michigan)

metastases may be osteolytic but commonly are osteoblastic. Multiple, peripheral, unilateral, endocrinologically active bronchial carcinoid adenomas have been described, but are very rare compared to gastrointestinal carcinoids where 10 to 30% of the tumors are multiple.[304]

The bronchoscopic appearance of the tumor is that of a proximally located, white to pink, polypoid, lobulated, or rarely, pedunculated mass covered with bronchial epithelium which has undergone squamous metaplasia. Examination of sputum cytology is therefore of little value.

Carcinoid adenomas may be confused with oat cell carcinomas in marginally adequate bronchial surface biopsies. Ulceration is uncommon. Many adenomas are highly vascular and opinion is divided as to the advisability and necessity for transbronchoscopic biopsy.[304,305] Wilkins experienced a 2.6% mortality with biopsy in his series, and considers a history of hemorrhage, a lesion occluding a main bronchus, and evidence of respiratory insufficiency to be contraindications to biopsy. Transbronchoscopic biopsy should be undertaken with the realization that endoscopic removal is hazardous and nearly always inadequate because of the high recurrence rate.

Carcinoid Syndrome

Bronchial carcinoids and oat cell carcinomas are believed to arise from Kultschitzky (K or argentaffin) cells derived from the neuroectoderm. Electron microscopic studies have shown these cells to be present in normal bronchial mucous glands, between columnar cells lining peripheral bronchioles, and especially between surface bronchial epithelial cells at the bifurcations of major bronchi.[306] Within the cells are so-called neurosecretory granules containing a 5-hydroxytryptamine (serotonin)-formaldehyde complex, which in fresh preparations is responsible for their silver reduction staining characteristic, the argentaffin reaction.[307] Carcinoid tumors may also occur in the anterior-superior mediastinum where they arise within the anatomic compartment of thymus gland. The "epithelial thymoma" associated with Cushing's syndrome is thought by some to be a mediastinal carcinoid.[308] Cells of this enterochromaffin system also give rise to the functioning carcinoid tumors of the gastrointestinal tract. The same ectopic hormones (ACTH, MSH, ADH, calcitonin, insulin) as well as serotonin and bradykinin may be elaborated by bronchial carcinoids and oat cell carcinomas.

In 1970, Wilson collected 3718 cases of abdominal carcinoid tumors and found 136 patients (3.7%) with symptomatic endocrinologic activity.[309] These figures can be compared with Fontanna's 1963 report in which the carcinoid syndrome occurred in 2% of 125 patients with bronchial carcinoid and in 7% of patients with gastrointestinal carcinoid. That functioning bronchial carcinoid adenomas are uncommon was indicated by Fontanna's review of the literature which revealed only 21 cases of endocrinologically active bronchial adenoma.[310] Oat cell carcinomas have produced the carcinoid syndrome in at least 2 patients. The typical carcinoid syndrome results from tumors in the jejunum or ileum. These tumors secrete 5-hydroxytryptamine (serotonin or 5-HT), rarely elaborate 5-hydroxytryptophan (5-HTP), have a high tumor serotonin content, rarely metastasize to bone and skin, and produce the syndrome when liver metastases are present. In comparison, bronchial carcinoids may secrete large amounts of 5-HTP, usually contain less serotonin, more commonly metastasize to bone and skin, and may cause the syndrome in the absence of metastases.[311] Bronchial and mediastinal carcinoids also have been responsible for ectopic production of ACTH. They are occasionally associated with multiple endocrine adenomatosis, or Wermer's syndrome, characterized by neoplasms or hyperplasia affecting the parathyroids, pancreatic islets, pituitary, adrenals, and thyroid.[307,312] The distinctive clinical features of hyperadrenocortisolism resulting from ACTH production by bronchial carcinoids are described under Bronchogenic Carcinoma and Ectopic Hormone Production.

When bronchial carcinoids are responsible for the carcinoid syndrome, the symptoms include severe and prolonged flushes with facial edema, anxiety and tremulousness, lacrimation, salivation, wheezing, diaphoresis, nausea and vomiting, explosive diarrhea, fever, tachycardia, hypotension, and oliguria. The duration and intensity of the flushing attacks (red-blue discoloration lasting hours to weeks and sometimes becoming permanent), and their prevention with the daily administration of 15 to 40 mg of prednisone is more characteristic of carcinoid tumors of the bronchus than those of the gut.[313] The associated facial edema may be misdiagnosed as "angioneurotic edema." Focal or diffuse collections of fibrous tissue deposited on the endocardium and valve cusps have produced stenosis or incompetence of the mitral and aortic valve. In contrast, gastrointestinal carcinoids metastatic to the liver have been associated with pulmonic stenosis and tricuspid insufficiency.

Oral or intravenous alcohol and injections of epinephrine, norepinephrine, dopamine, and histamine have been used as provocative tests to induce the carcinoid flush. Other diagnostic tests include quantitation of blood serotonin or measurement of its principal urinary metabolite, 5-hydroxyindolacetic acid (5-HIAA). Walnuts and bananas contain sufficient serotonin to falsely elevate urinary 5-HIAA above the normal daily 2-to 9-mg level. When these foods are excluded, a urinary 5-HIAA level above 25 mg per day is diagnostic of carcinoid. Values from 9 to 25 mg may be found in either carcinoid or nontropical sprue. Urine chromatography is used to distinguish 5-HIAA from other 5-hydroxyindoles because the syndrome may occur in patients without elevated 5-HIAA. 5-Hydroxytryptophan (5-HTP) is metabolized in other organs to serotonin (5-HT) and 5-HIAA; all 3 compounds may appear in the urine in varying concentrations. Bronchial carcinoids, oat cell carcinomas, and gastric carcinoids sometimes produce elevated urinary 5-HTP and very little or no 5-HIAA, perhaps because they lack a decarboxylase enzyme responsible for conversion of 5-HTP to serotonin. The carcinoid syndrome occurring in this circumstance is referred to as atypical. On the other hand, occasional patients with bronchial carcinoid tumors have positive tests for 5-HIAA but experience no symptoms of the carcinoid syndrome. The calcium infusion test has recently been used to provoke the flush and other manifestations of the syndrome. It is safe, easy to perform, and appears to be specific when combined with the simultaneous determination of the biochemical products of these neoplasms.[314]

The pathogenesis of the various symptoms experienced in the carcinoid syndrome is complex and controversial. It is now clear that serotonin is not the only biochemical mediator and that the syndrome can no longer be reduced to four lines of doggerel:

> This man was addicted to moanin'
> Confusion, edema, and groanin'
> Intestinal rushes; great tricolored blushes
> And died of too much serotonin'[315]

Carcinoid tumors have been shown to contain kinin-forming enzymes (kallikreins). During epinephrine-induced flushing, release or activation of kallikrein splits lysylbradykinin from kininogen, an alpha$_2$-globulin substrate in the blood. An aminopeptidase in the blood then rapidly converts lysylbradykinin to bradykinin. Bradykinin is a potent vasodilator which stimulates smooth muscle contraction in the gut and bronchus and can induce fibrosis. Despite these seemingly appropriate pharmacologic actions, it is not certain that bradykinin is responsible for elements of the syndrome other than the flush. Released serotonin, histamine, and catecholamines also play varying roles in a syndrome best considered to result from the combined effects of several mediators.

Management

Thoracotomy with the goal of complete excision is the treatment of choice for all 3 types of bronchial adenoma. Lobectomy with removal of contiguous lymph nodes, with or without a bronchial sleeve resection, is the most common operation. Pneumonectomy is indicated only when an appropriate bronchial reconstruction is impossible or if suppurative changes in the lung parenchyma distal to the site of obstruction are so severe as to preclude reasonable function postoperatively. Wedge resections have been done for peripheral adenomas but there are insufficient data to indicate whether this operation is an adequate one. Transpleural bronchotomy and local resection may be useful in selected cases of carcinoid and mucoepidermoid tumors when the lesion is found to be predominantly endobronchial, free of metastases, and without distal pulmonary suppuration.[304] Hypotension and bronchospasm add to the anesthetic risk in the carcinoid syndrome. Premedication with serotonin or bradykinin antagonists, the use of methoxamine (Vasoxyl) for hypotension, and avoidance of cyclopropane and thiopental have been suggested.[296]

Bronchial adenomas are relatively radioresistant, cylindromas perhaps less so than carcinoids and mucoepidermoid tumors. While cure cannot be achieved by irradiation therapy, long-term palliation may be achieved in the poor-risk or nonresectable case; endoscopic removal is inadequate but has also been used in such circumstances. Antitumor chemotherapy has received little attention but responses of limited duration have been achieved with cyclophosphamide (Cytoxan). This agent appears to have more antitumor effect than nitrogen mustard or 5-fluorouracil and severe exacerbation of carcinoid symptoms may occur within a few hours of its intravenous administration.[316]

Considerable work has been directed toward counteracting the pharmacologic symptoms of the carcinoid syndrome. The peripheral antagonists of serotonin, methysergide (Sansert), and cyproheptadine (Periactin) help control diarrhea when opiates and diphenoxylare hydrochloride with atropine (Lomotil) fail. Parachlorophenylalanine (PCAC) inhibits the formation of 5-HTP, the immediate precursor of serotonin, and has given good to excellent control of gastrointestinal symptoms. Phenothiazines antagonize the peripheral actions of kinins but are less useful in controlling the bronchial carcinoid flush than are corticosteroids. The latter may act by preventing the activation or release of vasoactive substances by the tumor. Alpha-adenergic blocking agents such as phentolamine may help to prevent catecholamine activation of the kinin system, thus ameliorating the flushing attacks.[311]

Survival figures for patients with bronchial adenomas show considerable variation best explained by differences in the incidence of lymph node metastases found at operation. Goodner studied 21 carcinoid patients, and only 12, or 57%, survived 5 years. Among the survivors only 7, or 33%, were free of disease. Metastases were demonstrated in 44% of the entire series.[317] O'Grady reported a 95% 5-year survival for 29 patients with bronchial carcinoid adenomas; none of the patients were found to have lymph node metastases.[302] The prognosis for patients with adenoid cystic carcinomas has been more discouraging: there was one 5-year survivor among the nine patients with cylindromas in these 2 studies.

TUMORS OF THE MEDIASTINUM, CHEST WALL, AND DIAPHRAGM, AND UNUSUAL TUMORS OF THE LUNG PARENCHYMA

MEDIASTINAL TUMORS

Anatomy and Distribution

The mediastinum is the midthoracic extrapleural space bordered on either side by the parietal pleura and lungs, anteriorly by the sternum, posteriorly by the ribs and paravertebral gutter, superiorly by the thoracic inlet, and inferiorly by the diaphragm. The loose areolar tissue of the mediastinum contains the heart, thoracic aorta and its proximal branches, the vena cavae, azygos and proximal innominate vein, thoracic duct, lymph nodes and lymphatics, esophagus, trachea, thymus, and the vagus, phrenic, posterior intercostal, and sympathetic nerves. Specific lesions tend to occur predominantly in one of three mediastinal compartments (Table 15-2). The anterior mediastinum is bounded by the sternum, the first rib, and an oblique line drawn from the diaphragm along the anterior border of the heart until it meets the boundary of the posterior mediastinum (Fig. 15-24). The posterior mediastinum begins at the posterior ribs and paravertebral gutter and is bounded anteriorly by a line drawn along the anterior surface of the vertebral bodies from the diaphragm to the first rib. The triangular middle mediastinum constitutes the remainder of the area.

Mediastinal abnormalities are about evenly divided between those in male and female, patients those that are symptomatic and those that are not, and those in the anterior, middle, and posterior compartments. When primary mediastinal new growths are considered, the incidence of malignant tumors in infants and children is approximately the same as that in adults (20 to 30%), neurogenic tumors, lymphomas, and teratomas making up the majority of pediatric mediastinal malignancies.[318,319] Thymic neoplasms, common in adults, are unusual in the pediatric age group. Metastatic carcinoma and lymphomas are responsible for the majority of mediastinal malignancies in adults. When these are excluded, at least 33 separate abnormalities may produce a mediastinal mass.[320–322] Faced with such potential confusion, it is important to realize that nearly three-fourths of all primary mediastinal disease is caused by four conditions: (1) neurogenic tumors, 30%; (2) teratodermoids, 20%; (3) thymomas, 10%; and (4) bronchogenic cysts, 10%. The majority of the remaining abnormalities are caused by extrathoracic structures and abnormal growths which project into the mediastinum, hernias through the esophageal, Morgagni, and Bochdalek foramina and substernal thyroid adenomas.

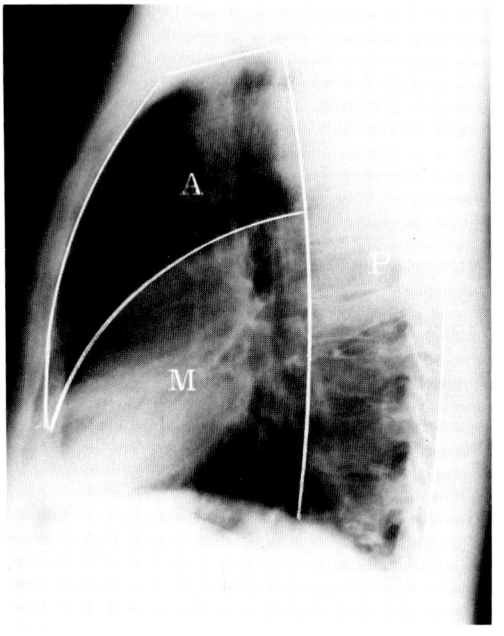

FIG. 15-24. Diagnosis is facilitated if the mediastinum is divided into anterior (*A*), middle (*M*), and posterior (*P*) compartments.

Distinguishing Mediastinal From Pulmonary and Pleural Lesions

Some difficulty may be encountered in differentiating mediastinal abnormalities from those that arise in lung or pleura. Because the mediastinum is extrapleural, a growth or fluid collection extending to the lateral confines of the space will invaginate the overlying mediastinal and visceral pleura, producing a sharp convex contour facing the lung; this is another manifestation of the extrapleural sign used to identify chest wall lesions, such as rib metastases, which displace the lateral pleural surfaces in a similar fashion. The two layers of pleura, mediastinal and visceral, smooth out minor surface irregularities in the mass, giving it better definition than a pulmonary lesion.[320] The tapering upper and lower borders of the mass form an obtuse angle with the line which represents the continuation of the mediastinal pleural above and below the mass (Fig. 15-25).

Mediastinal and pulmonary masses may also be differentiated by the presence of an air bronchogram and their respiratory motion. The presence of an air bronchogram or a mass which moves synchronously with the adjacent lung markings at fluoroscopy, indicates an abnormality of the lung parenchyma. Teratodermoids and thymomas in the anterior mediastinum may move synchronously with cardiac pulsation, while substernal thyroid adenomas and masses attached to the esophagus move with swallowing. The enlarged thymus of an infant may shrink with inspiration and a brief course of steroids (prednisone, 1.5 mg/kg body weight/day for 5 days) may be helpful in diagnosis, causing a rapid decrease in thymus size if a mass is due to thymic hyperplasia.

An anterior mediastinal mass may be distinguished from an enlarged heart, pericardial sac, or dilated pulmonary artery by the hilum overlay and hilum convergence signs.[320] The hilum overlay sign suggests a mediastinal mass rather than an enlarged cardiac silhouette when the first bifurcation of either the right or left pulmonary arteries in the frontal projection is seen more than 1 cm medial to the lateral edge of density in question (Fig. 15–26). If the pulmonary arteries appear to arise from the lateral edges of a large mediastinal shadow it is probably an enlarged heart or pericardial sac. A corollary of the

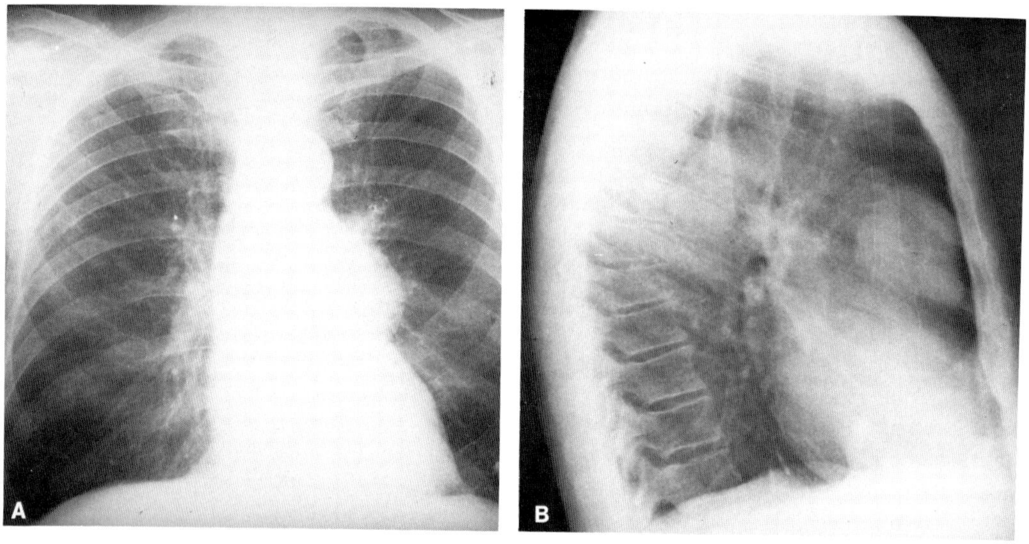

FIG. 15-25. Thymoma of the anterior mediastinum. **A.** The mediastinal mass invaginates the overlying pleural surfaces producing a sharp convex contour facing the lung. The smoothly tapering upper margin of the mass forms an obtuse angle with the line which would represent the continuation of the vertically directed mediastinal pleura. **B.** In this lateral chest roentgenogram, the lucency produced by the air-containing lung interposed between the thymoma and the sternum represents the sulcus sign. The sulcus sign is seen less frequently with teratodermoid tumors because they tend to be larger than thymomas.

FIG. 15-26. Embryonal cell carcinoma of the anterior mediastinum. The bifurcation of the left pulmonary artery (*arrows*) arises more than a centimeter medial to the lateral edge of the density. Such a demonstration of the hilum overlay sign is helpful in distinguishing a mediastinal mass from those arising from an abnormal cardiac or pulmonary artery shadow.

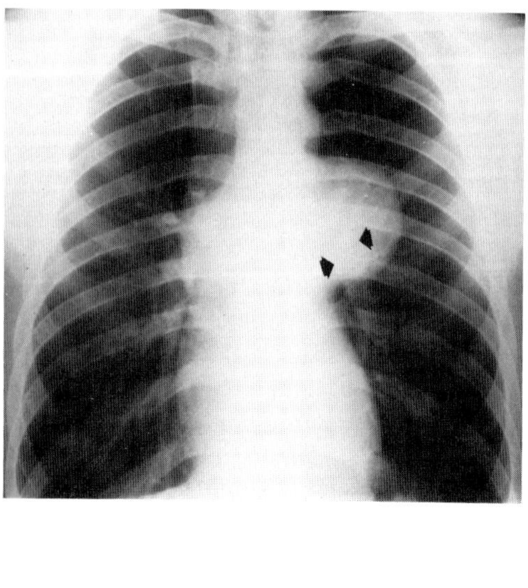

hilum overlay sign is the hilum convergence sign: a mass, in or overlapping a hilum, is suggested when the pulmonary artery branches are traced to their central convergence and found to emanate from the heart rather than the lateral edge of the mass. If the arteries converge into the lateral borders of the mass itself, the lesion is an enlarged pulmonary artery.

Failure of Symptoms and Physical Findings to Separate Benign and Malignant Mediastinal Abnormalities

The diverse symptoms experienced by patients with mediastinal disease can be assorted into five overlapping categories: (1) the absence of symptoms, common with benign developmental tumors or cysts; (2) symptoms caused by compression or infiltration of adjacent structures; (3) systemic symptoms suggesting that mediastinal involvement is secondary to disseminated infection or malignancy; (4) symptoms produced by local infection occurring within a confined space; and (5) catastrophic events following the rupture of a hollow viscus or blood vessel into the mediastinum.

Because the space for accommodating expanding lesions is limited, tumors and cysts, whether benign or malignant, sometimes produce similar evidence and degree of dysfunction despite a very different prognosis. For example, obstruction of the superior vena cava or internal jugular vein and hoarseness secondary to paralysis of the recurrent laryngeal nerve may be seen with benign as well as with malignant substernal thyroid adenomas. Cancer or achalasia of the esophagus may be responsible for esophageal dilatation, seen as a widening of the right mediastinum, and both may predispose to aspiration and pulmonary infection. Benign neurogenic tumors with a "dumbbell" or "hourglass" configuration extend through an intervertebral foramen, producing spinal cord compression with neurologic loss; aortic aneurysms and benign neurogenic tumors may give rise to local and referred pain, bone erosion, and pleural effusion, signs that may be mistakenly ascribed to malignancy. In addition, benign ganglioneuromas of the stellate ganglion have caused Horner's syndrome, findings usually associated with malignant Pancoast tumors of the lung. Moreover, roentgenographic evidence of rapid enlargement of a mediastinal mass does not confirm malignancy since it may result from hemorrhage into a benign new growth, a complication which may be fatal, especially if it occurs with a substernal goiter. When myasthenia gravis is associated with a thymoma, the tumor may behave in a benign or malignant fashion. These examples indicate that mediastinal new growths, benign or malignant, usually necessitate resection. Prompt thoracic exploration is needed in order to confirm diagnoses, to obviate malignant degeneration of benign tumors, and to prevent eventual compromise of vital structures.

The first clue to the diagnosis of mediastinal disease may be provided by physical findings such as tracheal deviation in the presence of an old thyroidectomy scar or goiter in the neck (substernal thyroid); increased parasternal percussion dullness associated with diplopia, ptosis, and proximal limb weakness typical of myasthenia gravis (thymoma); or dilated superficial veins of the thorax which accompany cough and retrosternal pressure sensations with hoarseness related to a paralyzed left vocal cord indicating recurrent laryngeal nerve involvement (metastatic lung cancer). More often, findings in the extrathoracic physical examination direct attention to diseases that may be responsible for hilar or mediastinal lymphadenopathy already documented by the chest roentgenogram. Common examples include hepatosplenomegaly and peripheral lymphadenopathy with mediastinal lymphoma or the same findings accompanied by skin papules, chronic iridocyclitis, and bone cysts in sarcoidosis.

Clubbing of the digits and hypertrophic osteoarthropathy have been reported with a variety of mediastinal conditions, benign and malignant; however, the combination of a mediastinal mass and nail or periosteal changes should prompt a thorough search for a small unrecognized primary lung cancer. This is one of the few situations in which bronchoscopy is helpful in the diagnosis of mediastinal disease.

Diagnostic Studies Used to Evaluate Mediastinal Masses

The roentgenographic investigation of every patient with mediastinal disease should begin with chest x-ray films in two projections and a *contrast study of the esophagus*. The esophagogram, an overpenetrated Bucky chest roentgenogram, and laminograms often do much to identify tumor borders and the presence and extent of metastases. On the Bucky film, special attention should be paid to widening of the paravertebral line where neoplasm, pus, or blood may push the mediastinal parietal pleura laterally (Fig. 15-27). Skin tests for tuberculosis and serologic tests for histoplasmosis and syphilis should be performed because granulomatous mediastinitis and aneurysms both may present with discrete, masslike roentgenographic abnormalities.

The presence of a posterior mediastinal mass indicates the need for coned-down roentgenographic views of the spine in the anteriorposterior, lateral, and oblique projections in order to identify erosion of the posterior ribs, vertebral bodies, pedicles, and transverse processes.

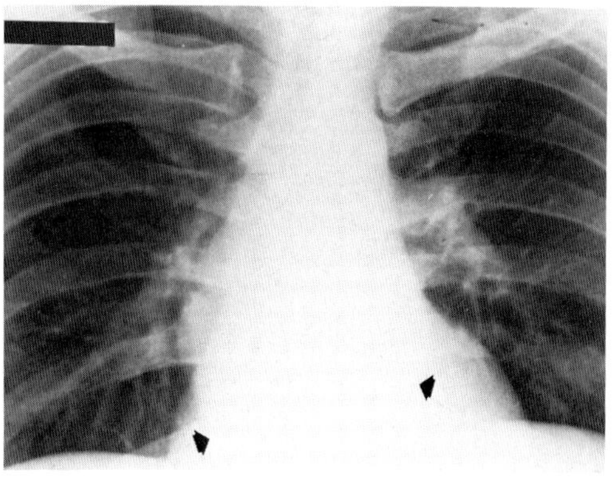

FIG. 15-27. Pott's disease of the thoracic spine. The appearance of a posterior mediastinal mass is produced by widening of the paravertebral line caused by a very large paravertebral tuberculous abscess.

Myelography is also indicated if there is evidence of spinal cord compression, widening of one of the intervertebral foramina suggesting a dumbbell-shaped neurogenic tumor, or when a meningocele is suspected because of the presence of anomalies of the vertebrae or ribs in a patient with generalized von Recklinghausen's disease. When a paravertebral mass is present in a hypertensive patient with excessive sweating and signs of hypermetabolism, measurements of urinary catecholamines, metanephrines, and VMA (vanillylmandelic acid) should be obtained, although pheochromocytoma is one of the least common posterior mediastinal tumors. Needle aspiration, cytologic studies, or cutting needle biopsy of mediastinal lesions abutting the chest wall are seldom of value because mediastinal exploration and tumor resection will be indicated regardless of the result.

When an anterior mediastinal mass is present at the right cardiophrenic angle, a barium enema may distinguish a hernia through the foramen of Morgagni from a pericardial cyst or thoracic malignancy. The most common content of such a hernia is greater omental fat and the contrast study demonstrates the high position of the transverse colon, sometimes with indentation of the barium column caused by traction exerted by the hernia. Diagnostic pneumoperitoneum is useful in verifying the position of the diaphragm and its relation to intra-abdominal structures which may herniate into the mediastinum. Pneumoperitoneum is diagnostic in a Morgagni hernia (Fig. 15-28). Computed tomography is quite useful in assessing mediastinal disease, particularly when fat (omental herniation in Morgagni hernia) or great vessels are involved. Computed tomography is discussed further in the section on lung cancer.

An upper gastrointestinal contrast study with small bowel follow-through may demonstrate herniation of the small gut through the foramen of Morgagni and, in the proper clinical setting, hypotonic duodenography may identify pancreatic carcinoma as the cause of bilateral hilar and mediastinal adenopathy. The upper gastrointestinal series will also confirm the presence of a hiatal hernia suggested by the patient's symptoms, the consistent absence of a subdiaphragmatic gastric air bubble, or the presence of an air-fluid interface within the thorax behind the heart (Fig. 15-29).

Lymphangiograms, pneumomediastinum, and bronchograms are of limited value in the identification of mediastinal masses, although bronchograms are sometimes used to corroborate the suspicion that a paramediastinal density is caused by a collapsed lobe or segment pancaked against the mediastinum. The introduction of air into the mediastinum for the investigation of anterior and central lesions has not been widely used in the United States where laminography and mediastinoscopy are more extensively used.

Mediastinoscopy, fluoroscopy, and venography have been discussed in the sections entitled Therapeutic Planning for Patients With Bronchogenic Carcinoma and Distinguishing Mediastinal from Pulmonary and Pleural Lesions. It is important to realize that the apparent pulsation of a mass at fluoroscopy does not reliably distinguish aneurysm from tumor, since clot within an aneurysm may dampen expansile movement, and a tumor adjacent to or surrounding a vessel may appear to pulsate. Venography, including azygography, has sometimes been substituted for the venous phase of a pulmonary angiogram, in the evaluation of venous obstruction and collateral circulation in patients with fibrosing mediastinitis or mediastinal new growths.

Three radionuclide scanning techniques may

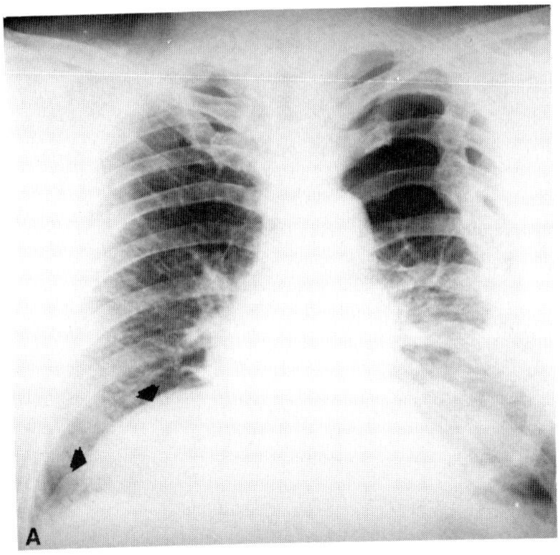

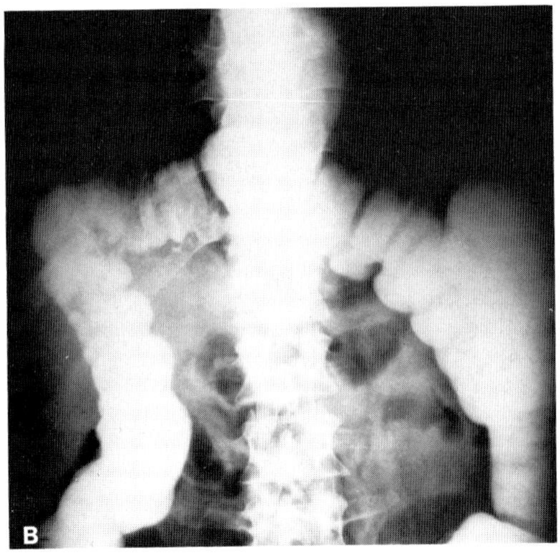

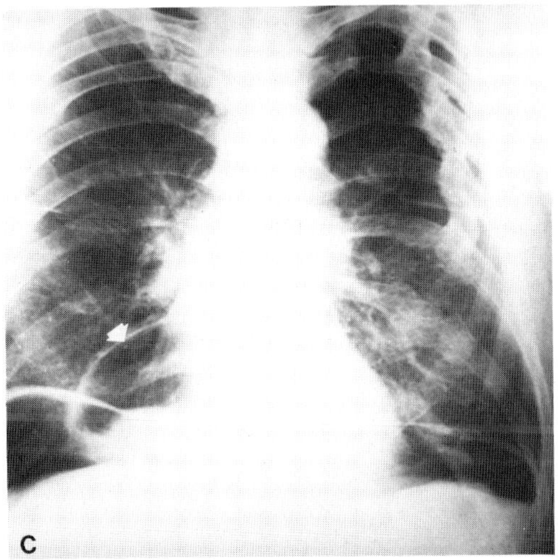

FIG. 15-28. Morgagni hernia of the anterior mediastinum. **A.** The arrows indicate the superior margin of an abnormal density at the right cardiophrenic angle. **B.** This roentgenogram was taken with the patient standing upright following a barium enema. It demonstrates the high position of the transverse colon caused by traction exerted by the herniation of omentum through the foramen of Morgagni. **C.** Pneumoperitoneum demonstrates the Morgagni hernia (*arrow*) which was suspected from the chest roentgenogram shown in *A*. Both hemidiaphragms are also outlined by abdominal air. (Chest roentgenograms courtesy of Dr. Robert A. Green, Ann Arbor, Michigan)

be used to study mediastinal masses. A positive iodine-131 thyroid scintiscan can provide a diagnosis when it outlines a substernal thyroid; however, a thyroid adenoma is not excluded by a negative scan. If a mediastinal mass is presumed to be an extension or metastasis from a previously diagnosed, well-differentiated thyroid cancer, thyroid stimulating hormone is first given in an effort to make the tumor tissue avid for radioiodine. The radioactive angiocardiogram, a modern version of the blood pool scan, consists of observation of the progress of a tracer bolus of technetium-99m-pertechnetate (dynamic phase), which gives useful information about the patency of the superior vena cava or the presence of pericardial fluid, and the examination of the blood pool (static phase), which demonstrates whether a given mass contains blood.[323] Concentration of the pertechnetate ion in the thyroid also delineates that organ. The use of gallium scans to evaluate the mediastinum for metastases is discussed under Lung Cancer.[238–240]

Scalene lymph node biopsy and angiocardiography are two of the most useful diagnostic procedures employed before thoracotomy in patients with mediastinal masses. Scalene lymph node biopsy is indicated when systemic symptoms or physical findings pointing to metastatic cancer, generalized lymphoma, or sarcoidosis are associated with mediastinal lymphadenopathy. If metastatic mediastinal involvement in-

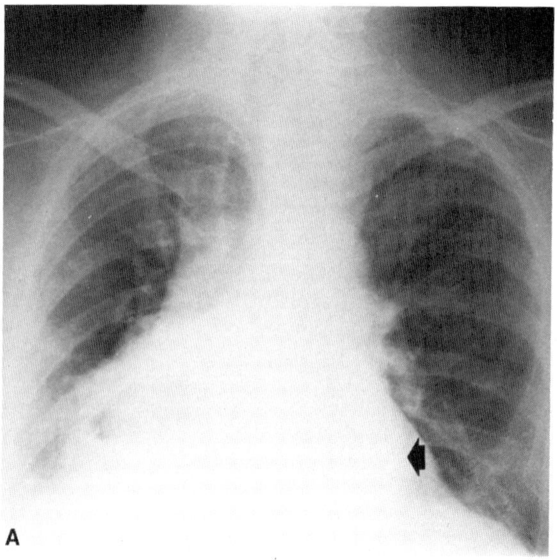

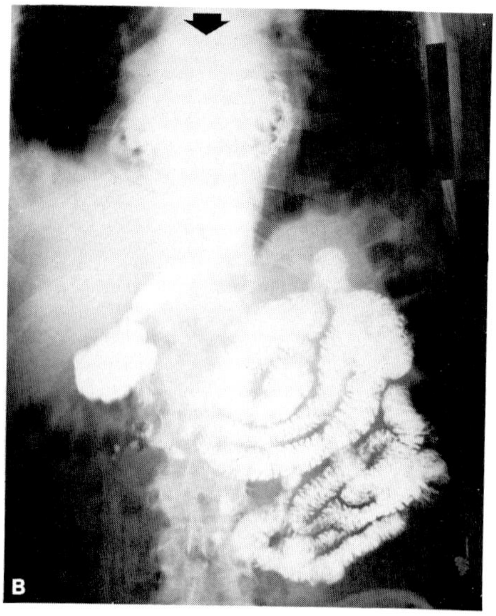

FIG. 15-29. Hiatal hernia in the middle mediastinum. **A.** The arrow indicates the left lateral margin of the herniated stomach. An air fluid level is seen on the right. **B.** The upper gastrointestinal contrast study confirmed the diagnosis made from the patient's symptoms and chest roentgenogram. The superior margin of the stomach is indicated by the arrow.

cludes roentgenographically visible paratracheal lymphadenopathy, the yield from scalene node dissection will be high, even in the absence of palpable scalene lymph node enlargement. Angiocardiography is important because mediastinal disease may mimic the clinical and roentgenographic findings of a cardiovascular abnormality. The confusion is usually due to a misleading history of chest trauma which falsely suggests a posttraumatic aneurysm; to the presence of a cardiovascular lesion in addition to a mediastinal mass; or to symptoms and signs of cardiovascular disease caused by the location or size of a mediastinal mass. For example, acquired pulmonic stenosis, the most common cardiac manifestation of a mediastinal mass, has been reported with thymoma, teratoma, lymphoma, and lymphatic cysts. To-and-fro murmurs related to vessel compression by a mass are common. Pericardial effusions secondary to local neoplastic invasion are not rare, and rupture of a teratoma into the pericardial sac can produce tamponade which is then confused with a ruptured aneurysm. Angiocardiography is often performed before thoracotomy because even the most unlikely masses may prove to be aneurysms and because vascular invasion by malignancy may dictate the need for preoperative irradiation, the type of surgery to be done, or may preclude surgery altogether.

Roentgenologic Features Which Distinguish Specific Categories of Mediastinal Disease

The density, projection, and configuration of a mass, the presence or absence of calcification or gas within a mass, and associated pulmonary parenchymal abnormalities provide clues to the origin of a mediastinal mass. As a very general rule, benign lesions tend to displace adjacent structures, whereas malignant growths infiltrate and destroy. Care must be taken to avoid confusing an effusion or hematoma loculated medial to the parietal pleura with a mediastinal tumor mass.

The density of a mass may be helpful in establishing a diagnosis, although it is often difficult to distinguish water densities within the mediastinum (pericardial spring water cyst) from a fat density in the same area (omentum in a Morgagni hernia). Configuration can be nearly diag-

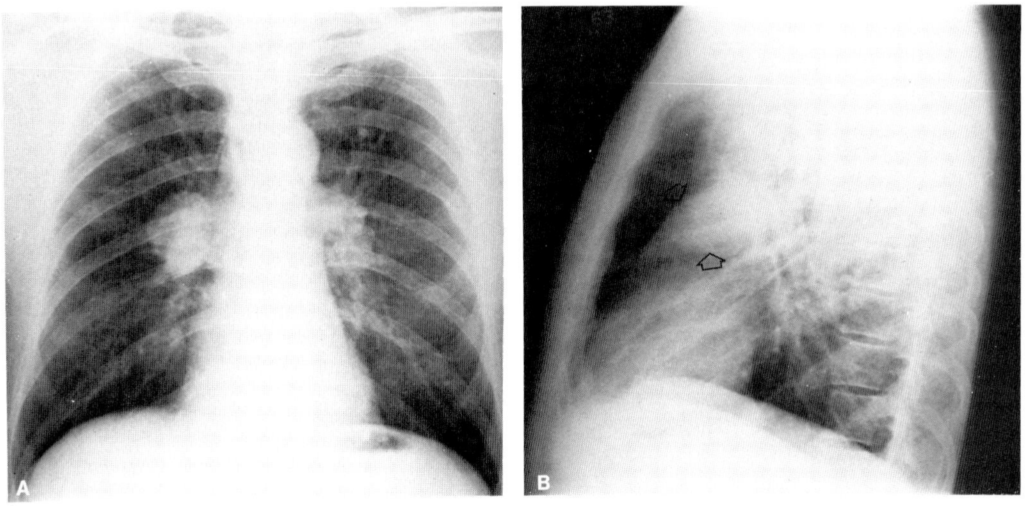

FIG. 15-30. A and **B.** Bronchogenic cyst of the anterior mediastinum.

nostic: the wavy, calcified margin of an aneurysm or a teardrop-shaped pericardial or bronchogenic cyst interposed within a long fissure, which may change in outline with positioning of the patient (Fig. 15-30). Lack of definition of the margin of a mass supports the diagnosis of malignancy, although many malignant tumors have sharp margins (Fig. 15-26).

The unilateral or bilateral and right or left projection of a mass does not establish a diagnosis, but may be suggestive: neurogenic tumors are usually unilateral, seldom crossing the midline; lymphoma and extramedullary hematopoiesis cause bilateral lobulated masses; a large Zenker's inferior pharyngeal diverticulum originates posteriorly and descends between the esophagus and vertebrae but usually veers to the left; most pericardial cysts and Morgagni hernias occur at the right cardiophrenic angle; esophageal epiphrenic diverticuli are found on the right in the distal esophagus; most Bochdalek hernias project into the left posterior thorax, sometimes occupying the entire space between mediastinum and lateral chest wall.

Calcification in the rim of a density suggests a cystic structure and may occur in a thymoma, thyroid adenoma, or aneurysm. Central calcification in an anterior mediastinal mass is most likely to be found in a benign thyroid adenoma or teratodermoid containing teeth or bone; stippled calcification does not exclude malignancy since it is sometimes present in thyroid carcinoma and neurosarcoma. Eggshell calcification within lymph nodes is typical of silicosis and phleboliths are pathognomonic of hemangiomas.

Masses containing gas or an air fluid level should bring to mind esophageal hiatal, Morgagni, or Bochdalek hernias; dilated esophagus from cancer, achalasia, or inflammatory stricture; epiphrenic or Zenker's diverticulum; infected bronchogenic cyst; mediastinal abscess; and enteric cyst (duplication of the gastrointestinal tract). The last is usually recognized in infancy because of its association with hemivertebrae, scoliosis, peptic ulceration, and hemorrhage.

When a mediastinal mass develops in a patient with a pulmonary parenchymal abnormality, diagnostic studies must be selected to determine whether it represents: (1) granulomatous infection with mediastinal lymph node enlargement; (2) aspiration secondary to esophageal disease; (3) metastasis from lung to mediastinum or from an extrathoracic primary tumor to lung and mediastinum; (4) mediastinal lymphoma with direct extension to lung; and rarely (5) primary mediastinal malignancy causing bronchial obstruction and volume loss (*e.g.*, teratocarcinoma, invasive thymoma).

Non-Neoplastic Causes of Mediastinal Widening

Granulomatous and fibrous mediastinitis, acute pyogenic mediastinal infections, aortic rupture, atherosclerotic buckling or aneurysmal dilatation of vessels, mediastinal lipomatosis, and esophageal dilatation are the relatively common non-neoplastic conditions which must be considered in the differential diagnosis of localized or diffuse mediastinal widening. In mediastinal lipomatosis, fat deposition causes bilateral mediastinal enlargement in some patients with endogenous or exogenous glucocorticoid excess. The fat is deposited in the upper mediastinum and at both cardiophrenic angles. There are no symptoms related to the mediastinal widening and no treatment is necessary unless Cushing's disease is the cause. Computed tomography is the procedure of choice when mediastinal lipomatosis is suspected.[255,256]

Acute Mediastinitis is often a sequela of esophageal perforation secondary to carcinoma of the esophagus or lung. The other common causes are foreign body penetration of the esophagus or bronchi by bone spicules, difficult esophagoscopy, endotracheal intubation, bronchoscopy, and crushed chest injury.

Mediastinitis from odontogenic or deep cervical infections is very rare. When such an infection dissects downward into the mediastinum, it does so in the perivascular or, more commonly, the retrovisceral space. The latter is a potential space behind the esophagus and anterior to the prevertebral layer of cervical fascia. The infection therefore begins in the posterior mediastinum. Much less often, tracheostomy or thyroid gland surgery may be complicated by mediastinitis beginning in the anterior mediastinum as a consequence of infection which spreads down the pretracheal space.[324,325]

The esophageal obturator airway, a device used by rescue squad workers to provide ventilation in emergency situations which would otherwise necessitate endotracheal intubation, may cause esophageal perforation, mediastinitis, and pyopneumothorax. The American Heart Association's certification course in advanced life support includes a manikin for instruction in the use of the esophageal airway. The device is associated with more complications than were originally recognized, including airway obstruction and inadequate ventilation of edentulous patients.[326,327] The perforation of the esophagus produced by this airway occurs at approximately 30 cm from the teeth and is posterolateral at the maximum depth of the airway within the esophagus.

The symptoms of the mediastinitis include prostration, excitability due to a sensation of impending doom, tachycardia, rigors, high fever, chest pain made worse by respiration, tenderness over the sternoclavicular joints, and pain referred to the ear. The examiner may identify the crepitance of subcutaneous emphysema and Hamman's sign, a crunching sound synchronous with cardiac pulsation heard over the anterior mediastinum and related to mediastinal emphysema. The chest roentgenogram may show localized or diffuse mediastinal widening with smooth borders and mediastinal or subcutaneous air, pneumothorax, or hydropneumothorax (Fig. 15-31). Extravasation of a water-soluble contrast material into the mediastinum and pleural space will confirm the diagnosis. Treatment includes immediate closure of the ruptured viscus, drainage, antibiotics, and intravenous rather than oral feeding.[328–330]

Boerhaave's syndrome, a more severe variant of the Mallory–Weiss syndrome, results when forceful vomiting is followed by a through-and-through tear of the lower posterior or left lateral esophageal wall. The mediastinitis that develops causes severe pain in the lower chest, epigastrium, or back which may be confused with pain resulting from intraabdominal pathology. Pleural effusion and pneumothorax may be present and are more common on the left. Extravasation of ingested contrast material and thoracentesis with withdrawal of gastric contents establish the diagnosis.

Acute hemorrhagic infection of mediastinal lymph nodes and soft tissues coexistent with hemorrhagic pneumonitis is characteristic of anthrax, a disease seen in persons exposed to imported wool, fur, or animal hides contaminated with *Bacillus anthracus*. Penicillin is the treatment of choice; tetracycline is a less effective alternative.

Aortic Rupture. The possibility of aortic rupture should be considered in all seriously injured auto accident victims, since a third of those with aortic damage have little or no evidence of blunt chest trauma, and widening of the mediastinum is often appreciated only in retrospect. Physical findings such as hoarseness (recurrent laryngeal nerve damage), a systolic murmur medial to the left scapula, superior vena caval obstruction, hypertension in the upper extremities, and weak femoral pulses are uncommon, but should be looked for. When there is rib fracture, hemothorax, or other evidence of chest trauma, and the initial chest roentgenogram shows a normal mediastinum, the chest x-ray films should be repeated at frequent intervals. If mediastinal widening becomes apparent, aortography should be performed immediately. When facilities for an aortogram are not available, a forward or venous aortogram done with intravenous catheters advanced as proximally as possible may produce a satisfactory substitute.[331] The aortogram may identify a rare second aortic tear, may prevent an unnecessary thoracotomy for mediastinal hematoma in an unstable patient with dire extrathoracic injuries, or may permit localization of an aortic disruption which might be difficult to find by direct palpation when the intact adventitia preserves the aortic contour. Traumatic aneurysms of the thoracic aorta occur most commonly in the posterior portion of the descending aortic arch distal to the origin of the left subclavian artery (see also Chap. 11).

Aortic Dissection. Aortic dissections begin in the 5 cm of aorta above the valve or distal to the origin of the left subclavian artery. Hypertension, Marfan's syndrome, pregnancy, coarctation and bicuspid aortic valve are predisposing factors. Type I dissections in the DeBakey classification begin in the ascending aorta and encompass the arch, extending to the descending and abdominal aorta. A Type II rent begins in the ascending aorta and stops at the left subclavian artery. Aortic regurgitation, or hemopericardium, may occur when proximal dissection involves the aortic root.[332]

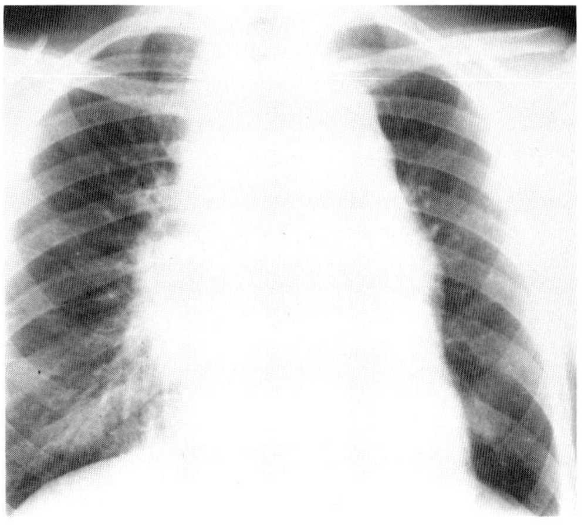

FIG. 15-31. Acute pyogenic mediastinitis secondary to foreign body perforation of the esophagus.

Immediate medical management with a continuous intravenous drip of methaphan (Arfonad) or nitroprusside is begun in order to maintain the systolic blood pressure between 100–120 mmHg regardless of the type of dissection. Propranolol is used to depress myocardial contractility.

Type I dissections usually are treated by surgery because complications such as carotid occlusion and hemopericardium are common. In Type II dissections surgery is usually reserved for patients with left pleural effusion, radiographic evidence of progressive dissection, or pain unrelieved by medical treatment.

Aortic dissection should be considered whenever pain ascribed to myocardial infarction, is maximal at onset, radiates to the back, and is associated with increased blood pressure. The most common plain chest x-ray film abnormalities with dissection are in the region of the aortic knob: increased aortic diameter; a double density produced by the superimposition of the false channel superior and posterior to the aortic arch, particularly if intimal calcification is present in the arch; and deviation of the trachea to the right. There may be a discrepancy between the diameters of the ascending and descending aorta. The lateral margin of the descending aorta is sometimes poorly defined because of extravasation of blood. Computed tomography has not been useful in the diagnosis of aortic dissections and aortography is necessary in order to identify the true and false lumen.[333]

Granulomatous and Fibrous Mediastinitis. In most patients, fibrous mediastinitis represents a later stage of granulomatous mediastinitis, and although early reports emphasized tuberculosis and syphilis, histoplasmosis may now be the leading cause.[334–336] Sarcoidosis, silicosis, actinomycosis, and fibrosis following hemorrhage from trauma are responsible for a handful of cases. Sansert (methysergide) may induce extensive mediastinal, pleural, pulmonary, and retroperitoneal fibrosis when used in patients with migraine headaches, but there remain a very few cases where mediastinal fibrosis complicates retroperitoneal fibrosis which is truly idiopathic.[337]

The roentgenographic picture and symptomatic complications produced by granulomatous and fibrous mediastinitis are similar, although intrusion on mediastinal structures is more common with sclerotic change. These conditions are usually seen in those under 40 years of age and in areas where histoplasmosis is endemic, they account for 10% of primary mediastinal masses with superior vena caval (SVC) obstruction.[334]

In most patients, symptoms evolve from compromise of the vena cava, airways, esophagus, or pulmonary vasculature and only a few patients complain of atypical retrosternal or interscapular pain. Oppression and throbbing in the head when bending forward, dyspnea on exertion, headache, dizziness, and edema of the face with distended neck veins are characteristic of the patient with SVC obstruction (see Lung Cancer, Clinical Manifestations). Hemoptysis (pulmonary vein stenosis), intractable right heart failure (pulmonary artery stenosis), dysphagia, or an asthmalike syndrome from tracheobronchial stricture may occur. Phrenic, recurrent laryngeal, and vagus nerve palsies have been described. Some patients are asymptomatic.

A previous history of pulmonary disease or symptoms is often elicited; moreover, these episodes have often occurred within months with granulomatous mediastinitis but may have preceded fibrous mediastinitis by years.[335]

In these two closely related processes, microscopic evidence of inflammatory activity blends imperceptibly from one category in to another. Acute granulomatous response and hyalinized collagenous tissue devoid of epithelioid and giant cells represent the two extremes of a continuum. Both can produce local or generalized mediastinal enlargement, the widening usually appearing high in the anterior mediastinum above the tracheal bifurcation. The most common radiologic picture in the granulomatous form is a rounded mass projecting above and to the right of the right hilum.[338]

The disease has been attributed to the seepage of an unidentified antigen with fibroblastic properties from within mediastinal lymph nodes, in a manner similar to the fibrous accretion stimulated at the periphery of an enlarging parenchymal histoplasmoma. (It is noteworthy that coccidioidomycosis, which produced impressive mediastinal lymphadenopathy in the acute and subacute stage more often than does histoplasmosis, is rarely, if ever, the cause of mediastinal fibrosis.)

Pulmonary hypertension generally results from involvement of pulmonary veins near the left atrium, but pulmonary hypertension and cor pulmonale may also result from constriction of only the right main pulmonary artery or of both the right and left pulmonary arteries.[339]

Characteristically, the signs of SVC obstruction which predominate early in the clinical course undergo some gradual spontaneous improvement as elaborate collateral channels enlarge. Secondary complications of venous obstruction and development of collaterals include hemorrhage from esophageal varices, recurrent superficial thrombophlebitis, postphlebitic syndrome of the arms, and chylothorax. Restrictive respiratory insufficiency from pleural fibrosis and reduced airflow rates from bronchial involvement also occur.[340]

Skin tests, serologic tests, tomograms, pulmonary arteriograms, venography, bronchoscopy, CT, and aortography may all play a role in this diagnosis. Scalene lymph node biopsy and mediastinoscopy are dangerous when SVC obstruction is present, but may be used in the absence of venous hypertension. Management of venous obstruction requires elevation, elastic support of the limbs, careful skin care, diuretics, and treatment of infection and superficial thrombophlebitis. The antiinflammatory action of glucocorticoids has been reported to be of benefit in the early reactive stage of idiopathic retroperitoneal fibrosis but there is no accumulated evidence of their effectiveness when the mediastinum is involved. Their use could lead to disseminated infection if tuberculosis or fungal infection are the cause of mediastinal granuloma.[340] Treatment for tuberculin-positive patients found to have granulomatous or fibrotic mediastinitis includes isoniazid chemoprophylaxis.

There are those who advocate resection of mediastinal lymph nodes that enlarge dramatically over several months in serologically positive patients with subacute histoplasmosis.[341] They feel that with such action, involvement of vital structures is avoided and that removal of succulent lymph nodes, the precursors of the fibrotic stage, and disruption of the lymphatic network prevents fibrosis. Patients treated in this fashion have done very well compared with those with fibrotic disease for whom surgery is seldom useful. This approach is difficult to evaluate because many of these patients would have spontaneous involution of lymphadenopathy and there has been no control group because the number of appropriate patients is small.

With the exception of patients with stenosis of the pulmonary arteries or veins, those with the fibrotic stage of the disease have a generally good prognosis. Signs and symptoms of SVC obstruction can be expected to improve as decompression by collateral channels occurs and the main indication for venous bypass surgery is the appearance of disabling complications: bleeding esophageal varices, chylothorax, and recurrent phlebitis.[341,342] Attempts to replace or bypass the superior vena cava are complicated by frequent postoperative thrombosis of any autograft, homograft, or prosthesis used. It has been claimed that better results are achieved if a Teflon or autogenous vein graft slightly larger than the replaced caval segment is used and if a temporary proximal arteriovenous fistula is created to increase blood flow through the graft.[334,340] Measurement of pre- and postoperative venous pressures provides an imprecise but objective estimate of the results of surgery. The patient's clinical status may improve with the subsequent development of collateral circulation, even if the graft eventually fails. These facts emphasize that bypass surgery, with and without complete surgical resection of the mediastinal granulomatous or fibrotic masses, is not necessary or even advisable in a majority of these cases.

Tumors of the Anterior Mediastinum

Thymomas, benign teratodermoids, teratocarcinomas, and malignant germ cell tumors including seminoma (germinoma), choriocarcinoma, and embryonal carcinoma comprise most of the primary neoplasms of the anterior mediastinum (Table 15-12). Teratomas and thymomas occur with about equal frequency and are much more common than germ cell tumors. Up to a fifth of teratomas undergo malignant degeneration and although the most common malignant change is adenocarcinoma (teratocarcinoma), a few of these neoplasms either contain some germ cell elements or present as primary mediastinal germ cell tumors. Some authors believe that teratodermoids and their malignant germ cell derivatives originate in embryonic maldevelopment of the thymus, thus explaining their predominance in the anterior mediastinum.

Thymoma. The normal thymus is composed of lobules, each of which is made up of epithelial cells (also referred to as reticular cells), lymphocytes (small cells), and Hassall's corpuscles, structures derived from epithelial cells and unique to the thymus. Thymomas consist of varying mixtures of lymphocytes and epithelial cells, with one or the other predominating in different areas of a single tumor. While the lymphocytes are generally monotonous and uniform in appearance, the epithelial cells vary greatly in size and shape, forming patterns which have been called spindle cell, rosette, and protoplasmic (organoid or endocrine-like).[343–345] The simplest classification of thymomas (small

TABLE 15-12. Abnormalities of the Mediastinum

Anterior Mediastinum	Middle Mediastinum	Posterior Mediastinum
Lymphoma	Lymphoma	Neurogenic tumor (inc. chemodectoma)
Thymoma	Metastatic carcinoma	Aortic aneurysm
Teratodermoid Teratocarcinoma	Sarcoidosis	Infectious spondylitis
Choriocarcinoma Seminoma	Infectious granuloma	Lymphoma
Embryonal carcinoma	Hiatal hernia	Meningocele
Substernal thyroid	Mediastinitis, abscess	Extramedullary hematopoiesis
Pericardial cyst or tumor	Aneurysm (aorta or major arteries)	Hematoma
Aneurysm (aorta, sinus of valsalva)	Bronchogenic and enteric cysts	Mediastinitis, abscess
Mediastinitis, abscess	Leiomyoma of the esophagus	Pheochromocytoma
Mesenchymal tumors (fibroma, lipoma, etc.)	Epiphrenic diverticulum of the esophagus	Hernia, Bochdalek
Hernia, Morgagni	Neurogenic tumor (vagus or phrenic)	Thoracic duct cyst
Parathyroid tumor	Chemodectoma	Angiofollicular lymph node hyperplasia (Castleman's tumor)
Hemangioma, lymphangioma	Hematoma	
Chemodectoma	Angiofollicular lymph node hyperplasia (Castleman's tumor)	
Hematoma		
Zenker's diverticulum		
Angiofollicular lymph node hyperplasia (Castleman's tumor)		

cell, epithelial, and spindle cell) is based on the relative number of lymphocytes and epithelial cells and the variation in shape of epithelial cells. This system is probably adequate because no sharp line of histologic demarcation is found among the types.[346] No constant relationship has been found between the occurrence of myasthenia gravis and any histologic feature with the exception that myasthenia gravis is less often associated with a spindle cell pattern.[345,347]

The "granulomatous thymoma" is excluded from this classification because no consensus has been reached about whether it represents Hodgkin's disease of the thymus or whether it is a primary thymic tumor which imitates the granulomatous and sclerosing histologic findings of Hodgkin's disease. Recently this tumor has been more generally recognized as a special type of Hodgkin's disease and it is now usually referred to as nodular sclerosing form of the lymphoma. It tends to occur in younger persons, particularly females, and remains more localized than most cases of Hodgkin's disease of the mixed cellularity or lymphocyte-depletion types, often involving the anterior superior mediastinal lymph nodes without visible disease in hilar or paratracheal lymph nodes. It responds to resection and irradiation and there is a high percentage of long-term survivors.[343,348]

Thymic tumors may have patterns which can be confused with other tumors which metastasize to the anterior mediastinum: small cell thymoma with lymphosarcoma; epithelial thymoma with reticulum cell sarcoma and Hodgkin's disease; and spindle cell thymoma with nerve sheath tumors or fusiform-celled undifferentiated carcinomas of lung or thyroid.

Although the most common histologic change within the thymus in patients with myasthenia gravis is simply general hyperplasia and an increase in germinal follicles, between 8 and 15% of patients with myasthenia gravis have thymomas. Roughly 50% of patients with thymomas have myasthenia gravis.[349] The presence of myasthenia usually leads to the recognition of the thymoma, although myasthenia has been reported to develop years after resection of a thymoma.

Thymomas are most often recognized in middle life and those in women are more commonly associated with myasthenia gravis. Thymomas also have been linked to agammaglobulinemia, aregenerative anemia, Cushing's disease, and idiopathic granulomatous myocarditis. Most but not all cases of agammaglobulinemia or aregenerative anemia have occurred with spindle cell thymomas. Removal of the thymoma has resulted in early or delayed improvement in the anemia in about half of the affected patients.[343,344] Cushing's disease has a high incidence of associated neoplasia and perhaps a third of the tumors are epithelial thymomas. Some of the thymic tumors occurring with Cushing's disease are thought to represent mediastinal carcinoid.[350]

When these related diseases are excluded, the symptoms and physical findings produced by thymomas are those common to other anterior mediastinal tumors. Asymptomatic patients are common (30%). Dyspnea may result when the patient lies supine and the tumor falls against the trachea. Local compression or invasion may obstruct the superior vena cava or innominate vein and cause paralysis of the recurrent laryngeal, phrenic, and vagus nerves, producing hoarseness, diaphragmatic paralysis, and gastric dilatation. Loss of lung volume as a result of bronchial infiltration and stenosis has occurred. Pleural and pericardial effusions sometimes result from central venous obstruction or regional invasion. Interposition of the tumor between the heart and chest wall can muffle heart sounds and cause electrocardiogram changes which suggest acute anterior myocardial infarction. Examination of the anterior thorax may show tracheal deviation, venous distension, widening of the parasternal area of percussion dullness, and decrease in breath sounds and fremitus.

Thymomas tend to be smaller than teratodermoid tumors. They are therefore somewhat more likely to show unilateral projection on the posteroanterior chest roentgenogram with the lateral view demonstrating an air lucency intervening between the anterior edge of the tumor and the posterior surface of the sternum—the sulcus sign (Fig. 15-25). There may be calcification in the margin of some thymic cysts, but the bone densities sometimes seen with teratomas are not present.

The malignant potential of a thymoma is not determined by its histologic appearance or the presence of a capsule but by the thoracic surgeon's visual estimate of the extent of invasion and the tumor's behavior during subsequent years of patient observation. Thymomas may become inoperable because of local extension or pleural seeding but distant metastases do not occur and pleural, pericardial, phrenic nerve, and innominate vein invasion are not absolute contraindications for surgery.[346,351–353] Irradiation is subordinate to surgery in the treatment of thymomas although palliation by irradiation can be expected when complete removal of the tumor is not possible.[353] Preoperative irradiation is no longer recommended in patients with thymoma and myasthenia gravis.[351] In some centers, all thymomas are treated with a full course of postoperative irradiation because even those which are initially characterized as completely encapsulated and benign and thought to be completely excised may recur as highly aggressive malignant thymomas.[348]

One representative study found the 5-yr survival with invasive thymomas to be 23% while that for noninvasive thymomas was 80%.[344] The presence or absence of myasthenia and the invasiveness of the tumor both play a role in postoperative survival. Because the medical management of myasthenia has improved with high-dose corticosteroids, survival may now more often be determined by invasiveness. Local invasion is an indication for postoperative irradiation therapy.[351-353]

Thymectomy is followed by improvement in about two-thirds of myasthenic patients without thymoma, and there is now a tendency to recommend surgery for most patients who remain incapacitated for 6 months despite drug therapy.

Teratodermoid Tumors. The mediastinum is second only to the ovary or testis as the location for teratodermoid tumors. Dermoids are composed of epidermis and dermal glands with hair and sebaceous material as the most common elements. The inclusive term *teratodermoid* is used because endodermal structures (bronchial or intestinal epithelium) and mesodermal structures (smooth muscle, lymphoid tissue, bone) are so common. These tumors are usually recognized in adolescence or young adulthood and a fifth are malignant.

Adenocarcinoma is the most common malignancy found with teratodermoids. The extragonadal germ cell tumors of the mediastinum include seminoma, choriocarcinoma and embryonal carcinoma.[354,355] All three of these unusual neoplasms are more common in young men, but they also develop in women. Mixed histologic patterns in which embryonal carcinoma co-exists with seminoma, choriocarcinoma, or teratocarcinoma are common. One theory suggests that these tumors originate in the endoderm of the yolk sac and that the cells reach the gonad by migrating along the urogential ridge which extends from the sixth cervical vertebra to the third lumbar vertebra. This theory would explain the presence of germ cell tumors in the mediastinum and retroperitoneal area.[355]

The criteria for primary origin of these tumors in the mediastinum include an absence of palpable testicular masses and of retroperitoneal and paraaortic metastases as documented by a normal intravenous pyelogram and lymphangiogram.[356] Benign cystic teratodermoids, the most common tumors in this group, have an equal sex incidence.

The symptoms and physical findings identified with teratodermoids are, with few exceptions, similar to those described with thymomas. Because the majority are benign, most produce no symptoms or only minor pressure-effects. Infection of a cystic mass sometimes results in rupture into the pleural or pericardial space or a bronchus, with the latter leading to expectoration of hair or sebaceous material or causing lipoid granuloma in the lung. Hemorrhage within the mass may cause severe pain and sudden increase in size. Gynecomastia secondary to the elaboration of chorionic gonadotropin may occur with malignant mediastinal germ cell tumors even when very minute areas of choriocarcinoma escape recognition among other germ cell elements.

Teratomas commonly contain opacities produced by linear calcification of the margin of a cystic lesion or the presence of bone or teeth. When the masses are cystic, fatty material may layer out on top of fluid contained in the cyst, causing a fat layer to be visible on the chest roentgenogram. The tumors vary in size from small, barely visible densities to huge tumors which nearly fill the chest. Malignancy is suggested by rapid growth, bosselated margins to a solid, rather than cystic structure, the appearance of satellite nodules, and positive serum or urine tests for chorionic gonadotropin.

Benign teratodermoid tumors do not recur following surgical resection. Malignant teratoid tumors are managed by surgery, irradiation, or chemotherapy.[357] When feasible, the tumors are resected. Seminoma is then treated with irradiation with tumor doses of 2000 to 3000 rad delivered over 2 to 3 weeks. Since the majority of seminoma patients who die have metastases to bone and lymph nodes rather than local recurrence, early systemic chemotherapy with a single alkylating agent such as cyclophosphamide is currently indicated. Embryonal carcinoma is not radiosensitive and tumor doses in excess of 4000 rad are usually without benefit; therefore, multiple chemotherapy with drugs such as methotrexate, dactinomycin, and chlorambucil is preferred. Other alkylating agents such as nitrogen mustard or cyclophosphamide are sometimes substituted for chlorambucil and vincristine may be used instead of methotrexate in this triple regimen. Mithramycin alone is also deserving of trial in the treatment of pure embryonal carcinoma and is active against seminoma. Radiation therapy is unlikely to benefit choriocarcinoma of the mediastinum unless the tumor is one with mixed germ cell elements and combination chemotherapy with methotrexate, 5-fluorouracil, cyclophosphamide, and vincristine appears to be the preferred treatment.[358] Chorionic gonadotropin levels can be used to monitor the response of choriocarcinoma to treatment.

With treatment as outlined, patients with mediastinal seminoma have about a 50% 10-year survival. Survival with the other germ cell tumors and with the more common teratocarcinoma is usually measured in months. Death by local recurrence is characteristic of embryonal carcinoma; widespread metastases are common with tumors of the other cell types.

Mesenchymal and Vascular Tumors of the Anterior Mediastinum. Mesenchymal tumors, lipomas, fibromas, myomas, and mesotheliomas, comprise less than 5% of mediastinal tumors and have a relatively high incidence of malignancy (50%), each benign type having its malignant counterpart. Hybrid forms such as fibromyoma and fibrolipoma may have a greater tendency to undergo malignant transformation. With the exception of fibrosarcomas, which are more common in the posterior mediastinum, most of these tumors occur in the anterior compartment. Lipomas can sometimes be recognized because they are less dense than other mediastinal tumors. They are usually unilateral and because of their pliability, they are asymptomatic, often spreading out over an entire hemidiaphragm as if they had been poured into place. As do other tumors in this group, fibromas tend to reach large size while remaining asymptomatic; benign as well as malignant fibromas may be associated with pleural effusions.[359] Mediastinal fibrosarcoma has no predilection for any one mediastinal compartment. Well-differentiated liposarcomas grow slowly and considerable long-term palliation can be achieved by reexcision of symptomatic tumor bulk. Although lymphangiomas and hemangiomas or their rare malignant counterparts occur most frequently in the anterior mediastinum, the most common vascular "tumor" in this area is an aortic aneurysm. As with lipomas, the consistency of benign vascular tumors is such that symptoms are infrequent. Phleboliths or the erosion of adjacent ribs may occur with hemangiomas but these tumors are not visualized with angiography. Malignant connective tissue tumors destroy by local invasion rather than widespread metastases. Their primary treatment is surgical since they respond poorly to irradiation or chemotherapy.

Substernal Goiter. Totally intrathoracic goiters with no palpable goiter in the neck arise from aberrant thyroid tissue in the mediastinum and are extremely rare. ("Bobbing" goiters, which disappear in the neck and reappear when the Valsava maneuver is performed with the neck flexed forward, are more common.) The most common anterior mediastinal thyroid mass arises from the growth of a benign nontoxic adenoma in one of the lower poles of the thyroid and is often preceded by a history of palpable goiter in the neck and/or thyroidectomy. Histologically the lesions consist of multiple degenerating colloid and fetal adenomas in a colloid thyroid. The majority lie anterior to the trachea and cause the trachea to be deviated to the right or left; occasionally the trachea may be displaced anteriorly and separated from the esophagus when the adenoma lies between these two structures. The borders of the mass may be smooth or lobulated but are sharply defined. Calcification is sometimes present.

Patients with cervical goiter may have substernal extension. Breathlessness is common and tracheal obstruction is frequently demonstrable on flow–volume loops, but this mechanism of respiratory failure is easily overlooked.[360,361] Hoarseness and brassy cough are the most typical findings with large substernal thyroid masses. Complications include stridor aggravated by recumbency with the usual mass anterior to the trachea, dysphagia when the adenoma is posterior to the trachea, and recurrent laryngeal nerve paralysis and superior vena caval or internal jugular compression which can occur with either benign or malignant adenomas.

Toxic nodules and carcinoma are distinctly uncommon. Tracheal collapse may first be recognized after extubation following surgical removal of the mass and is caused by destruction of tracheal rings from long-standing pressure.

The diagnosis of substernal thyroid is made if the mass moves with swallowing at fluoroscopy or if the radionuclide scan is positive.

Until recently, information on the frequency of positive thyroid scans in mediastinal goiter was limited and conflicting. Review of 27 cases of tissue-documented mediastinal goiter (24 nontoxic goiters, 3 carcinomas) show that the ^{131}I scan was positive in all.[362] If the ^{131}I uptake is less than 5% and if the scan is equivocal, a repeat scan may be positive after a larger dose of ^{131}I or thyroid-stimulating hormone is administered. Many mediastinal goiters do not necessitate surgery. Thyroid scans should be done more frequently in patients with mediastinal masses because mediastinal goiters have been described in all mediastinal compartments. Angiography may be required to exclude buckling or aneurysmal dilatation of the innominate artery when these tests are negative. When a small retrosternal gland produces no symptoms and is shown to concentrate radioiodine in a euthyroid patient who is a relatively poor surgical candidate, it is safe to observe the adenoma. Surgery is usually recommended in order to avoid future symptoms of compression, or the potentially serious acute complication of hemorrhage into the mass in a patient who may have become a greater surgical risk with advancing age.

Reactive Lymphoid Disorders. A variety of nonmalignant lymphoid disorders with greatly different prognoses involve the mediastinum and lung. They are uncommon but those that cause mediastinal lymphadenopathy often are radiographically indistinguishable from malignant lymphomas. The nonmalignant lymphoid diseases that cause infiltrates in the lung parenchyma rarely cause enlargement of mediastinal, tracheobronchial, or bronchopulmonary lymph nodes. It is helpful, therefore, to separate the "reactive" lymphoid disorders into those that cause thoracic lymph node enlargement and those that cause changes in the lung itself. The classification by radiologic appearance (below) is subject to several oversimplifications: malignant lymphoma commonly involves the lung by direct extension into the parenchyma from enlarged mediastinal lymph nodes; infectious mononucleosis has rarely been reported to cause pulmonary infiltrations in addition to the more common mediastinal node enlargement; lymphomatoid granulomatosis may rarely produce lymphadenopathy. Castleman's disease and the two somewhat related reactive lymphadenopathies, angioimmunoblastic lymphadenopathy and histiocytosis with giant lymph node hyperplasia, are the conditions in this group most likely to be mistaken for neoplasm. They are described below. Pseudo-lymphoma and lymphocytic interstitial pneumonia appear under Inflammatory Pseudo-tumors. Detailed discussion of the other "reactive" lymphoid disorders is beyond the scope of this chapter[363–367] (see also Chap. 13).

Tumors of the Middle Mediastinum

When metastatic lung cancer is excluded, middle mediastinal masses at the level of the tracheal bifurcation are diagnosed as sarcoidosis, malignant lymphoma, metastatic carcinoma, lymph node enlargement from granulomatous infection, bronchogenic cysts, and localized pulmonary artery dilation in about that order of frequency. Infectious mononucleosis, collagen disease, erythema nodosum, and the other reactive lymph node disorders are unusual causes of an abnormal mediastinum (see also Reactive Lymphoid Disorders above).

Lymphoma and Metastatic Cancer. Lymph node enlargement with malignant lymphomas is most common in the middle and anterior mediastinum but also occurs in the posterior mediastinum. Hodgkin's disease is by far the most common cause, followed by lymphosarcoma. These diseases seldom present with isolated asymptomatic mediastinal disease if painless enlargement of peripheral lymph nodes, hepatosplenomegaly, constitutional symptoms, and cutaneous or retroperitoneal disease are carefully sought. Extranodal sites of involvement in the gastrointestinal tract, pharynx, and bone should

Lymphoid Disorders of Mediastinum and Lung

- Lymphadenopathy
  - Lymphadenitis
    - Mononucleosis
    - Specific granulomas
      - Coccidioidomycosis
      - Histoplasmosis
      - Tuberculosis
      - Other granulomas-sarcoidosis
    - Collagen disease
  - Giant lymph node hyperplasia (Castleman's disease)
  - Angioimmunoblastic lymphadenopathy
  - Massive histiocytosis with lymph node hyperplasia
  - Malignant lymphoma
- Parenchymal Lung Disease
  - Pseudolymphoma
  - Interstitial lymphoid pneumonitis
  - Lymphomatoid granulomatosis
  - Benign lymphocytic angiitis

be looked for in lymphosarcoma. Pulmonary parenchymal lesions are very common in Hodgkin's disease but are almost never seen in the untreated patient until hilar lymphadenopathy is also present. When the mass of nodes in the middle mediastinum extends into the lung field as a continuous density on the frontal view, sarcoidosis and infectious granuloma are less likely, and lymphoma and metastatic disease are prime considerations.[354] Superior vena caval obstruction may occur with Hodgkin's disease. When massive, bilateral, irregular mediastinal enlargement is present, the diagnosis of mediastinal lymphoma is usually made by biopsy of peripheral or scalene lymph nodes, and mediastinoscopy or limited anterior exploratory thoracotomy are only occasionally necessary.

Parenchymal pulmonary nodules, diffuse lung infiltrates, and pleural effusions occur in up to 25% of patients with non-Hodgkins lymphoma,[367a,b] and are more common in Hodgkins disease.[367c]

Should lymphoma be limited to the mediastinum, the most common histologic variant is nodular sclerosing Hodgkin's disease, which does not often cause enlargement of the paratracheal lymph nodes. When there is no evidence of extrathoracic Hodgkin's disease, this fact may have subtle importance in the differential diagnosis, since both sarcoidosis and tuberculosis have a definite predilection for paratracheal lymph nodes, especially the azygous node which lies at the right lateral tracheal wall just above the proximal end of the right mainstem bronchus. When a mediastinal abnormality is being investigated, histologic examination of lymph nodes obtained by scalene biopsy or by mediastinoscopy must always include special stains for acid fast bacilli and fungi.

Lung cancer is the most frequent metastatic tumor to produce a unilateral mediastinal mass, and generalized mediastinal enlargement caused by a very small or invisible endobronchial primary is not uncommon. Metastatic carcinoma from the pancreas, stomach, prostate, kidney, and testicle tend to produce bilateral hilar and mediastinal lymph node enlargement. By the time metastases from these tumors are so extensive that the mediastinum is involved, the inventory of systems and physical examination usually suggest the location of the primary. Advanced lung cancer is often responsible for a similar roentgenographic pattern in which both mediastinal margins are widened but, again, only when the primary tumor's location is obvious from the chest roentgenogram or the *type and chronology of symptoms*. In this circumstance, the scalene lymph node biopsy may show cancer consistent with either a thoracic or extrathoracic primary (*e.g.*, adenocarcinoma) but the patient's best interest is not served by an exhaustive search for that tumor.

Bronchogenic Cysts. Most bronchogenic cysts develop in the paratracheal area or main carina and project into the posterior part of the middle mediastinum, but not so far posterior as neurogenic tumors.[368] These cysts are common, however, and may occur anywhere in the mediastinum, lung supraclavicular fossa, and the cervical, paraspinal, and presternal area.[369] They represent pinched off buds of the primative foregut or trachea and are lined with pseudo-stratified columnar epithelium with mucous glands, cartilage, and smooth muscle in the cyst wall. Because they contain fluid, they have a relatively uniform density, smooth borders, and a rounded, fusiform, or teardrop configuration (Fig. 15-30). Bronchogenic cysts in older children and in adults tend to be attached to main or lobar bronchi and are asymptomatic, except in rare circumstances when infection produces the signs and symptoms of mediastinal abscess, including an air fluid level on the chest roentgenogram. Carinal cysts interposed between trachea and esophagus are more serious, sometimes producing dysphagia, dyspnea, noisy respiration, and weight loss in infants. Malignant degeneration is rare but bronchogenic carcinoma originating in a cyst wall has been reported.

Pericardial Cysts. The relatively common pericardial cyst is developmental in origin, perhaps resulting from sequestration of part of the pleuroperitoneal cavity by the developing diaphragm. The thin, fibrous wall lined with mesothelial cells is adherent to the parietal pericardium and occasionally communicates with the pericardial sac. Filled with clear fluid, three-quarters of these "springwater cysts" occur as rounded densities at the right cardiophrenic-sternodiaphragmatic angle. Echography can be used to identify a pericardial cyst that actually abuts the chest wall and has no normally aerated lung between the chest wall and the cyst. Computed tomography may also help to distinguish a pericardial cyst from omental fat seen in a Morgagni hernia. If a diagnosis of neoplasm or Morgagni hernia has been excluded by previous chest roentgenograms, CT, gastrointestinal contrast studies, or pneumoperitoneum, the diagnosis may be confirmed and the cyst managed by aspiration of the crystal-clear fluid, thus avoiding the resectional surgery which is usually recommended.[370] Infection is rare and malignancy nonexistent. These cysts are asymptomatic even when quite large and when they can be shown to exist on remote chest x-ray films and diagnosed and managed by aspiration, major thoracic surgery seems unnecessary unless progressive enlargement on the comparison roentgenograms casts doubt on the diagnosis.

Other Masses of the Middle Mediastinum. Benign intramural leiomyomas in the distal two-thirds of the esophagus and sarcomas, the most common of which is fibrosarcoma in the upper third of the esophagus, are more likely to be seen as middle mediastinal masses on the routine lateral chest roentgenogram than is carcinoma of the esophagus. The latter is seldom large enough to permit recognition without an esophagogram. When the esophagus is dilated from achalasia or from neoplastic obstruction at the gastroesophageal junction, it may be visible on the frontal projection as a smooth, laterally convex density which extends to the diaphragm, enlarging the mediastinum to the right (Fig. 15-32). Esophageal hiatal hernia and epiphrenic diverticulum also occur in the middle mediastinum.

Aneurysms of the thoracic aorta may project into the middle mediastinum. Atherosclerotic aneurysms are the most common in this compartment because they tend to involve the descending thoracic aorta. However, traumatic, poststenotic (coarctation), mycotic, syphilitic, and dissecting aneurysms may also extend to this level.

Tumors of the Posterior Mediastinum

Neurogenic Tumors. Neurogenic tumors are the most common primary neoplasm of the mediastinum and are nearly always found posteriorly. In an analysis of 34 reports including 3364 primary mediastinal tumors, they represented 19.4% of the total; lymphomas were next in frequency (15.8%), followed by bronchogenic and pericardial cysts (14.2%), teratodermoid tumors (12.8%), and thymomas (11.5%). A fifth of the entire group of neural tumors were malignant.[371]

A simplified classification of neurogenic tumors based on cell of origin is given in Figure 15-33. Fisher and Vuzevski have presented electron-microscopic evidence indicating that schwannomas and neurofibromas have similar ultrastructural characteristics and that their structural differences are related to quantitative variation in collagen content.[372] With light microscopy, neurofibromas differ from schwannomas in that the nerve fibers are intimately mixed with the Schwann cells, whereas in the schwannoma the proliferation of Schwann cells displaces the nerve fibers which are found on the surface of the tumor. Either tumor may arise from spinal somatic nerves, the sympathetic nerve chain, or the vagus nerve. If both are

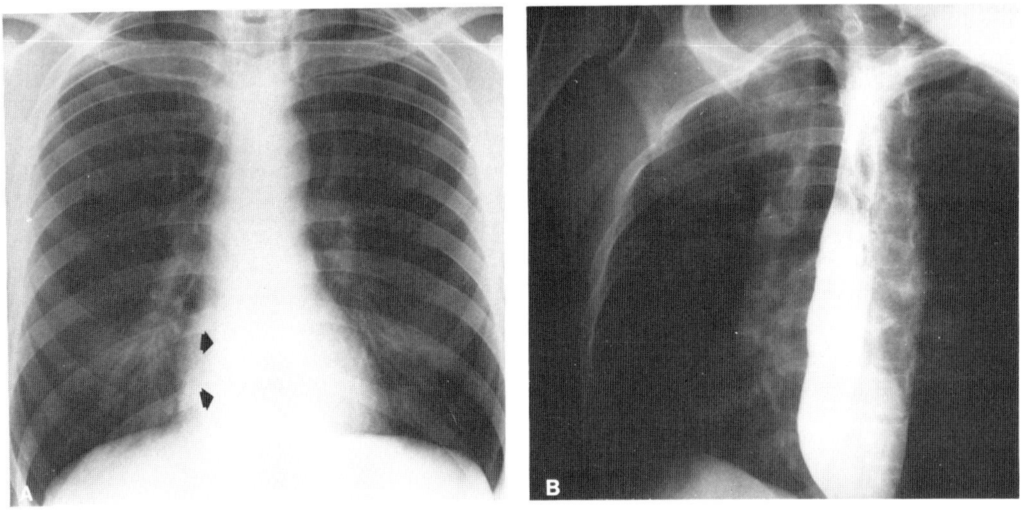

FIG. 15-32. Achalasia. **A.** The right mediastinal margin shows a widening which can be followed to the diaphragm (*arrows*). **B.** The barium swallow demonstrates a dilated esophagus having a distal "bird's beak" configuration. This study was done following recovery from an episode of massive aspiration.

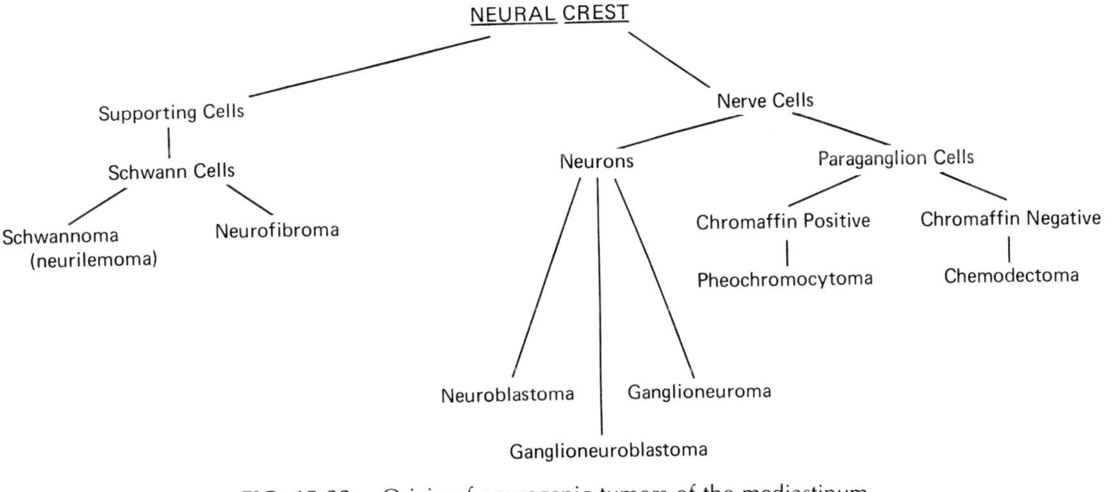

FIG. 15-33. Origin of neurogenic tumors of the mediastinum.

derived from the Schwann cell, the malignant form of either should be termed a malignant schwannoma (also: neurofibrosarcoma). Opinions differ as to whether the malignant form arises *de novo* or from malignant degeneration of benign schwannomas; regardless, the malignant type is uncommon, the ratio of benign to malignant schwannomas being 10.8:1.[371,373] Neurofibromas and schwannomas account for approximately half of mediastinal neural tumors; the malignant tumors of this type occur in children, the benign tumors in the third and fourth decade. Both are associated with von Recklinghausen's disease in which a somewhat higher incidence of malignant schwannoma (6%) is found.[371,373] The presence of a posterior mediastinal mass in this disease does not imply a nerve sheath tumor, however, since meningoceles in this site are more common.

Ganglioneuroma, neuroblastoma, and the uncommon hybrid, ganglioneuroblastoma, are nerve cell tumors representing proliferations of ganglion cells from undifferentiated elements that have migrated to the neural crest to form components of the paraganglionic autonomic nervous system.[374] The benign ganglioneuroma is the most common tumor in this group, making up 23% of all thoracic neural tumors. It has an equal sex incidence and half of the patients are less than 20 years old. The ganglioneuroma is the most common tumor in patients under the age of 16 years in whom it comprises a third of all thoracic neural tumors. The malignant neuroblastoma, a tumor of early childhood, represents at least a quarter of the primary mediastinal neurogenic tumors in children (four-fifths of neuroblastomas originate in the abdominal or retroperitoneal areas, a fifth in the mediastinum where their prognosis is considerably better).

Pheochromocytoma arising from chromaffin cells of the sympathoadrenal system and chemodectomas originating in chemoreceptor tissue are the least common neurogenic tumors of the posterior mediastinum. Both are rare. The great majority of pheochromocytomas are benign. The slow-growing, rarely metastasizing chemodectoma is most commonly found in the aortic body but may be located in a perplexing variety of sites throughout the body including all three mediastinal compartments.[375] Recent reports stress the secretion of catecholamines by chemodectomas whereby they produce a syndrome indistinguishable from pheocromocytoma. The extreme vascularity of both these tumors makes thoracic aortography a worthwhile investigation when intermittent or sustained hypertension, perspiration, palpitation, chest pain, and intense headaches suggest the diagnosis. Urinary assays for catecholamines, metanephrines, and vanillylmandelic acid (VMA) are diagnostic of these tumors. The other sympathetic nerve tumors may also produce neurohormones without correlation with differentiation of the tumor and urinary homovanillic acid (HVA) and vanillylmandelic acid (VMA) should be quantitated whenever neural tumors are suspected, especially in children.[376]

Patients with nerve sheath tumors and ganglioneuromas comprise 90% of those with mediastinal neurogenic tumors; half of these patients are asymptomatic when their tumors are first recognized on routine chest roentgenogram.[374] In those patients with symptoms, the most common complaint is a vague, sometimes intermittent discomfort in the chest. "Root pain" is relatively uncommon and symptoms related to pressure on the brachial plexus or stellate ganglion (Horner's syndrome) are less common still. Large tumors, especially ganglioneuromas, may be responsible for cough, repeated respiratory infections, sputum production, and shortness of breath. Distention of the veins of the neck from mediastinal venous compression and dysfunction of the phrenic, recurrent laryngeal, and vagus nerves occurs, but rarely. Origin of a tumor from the vagus nerve may result in abdominal pain and cramps. Symptomatic hypoglycemia has been reported with malignant schwannomas. Nerve sheath tumors, neuroblastomas, and less commonly, ganglioneuromas may cause spinal cord compression with disturbances in sensation and gait when they protrude through an intervertebral foramen.

The childhood neuroblastomas are known for their predisposition to present with recent and prominent systemic symptoms such as anorexia, weight loss, dyspnea, pleuritic pain, and fever reminiscent of sepsis. Bone marrow biopsies often show neuroblastoma tumor cells, particularly when anemia is present. Since neuroblastoma frequently involves bone, roentgenographic and radionuclide skeletal surveys should also be performed to identify metastatic disease. The metabolic activity of neuroblastoma may be used to visualize the tumor's distribution. Radioactive selenomethionine has been administered and scans performed at 3 to 6 hours show a fairly high incidence of radioactivity in the primary tumor as well as in metastases.[377] *Café au lait* patches or neurofibromas on the skin are uncommon but helpful clues pointing to thoracic neurofibromas or schwannomas. Malignant schwannomas are much more likely to arise from malignant degeneration of a benign tumor associated with Von Reckinghausen's disease than from a solitary benign neurilemoma.

With the exception of the neuroblastomas,

neurogenic tumors have a predilection for upper thoracic sites and are more common on the right than on the left side of the mediastinum. Calcification may occur in neurofibromas, schwannomas, ganglioneuromas, and neuroblastomas. The calcium appears as curvilinear or strandlike densities in cystic tumors, or has a blotchy appearance in solid tumors. Bone changes seen on the roentgenogram are caused by pressure from an expanding tumor and consist of erosion of the inferior margins of ribs, the vertebral pedicles, or lateral portion of the vertebral bodies.[374] The vertebral ends of the ribs may be spread, widening rib interspaces until one or more ribs is dislocated from the spine. Dumbbell-shaped tumors expand the intervertebral foramina[378] If there is widening of a intervertebral foramen, a myelogram is needed whether or not there are symptoms. Actual destruction of bone occurs with neuroblastomas. Scoliosis is common with any of these tumors. The ganglioneuroma is particularly likely to reach a large size before discovery, appearing on the posteroanterior roentgenogram as a dense, more oval than round, laterally circumscribed mass having its longest axis parallel to the spine along the sympathetic chain. In the PA view, the broad-based medial border merges imperceptably with the density of the mediastinum, while in the lateral projection the borders of the ganglioneuroma are often poorly defined. In contrast, a more nearly round mass with a narrow based mediastinal attachment in the PA view is more likely to represent a schwannoma, especially if the tumor margins are relatively well circumscribed in the lateral chest x-ray film (Fig. 15-34).

The primary treatment for mediastinal neurogenic tumors is surgical but postoperative irradiation is used routinely for neuroblastomas, and radiation therapy may be helpful in combination with surgery in initial treatment, or for palliation of unresectable malignant schwannomas. The prognosis for benign nerve sheath tumors and ganglioneuromas is uniformly good, because it is rare for either tumor to recur following surgery.[374] Schwannomas are typically encapsulated and easily enucleated; ganglioneuromas are characteristically densely adherent to surrounding structures; nevertheless, even when resection of a ganglioneuroma is necessarily incomplete, long-term survival can be expected.[374,379] It is common practice to resect the intraspinous portion of a dumbbell tumor first so that spinal cord damage from postoperative swelling or hemorrhage is minimized. Thoracotomy to remove the main bulk of tumor is then done at a later date. Some centers care for these cases as a team, using a neurosurgeon and a thoracic surgeon so that both portions of the tumor can be removed in a one stage procedure.[378,380]

The poor prognosis of malignant schwannomas of the mediastinum was documented in Ingel's 1971 review in which 29 of 40 patients (72.5%) died from their malignancy after surgical removal of the tumor.[371] The average survival time was 2 years. These tumors may involve the spinal subarachnoid space from centripetal growth entirely within the nerve sheath or they may extend into the surrounding tissues to form a nodular tumor which then metastasizes widely through the bloodstream. Wide radical resection to remove a long segment of nerve in either direction is required.

The behavior of neuroblastoma is sometimes unpredictable. Spontaneous cures have been reported in 1 to 3% of patients whose neuroblastomas have matured into ganglioneuromas with loss of their malignant potential. The results with treatment of mediastinal neuroblastoma (56% survival) are twice as good as those achieved with neuroblastomas overall (30% survival), and are nearly three times as good as those with retroperitoneal neuroblastomas (19% survival).[379]

An aggressive surgical approach for local extension of the tumor into the intraspinal, cervical, and subdiaphragmatic areas or the contralateral thorax appears justified.[379] When these tumors appear nonresectable and bone metastases are present, the usual treatment had included preoperative irradiation followed by surgery 6 to 8 weeks later with a second course of irradiation being given postoperatively.[381] Grosfeld and associates, however, found no evidence that control of the primary tumor in disseminated mediastinal neuroblastoma with bone involvement improved survival.[379] In more favorable cases, surgery followed by irradiation

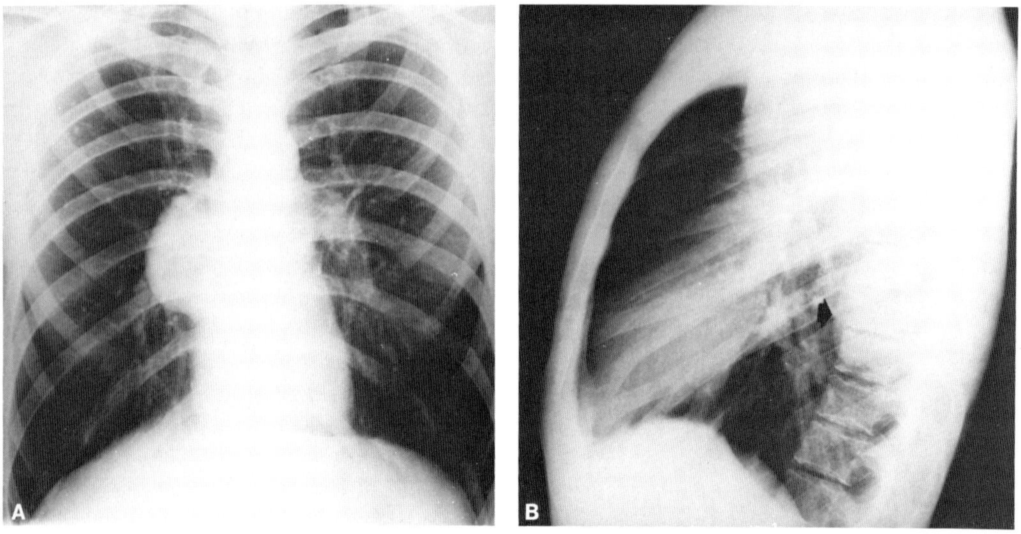

FIG. 15-34. **A** and **B.** Benign schwannoma of the posterior mediastinum. The tumor's narrow attachment to the mediastinum and the sharp definition of its margins in the lateral chest roentgenogram (*arrow*) are characteristic.

appears to be the treatment of choice. Cure should not be expected with surgery or chemotherapy alone or in combination. Cure has been achieved in some children, including some with liver metastases, with either x-ray therapy alone or x-ray therapy combined with chemotherapy. Cyclophosphamide alone or in combination with vincristine probably prolongs survival when used in those requiring palliation.[382]

Angiomatous Lymphoid Hamartoma (synonyms: giant lymph node hyperplasia, Castleman's disease, angiofollicular lymph node hyperplasia) is a pathologic entity of questionable origin first described by Castleman in 1954.[383] Approximately 60% of these benign, tumorlike masses of lymphoid tissue have occurred within anterior mediastinal, hilar, tracheobronchial, or posterior mediastinal lymph nodes. The remainder of the 65 tumors reported by 1972 appeared in a variety of sites including the retroperitoneal area, pulmonary parenchyma, skin, and muscle. The ages of the patients were evenly divided between the second, third, and fourth decades and although a few patients developed mild, nonspecific complaints of lassitude, pressure sensations, or chronic cough, the majority were asymptomatic. There was no predisposition to either sex.

The radiographic appearance of these round to oval, relatively well circumscribed, 4 to 5 cm masses with regular or lobulated margins, is nonspecific and incorrect preoperative diagnoses have included bronchogenic cancer, thymoma, bronchial cyst, and neurogenic tumor. When the tumor is adjacent to a rib in the posterior mediastinum, rib erosions and reactive sclerosis may develop.

The absence of symptoms of concomitant inflammatory disease in the majority of patients and the not unusual finding of pathologic changes limited to a single member of an aggregate of lymph nodes makes an exaggerated inflammatory response in a lymph node an unlikely cause of these tumors.[384]

The intrathoracic tumor's cut surface is pale yellow in contrast to its highly vascular red-brown capsule which is formed from a well-developed arterial supply arising from either the intercostal or the bronchial arteries. The microscopic appearance is characterized by the presence of lymphatic follicles and the number of penetrating blood vessels to the follicles seems to be directly related to the degree of obliteration of the normal follicular architecture.[385] The proliferation and sclerosis of the tumor's stromal blood supply, the distinctive and large systemic arterial blood supply to the tumor's capsule, and the failure of the tumor's blood supply to follow the normal distribution in a lymph node caused Tung to postulate that this lesion represents a vascular hamartoma in a lymph node, thus, angiomatous lymphoid hamartoma.[385] The benign nature of the growth is confirmed by the lack of evidence of recurrence after local excision.

Sinus histiocytosis with massive lymphadenopathy is another benign reactive disorder in which cervical but also mediastinal and hilar lymph nodes are enlarged; patients are usually young blacks.[366] In contrast, angioimmunoblastic lymphadenopathy is seen in middle-aged patients, has a variable prognosis, and may be a variant of giant lymph node hyperplasia.[386]

Extramedullary Hematopoiesis. Large tumors of heterotrophic bone marrow may project as bilateral, homogeneous, posterior mediastinal masses immediately adjacent to the spine in patients with hereditary spherocytosis, sickle cell anemia, thalassemia, and bone marrow dysfunction from chemical exposure, replacement, or sclerosis. The outline of such masses is usually lobulated, but may be smooth. Extramedullary blood formation as a cause for a posterior mediastinal mass is suggested by: (1) the history of a severe congenital hemolytic anemia; (2) a peripheral blood smear showing leukoerythroblastosis (both erythroid and myeloid immature elements); and (3) the presence of an enlarged spleen, peripheral lymph nodes, or liver: the other organs known to participate in extramedullary hematopoiesis. A prolonged stimulus is usually necessary before the mass becomes visible on the chest roentgenogram, and the finding is therefore more common among older children and adolescents. Diagnosis of this compensatory change within lymph nodes is confirmed by needle aspiration.

Bochdalek Hernia. Bochdalek hernia (congenital posterolateral diaphragmatic hernia, pleuroperitoneal hiatus hernia) is the most common congenital diaphragmatic hernia.[387,388] Although any portion or all of the diaphragm may be absent, most defects are posterolateral on the left side and result from failure of fusion of the fetal pleuroperitoneal membrane. The abnormality is a relatively common cause of severe cardiorespiratory distress in infants and children but is rarely reported in adults. Of the 50 adult cases reported in the literature and reviewed by Ahrend and Thompson in 1971, a fourth were asymptomatic and the remainder presented with abdominal pain or vague remitting gastrointestinal symptoms with or without intestinal obstruction.[389] The omentum, stomach, and colon are most commonly involved in incarcerated Bochdalek hernias and the wide variety of difficult-to-interpret roentgen shadows which result may occasionally be confused with masses arising in the posterior mediastinum. Traumatic diaphragmatic hernias from blunt and penetrating injuries are more common than Bochdalek hernias in adult patients[390] (see also Chap. 11).

Miscellaneous Lesions of the Posterior Mediastinum. Sarcomas, plasmacytomas, Ewing's tumors, spinal tumors, aneurysmal bone cysts, and metastatic carcinoma rarely may produce posterior mediastinal paravertebral masses with fusiform configuration, although tumors in bones generally cause only local destructive changes. Granulomatous or pyogenic osteomyelitis are more common causes of such fusiform masses (see Fig. 15-21*B* and Fig. 15-27).[391] A similar roentgenologic abnormality may result from hematomas associated with spinal fractures.

TUMORS OF THE CHEST WALL

Primary tumors of the chest wall originate in the soft tissue, cartilage, or bone, and therefore show great dissimilarities in clinical behavior and histologic appearance. Primary skeletal neoplasms tend to originate in the long bones of the extremities and benign and malignant cartilaginous or bony tumors occurring in the chest wall make up less than 10% of these tumors. Benign tumors are approximately one and a half times more common than malignant primary tumors of the chest wall and both are more common in

TABLE 15-13. The More Common Primary Tumors of the Chest Wall

Soft Tissue	Cartilage	Bone
Benign	Benign	Benign
Lipoma	Osteochondroma	Simple bone cysts
Hemangioma	Chondroma	Osteoma
Cystic hygroma		Osteoblastoma
		Osteoid osteoma
Malignant	Malignant	Malignant
Fibrosarcoma	Chondrosarcoma	Osteogenic sarcoma
		Ewing's sarcoma
		Nonneoplastic
		Fibrous dysplasia

males. Their diagnosis is complicated by disease of the thoracic wall which occurs in lymphoproliferative disorders (reticulum cell sarcoma, Hodgkin's disease), hematopoietic malignancy (plasma cell myeloma), metastatic carcinoma or sarcoma, and nonneoplastic disease of uncertain histogenesis (fibrous dysplasia). Primary tumors of the chest wall are uncommon and this discussion is limited to those which are seen with some frequency (Table 15-13). Additional information is found in reviews listed in the bibliography.[392–395]

Metastatic neoplasms involving the thorax by direct extension and by bloodborne or lymphatic spread are far more common than are primary chest wall neoplasms. The tumors which most commonly metastasize to the thoracic wall are the neuroblastoma in childhood, carcinoma of the breast in women, and carcinomas of the prostate, lung, and kidney in men. Because of their rich blood supply, the ribs are especially prone to metastatic involvement which tends to be posterior in proximity to the vertebral veins. In contrast, the majority of primary rib tumors develop anteriorly.

No tumor involves the thoracic skeleton more frequently than does multiple myeloma: vertebrae, ribs, clavicles, sternum and scapula show lytic lesions in that order of frequency. In occasional patients, myeloma presents as an apparently solitary, destructive rib lesion with an associated soft tissue mass which protrudes into the thorax to produce an extrapleural sign on the chest roentgenogram (Fig. 15-35). The solitary plasmacytoma is also the most common malignant tumor of the sternum in some series. In most of these cases disseminated disease will eventually develop.[395a] Multiple myeloma is also associated with more frequent pulmonary infections, diffuse pulmonary plasma cell infiltrates, lung amyloid, and occasionally pleural effusions.

Conditions Mimicking Chest Wall Tumors

A partial list of the large number of conditions which may cause clinical and radiographic confusion with primary chest wall tumors is given below. Tietze's syndrome or costal chondritis is relatively common, nonsuppurative, tender swelling in the anterior chest wall which affects both sexes equally in the second to fourth decades. The majority of patients experience unilateral relapsing pain, tenderness, and swelling of the second or third costosternal junctions. Single swellings are the rule, but multiple bilateral lesions have been described in 20% of the reported cases.[396] The condition sometimes relapses over weeks to months and often appears to be related to antecedent viral upper respiratory tract infection or minor chest wall trauma, including coughing. There are no systemic symptoms, and other joints are not affected. Examination discloses a firm, tender, bullous or fusiform swelling which elevates an upper costosternal or sternoclavicular joint 0.5 to 3 cm above the chest wall. Erythema of the overlying skin is usually absent but a local increase in warmth may be appreciated. There is no regional lymphadenopathy. Most patients with this syndrome are reported to have no abnormalities on conventional chest roentgenograms, but some authors describe hypertrophy and excess calcification of the involved costal cartilage, best demonstrated in tangential views.[397] Although the diagnosis of Tietze's syndrome should be made on a clinical basis, histologic study reveals the striking absence of inflammatory changes in the cartilage and overlying soft tissues. For the most part, this condition is self-limited and treatment consists of the use of local heat and analgesics or infiltration of the affected area with procaine or corticosteroids. Refractory cases lasting months to years have been managed by surgical resection of the cartilage.

Painful inflammation and swelling of one or more costochondral cartilages occurs in nearly half the patients with relapsing polychondritis.[398] Unlike Tietze's syndrome, this systemic disease causes inflammatory destruction of cartilage in the ears, nose, trachea, larynx, and peripheral joints, threatening life by respiratory involvement. The disease may occasionally involve a single cartilaginous focus and may pursue a smoldering course over many years.

Hyperparathyroidism is included among the conditions which cause roentgenographic confusion with chest wall tumors because some affected patients have roentgenographic findings which resemble multiple myeloma, fibrous dysplasia, or chondromas.

Actinomycosis of the chest wall, tuberculous cold abscess, syphilitic gumma, and bone erosion by aortic aneurysm have been confused with chest wall neoplasms. In addition, a high index of suspicion is now required if pyogenic osteomyelitis of sternoclavicular or costochondral articulations is to be promptly recognized in patients who inject illicit drugs.[391] Ewing's sarcoma of bone often produces fever and rapid progression of local soft tissue findings, resulting in confusion with inflammatory conditions. Attempts to incise and drain this childhood neoplasm are therefore not uncommon.

The most common nonneoplastic conditions misdiagnosed as cartilaginous tumors are the effect of trauma: malunited fractures or separations of costal cartilage.[394]

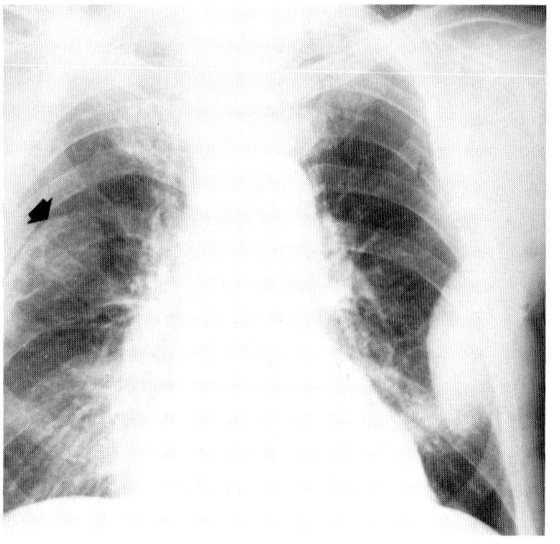

FIG. 15-35. Multiple myeloma involving the thoracic skeleton. The two extrapleural densities seen at the left lateral chest wall are the result of rib involvement. The arrow indicates expansion and destruction in the right seventh posterior rib. (Chest roentgenogram courtesy of Dr. Alan H. Wolson, Ann Arbor, Michigan)

Conditions Causing Both Clinical and Radiologic Confusion with Chest Wall Tumors
Rib anomalies and fractures
Relapsing polychondritis
Osteomyelitis
Tietze's syndrome
Center of ossification
Aseptic necrosis
Spontaneous resorption of ribs
Hyperparathyroidism
Paget's disease
Metastatic neoplasm
Infantile cortical hyperostosis

Clinical Presentation of Primary Chest Wall Neoplasms

The presence or absence of pain is of limited value in distinguishing malignant from benign chest wall neoplasms.[399] Primary cartilaginous tumors of the chest wall often produce indolent symptoms even when malignant. When all neo-

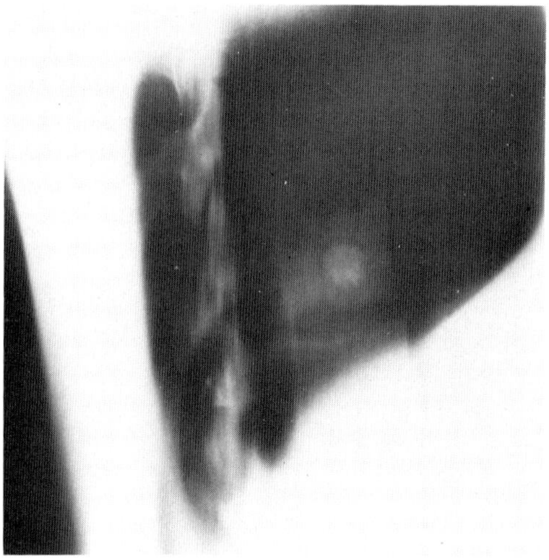

FIG. 15-36. Osteoid osteoma of the thoracic spine. This benign growth caused severe pain and was confused with malignancy until operation. The radiolucent nidus surrounded by an area of reactive thickened bone is characteristic.

plasms of the chest wall are considered, pain is more common with those that are malignant, but approximately half of the patients with pain have benign tumors. Osteoid osteoma, a benign growth that is uncommon in the thoracic skeleton, is particularly likely to produce clinical confusion with osteomyelitis or malignancy because it causes severe progressive pain with nighttime exacerbation. The roentgenographic picture of a round or oval radiolucent nidus less than 1 cm in diameter surrounded by an area of reactive thickened bone is often diagnostic (Fig. 15-36). With other chest wall tumors, pain appearing before the recognition of a mass often indicates nerve or pleural involvement and therefore favors malignancy. On the other hand, asymptomatic tumefactions detected on routine chest roentgenograms are seldom malignant.[400] The character of the pain depends on the nature of the tumor's growth: local dull pain is most common but pleuritic pain accompanied by dyspnea, pressure sensations, and palpitation may develop when extension is primarily intrathoracic. Incorrect diagnoses may result when tumors of the lower ribs irritate intercostal nerves, causing pain to be referred to the abdomen or groin. In other cases, encroachment on the cervical sympathetic nerves or on the brachial plexus produces signs and symptoms in the face, eye, neck, shoulder, and arm.

In addition to posteroanterior, lateral, and Bucky roentgenograms, fluoroscopy, tomograms and x-ray studies after the induction of pneumothorax may help delineate a primary chest wall tumor from adjacent structures. Malignancy is suggested by rapid growth of ill-defined destructive lesions, especially those penetrating the cortex, transgressing the periosteum, forming associated soft tissue tumors, or involving adjacent bones. Benign tumors often show roentgen stability on comparison films. A sclerotic margin is more common with benign tumors but may also occur with slowly growing malignant tumors. Benign tumors are more circumscribed, and tend to expand bone without destruction; however, size as well as histology determine whether or not the cortex of the diseased bone remains intact. Serum calcium and phosphorus determinations and acid and alkaline phosphatase levels have some diagnostic value (*e.g.*, the latter tends to be elevated in osteogenic sarcoma). Radionuclide scans of the bones are sometimes useful in localizing tumors or assessing their extent. They have particular application in Ewing's sarcoma where there is a tendency to metastasize to other bones.

General Principles in the Management of Primary Chest Wall Tumors

Nearly all tumors of the sternum are malignant. Primary tumors of the thoracic vertebrae are usually benign; primary malignant tumors of the scapula are fairly common, but metastatic disease is uncommon in the scapula.[401] The great majority of the primary chest wall neoplasms arise in the ribs where there is an approximately equal division between benign and malignant growths.[395,402] The relative frequency of malignant neurogenic tumors involving the chest wall in von Reckling-hausen's disease has been discussed. In addition, women who have received irradiation for breast cancer have developed skeletal and extraskeletal (soft tissue) osteosarcoma and fibrosarcoma.[403] Extraskeletal osteosarcomas arising in somatic soft tissues from pleuripotential fibroblastic cells are otherwise quite rare. A long latent period of 7 to 23 years between irradiation exposure and the development of either of these tumors has been characteristic.

Tumors of the thoracic skeleton should not be observed without biopsy unless they are multiple. The only circumstance in which single cartilaginous tumors of the chest wall are not resected is in childhood when biopsy has shown them to be benign. The rate of growth of benign cartilaginous tumors slows after adolescence and no new ones should form during adult life. Operation is performed if the growth rate accelerates, if the tumor continues to grow after adolescence, or if a tumor appears in an adult.[394] There is a tendency to underdiagnose the malignancy of cartilaginous tumors and it is not unusual to find chondrosarcoma when reviewing histologic sections interpreted as benign chondroma before tumor recurrence.[394] Pathologic interpretation from a small tissue specimen is hazardous and needle or punch biopsies can prove to be inadequate.[404] (For example, although most chondrosarcomas are malignant from the start, they can develop in the margin of an enlarging osteochondroma.) Surgical biopsies should be performed by an experienced surgeon capable of performing a wide chest wall resection and reconstruction should the tumor prove to be malignant. The biopsy site must be excised to avoid implantation of tumor in skin or soft tissues.

The principal treatment of chest wall neoplasms is surgical and, with the exception of Ewing's sarcoma and reticulum cell sarcoma which are treated with irradiation, all primary malignant tumors should be widely excised. When the malignant tumor occurs in a rib, the entire rib should be removed because of the danger of intramarrow or periosteal extension.[404] Soft tissue extension is an indication to excise a rib above and below the mass. The pleura is entered some distance from the mass, and if pleura, lung, and pericardium are involved, these too are removed along with intercostal muscles above and below the tumor.[393] Large defects in the chest wall may be covered by synthetic materials such as Marlex mesh, by division of costal cartilage and the shifting of a rib, though the use of periosteal strips or fascia lata, and by elevation of the lateral attachment of the diaphragm to cover defects which are low and lateral on the thorax. Such reconstructions usually result in little functional impairment. When the manubrium is involved, the medial ends of the clavicles should be removed. For tumors in the lower portion of the sternum, all of the sternum except the manubrium should be sacrificed together with the adjacent costal cartilages.[405] Primary high-grade malignancies of the scapula must be treated by forequarter amputation. Vertebral neoplasms involving the transverse and spinous processes and pedicles can be surgically removed but those in the body of a vertebra are managed by curettage followed by irradiation.[401]

The most common error made in the treatment of chest wall neoplasms is the failure to perform a sufficiently wide excision. Chondrosarcoma and fibrosarcoma, the most common sarcomas to occur in the chest wall, usually kill by repeated local recurrences. Reexcision of these recurrences is frequently necessary and may significantly prolong life because hematogenous and lymphatic invasion are less common and occur later than with many extrathoracic malignancies. These sarcomas eventually metastasize by way of the blood stream but since lymphatic metastases also occasionally occur, regional lymph nodes should be removed if they are palpable or are close to the tumor. A solitary pulmonary metastasis does not preclude radical surgical treatment of a fibrosarcoma of low grade malignancy, since associated pulmonary resection can be curative. The uncommon rhabdomyosarcomas, malignant synoviomas, spindle cell sarcomas, and epithelial tumors of the chest wall commonly metastasize by way of the lymphatics, and their removal should be accompanied by regional lymph node dissection.

Threlkel studied 23 patients with malignant chest wall tumors of various types, and found that of the 6 who survived 5 years or more (26%), 2 required reexcision beyond the seventh year.[400] A similar survival experience emphasizing the need for long-term evaluation of surgically treated patients for recurrent tumor was reported in O'Neal's thorough review of cartilaginous neoplasms.[394]

Soft Tissue Tumors of the Chest Wall

The more common thoracic soft tissue tumors include the lipoma, neurogenic tumors, fibrosarcoma, hemangioma, and cystic hygroma. The common benign lipoma has a characteristic spongy (fatty) consistency and transilluminates well. A lipoma presents no difficulty in diagnosis unless it arises near the parietal pleura, causing a soft tissue mass which indents the lung. There is general agreement that the very rare liposarcoma almost always arises *de novo* and not from a preexisting lipoma. Liposarcomas are probably more common about the shoulders in older men, and while they rarely metastasize, local recurrences occur in about half of the patients treated surgically.

Fibrosarcoma, the most common malignant soft tissue tumor of the chest wall, rivals the chondrosarcoma in frequency in some series.[399] It tends to occur in young adults, also about the region of the shoulder. These growths vary widely in their behavior and although hematogenous metastases are not uncommon (25%), those of low-grade malignancy are some of the more curable chest wall tumors if procrastination in performing a definitive wide surgical excision is avoided. The difficulties encountered in the management of this tumor are illustrated in one reported case in which 16 operations and irradiation therapy were needed for local control. In each instance, the pathologist indicated that the resection had apparently encompassed the tumor.[404] Soft tissue sarcomas often have a pseudocapsule and the inclination to shell out the neoplasm must be resisted. Radiotherapy has some palliative effect on liposarcomas, fibrosarcomas, and rhabdomyosarcomas but chemotherapy is of little value. Recurrences should be reexcised.

Hemangiomas of the chest wall which develop in striated muscle may produce roentgenographic evidence of rib hypertrophy and notching. The roentgenologic demonstration of phleboliths is uncommon, but pathognomonic. These neoplasms grow slowly until adulthood and rarely, if ever, undergo malignant change. However, they may form a pulsatile mass with a bruit and be mistaken for metastases from thyroid or renal carcinoma.

Cystic hygromas (cavernous lymphangiomas) are uncommon, thin-walled, cystic, multilocular tumors which usually occur in the region of the neck in small children. These benign tumors may extend into the mediastinum and chest wall and are difficult to remove surgically because of their intimate association with adjacent structures. Despite these technical difficulties, cystic hygromas seldom recur.

Cartilaginous Tumors of the Chest Wall

Benign cartilaginous tumors of the chest wall are less common than the malignant chondrosarcoma, and most occur anteriorly near the costochondral junctions in young people. The most common benign tumor is the osteochondroma (osteocartilaginous exostosis) which frequently presents as a mass arising from the scapula or a rib in patients in the second decade (Fig. 15-37). Growth begins in childhood and ceases when general body growth is complete. The tumor may be sessile or may develop on a broad stalk, the cortex of which is continuous with the underlying bone. Microscopically, the bony portion of the tumor is similar to the underlying cancellous bone. Overlying the bony portion is a cartilaginous cap some of which may be calcified so as to present a radiodense margin resembling a cauliflower. Malignant transformation of the cartilaginous portion to chondrosarcoma probably occurs in less than 1% of cases unless multiple tumors are present in hereditary multiple exostosis. In this condition, evolution to chondrosarcoma is relatively common.[394] "Osteochondrosarcoma" is a misnomer because the bone in these tumors is not neoplastic. Osteochondromas should be resected with a wide margin since chondrosarcoma may be identified in but a small portion of the cartilaginous cap.

Chondromas are somewhat less common in the thorax than are osteochondromas. Roentgenographically, they appear as well-demarcated expansion of a rib near a costochondral junction.

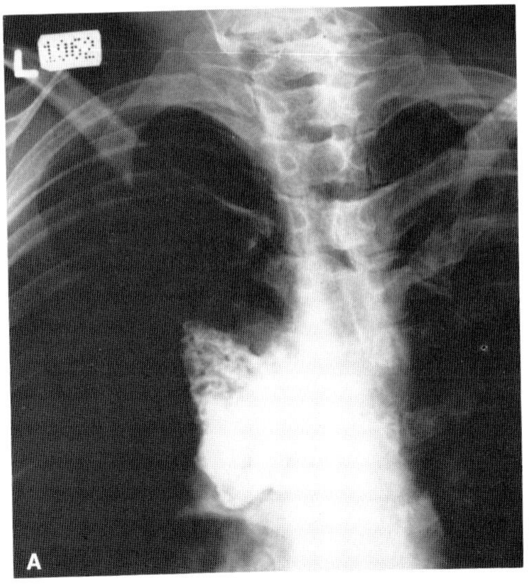

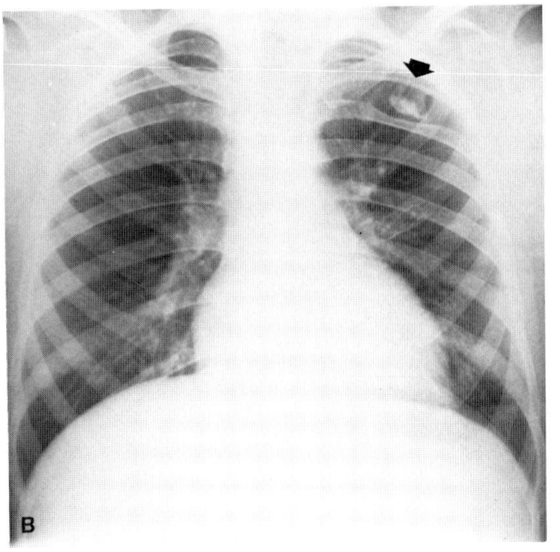

FIG. 15-37. Osteochondromas of the ribs. **A.** Calcification of the cartilaginous cap overlying the bony portion of these benign tumors sometimes causes them to resemble a cauliflower. **B.** This small osteochondroma caused pain by erosion of an adjacent posterior rib. (Chest roentgenograms courtesy of Dr. Walter M. Whitehouse, Ann Arbor, Michigan)

A central, sharply circumscribed, lucent area often contains flocculent calcifications. These benign and usually asymptomatic tumors consist of well-differentiated mature cartilage which is less well formed than normal cartilage. The terms "enchondroma" and "juxtacortical chondroma" refer to the growth's site of origin: the former arises in the medullary portion of bone, the latter in the subperiosteum. Nomenclature which includes the subclassifications of myxochondroma and chondromyxosarcoma is unnecessarily complex since the mucoid substance is not neoplastic but is a product of degeneration. Chondromas sometimes reach very large size and may be roentgenographically indistinguishable from the chondrosarcomas to which they occasionally give rise.[406] Wide surgical excision is recommended.

Chondrosarcoma, the most common primary malignant tumor of the chest wall, accounts for a third to a half of all malignant neoplasms of the thoracic cage and ranks just behind the solitary plasmacytoma as a cause of single malignant rib lesions. A primary type arising *de novo*, usually in postadolescent boys, is less common in the thorax than is a secondary form developing from benign osteochondromas, chondromas, and Paget's disease in the older age group.[393,405] In this circumstance, a history of a long-standing benign mass in the same area may be elicited. Chondrosarcoma, Ewing's sarcoma, and the less common osteogenic sarcoma of the chest wall are all more common in males. Chondrosarcomas radiographically present as large, flocculently calcified masses which seem to arise from the periosteum of upper anterior ribs, scapula, or sternum in such a way that the underlying bone often shows minimal destruction (Fig. 15-38). When large chondrosarcomas with spotty calcification display largely intrathoracic growth, rib detail x-ray films, conventional tomograms, and CT may be required to exclude irregularly calcified teratomas or substernal thyroid adenomas. Blood-borne metastases from chondrosarcoma, most common in lung and epidural space implicating an intercostal vein to vertebral vein pathway, are much less common, and often appear later than those from osteogenic sarcoma. Several local recurrences are sometimes treated with reexcision before dissemination occurs. On microscopic examination, the metastases may resemble fibrosarcoma

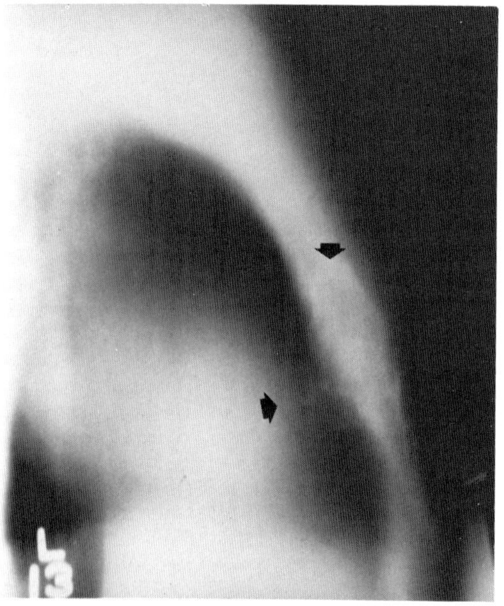

FIG. 15-38. Chondrosarcoma of the sternum. The vertical arrow indicates the area of bone expansion and destruction demonstrated in this laminogram of the sternum. The horizontal arrow points to the margin of the associated anterior mediastinal extension of the partially calcified tumor mass (poorly visualized in this laminographic cut). (Chest roentgenogram courtesy of Dr. Alan H. Wolson, Ann Arbor, Michigan)

and appear more malignant than the primary tumor.

Treatment is by radical surgical excision. There is no consensus as to the value of preoperative irradiation for chondrosarcoma or osteogenic sarcoma of the chest wall.[393] Although these tumors are considered relatively radioresistant, irradiation therapy has been of some use for palliation. Chemotherapy for chondrosarcoma has been generally ineffective but Adriamycin is deserving of trial in widespread metastatic disease. O'Neal reviewed 60 patients with chondrosarcoma who underwent radical surgical resection for anticipated cure, and found 6 patients (10%) to be alive two or more years later.[394]

Bony Tumors of the Chest Wall

Benign osseous tumors in the thorax are rare. Unlike benign cartilaginous tumors, they are not premalignant. Simple bone cysts (unicameral bone cysts) occur in the anterior portions of the ribs or in the clavicles but are more likely to be seen on a chest roentgenogram in the head of the humerus. They cause a circumscribed, uniformly radiolucent defect which may expand and thin the cortex without producing symptoms unless pathologic fracture occurs. Giant cell tumors, 10% of which are malignant, may be found in the head or tubercle of a rib; osteomas usually occur in the scapula, osteoblastomas in the vertebrae. The severe pain which may occur with the benign osteoid osteoma in a scapula or vertebra has been mentioned.

Osteogenic sarcomas of the thorax are much less common than chondrosarcomas and O'Neal, who studied 60 primary chest wall malignancies and found no osteogenic tumors, concluded that reported cases which are free of suspicion of being chondrosarcomas are rare.[394] In the thorax, osteogenic sarcomas tend to occur in older patients and the scapula is a common site. Osteogenic sarcoma, Ewing's sarcoma, and reticulum cell sarcoma are sometimes roentgenographically indistinguishable.[400] Osteogenic sarcoma produces bone destruction (osteolytic form), or more commonly, destruction and reactive new bone formation (osteolytic-osteosclerotic form). Cortical destruction usually occurs with little bone expansion and extension of the tumor into soft tissues is often associated with the deposition of horizontal bone spicules arranged perpendicular to the cortex: "sunburst spiculation." Hematogenous spread to the lung occurs early and although the treatment of this relatively radioresistant tumor is radical surgical excision, most cures of thoracic lesions have followed postoperative irradiation.[407] Cade advocated radical preoperative irradiation therapy (7000 to 8000 rad for osteogenic sarcoma of the long bones) followed in 3 months by resection in those patients still thought to be free of metastases. This delayed surgical treatment did not decrease the survival rate.[408] The disappointing survival, however, will not be much improved by pre- or postoperative irradiation which seeks to ablate the primary tumor because the poor results are largely due to distant microfoci of disease present in 80% of patients at the time of diagnosis. Therefore, systemic chemotherapy seems more promising. High-dose methotrexate with citrovorum factor rescue and cyclic Adriamycin is being investigated in patients who have undergone surgery for osteogenic sarcoma.[409]

Ewing's sarcoma comprises 10 to 15% of all primary malignant tumors of the ribs, but may also involve the scapulae and, less commonly, the sternum. Most of the patients (90%) are under 30 years of age; the peak incidence occurs between 10 and 20 years. This aggressively malignant tumor probably arises from the reticuloendothelial system and its microscopic appearance, uniform basophilic cells approximately twice the size of lymphocytes arranged in pseudo-rosettes in a vascular stroma, may be confused with neuroblastoma, reticulum cell sarcoma, and undifferentiated small cell carcinoma of the lung.[393] Systemic symptoms of fever, weight loss, and malaise are often prominent and are associated with rapidly progressive local changes of increased heat, pain, and tenderness. Roentgenograms usually show a predominantly destructive process with little reactive change; characteristically, there is rapid extension to involve a large portion of the shaft of the involved bone (Fig. 15-39). A soft tissue mass is present in most cases. Multiple areas of periosteal new bone formation may produce an onion-peel appearance that can also occur with osteosarcoma and osteomyelitis; deposition of horizontal bone spicules in the soft tissue mass sometimes results in a sunburst or hair-on-end picture, resembling osteosarcoma or chondrosarcoma. Metastases to the lungs and other bones are identified within the first 2 years of observation in 85% of patients, and radiotherapy with a tumor dose of 4000 to 6000 rad given to the entire length of the involved bone and adjacent soft tissues has resulted in tumor recurrence in approximately a third of the patients. Better results have been obtained in patients with localized disease when the same irradiation treatment was administered with concomitant multicourse high-dose cyclophosphamide-vincristine chemotherapy.[410]

Fibrous Dysplasia of the Thoracic Skeleton

Fibrous dysplasia is a common nonneoplastic condition of bone of unknown cause in which "primitive fibrous tissue proliferates in the medullary cavity and erodes the cortex from within, often producing expansion or distortion of the bone."[411] Histologic examination reveals irregularly oriented spicules of woven bone in a stroma of fibrous tissue.

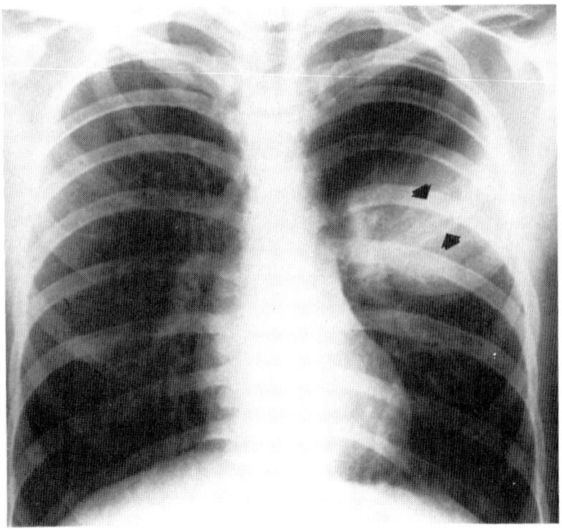

FIG. 15-39. Ewing's sarcoma. The involved rib (*arrows*) shows a predominately destructive process with little reactive change. Characteristically a long section of the shaft of the rib displayed a moth-eaten appearance. (Chest roentgenogram courtesy of Dr. Alan H. Wolson, Ann Arbor, Michigan)

Fibrous dysplasia is the most commonly encountered noncartilaginous abnormality in the ribs of young adults between the ages of 20 and 30 years. Monostotic lesions are more common than are polyostotic defects.[395,411] In most cases, fibrous dysplasia involves a single rib, but other bones may be affected, and a small number of patients with the polyostotic form, usually females, show skin pigmentation, precocious puberty, or hyperthyroidism (Albright's syndrome).[393]

In contrast to the primary rib tumors fibrous dysplasia is most often found in the posterior aspects of the ribs. Pain is rare, the presence of a mass variable, but pathologic fractures are common. There is considerable variation in the roentgenographic appearance because of the differing proportions of fibrous or osseous tissue formed. The bone may be osteoblastic and have a homogeneous ground-glass appearance or areas of endosteal sclerosis may produce a multilocular cystic change (Fig. 15-40).

The disease usually stabilizes at puberty and

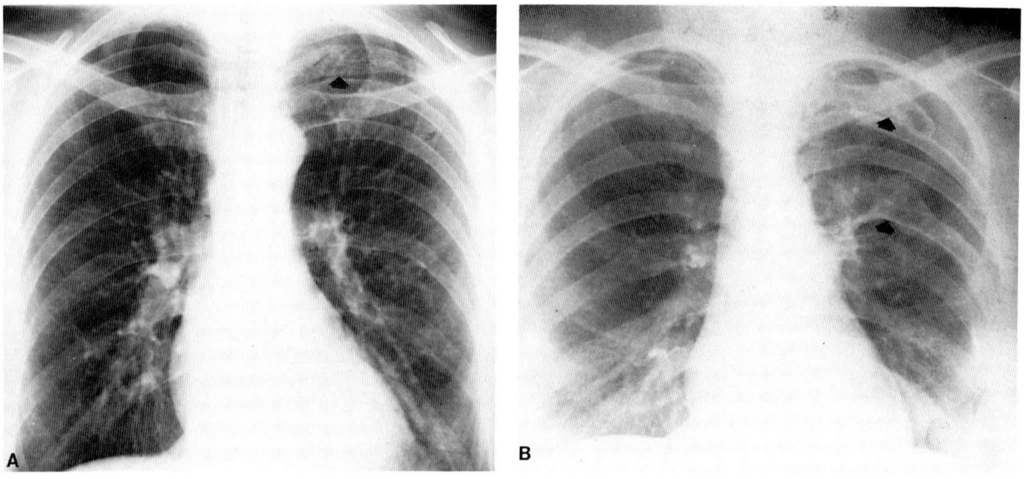

FIG. 15-40. Fibrous dysplasia. **A.** The left fourth posterior rib (*arrow*) is minimally expanded and is somewhat more dense than its counterpart on the right. **B.** Areas of endosteal sclerosis have produced a multilocular cystic appearance in these diseased ribs on the left (*arrows*). (Chest roentgenograms courtesy of Dr. Walter M. Whitehouse, Ann Arbor, Michigan)

may even regress, but a few cases have continued growth into adulthood. Sarcomatous degeneration has been reported, but is rare; nevertheless, irradiation should be avoided so as to minimize this risk.[411] When lesions are multiple, the patient should be observed for malignant change. Single lesions should be excised.[412]

Primary Tumors of the Pleura

These relatively rare tumors are considered in detail in Chap. 12, Pleural Diseases, Mesothelioma.

TUMORS OF THE DIAPHRAGM

In 1965, Weiner and Chow were able to identify only 71 reported cases of primary diaphragmatic tumor.[413] Furthermore, metastatic carcinoma is very rare in striped muscle, and although a number of authors have assumed that secondary tumor deposits in the diaphragm were common, Brennan found that this was not the case.[414] In his series of 151 autopsies on patients dying from malignant disease, 12 (7.9%) were found to have involvement of the diaphragm as compared with 5(3.4%) who had metastases to the spleen. Metastases to the diaphragm from carcinomas of the bronchus, even of the lower lobe, involved the diaphragm in only 2% of the cases. Nevertheless, the diaphragm more often harbors a secondary than a primary neoplasm.

Primary diaphragmatic tumors arise exclusively from mesodermal elements, and the most common benign neoplasms, lipomas, mesenteric or bronchogenic cysts, neurofibromas, and angiofibromas, are about one and a half times more common than the sarcomas. Fibrosarcoma is the most frequently encountered malignant tumor.

A majority of diaphragmatic tumors are symptomatic but the symptoms often first appear only when the growth has reached large size. Pain in the lower chest or flank, aggravated by deep inspiration, is the most frequent complaint. Cough is also common.[413] Dyspnea has been described in nearly a fourth of affected patients and is often explained by lung compression rather than interference with diaphragmatic motion, or by the presence of pleural effusion since the tumors usually move synchronously with the diaphragm causing little disturbance in function, and pleural effusions are surprisingly uncommon (less than 10%).[414,415] Most diaphragmatic tumors project upward into the thorax rather than into the peritoneal space, but left-sided neoplasms may produce gastrointestinal symptoms by compressing the stomach. Tumors of the right diaphragm may displace the liver and are therefore sometimes associated with a palpable abdominal mass. Shift of the mediastinum with displacement of the cardiac apical impulse also occurs. Hiccoughs have been recorded in but a single patient.[413] Clubbing of the digits and hypertrophic osteoarthropathy have been limited to patients with benign or malignant primary neurogenic tumors arising from the intradiaphragmatic portion of the phrenic nerve. Diaphragmatic motion has been normal in these patients. Severe hypoglycemia was associated with a large fibrous diaphragmatic tumor which contained insulin activity.[416]

On the chest roentgenogram, the most common appearance is a localized, convex, sharply defined, but occasionally lobulated shadow which is confluent with the diaphragm. Smaller tumors may produce an extrapleural sign: the lung is smoothly invaginated and the angle formed by the outline of the mass with the outline of the diaphragm is obtuse. It may be impossible to determine whether a tumor is infra- or supradiaphragmatic without pneumoperitoneum, a study which clearly outlines those neoplasms having primarily infradiaphragmatic growth. When the mass is above the diaphragm, pneumothorax may be helpful in establishing its extrapulmonary location. Before considering these examinations, preexisting chest roentgenograms should be reviewed because long-standing, bizarre, nonneoplastic roentgenologic variations in the contour of the diaphragm caused by pleural inflammatory disease, loculated effusions, fibrin deposits, herniated abdominal contents, sequestration of the lung, and eventration of the diaphragm are much more common than diaphragmatic tumors.

Fluoroscopy will identify a paralyzed diaphragm, and often indicates the organ responsible for an abnormal diaphragmatic shadow. Paradoxic movement of the diaphragm demonstrated at fluoroscopy with the sniff test may occur with traumatic herniation, eventration, or from neoplastic invasion of the phrenic nerve.[417] Some diaphragmatic tumors cause fixation of the diaphragm without paradoxic motion, a finding which may also occur with inflammatory disease. Fluoroscopy and an upper gastrointestinal contrast study should be performed early with special attention directed to the movement of the diaphragm.

When a diaphragmatic tumor is suspected in the presence of a pleural effusion, thoracentesis with cytologic examination of the pleural fluid, pleural biopsy, and a postevacuation x-ray film may be useful. Intravenous pyelograms, barium enema, and CT may be necessary to exclude a neoplasm of the kidney or adrenal, and herniation of the colon. Roentgenologic evidence of calcification is extremely rare in primary tumors of the diaphragm and strongly suggests that the abnormality is related to inflammatory disease or to asbestosis. Mesothelioma must be excluded if the patient's history includes asbestos exposure. The presence of calcium in an abnormal diaphragmatic contour should also prompt skin tests for tuberculosis, and complement fixation, hemagglutination, or bentonite flocculation tests for echinococcosis.

Treatment of primary diaphragmatic tumors is by excision, and removal of malignant tumors may involve resection of the entire hemidiaphragm and adjacent thoracic wall, pericardium, and lung. Closure of the defect between the pleural and peritoneal cavities may be conducted using fascia lata grafts, synthetic material, or extracostal skin and muscle flaps.[418]

UNUSUAL TUMORS OF THE LUNG

The tracheobronchial tree and lung may harbor a large number of uncommon-to-very-rare benign and malignant tumors and tumor-like growths of disparate histology. The symptoms produced by these neoplasms are determined by their location within the airways or the lung parenchyma and the classification given below takes cognizance of the importance of predominant sites of growth. Cough, wheezing, hemoptysis, and recurrent or persistent suppuration with eventual irreversible lung damage occur with rare benign or malignant neoplasms which are endobronchial; the strategic location of these tumors ensures that clinical innocence does not proceed from histologic benignity. The uncommon tumors which develop entirely outside the bronchial tree in the lung parenchyma occasionally attain sufficient size to cause dyspnea or pressure phenomena; more often, they are found as asymptomatic solitary pulmonary nodules on routine roentgenograms.

Classification of Unusual Tumors of the Lung by Site of Predominant Location

Tumors of the Trachea or Major Bronchial Tree
- Papilloma, Fibroma, Chondroma, osteochondroma (Sarcomatous counterparts)
- Lipoma
- Granular cell myoblastoma
- Polyp
- Tracheal tumors
  - Hemangioma
  - Lymphangioma
  - Tracheopathia osteoplastica
- Specific granulomatous pseudotumors
  - Tuberculosis
  - Syphilis
- Amyloid pseudotumors
- Bronchial mucocoele

Tumors of the Trachea and Major Bronchi or Distal Bronchi and Lung Parenchyma
- Leiomyoma (leiomyosarcoma)
- Nerve sheath tumors (malignant schwannoma)
- Carcinosarcoma

Tumors of the Distal Tracheobronchial Tree and Lung Parenchyma
- Hemangiopericytoma
- Sclerosing hemangioma
- Blastoma (embryoma)
- Inflammatory pseudotumors
  - Plasma cell granuloma
  - Pseudolymphoma
- Histiocytoma (xanthoma)
- Endometriosis

The benign endobronchial tumors in this group can sometimes be removed with a rigid bronchoscope and bronchoscopic snare or the bronchoscopic resectoscope using a combined cutting and coagulating current. When an upper-lobe bronchus is involved, artificial pneumothorax may bring the bronchus into alignment with the bronchoscope. Other benign growths may be managed by bronchotomy or bronchial sleeve resection and bronchial reanastomosis. The decision to perform a lobectomy to remove both a benign obstruction and the distal damaged lung should be made with the recognition that the chronic suppurative disease may show dramatic improvement if the obstruction can be relieved endoscopically. The bronchiectatic lobe can be removed later should it continue to cause symptoms despite conscientious medical treatment. Nevertheless, benign bronchial obstruction with destruction of the distal lung is often a delayed diagnosis, and references to lobectomy and pneumonectomy are common in reports of uncommon benign endobronchial tumors.[419,420]

Uncommon Tumors of the Trachea or Major Bronchi

Tracheal tumors are rare.[421] Benign tumors of the trachea tend to develop in children, malignant squamous cell and adenoid cystic carcinomas in adult patients. Squamous cell carcinoma is several times more common than adenoid cystic carcinoma, the second most common malignancy.[422] Other malignancies which have been reported to develop in the trachea include oat cell carcinoma, mucoepidermoid carcinoma, lymphoma, plasmacytoma, sarcomas, melanomas, hemangioendothelioma, and chemodectoma. Carcinoma of the thyroid and esophagus involves the trachea secondarily.

Progressive shortness of breath made worse by exertion, hemoptysis, cough, wheezing, change in voice, and dysphagia are the most common symptoms. When unexplained, these complaints should prompt anteriorposterior and lateral roentgenograms of the trachea. The chest x-ray film is normal in 75% of the patients with tracheal tumors and impressive narrowing of the lumen is usually present before diagnosis. The esophagus is commonly displaced by an extrinsic mass when a tracheal tumor is found. A barium swallow should be performed, followed by direct examination of the esophagus when bronchoscopy is done. Benign and malignant tra-

lumen, symptoms develop gradually. Se- distal suppurative disease is therefore the common complication, although degenera- to chondrosarcoma may rarely occur, as chondromas and osteochondromas of the t wall. Bronchial sleeve resection or bron- omy are used to insure complete removal.

oma. The majority of pulmonary lipomas r in middle-aged or elderly men and they in the larger bronchi, perhaps from adipose e present normally in the submucosa.[428] nchial lipomas are solitary in contrast to sub- neous lipomas which are frequently multi- Only 18 of the 51 cases of endobronchial na reported by 1970 were managed by nchoscopic removal.[429] The frequency with ch major resectional surgery was performed nese patients was related to concern over the ihood of a malignant tumor in the absence of eoperative bronchoscopic biopsy and the de- to remove lung damaged by infection. In e patients treated by bronchoscopic removal he lipoma, roentgenographic evidence of nic suppuration often disappeared. Lipoma ne pulmonary parenchyma is even less com- (20%) than lipoma of the bronchus %).[430] Thoracotomy is required to exclude nchogenic carcinoma.

ranular Cell Myoblastoma. Granular cell oblastomas are uncommon tumors of uncer- origin which usually occur in the skin, gue, voluntary muscles, or breast. By 1978, cases of solitary and 2 cases of multiple nors had been reported in the tracheobron- al tree, usually in the lower trachea or main- n bronchi.[431] The tumors are nonencapsu- d and consist of large ovoid or polygonal cells h abundant granular eosinophilic cytoplasm l nuclei with prominent small nucleoli. There ittle supporting stroma. Granular cell myo- stomas were once thought to arise from the mitive myoblast, but are now believed to ginate from Schwann cells or histiocytes. Al- ugh there have been no reports of metastases m endobronchial granular cell myoblastomas, re may be local invasion of the bronchus and lung and there are a few cases in which malignant tumors of this type have metastasized from other primary sites. Uncertainty over the extent of local invasion and future biologic behavior of these tumors makes endoscopic removal suboptimal treatment.[431]

Bronchial Mucocele refers to a grossly dilated, mucus-filled bronchus which retains its normal connection to the distal bronchial tree. The majority have been recognized in the left upper lobe of the lung in asymptomatic patients with little or no history to suggest previous pulmonary inflammatory disease. The accumulation of mucus within the dilated bronchus has resulted from bronchial obstruction from complete congenital atresia, from congenital membranous obstruction, or from post-inflammatory stricture or neoplasm which separate the mucocele from the proximal bronchial tree.[432,433]

Whereas obstructions to lobar bronchi cause varying degrees of volume loss in the involved lobe, the majority of bronchial mucoceles produced by segmental bronchial atresia have been accompanied by a striking degree of focal hyperinfation from collateral air drift into the obstructed segment.[433] The mucocele which sometimes is seen well only on laminograms, appears as an oblong, sharply marginated opacity which may have a branching pattern.[434] Gradual enlargement of the blocked segment may lead to confusion with a bronchogenic cyst, intralobar pulmonary sequestration, pulmonary venous varix, or mucoid impaction from allergic bronchopulmonary aspergillosis. The latter occurs in patients experiencing an exacerbation of symptomatic asthma, chronic bronchitis, or cystic fibrosis.

Bronchial mucocele differs from allergic bronchopulmonary aspergillosis in that atelectasis, coexistent pneumonia, hemoptysis, pleuritic pain, purulent sputum, and the expectoration of mucous plugs are not characteristic.[433]

Although surgery has been recommended for bronchial mucoceles, there are surprisingly few infections in patients with bronchial atresia and some mucoceles show no change over a period of many years.[434]

cheal tumors should be managed by surgery when possible.[423] Oat cell carcinoma and lymphoma should be treated by irradiation and chemotherapy.

A good clinical history and physical examination are necessary if benign growths within the airways are to be separated from malignancy and inflammatory disease of the lung. The physical findings and roentgenographic presentation of endobronchial obstructing lesions are discussed under lung cancer and bronchial adenomas.

Squamous Papilloma. The larynx is the usual site for development of papillomas, the most common tumor of the respiratory tree in infants and children. Involvement of the lower respiratory tract and adult bronchoalveolar disease without preceding laryngeal papillomatosis is rare.[424] When the disease begins in childhood, it is usually self-limited, with approximately 2 to 3% showing extension beyond the larynx; in adults, the course may be more protracted and malignant transformation to well-differentiated, locally invasive squamous carcinoma has been reported.[424,425]

The pathogenesis and method of spread are unknown, but current opinion favors a viral causation and multicentric origin rather than aerogenous dissemination by implantation. The sessile or polypoid papillomas are formed by squamous epithelium supported upon folds of connective tissue. They should not be confused with single, nonrecurring, noninflammatory tracheobronchial polyps which duplicate the various fibrous, myxomatous, and vascular histology of a nasal polyp.[426]

The clinical presentation is that of hoarseness and respiratory distress which may require tracheostomy and repeated endoscopy for surgical removal of laryngeal and tracheobronchial papillomas. In the rare patient with involvement of the distal bronchi and lungs, cavities lined by thick papillomatous growths resembling condylomata acuminata may develop. Al-Saleem recommends that patients needing tracheostomy for extensive papillomatosis show no recurrence for 3 to 6 months before decannulization.[424] Irradiation should be avoided because the only ma-

lignant change reported in ju
tosis has followed x-ray thera

Other Tracheal Tumors. Bron
nostic in hemangioma and lym
trachea. Both tumors are seen i
should be avoided. Hemangio
ratory distress are cured by
phangiomas by resection.[419] In
teoplastica, multiple, small ben
bony and cartilaginous tumor
found to extend from beneath
the main carina and mainste
The diameter of the airways
verely reduced, and subsequen
usual cause of death. Bronchos
the osseous growths is often
major tracheal resection and
must sometimes supplant cons
ment.

Fibroma and Fibrosarcoma. Fi
common intrabronchial mes
may occur even more rarely in
lung, or the pleura. These tum
of spindle-shaped cells lying i
staining stroma and are differ
brosarcoma by the absence of
pleomorphism, or excessive nu
figures. Fibromas can often be r
choscopy.

By 1972, 48 cases of bronchop
sarcoma had been reported. T
tumors, their intrapulmonary o
location, and the number of mit
value in predicting biologic be
endobronchial fibrosarcomas hav
mitotic figures per ten microsco
fields behave in a benign fashio
part. In contrast, and contrary t
belief, small intrapulmonary
without pleural involvement ar
malignant tumors. Treatment is

Chondromas and Osteochondromas
and osteochondromas are found
and major bronchi where they a
laginous rings. Because they gro
usually do not exceed the diamet

chial lumen, symptoms develop gradually. Severe distal suppurative disease is therefore the most common complication, although degeneration to chondrosarcoma may rarely occur, as with chondromas and osteochondromas of the chest wall. Bronchial sleeve resection or bronchotomy are used to insure complete removal.

Lipoma. The majority of pulmonary lipomas occur in middle-aged or elderly men and they arise in the larger bronchi, perhaps from adipose tissue present normally in the submucosa.[428] Bronchial lipomas are solitary in contrast to subcutaneous lipomas which are frequently multiple. Only 18 of the 51 cases of endobronchial lipoma reported by 1970 were managed by bronchoscopic removal.[429] The frequency with which major resectional surgery was performed in these patients was related to concern over the likelihood of a malignant tumor in the absence of a preoperative bronchoscopic biopsy and the desire to remove lung damaged by infection. In those patients treated by bronchoscopic removal of the lipoma, roentgenographic evidence of chronic suppuration often disappeared. Lipoma of the pulmonary parenchyma is even less common (20%) than lipoma of the bronchus (80%).[430] Thoracotomy is required to exclude bronchogenic carcinoma.

Granular Cell Myoblastoma. Granular cell myoblastomas are uncommon tumors of uncertain origin which usually occur in the skin, tongue, voluntary muscles, or breast. By 1978, 46 cases of solitary and 2 cases of multiple tumors had been reported in the tracheobronchial tree, usually in the lower trachea or mainstem bronchi.[431] The tumors are nonencapsulated and consist of large ovoid or polygonal cells with abundant granular eosinophilic cytoplasm and nuclei with prominent small nucleoli. There is little supporting stroma. Granular cell myoblastomas were once thought to arise from the primitive myoblast, but are now believed to originate from Schwann cells or histiocytes. Although there have been no reports of metastases from endobronchial granular cell myoblastomas, there may be local invasion of the bronchus and lung and there are a few cases in which malignant tumors of this type have metastasized from other primary sites. Uncertainty over the extent of local invasion and future biologic behavior of these tumors makes endoscopic removal suboptimal treatment.[431]

Bronchial Mucocele refers to a grossly dilated, mucus-filled bronchus which retains its normal connection to the distal bronchial tree. The majority have been recognized in the left upper lobe of the lung in asymptomatic patients with little or no history to suggest previous pulmonary inflammatory disease. The accumulation of mucus within the dilated bronchus has resulted from bronchial obstruction from complete congenital atresia, from congenital membranous obstruction, or from post-inflammatory stricture or neoplasm which separate the mucocele from the proximal bronchial tree.[432,433]

Whereas obstructions to lobar bronchi cause varying degrees of volume loss in the involved lobe, the majority of bronchial mucoceles produced by segmental bronchial atresia have been accompanied by a striking degree of focal hyperinfation from collateral air drift into the obstructed segment.[433] The mucocele which sometimes is seen well only on laminograms, appears as an oblong, sharply marginated opacity which may have a branching pattern.[434] Gradual enlargement of the blocked segment may lead to confusion with a bronchogenic cyst, intralobar pulmonary sequestration, pulmonary venous varix, or mucoid impaction from allergic bronchopulmonary aspergillosis. The latter occurs in patients experiencing an exacerbation of symptomatic asthma, chronic bronchitis, or cystic fibrosis.

Bronchial mucocele differs from allergic bronchopulmonary aspergillosis in that atelectasis, coexistent pneumonia, hemoptysis, pleuritic pain, purulent sputum, and the expectoration of mucous plugs are not characteristic.[433]

Although surgery has been recommended for bronchial mucoceles, there are surprisingly few infections in patients with bronchial atresia and some mucoceles show no change over a period of many years.[434]

cheal tumors should be managed by surgery when possible.[423] Oat cell carcinoma and lymphoma should be treated by irradiation and chemotherapy.

A good clinical history and physical examination are necessary if benign growths within the airways are to be separated from malignancy and inflammatory disease of the lung. The physical findings and roentgenographic presentation of endobronchial obstructing lesions are discussed under lung cancer and bronchial adenomas.

Squamous Papilloma. The larynx is the usual site for development of papillomas, the most common tumor of the respiratory tree in infants and children. Involvement of the lower respiratory tract and adult bronchoalveolar disease without preceding laryngeal papillomatosis is rare.[424] When the disease begins in childhood, it is usually self-limited, with approximately 2 to 3% showing extension beyond the larynx; in adults, the course may be more protracted and malignant transformation to well-differentiated, locally invasive squamous carcinoma has been reported.[424,425]

The pathogenesis and method of spread are unknown, but current opinion favors a viral causation and multicentric origin rather than aerogenous dissemination by implantation. The sessile or polypoid papillomas are formed by squamous epithelium supported upon folds of connective tissue. They should not be confused with single, nonrecurring, noninflammatory tracheobronchial polyps which duplicate the various fibrous, myxomatous, and vascular histology of a nasal polyp.[426]

The clinical presentation is that of hoarseness and respiratory distress which may require tracheostomy and repeated endoscopy for surgical removal of laryngeal and tracheobronchial papillomas. In the rare patient with involvement of the distal bronchi and lungs, cavities lined by thick papillomatous growths resembling condylomata acuminata may develop. Al-Saleem recommends that patients needing tracheostomy for extensive papillomatosis show no recurrence for 3 to 6 months before decannulization.[424] Irradiation should be avoided because the only malignant change reported in juvenile papillomatosis has followed x-ray therapy.[424]

Other Tracheal Tumors. Bronchoscopy is diagnostic in hemangioma and lymphangioma of the trachea. Both tumors are seen in infancy. Biopsy should be avoided. Hemangiomas causing respiratory distress are cured by irradiation, lymphangiomas by resection.[419] In tracheopathia osteoplastica, multiple, small benign, submucosal, bony and cartilaginous tumor excrescences are found to extend from beneath the vocal cords to the main carina and mainstem bronchi.[419,420] The diameter of the airways may become severely reduced, and subsequent infection is the usual cause of death. Bronchoscopic removal of the osseous growths is often impossible and major tracheal resection and reconstruction must sometimes supplant conservative management.

Fibroma and Fibrosarcoma. Fibroma, the most common intrabronchial mesodermal tumor, may occur even more rarely in the trachea, the lung, or the pleura. These tumors are composed of spindle-shaped cells lying in a dense, dark-staining stroma and are differentiated from fibrosarcoma by the absence of hypercellularity, pleomorphism, or excessive numbers of mitotic figures. Fibromas can often be removed at bronchoscopy.

By 1972, 48 cases of bronchopulmonary fibrosarcoma had been reported. The size of these tumors, their intrapulmonary or endobronchial location, and the number of mitoses are of some value in predicting biologic behavior.[427] Small endobronchial fibrosarcomas having three or less mitotic figures per ten microscopic high-power fields behave in a benign fashion for the most part. In contrast, and contrary to a widely held belief, small intrapulmonary fibrosarcomas without pleural involvement are more highly malignant tumors. Treatment is surgical.

Chondromas and Osteochondromas. Chondromas and osteochondromas are found in the trachea and major bronchi where they arise from cartilaginous rings. Because they grow slowly, and usually do not exceed the diameter of the bron-

Tumors of the Trachea and Major Bronchi or Distal Bronchi and Lung Parenchyma

Leiomyoma. Miller's identification of 22 cases of pulmonary leiomyoma reported by 1969 indicates that this benign tumor is approximately half as common as leiomyosarcoma.[419,427] Ten of the 22 leiomyomas were found in a major bronchus. Benign smooth muscle tumors appear to be more common in females; half are seen in patients over 40 years of age.[435] Cough and symptoms of infection are the usual complaints of patients with endobronchial leiomyomas. Peripheral parenchymal tumors of this type have no roentgenographic features which distinguish them from other benign or malignant, primary or metastatic growths. One patient with an endobronchial leiomyoma was adequately treated by bronchoscopic removal of the tumor but bronchial sleeve resection or lobectomy are often necessary. A metastasis from a well-differentiated leiomyosarcoma of the uterus may histologically resemble a benign leiomyoma.

Leiomyosarcoma and Fibrosarcoma. The number of mitoses, the size, and the endobronchial or intrapulmonary location serve as guides to the biologic behavior of bronchopulmonary leiomyosarcomas as well as fibrosarcomas. These two tumors are sometimes collectively referred to as spindle cell sarcomas. In contrast to leiomyomas which are more common in women, most leiomyosarcomas are found in middle-aged to elderly adult men.[427] The most common presenting symptoms, regardless of the location of the leiomyosarcoma, are cough, hemoptysis, and chest pain. The roentgenographic appearance is usually that of a large (often greater than 10 cm), sharply circumscribed mass with a regular or lobulated margin. Cavitation may, in rare cases, be present in leiomyosarcomas. Small endobronchial leiomyosarcomas confined to the walls of large bronchi behave much like comparably located fibrosarcomas: metastases are uncommon and long-term survival may result following surgery. Despite the high incidence of metastases from small parenchymal leiomyosarcomas, Guccion reported a collective 5-year survival rate of 44% after surgery.[427] Large intrapulmonary leiomyosarcomas which are inoperable or are only partially resectable because of chest wall invasion have a less favorable prognosis.

Nerve Sheath Tumors. Schwannomas and neurofibromas are much less common within the lung than in the paravertebral gutter (see Tumors of the Posterior Mediastinum). Malignant schwannoma of the lung is an even rarer tumor which may have a microscopic appearance resembling leiomyosarcoma and fibrosarcoma, the other spindle cell sarcomas of the lung. The diagnosis of malignant schwannoma of the lung is afforded additional support if the patient has generalized von Recklinghausen's disease.

Carcinosarcoma and Blastomas. Carcinosarcoma and blastoma are rare, primary, mixed malignancies of the lung that contain both carcinoma and sarcoma. Both are more common in elderly men. In carcinosarcoma, there is a histologic transition from squamous, adeno-, or undifferentiated large cell carcinoma to components of sarcoma which may include fibrosarcoma, osteogenic sarcoma, chondrosarcoma, or various mixtures.[436,437] The pulmonary blastoma (embryoma) is composed of epithelial-lined tubules resembling embryonic bronchial structures distributed in an abundant stroma of immature sarcoma.[438] Blastomas are thought to arise from pleuripotential, immature pulmonary mesenchyme and seldom have a significant endobronchial component. Chondrosarcomas, on the other hand, show both intrabronchial and extrabronchial growth. Metastases to regional lymph nodes and extrathoracic sites occur with both tumors.

Although the validity of a separate classification of carcinosarcoma in any organ system is debatable, experimental evidence indicates that these tumors are real entities and not just "collision tumors."[436] The preferred treatment of both tumors is resection; however, in some patients with metastases, palliation may be obtained with roentgen therapy. The biologic behavior of these tumors is quite unpredictable, but survival appears to be similar to that for patients with bronchogenic carcinoma.

Tumors of the Distal Tracheobronchial Tree and Lung Parenchyma

Sarcoma. Primary sarcoma of the lung is a rare tumor. It occurs predominantly during the third and fourth decades and responds more favorably to resection than does bronchogenic carcinoma. The 5-year survival rate following surgery is better than 50%. The tumors include leiomyosarcoma, rhabdomyosarcoma, and the most common, fibrosarcoma. The histologic features frequently create confusion, and the evidence that the tumors are not metastatic may only be persuasive with prolonged observation[427,438a] (see also Leiomyoma, above).

Hemangiopericytoma. The histologic features of the hemangiopericytoma are distinctive and include a profuse proliferation of capillaries surrounded by a characteristic tumor cell, the pericyte, a modified smooth muscle cell which functions to alter the size of the capillary lumen.[439,440] This tumor has a universal distribution (wherever capillaries exist); in the thorax, it is somewhat more common in the mediastinum than in the lung or pleura. There is no predilection for sex or age and the malignant potential of individual hemangiopericytomas can only be determined by extended observation. A tumor which is regarded as benign on the basis of encapsulation and microscopic appearance may subsequently prove to be malignant with very late identification of metastases. A tumor which metastasizes, however, is more likely to show diffuse local spread at the time of surgery, while one that is encapsulated more often follows a benign course.

The roentgenographic appearance is that of a well-demarcated, homogeneous mass which, rarely, may be seen to pulsate on fluoroscopic examination. The rich vascular supply produces a tumor "stain" with angiography, a finding which may be helpful in diagnosis or in identifying recurrences, since among lung and mediastinal tumors only the pheochromocytoma and chemodectoma are likely to show extreme vascularity with angiography.

Treatment is primarily surgical. Radiotherapy affords some measure of control.

Sclerosing Hemangioma. Sclerosing hemangiomas are tumors of uncertain histogenesis demonstrating proliferation of vessels with a marked tendency to sclerosis, hemorrhage in various stages of organization, and infiltration of the supporting tissues and air spaces with histiocytes containing various amounts of fat and hemosiderin.[441] Such tumors were first described in the skin and are very rare in the lung where they occur in the lower lobes, usually in women in the third and fourth decades. The tumors contain abundant fat but are not associated with hypercholesterolemia or generalized xanthomatosis. Their lipid content is so great that Liebow believes that many nonmetabolic xanthomas (fibrous histiocytomas, see below) are in fact sclerosing hemangiomas.[441]

Sclerosing hemangiomas differ from so-called postinflammatory tumors in that the latter are composed predominantly of plasma cells and other leukocytic elements and contain no clearly hemangiomatous components. Sclerosing hemangiomas grow slowly and are often clinically silent since they are not associated with obstructive pneumonitis. Prognosis after local resection or lobectomy is excellent.

Inflammatory Pseudo-tumors. Pseudo-tumors are produced by the accumulation of plasma cells or lymphocytes in the lung. Two types of local plasma cell collection occur. Both are rare.

True primary plasma cell parenchymal *tumors* (plasmacytomas) may be single or multiple, may consist of myeloma cells and elaborate M-type proteins, and usually progress to disseminated disease. In contrast, the plasma cell *granuloma* represents a benign collection composed mainly of plasma cells, but with varying numbers of lymphocytes, leukocytes, and fibroblasts in an area of focal infection. The plasma cell granuloma is an inflammatory pseudo-tumor which may present as an asymptomatic mass or may expand to cause radiographic findings and symptoms related to bronchial compression.[442] Thoracotomy usually is performed to exclude bronchogenic carcinoma but efforts to identify a specific infectious agent are seldom successful.

Primary lymphomatous lesions in the lung parenchyma may be separated into four categories: lymphocytic lymphoma, histiocytic lymphoma, Hodgkin's disease, and the benign inflammatory pseudo-tumor, pseudo-lymphoma.

In 1963, Saltzstein set forth the criteria for the diagnosis of pseudolymphoma: (1) mixed cellular pulmonary infiltrate with mature lymphocytes predominating; (2) lymph nodes free of malignant lymphoma; and (3) the presence of true germinal centers within the infiltrate.[443] He considered the third criterion the most important in distinguishing benign from malignant disease but cautioned that an unequivocal histologic diagnosis of benignancy was not possible in all cases. (Malignant lymphocytic lymphomas in the lung have a uniform cellular infiltrate of immature lymphocytes, contain no germinal centers, and frequently involve lymph nodes.)

In contrast to patients with malignant lymphoma, patients with pseudo-lymphoma are asymptomatic or have mild pleuritic pain and fatigue. Rales may be heard over the involved area. There are no other gross signs or symptoms and the hemogram, bone marrow examination, and bronchoscopy are normal.

On the chest roentgenogram, pseudo-lymphoma usually appears as a segmental or lobar consolidation extending from the hilum toward the lung periphery. The infiltrates rarely project all the way to the pleura along the lateral chest wall and their peripheral margins are faint, irregular, and indistinct.[444] The abnormality occasionally presents as a solitary pulmonary nodule.

Carrington and Liebow described a third variant of pseudo-lymphoma, lymphocytic interstitial pneumonia (LIP), characterized by diffuse, unilateral or bilateral infiltration of lymphoid tissue which caused patchy, linear, and nodular densities most prominent in the lower lung fields.[445,363–367] Steroid therapy has produced improvement in some patients with this roentgen pattern. Lymphocytic interstitial pneumonia is discussed further in Chap. 13. Although air bronchograms occur in both malignant lymphoma and pseudo-lymphoma, hilar adenopathy, pleural effusion, and atelectasis common in malignant lymphoma are not seen in pseudo-lymphoma.

Monoclonal and polyclonal gammopathies have been associated with lymphocytic interstitial pneumonia and nodular pseudo-lymphoma but the pathophysiologic implications of this finding are unresolved.[446]

The treatment of pulmonary lymphocytic tumors including pseudo-lymphoma has been primarily surgical, with radiotherapy being reserved for palliation of the malignant forms.[443,446]

Histiocytoma (Xanthoma). The pathogenesis and differentiation of the histiocytoma or xanthoma from sclerosing hemangiomas is not precise (see above.).[441,447] Histiocytomas are loosely encapsulated, golden yellow tumors consisting of two types of cells with transitional forms. Irregular spindle cells are interspersed with variously sized clusters of typical foam cells containing fat. These tumors develop in other connective tissue sites and of the few which have behaved in a malignant fashion, most arose in the retroperitoneal area and some metastasized to lung. Bronchial invasion by a histiocytoma originating in the lung has been described but the tumors appear to have minimal malignant potential. Grossman feels that the histiocytoma should be considered as an entity separate from the pulmonary inflammatory pseudo-tumor with which it is sometimes classified.[447] Treatment is surgical.

Endometriosis. Bronchopulmonary endometriosis may present as hemoptysis which develops with the onset of menstruation, as solitary or multiple asymptomatic pulmonary nodules, or least commonly, as an endobronchial obstructing lesion associated with atelectasis.[448] Disease within the bronchi or pulmonary parenchyma probably results from hematogenous embolization since most patients have histories of pelvic surgery (cesarean section, dilation and curettage, hysterectomy). In a review of 11 reported cases of histologically examined pulmonary endometriosis, Jelihovsky and Grant found that 6 of the women had died during pregnancy or shortly after delivery and suggested that these deposits of decidua without endometrial glands had resulted from agonal embolization.[449] In the other 5 cases, larger single lesions with endometrial glands were found in surgically resected specimens. Three of the 5 had experienced cyclical hemoptysis or recurrent pneumothorax. Radiographic examination may show solid or cystic nodular disease of the lung.[450]

The syndrome of recurring catamenial spontaneous pneumothorax is not common but is seen more frequently than is endometriosis of the lung parenchyma. Features common to most reported cases include involvement of the right hemithorax; close temporal relationship to the onset of menstrual flow; rapid spontaneous resolution of the pneumothorax; failure to occur at other times in the menstrual cycle; and onset of the disease in women aged 30 to 40 years when pelvic endometriosis is commonly seen. Pneumothorax has not been seen in affected women when pregnant or when progestogen-mestranol (Enovid) are given continously (without cyclic interruption) in dosage sufficient to suppress both ovulation and menstruation.[451]

Half of the patients with recurrent catamenial pneumothoraces have had pelvic, diaphragmatic, or pleural endometriosis but hemothorax is seen in the minority.[451,452] Not all patients with recurrent pneumothorax have been shown at thoracotomy to have perforations in the right hemidiaphragm. Rossi has outlined a number of additional objections to the older postulate that held that during menstruation there is passage of air via the genital tract into the peritoneal cavity and thence through diaphragmatic defects into the pleural cavity.[452]

Prostaglandin F_2 has been shown to cause bronchiolar and vascular constriction. There is pronounced increase in this substance in the sloughing endometrium and in the plasma of some women at the time of menstruation during ovulatory cycles; the prostaglandin content of menstrual fluid is reduced in anovulatory cycles. Whether prostaglandin F_2 is somehow related to the recurrence of spontaneous pneumothorax is unknown.[452] It has been demonstrated that some patients with this syndrome may suffer additional pneumothoraces if pleural abrasion rather than parietal pleurectomy is performed at thoracotomy.

NEOPLASMS METASTATIC TO THE LUNG AND THORAX

CLINICAL PRESENTATIONS

Metastatic malignancy is tumor that has been transported from the primary to a new site. Characteristic patterns of invasion and predilection for spread to certain tissues suggest the mechanism of spread for some tumors. Invasion of lymphatic vessels with involvement of regional lymph nodes is common for malignant melanoma; invasion of blood vessels and spread through the vascular system is more characteristic of renal carcinoma. Whether cells gain entry to the circulation through invasion of blood vessels or lymphatics, circulating tumor cells and tissue susceptibility must function in concert to permit a new tumor site to become established. Airway spread of tumor has been suggested for bronchoalveolar carcinoma, but this remains speculative. Thoracic metastasis may result from tumors whose primary is in the thorax or elsewhere.

Chest Wall Metastases

Enlarged supraclavicular or axillary lymph nodes, intracutaneous or subcutaneous nodules, or bone tenderness may be the earliest clinical manifestations of metastatic tumor. Superficial masses should be biopsied if the diagnosis is in doubt. Roentgen examination of the ribs and spine commonly demonstrate osteolytic (multiple myeloma, lung, renal, breast, prostate carcinoma) or osteoblastic (prostate, thyroid) lesions. Radioisotope bone scans are more sensitive,[241] and demonstrate increased uptake in most metastatic lesions except multiple myeloma which characteristically has reduced uptake.

Pleural Metastases

Pleural metastases occasionally present with pleuritic chest pain, or are clinically silent but show roentgenographic evidence of pleural nodules. Commonly, patients present with pleural effusion, frequently bilateral. This problem is discussed in detail in Chapter 12 on pleural disease and neoplasms.

Diffuse Pulmonary Metastasis (Lymphangitic Spread)

Dyspnea is an infrequent presenting feature of neoplastic diseases. When this occurs, particularly in a patient with cor pulmonale and pulmonary infiltrates, the possibility of extensive pulmonary vascular or lymphatic tumor involvement must be considered.[453–457] These patients characteristically have severe arterial hypoxemia with a high alveolar–arterial oxygen gradient, but the dyspnea is not completely relieved by correction of arterial oxygen with supplemental oxygen, suggesting more complex factors are responsible (see Chap. 2). Pleural effusions are commonly present. Chest roentgenograms demonstrate reticular parenchymal infiltrates, generally most marked in the lung bases, with dilated linear subpleural septal lymphatics (Kerley B lines).[458,459] Nodular lesions may also be present. At this stage, particularly in patients who are immune suppressed because of chemotherapy or use of corticosteroids, the differential diagnosis must include infections, cytotoxic drug induced interstitial lung disease, and diffuse pulmonary hemorrhage (see Chapter 8, on infections of the compromised host and Chapter 13, on diffuse parenchymal lung disease).

About half such patients survive less than 3 months and 90% less than 6 months, but 10% (particularly those with carcinoma of the breast) may respond to therapy, show improvement, and survive for several years.[457]

The pathogenesis generally includes widespread invasion of lymphatics with involvement of hilar lymph nodes and peripheral or central obstruction of lymphatic channels. The most persuasive studies suggest that vascular emboli precede the perivascular invasion of lung lymphatics in most patients.[453,457] Typical "lymphangitic spread" is seen most commonly with adenocarcinomas of the breast, stomach, lung pancreas, colon, endometrium, and ovary; carcinoma of the prostate, cervix, and rare tumors may occasionally present in this way.[453–457]

Pulmonary tumor emboli may mimic thromboembolism.[456] This presentation is discussed in detail in Chapter 10 under Tumor Emboli.

Hilar node involvement is discussed above, under Tumors of the Middle Mediastinum.

Nodular (Discrete) Metastasis

Early pulmonary metastases produce few symptoms other than dry cough because they usually have an extrabronchial origin in the periphery of the lung. Hemoptysis is rare. Pain is rarely mentioned in surgical series because like weight loss, it suggests widespread metastases. Clubbing and osteoarthropathy have been described. Studies of sputum cytology have shown cancer cells in 5 to 25% of these patients. Large, or rapidly growing metastatic lesions may cavitate. Endobronchial and peribronchial metastasis, most common from cancer of the breast, may be identified predominantly by their histologic similarity to the primary tumor.[460,461]

It is sometimes impossible to distinguish a metastasis from a coincident primary bronchogenic cancer. The likelihood that a solitary nodule seen on a chest roentgenogram is a metastasis is less than 1% if the patient has no history of malignancy.[462] When there is a history of malignancy, the overall chance that a new pulmonary nodule is a metastasis is greatly influenced by the disease free interval and the location of the earlier primary. If the primary was in the upper airway, prostate, stomach or breast, the solitary nodule is probably a new lung cancer. Multiple primary lung cancers are being recognized more frequently.[463,198a] When the first malignancy was in the large bowel, kidney or testicle, there is an even chance for a metastatic or new cancer. Previous treatment for a sarcoma or melanoma make a metastasis much more likely than a primary lung cancer.

MANAGEMENT

In general, the most important aspects of management are concerned with optimal management of the specific tumor type, and supportive care.

Management of a few of these patients has changed with the development of effective chemotherapy for their tumors. Better understanding of prognostic factors also has become important. These include the following: (1) tumor doubling time; (2) disease free interval from ablation of the primary tumor to recognition of metastases; (3) number and distribution of metastases; (4) size of metastases; and (5) biologic variables such as whether the venous drainage of the primary tumor is to the liver, the lung or to both.

Studies of patients treated by pulmonary resection for lung metastases from extrathoracic carcinomas and sarcomas show that 20 to 30% live 5 years; considerably higher than those who survive lung resection for primary lung cancer. It must be emphasized that these results are achieved in small groups culled from the best candidates among thousands of patients with malignancy in major cancer treatment centers. The relatively large percentage of patients with sarcoma in these series is one indication of the rigorous selection.

Surgical Resection

The minimal criteria for operability of pulmonary metastases are as follows: (1) complete control of the primary tumor; (2) absence of extrathoracic metastases; and (3) whole-lung tomograms which show that all the metastases can be resected. Bilateral metastases are seldom removed. Exceptions include metastases with long TDT and those for which chemotherapy is effective when combined with surgery. At present these are limited to seminoma and osteogenic sarcoma.[464,465] Metastatic choriocarcinoma or hydatidiform mole are treated best with chemotherapy even when presenting as a solitary pulmonary nodule.[466]

When thoracotomy is considered for pulmonary metastatic disease, the preoperative diagnostic evaluation should begin with review of the surgical pathology reports from the operation done to control the primary malignancy. The surgeon's dictated summary also may contain clues as to the likelihood of local recurrence or extrathoracic metastases. Benign pulmonary disease causes a fifth of the new nodules in patients whose primary malignancy has been controlled, and tests to exclude the coincidental appearance of benign disease are often needed. Earlier chest roentgenograms should always be obtained. They either confirm that a nodule is new or make it possible to calculate the doubling time of metastases that were overlooked when smaller. Lung tomography and liver function tests are mandatory. A high percentage of the patients whose tomograms show more than one nodule have even more extensive disease at thoracotomy. Pulmonary function tests are particularly useful in this group. The lower limit of detectability of parenchymal nodules by conventional tomography is approximately 6 mm compared with 3 mm using CT. Substitution of CT for conventional tomography as the primary screening method when evaluating patients for early metastases may not be justified, because although CT identifies half again as many nodules, more than half of these additional nodules are benign.[467,468] Mediastinoscopy and mediastinal tomograms should be considered for patients with histories of carcinoma or melanoma before surgery is done to remove a pulmonary metastasis. More than a third have tertiary metastases in mediastinal lymph nodes.

Mediastinoscopy is seldom done before resecting metastatic sarcomas because they invade blood vessels but do not metastasize to the mediastinal lymph nodes. Sarcomas almost never present with lung metastases before recognition of the primary malignancy.[469] Metastases from sarcomas are commonly limited to the lungs and respiratory failure is the most common cause of death. The median survival after recognition of the first pulmonary metastasis is 5 months.[469] In most studies, the median and 5-year survival of patients operated upon for sarcomatous pulmonary metastases is lower than that of comparable patients with carcinoma. There are few guidelines for resection of pulmonary metastases from sarcomas because the number of treated patients is small and there are 10 or more commonly recognized histologic types. Some centers are now treating bilateral metastatic osteogenic sarcoma by surgery combined with high-dose methotrexate, citrovorum factor rescue, Adriamycin, and cyclophosphamide. Patients with metastatic Ewing's sarcoma are seldom candidates for operation because extensive bilateral pulmonary dissemination is the rule.

Renal adenocarcinoma often metastasizes to the lung. There is no effective systemic therapy for this malignancy. Nephrectomy alone is probably justified when unilateral pulmonary metastases are present at the time the primary cancer is diagnosed. Opinions differ as to whether unilateral pulmonary metastases should be removed when they appear after the primary is thought to be controlled.[470] A renal tumor is often not suspected clinically when these patients present with pulmonary metastases; therefore, patients found to have clear cell tumors of the lung should have an intravenous pyelogram. Primary clear cell carcinoma of the lung and benign clear cell tumors of the lung (sugar tumors) may resemble metastatic hypernephroma histologically. Both are rare.[470] Other malignancies which sometimes produce clear cell metastases in the lung include adrenal carcinoma, carcinomas from the female urogenital tract, seminomas and liposarcomas.

Patients with metastasis from malignant melanoma should meet stringent selection criteria before being operated upon because results are uniformly poor. Melanoma and breast cancer often produce early tertiary metastases to the mediastinal lymph nodes. These lymph nodes should be examined before a pulmonary deposit is removed. An occasional patient with malignant melanoma has a long survival after a solitary pulmonary metastasis is removed following a long disease free interval.

Tumor doubling time is discussed in the section on lung cancer under Predictive Criteria. TDT refers to doubling of volume. When the radius of a nodule has increased by 1.25, the nodule has twice the volume. An example of the less tedious method of obtaining TDT is given by Joseph and his co-workers.[471] Most authors who have calculated TDT agree that the faster the tumor's growth rate, the shorter the survival and the shorter the time interval between treatment of the primary tumor and onset of metastases.[471,472] Calculation of the volume doubling time of metastasis permits some observations which otherwise would be possible only from the disease free interval. Only if the TDT is related to the late, rare, and exclusively pulmonary spread and also to the production of metastases from metastasis, will TDT *per se* have a real correlation with the cure rate after resection of pulmonary metastases.[473] Nevertheless, a long TDT lengthens survival even if the final cure rate is the same, although the prolongation of life is not exactly proportional to the TDT. Workers who have applied TDT as a criterion for patient selection urge that all patients with a TDT greater than 40 days be considered for resection even of multiple or bilateral metastases.[471] More than 1 month of observation is needed in order to accurately calculate the TDT of more than half of all pulmonary metastases; therefore, some would introduce a 1- to 2-month observation period before resecting lung deposits of unknown growth rate.[474]

The size of the metastasis to be removed is also important. When solitary metastases with the same TDT are compared, size has marked prognostic importance, probably because size reflects the extent of undetected remaining disease. The influence of size also can be appreciated from the following: Compare the survival time from resection of solitary metastatic nodules with the same TDT in two patients. One metastasis is small, the other large. Bias can only be avoided by crediting the large metastasis with the time spent growing from small to large.[458]

The surgical technique used to treat pulmonary metastases is important.[473] Patients with bilateral metastases should have the first operation on the least involved lung so that pulmonary function is preserved and the extent of disease known should a major resection be needed when the more involved lung is explored. Mediastinal and hilar lymph nodes are evaluated by frozen section before lung is removed. The lung is examined in both inflated and deflated positions and all lesions are marked with sutures before any are resected so that atelectasis or intraparenchymal hemorrhage is not mistaken for metastases. Wedge and segmental resections are used more often than when operating for bronchogenic cancer.

REFERENCES

1. US Public Health Service: Smoking and Health. Washington, DC, US Department of Health, Education and Welfare, 1979
2. SILVERBERG E: Cancer statistics, 1979. Cancer 29:6, 1979
3. SCHNEIDERMAN MA, LEVIN DL: Trends in lung cancer: Mortality, incidence, diagnosis, treatment, smoking and urbanization. Cancer 30:1320–1325, 1972
4. BIOMETRY BRANCH, National Cancer Institute, National Institutes of Health: The Third National Cancer Survey, Advanced Three Year Report, 1969–1971 Incidence. Washington, DC, US Department of Health, Education, and Welfare Publication No. 74–637, 1974
5. US Public Health Service: Smoking and Health. Report of the Advisory Committee to the Surgeon General of the Public Health Service, p 131. Washington DC, US Department of Health Education and Welfare, 1964
6. US Public Health Service: The Health Consequences of Smoking. Washington DC, US Department of Health, Education and Welfare, 1973

6a. HIRAYAMA T: Nonsmoking wives of heavy smokers have a higher risk of lung cancer: A study from Japan. Br Med J 282:183, 1981

7. WYNDER EL: Etiology of lung cancer: Reflections on two decades of research. Cancer 30:1332–1338, 1972
8. GSELL OR, ABELIN T: Cigar and pipe smoking in relation to lung cancer and excess mortality. J Natl Cancer Institute 48:1795–1803, 1972
9. HAMMOND EC: Smoking in relation to the death rate of 1 million men and women. Natl Cancer Institute Monogr 19:127–204, 1966
10. WYNDER EL, MABUCHI K, BEATTIE EJ: The epidemiology of lung cancer. JAMA 213:2221–2228, 1970
11. AUERBACH O, HAMMOND EC, GARFINKEL MA: Changes in bronchial epithelium in relation to cigarette smoking, 1955–1960 vs 1970–1977. N Engl J Med 300:381, 1979
12. GORI GB, LYNCH CJ: Toward less hazardous cigarettes. Current advances. JAMA 240:1255, 1978
13. BELCHER JR: World-wide differences in the sex ratio of bronchial carcinoma. Br J Dis Chest 65:205–216, 1971
14. COX JD, YESNER RA: Adenocarcinoma of the lung: Recent results from the Veterans Administration Lung Group. Am Rev Respir Dis 120:1025, 1079
15. VINCENT RG, PICKREN JW, WARREN WL et al: The changing histopathology of lung cancer: A review of 1682 cases. Cancer 39:1647, 1977
16. DELARUE NC, ANDERSON W, SANDERS D et al: Bronchioloalveolar carcinoma: A reappraisal after 24 years. Cancer 29:90–97, 1972
17. WYNDER EL, BERG JW: Cancer of the lung among non-smokers. Special reference to histologic patterns. Cancer 20:1161–1171, 1967
18. COHEN S, HOSSAIN S: Primary carcinoma of the lung: A review of 417 histologically proved cases. Dis Chest 49:67–74, 1966
19. ROHWEDDER JJ, WEATHERBEE L: Multiple primary bronchogenic carcinoma with review of the literature. Am Rev Respir Dis 109:435–445, 1974
20. WALLER RE: The combined effects of smoking and occupational or urban factors in relation to lung cancer. Ann Occup Hyg 15:67–71, 1972
21. SANDERMAN FW: Carcinogenic effects of metals. Fed Proc 37:40, 1978
22. ROOKE GB: Carcinoma of the lung in Lancashire coalminers. Thorax 34:229, 1979

22a. FIGUEROA WG, RASZKOWSKI R, WEISS W: Lung cancer in chloroethyl methyl ether workers. N Engl J Med 21:1096, 1973

22b. MORGAN WKC: Industrial carcinogens: The extent of the risk. Thorax 34:431, 1979

23. MOK CK, NANDI P, ONG GB: Coexistent bronchogenic carcinoma and active pulmonary tuberculosis. J Thorac Cardiovasc Surg 76:469, 1978
24. BALO J, JUHASZ E, TEMES J: Pulmonary infarcts and pulmonary carcinomas. Cancer 9:918–922, 1956
25. LIEBOW AA: Bronchiolo-alveolar carcinoma. In Dock W, and Snapper I (eds): Advances in Internal Medicine, Vol X, p 338. Chicago, Year Book Medical Publishers, 1960
26. DONALDSON JC, KAMINSKY DB, ELLIOTT RC: Bronchiolar carcinoma. Report of 11 cases and review of the literature. Cancer 41:250, 1978
27. DAVIS AL: Bronchogenic carcinoma in chronic obstructive pulmonary disease. JAMA 235:621, 1976
28. COHEN BH et al: A common familial component in lung cancer and chronic obstructive pulmonary disease. Lancet 2:523, 1977
29. YESNER R: Spectrum of lung cancer and ectopic hormones. In Sommers SC, Rosen PP (eds): Pathology Annual, Vol 13, pp 217. New York, Appleton-Century-Crofts, 1978
30. FEINSTEIN AR et al: Observer variability in the histologic diagnosis of lung cancer. Am Rev Respir Dis 101:671, 1970
31. FEINSTEIN AR, GELFMAN NA, YESNER R: The diverse effects of histopathology on manifestations and outcome of lung cancer. Chest 66:225–229, 1974
32. SMITH L: Oat cell carcinoma as a malignant apudoma. J Thorac Cardiovasc Surg 70:147, 1975
33. CARTER D: Pathology of early squamous cell carcinoma of the lung. In Sommers SC, Rosen PP

(eds): Pathology Annual, Vol 13. pp 131–147. New York, Appleton-Century-Crofts, 1978

34. CAMPOBASSO O: Characteristics of peripheral lung tumors that suggest the bronchioloalveolar origin. Br J Cancer 22:655–662, 1968
35. GREENBERG SD, SMITH MN, SPJUT HJ: Bronchiolo-alveolar carcinoma—cell of origin. Am J Clin Pathol 63:153, 1975
36. JACQUES J, CURRIE W: Bronchiolo-alveolar carcinoma. Cancer 40:2171, 1977
37. MILLER WT, HUSTED J, FREIMAN D et al: Bronchiolo-alveolar carcinoma: Two clinical entities with one pathologic diagnosis. Am J Roentgenol 130:905, 1978
38. ZHEUTLIN N, LASSER EC, RIGLER LG: Bronchographic abnormalities in alveolar cell carcinoma of the lung. Dis Chest 25:542, 1954

38a. HOMMA H et al: A case of alveolar cell carcinoma accompanied by fluid and electrolyte depletion through production of voluminous lung liquid. Am Rev Respir Dis 111:857, 1975

39. MARIO M, GALY P: Bronchiolo-alveolar cell carcinoma. Clinicopathologic relationships, natural history, and prognosis in 29 cases. Am Rev Respir Dis 107:621–629, 1973
40. FISHMAN HC et al: Massive intrapulmonary venoarterial shunting in alveolar cell carcinoma. Am Rev Respir Dis 109:124–127, 1974
41. LUDINGTON LG et al: Bronchiolar carcinoma (alveolar cell) another great imitator; a review of 41 cases. Chest 61:622–628, 1972
42. BURDON JGW, SINCLAIR RA, HENDERSON MM: Small cell carcinoma of the lung. Prognosis in relation to histologic type. Chest 76:302, 1979
43. HANSEN HH, DOMBERNOWSKY P, HANSEN M et al: Chemotherapy of advanced small cell anaplastic carcinoma: Superiority of a four-drug combination to a three-drug combination. Ann Intern Med 89:117, 1978
44. RAZZUK MA et al: Observations on ultrastructural morphology of bronchial carcinoma. J Thorac Cardiovasc Surg 59:581, 1970
45. HYDE L, HYDE CI: Clinical manifestations of lung cancer. Chest 65:299–306, 1974

45a. PARISH JM, MARSCHKE RF, DINES DE, LEE RE: Etiologic considerations in superior vena caval syndrome. Am Rev Resp Dis 123(Suppl):63, 1981

46. LOKICH J, GOODMAN R: Superior vena cava syndrome. JAMA 231:58, 1975
47. HOWARD N: Phlebography in superior vena caval obstruction. Radiology 81:380–384, 1963

47a. SCHRAUFNAGEL DE, HILL R, LEECH JA, PARE JAP: Superior vena caval obstruction: Is it a medical emergency? Am J Med 70:1169, 1981

48. PEREZ CA, PRESANT CA, VAN AMBURG AL: Management of superior vena cava syndrome. Semin Oncol 5:123, 1978
49. LEVITT SH, JONES TK, KILPATRICK SJ et al: Treatment of malignant superior vena caval obstruction: A randomized study. Cancer 24:447–451, 1969

49a. SCHECTER A, REICHEL J: Prolonged survival in bronchogenic carcinoma complicated by superior vena caval obstruction. Lung 159:13, 1981

50. GREEN RA: Respiratory system. In Judge RD, Zuidema GD (eds): Physical Diagnosis: A Physiologic Approach to the Clinical Examination, 2nd ed, pp 153–158. Boston, Little, Brown & Co, 1968
51. GAUTAM HP, KNIGHT EOW: Spontaneous pneumothorax due to perforated bronchial carcinoma. Br J Dis Chest 64:110–111, 1970

51a. DINES DE et al: Malignant pulmonary neoplasms predisposing to spontaneous pneumothorax. Mayo Clinic Proc 48:542, 1973

52. LIGHT RW, MACGREGOR MI, LUCHSINGER PC et al: Pleural effusions: The diagnostic separation of transudates and exudates. Ann Intern Med 77:507–513, 1973
53. PANCOAST HK: Importance of careful roentgenray investigations of apical chest tumors. JAMA 83:1407–1411, 1927
54. PAULSON DL: Carcinomas in the superior pulmonary sulcus. J Thorac Cardiovasc Surg 70:1095, 1975
55. DECKER DA, DINES DE, PAYNE WS et al: The significance of a cytologically negative pleural effusion in bronchogenic carcinoma. Chest 74:640, 1978
56. CUNNINGHAM JJ: Grey scale echography of the lung and pleural space: Current applications of oncologic interest. Cancer 41:1329, 1978
57. FRACCHIA AA, KNAPPER WH, CAREY JT et al: Intrapleural chemotherapy for effusion from metastatic breast carcinoma. Cancer 26:626–629, 1970
58. BAYLY TC, KISNER DC, SYBERT A et al: Tetracycline and quinacrine in the control of malignant pleural effusions: A randomized trial. Cancer 41:1188, 1978
59. MILLER JI, MANSOUR KA, HATCHER CR JR: Carcinoma of the superior pulmonary sulcus. Ann Thorac Surg 28:44, 1978
60. PAULSON D: Editorial: Carcinoma of the superior pulmonary sulcus. Ann Thorac Surg 28;3, 1978
61. CROFT PB, WILKINSON M: The incidence of carcinomatous neuromyopathy in patients with various types of carcinoma. Brain 88:427–434, 1965
62. CROFT PB, WILKINSON M: The course and prognosis in some types of carcinomatous neuromyopathy. Brain 92:1–8, 1969
63. WILKINSON PC, ZEROMSKI J: Immunofluorescent detection of antibodies against neurons in sensory carcinomatous neuropathy. Brain 88:529–537, 1965
64. TROJABORG W, FRANTZEN E, ANDERSEN I: Periph-

eral neuropathy and myopathy associated with carcinomas of the lung. Brain 92:71–82, 1969

65. CROFT PB, URICH H, WILKINSON M: Peripheral neuropathy of the sensorimotor type associated with malignant disease. Brain 90:31–66, 1967
66. BROWN JC, JOHNS RL: Diagnostic difficulties encountered in the myasthenic syndrome sometimes associated with carcinoma. J Neurol Neurosurg Psychiatry 37:1214, 1974
67. OH SJ, KIM KW: Guanidine hydrochloride in Eaton–Lambert syndrome. Neurology 23:1084, 1973
68. GUTMAN L, CROSBY TW, TAKAMORI M et al: The Eaton–Lambert syndrome and autoimmune disorders. Am J Med 53:354–356, 1972
69. CARR-LOCKE DL: Autonomic neuropathy and inappropriate secretion of antidiuretic hormone: Occurrence in a patient with bronchogenic carcinoma. JAMA 241, 2298, 1979
70. AHMAD M: Autonomic neuropathy and carcinoma of the lung. Can Med Assoc J 113:410, 1975
71. MACGEE EE: Surgical treatment of cerebral metastases from lung cancer: The effect on quality and duration of survival. J Neurosurg 35:416–420, 1971
72. RASKIND R, WEISS SR, WERMUTH RE: Single metastatic brain tumors: Treatment and follow-up in 41 cases. Am Surg 35:510–515, 1969
73. BURGESS RE, BURGESS VF, DIBELLA NJ: Brain metastasis in small cell carcinoma of the lung. JAMA 242:2084, 1979
74. NEWMAN SJ, HANSEN HH: Frequency, diagnosis, and treatment of brain metastases in 247 consecutive patients with bronchogenic carcinoma. Cancer 33:492, 1974
75. GILBERT H, APUZZO M, MARSHALL L et al: Neoplastic epidural spinal cord compression: A current perspective. JAMA 240:2771, 1978
76. ODELL WD, WOLFSEN AR: Humoral syndromes associated with cancer. Annu Rev Med 29:379, 1978
77. HANSEN HH, MUGGIA FM: Staging of inoperable patients with bronchogenic carcinoma with special reference to bone marrow examination and peritoneoscopy. Cancer 30:1395, 1972
78. GORDON GS, ROOF BS, HALDEN A: Skeletal effects of cancers and their management. In Holland JF, Frei E (eds): Cancer Medicine, p 1080. Philadelphia, Lea & Febiger, 1973
79. MEYERS WPL: Differential diagnosis of hypercalcemia and cancer. Cancer 27:258, 1977
80. BESARAB A, CARO JF: Mechanisms of hypercalcemia in malignancy. Cancer 41:2276, 1978
81. GUZZO CE, PACHAS WN, PINALS RS et al: Urinary hydroxyproline excretion in patients with cancer. Cancer 24:382, 1969
82. AZZOPARDI JG, WHITTAKER RS: Bronchial carcinoma and hypercalcemia. J Clin Pathol 22:718, 1969
83. CHAKMAKJIAN ZH, BETHUNE JE: Sodium sulfate treatment of hypercalcemia. N Engl J Med 275:862, 1966
84. POWELL D, SINGER MD, MUVRY TM et al: Nonparathyroid humoral hypercalcemia in patients with neoplastic diseases. N Engl J Med 289:176, 1973
85. SUKI WN et al: Acute treatment of hypercalcemia with furosemide. N Engl J Med 283:836, 1970
86. MASSRY SG, MUELLER E, SILVERMAN AG et al: Inorganic phosphate treatment of hypercalcemia. Arch Intern Med 121:307, 1968
87. PERLIA CP et al: Mithramycin treatment of hypercalcemia. Cancer 25:389, 1970
88. GILBY ED, BONDY PK, FORSLING M: Impaired water excretion in oat cell lung cancer. Br J Cancer 34:323, 1976
89. SCHWARTZ WB, BENNETT W, CURELOP S: A syndrome of renal sodium loss and hyponatremia probably resulting from inappropriate secretion of antidiuretic hormone. Am J Med 23:529, 1957
90. BARTTER FC, SCHWARTZ WB: The syndrome of inappropriate secretion of antidiuretic hormone. Am J Med 42:790, 1967
91. BARTTER FC: The syndrome of inappropriate secretion of antidiuretic hormone. J R Coll Physicians Lond 4:264, 1970
92. FICHMAN M, BETHUNE J: Effects of neoplasms on renal electrolyte function. Ann NY Acad Sci 230:460, 1974
93. DEFRONZO RA, BRAINE H, COLVIN OM et al: Water intoxication in man after cyclophosphamide therapy. Ann Intern Med 78:861, 1973
94. MUNRO AHG, COMPTON GK: Inappropriate antidiuretic hormone secretion in oat cell carcinoma of the bronchus: Aggravation of hyponatremia by intravenous cyclophosphamide. Thorax 27:640, 1972
95. HANTMAN D, ROSSIER B, ZOHLMAN R et al: Rapid correction of hyponatremia in the syndrome of inappropriate secretion of antidiuretic hormone. Ann Intern Med 78:870, 1973
96. GRANTHAM J, BROWN RW, SCHLOERK PR: Asymptomatic hyponatremia and bronchogenic carcinoma: The deleterious effects of diuretics. Am J Med Sci 249:61, 273–279, 1965
97. FORREST JN, COX M, HONG C et al: Superiority of demeclocycline over lithium in the treatment of chronic syndrome of inappropriate secretion of antidiuretic hormone. N Engl J Med 298:173, 1978
98. LIDDLE GW, GIVENS JR, NICHOLSON WE et al: The ectopic ACTH syndrome. Cancer Res 25:1057, 1965
99. AMATRUDE TT, UPTON GV: Hyperadrenocorticism

and ACTH-releasing factor. Ann NY Acad Sci 230:168, 1974

100. AYRAZIAN LF, SCHNEIDER B, GEWIRTZ G et al: Ectopic production of big ACTH in carcinoma of the lung: Its clinical usefulness as a biologic marker. Am Rev Respir Dis 111:279–287, 1975

101. YALOW RS, EASTRIDGE CE, HIGGINS G et al: Plasma and tumor ACTH in carcinoma of the lung. Cancer 44:1789, 1979

102. HYMES AC, DOE RP: Adrenal function in cancer of the lung with and without Cushing's syndrome. Am J Med 33:398, 1962

103. HAUGER-KLEVENE JH: Asymptomatic production of ACTH. Radio immunoassay in squamous cell, oat cell, and adenocarcinoma of the lung. Cancer 22:1262, 1968

104. UPTON GV, AMATRUDA TT: Evidence for the presence of tumor peptides with corticotropin-releasing factor-like activity in the ectopic ACTH syndrome. N Engl J Med 285:419, 1971

105. AMATRUDA TT JR, UPTON GV: Hyperadrenocorticism and ACTH-releasing factor. Ann NY Acad Sci 230:168, 1974

106. MASON AMS, RATCLIFFE JG, BUCKLE RM et al: ACTH secretion by bronchial carcinoid tumors. Clin Endocrinol (OXF) 1:3, 1972

107. OKIKE N, BERNATZ PE, WOOLNER LB: Carcinoid tumors of the lung. Ann Thorac Surg 22:270, 1976

108. RODGERS-SULLIVAN RF, WEILAND LH, PALUMBO PJ et al: Pulmonary tumorlets associated with Cushing's syndrome. Am Rev Respir Dis 117:799, 1978

109. LIDDLE GW, NICHOLSON WE, ISLAND DP: Clinical and laboratory studies of ectopic humoral syndromes. Recent Prog Horm Res 25:283, 1969

110. MILLER AB, FOX W, TALL R: Five-year follow-up of the Medical Research Council cooperative trial of surgery and radiotherapy for the primary treatment of small-celled or oat-celled carcinoma of the bronchus. Lancet 2:501, 1969

111. GORDEN P, BECKER CE, LEVEY GS et al: Efficacy of aminoglutethimide in the ectopic ACTH syndrome. J Clin Endocrinol Metab 28:921, 1968

112. CAREY RM, ORTH DN, HARTMANN WH: Malignant melanoma with ectopic production of adrenocorticotropic hormone: Palliative treatment with inhibitors of adrenal steroid biosynthesis. J Clin Endocrinol Metab 36:482, 1973

113. GALL EA, BENNETT GA, BAUER W: Generalized hypertrophic osteoarthropathy: A pathologic study of seven cases. Am J Pathol 27:349, 1951

114. HOLLING HE: Pulmonary hypertrophic osteoarthropathy. Ann Intern Med 66:232, 1967

115. EPSTEIN O, ADJUKIEWICZ AB, DICK R et al: Hypertrophic osteoarthropathy. Am J Med 67:88, 1979

116. ROSENTHAL L, KIRSH J: Observations on radionuclide imaging in hypertrophic pulmonary osteoarthropathy. Radiology 120:359, 1976

117. CALABRO JJ: Cancer and arthritis. Arthritis Rheum 10:553, 1967

118. STENSETH JH, CLAGETT OT, WOOLNER LB: Hypertrophic pulmonary osteoarthropathy. Dis Chest 52:62, 1967

119. SCHUMACHER HR: Articular manifestations of hypertrophic pulmonary osteoarthropathy in bronchogenic carcinoma: A clinical and pathologic study. Arthritis Rheum 19:629, 1976

120. FISCHER DS, SINGER DH, FELDMAN SM: Clubbing, a review, with emphasis on hereditary acropachy. Medicine 43:459, 1964

121. GINSBURG J, BROWN JB: Increased oestrogen excretion in hypertrophic pulmonary osteoarthropathy. Lancet 2:1274, 1961

122. FUSCO FO, ROSEN SW: Gonadotropin-producing anaplastic large-cell carcinomas of the lung. N Engl J Med 275:507, 1966

123. DUPONT B, HOYER I, BORGESKOV S et al: Plasma growth hormone and hypertrophic osteoarthropathy in carcinoma of the bronchus. Acta Med Scand 188:25, 1970

124. SEMPLE T, MCCLUSKIE RA: Generalized hypertrophic osteoarthropathy in association with bronchial carcinoma: A review based on 24 cases. Br Med J 1:754, 1955

125. BECK C, LARKINS RG, MARTIN TJ et al: Stimulation of growth hormone release from superfused rat pituitary by extracts of hypothalamus and of human lung tumors. J Endocrinol 59:325, 1973

126. WEINTRAUB BD, ROSEN SW: Ectopic production of human chorionic somatomammotropin by nontrophoblastic cancers. J Clin Endocrinol Metab 32:94, 1971

127. ROSEN SW: Ectopic gonadotropin in bronchogenic carcinoma. JAMA 210:908, 1969

128. FAIMAN C, COLWELL JA, RYAN RJ et al: Gonadotropin secretion from a bronchogenic carcinoma. Demonstration by radioimmunoassay. N Engl J Med 277:1395, 1967

129. BECKER KL, COTTRELL J, MOORE CF et al: Endocrine studies in a patient with gonadotropin-secreting bronchogenic carcinoma. J Clin Endocrinol Metab 28:809, 1968

130. CHARLES MA, CLAYPOOL R, SCHAAF M et al: Lung carcinoma associated with production of three placental proteins. Arch Intern Med 132, 1973

131. ROSEN S, BECKER CE, SCHLAFF S et al: Ectopic gonadotropin production before clinical recognition of bronchogenic carcinoma. N Engl J Med 279:640, 1968

132. COTTRELL JC, BECKER KL, MATTHEWS MJ et al: The histology of gonadotropin-secreting bronchogenic carcinoma. Am J Clin Pathol 52:720, 1969

133. LEVINE RJ, METZ SA: A classification of ectopic

hormone-producing tumors. Ann NY Acad Sci 230:533, 1974

134. UNGER RH, LOCHNER JV, EISENTRAUT AM: Identification of insulin and glucagon in a bronchogenic metastasis. J Clin Endocrinol Metab 24:823, 1964

135. SILVA O, BECKER KL, PRIMACK A et al: Ectopic secretion of calcitonin by oat-cell carcinoma. N Engl J Med 290:1122, 1974

136. BECKER KL, NASH DR, SILVA O et al: Urine calcitonin levels in patients with bronchogenic carcinoma. JAMA 243:670, 1980

137. GENEST J, ROJO-ORTEGA JM, KURCHEL O et al: Malignant hypertension with hypokalemia in a patient with a renin producing pulmonary carcinoma. Trans Assoc Am Physician 88:192, 1975

138. SAID SI, FALOONA GR: Elevated plasma and tissue levels of vasoactive intestinal polypeptide in the watery-diarrhea syndrome due to pancreatic, bronchogenic and other tumors. N Engl J Med 293:156, 1975

139. SANDLER M, KARIM SMM, WILLIAMS ED: Prostaglandins in aminopeptide-secreting tumors. Lancet 2:1053, 1968

140. HORAI T, NISHIHARA H, TATEISH R et al: Oat cell carcinoma of the lung simultaneously producing ACTH and serotonin. J Clin Endocrinol Metab 37:212, 1973

141. VINCENT RG, CHU TM, FERGEN TB et al: Carcinoembryonic antigen in 228 patients with carcinoma of the lung. Cancer 36:2069, 1975

142. FORD CHJ, NEWMAN CE, LARKIN J: Role of carcinoembryonic antigen in bronchial carcinoma. Thorax 32:582, 1977

143. COOMBES RC, ELLISON ML, NEVILLE AM: Biochemical markers in bronchogenic carcinoma: Review. Br J Dis Chest 72:263, 1978

144. STEELE JD, BUELL P: Asymptomatic solitary pulmonary nodules. J Thorac Cardiovasc Surg 65:140–151, 1973

145. STEELE JD: The solitary pulmonary nodule. J Thorac Cardiovasc Surg 46:21–39, 1963

146. STEELE JD: The Solitary Pulmonary Nodule, p 14. Springfield, Charles C Thomas, 1964

147. DAVIS EW, KATZ S, PEABODY JW: The surgical implications of solitary tumors of the lung. Am J Surg 89:402–407, 1955

148. HOLIN SM, DWORK RE, GLASER S et al: Solitary pulmonary nodules found in a community wide chest roentgenographic survey. Am Rev Tuberculosis 70:427–439, 1959

149. WEISS W, BOUCOT KR: The prognosis of lung cancer originating as a round lesion. Am Rev Respir Dis 116:827, 1977

150. STEELE JD, BUELL P: Asymptomatic solitary pulmonary nodules. J Thorac Cardiovasc Surg 65:140, 1973

151. COMSTOCK GW, VAUGHAN RH, MONTGOMERY G: Outcome of solitary pulmonary nodules discovered in an x-ray screening program. N Engl J Med 254:1018, 1956

152. MITCHELL RS: Late results of treatment of the solitary dense tuberculous pulmonary focus (tuberculoma) without resection or chemotherapy. Ann Intern Med 39:471, 1953

153. MAY IA, ROSE K, DUGAN DJ: The solitary pulmonary lesion. Calif Med 80:9, 1954

154. GOOD CA, CLAGETT OT, WEED LA: Granuloma of the lung: A problem of differential diagnosis. Trans Natl Tuberculosis Assoc 47:294, 1951

155. GOOD CA, HOOD RT, MCDONALD JR: Significance of the solitary mass in the lung. Am J Roentgenol Radium Ther Nucl Med 70:543, 1953

156. HODGSON CH, MCDONALD JR: The diagnosis and management of solitary circumscribed lesions of the lungs. Dis Chest 24:289, 1953

157. HOOD RT JR, GOOD CA, CLAGETT OT et al: Solitary circumscribed lesions of the lung: Study of 156 cases in which resection was performed. JAMA 152:1185, 1953

158. STEELE JD: The Solitary Pulmonary Nodule, p 19. Springfield, Charles C Thomas, 1964

159. DAVIES DF: A review of detection methods for the early diagnosis of lung cancer. J Chronic Dis 19:819–845, 1966

159a. SIEGELMAN SS et al: C.T. of the solitary pulmonary nodule. Am J Roentgen 135:1, 1980

160. HATTIORI S, MATSUDA M, SUGIYAMA T et al: Cytologic diagnosis of early lung cancer: Brushing method under x-ray television fluoroscopy. Dis Chest 45:129, 1964

161. STEELE JD: The Solitary Pulmonary Nodule, p 8. Springfield, Charles C Thomas, 1964

162. DAHLGREN S, NORDENSTRÖM B: Transthoracic Needle Biopsy. Chicago, Year Book Medical Publishers, 1966

163. ZAVALA DC, ROSSI NP, BENDELL GN: Bronchial brush biopsy. Ann Thorac Surg 13:519–528, 1972

164. ZAVALA DC, BEDELL GN: Percutaneous lung biopsy with a cutting needle. Am Rev Respir Dis 106:186–193, 1972

165. LALLI AF, MCCORMACK LJ, ZELCH M et al: Aspiration biopsies of chest lesions. Radiology 127:35, 1978

166. STEEL SJ, WINSTANLEY DP: Trephine biopsy of the lung and pleura. Thorax 24:576, 1969

167. SCHACTER EN, BASTA W: Subcutaneous metastasis of an adenocarcinoma following a percutaneous pleural biopsy. Am Rev Respir Dis 107:283–289, 1973

168. RICHARDSON RH, ZAVALA DC, MUKERJEE PK et al: The use of fiberoptic bronchoscopy and brush biopsy in the diagnosis of suspected pulmonary malignancy. Am Rev Respir Dis 109:63–72, 1974

169. STRINGFIELD JT, MARKOWITZ DJ, BENTZ RR et al: The effect of tumor size and location on diag-

nosis by fiberoptic bronchoscopy. Chest 72:474, 1977

170. COLLINS VP, LOEFFLER RN, TIVEY H: Observations on growth rates of human tumórs. Am J Roentgenol Radium Ther Nucl Med 76:988–1000, 1956

171. MEYER JA: The concept and significance of growth rates in human pulmonary tumors. Ann Thorac Surg 14:309–322, 1972

172. SPRATT JS JR, SPJUT HJ, ROPER CL: The frequency distribution of rates of growth and estimated duration of primary pulmonary carcinomas. Cancer 16:687, 1963

173. GARLAND LH, COULSON W, WOLLIN E: The rate of growth and apparent duration of untreated primary bronchogenic carcinoma. Cancer 16:694, 1963

174. NATHAN HM: Management of solitary pulmonary nodules: An organized approach based on growth rate and statistics. JAMA 227:1141–1144, 1974

175. VANCE JW et al: The solitary circumscribed pulmonary lesion due to bronchogenic carcinoma: A 3 year follow-up study of 94 surgically treated patients. Dis Chest 36:231, 1959

176. TALA P, VIRKKULA L: The malignant solitary pulmonary lesion: A follow-up study of 117 surgically treated patients. Thorax 15:252, 1960

177. O'CONNOR TM, LEPLEY D JR, WEISEL W et al: The malignant solitary pulmonary nodule follow-up study. Arch Surg 86:985, 1963

178. BATESON EM: The solitary circumscribed bronchogenic carcinoma: A radiological study of 100 cases. Br J Radiol 37:598, 1964

179. STEELE JD, KLEITSCH WP, DUNN JE JR et al: Survival in males with bronchogenic carcinomas resected as asymptomatic solitary pulmonary nodules. Ann Thorac Surg 2:368, 1966

180. JACKMAN RJ, GOOD CA, CALGETT OT et al: Survival rates in peripheral bronchogenic carcinomas up to four centimeters in diameter presenting as solitary pulmonary nodules. J Thorac Cardiovasc Surg 57:1–8, 1969

181. MELICK DW, GRANT AR: Surgery in primary pulmonary coccidioidomycosis and in combined diseases of coccidioidomycosis and tuberculosis. Dis Chest 54:22–28, 1968

182. READ CT: Pulmonary coin lesion in the southwest: Solitary pulmonary nodules. Arizona Med 29:775, 1972

183. GOODWIN RA JR, SUELL JD JR: The enlarging histoplasmoma: Concept of a tumor-like phenomenon encompassing the tuberculoma and coccidioidoma. Am Rev Respir Dis 100:1–11, 1969

184. SUTARIA MK, POLK JW, REDDY P: Focalized pulmonary histoplasmosis (Coin Lesion): A report of 58 cases. Chest 61:361–364, 1972

185. BATESON EM: So-called hamartoma of the lung—a true neoplasm of fibrous connective tissue of the bronchi. Cancer 31:1458–1467, 1973

186. KOUTRAS P, URSCHEL HC, PAULSON DL: Hamartoma of the lung. J Thorac Cardiovasc Surg 61:768, 1971

187. DOPPMAN J, WILSON G: Cystic pulmonary hamartoma. Br J Radiol 38:629, 1965

188. BATESON EM: An analysis of 155 solitary lung lesions illustrating the differential diagnosis of mixed tumors of the lung. Clin Radiol 16:51–65, 1965

189. BYNUM LJ, WILSON JE: Radiographic features of pleural effusions in pulmonary embolism. Am Rev Respir Dis 117:829, 1978

190. MOYER JH, GLANTZ G, BIEST AN: Pulmonary arteriovenous fistulas: Physiologic and clinical considerations. Am J Med 32:417–435, 1962

191. FONTANA RS: Early diagnosis of lung cancer. Am Rev Respir Dis 116:399, 1977

192. MELAMED M, FLEHINGER B, MILLER D et al: Preliminary report of the lung cancer detection program in New York. Cancer 39:369, 1977

193. CORTESE DA et al: Clinical application of a new endoscopic technique for detection of in situ bronchial carcinoma. Mayo Clin Proc 54:635, 1979

194. DOIRON DR, PROFIO E, VINCENT RG et al: Fluorescence bronchoscopy for detection of lung cancer. Chest 76:27, 1979

195. HIGGANS GA, LAWTON R, HEILBRUNN A et al: Prognostic factors in lung cancer: Surgical aspects. Ann Thorac Surg 7:472, 1969

196. WEISS W, COOPER DA, BOUCOT KR: Operative mortality and 5-year survival rates in men with bronchogenic carcinoma. Ann Intern Med 71:59, 1969

197. DELARUE NC, STRASBERG SM: The rationale of intensive preoperative investigation in bronchogenic carcinoma. J Thorac Cardiovasc Surg 51:391, 1966

197a. VINCENT RC, TAKITA H, LANE WW et al: Surgical therapy of lung cancer. J Thorac Cardiovasc Surg 71:581, 1976

198. RUBINSTEIN I, BAUM GL, KALTER Y et al: The influence of cell type and lymph node metastases on survival of patients with carcinoma of the lung undergoing thoracotomy. Am Rev Respir Dis 119:253, 1979

198a. SHIELDS TW et al: Long-term survivors after resection of lung carcinoma. J Thorac Cardiovasc Surg 76:439, 1978

199. WEISS W: Operative mortality and five-year survival rates in men with bronchogenic carcinoma. Chest 66:483, 1974

200. PAULSON DL: Carcinoma of the Lung: Current Problems in Surgery. Chicago, Year Book Medical Publishers, 1967

201. TAYLOR AB: United Birmingham Hospitals, Annual Cancer Report 2:36, 1954

202. LAWRENCE GH, WALKER JH, PINKERS L: Extended resection of bronchogenic carcinoma: A reappraisal and suggested plan of management. N Engl J Med 263:615, 1960
203. DILLON ML, POSTLETHWAIT RW: Carcinoma of the lung. Ann Thorac Surg 11:193, 1971
204. GUTTMANN RJ: Results of radiation therapy in patients with inoperable carcinoma of the lung whose status was established at thoracotomy. Am J Roentgenol Radium Ther Nucl Med 93:99, 1965
205. HARKEN DE, BLACK H, CLAUSS R et al: A simple cervicomediastinal exploration for the tissue diagnosis of intrathoracic disease, with comments on the recognition of inoperable carcinoma of the lung. N Engl J Med 25:1041, 1954
206. KIRSCH MM et al: Treatment of bronchogenic carcinoma with mediastinal metastases. Ann Thorac Surg 12:11, 1971
207. NARAKE T, SUENASU K, ISHIKAWA S: Lymph node mapping and curability at various levels of metastasis in resected lung cancer. J Thorac Cardiovasc Surg 76:832, 1978
208. DELARUE NC, SAUNDERS DE, SILBERBERG SA: Complementary value of pulmonary angiography and mediastinoscopy in individualizing treatment for patients with lung cancer. Cancer 26:1370, 1970
209. BERGH NP, RYDBERG B, SCHERSTEN T: Mediastinal exploration by the technique of Carlens. Dis Chest 46:399, 1964
210. FEINSTEIN A: A new staging system for cancer and reappraisal of "early" treatment and "cure" by radical surgery. N Engl J Med 279:748, 1968
211. FEINSTEIN A: Symptomatic patterns, biologic behavior, and prognosis in cancer of the lung: Practical application of boolean algebra and clinical taxonomy. Ann Intern Med 61:27, 1964
212. SENIOR RM, ADAMSON JS: Survival in patients with lung cancer: An appraisal of Feinstein's symptom classification. Arch Intern Med 125:975, 1970
213. LINE DH, DEELEY TJ: The necropsy findings in carcinoma of the bronchus. Br J Dis Chest 65:238, 1971
214. MACDONALD I: The individual basis of biologic variability in cancer. Surg Gynecol Obstet 106:227, 1958
215. CARR DT: The staging of lung cancer. Am Rev Respir Dis 117:819, 1978
216. MOUNTAIN CF, CARR DT, ANDERSON WAD: A system for the clinical staging of lung cancer. Am J Roentgenol Radium Ther Nucl Med 120:130, 1974
217. PEACE PK, PRICE JL: Preoperative tomographic assessment of the mediastinum in bronchial carcinoma. Thorax 28:367–370, 1973
218. JAMES EC, ELLWOOD RA: Mediastinoscopy and mediastinal roentgenology. Ann Thorac Surg 18:531, 1974
219. FRYJORDET A, KLEVMARK B: Investigations of operability in cases of bronchial carcinoma. Evaluation of 515 patients. Scand J Thorac Cardiovasc Surg 5:97–102, 1971
220. RINKER CT et al: Combined superior vena cava cavography and azygography in patients with suspected lung carcinoma. Radiology 88:441–445, 1967
221. WOLFEL DA, LINDBERG EJ, LIGHT JP: The abnormal azygogram—an index of inoperability. Am J Roentgen Radium Ther Nucl Med 97:933–938, 1966
222. SACKNER MA: Bronchofiberscopy. Am Rev Respir Dis 111:62, 1975
223. ANDERSON HA, FABER LP (eds): Diagnostic and therapeutic applications of the bronchoscope. Chest (Suppl) 73:685, 1978
224. STRADLING P: Diagnostic Bronchoscopy: An Introduction. London, E & S Livingstone, 1968
225. IKEDA S: Atlas of Flexible Bronchofiberscopy. Baltimore, University Park Press, 1974
226. IKEDA S: Flexible fiberoptic bronchoscope. Ann Otol Rhinol Laryngol 79:916, 1970
227. ERICKSON AD et al: Cerebral air embolism complicating transbronchial lung biopsy. Ann Intern Med 90:937, 1979
228. CREDLE WF JR, SMIDDY JF, ELIOTT RC: Complications of fiberoptic bronchoscopy. Am Rev Respir Dis 109:67, 1974
229. CARLENS E: Mediastinoscopy: A method for inspection and tissue biopsy in the superior mediastinum. Dis Chest 36:343–352, 1959
230. PEARSON FG, NELEMS JM, HENDERSON RD et al: The role of mediastinoscopy in the selection of treatment for bronchial carcinoma with involvement of superior mediastinal lymph nodes. J Thorac Cardiovasc Surg 64:383–390, 1972
231. LACQUET LK, MARTENS A, KLEEF JV et al: Mediastinoscopy and bronchial carcinoma: Experience with 600 mediastinoscopies. Thorax 30:141, 1975
232. SHIELDS TW: Preoperative radiation therapy in the treatment of bronchial carcinoma. Cancer 30:1388, 1972
233. DEELEY TJ: Review article. The treatment of carcinoma of the bronchus. Br J Radiol 40:801, 1967
234. PAULSON DL, REISCH JS: Long-term survival after resection for bronchogenic carcinoma. Ann Surg 184:324, 1976
235. BOWEN TE, ZAITCHUK R, GREEN DC et al: Value of anterior mediastinotomy in bronchogenic carcinoma of the left upper lobe. J Thorac Cardiovasc Surg 76:269, 1978
236. ACOSTA JL, MANFREDI F: Selective mediastinoscopy. Chest 71:150, 1977

237. HUTCHINSON CM, MILLS NL: The selection of patients with bronchogenic carcinoma for mediastinoscopy. J Thorac Cardiovasc Surg 71:768, 1974

238. DEMEESTER TR, GOLOMB HM, KIRCHNER P et al: The role of gallium-67 scanning in the clinical staging and preoperative evaluation of patients with carcinoma of the lung. Ann Thorac Surg 28:451, 1979

239. ALAZRAKI NP, RAMSDELL JW, TAYLOR A et al: Reliability of gallium scan chest radiology compared to mediastinoscopy for evaluating mediastinal spread in lung cancer. Am Rev Respir Dis 117:415, 1978

240. FOSBURG RG, HOPKINS GB, KAN MK: Evaluation of the mediastinum by gallium-67 scintigraphy in lung cancer. J Thorac Cardiovasc Surg 77:76, 1979

241. HOOPER RG, BEECHLER CR, JOHNSON MC: Radioisotope scanning in the initial staging of bronchogenic carcinoma. Am Rev Respir Dis 118:279, 1978

242. KRUGER HE, VESSAL K: Lung scanning as a screening method for cancer of the lung. Cancer 23:508–512, 1969

243. JAMES AE, WHITE RI, COOPER M et al: Pretreatment diagnostic evaluation with reference to pulmonary scans in lung cancer. J Thorac Cardiovasc Surg 61:530–540, 1971

244. MAYNARD CD, COWAN RJ: Role of the scan in bronchogenic carcinoma. Semin Nucl Med 1:195–205, 1971

245. ROUVIERE H: TOBIAS MJ (trans): Anatomy of Human Lymphatic System. Ann Arbor, Edwards Brothers, 1938

246. NOHL-OSER HC: An investigation of the anatomy of the lymphatic drainage of the lungs as shown by the lymphatic spread of bronchial carcinoma. Ann R Coll Surg Engl 51:157–176, 1972

247. BRANTIGAN JW, BRANTIGAN CO, BRANTIGAN OC: Biopsy of nonpalpable scalene nodes in carcinoma of the lung. Am Rev Respir Dis 107:962–973, 1973

248. KREEL L: Computed tomography of the thorax. Radiol Clin North Am 16:575, 1978

249. HEITZMAN ER, PROTO AV, GOLDWIN RL: The role of computerized tomography in the diagnosis of diseases of the thorax. JAMA 241:933, 1979

250. New Policy Outlines Role of CT. American College of Radiology Bulletin 33:2, 1977

251. KOLLINS SA: Computed tomography of the pulmonary parenchyma and chest wall. Radiol Clin North Am 15:297, 1977

252. HEITZMAN ER, GOLDWIN RL, PROTO AV: Radiologic analysis of the mediastinum utilizing computed tomography. Radiol Clin North Am 15:309, 1977

253. CROWE JK, BROWN LR, MUHM JR: Computed tomography of the mediastinum. Radiology 128:75, 1978

254. UNDERWOOD GH, HOOPER RG, AXELBAUM SP et al: Computed tomographic scanning of the thorax in the staging of bronchogenic carcinoma. N Engl J Med 300:777, 1979

255. MATHEWS MJ, KANHOUWA S, PICKREN J et al: Frequency of residual and metastatic tumor in patients undergoing curative surgical resection for lung cancer. Cancer Chemotherapy Report 4(3):63, 1973

256. BUTLER AP, LEO JS, LIN JP et al: The value of routine cranial computed tomography in neurologically intact patients with primary carcinoma of the lung. Radiology 131:399, 1979

257. BELL JW: Abdominal exploration in one-hundred lung carcinoma suspects prior to thoracotomy. Ann Surg 167:199–203, 1968

258. YASHAR J: Transdiaphragmatic exploration of the abdomen during surgery for bronchogenic carcinoma. J Thorac Cardiovas Surg 52:599–603, 1966

259. DOMBERNOWSKY P, HIRSCH F, HANSEN HH et al: Peritoneoscopy in the staging of 190 patients with small-cell anaplastic carcinoma with special reference to subtyping. Cancer 41:2008, 1978

260. DURRANT KR et al: Comparison of treatment policies in inoperable bronchial carcinoma. Lancet 1:715–719, 1971

261. LAING AH, BERRY RJ, NEWMAN CR et al: Treatment of inoperable carcinoma of the bronchus. Lancet 2:1161, 1975

262. PATTON AJ, KARDINAL CG: Bronchogenic carcinoma: A plea for conservative management. Mo Med 74:19, 1974

263. ROHWEDDER JJ: Conservative treatment of bronchogenic carcinoma. Compr Therapy 5:66, 1979

264. WILLIAMS IP, CLEIN GP, FORD HT et al: Symptomatic treatment of carcinoma of the bronchus using combination chemotherapy. Br J Dis Chest 72:131, 1978

265. DESPREZ R: Editorial comment. In Rogers DE et al (eds): 1979 Year Book of Medicine, p 168. Chicago, Year Book Medical Publishers, 1979

266. GREEN RA, HUMPHREY E, CLOSE H et al: Alkylating agents in bronchogenic carcinoma. Am J Med 46:516–525, 1969

267. DEELEY TJ: Radiotherapy for carcinoma of the bronchus. Cancer Treat Rev 1:39, 1974

268. MILLER AB, FOX W, TALL R: Five year follow-up of the Medical Research Council cooperative trial of surgery and radiotherapy for the primary treatment of small-celled or oat-celled carcinoma of the bronchus. Lancet 2:501, 1969

269. HYDE L, WOLF J, MCCRACKEN S et al: Natural course of inoperable lung cancer. Chest 64:309, 1973

270. BRASHEAR RE: Should asymptomatic patients

with inoperable bronchogenic carcinoma receive immediate radiotherapy? NO. Am Rev Respir Dis 117:411, 1978
271. PHILLIPS TL, MILLER RJ: Should asymptomatic patients with inoperable bronchogenic carcinoma receive immediate radiotherapy? YES. Am Rev Respir Dis 117:405, 1978
272. PEREZ CA: Radiation therapy in the management of carcinoma of the lung. Cancer 39:901, 1977
273. ROSWIT B et al: The survival of patients with inoperable lung cancer: A large-scale randomized study of radiation therapy versus placebo. Radiology 90:688–695, 1968
274. GUTTMANN R: Radical supervoltage therapy in inoperable carcinoma of the lung. In Deeley TJ (ed): Modern Radiotherapy Series, Carcinoma of the Bronchus, p 193. London, Butterworth & Co, 1971
275. BRODER LE, COHEN MH, SELAWRY OS: Treatment of bronchogenic carcinoma. II. Small cell. Cancer Treat Rev 4:219, 1977
276. WEISS R: Small cell carcinoma of the lung: Therapeutic managment. Ann Intern Med 88:522, 1978
277. SERRAH-DAVIES E: Does postoperative irradiation improve survival in lung cancer? JAMA 196: 345–347, 1966
278. BUCHBERG A, LUBLINER R, RUBEN EH: Carcinoma of the lung: Duration of life of individuals not treated surgically. Dis Chest 20:257, 1951
279. SELAWRY O: Monochemotherapy of bronchial carcinoma with special reference to cell type. Cancer Chemotherapy Report 4(Part 3): 177–188, 1973
280. SHIELDS TW: Status report of adjuvant cancer chemotherapy trial in the treatment of bronchial carcinoma. Cancer Chemotherapy Report (Part 3)4:119–124, 1973
281. BRUNNER KW, MARTHALER T, MULLER W: Effects of long term adjuvant chemotherapy with cyclophosphamide for radically resected bronchogenic carcinoma. Cancer Chemotherapy Report 4(Part 3):125–132, 1973
282. SCHABEL FM: The use of tumor growth kinetics in planning curative chemotherapy of advanced solid tumors. Cancer Res 29:2384–2389, 1969
283. HOLMES EC, GOLUB SH: Immunologic defects in lung cancer patients. J Thorac Cardiovasc Surg 71:161, 1976
284. LIEBLER GA, CONCANNON JP, MAGOVERN GA et al: Immunoprofile studies for patients with bronchogenic carcinoma. J Thorac Cardiovasc Surg 4:506, 1977
285. MCKNEALLY MF, MAVER C, KANSEL HW et al: Regional immunotherapy with intrapleural BCG for lung cancer. J Thorac Cardiovasc Surg 72:333, 1976
286. EDWARDS FR, WHITWELL F: Use of BCG as an immunostimulant in the surgical treatment of carcinoma of the lung. Thorax 29:654, 1974
287. RUCKDESCHEL JC, CODISH SD, STRANAHAN A et al: Postoperative empyema improves survival in lung cancer. Documentation and analysis of a natural experiment. N Engl J Med 287:1013, 1972
288. ANTHONY HM, MEARNS AJ, MASON MK et al: Levamisole and surgery in bronchial carcinoma patients. Increase in deaths from cardiorespiratory failure. Thorax 34:4, 1979
289. AMERY WK, SPREAFICO F, ROJAS AF et al: Adjuvant treatment with levamisole in cancer: A review of experimental and clinical data. Cancer Treat Rev 4:167, 1977
290. LIPSON SD, CHRETIEN PB, MUKUCH R et al: Thymosin immunotherapy in patients with small cell carcinoma of the lung. Cancer 43:863, 1979
291. ISRAEL L, EDELSTEIN R, DEPIERRE A et al: Daily intravenous infusion of *Corynebacterium parvum* in twenty patients with disseminated cancer: A preliminary report of clinical and biologic findings. J Natl Cancer Institute 55:29, 1975
292. ROJAS AF, FEIRSTEIN JN, MICHIEWICZ E et al: Levamisole in advanced human breast cancer. Lancet 1:211, 1976
293. SMITH RT: Possibilities and problems of immunologic intervention in cancer. N Engl J Med 287:439, 1972
294. BAST RC, ZBAR B, BOROS T et al: BCG and cancer. N Engl J Med 290:1413, 1974
295. BAST RC, ZBAR B, BOROS T et al: BCG and cancer (second of two parts). N Engl J Med 290:1458, 1974
296. TOOLE AL, STERN H: Carcinoid and adenoid cystic carcinoma of the bronchus. Ann Thorac Surg 13:63, 1972
297. SALYER DC, SALYER WR, EGGLESTON JC: Bronchial carcinoid tumors. Cancer 36:1522, 1975
298. KENNEDY A: The diagnosis of pulmonary carcinoid tumors. Br J Dis Chest 73:71, 1979
299. LAWSON RM, RAMANATHAN L, HURLEY G et al: Bronchial adenoma: Review of an 18-year experience at the Brompton Hospital. Thorax 31:245, 1976
300. OKIKE N, BERNATZ PE, WOOLNER LB: Carcinoid tumors of the lung. Ann Thorac Surg 22:270, 1976
301. TOLIS GA, FRY WA, HEAD L et al: Bronchial adenomas. Surg Gynecol Obstet 134:605, 1972
302. O'GRADY WP, MCDIVITT RW, HOLMAN CW et al: Bronchial adenomas. Arch Surg 101:558, 1970
303. ARRIGONI MG, WOOLNER LB, BERNATZ PE: Atypical carcinoid tumors of the lung. J Thorac Cardiovasc Surg 64:413, 1972
304. BATSON JR, GALE JW, HICKEY RC: Bronchial adenomata. Arch Surg 64:413, 1972
305. WILKINS EW, DARLING RC, SOUTTER L et al: A con-

tinuing clinical survey of adenomas of the trachea and bronchus in a general hospital. J Thorac Cardiovasc Surg 46:279, 1963

306. BENSCH KG, CORRIN B, PARIENTE R et al: Oat-cell carcinoma of the lung: Its origin and relationship to bronchial carcinoid. Cancer 22:1163, 1968
307. WEISS L, INGRAM M: Adenomatoid bronchial tumors. A consideration of the carcinoid tumors and the salivary tumors of the bronchial tree. Cancer 14:161, 1961
308. ROSAL J, HIGA E: Mediastinal endocrine neoplasm of probably thymic origin related to carcinoid tumor. Clinicopathologic study of 8 cases. Cancer 29:1061, 1972
309. WILSON H: Carcinoid tumors. Current Problems in Surgery, p 36. Chicago, Year Book Medical Publishers, 1970
310. FONTANNA RS, TYCE GM, FLOCK EV et al: Serotonin and the carcinoid syndrome in patients with bronchial tumors. Ann Otol Rhinol Laryngol 72:1024, 1963
311. OATS JA, BUTLER TC: Pharmacologic and endocrine aspects of carcinoid syndrome. Adv Pharmacol 5:109, 1967
312. ROSAL J, HIGA E, DAVIE J: Mediastinal endocrine neoplasm in patients with multiple endocrine adenomatosis. Cancer 29:1075, 1972
313. MELMON KL, SJOERDSMA A, MASON DT: Distinctive clinical and therapeutic aspects of the syndrome associated with bronchial carcinoid tumors. Am J Med 39:568, 1965
314. KAPLAN EL, JAFFE BM, PESKIN GW: A new provocative test for the diagnosis of the carcinoid syndrome. Am J Surg 123:173, 1972
315. BEAN WB: Vascular lesions caused by humoral mechanisms, p 1171. In Bean (ed): Vascular Spiders and Related Lesions of the Skin. Springfield, Charles C Thomas, 1958
316. MENGEL CE, KELLY MG, CARBONE PP et al: Clinical and biochemical effects of cyclophosphamide in patients with malignant carcinoid. Am J Med 38:396, 1965
317. GOODNER JT, BERG JW, WATSON WL: The nonbenign nature of bronchial carcinoids and cylindromas. Cancer 14:539, 1961
318. WYCHULIS AR, PAYNE WS, CLAGETT OT et al: Surgical treatment of mediastinal tumors, a 40 year experience. J Thorac Cardiovasc Surg 62:379, 1971
319. BENTON C, SILVERMAN FN: Some mediastinal lesions in children. Semin Roentgenol 4:91, 1969
320. FELSON B: The mediastinum. Semin Roentgenol 4:41, 1969
321. HEITZMAN ER: The Mediastinum: Radiological Correlations With Anatomy and Pathology. St. Louis, C. V. Mosby, 1978
322. KELLEY M, MANNES EJ, RAVIN CE: Mediastinal masses of vascular origin: A review. J Thorac Cardiovasc Surg 78:559, 1978
323. BRONTE FJ, CURRY TS III: Radionuclide scanning in the diagnosis of mediastinal masses. Semin Roentgenol 44:33, 1969
324. MONCADA R, WARPEHA R, PICKLEMAN I et al: Mediastinitis from odontogenic and deep cervical infections. Chest 73:497, 1978
325. Case records of Massachusetts General Hospital: Case 15–1978: Weekly clinicopathological exercises. N Engl J Med 298:894, 1978
326. KEY GK: Use of the esophageal obturator airway. Postgrad Med 67:189, 1980
327. BRYSON K, BENUMOF JL, WARD CF: The esophageal obturator airway: Clinical comparison with a mask and oropharyngeal airway. Chest 74:537, 1978
328. BERRY BE, OCHSNER JL: Perforation of the esophagus. A 30-year review. J Thorac Cardiovasc Surg 65:1, 1973
329. KELLY DL, NEUGEBAUER MK, FOSBURG RG: Spontaneous intramural esophageal perforation. J Thorac Cardiovasc Surg 63:504, 1972
330. BUNTAIN WL, LYNN HB: Traumatic pneumatic disruption of the esophagus. J Thorac Cardiovasc Surg 63:553, 1972
331. WILSON RF, ARBULU A, BASSETT JS et al: Acute mediastinal widening following blunt chest trauma. Arch Surg 104:551, 1972
332. DEBAKEY ME, NOON G: Aneurysms of the thoracic aorta. Mod Concepts Cardiovasc Dis 10:33, 1975
333. EARNEST F, MUHUN JR, SHEEDY PF: Roentgenographic findings in thoracic aortic dissection. Mayo Clin Proc 5:43, 1979
334. HACHE L, WOOLNER LB, BERNATZ PE: Idiopathic fibrous medastinitis. Dis Chest 41:9, 1962
335. SCHOWENGERDT CG, SUYEMOTO R, MAIN FB: Granulomatous and fibrous mediastinitis: A review and analysis of 180 cases. J Thorac Cardiovasc Surg 57:365, 1969
336. WIEDER S, RABINOWITZ JG: Fibrous mediastinitis: A late manifestation of mediastinal histoplasmosis. Radiology 125:305, 1977
337. LIGHT AM: Idiopathic fibrosis of mediastinum: A discussion of three cases and review of the literature. J Clin Pathol 31:78, 1978
338. FEIGNIN DS, EGGLESTON JC, SIEGELMAN SS: The multiple roentgen manifestations of sclerosing mediastinitis. Johns Hopkins Med J 144:1, 1979
339. ARNETT EN, BACOS JM, MACHER AM: Fibrosing mediastinitis causing pulmonary arterial hypertension without pulmonary venous hypertension. Am J Med 63:634, 1977
340. LONGMIRE WP, GOODWIN WE, BUCKBERG GD: Management of sclerosing fibrosis of the mediastinal and retroperitoneal areas. Ann Surg 165:1013, 1967

341. ZAJTCHUK R, STREVEY TE, HEYDORN WH et al: Mediastinal histoplasmosis: Surgical considerations. J Thorac Cardiovasc Surg 66:300, 1973
342. GARCIA JM, RAMIREZ R, BACOS J et al: Technique for reconstruction of superior vena cava in fibrosing mediastinitis. J Thorac Cardiovasc Surg 65:547, 1973
343. LATTES R: Thymoma and other tumors of the thymus. Cancer 15:1224, 1962
344. LEGG MA, BRADY WJ: Pathology and clinical behavior of thymomas: A survey of 51 cases. Cancer 18:1131, 1965
345. COSSMAN J, DEEGAN MJ, SCHMITZER B: Thymoma: An immunologic and electron microscopic study. Cancer 41:2183, 1978
346. CONKLE DM, ADKINS RB: Primary malignant tumors of the mediastinum. Ann Thorac Surg 14:553, 1972
347. GEREIN AN, STRIVSTAVA SP, BURGESS J: Thymoma: A ten year review. Am J Surg 136:49, 1978
348. BENJAMIN SP, MCCORMACK LJ, EFFLER DB et al: Primary tumors of the mediastinum. Chest 62:297, 1972
349. BURKELL CC, CROSS JM, KENT HP et al: Mass lesions of the mediastinum. Curr Probl Surg: 2–57, June 1969
350. ROSAL J, HIGA E: Mediastinal endocrine neoplasm of probable thymic origin related to carcinoid tumor: Clinicopathologic study of 8 cases. Cancer 29:1061, 1972
351. WILKINS EW, CASTLEMAN B: Thymoma: A continuing survey at the Massachusetts General Hospital. Ann Thorac Surg 28:252, 1979
352. BOLOOKI H, SCHWARTZMAN RJ: High-dose steroids for perioperative management of patients with myasthenia gravis undergoing thymectomy. J Thorac Cardiovasc Surg 75:754, 1978
353. MARKS RD, WALLACE KM, PETTIT HS: Radiation therapy control of nine patients with malignant thymoma. Cancer 41:117, 1978
354. HOCHHOLZER L, THEROS EG, ROSEN SH: Some unusual lesions of the mediastinum: Roentgenologic and pathologic features. Semin Roentgenol 4:47, 1969
355. RECONDO J, LIBSHITZ HI: Mediastinal extragonadal germ cell tumors. Urology 11:369, 1978
356. MEARES EM, BRIGGS EM: Occult seminoma of the testes masquerading as primary extragonadal germinal neoplasms. Cancer 30:300, 1972
357. MARTINI N et al: Primary mediastinal germ cell tumors. Cancer 33:763, 1974
358. SICKLES EA, BELLIVEAU RE, WIERNIK PH: Primary mediastinal choricarcinoma in the male. Cancer 33:1196, 1974
359. BARUA NR, PATEL AR, TAKITA H et al: Fibrosarcoma of the mediastinum. J Surg Oncol 12:11, 1979
360. JAUREQUI R, LILKER ES, BAYLEY A: Upper airway obstruction in euthyroid goiter. JAMA 238:2163, 1977
361. WARREN CP: Acute respiratory failure and tracheal obstruction in the elderly with benign goiters. Can Med Assoc J 121:191, 1979
362. IRWIN RS, BRAMAN SS, ARVANITIDIS AN et al: Thyroid scanning in preoperative diagnosis of mediastinal goiter. Ann Intern Med 89:73, 1978
363. ISRAEL HL, PATCHEFSKY AS, SALDANA MJ: Wegener's granulomatosis, lymphomatoid granulomatosis, and benign lymphocytic angiitis and granulomatosis of lung. Ann Intern Med 87:691, 1977
364. FEIGN DS, SIEGELMAN SS, THEORS EG et al: Nonmalignant lymphoid disease of the chest. J Roentgenol 129:221, 1977
365. FILLY R, BLANK N, CASTELLINO RA: Radiographic distribution of intrathoracic disease in previously untreated patients with Hodgkin's disease and non-Hodgkin's lymphoma. Radiology 120:277, 1976
366. ROSAI J, DORFMAN RF: Sinus histiocytosis with massive lymphadenopathy: A pseudolymphomatous benign disorder. Analysis of 34 cases. Cancer 30:1174, 1970
366a. GORDONSON J, QUINN M, KAUFMAN R et al: Mediastinal lymphadenopathy and undifferentiated connective tissue disease. Am J Roentgenol 131:325, 1978
367. SALDANA MJ, PATCHEFSKY AS, ISRAEL HI et al: Pulmonary angiitis and granulomatosis. Hum Pathol 8:391, 1977
367a. MANOHARAN A et al: Intrathoracic manifestations in non-Hodgkin's lymphoma. Thorax 34:29, 1979
367b. JENKINS PF et al: Non-Hodgkin's lymphoma, chronic lymphatic leukemia and the lung. Br J Dis Chest 75:22, 1981
367c. MACDONALD JB: Lung involvement in Hodgkin's disease. Thorax 32:664, 1977
368. ROGERS LF, OSMER JC: Bronchogenic cyst: A review of 46 cases. Am J Roentgenol Radium Ther Nucl Med 91:273, 1964
369. MAGNUSSEN JR, THOMPSON JN, DICKINSON JT: Presternal bronchogenic cysts. Arch Otolaryngol 103:52, 1977
370. CROFTON J, DOUGLAS A: Respiratory Diseases, 2nd ed, p 615. Oxford, Blackwell Scientific Publications, 1971
371. INGELS GW et al: Malignant schwannomas of the mediastinum. Cancer 27:1190, 1971
372. FISHER ER, VUZEVSKI VD: Cytogenesis of schwannoma (neurilemomoma), dermatofibroma, and dermatofibrosarcoma as revealed by electron microscopy. Am J Clin Pathol 49:141, 1968
373. D'AGOSTINO AN, SOULE EH, MILLER RH: Primary malignant neoplasms of nerves (malignant neurilemomas) in patients without manifestations of

multiple neurofibromatosis (von Recklinghausen's disease). Cancer 16:1003, 1963

374. CAREY LS, ELLIS FH, GOOD CA et al: Neurogenic tumors of the mediastinum: A clinicopathologic study. Am J Roentgenol Radium Ther Nucl Med 84:189, 1960
375. EQUIST RW, TORMEY DC, JENIS EH et al: Malignant chemodectoma of the superior mediastinum with elevated homovanillic acid. Chest 66:209, 1974
376. GALE AW et al: Neurogenic tumors of the mediastinum. Ann Thorac Surg 17:434, 1974
377. D'ANGIO GJ, LOKEN M, NESBIT M: Radionuclear (^{75}Se) identification of tumor in children with neuroblastoma. Radiology 93:615, 1969
378. AKWARI OE, PAYNE WS, ONOFRIO BM et al: Dumbbell neurogenic tumors of the mediastinum: Diagnosis and management. Mayo Clin Proc 53:353, 1978
379. GROSFEDL JL, WEINBERGER M, KILMAN JW et al: Primary mediastinal neoplasms in infants and children. Ann Thorac Surg 12:179, 1971
380. DAVIDSON KG, WALBAUM PR, MCCORMACK RJM: Intrathoracic neural tumors. Thorax 33:359, 1978
381. HARRISON JH, MAHONEY EM: Genitourinary tract cancer. In Holland JF, Frei E (eds): Cancer Medicine, p 1653. Philadelphia, Lea & Febiger, 1974
382. PRIEBE CJ JR, CLATWORTHY HW JR: Neuroblastoma: Evaluation of the treatment of 90 children. Arch Surg 95:538, 1967
383. CASTLEMAN B: Massachusetts General Hospital case records: Weekly clinicopathologic exercises—case 40011—hyperplasia of mediastinal lymph nodes. N Engl J Med 250:26, 1954
384. LATTES R, PACHTER MR: Benign lymphoid masses of probably hamartomatous nature: Analysis of 12 cases. Cancer 15·197, 1962
385. TUNG KSK, MCCORMACK LJ: Angiomatous lymphoid hamartoma. Cancer 20:525, 1967
386. MOORE SB, HARRISON EG, WEILAND LH: Angioimmunoblastic lymphadenopathy. Mayo Clin Proc 51:273, 1976
387. EHRLICH FE, SALZBERG AM: Pathophysiology and management of congenital posterolateral diaphragmatic hernias. Am Surg 44:26, 1978
388. ORRINGER MB, KIRSH MM, SLOAN H: Congenital and traumatic diaphragmatic hernias exclusive of the hiatus. Curr Probl Surg: 1–64, 1975
389. AHREND TR, THOMPSON BW: Hernia of the foramen of Bochdalek in the adult. Am J Surg 122:613, 1971
390. BRYER JV, HEGARTY MM, HOWE C et al: Traumatic diaphragmatic hernia. Br J Surg 65:69, 1978
391. JARA FM, YAP A, TOLEDO-PEREYRA LH et al: The role of surgery in primary osteomyelitis of the chest wall. J Thorac Cardiovasc Surg 77:147, 1979
392. OCHSNER A SR, OCHSNER A JR: Tumors of the thoracic wall. In Spain DM (ed): Tumors of the Chest, p 209. New York, Grune & Stratton, 1960
393. TEITELBAUM SL: Tumors of the chest wall: Collective Review. Surg Gynecol Obstet 129:1059, 1969
394. O'NEAL LW, ACKERMAN LV: Cartilaginous tumors of ribs and sternum. J Thorac Surg 21:71, 1951
395. HOCHBERG LA: Primary tumors of the rib: Review of the literature and presentation of eleven cases not reported previously. Arch Surg 67:566, 1953
395a. KINTZER JS, ROSENOW EC, KYLE RA: Thoracic and pulmonary abnormalities in multiple myeloma. Arch Int Med 138:727, 1978
396. LEVEY GS, CALABRO JJ: Tietze's syndrome: Report of two cases and review of the literature. Arthritis Rheum 5:261, 1962
397. SKORNECK AB: Roentgen aspects of Tietze's syndrome. Am J Roentgenol Radium Ther Nucl Med 83:748, 1960
398. MCADAM LP, O'HANLAN MA, BLUESTONE R et al: Relapsing polychondritis. Medicine 55:193, 1976
399. OMELL GH, ANDERSON LS, BRAMSON RT: Chest wall tumors. Radiol Clin North Am 11:197, 1973
400. THRELKEL JB, ADKINS RB JR: Primary chest wall tumors. Ann Thorac Surg 11:450, 1971
401. OCHSNER A JR, OCHSNER A: Tumors of the chest wall. Surg Clin North Am 46:1447, 1966
402. TEITELBAUM SL: Twenty years experience with intrinsic tumors of the bony thorax at a large institution. J Thorac Cardiovasc Surg 63:776, 1972
403. ALPERT LI, ABACI I, WERTHAMER S: Radiation-induced extraskeletal osteosarcoma. Cancer 31:1359, 1973
404. BRINDLEY GV JR: Primary malignant tumors of the chest wall (Excluding primary cutaneous neoplasms). Ann Surg 153:684, 1961
405. ARNOLD PG, PAIROLERO PC: Chondrosarcoma of the manubrium. Resection and reconstruction with pectoralis major muscle. Mayo Clin Proc 53:54, 1978
406. PANDEY S: Giant chondromas arising from the ribs. J Bone Joint Surg 57:519, 1975
407. OCHSNER A SR, OCHSNER A JR: Tumors of the thoracic wall. In Spain DM (ed): Tumors of the Chest, p 232. New York, Grune & Stratton, 1960
408. CADE S: Osteogenic sarcoma: A study based on 113 patients. J R Coll Surg Edinb 1:79, 1955
409. ROSEN G et al: High-dose methotrexate with citrovorum factor rescue and Adriamycin in childhood osteogenic sarcoma. Cancer 33:1151, 1974
410. FERNANDEX CH, LINDBERG RD, SUTOW WW et al: Localized Ewing's sarcoma—treatment and results. Cancer 34:143, 1974
411. Fibrous dysplasia of bone. Br Med J 1:685, 1971

412. OCHSNER A SR, OCHSNER A JR: Tumors of the thoracic wall. In Spain DM (ed): Tumors of the Chest, p 212. New York, Grune & Stratton, 1960
413. WIENER MF, CHOW WH: Primary tumors of the diaphragm. Arch Surg 90:143, 1965
414. BRENNAN JL: Metastatic tumors of the diaphragm. Br J Surg 58:458, 1971
415. OCHSNER A SR, OCHSNER A JR: Tumors of the diaphragm. In Spain DM (ed): Tumors of the Chest, p 240. New York, Grune & Stratton, 1960
416. MILLER DR et al: Hypoglycemia due to nonpancreatic mesodermal tumors—Report of two cases. Ann Surg 150:684, 1959
417. FELSON B: Fundamentals of Chest Roentgenology, p 222. Philadelphia, WB Saunders, 1960
418. MEREDITH JH, BRADSHAW HH: Leiomyoma of the diaphragm. J Thorac Cardiovasc Surg 37:641, 1959
419. MILLER DR: Benign tumors of lung and tracheobronchial tree. Ann Thorac Surg 8:542, 1969
420. CALDAROLA VT, HARRISON EG, CLAGETT OT et al: Benign tumors and tumorlike conditions of the trachea and bronchi. Ann Otol Rhinol Laryngol 73:1042, 1964
421. WEBER AL, GRILLO HC: Tracheal tumors: A radiological, clinical and pathological evaluation of 84 cases. Radiol Clin North Am 16:227, 1978
422. ROSTOM AY, MORGAN RL: Results of treating primary tumors of the trachea by irradiation. Thorax 33:387, 1978
423. BIRT BD: The management of malignant tracheal neoplasms. J Laryngol Otol 84:723, 1970
424. AL-SALEEM T, PEALE AR, NORRIS CM: Multiple papillomatosis of the lower respiratory tract. Cancer 22:1173, 1968
425. KAUFMAN G, KLOPSTOCK R: Papillomatosis of the respiratory tract. Am Rev Respir Dis 88:839, 1963
426. TEDESCHI LG, LIBERTINI R, CONTE B: Endobronchial polyp. Chest 63:110, 1973
427. GUCCION JG, ROSEN SH: Bronchopulmonary leiomyosarcoma and fibrosarcoma: A study of 32 cases and reviews of the literature. Cancer 30:836, 1972
428. POLITIS J, FUNAHASKI A, GEHLSEN JA et al: Intrathoracic lipomas: Report of three cases and review of the literature with emphasis on endobronchial lipoma. J Thorac Cardiovasc Surg 77:550, 1979
429. JENSEN MS, PETERSEN AH: Bronchial lipoma: Three cases and review of the literature. Scand J Thorac Cardiovasc Surg 4:131, 1970
430. PLACHTA A, HERSHEY H: Lipoma of the lung: Review of the literature and report of a case. Am Rev Respir Dis 86:912, 1962
431. VALENSTEIN S, TURNER RJ: Granular cell myoblastoma of the bronchus: Case report and review of the literature. J Thorac Cardiovasc Surg 76:465, 1978
432. Bronchial mucocele. Br Med J 3:721, 1971
433. TALNER LB, GMELICH JT, LIEBOW AA et al: The syndrome of bronchial mucocele and regional hyperinflation of the lung. Am J Roentgenol 110:675, 1970
434. LEMIRE P, TREPANIER A, HERBERT G: Bronchocele and blocked bronchiectasis. Am J Roentgenol 110:687, 1970
435. TAYLOR TL, MILLER DR: Leiomyoma of the bronchus. J Thorac Cardiovasc Surg 57:284, 1969
436. STACKHOUSE EM, HARRISON EG, ELLIS FH JR: Primary mixed malignancies of lung: Carcinosarcoma and blastoma. J Thorac Cardiovasc Surg 57:385, 1969
437. KAKOS GS, WILLIAMS TE, ASSOR D et al: Pulmonary carcinosarcoma. J Thorac Cardiovasc Surg 61:777, 1971
438. DIXON DS, BRESLOW A: Pulmonary blastoma. Am Rev Respir Dis 108:968, 1973
438a. CAMERON EJW: Primary sarcoma of the lung. Thorax 30:516, 1975
439. FELDMAN F, SEAMAN WB: Primary thoracic hemangiopericytoma. Radiology 82:998, 1964
440. MCMASTER MJ, SOULE EH, IVINS JC: Hemangiopericytoma: A clinicopathologic study and long-term followup of 60 patients. Cancer 36:2232, 1975
441. LIEBOW AA, HUBBEL DS: Sclerosing hemagioma (histiocytoma, xanthoma) of the lung. Cancer 9:53, 1956
442. TCHERTKOFF V, BOCK YL: Plasma cell granuloma of the lung: Case report and review of the literature. Dis Chest 44:440, 1963
443. SALTSTEIN SL: Pulmonary malignant lymphomas and pseudolymphomas: Classification, therapy, and prognosis. Cancer 16:928, 1963
444. HUTCHINSON WB, FRIEDENBERG MJ, SALTZSTEIN S: Primary pulmonary pseudolymphoma. Radiology 82:48, 1964
445. CARRINGTON CB, LIEBOW AA: Lymphocytic interstitial pneumonia. Am J Pathol 48:36a, 1966
446. REICH NE, MCCORMACK LJ, VAN ORDSTRAND HS: Pseudolymphoma of the lung. Chest 65:424, 1974
447. GROSSMAN RE, BEMIS EL, PEMBERTON AH et al: Fibrous histiocytoma or xanthoma of the lung with bronchial involvement. J Thorac Cardiovasc Surg 65:653, 1973
448. BUTLER H, LAKE KB, VANDYKE JJ: Bronchial endometriosis and bronchiectasis: A possible relationship. Arch Intern Med 138:991, 1978
449. JELIHOVSKY T, GRANT AF: Endometriosis of the lung: A case report and review of the literature. Thorax 23:434, 1968
450. ASSOR D: Endometriosis of the lung: Report of a case. Am J Clin Pathol 57:311, 1972
451. DAVIES R: Recurring spontaneous pneumothorax

concomitant with menstruation. Thorax 23:370, 1968

452. ROSSI NP, GOPLERUD CP: Recurrent catamenial pneumothorax. Arch Surg 109:173, 1974
453. JANOWER ML, BLENNERHASSET JB: Lymphangitic spread of metastatic cancer to the lung: A radiologic-pathologic classification. Radiology 101:267, 1971
454. GILBERG K, RAKOWSKI H: Pulmonary lymphangitic spread of cancer of the cervix. N Engl J Med 289:921, 1973
455. YANG SP, LIN CC: Lymphangitic carcinomatosis of the lungs: The clinical significance of its roentgenologic classification. Chest 62:179, 1972
456. GONZALEZ-VITALE JC, GARCIA-BUNNEL R: Pulmonary tumor emboli and cor pulmonale in primary carcinoma of the lung. Cancer 38:2106, 1976
457. THURLBECK WM: Neoplasia of the pulmonary vascular bed. In Moser KM (ed): Pulmonary Vascular Diseases, Chpt II. New York, Marcel Dekker, 1979
458. LEVIN B: Subpleural interlobular lymphectasia reflecting metastatic carcinoma. Radiology 72:682, 1959
459. ALTEMUS R: Localized interlobular septal lines in bronchogenic cardinoma. J Thorac Cardiovasc Surg 57:380, 1969
460. BAUMGARTNER WA, MARK JBD: Metastatic malignancies from distant sites to the tracheobronchial tree. J Thorac Cardiovasc Surg 79:499, 1980
461. DEBEER RA, GARCIA RL, ALEXANDER SC: Endobronchial metastasis from the cancer of the breast. Chest 73:94, 1978
462. WEISS L, GILBERT HA: Treatment of pulmonary metastases. In Weiss L, and Gilbert HA (eds): Pulmonary Metastasis, Introduction, pp 194. Boston, GK Hall, 1978
463. MARTINI N, MALAMED MR: Multiple primary lung cancers. J Thorac Cardiovasc Surg 70:606, 1975
464. BAINS MS, MCCORMACK PM, CVITKOVIC E et al: Results of combined chemo-surgical therapy for pulmonary metastases from testicular carcinoma. Cancer 41:850, 1978
465. ROSEN G, HUVOS AG, MOSENDE C et al: Chemotherapy and thoracotomy for metastatic osteogenic sarcoma. Cancer 41:841, 1978
466. SHIRLEY RL, GOLDSTEIN DP, COLLINS JJ: The role of thoracotomy in the management of patients with chest metastases from gestational trophoblastic disease. J Thorac Cardiovasc Surg 63:545, 1972
467. SCHANER EG, CHANG AE, DOPPMAN JL et al: Comparison of computed and conventional whole lung tomography in detecting pulmonary nodules: A prospective radiographic-pathologic study. Am J Roentgenol 131:55, 1978
468. MUHM JR, BROWN LR, CROWE JK: Detection of pulmonary nodules by computed tomography. Am J Roentgenol 128:267, 1977
469. MCKENNA RJ, MCKENNA RJ JR: Patterns of pulmonary metastases—an orthopedic hospital experience. In Weiss L, and Gilbert HA (eds): Pulmonary Metastasis, pp 168. Boston, GK Hall, 1978
470. KATZENSTEIN AL, PURVIS R JR, GMELICH J et al: Pulmonary resection for metastatic renal adenocarcinoma. Cancer 41:712, 1978
471. JOSEPH WL, MORTON DL, ADKINS PC: Prognostic significance of tumor doubling time in evaluating operability in pulmonary metastatic disease. J Thorac Cardiovasc Surg 61:23, 1971
472. MALAISE EP, CHAVAUDRA M, COURDI A et al: Tumor growth rate and pulmonary metastasis. In Weiss L, and Gilbert HA (eds): Pulmonary Metastasis, p 200. Boston GK Hall, 1978
473. DONGEN JA, SLOOTEN EA: The surgical treatment of pulmonary metastases. Cancer Treat Rev 5:29, 1978
474. VINCENT RG, CHOKSKI LB, TAKITA H et al: Surgical resection of the solitary pulmonary metastases. In Weiss L, Gilbert HA (eds): Pulmonary Metastasis, p 232. Boston, GK Hall, 1978

Index

Numerals followed by an "f" indicate a figure; "t" following a page number indicates a table.